ANESTHESIA AND PERIOPERATIVE CARE OF THE COMBAT CASUALTY

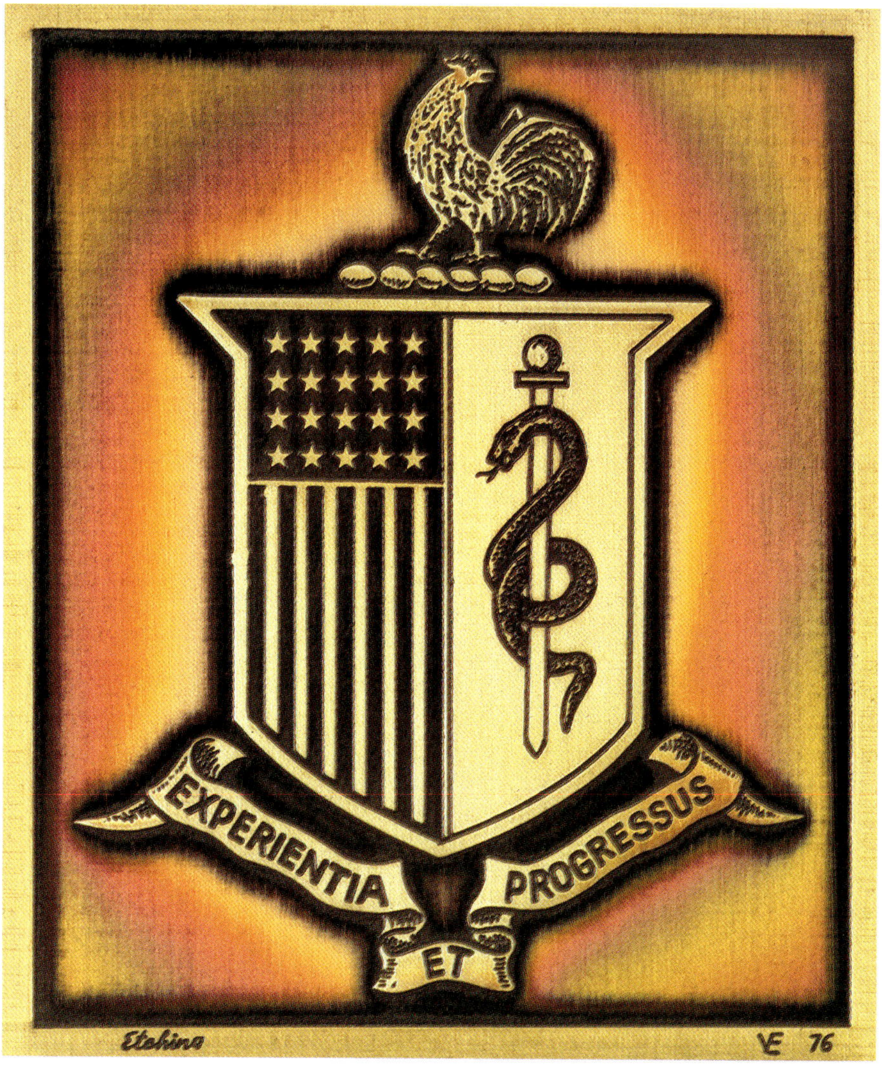

The Coat of Arms
1818
Medical Department of the Army

A 1976 etching by Vassil Ekimov of an
original color print that appeared in
The Military Surgeon, Vol XLI, No 2, 1917

The first line of medical defense in wartime is the combat medic. Although in ancient times medics carried the caduceus into battle to signify the neutral, humanitarian nature of their tasks, they have never been immune to the perils of war. They have made the highest sacrifices to save the lives of others, and their dedication to the wounded soldier is the foundation of military medical care.

Textbook of Military Medicine

Published by the

Office of The Surgeon General
Department of the Army, United States of America

Editor in Chief
Brigadier General Russ Zajtchuk, MC, U.S. Army
Director, Borden Institute
Commanding General
U.S. Army Medical Research and Materiel Command
Professor of Surgery
F. Edward Hébert School of Medicine
Uniformed Services University of the Health Sciences

Officer in Charge and Managing Editor
Colonel Ronald F. Bellamy, MC, U.S. Army
Borden Institute
Associate Professor of Military Medicine,
Associate Professor of Surgery,
F. Edward Hébert School of Medicine
Uniformed Services University of the Health Sciences

The TMM Series

Part I. *Warfare, Weaponry, and the Casualty*

Medical Consequences of Nuclear Warfare (1989)

Conventional Warfare: Ballistic, Blast, and Burn Injuries (1991)

Military Psychiatry: Preparing in Peace for War (1994)

War Psychiatry (1995)

Medical Aspects of Chemical and Biological Warfare

Military Medical Ethics

Part II. *Principles of Medical Command and Support*

Medicine and War

Medicine in Low-Intensity Conflict

Part III. *Disease and the Environment*

Occupational Health: The Soldier and the Industrial Base (1993)

Military Dermatology (1994)

Mobilization and Deployment

Environmental Hazards and Military Operations

Part IV. *Surgical Combat Casualty Care*

Anesthesia and Perioperative Care of the Combat Casualty (1995)

Combat Injuries to the Head, Face, and Neck

Combat Injuries to the Trunk

Combat Injuries to the Extremities and Spine

Rehabilitation of the Injured Soldier

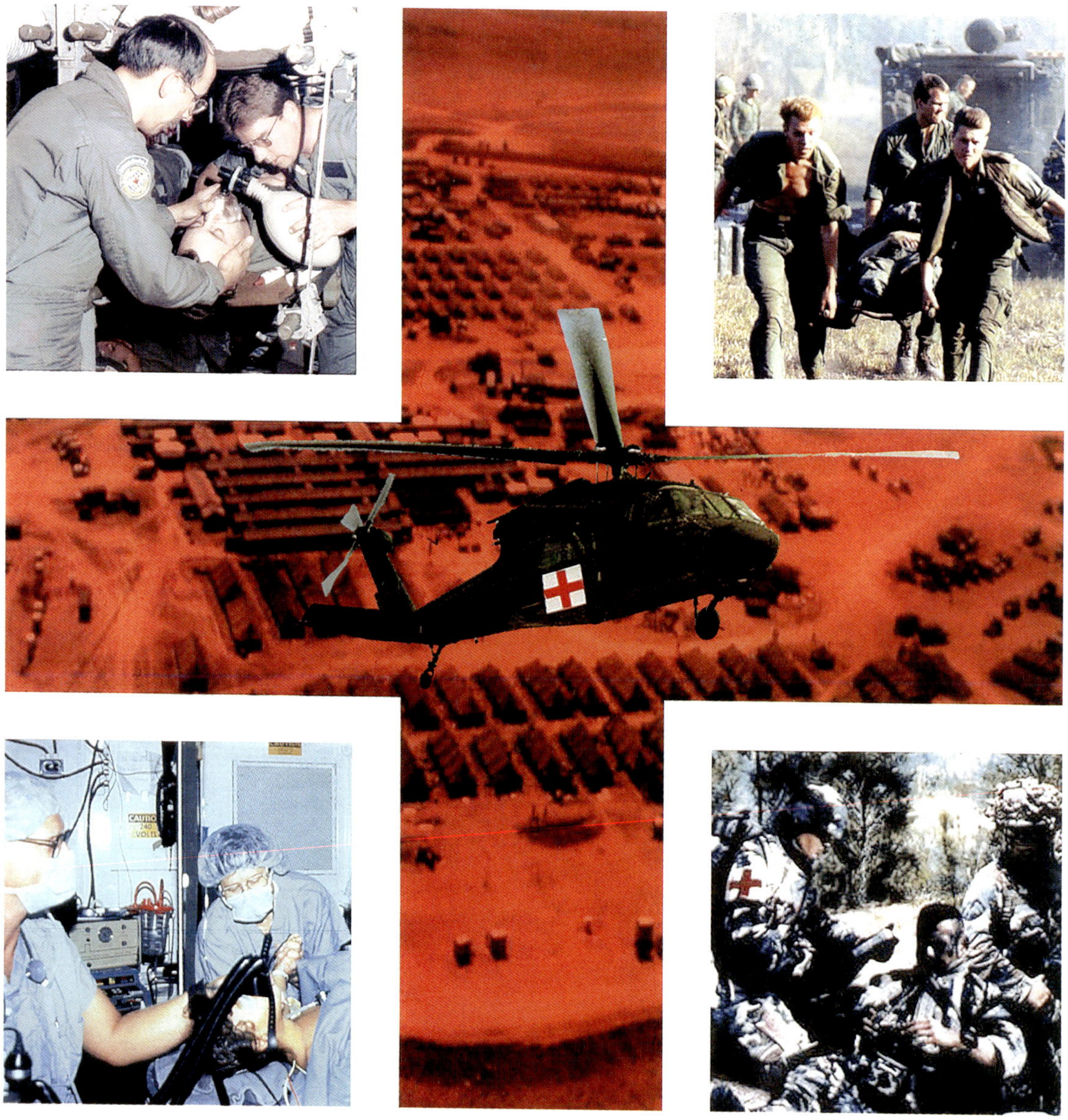

The care of the combat casualty is a multifaceted endeavor in which the acts of individual medical personnel are inextricably linked. A continuum of care must exist from the most junior medic in the field through evacuation to the most senior specialist in a deployable hospital. The essential prerequisites at all echelons of care are courage, endurance, skill, knowledge, and above all, devotion to the well-being of the casualty.

ANESTHESIA AND PERIOPERATIVE CARE OF THE COMBAT CASUALTY

Specialty Editors

BRIGADIER GENERAL RUSS ZAJTCHUK
Medical Corps, U.S. Army

CHRISTOPHER M. GRANDE, M.D.
Executive Director
International Trauma Anesthesia and Critical Care Society

Office of The Surgeon General
United States Army
Falls Church, Virginia

Walter Reed Army Medical Center
Washington, D.C.

United States Army Medical Department Center and School
Fort Sam Houston, Texas

Uniformed Services University of the Health Sciences
Bethesda, Maryland

1995

Editorial Staff: Lorraine B. Davis
Senior Editor

Colleen Mathews Quick
Associate Editor / Writer

Nancy Michel
Copyeditor

This volume was prepared for military medical educational use. The focus of the information is to foster discussion that may form the basis of doctrine and policy. The volume does not constitute official policy of the United States Department of Defense.

Dosage Selection:

The authors and publisher have made every effort to ensure the accuracy of dosages cited herein. However, it is the responsibility of every practitioner to consult appropriate information sources to ascertain correct dosages for each clinical situation, especially for new or unfamiliar drugs and procedures. The authors, editors, publisher, and the Department of Defense cannot be held responsible for any errors found in this book.

Use of Trade or Brand Names:

Use of trade or brand names in this publication is for illustrative purposes only and does not imply endorsement by the Department of Defense.

Neutral Language:

Unless this publication states otherwise, masculine nouns and pronouns do not refer exclusively to men

---

Published by the Office of The Surgeon General at TMM Publications
Borden Institute
Walter Reed Army Medical Center
Washington, DC 20307-5001

Library of Congress Cataloging–in–Publication Data
Anesthesia and perioperative care of the combat casualty / prepared under the direction of Russ Zajtchuk.
p. cm. — (Textbook of military medicine. Part IV, Surgical combat casualty care ; [v. 1])
Includes bibliographical references and index.
1. Surgery, Military. 2. Anesthesiology. 3. Therapeutics Surgical. 4. War wounds—Surgery. I. Zajtchuk, Russ. II. Series.
[DNLM: 1. Anesthesia. 2. Preoperative Care. 3. Intraoperative Care. 4. Military Medicine. 5. Postoperative Care. UH 390 T355 pt.4 1995 v. 1]
RD153.A54 1995
617.9'6799—dc20
DNLM/DLC
for Library of Congress 95-41596
CIP

PRINTED IN THE UNITED STATES OF AMERICA

04, 03, 02, 01, 00, 99, 98 5 4 3 2

Contents

Foreword

This is an exciting time to be in the U.S. Army Medical Department. Not since the end of World War II have such fundamental changes occurred: decreased resources and personnel; increased emphasis on support of forces deployed in the field; uncertainty as to the nature of the next war in which we will be providing medical support—a consequence of the dissolution of the Cold War; and overlaying all, the fundamental changes likely to be wrought by applications of advanced technology. These factors will change the provision of combat casualty care in ways that we can only speculate about. But we must not make changes simply for the sake of change; we must keep faithful to the fundamental principles of military medicine. The *Textbook of Military Medicine* is a repository of the science and art of military medicine, and as such is our anchor in this vast sea of change. By keeping the historical, factual, and scientific bases of military medicine readily accessible in this series of textbooks, the lessons learned in previous wars will not need to be relearned—at the casualty's expense—in future wars.

The U.S. Army does not recognize any one group of practitioners as preeminent in the management of combat casualties. Rather, combat casualty care occurs along a spectrum ranging from buddy aid on the battlefield to definitive care at hospitals in the continental United States. For this reason, this textbook, *Anesthesia and Perioperative Care of the Combat Casualty*, is not restricted merely to the technical aspects of providing anesthetics; instead, it encompasses the constellation of actions that, taken together, ensure an optimal outcome for the casualty.

The probability of massive wars of prolonged duration has decreased. These wars were dominated by attrition of personnel, in which conserving the fighting strength was the major focus of the U.S. Army Medical Department. In future wars, however, the medical department will probably be judged more by its ability to save lives. Thus this book, with its emphasis on lifesaving intervention, is especially timely. Nevertheless, the true contribution of anesthesia in military medicine is probably not found in mortality and morbidity statistics but in something more difficult to measure and perhaps even more important: the alleviation of pain and suffering.

I strongly recommend that all commanders and medical officers read this volume with an open mind. Massive changes are occurring in military medicine. Medical officers of the future will encounter numerous changes in doctrine and advanced technology; our willingness to respond to these opportunities will be necessary to ensure that our soldiers receive nothing less than the best combat casualty care.

Lieutenant General Alcide M. LaNoue
The Surgeon General
U.S. Army

December 1995
Washington, D.C.

Preface

The extent to which the specialty of anesthesiology has come of age is apparent when we consider that no official history was published on the science and practice of providing anesthesia in World War II. Information on anesthesia was contained in single chapters in other specialty volumes. Now we have a 31-chapter volume, *Anesthesia and Perioperative Care of the Combat Casualty*. This textbook is not limited to the purely technical aspects of anesthesia practice. Instead, except for details of surgical technique and rehabilitation, it portrays the entire expanse of modern combat casualty care. In a real sense, this volume of the *Textbook of Military Medicine* can be viewed as a treatise on combat casualty care for the military anesthesia provider. Throughout the textbook, the term "military anesthesia provider" has been used whenever possible to underline the fact that in the U.S. Army Medical Department, as well as in the other services, the provision of anesthesia is the joint effort of officers drawn from two corps: medical and nursing.

Because military medicine is organized by echelon, the provision of combat casualty care is best understood as a continuum to which each echelon makes an essential contribution. This is the fundamental difference between combat casualty care in military medicine and trauma management in civilian hospitals, and this approach must be clearly understood in advance by all healthcare providers in the military medical services. The best efforts of hospital-based practitioners will be to no avail if lifesaving first aid on the battlefield is inadequate or if evacuation from the battlefield is not timely. Likewise, the best battlefield first aid or the most expeditious evacuation will be wasted unless hospital care is correspondingly excellent. An optimal outcome for the casualty is ensured only by the entire constellation of actions that compose combat casualty care.

The *Textbook of Military Medicine* is honored to publish illustrations of combat casualties from two sources that were compiled during the Vietnam War: the Wound Data and Munitions Effectiveness Team (WDMET) collection, a vast databank that was compiled at the direction of General Creighton Abrams, which contains information on nearly 8,000 casualties; and the Swan Vietnam Surgical Slide Set, which was compiled by Colonel Kenneth Swan, Medical Corps, U.S. Army Reserve, in 1970. This volume contains more than 100 never-before-published illustrations from these sources.

This book's long gestation began while Donald P. Jenkins, Ph.D., was Managing Editor. During the book's formative years, Colonel Brian C. Condon, Medical Corps, U.S. Army (retired), in his capacity then as Anesthesia Consultant to The U.S. Army Surgeon General, and Christopher M. Grande, M.D., of the International Trauma Anesthesia and Critical Care Society, recruited authors and guided the development of their chapters. More recently, however, at my request, Captain W. Clayton Petty, Medical Corps, U.S. Navy, and Colonel Denver E. Perkins, Medical Corps, U.S. Army, provided the professional advice and the de novo chapters that made publication possible. The U.S. Army Medical Department owes each of these individuals a debt of gratitude.

Brigadier General Russ Zajtchuk
Medical Corps, U.S. Army

December 1995
Washington, D.C.

The current medical system to support the U.S. Army at war is a continuum from the forward line of troops through the continental United States; it serves as a primary source of trained replacements during the early stages of a major conflict. The system is designed to optimize the return to duty of the maximum number of trained combat soldiers at the lowest possible level. Far-forward stabilization helps to maintain the physiology of injured soldiers who are unlikely to return to duty and allows for their rapid evacuation from the battlefield without needless sacrifice of life or function.

Medical Force 2000 (MF2K)
PATIENT FLOW IN A THEATER OF OPERATIONS

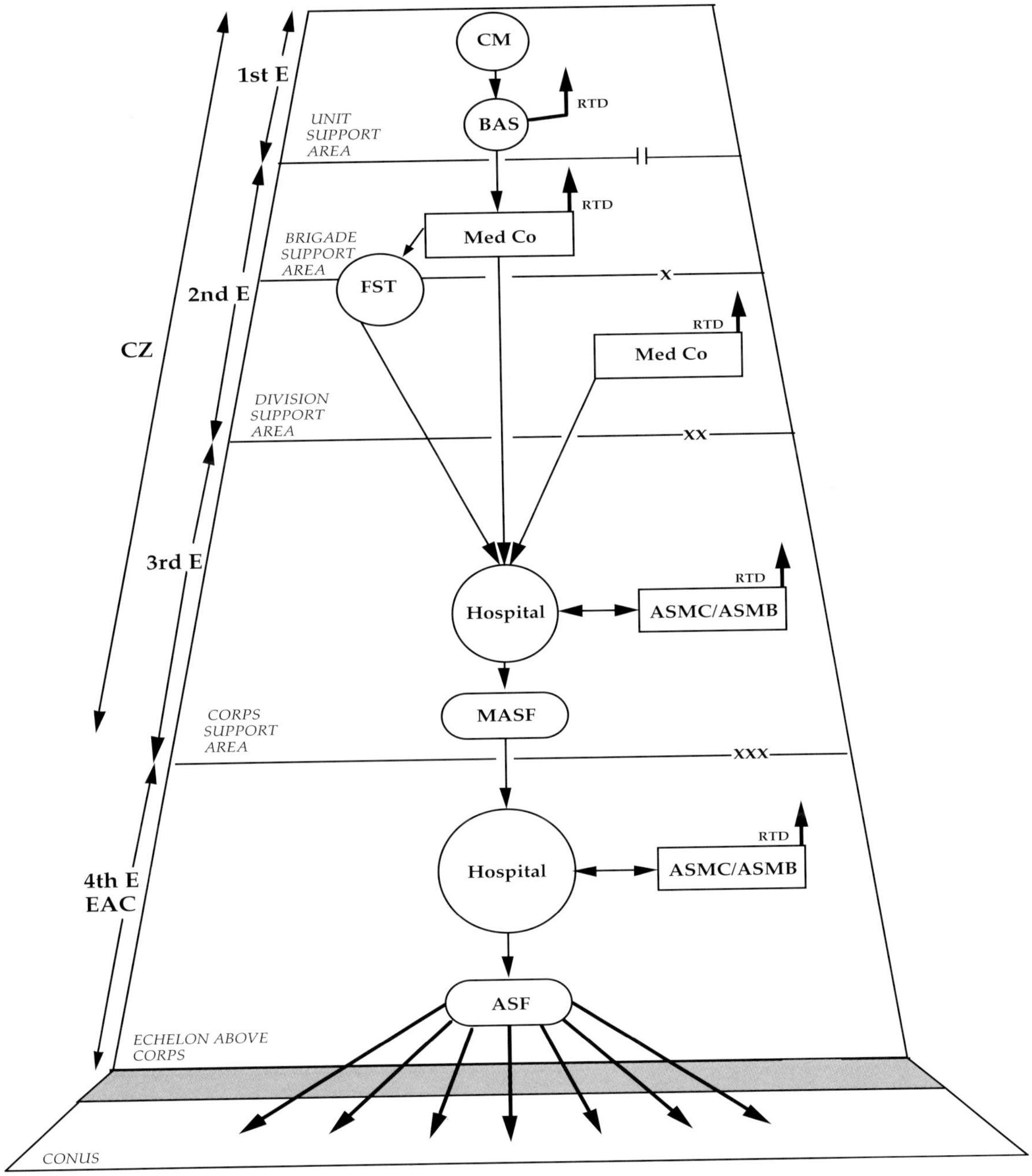

ASF:	Aeromedical Staging Facility, USAF	E:	Echelon
ASMB:	Area Support Medical Battalion	EAC:	Echelon Above Corps
ASMC:	Area Support Medical Company	FST:	Forward Surgical Team
BAS:	Battalion Aid Station	MASF:	Mobile Aeromedical Staging Facility, USAF
CM:	Combat Medic	Med Co:	Medical Company
CONUS:	Continental United States	RTD:	Return to Duty
CZ:	Combat Zone		

Chapter 1

COMBAT TRAUMA OVERVIEW

RONALD F. BELLAMY, M.D.*

*Colonel, Medical Corps, U.S. Army; Managing Editor and Officer in Charge, Textbook of Military Medicine, Borden Institute, Walter Reed Army Medical Center, Washington, D. C. 20307-5001

INTRODUCTION

For military anesthesiologists to assume responsibilities that transcend their traditional role in field hospitals, they will need a broad understanding of the problems of medical support in the theater of operations. The military anesthesiologist who is aware of what it is that makes military medicine unique and who is well versed in the management of trauma will be able to make important contributions to many of the problems that arise in combat casualty care. This chapter gives an epidemiologically oriented overview of that vast expanse of human misery treated by the specialty of military medicine, with special emphasis on combat trauma sustained in conventional land warfare. The stage will then be set for the ensuing chapters, with their detailed discussions of resuscitation, with special emphasis on emergency lifesaving interventions; the practice of anesthesia in the combat zone; anesthetic management of specific types of combat injuries; and critical-care medicine.

ATTRITION IN WAR

The military anesthesiologist's principal wartime role in the theater of operations will be, of course, to care for casualties with combat trauma, but it needs to be emphasized that such injuries constitute only one of the sources of attrition that can potentially destroy an army. The important sources of personnel attrition in the combat zone are (*a*) enemy action, which by definition includes not only battle injuries but also being captured; (*b*) disease; (*c*) nonbattle injury, which also includes the effect of a hostile environment; (*d*) desertion; and (*e*) administrative action that results in a soldier's being transferred from the unit in question (Figure 1-1). Not all the sources of attrition have medical implications; for the purpose of this chapter, only battle injury, disease, and nonbattle injury will be considered.

It should be noted that the word "casualty" was not used in the preceding paragraph. In the past, in most armies, a casualty was defined as a soldier who had been either physically injured by enemy action or captured. It was therefore inappropriate to refer to "disease casualties" or "psychiatric casualties." The U.S. Army Medical Department (AMEDD) has recently changed the definition of casualty: a combat-zone soldier who is noneffective for any medical reason.[1] This chapter uses the word casualty in its traditional meaning whenever historical data are studied.

Although it is usual to classify battle injury as injury that has resulted from the hostile actions of a military enemy, many battle injuries are actually inflicted by the casualty's own side in the confusion of the fighting. Perhaps because of the pejorative and emotional connotation that surrounds such casualties of so-called "friendly fire," their numerical importance as a source of attrition has been somewhat downplayed in the past. Although unofficial guidance on casualties of friendly fire suggests that 0.5% of battle casualties may fall into this category, more recent studies indicate that the actual prevalence is more like 10% to 20%.[2]

Historical Aspects

When viewed from the perspective of military history, disease and its common companion, a hostile environment, have been far greater threats to soldiers' health than hostile acts of a military en-

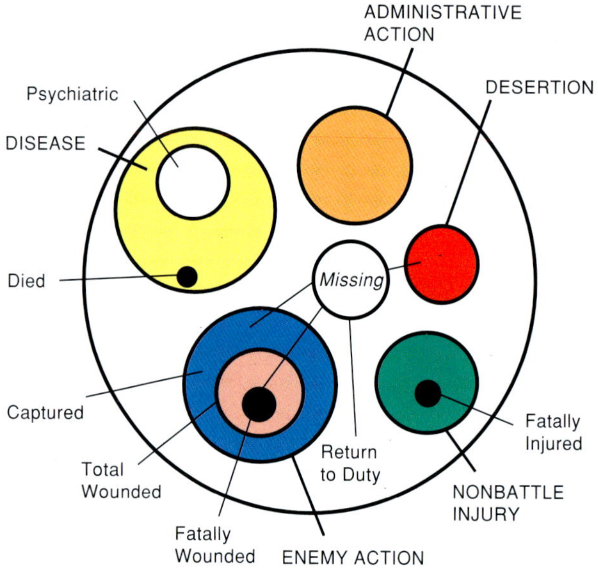

Fig. 1-1. Possible sources of attrition in a military unit. The major categories are enemy action, disease, nonbattle injury, desertion, and administrative action. Psychiatric casualties are placed in the disease category. Soldiers who are missing in action can ultimately be placed in the captured, fatally wounded, or desertion categories, or they can be returned to duty.

TABLE 1-1

ATTRITION IN THE GRANDE ARMÈE IN THE RUSSIA CAMPAIGN OF 1812

Source of Attrition	Number Affected
Died of hunger, exhaustion, cold, or disease	200,000
Killed in battle	100,000
Prisoners of war	100,000
Deserters	50,000
In hospital	50,000

Data source: Bodart G. *Losses of Life in Modern Wars.* Oxford, England: Clarendon Press; 1916: 127.

emy. There is no better example of this than the disaster that befell Napoleon's Grande Armèe in 1812. Napoleon started his invasion of Russia in June with more than 600,000 soldiers and finished in December with about 100,000. One assessment of what happened to the missing 500,000 is given in Table 1-1.[3] Most of these losses were from the group of armies under Napoleon's personal command: of 450,000 soldiers, only 25,000 are believed to have survived.[4] It is part of the mythology surrounding the campaign of 1812 that it was the cold of the Russian winter more than any other factor that destroyed the Grande Armèe, but this explanation was a self-serving fabrication of Napoleon's. More than two thirds of the Grande Armèe had been lost before the end of the summer of 1812 and before the major battle of the campaign, at Borodino on 7 September 1812. Heat and disease (primarily typhus and dysentery) during the summer, not cold and starvation during the autumn, caused the catastrophic attrition.[5] Disease wiped out the Grande Armèe because Napoleon's logistical support was predicated on an unrealistically optimistic appraisal of the campaign's duration (eg, food was available for only 3 wk) and, worse, his medical support was inadequate—even given the primitive nature of military medicine in the early 19th century.

The attrition of the Grande Armèe in Russia was by no means unique in the history of warfare, but lest it be thought that this experience is totally irrelevant to the modern age, the following example of attrition from World War II may be instructive. For brilliance of leadership, the North African campaign of the renowned German general Erwin Rommel is held in the greatest esteem by military authorities. Rommel ultimately lost, but his defeat is usually attributed to the overwhelming materiel and personnel strength of his adversaries. What is not generally appreciated is that Rommel's manpower problems were much of his own making. Table 1-2 shows the sources of attrition in Rommel's main fighting force—Panzerarmee Afrika—for the 15-month period starting in October 1941.[6]

For every German soldier that Rommel lost to battle injury, almost three were lost to disease. While the destruction of the Grande Armèe was fundamentally due to Napoleon's callous indifference to the needs of his soldiers, the attrition of Panzerarmee Afrika, although partially due to the hostile environment of the North African desert, was primarily the result of Rommel's ignorant indifference to his own and his soldiers' health. He never recognized what disease was doing to the strength of his army, and he clearly never understood that it is the commander and not the military medical service who is ultimately responsible for the health of the soldier.[7] It is not a little ironic that leaders such as Napoleon and Rommel are held in such high regard by the military profession when, in fact, they were a worse threat than the enemy to their own men.

Importance of Attrition due to Battle Injury

The relative importance of losses due to battle injury and from disease and nonbattle injury is determined by a variety of factors, including

- the presence of endemic diseases,
- the climate and the environment,

TABLE 1-2

ATTRITION IN PANZERARMEE AFRIKA* OCTOBER 1941–DECEMBER 1942

Source of Attrition	Number Affected
Killed	4,524
Wounded†	16,824
Missing‡	13,024
Sick§	88,320

*Average strength 43,000
†About 95% required evacuation to Europe
‡About 50% were probably captured; the remainder were killed
§Required admission to a hospital; at least 28,000 required evacuation to Europe
Data source: Fischer H. *Der deutsche Sanitätsdienst 1921–1945.* Vol 3. Osnabrück, Germany: Biblio Verlag; 1983: 1517, 1535.

- the duration of the deployment, and
- the nature of the tactical mission and the intensity of the fighting.

It is certainly possible for battle injury to be the major source of attrition in short but fiercely fought campaigns. The Battle of Cannae in 216 BC, in which a Roman army of some 86,000 was totally destroyed by Hannibal, with the loss of 50,000 killed and 25,000 captured, is a good example of circumstances in which battle injury is the predominant source of attrition in a campaign.[8] A more recent example of the importance of the intensity of the fighting as a determinant of attrition is the German airborne attack on the Island of Crete. Over a 10-day period in May 1941, a German force of about 22,000 lost no fewer than 6,000 men: 4,000 killed and 2,000 wounded. The first day alone saw 4,000 casualties among the 8,000 airborne troops who had arrived on Crete.[9] Needless to say, losses due to disease during this period were a minor component of the overall attrition.

Thus, given (*a*) intense fighting, (*b*) military leadership that recognizes its responsibility for the health of the men, (*c*) a knowledgeable and efficient medical service, and (*d*) the good fortune to fight in a climate and an environment that are not especially hostile, disease and nonbattle injury may not be the predominant sources of attrition. The British experience in the early weeks of the Normandy invasion in the summer of 1944 may be taken as an example. Figure 1-2 shows the partition of the British army's losses (rounded off to the nearest 500) during the 7 weeks after the landing on D day, 6 June 1944. Battle injury caused approximately 56% of the total British attrition due to medical reasons (missing and prisoner casualties are not considered).[10] Given enlightened leadership and an effective medical service, attrition due to battle injury is likely to be of greater importance than would be suggested from considerations based on the U.S. experience in, for example, the Spanish–American War—in which battle injury caused fewer than 7% of the total deaths.[11]

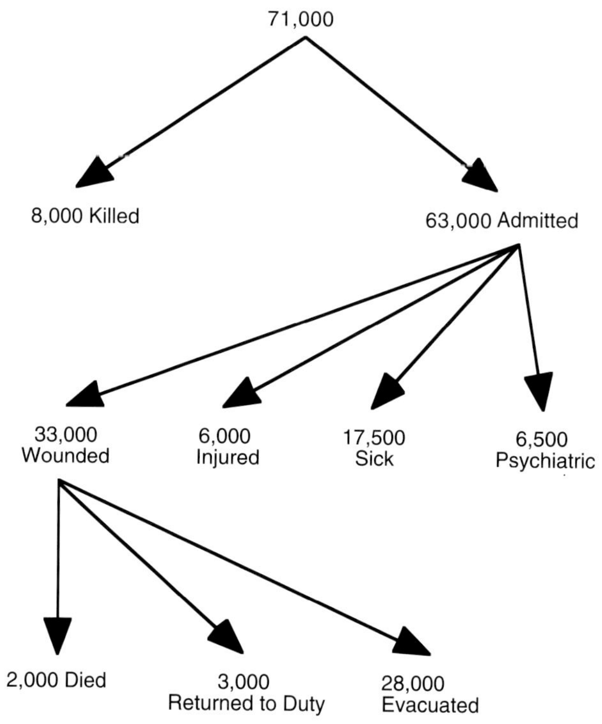

Fig. 1-2. Partition of the medical sources of attrition for the British army in Normandy, 6 June through 31 July 1944. Battle injury was the major source of attrition in the high-intensity campaign. Data source: Crew FAE. *Campaigns. North-West Europe*. Vol 4. London, England: The Army Medical Services, Her Majesty's Stationery Office; 1962: 597, 608, 610.

Magnitude of Attrition

To determine the medical assets (eg, the number of anesthesiologists) required in a war, an estimate of the expected number of battle, nonbattle, and disease casualties is needed. Although the medical threat from disease and the environment can be forecasted if the prevalence of endemic diseases in the theater of operation and its climate are known with some accuracy, the estimation of battle casualty rates is at best an art. Battle casualty rates, like those for disease and nonbattle injury, are usually given as an *incidence* (ie, the number of casualties per 1,000 soldiers per day, or the percentage of a unit of known size per day). The current practice is to use computer models that incorporate historical data to estimate rates for a unit of given size carrying out a specified tactical mission (eg, an airborne battalion assaulting a fortified position, or a division engaged in an opposed river crossing). The major deficiency of this empirical approach is that the data are from unique historical events and may not be applicable to a hypothetical future combat operation. What would have been the result if data gathered during the assault of the Siegfried line (1944–1945) had been used to predict the number of casualties before U.S. forces attacked the Saddam line in Kuwait in February 1991? A prediction based on the historical data would have overestimated by several hundredfold the actual number of casualties for this simple reason: the defense of the Siegfried line was conducted by well-trained and highly motivated German professionals, while the Saddam line was defended by ineffective Iraqi draftees.

Intensity

Because it is difficult to predict casualty rates for all warfighting scenarios, descriptive terms such as "intensity" have commonly been used as qualitative indicators of expected attrition. Using this approach, it is possible to conceive of a hypothetical spectrum of combat intensities extending from peacekeeping operations to global nuclear war.[12] Between the extremes are various intensities of conventional war. The "low"-intensity end of the spectrum is typified by the Vietnam War, with its multitude of tiny search-and-destroy missions; the 1944 Normandy invasion and the gigantic air-land battle that occurred in the summer of 1943 at Kursk in central Russia are both examples of the "high"-intensity end.

The concept of intensity is meaningful only when viewed as a quasi-statistical term that depends on both the duration of the combat and the size of the population at risk. The term is meaningless when applied to a single soldier or to a short, small-unit combat action. For a soldier who is killed in action, the combat was of maximum intensity regardless of whether his death occurred in a low-intensity peacekeeping operation or a high-intensity global nuclear war. The combat action in Mogadishu, Somalia, on 3 October 1993 (during which 18 U.S. Army Rangers were killed and 70 were wounded during a company-sized operation) was no doubt considered very intense by the participants. However, a single such action during a several-month-long deployment by a brigade- or division-sized unit would qualify the entire operation as one of very low intensity. On the other hand, if the combat action in Mogadishu had been repeated daily over months by hundreds of company-sized units, the level of attrition would have been that of a high-intensity war.

The purpose of the Venn diagrams in Figure 1-3 is to contrast the trauma-generating potential of three very different sources: a modern U.S. city, a low-intensity war, and a high-intensity war. The city is represented by San Francisco in 1977.[13] From a population of about 550,000, the probability of becoming a casualty (defined as either being killed at the scene or sustaining an injury that required admission to a hospital) was about 1 in 78. Of all trauma victims, 6% were fatally injured. The low-intensity war is represented by the U.S. Army in the Vietnam War for the year 1969.[14–16] The average troop strength was about 326,000 and the overall probability of becoming a battle casualty was slightly more than 1 in 10; for soldiers who were casualties, the probability of dying was about 1 in 5. The Iraqi army (but not the U.S. Army) experienced high-intensity attrition during the Persian Gulf War.[17] Approximately 500,000 Iraqis were deployed in the Kuwaiti theater of operation, of whom about 100,000 were killed and 100,000 were taken prisoner. The Venn diagram that portrays the Iraqi experience makes clear the truth of the famous observation by the noted Russian military surgeon Nikolai Ivanovich Pirogov (1810–1881) that "war is an epidemic of injuries."[18]

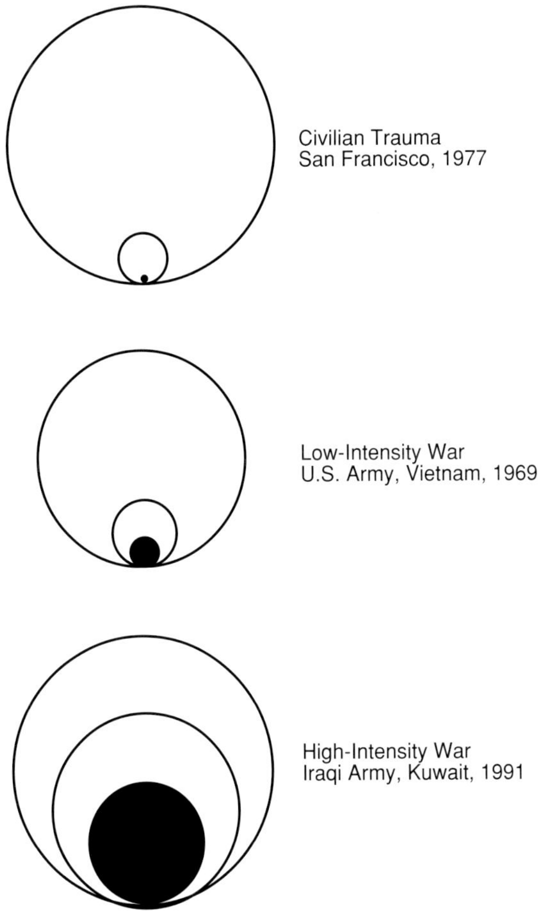

Fig. 1-3. The largest circle in each Venn diagram is proportional to the population at risk; the inner circle is proportional to the number of casualties, and the black circles are proportional to the number of fatalities. The Iraqi data are provisional. We have assumed that 100,000 have been killed and 100,000 wounded or taken prisoner.

Battle Casualty Rates

Casualty rates can be calculated for the three examples shown in Figure 1-3, but it should be understood that such overall average rates ignore not only day-to-day (ie, stochastic) fluctuations but also unique events (eg, battles) and disasters (eg, earthquakes). They are statistical generalizations and are useful only for illustrative purposes. Calculated casualty rates are about 0.0035% per day for the city, 0.025% per day in the low-intensity war, and 0.7% per day in the high-intensity war. The respective rates for civilian trauma and low-intensity war, and the respective rates for low-intensity and high-intensity wars, each differ by about one order of magnitude. Although the city selected—San Francisco in 1977—had a notably benign milieu given the violence-plagued U.S. cities of the last decade of the 20th century, an increase of the rate much beyond 0.004% or 0.005% per day is unlikely. By way of comparison, the overall attrition rate for Napoleon's Grande Armèe in Russia was from 1% to 3% per day; for Panzerarmee Afrika, attrition due to enemy action averaged about 0.15% per day; and for battle injury in the British army in Normandy, the average rate was about 0.18% per day. A battle casualty rate of 0.17% per day characterized German attrition in the first 100 days of their attack on the Soviet Union in 1941.[9] In actual numbers, this rate meant about 5,500 casualties *per day*—more than 10-fold higher than the *total* U.S. Army losses in the Persian Gulf War. It should be understood that these rates are meaningful only for large populations of soldiers engaged in combat for prolonged periods. They are presented for illustrative purposes and are not equivalent to the official projected rates found in U.S. Army Field Manual 8-55, *Planning for Health Service Support*.[1]

Although there is no completely successful approach to predicting attrition, some well-documented empirical observations on attrition have been made:

- Battle casualty rates are inversely proportional to the size of the unit; for example, a battalion will have a higher rate than a division.[12] There is an obvious explanation for this fact: the smaller the combat unit, the fewer the combat support and combat service support personnel who, by virtue of their duties, are not exposed to direct enemy fire.
- When combat units are actually in contact with the enemy, division battle casualty rates in high-intensity war have usually been about 1% per day, although on rare occasions rates of up to 10% per day have been observed. Corresponding brigade and battalion rates are 3% and 10% per day, respectively. Army rates can be expected to be less than 1% per day.[19]
- Disease and nonbattle injury rates occur at a constant rate, which ranges from 0.1% to 0.3% per day to 0.5% per day when (*a*) combat operations interfere with the provision of effective preventive medicine or (*b*) the environment is especially hostile.[19]

To put the estimation of casualty rates in practical perspective, consider the following example. A brigade-sized force (about 3,000 men) is engaged in day-long, high-intensity combat. Given a battle casualty rate of 3% per day, 100 casualties may be expected. In addition, 15 soldiers can be expected to be lost because of disease. Not all the combat casualties will require anesthetic management, because some of them will have been killed and some will have minor wounds not requiring an anesthetic.

THE NATURE OF COMBAT INJURY

Combat injury and civilian trauma differ in significant respects. The nature of combat injury depends on several factors: (*a*) the mechanisms of injury, of which penetrating injury is the predominant; (*b*) the source of penetrating missiles, of which fragments and bullets predominate; (*c*) the distribution of missile wounds on the body surface; and (*d*) the relation between mortality and wound location: specifically, which internal organs have been struck.

Mechanisms of Injury

The mechanisms of injury found in conventional land warfare—penetrating, blast, blunt, and thermal—do not differ from the mechanisms that cause injury in civilian life. What is different is the relative prevalence of the mechanisms. While a blunt mechanism is the most important source of injury for civilians, trauma inflicted during combat is overwhelmingly penetrating in nature (Figure 1-4). Data

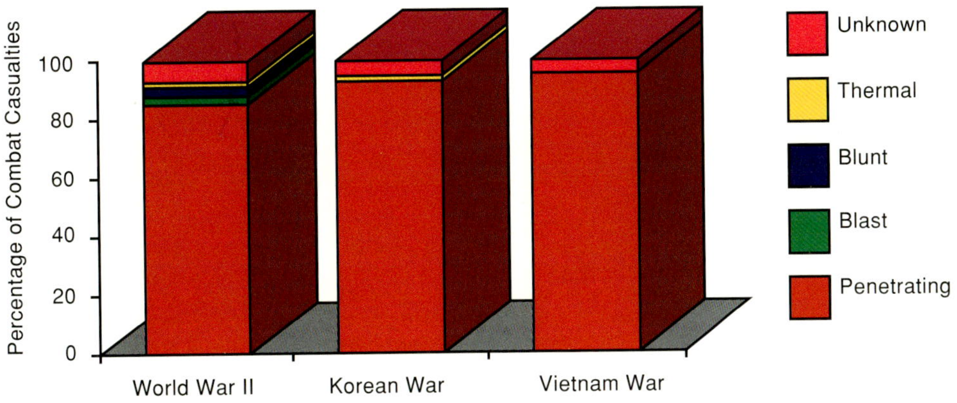

World War II: for 600,000 casualties surviving to receive medical care[1]
Korean War: all combat casualties[2]
Vietnam War: January 1965 to June 1970; for casualties surviving to receive medical care[3]; injuries were either penetrating or other than penetrating

Fig. 1-4. Mechanism of injury in US Army combat casualties. Penetrating missiles were the source of injury in 85% to 95% of casualties. Data sources: (1) Reister FA. *Medical Statistics in World War II*. Washington, DC: Department of the Army, Office of The Surgeon General; 1975: Table 7, p 90 and Table 17, p 202. (2) Reister FA. *Battle Casualties and Medical Statistics: US Army Experience in Korea*. Washington, DC: Department of the Army, The Surgeon General; 1973: 45. (3) Neel S. Medical Support of the US Army in Vietnam 1965–1970. Washington, DC: Department of the Army; 1973: 54.

compiled from the U.S. Army's records for World War II,[20] the Korean War,[21] and the Vietnam War[22] indicate that penetrating missiles are the mechanism of injury in about 90% of all battle casualties (ie, soldiers who are injured as a result of the hostile actions of a military enemy).

It is commonly thought that "blast" is a frequent cause of combat trauma, but this is a misconception. It no doubt springs from popular images of people being blown apart by powerful explosions. Although it is true that soldiers in close proximity to the detonation of a large explosive munition may sustain blast and thermal injuries, penetrating missile wounds constitute the major medical treatment problem. This phenomenon is especially apparent when an extremity is amputated by the detonation of a buried antipersonnel mine. Much of the damage is done by penetrating missiles that arise secondarily from the ground, the soldier's boot, and even his foot. The secondary missiles, in conjunction with the "blast wind" (ie, the mass of air displaced by the explosion) are responsible for the gross mutilation that is characteristic of such injuries. Primary blast injury—due to overpressure from a blast wave—is distinctly uncommon in surviving casualties except in the form of perforated tympanic membranes. It is possible that, in future wars, the development of enhanced blast weapons such as fuel air explosives will increase the possibility of more-serious blast overpressure injuries involving the lung and solid abdominal viscera.[23]

Blunt trauma, the mechanism of injury responsible for most civilian trauma, is much less common as a cause of battle injury. When combat blunt trauma is found, it is usually in the context of a tactical vehicle detonating an antitank mine.[24] Even in these circumstances, blunt injury is the cause of only a small proportion (8%) of tank-crew casualties.[25]

The infrequent use of flame and incendiary weapons in modern warfare would be expected to make thermal injury uncommon. When soldiers are burned, the thermal injuries are usually caused by secondary explosions and fires arising from the fuel of battle-damaged armored fighting vehicles and aircraft. During World War II, about 40% of tank-crew casualties who survived to receive care were burned.[25] Half of these men had burns as their only injury. The other half had burns in addition to penetrating missile wounds. Most of the remaining 60% of tank-crew casualties had penetrating trauma. The design of the armored vehicles used by the U.S. military, such as the Abrams main battle tank, has minimized the potential for secondary explosions and fires, further decreasing the likelihood for thermal injury.

Unique circumstances, however, may generate large numbers of burned casualties. For example, at least 14% of all British army casualties in the Falklands War sustained burns because of a single combat action: two British troopships were set on fire by enemy action before the soldiers could disembark.[26]

Nonbattle Injury

The preceding treatment of mechanisms deals exclusively with injuries sustained as the result of the hostile actions of a military enemy. There is another category of trauma that may afflict soldiers in the combat zone: nonbattle injury. Nonbattle injuries show some similarity to civilian trauma in that blunt and thermal trauma are common. Vehicular accidents, especially those involving rotorwing aircraft, are common, but most serious cases of nonbattle injury result from accidents with weapons such as explosive munitions. Thus, penetrating missile wounds are also commonly found in soldiers with nonbattle injuries.

The lethality of nonbattle injuries in the Vietnam War can be calculated: dead at the site of the accident, 5.0%; died in hospital, 1.2%.[27] As will be discussed later in this chapter, the mortality of nonbattle injuries is significantly lower than the mortality of battle injuries.

Service-Specific Aspects of Combat Injury

The mechanisms of injury and the rates of attrition are service-specific. During World War II, the overall U.S. Navy casualty rate was about 0.06% per day.[28] The probability of a fatal outcome following a combat injury on a ship was much higher than that observed in conventional land warfare: 48% of casualties were either killed or missing. Penetrating injuries were found in 39% of surviving naval casualties; this mechanism of action is therefore much less common aboard ship than in land warfare. Burns were the mechanism of injury in 22% of the casualties. Combined penetrating and thermal trauma occurred in 11% of casualties.

As befits the nature of air warfare in the last half of the 20th century, aircrew (air force and navy) casualties are uncommon, and their medical outcome is closely related to the magnitude of the aircraft's battle damage. When the damage is sufficiently severe to cause the loss of the aircraft, about two thirds of the crew can be expected to become casualties. Data indicate that one half of airmen who are injured are killed, and about two thirds of survivors have orthopedic injuries due to blunt trauma.[29]

Sources of Penetrating Missiles

Bullets from small arms and fragments from explosive munitions are the two sources of penetrating wounds on the modern battlefield. In the major wars of this century, wounds made by explosive munitions have been numerically much more important, being found in more than two thirds of all casualties. Three examples illustrate this statement. One study of British casualties in Normandy found that 69% of the casualties had wounds made by explosive munitions.[9] Similarly, in the Israeli army in the Lebanon War of 1982, explosive munitions caused about 80% of the casualties.[30] The U.S. experience in the Vietnam War was no different: about 76% of all army casualties had penetrating missile wounds caused by fragments from explosive munitions.[16] However, an analysis of the Vietnam data provides this interesting insight: the relative numerical importance of bullet and fragments as the sources of penetrating wounds depends on *how* the war is fought. In the early part of the war, the percentage of soldiers with gunshot wounds was unusually high, sometimes exceeding 50%. The reason is that during the early part of the Vietnam War, U.S. Army units engaged in search-and-destroy operations in which both they and their opponents were usually armed with small arms.[22] A high proportion of casualties with gunshot wounds is one characteristic of low-intensity warfare, unlike what is found in high-intensity warfare involving armored fighting vehicles, artillery, and aircraft.

Explosive Munitions

The explosive munitions that cause fragmentation injuries are shells, rockets, bombs, mortars, mines, hand grenades, and ad hoc devices such as booby traps.[31] The basic design consists of a container, a fuze, and an explosive. Until recently, the container (ie, the shell), being broken apart by the detonation of the explosive, provided the fragments. Because the shell broke into irregular pieces of assorted sizes (some weighing a pound or more) and a range of velocities, it is customary to refer to such weapons as "random"-fragmentation munitions. With explosive munitions of more recent vintage, the container is designed to break up into small pieces of uniform size and shape; therefore, the fragments' initial velocities are constrained to a narrow range. A typical design produces hundreds to thousands of 50- to 1,000-mg fragments, which are expelled with very high initial velocities (4,000–6,000 fps). In the most modern designs, preformed fragments are placed in the container and are expelled by the detonation of an explosive charge. The Vietnam War–era Claymore mine, with its 700 steel ball bearings (0.75 g each), is a good example of an explosive munitions containing preformed fragments. In the armaments industry, the two latter categories of explosive munitions are referred to as "improved"-fragmentation munitions.

The penetrating wounds produced by random- and improved-fragmentation munitions show characteristic differences. The older explosive munitions, especially the shells, were capable of causing massive mutilating injuries such as decapitation. Improved-fragmentation munitions characteristically produce multiple wounds; frequently, the casualty will be riddled with many small fragments.

Another characteristic of modern explosive munition design is that the individual munitions are frequently clustered (ie, packaged together) in a carrier (a bomb, shell, or rocket) for delivery to the enemy position. The individual submunitions are disseminated from their carrier before being detonated. Such cluster munitions greatly increase the casualty-generating potential of a given weight of munition.

A recently developed cluster munition consists of shaped-charge warheads with easily fragmentable side walls. A shaped-charge warhead is a sophisticated device that was developed during World War II as an antiarmor weapon. The hot, rapidly moving gas produced by the explosion of the shaped-charge warhead is focused in much the same way that a lens focuses light. By combining the antiarmor effect of the shaped-charge warhead with antipersonnel fragmentation effects, a dual-purpose submunition can be made.

Small Arms

The most commonly used military small arms are the assault rifle and the machine gun.[31] Their essential characteristic is that they are fully automatic; that is, they will fire as long as the trigger is pulled and there are rounds in the magazine. This behavior distinguishes military from civilian small arms: the latter class of weapons, although usually but mistakenly referred to as "automatic," are actually "semiautomatic." In a semiautomatic small arm, the trigger must be pulled every time a bullet is fired. What is automatic in a semiautomatic small arm is the chambering (of rounds) and extraction (of cartridges).

The machine gun was perfected during World War I to the extent that it displaced the single-shot, bolt-action rifle as the dominant military small arm. The machine gun was responsible for some of the most notorious slaughters on the western front, including the killing of some 20,000 British soldiers on the first day of the Battle of the Somme in 1916.[32] The assault rifle was developed during the last years of World War II and may be looked on as an effort to give the individual soldier some of the potential firepower of the machine gun. The two best-known assault rifles today are the M16 series developed in the United States (the M16A2 is not technically fully automatic, as it is designed to fire three-round bursts) and the various designs of Kalashnikov such as the AK47 and the AK74.

The most commonly used machine gun and assault rifle bullets have calibers (in millimeters) of 5.45, 5.56, 7.62, and 12.7. The muzzle velocities range between 2,350 and 3,300 fps. Such velocities are substantially greater than those found in bullets fired by civilian handguns, which typically have muzzle velocities of 800 to 1,200 fps. Because the kinetic energy of a projectile is a function of its velocity squared, bullets fired from military small arms almost always have muzzle kinetic energy substantially greater (3-fold or more) than that of bullets fired by civilian handguns.

The *potential* for massive energy transfer and resultant tissue damage is increased by the high kinetic energy of military bullets. Whether the potential is actually realized, however, depends on aspects of the bullet's construction and the biophysical characteristics of the target tissue. The latter factor is apparent when comparing wounds made in bone and lung. Energy transfer is maximized when a missile strikes bone, but is minimized in lung with its low density and high viscoelasticity. A bullet's construction becomes an important determinant of energy transfer when it potentiates deformation or fragmentation. Bullets fired by military small arms are required by international law to be covered by a metal jacket, which is supposed to minimize deformation. Consequently, deformation of military bullets is less commonly seen than with unjacketed bullets used by civilians. Nevertheless, military bullets can cause extensive tissue damage because they may break up or fragment along their trajectory in the body. The fragmentation occurs because the bullet's metal jacket can easily be disrupted. Fragmentation is commonly seen with the M193 and M855 rounds fired by the

M16 series of assault rifles, but also occurs with 7.62-mm x 51-mm North Atlantic Treaty Organization (NATO) and M1943 Kalashnikov rounds, when manufactured with thinner-than-usual or nonsteel jackets, respectively.

Another factor that tends to increase energy transfer from military small-arm bullets is their propensity to yaw and tumble in tissue. This instability is more common than with bullets designed to be fired from civilian handguns, and is caused by the characteristic long, pointed shape of military bullets, which, by maximizing the separation between the bullet's centers of pressure and mass, predisposes to yaw and tumbling.

Massive energy transfer usually results in massive tissue damage. Nevertheless, it is important to recognize that neither the magnitude of the energy transfer nor the magnitude of tissue damage is necessarily synonymous with the magnitude of the medical treatment problem. A tiny wound of the parietal cortex made by a small fragment with several hundred joules of energy gives rise to a far different medical problem than does a massive above-the-knee amputation caused by the transfer of tens of thousands of joules of energy from an exploding antipersonnel mine.

The lethality of penetrating missile wounds sustained in combat is well defined.[30] The probability of a fatal outcome from a fragment wound made by a random-fragmentation munition is about 1 in 5 for shells and about 1 in 10 for hand grenades. Paradoxically, the lethality of improved-fragmentation munitions is lower: 1 in 7 for shells and as low as 1 in 20 for hand grenades. The probability of a fatal outcome from a single wound made at random by a bullet from a military small arm is about 1 in 3. Due to the fully automatic design of military small arms, multiple wounds can be expected; in fact, data from the Vietnam War show that a soldier killed by military small-arms fire was struck, on average, by 3.2 bullets.[15]

Distribution of Missile Wounds by Body Surface

An understanding of the medical treatment problems caused by bullets and fragments is furthered by understanding the distribution of penetrating missile wounds on the body surface. Unfortunately, data from previous wars giving the distribution of wounds are difficult to interpret for several reasons:

- First, the definitions of body regions lack consistency (eg, where does the shoulder become the thorax?).
- Second, diverse selection criteria are used (eg, some reports deal only with treated casualties, while others include dead as well as living casualties).
- Third, many casualties have wounds that involve multiple regions on the body. How to classify such casualties is a major methodological problem.

It is possible to simplify the analysis of the distribution of penetrating missile wounds by assuming that, to a first approximation, hits on the body are random and thus are distributed as a function of body surface area (eg, a thigh gets more hits than a little toe because it has more surface area). If so, then the observed distribution should be approximated by the "Rule of Nines" (Table 1-3, first column).

Of course, most soldiers are not wounded while standing in the anatomical position, so using the Rule of Nines for estimating regional body surface areas is not likely to make for accurate predictions. During World War II, British analysts attempted to develop a model for the observed distribution of wounds by assuming that the exposed body surface area was very much altered by the position of the soldier at the time of wounding.[33] For example, the regional distribution of the surface area exposed to a frontal attack is very much different for a soldier crouching or in the prone position, compared with one standing in the anatomical position (see Table 1-3, second column).

Although the problem of multiple wounds is not addressed, the most useful treatment of the distribution of penetrating missile wounds is Beebe and DeBakey's analysis of the World War II data of the U.S. Army.[11] The distribution observed in World War II for the total population of casualties for ground warfare (see Table 1-3, third column) shows a major deviation from the predicted distribution in the unexpectedly high proportion of head wounds. Although the observed distribution represents the effect of aimed fire to a limited extent, the increased propensity of missiles to strike the head is primarily due to the head's increased exposure (for tactical reasons) compared with other body parts. The fourth column of Table 1-3 shows the distribution observed for casualties who survived long enough to enter the medical system. It also shows an unexpectedly high number of casualties with head wounds, but the departure from the predicted distribution is less than that seen in the total casualty population. No doubt the decrease in the percentage of casualties with head wounds who survive to

TABLE 1-3

DISTRIBUTION OF MISSILE WOUNDS BY BODY SURFACE AREA (PERCENTAGE)

Body Region	Rule of Nines	Predicted[1]	WWII[2] All	WWII[2] Living
Head, Face, and Neck	9	12	21	15
Chest and Abdomen	37*			
Chest		16	13	10
Abdomen		11	11.5	5
Extremity				
Upper	18	22	23.5	28
Lower	36	39	35	41.5

* The combined surface areas of the torso plus the genitals and the perineum
Definitions:
Rule of Nines: body surface area as used to quantitate the magnitude of a burn
Predicted: the standard anatomical distribution of regional surface areas has been adjusted by assuming that the soldier will be in a variety of combat-relevant postures (standing, crouching, and prone), weighted according to an assumed probablity
WWII: All: US Army ground casualties, both living and dead
Living: US Army ground casualties who survive to enter the medical system
Data sources: (1) Palmer A. Survey of battle casualties, Eighth Air Force, June, July, and August 1944. In: Beyer JC, ed. *Wound Ballistics*. Washington, DC: Department of the Army, Office of The Surgeon General; 1962: 573. (2) Beebe GW, DeBakey ME. *Battle Casualties*. Springfield, Ill: Charles C Thomas; 1952: 92, 186.

receive treatment is indicative of the high immediate lethality of such wounds.

The data in Table 1-3 are consistent with the conclusion that the regional distribution of penetrating missile wounds is an approximate function of the distribution of body surface area except that the head, face, and neck receive about twice as many wounds as expected. The discrepancy is lessened when adjustments are made for the position assumed by the soldier during combat and when only treatable casualties are considered. Either way, about two thirds of all casualties can be expected to have wounds of the extremities.

Wound Depth

The data in Table 1-3 give only the location on the body surface of a penetrating wound and do not tell whether there is an associated internal injury. Both a superficial wound involving only the abdominal wall and a wound made by a missile that perforates through the entire abdomen and injures several intraabdominal viscera are classified as *abdominal*, but only the latter wound is likely to be associated with mortality or significant morbidity. Thus, regional wound distributions need to be interpreted in terms of the depth of the wound tract. A therapeutically useful distinction can be made between penetrating missile wounds that involve only soft tissue (ie, skin, fat, or skeletal muscle) and those that also involve bone, neurovascular structures, or viscera. The distinction between soft-tissue and visceral wounds can also be applied to resolving the problem of classifying casualties with multiple wounds because many have multiple soft-tissue wounds only, or have, in addition to the soft-tissue wounds, an injury of a solitary internal organ. The classification of penetrating wounds in this chapter uses the distinction between soft-tissue and visceral wounds and utilizes two resources: the Wound Data and Munitions Effectiveness Team (WDMET) study[15] from the Vietnam War and the Abbreviated Injury Scale (AIS)[34] developed by the Association for the Advancement of Automotive Medicine.

The WDMET study consists of detailed descriptions of about 8,000 U.S. Army and U.S. Marine casualties wounded during an 18-month period from 1967 to 1969. Teams of data collectors accompanied company- and battalion-sized units during tactical operations such as search-and-destroy missions. Data were collected on the tactical situation, the weapons that caused the wounds, field first aid and the circumstances of evacuation, the detailed anatomy of wounds (including autopsy reports for those who were fatally wounded), and initial care in hospitals. The WDMET study is uniquely valuable because an effort was made to describe all casualties occurring during a given combat action, including the killed-in-action and carded-for-record-only categories, in addition to casualties who were hospitalized.

The AIS was introduced in 1976 for the purpose of standardizing the assessment of trauma resulting from automobile accidents. The potential lethality of a given injury was assigned a numerical rating: 1 (minor), 2 (moderate), 3 (serious), 4 (severe), 5 (critical), and 6 (not survivable). Nine anatomical regions were recognized: head, face, neck, thorax, abdomen, spine, upper extremity, lower extremity including the pelvis, and external. The last region is the skin and superficial soft tissue. Although the AIS initially emphasized blunt trauma, subsequent modifications have included entries for penetrating trauma.

Combat casualties from the WDMET database were classified according to the AIS with these exceptions: following the methodology used by the Injury Severity Score (ISS), the pelvic bones were considered part of the extremities, and the spine was amalgamated into the neck, thorax, and abdomen anatomical regions.[35] The following anatomical definitions were used:

- external, which includes skin, fat, and skeletal muscle anywhere on the body;
- head, which includes the skull and its contents;
- face, which includes the facial bones, eyes, and the oral and nasal cavities;
- neck, which includes the viscera and the cervical spine;
- chest, which includes the rib cage, thoracic spine, and thoracic viscera;
- abdomen, which includes the abdomen, pelvis, and the lumbar spine; and
- extremity, which includes bones and neurovascular structures.

It should be noted that the word "extremity" as used in this analysis does not have the same meaning that it has in Table 1-3; in those data, not only fractures and neurovascular injuries but also wounds of the soft tissues are included in the term "extremity."

A casualty with two or more wounds was assigned to a specific body region rather than the multiple category only if the AIS value for an injury in one region exceeded the AIS values for all injuries in the other regions. Only casualties who had two or more injuries of equal AIS value in different body

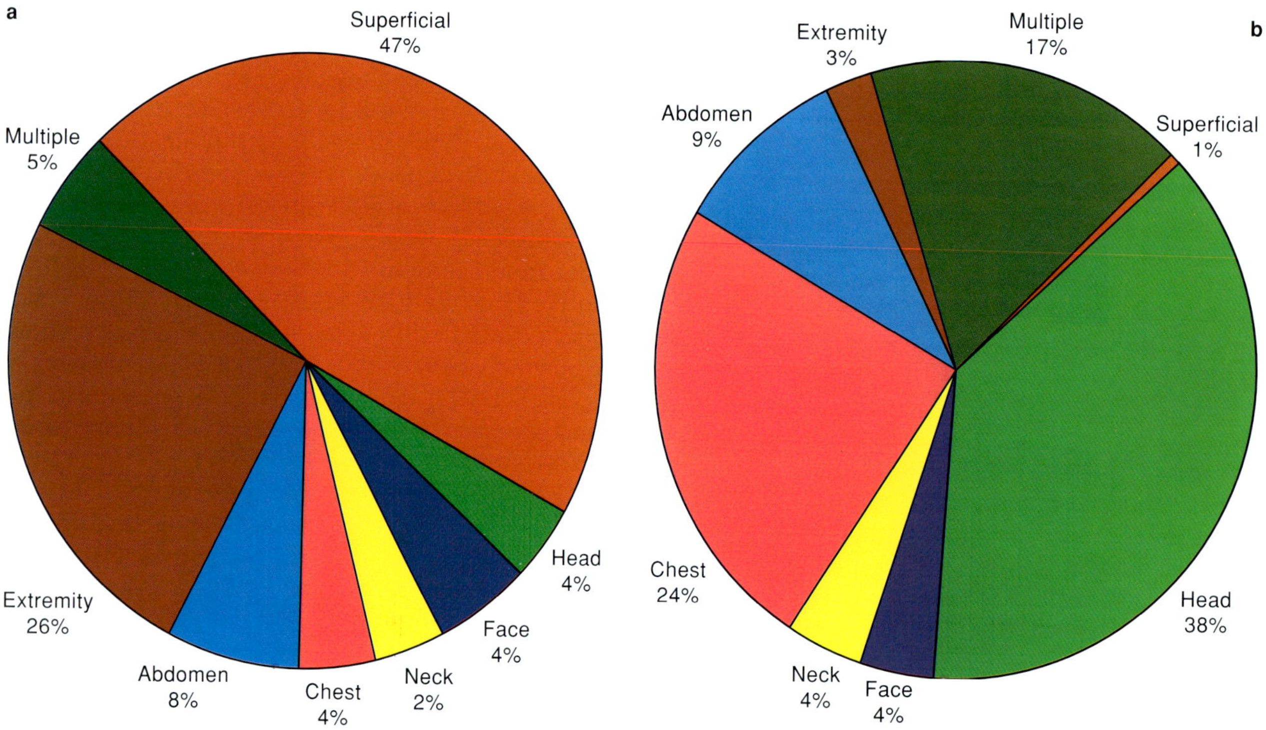

Fig. 1-5. Distribution of nonfatal (**a**) and fatal (**b**) wounds by body region. Superficial wounds (involving the skin, fat, and skeletal muscle) and injuries to the bones of the extremities are the most common sites of nonfatal wounds. The head and chest are the most common sites of fatal injuries. The multiple wounds category is restricted to casualties whose injuries were (1) of equal value according to the Abbreviated Injury Scale and (2) to at least two different body regions. Data source: Wound Data and Munitions Effectiveness Team database.

regions were classified as multiple. Thus, a casualty with AIS injuries of 5 for both the brain and the lung was classified as multiple, while a casualty with an AIS injury of 4 in the liver and 3 for the extremity was placed in the abdominal category. The analysis of the WDMET data in terms of the AIS for casualties who were fatally wounded and for those who survived is shown in Figure 1-5. About two thirds of fatally wounded casualties had wounds of either the head or the chest. Wounds of the soft tissues and the extremity skeleton were found in about three fourths of living casualties. This last finding is consistent with the military surgery experience of the 20th century, which is that at least two thirds of operations performed on combat casualties involved the management of soft-tissue wounds and fractures.

MEDICAL OUTCOME OF COMBAT INJURY

The medical outcome of combat trauma is usually discussed in terms of *mortality* and *morbidity*. Mortality is easily measured because it is not difficult to recognize when someone is dead. Much more difficult is arriving at an all-embracing definition of morbidity. When is an injury present, and how severe must it be to for the soldier to be classified as a casualty? These are not idle questions. One of the major problems of interpreting combat casualty data from the Vietnam War is that in addition to such casualty categories as killed in action, died of wounds, and wounded in action, there is a fourth category: carded for record only. Casualties who are carded for record only have very minor wounds that require either no treatment or treatment that does not require admission to a medical treatment facility. Should these soldiers be included in any assessment of medical outcome? Inclusion of casualties who are carded for record only has a marked effect on mortality and morbidity data because the population is not numerically insignificant: they constituted the largest single group of the U.S. Army's combat casualties in the Vietnam War. Such casualties have been excluded from the following analysis because their conditions do not constitute medical problems.

Combat mortality is quantitated in terms of two indicators: killed in action and died of wounds.[1] They differ not only in terms of *time* of death but, more importantly, in *where* death occurred. The locations of death for fatally wounded U.S. soldiers in World War II, the Korean War, and the Vietnam War, combined, are shown in Figure 1-6.[11,20,21] About 90% of fatally wounded U.S. soldiers expired on the battlefield; only about 10% expired after having entered the medical system. Expiring before entering the medical system is tantamount to dying before receiving effective medical care; in AMEDD, this means dying before reaching the battalion aid station, the lowest level at which a medical treatment facility is found. Thus, casualties who are killed in action expire *before* reaching any medical treatment facility, while casualties who die of wounds expire *after* reaching a medical treatment facility.

Mortality outcome data are given not only as the gross number of casualties who are classified as killed in action or died of wounds but also as nor-

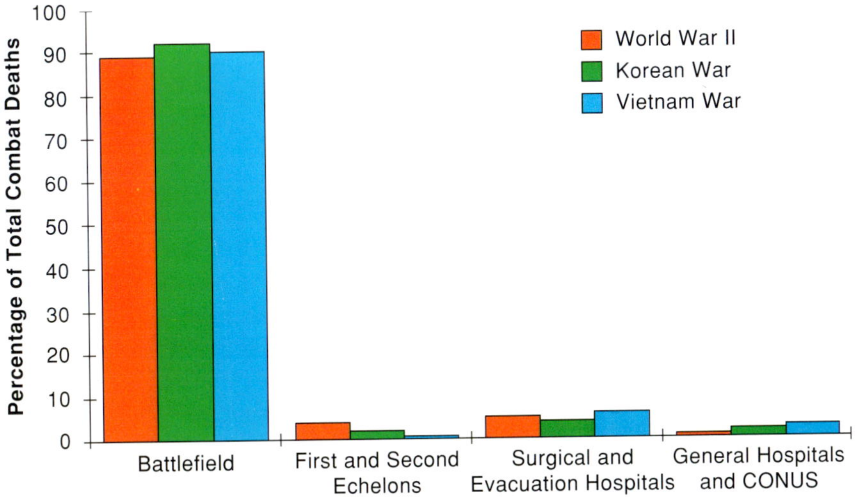

Fig. 1-6. The site of death for 90% of fatally wounded combat casualties is the battlefield. CONUS: continental United States. Data sources: (1) Beebe GW, DeBakey ME. *Battle Casualties*. Springfield, Ill: Charles C Thomas; 1952: 21, 92, 125, 186. (2) Reister FA. *Medical Statistics in World War II*. Washington, DC: Department of the Army, Office of The Surgeon General; 1975: 13; 90, Table 7; 202, Table 17. (3) Reister FA. *Battle Casualties and Medical Statistics: US Army Experience in Korea*. Washington, DC: Department of the Army, The Surgeon General; 1973: 12, 17, 45.

malized statistics: as the percentage of the total casualty population, or the percentage of the *admitted/hospitalized* population (ie, casualties who were admitted to a medical treatment facility, the vast majority of whom were then hospitalized), respectively.

Killed in Action

The formula for calculating the percentage of casualties classified as killed in action is

$$\frac{\text{total number classified as killed in action}}{\text{total number of casualties}} \bullet 100$$

The magnitude of the percentage of the population who are killed in action depends on at least three factors:

1. The lethality of the weapons. A war fought with assault rifles is likely to have a greater percentage of casualties who are killed in action than a war fought with BB guns.
2. The feasibility and effectiveness of first aid.
3. The length of time required for evacuation from the battlefield to a medical treatment facility. The longer a casualty remains on the battlefield, he is not only more likely to die from his original wound but he is also more likely to receive a new and possibly more-lethal wound.

Exhibit 1-1 shows sample calculations of percentages of killed in action for the U.S. Army in the Vietnam War.[16] Depending on which data and definitions are used, the percentages range between 14.6% and 24.2%. The higher figure is probably a better indicator of the probability of a fatal outcome when wounded by enemy action, because it excludes the casualties who are carded for record only and includes all killed and missing soldiers.

Data from 604 soldiers recorded in the WDMET study as having been killed in action suggest that most fatally wounded casualties die very rapidly, with perhaps 70% being apparently dead within 5 minutes of wounding (Figure 1-7). This observation has important implications for interpreting the relation between mortality and the time for evacuation. One of the major criteria for judging the effectiveness of the medical service in the field is the time taken to evacuate casualties. During the Vietnam War, the time from wounding until a U.S. Army casualty left the battlefield was unprecedentedly short (median time 29 min).[15(T4-1-7)] Because most casualty evacuation in Vietnam was by helicopter and most evacuation flights lasted less than half an hour (usually 5–20 min), it seems quite likely that most casualties were received by hospitals within 1 hour of wounding. Nevertheless, this evacuation time, which is so much faster than that of any previous war (eg, in Italy in 1944, the average time was 11.4 h from wounding to operation[36]), is still not swift enough, when considered in the context of Figure 1-7, to save more than a tiny fraction of fatally wounded casualties.

Died of Wounds

The formula for calculating the percentage of casualties classified as died of wounds is

$$\frac{\text{total number classified as died of wounds}}{\text{total number of admitted or hospitalized casualties}} \bullet 100$$

The magnitude of the percentage of the population who die of wounds depends on at least two factors:

1. Adequacy of surgical care. For example, if no neurosurgical care can be given, the number of casualties with head wounds who die will increase.
2. Casualty load and triage considerations. For example, during a mass casualty situation, it may be necessary to place certain casualties in the expectant category, resulting in a greater number of casualties who will die of wounds.

Exhibit 1-1 also shows sample calculations of percentages of casualties who died of wounds for the U.S. Army in the Vietnam War. Depending on which data and definitions are used, the percentage who died of wounds can be calculated to be 2.2%, 3.1%, or 3.4%. The first figure included the casualties who were carded for record only in the denominator and is invalid, since FM 8-55 states that the died-of-wounds population is part of the wounded-in-action population, but the carded-for-record-only population is not.[1] The population base for the 3.1% figure includes only admitted/hospitalized casualties and is, therefore, a more valid indicator of mortality in casualties who need medical treatment. Hospital mortality (ie, excluding the casualties who died while at the first or second echelons) was 3.4%.

The time of death for casualties who died of wounds as found in the WDMET data is shown in Figure 1-7. These data are similar to those of the British experience in the Normandy campaign, in which 50% of deaths occurred in the first 24 hours,

EXHIBIT 1-1

KILLED IN ACTION AND DIED OF WOUNDS DURING THE VIETNAM WAR, 1961–1979

Dead:	
1. Killed in action	27,129*
2. Died of wounds	3,529†
3. Died while missing in action	5,998‡
Wounded in Action (WIA) but Survived:	
4. WIA, admitted to hospital	96,924
5. WIA, admitted to nonhospital medical treatment facility, or quarters	13,716
6. Carded for record only	44,858

*Records of the Office of The Adjutant General (OTAG) state that there were 30,562 casualties classified as killed in action.
†104 casualties died at the first or second echelons (ie, before reaching a hospital).
‡Records of OTAG state that 5,998 soldiers were classified as died while missing; these casualties are in addition to those killed in action. Most were probably killed in helicopters that were destroyed in combat actions.
Data source: The Office of The Surgeon General as collated in: US Army Patient Administration Systems and Biostatistics Activity. Battle Injury Dispositions by Causative Agent—Active Duty Army Personnel with Initial Admission in Vietnam. Fort Sam Houston, Tex: Academy of Health Sciences, Department of the Army: 2 June 1981. Unpublished data.

Sample Calculations

(The numerals on the left side of the equation refer to the categories shown above)

Percentage Killed in Action:

14.6: Defined as number classified as killed in action divided by the total number of casualties exclusive of the missing: categories 1÷(1+2+4+5+6) = (27,129÷186,156) • 100

17.2: Defined as number classified as killed in action plus died while missing divided by total number of casualties: categories (1+3)÷(1+2+3+4+5+6) = (33,127÷192,154) • 100

18.6: Defined as number classified as killed in action according to OTAG plus died while missing divided by total number of casualties: categories (1+3)÷(1+2+3+4+5+6) = (36,460÷195,587) • 100

24.2: Defined as number classified as killed in action according to OTAG plus died while missing divided by total number of casualties minus the carded for record only: categories (1+3)÷(1+2+3+4+5) = (36,460÷150,729) • 100

Percentage Died of Wounds:

2.2: Defined as number classified as died of wounds divided by total number of casualties minus killed and missing: categories 2÷(2+4+5+6) = (3,529÷159,027) • 100

3.1: Defined as number classified as died of wounds divided by total number of casualties admitted to hospital, nonhospital medical treatment facility, and placed on quarters: categories 2÷(2+4+5) = 3,529÷114,169 • 100

3.4: Defined as number classified as died of wounds minus 104 (number dead at first or second echelons) divided by the total number of casualties admitted to hospital: categories 2÷(2+4) = (3,529 – 104)÷(100,453 – 104) • 100

80% within 3 days, and all but 5% by the end of the first week.[10] Because medical care can play an important role in determining the outcome in casualties who are at risk of dying of wounds, the lethality associated with wounds of specific body regions has changed during wars in which the U.S. Army has been involved. During World War I, casualties with wounds of the extremities who developed anaerobic infection were the largest component of the died-of-wounds category.[11] During World War

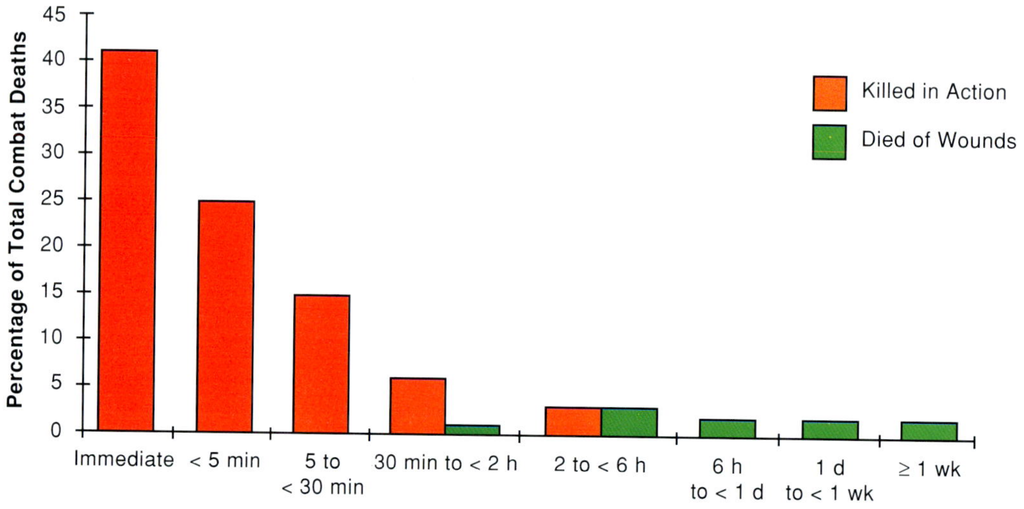

Fig. 1-7. When the time to death after wounding is plotted for battlefield casualties who are killed in action and who die of wounds, most are seen to die in less than 10 minutes, demonstrating that the "Golden Hour" seen in civilian casualties does not apply. Data source: Wound Data and Munitions Effectiveness Team database.

II, the major cause of death in soldiers who died of their wounds was intraabdominal injury.[37] During the Vietnam War, soldiers who died from wounds of the head constituted the largest component of the died-of-wounds category.[38]

This last fact has important implications for understanding the reciprocal relation between the killed-in-action and died-of-wounds categories. It is likely that rapid evacuation of gravely wounded casualties from the Vietnam battlefield brought casualties to the hospital level who, in prior wars, would have expired on the battlefield (and thus would have been classified as killed in action). Thus, the percentage of casualties who were killed in action would be reduced, while the percentage of casualties who died of their wounds would be elevated. The converse will be true given prolonged evacuation from the battlefield: the great majority of the gravely wounded will die on the battlefield (and will thus be classified as killed in action). Relatively few will reach the hospital level, so the percentage of casualties who died of wounds will be strikingly low. This situation—a high percentage of casualties who were killed in action (31%) and a low percentage of casualties who died of wounds (1.1%)—characterized the British army's Falklands War experience, a war in which evacuation time may have been unusually long.[26]

In the past, the quality of medical care has all too often been assessed in terms of the died-of-wounds rate. However, this assessment may give very misleading results. The reciprocal relation between the number of soldiers who are killed in action and the number who die of wounds is shown schematically in Figure 1-8, in which two hypothetical scenarios with identical casualty populations are contrasted: one in which evacuation is sluggish and hospital care is mediocre, and one in which evacuation is quite prompt and hospital care is optimal. Because the died-of-wounds rate is higher in the second scenario, it is possible to conclude that the quality of care is worse. The correct conclusion becomes apparent only if the overall mortality is considered. Then it is obvious that the care given in the first scenario is inferior. The effectiveness of the entire field medical system is measured when overall mortality is studied.

Absence of a "Golden Hour" in Combat Trauma

Since D. D. Trunkey's report[39] on civilian trauma was published in 1983, it has become customary to assume that the times at which fatally injured trauma victims die fall into three distinct periods: *immediate* (within the first hour), *early* (2–3 h after injury), and *late* (several days to several weeks after injury). Trunkey's study showed that about half of all deaths occur in the immediate period, 30% in the early, and the remainder in the late. Based on this distribution, there is reason to believe that, given rapid evacuation to a trauma center and excellent care there, many of the deaths that occur in the early period can be prevented. The first hour after injury has been called the "Golden Hour," since care insti-

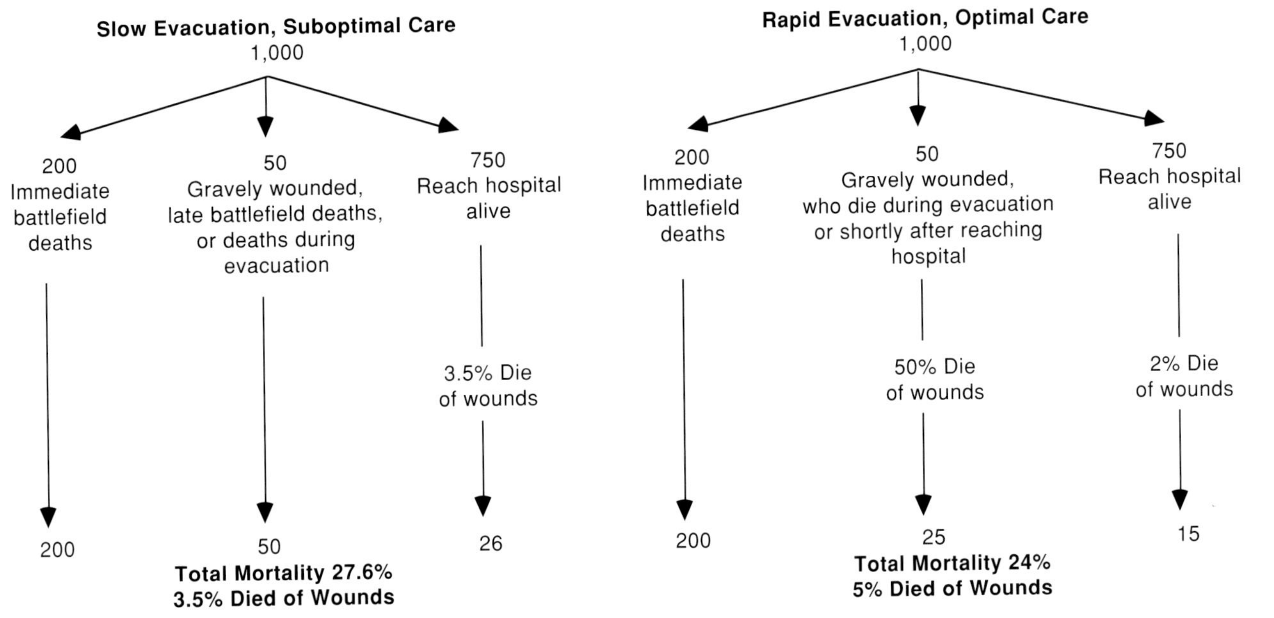

Fig. 1-8. These two hypothetical populations of combat casualties with identical Injury Severity Scores are evacuated at different speeds and receive different medical care. The difference in medical outcome appears paradoxical: the number of casualties who die of wounds is much higher in the rapidly evacuated group, although the total mortality is lower.

tuted within this interval is likely to be lifesaving for trauma victims who might otherwise die in the early period. Care started after the first hour is more likely to be futile. A similar, albeit less well-substantiated and -defined concept, is found in combat casualty care: the medical service has an hour to institute lifesaving first aid in the critically wounded soldier; otherwise, survival becomes increasingly unlikely.

The clinical evidence that was used to establish the trimodal distribution of trauma deaths is of civilian origin and, therefore, blunt trauma was the usual mechanism of injury. However, Figure 1-7 shows no evidence of a trimodal distribution of combat deaths: 80% to 90% of all deaths occur during what, by analogy, would be Trunkey's immediate period, with perhaps 70% occurring in the first 5 minutes. Although there are late deaths, it is difficult to recognize a distinct cluster of deaths after the initial peak. It is likely that this difference between the military and civilian experiences arises from the great predominance of penetrating trauma in the former, with penetrating injury's potential for rapid exsanguinating hemorrhage. Support for this view comes from a 1993 study[40] of a civilian trauma population who had a much higher percentage of penetrating trauma than the population in Trunkey's study. Most deaths in the 1993 study occurred during what would be Trunkey's immediate period, following which deaths became progressively less common until the onset of sepsis and multiple organ failure days afterward. The implication for combat casualty care, based on the observed distribution of deaths found in the WDMET data, is obvious: if there is a "golden" period, it is a golden 5 minutes.

Historical Trends in Combat Mortality

Historical trends in combat mortality and their supporting data are shown in Figure 1-9. The wars have been selected for illustrative purposes and do not constitute a systemic appraisal of combat mortality. As a general rule, at present, given optimal combat casualty care, 20% to 25% of battle casualties can be expected to be killed in action and 3% to 5% of survivors reaching the hospital level alive will die of their wounds. This conclusion depends on two important qualifications: (1) medical care must be state of the art and science and (2) the tactical situation must allow for application of the available medical resources. The latter qualification means that the army in question must not be losing badly. Losers may have terrible combat mortality. Two 20th-century battles illustrate this point: at the battle of Stalingrad, about 75% of German casualties were in the killed and died categories after mid-December 1942[41]; at the battle of

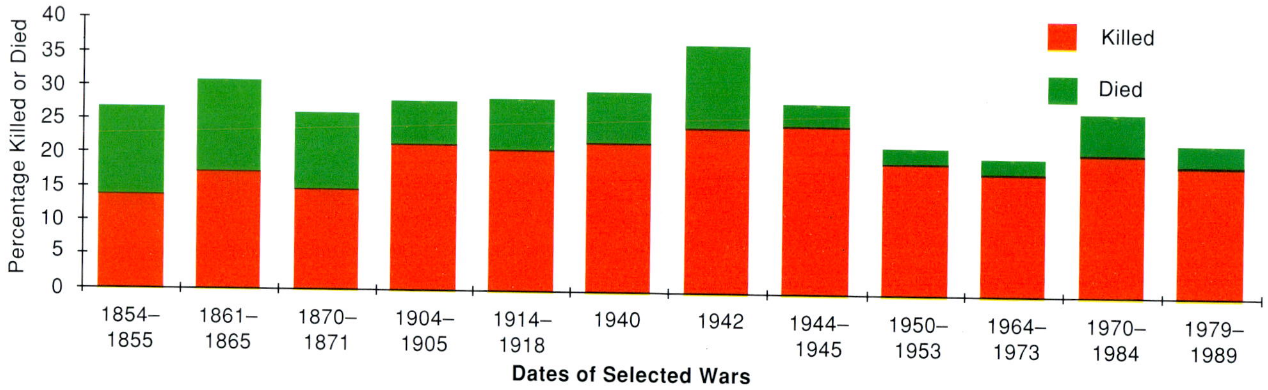

Fig. 1-9. *See legend on page 19.*

Okinawa, Japanese mortality was about 95% of all soldiers.[42] If there is one lesson that military history teaches, it is that the essential prerequisite for low combat mortality is to win!

Outcome of Specific Body-Region Injuries

The mortality of combat injuries can be understood best when wounds of separate body regions are studied. The following outcome data are from the WDMET study for soldiers wounded in the head, chest, abdomen, and extremities.[15] Casualties were placed in the *head* category when a projectile (bullet or fragment) reached the periosteum of the skull or deeper; in the *chest* category when a projectile reached the rib cage or deeper; in the *abdominal* category when a projectile perforated the peritoneum; and in the *extremity* category when a projectile injured the skeleton or a neurovascular structure in the upper or lower extremity. Injuries were classified as *primary* (ie, one body region had an AIS score greater than any other body region) or *multiple* (ie, two or more body regions had injuries of equal potential lethality according to the AIS). Casualty outcomes were defined as follows:

- killed: succumbed on the battlefield,
- died: succumbed while receiving care at a medical facility,
- hospitalized: admitted to a medical treatment facility, and
- survived: either returned to duty or was alive when evacuated from Vietnam.

Head

- Total mortality: 373/477 = 78%
- Hospital mortality: 37/141 = 26%

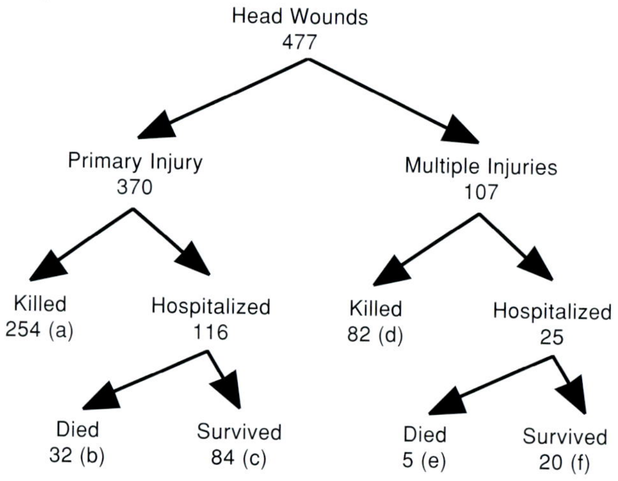

Primary Injury. Of the 254 casualties whose head wounds were their primary injury and who were killed (point *a* on the diagram), 184 (72.4%) sustained massive brain destruction (eg, injury to three or more lobes, avulsion of the brain, decapitation, crushing of the head), and 43 (17%) had isolated injury to the midbrain or brainstem. The remainder had an injury involving one or two lobes or a depressed skull fracture.

Of the 32 who died after being hospitalized (point *b* on the diagram), slightly fewer than one half were treated expectantly.

Of the 84 casualties who survived (point *c* on the diagram), 44 had an injury that involved only one cerebral lobe, 15 had injuries involving two lobes, and 12 had depressed skull fractures caused by tangential gunshot wounds.

Multiple Injuries. Of the 82 casualties with multiple injuries who were killed (point *d* on the diagram), 27 (33%) had massive brain destruction in addition to grossly mutilating injuries to other parts of the body. Most of the remainder had injuries to one or two lobes.

Fig. 1-9. Percentages of casualties who died or were killed in selected wars. The figure is based on the following supporting data:

1854–1855: British battle casualties in the Crimean War. Killed: 1,933; died: 1,599[1]; wounded: 12,100.[2] The high hospital mortality is characteristic of the preantisepsis era of military surgery. An additional 11,477 died of disease.

1861–1865: Union battle casualties in the American Civil War. Killed: 67,058; died: 43,012; wounded: 318,187.[3] An additional 233,789 died of disease. The killed figure does not include the missing in action, a significant proportion of which probably were also killed.

1870–1871: German battle casualties in the Franco–Prussian War. Killed: 17,300; died: 11,000; wounded: 96,200.[4]

1904–1905: Japanese battle casualties in the Russo–Japanese War. Killed: 47,500; died: 11,500; wounded: 173,400.[4] The first "modern" war in several senses: machine guns and high-explosive shells dominated the battlefield, and some military surgeons used antiseptic and aseptic techniques.

1914–1918: British battle casualties in France and Flanders. Killed: 381,261; died: 151,356; surviving wounded: 1,837,613; missing and assumed killed: 144,890.[5]

1940: German battle casualties during the conquest of France, May–June 1940. Killed: 21.9%; died: 7.8%.[6] Actual numerical data are not given, but according to Fischer[7] there were approximately 48,000 battle fatalities. The Germans ascribed the high mortality to the delayed evacuation of casualties from rapidly moving armored units.

1942: German battle casualties on the Russian front, January 1942. Killed: 24.4%; died: 12.3%.[6] Actual numerical data are not given, but the same source indicates that there were about 55,000 battle fatalities.[6] The high mortality is the result of the extraordinary difficulty of providing effective combat casualty care in the extreme cold during the massive Soviet counterattack that followed the collapse of the German attack on Moscow.

1944–1945: American battle casualties in Italy, January 1944–May 1945. Killed: 25,183; died: 2,770; total admissions (carded for record only category excluded): 76,351.[8] Reister's data are somewhat different from those given by Snyder and Culbertson[9]: killed: 16,648; hospitalized/died: 1,631; hospitalized/survived: 61,393; killed: 20.9%; died: 2.6%. The latter data do not include casualties who died of wounds prior to hospitalization nor some 9,000 additional soldiers who were killed but were presumably still classified as missing when the data were collated in 1945.

1950–1953: American battle casualties during the Korean War.[10]

1964–1973: US Marine Corps battle casualties during the Vietnam War. Killed: 11,490; died: 1,454; nonfatal wounds/hospital care required: 51,399.[11] The Marine Corps' mortality data appear to be more favorable than are the corresponding US Army data.

1970–1984: British army casualties from Northern Ireland, for soldiers killed or wounded by explosive devices. Killed: 174; died: 42; total injured: 828.[12] These data are useful for understanding mortality in "peacekeeping" operations (now officially known as operations other than war [OOTW]). Evacuation time from the site of wounding to surgical care was almost certainly shorter than that in any of the wars described. It is also probable that the wounds were, on average, more severe.

1979–1989: Russian battle casualties during the Afghanistan War. Two sources are available. The first[13] gives normalized statistics for killed (19.5%) and died (3.5%), but actual data are given for what may be different casualty categories: fatally wounded, 13,833, and wounded, 49,985. The second[14] has the following entries: killed: 9,511; died: 2,386; surviving wounded: 51,367. Using these data, killed in action would be 15.0% and died of wounds 4.4%. Which source is correct is not known. Both sources indicate that there were more than 400,000 admissions for disease.

Data sources: (1) Palmer A. *The Crimean War*. New York, NY: Dorset Press; 1987: 244. (2) Beebe GW, DeBakey ME. *Battle Casualties*. Springfield, Ill: Charles C Thomas; 1952: 77. (3) Livermore TL. *Number & Losses in the Civil War in America: 1861–65*. New York, NY: Kraus Reprint Co; 1969: 8. (4) La Garde LA. *Gunshot Injuries*. New York, NY: Wm Wood and Co; 1916: 413. (5) Mitchell TJ, Smith GM. *Casualties and Medical Statistics of the Great War*. London, England: The Army Medical Services. His Majesty's Stationery Office; 1931: 108. (6) Mueller-Hillebrand B. Statistics System. US Army Historical Division Study PC 011 Koenigstein Ts. 1949: 121, 136. Unpublished. Available at the National Archives, Washington, DC. (7) Fischer H. *Der Deutsche Sanitätsdienst 1921–1945*. Vol 2. Osnabrück, Germany: Biblio Verlag; 1983: 343. (8) Reister FA. *Medical Statistics in World War II*. Washington, DC: Department of the Army, Office of The Surgeon General; 1975: 76–79. (9) Snyder HE, Culbertson JW. Studies of Fifth US Army hospitalized casualty deaths. In: Beyer JC, ed. *Wound Ballistics*. Washington, DC: Department of the Army, Medical Department, Office of The Surgeon General; 1962: 473. (10) Reister FA. *Battle Casualties and Medical Statistics: US Army Experience in Korea*. Washington, DC: Department of the Army, The Surgeon General; 1973: 45. (11) Directorate for Information Operation and Control. Number of casualties incurred by US military personnel in connection with the conflict in Vietnam. Washington, DC: Department of Defense (OASD Comptroller), January 15, 1976: Table 1051..Unpublished. (12) Mellor SG, Cooper GJ. Analysis of 828 servicemen killed or injured by explosion in Northern Ireland 1970–1984: The Hostile Action Casualty System. *Br J Surg*. 1989;76:1006–1011. (13) Nechaev E. Soviet military experience in providing health care during Afghanistan War: Problems of further military medicine development. *Military Medical Journal* (Moscow). 1992;2:5–14. (14) Krivosheyev GF, ed. *Losses to the Armed Forces of the USSR in Battles, Combat Operations, and Military Conflicts: Statistical Investigations*. Moscow, Russia: Military Press; 1993: 402–404.

Of the 5 hospitalized casualties with multiple injuries who died (point *e* on the diagram), 2 were treated expectantly. Of the 20 hospitalized casualties who survived (point *f* on the diagram), 7 had single-lobe and 6 had double-lobe injuries.

In addition, the fatal head wounds of 7 casualties who were killed in action were insufficiently described to justify inclusion in the diagram. An additional 27 casualties, also not included, sustained systemic mutilation that almost certainly included a fatal brain injury. Eight casualties with gunshot wounds and 4 with fragment wounds of the scalp did not have evidence of skull or central nervous system (CNS) injury. They are not included, but one casualty with a gunshot wound of the scalp and a cerebral concussion is included.

Type of Penetrating Missile. The partition by outcome of casualties whose primary injury was in the head by type of penetrating missile is as follows: 53% of those who were fatally wounded and 5% of those who survived were injured by bullets; 28% of those who were fatally wounded and 14% of those who survived were injured by explosive munitions. These data indicate that the probability of being fatally wounded if struck in the head by a bullet approached 9 in 10. In fact, of the casualties who survived to be evacuated from Vietnam, only 3 in the entire population (477) had penetrating head wounds caused by a bullet in which the brain parenchyma was directly injured (as distinct from a depressed fracture of the skull with associated brain injury caused by a tangential bullet wound). Casualties with multiple injuries of which one component was in the head were likely to be victims of explosive munitions rather than small arms.

Chest

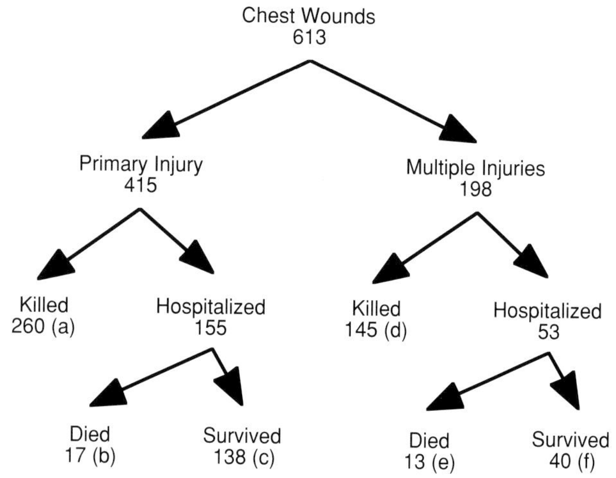

- Total mortality: 435⁄613 = 71%
- Hospital mortality: 30⁄208 = 14%

Primary Injury. Of 613 casualties who were classified as having chest wounds, the chest wound was the primary injury in 415. Of these, 260 were killed (point *a* on the diagram). The sites of fatal injury were heart or great vessels or both, 43%; lung, including trachea, 30%; and heart, great vessels, and lung, 27%.

Of the 155 casualties who were hospitalized with primary injury, 17 died (point *b* on the diagram): 8 deaths occurred intraoperatively, 7 died preoperatively, and 2 died postoperatively. Nine of these casualties had wounds of the lung only, 4 had wounds of the heart or great vessels, and 4 had wounds of the heart or great vessels and lung.

Of the 138 casualties who survived their primary injury (point *c* on the diagram), 61% had wounds of the lung, 34% had a significant chest-wall injury in addition to a lung injury, and 5% had a wound of the mediastinum, which, in two cases, involved a partial-thickness laceration of the myocardium.

Multiple Injuries. Of the 198 casualties with multiple injuries (but whose chest wounds were predominant), 145 were killed (point *d* on the diagram). Of these, 53% had wounds involving the lungs, 37% had mutilating wounds of the entire trunk, and 10% had wounds of the lung and/or the heart and the great vessels.

Of the 53 casualties with multiple injuries who were hospitalized, 13 died (point *e* on the diagram). Of these, 6 died before operation, 4 died intraoperatively, and 3 died postoperatively.

All of the 40 casualties who were hospitalized and survived had wounds of the lung or chest wall or both (point *f* on the diagram).

In addition, but not included in the diagram, 37 casualties had thoracic injuries in which the chest component was of lesser severity when compared to an injury in another body part. Of these casualties, 24 were killed, 4 died, and 9 survived. The thoracic injury was limited to the lungs in 82% of these casualties. An additional 18 casualties had nonpenetrating injuries, but they also are not included here.

Of the 155 casualties who were evacuated alive from the battlefield with primary thoracic injuries, 24 (15%) had a formal thoracotomy. Mortality in this group was 10 of 24 (42%). Three casualties with multiple injuries had a thoracotomy; all died.

Type of Penetrating Missile. The partition by outcome of casualties whose primary injury was in the chest by type of penetrating missile is as follows: 44% of those who were fatally wounded and 11% of those who survived were injured by bullets; 30% of those who were fatally wounded and 15% of those who survived were injured by explosive munitions. These data indicate that the probability of being fatally wounded if struck in the chest by a bullet is about 4 in 5. Most of the casualties in the multiple category who had thoracic wounds were injured by explosive munitions.

Abdomen

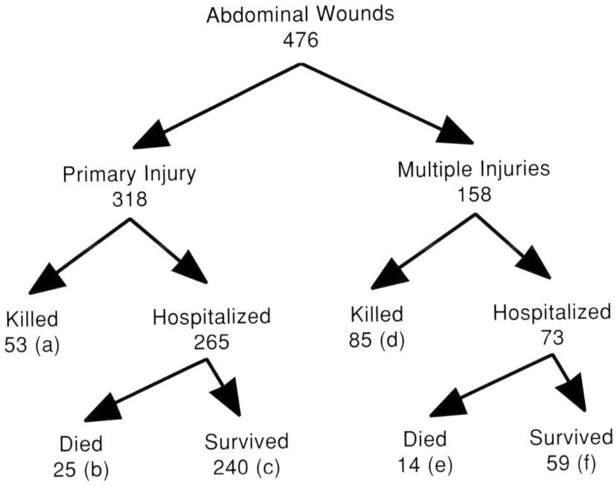

- Total mortality: $^{177}/_{476}$ = 37% (42% when casualties with negative laparotomies are excluded)
- Hospital mortality: $^{39}/_{338}$ = 11.5% (13.3% when casualties with negative laparotomies are excluded)
- Total mortality of casualties whose primary injury involves the abdomen: $^{78}/_{318}$ = 24.5% (28% when casualties with negative laparotomies are excluded)
- Hospital mortality of casualties whose primary injury involves the abdomen: $^{25}/_{265}$ = 9.4% (11% when casualties with negative laparotomies are excluded)

Primary Injury. Of the 318 casualties whose abdominal wounds were their primary injury, 53 were killed (point *a* on the diagram). In all casualties, death was due to hemorrhage: 42% exsanguinated from an intraabdominal vascular injury (45%, iliac vessels; 40%, aorta or inferior vena cava; 15%, miscellaneous); 25% had a mutilating abdominal injury; 18% had involvement of multiple intraabdominal organs exclusive of the named vessels; 11% had a liver injury; and 4% had an involvement of a single intraabdominal organ other than the liver.

Of the 265 casualties who were hospitalized with primary abdominal wounds, 25 died (point *b* on the diagram). Death was due to hemorrhage in 60% of casualties, intraabdominal sepsis in 25%, and pulmonary insufficiency in 15%. The sites of abdominal injury were as follows: multiple sites, exclusive of vessels, 38% (average number of injured organs was 4.4); intraabdominal vessels, 30% (the iliac vessels accounted for two thirds of these); liver, 21%; single organ exclusive of the liver, 12%.

Two hundred forty casualties survived their primary abdominal wounds (point *c* on the diagram). On average, survivors had 1.8 injured intraabdominal organs; one half of the survivors had an injury to only one organ. The most commonly injured organs were the colon including the rectum, 23%; the small bowel including the duodenum, 23%; and the liver, 14%. Only 1% of survivors in the primary category had a vascular injury.

Multiple Injuries. Of the casualties with abdominal wounds, 158 had multiple injuries. In this category, 85 casualties were killed (point *d* on the diagram). Of these, 71% had injuries to the chest; about one half had true thoracoabdominal wounds (ie, a single missile traversed both thorax and abdomen). The remaining casualties had various combinations of abdominal injuries in addition to wounds of the head or extremities.

Of the 73 casualties with multiple injuries who were hospitalized, 14 died (point *e* on the diagram). All casualties in this category had wounds of the lung in addition to their intraabdominal injuries.

Of the 59 hospitalized casualties who survived (point *f* on the diagram), 65% had extremity wounds in addition to their abdominal wounds; 25% had head wounds, all but one of which were treated by craniotomy; and 10% had chest wounds, one of which required a thoracotomy.

There were an additional 7 casualties in whom the abdominal component was of lesser severity than a wound to some other body part. All 7 were fatally wounded, and in all casualties the more serious wound was to the head. An unknown number of casualties had an injury that was subsequently shown to involve only the abdominal wall. The number of such casualties approximates but is greater than the number of casualties who had negative laparotomies (39 casualties in the primary category and 11 in the multiple categories, 15% of all laparotomies). Casualties who had a negative laparotomy were classified in the abdominal category even though no intraabdominal injury was present.

Type of Penetrating Missile. The partition by outcome of casualties whose primary injury was in the abdomen by the type of penetrating missile is as follows: 24% of those who were fatally wounded and 10% of those who survived were injured by bullets; 19% of those who were fatally wounded and 47% of those who survived were injured by explosive munitions. These data indicate that the probability of being fatally wounded if struck in the abdomen by a bullet was about 2 in 3. Most of the casualties in the multiple category who had abdominal wounds were injured by explosive munitions.

Extremities

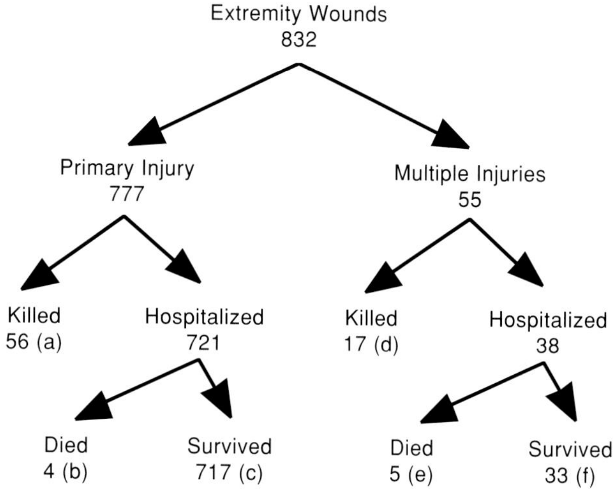

- Total mortality: $^{82}/_{832} = 9.9\%$
- Hospital mortality: $^{9}/_{759} = 1.2\%$

Primary Injury. Of 832 casualties classified with extremity wounds, 777 had these wounds as their primary injury. Of these casualties, 56 were killed (point *a* on the diagram) and in all, the cause of death was exsanguination. Thirty-five deaths were caused by amputations of an arm or leg, 17 exsanguinated from an isolated arterial wound (the femoral artery was the most common site), and 4 died who had sustained multiple extremity fractures.

Of the 777 casualties whose extremity wounds were the primary injury, 721 were hospitalized. Of these, 4 died (point *b* on the diagram). Two casualties died while being treated for femoral artery lacerations, one died of gas gangrene following a failed axillary artery repair, and one died in what was reported as "mysterious circumstances" following treatment for a forearm amputation.

Of the 721 hospitalized casualties, 717 survived (point *c* on the diagram). About 50% of the survivors had fractures of extremity long bones, and 20% had fractures involving the hands or feet. Major extremity amputations and isolated vascular injuries were each found in 8% of the casualties in this category.

Multiple Injuries. Of the 832 casualties with extremity wounds, 55 were classified as having multiple injuries; of these, 17 were killed (point *d* on the diagram). Most casualties with multiple injuries exsanguinated from major extremity amputations or femoral artery lacerations, in addition to hemorrhage from injured intraabdominal viscera. The remainder had injuries to the head or thorax in addition to the extremity wound.

Of the 55 multiply injured casualties in the extremity wound category, 38 were hospitalized, and of these, 5 died (point *e* on the diagram). Casualties in this category exsanguinated from femoral artery injuries in conjunction with bleeding from within the chest or abdomen.

Of the 38 hospitalized casualties with multiple injuries, 33 survived (point *f* on the diagram). In these casualties, the extremity injury coexisted with injuries to the head (including the face), chest, and abdomen, in that order.

Excluded from the extremity analysis were approximately 300 casualties in whom the extremity injury was of secondary severity. Most of these casualties fell into one of two categories: (1) grossly mutilating injuries in which the extremity injury coexisted with major disruption of the head or trunk, and (2) a long-bone fracture in addition to a severe and frequently fatal injury of the head, chest, or abdomen.

Type of Penetrating Missile. The partition by outcome of casualties whose primary injury was in the extremity as a function of the type of penetrating missile is as follows: 4% of those who were fatally wounded and 30% of those who survived were injured by bullets; 11% of those who were fatally wounded and 55% of those who survived were injured by explosive munitions. These data indicate that the probability of being fatally wounded if struck in an extremity by a bullet that injured bone or neurovascular structures was about 1 in 11. Explosive munitions were actually more deadly than bullets: the probability of a fatal outcome was about 1 in 6. The reason for the higher lethality of explosive munitions is no doubt related to the propensity of antipersonnel mines to cause amputations.

Morbidity

The ability of the medical service to perform its mission, which is summarized in such statements as "conserve fighting strength" and "maintain the fighting power of the command," depends on how effectively combat morbidity is reduced. Morbidity is more difficult to measure than mortality because the latter has a clear endpoint. Indices of morbidity that have been used are (1) the percentage of surviving wounded who return to duty, or alternatively, the percentage of surviving wounded who are separated from the army, and (2) the length of time a soldier who ultimately does return to duty remains noneffective following a combat injury (Table 1-4).[20–22,43] The morbidity data for the U.S. Army have not changed appreciably in the wars of this century. The explanation is probably to be found in two facts:

- The rate of healing of bone and soft tissue has not changed very much.
- The organization of the army in the theater of operations, as well as other administrative factors, does not allow rapid return to duty.

The latter observation may seem strange given the official emphasis placed on conserving fighting strength but was a well-known fact during both the Vietnam War and the Persian Gulf War. During the latter, there were many anecdotal reports that field medical facilities were told to evacuate all casualties regardless of how soon they were expected to return to duty. The reason for this decision is simply that extensive casualty-holding facilities within the combat zone constitute a considerable logistical burden. In a short conflict such as the Persian Gulf War, in which there may be little need for replacements, it is neither necessary nor cost-effective to hold wounded and sick soldiers in the combat zone.

TABLE 1-4

INDICES OF MORBIDITY

War	Days Noneffective	Disability Separation (% of Wounded)
World War I[1]	96	11
World War II[2]	118	18
Korea[3]	93	9
Vietnam[4]	86*	11*

*No final figures appear to have been published for indices of morbidity. Neel gives data that are specific for Vietnam, but how long the soldiers who had been evacuated from there remained noneffective is unclear. The figures given in this table were obtained by extrapolation using factors derived from the World War II and Korean War data given by Neel.

Data sources: (1) Love AG. *Statistics*. In: *Medical and Casualty Statistics*. In: *Medical Department of the United States Army in the World War*. Vol 15, Part 2. Washington, DC: Government Printing Office; 1925: 1181, 1183. (2) Reister FA. *Medical Statistics in World War II*. Washington, DC: Department of the Army, The Surgeon General; 1975: 13. (3) Reister FA. *Battle Casualties and Medical Statistics: US Army Experience in Korea*. Washington, DC: Department of the Army, Office of The Surgeon General; 1973: 712, 717. (4) Neel S. *Medical Support of the US Army in Vietnam 1965–1970*. Washington, DC: Department of the Army; 1973: 52–53.

What happened in Vietnam has a different explanation. Because there was a congressionally mandated limit on the number of troops within the combat zone, senior commanders were faced with the choice of either allowing the wounded to recover in country (and thereby reducing the number of effective soldiers in combat units) or evacuating the casualties from Vietnam and bringing in replacements, thereby maintaining the fighting strength. The latter course was usually chosen, although commanders recognized that evacuated soldiers usually were not returned to duty in Vietnam.

An army's commitment to return to duty is implicit in its evacuation policy (ie, the maximum number of days a casualty can be allowed to remain in the theater of operation before he must be evacuated).[1(p4-1–4-3)] For example, if the evacuation policy is set at 30 days, a casualty judged by the medical service to require more than 30 days to return to duty would be evacuated as soon as possible. The longer the evacuation policy, the greater the return to duty from the theater of operation but, conversely, the greater the medical deployment. Evacuation policies have ranged from as long as 180 days in the European Theater of Operations in 1944 to as short as 7 days during one phase of the Persian Gulf War.

Soldiers with soft-tissue wounds and fractures together constitute about three fourths of surviving casualties (see Figure 1-5). Because soft-tissue wounds heal much more quickly, on average, than do fractures or complicated wounds of the trunk or head, the population of casualties with soft-tissue wounds makes a disproportionately small contribution to the total number of man-days lost. As a general rule, about one third of the total man-days lost are due to soft-tissue wounds, one third are due to fractures, and one third are due to all other wounds (but especially to complicated abdominal or facial injuries).

The organization of the medical service in the field can have an important impact on the magni-

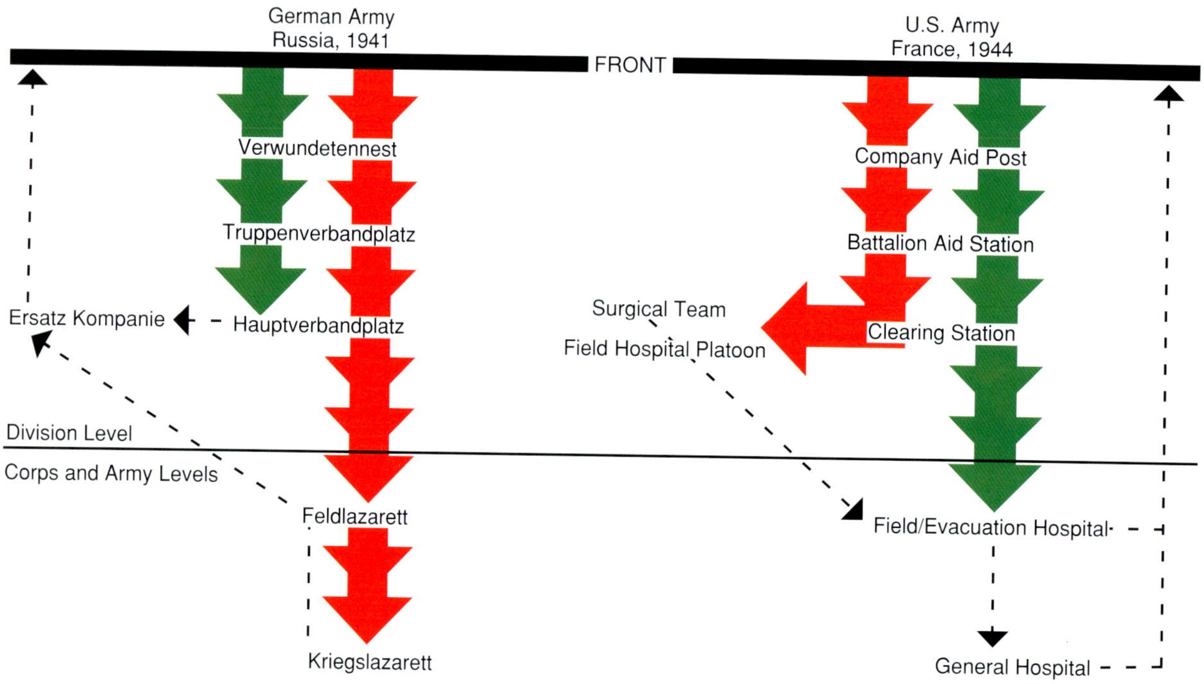

Fig. 1-10. A highly simplified and idealized diagram of evacuation patterns used by the German Army in Russia in July 1941 and by the US Army in France in summer and fall, 1944. The red lines indicate the flow of casualties with potentially fatal injuries; the green lines, the flow of casualties with nonlethal injuries. The German organization was designed to evacuate to the corps and army levels all casualties whose injuries made return to duty within a few weeks unlikely. Casualties with lesser injuries were retained within the division, where they were segregated to facilitate rapid return to duty. The American organization was designed to evacuate the great majority of casualties, including those with minor injuries, to the corps and army levels. Casualties with life-threatening injuries, however, received resuscitative surgery before leaving the division. Thus, the American organization emphasized the saving of lives; the German, the return to duty of the lightly wounded. Adapted with permission from Bellamy RF. Contrasts in combat casualty care. *Milit Med*. 1985;150:406.

tude and duration of noneffectiveness of combat casualties. Mortality can also be affected by the way the medical services are organized. These conclusions are illustrated by comparing the U.S. and German field medical organizations as they existed during two discrete periods of World War II: the German Army in Russia, summer 1941; and the U.S. Army in France, summer 1944 (Figure 1-10).[44]

The German organization emphasized early return to duty by treating the less-seriously wounded in the division area. To achieve this goal, a replacement company (Ersatz Kompanie) was attached to the main medical unit *organic to* (ie, an intrinsic part of) the division. Seriously wounded soldiers were evacuated from the division to corps- and army-level hospitals far to the rear.

The U.S. Army's medical system was almost the opposite in both casualty flow and goal. When needed, a small surgical hospital derived from corps assets was attached to the main medical unit organic to the division for the purpose of providing resuscitative surgical care for the most-gravely wounded soldiers. All other casualties, but especially those with less-severe injuries, were sent to hospitals in the corps or army area, from where it was difficult to effect a rapid return to duty.

As expected, the outcomes in terms of mortality and return to duty for these contrary ways of organizing the medical system were very different (Figure 1-11). The German system sacrificed the seriously wounded (German died of wounds, 10.6%) at the expense of soldiers who might be expected to return to duty (German return to duty, 87%), while the U.S. system strove to save lives (U.S. died of wounds, 3.1%) but somewhat ignored the organizational aspects that would accelerate the return to duty of the less severely injured (U.S. return to duty, 70%). It should be understood that the twin goals of saving lives and conserving fighting strength are not necessarily incompatible.

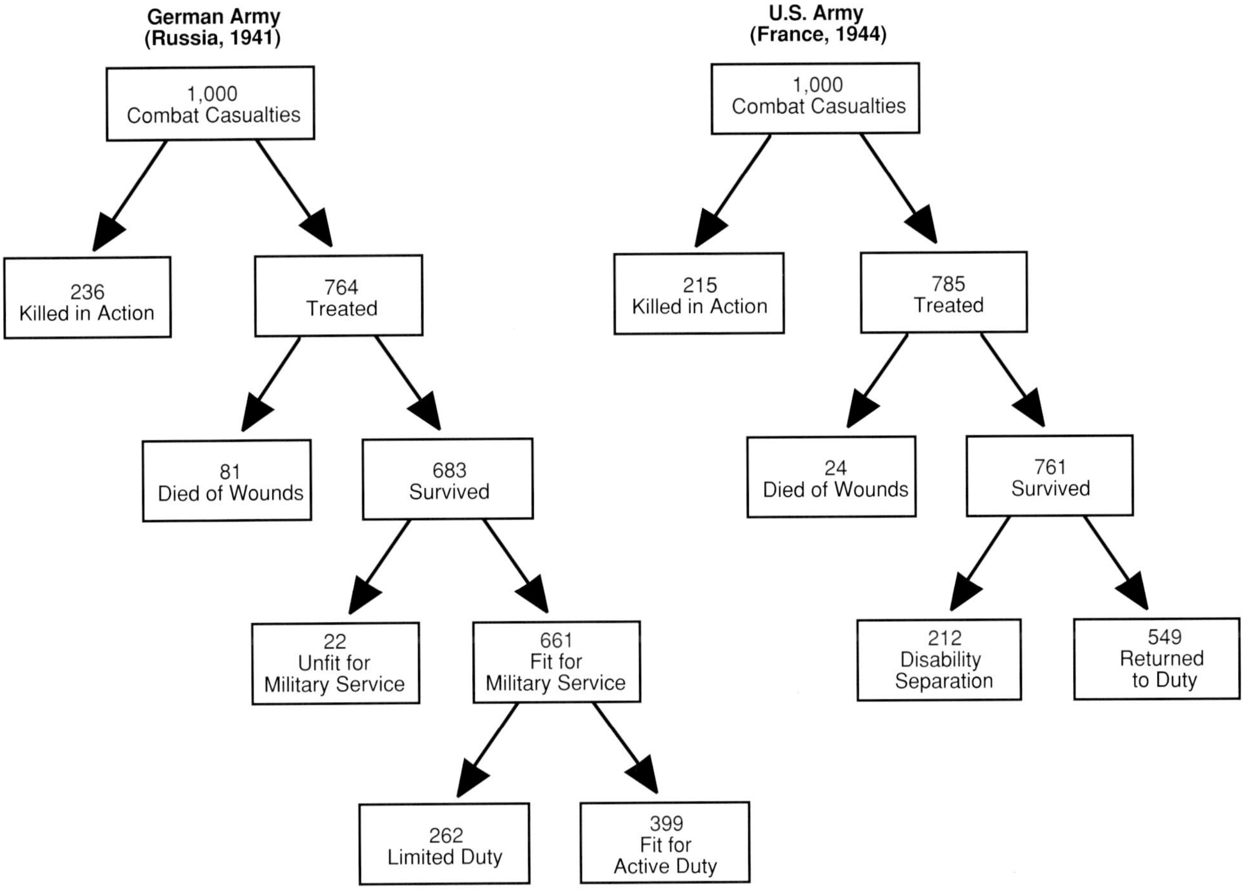

Fig. 1-11. The numerical counterpart of the functional differences shown in Fig. 1-10. The German system returned to duty a higher percentage of the surviving wounded than did the US Army but at the expense of a fatal outcome in almost one third of the casualties. Adapted with permission from Bellamy RF. Contrasts in combat casualty care. *Milit Med*. 1985;150:408.

Injury Severity Assessment

Approaches to injury severity assessment modeling fall into two categories: (1) those that measure physiological parameters and (2) those that quantitate the anatomical damage. The best known and most extensively used of the physiological injury severity scoring systems is the Trauma Score, which is calculated from measurements of respiratory rate, respiratory effort, systolic blood pressure, capillary refill, and the Glasgow coma scale.[45] The range of the Trauma Score is from 1 (dead) to 16 (normal). The probability of survival is a function of the Trauma Score; the ensuing curve has a sigmoid shape, with scores of 8 or 9 predicting a 50% probability of survival. The desirable feature of the Trauma Score, as with other physiologically based injury severity systems, is that it is simple to apply and, therefore, being readily repeatable, can easily demonstrate changes in the casualty's condition over time.

The purpose of the Trauma Score is to predict the probability of death and, thereby, the desirability of sending an injury victim to a trauma hospital. It does this well when assessed in terms of predictive power.[46] However, the questions that need to be asked in combat casualty care are not only "How likely is the casualty to die?" but also "Is the casualty noneffective?" and "Does the casualty therefore need to be evacuated?" A casualty with a penetrating missile wound of the abdomen, regardless of the actual Trauma Score, will require evacuation and laparotomy. A casualty with an open, comminuted fracture of the femur may be physiologically intact but will certainly need to be evacuated from the battlefield. A physiological injury severity index will not be helpful in making the determination. Accordingly, the actual use of such indicators of injury severity has been uncommon in combat casualty care. Military anesthesiologists interested in the important subject of the desirable features of a militarily useful triage methodology are referred elsewhere[47] in the literature.

Anatomical injury severity models differ from the physiological indices in this important respect: physiological indices are battlefield useable, but the anatomical indices are utterly useless for real-time application. The reason for this deficiency is the near impossibility of obtaining the needed detailed description of the anatomical injury at the time that triage and treatment decisions are made. Nevertheless, the anatomical models, applied retrospectively, may permit useful insight into *why* observed mortality and morbidity occurred.

The best known anatomical model is the Injury Severity Score,[48] which is, in essence, an algorithm for combining Abbreviated Injury Scale entries for different body regions. The major deficiencies of this approach are well known: first, the Abbreviated Injury Scale was developed to assess, and is most applicable to, blunt trauma; and second, the Injury Severity Score ignores the cumulative effect of multiple injuries within a given body region. Nevertheless, the application of injury severity scoring to combat casualties should have some heuristic value, in that the shape of the frequency distribution of injury severity may suggest how feasible it really is to reduce combat mortality.

Theoretical Distribution

Many frequency distribution curves are theoretically possible. One possible curve is the standard normal distribution (ie, the Gaussian curve) (Figure 1-12). With this distribution, most trauma victims

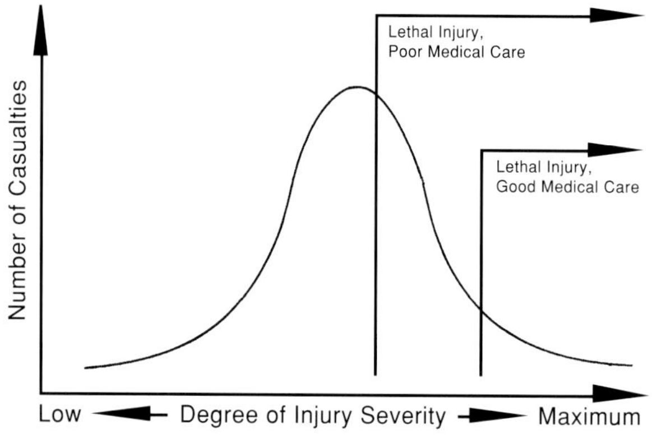

Fig. 1-12. Normal distribution of injury severity. In this hypothetical population, the degree of injury severity at which casualties would die if they receive poor medical care falls higher on the curve than it does if the medical care they receive is good.

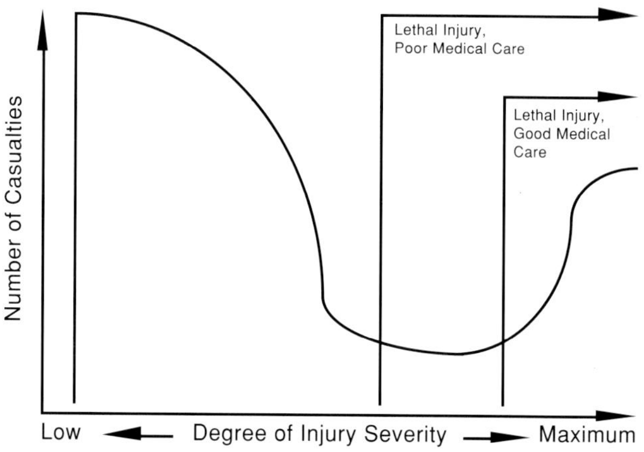

Fig. 1-13. If the distribution of injury severity is bimodal, then the quality of medical care has less effect on mortality than it would if distribution were normal.

will have injuries of intermediate severity; there are few minor or very severe injuries. A second possible curve has two peaks: this is known as a bimodal distribution (Figure 1-13). With this distribution, most trauma victims will have either minor or severe injuries; a few will have injuries of intermediate severity.

The bimodal distribution, because of its peculiar shape, seems intuitively unlikely; yet, some well-defined types of trauma have injury severity distributions of this shape. Figure 1-14 shows the distribution of injury severity found for domestic airplane crashes in which at least one life was lost.[49] The indices of injury severity used here are very simple: none, minimal, serious, fatal. A bimodal distribution is clearly apparent. Figure 1-15 shows the injury severity distribution, quantitated in terms of the Injury Severity Score, for a 1989 airplane crash on the M1 motorway in England.[50] Again, a bimodal distribution of injury severity is seen. Data published in 1994[51] indicate that the distributions of both the Trauma Score and the Glasgow coma scale in typical populations of trauma victims are also bimodal.

For didactic purposes, distributions shown in both Figures 1-12 and 1-13 are assumed to have a score above which all casualties will die even when they receive medical care. However, the score associated with death will be higher with good care and lower with poor. Figure 1-12 shows that improving medical care will markedly increase the number of survivors if the distribution is normal. By way of contrast, Figure 1-13 shows that a similar improvement in the quality of medical care will be associated with much less salvage if the distribution is

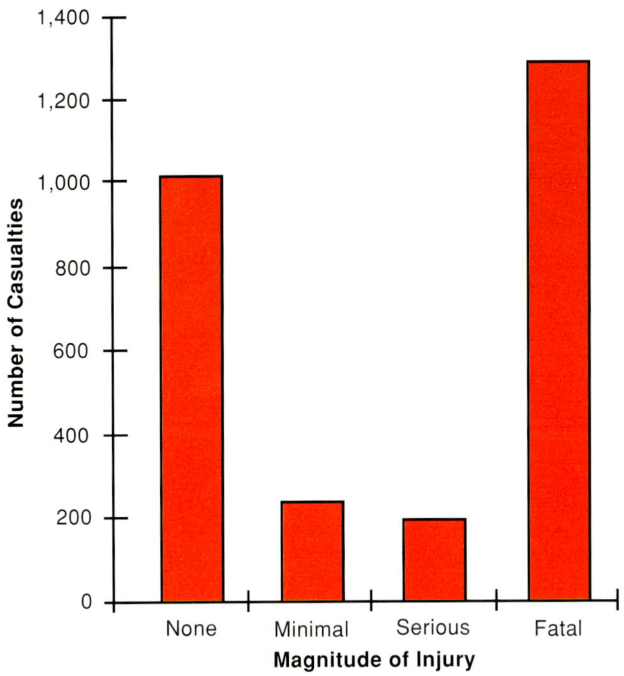

Fig. 1-14. Distribution of the magnitude of injury in all domestic airplane crashes during the period 1979 through 1984 in which one or more passengers were fatally injured. A bimodal distribution is apparent. Data source: National Transportation Safety Board.

bimodal. In terms of military medicine, care of poor quality might be thought of as military surgery as practiced in the early part of the 20th century, and good care might be military surgery as it is practiced at the end of the 20th century. Clearly, a major reduction in mortality would be expected if injury severity of combat casualties has a normal distribution, but a much smaller reduction would be expected if the real distribution has a bimodal shape.

Actual Distribution

Figure 1-16 shows the distribution of injury severity found for combat casualties in a sample taken from the WDMET database.[35] The distribution is clearly not normal in shape but it is also less obviously bimodal than is the distribution shown in Figure 1-15, primarily because of the peak in deaths in the Injury Severity Score interval 20–29. Most of the dead casualties who appear in this interval are soldiers who had sustained penetrating head wounds, the lethality of which is grossly underestimated by the Abbreviated Injury Scale. They are assigned an Abbreviated Injury Scale score of 5, but a more realistic assessment would be to assign them a score of 6 (Injury Severity Score = 75). Most of the dead casualties in the Injury Severity Score interval 20–29 should, therefore, be in the Injury Severity Score interval > 60.

Given this needed change, there is no doubt that the casualty population found in the WDMET study is best described by a bimodal injury severity distri-

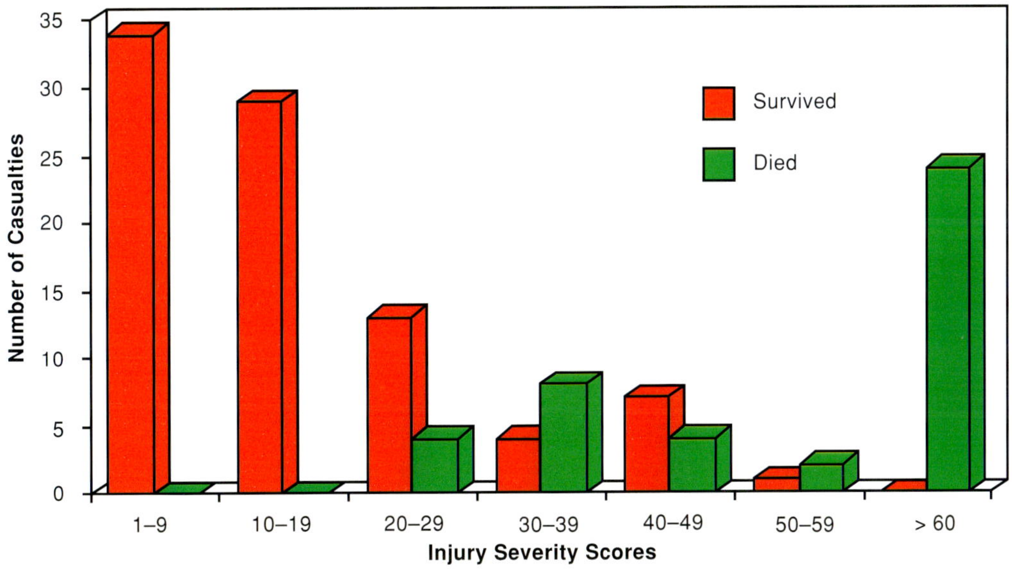

Fig. 1-15. Injury Severity Scores for the victims of the crash of a Boeing 737-400 onto the M1 Kegworth motorway in England, 1989. The bimodal distribution of injury severity is apparent. Data source: Rowles JM, Kirsh G, Macey AC, Colton CL. The use of injury scoring in the evaluation of the Kegworth M1 aircrash. *J Trauma*. 1992;32:441–447.

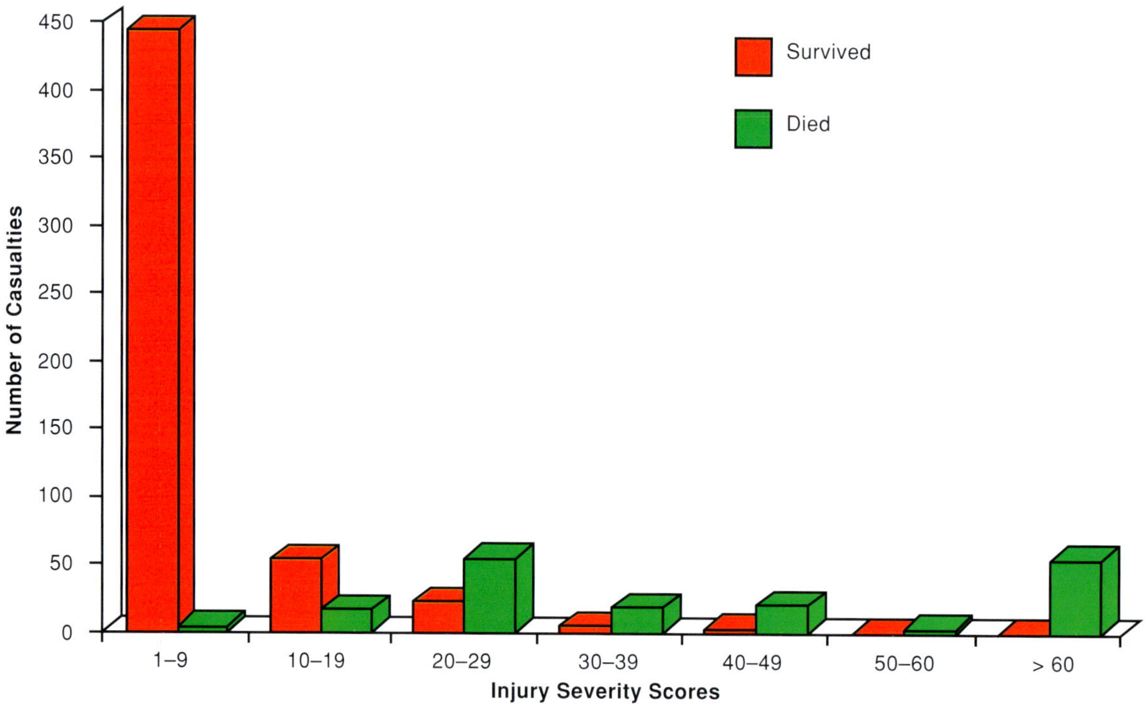

Fig. 1-16. Distribution of Injury Severity Scores in a population of casualties from the Vietnam War. A bimodal distribution is apparent, with most casualties falling into one of two populations: those with minor to moderately severe injuries, and those with nonsurvivable injuries. Data source: Wound Data and Munitions Effectiveness Team database.

bution. In simple terms, there are two major subpopulations: the larger one containing casualties with minor or moderate injuries, and the smaller containing those with critical and unsurvivable injuries. Only a small minority (perhaps 10%), those with serious or severe injuries who fall between the two major subpopulations at either end of the injury severity distribution, are likely to be helped by trauma care of the highest quality and sophistication. Survival of the casualties at either end of the injury severity distribution is not appreciably influenced by the quality of care. Those with minor or moderate injuries do not die if given even a modicum of care, and those with critical or unsurvivable injuries are beyond any conceivable help. What this means for military medicine is that it will not be easy to achieve a substantial decrease in combat mortality because of the small size of the population that is helped by surgical care of the highest quality. These considerations are consistent with the relatively small decrease in combat mortality observed in U.S. wars of this century.[52] It must be emphasized that this conclusion applies only to mortality and not to the morbidity of combat injuries. Modern military surgery has unquestionably reduced the morbidity of battle injuries—especially through the decrease in wound sepsis.

Pathophysiological Causes of Death

Medical interventions designed to reduce combat mortality must be predicated on a thorough understanding of the pathophysiological derangements that cause the death of injured soldiers. Figure 1-17, which is based on the WDMET study[15] and Arnold and Cutting's paper[38] on the causes of death in medical treatment facilities in Vietnam, provides the needed information. Mortality is classified as killed in action due to exsanguination (44%), CNS injury (31%), and combined injuries (13%); and died of wounds due to CNS injury (5%), multiple organ failure/sepsis (4%), and shock (3%).

Exsanguination was the most common cause of death for U.S. ground forces in Vietnam, accounting for about one half of the combat mortality in the WDMET study. The most common sites of injury were the heart, thoracic aorta, pulmonary artery, and intraparenchymal pulmonary vessels. However, in about 20% of the casualties who exsanguinated on the battlefield, the site of bleeding was

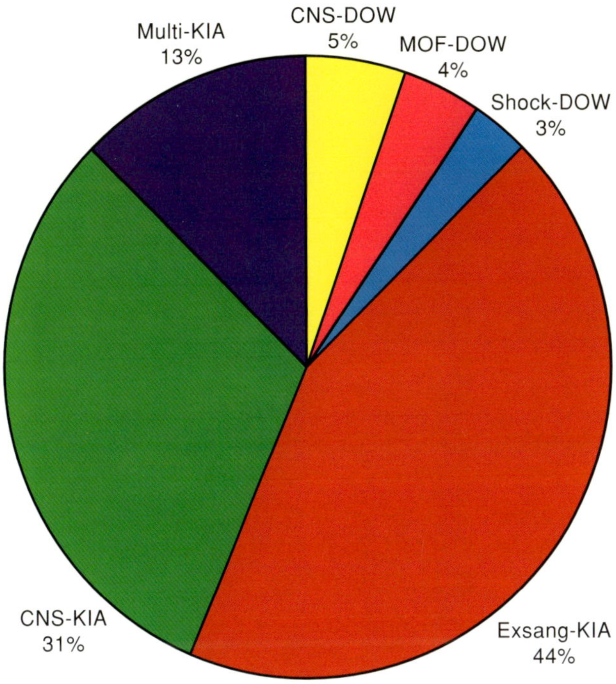

Fig. 1-17. The pathophysiological causes of death in the Vietnam War. Data from the Wound Data and Munitions Effectiveness Team database show that exsanguination and injury to the central nervous system were the most common causes of death. Key: CNS: central nervous system; DOW: died of wounds; Exsang: exsanguination; KIA: killed in action; MOF: multiple organ failure; Multi: multiple injuries. Data sources: (1) Wound Data and Munitions Effectiveness Team. *The WDMET Study*. 1970. (2) Arnold K, Cutting RT. Causes of death in United States military personnel hospitalized in Vietnam. *Milit Med*. 1978;143:161–164.

an artery in an extremity (femoral and brachial were the most common), in which first aid could, in theory, have been lifesaving.[53] Death from shock at the hospital level was uncommon, even though some 10% of all WDMET hospital admissions were judged by their surgeons as being in circulatory shock.[15(T4-7-9)] Of the hospitalized casualties who died of shock, roughly equal numbers were categorized as dying of continued bleeding (the sites were most commonly the liver or pelvis), uncontrollable coagulopathy, and "irreversible shock." Given that about 50% of the killed die by exsanguination, it would appear from the WDMET data that about 18% of all casualties are at risk of dying from exsanguination or shock, with the overall mortality in this group being 60%.

The difficulty of affecting the outcome in the remaining 80% of the casualties who die of exsanguination is suggested by the data given in Exhibit 1-2, which describe the clinical and anatomical features in 10 consecutive casualties in the WDMET study who were killed in action but who survived for 10 or more minutes after being fatally wounded. It should be apparent that stabilization by conventional first aid has little to offer to these gravely wounded soldiers even though (*a*) they lived long enough to receive battlefield first aid and (*b*) had injuries that are much more surgically treatable than are wounds of the heart or aorta. Only an intervention designed, in essence, to slow the process of dying until surgery can be carried out has any possibility of preventing death in this group. What is needed is a radically new approach to battlefield stabilization, perhaps based on yet-to-be-discovered biochemical and biophysiological interventions, which will make possible metabolic down-regulation with consequent temporary suspension of cardiopulmonary function without causing permanent tissue injury. Finding successful solutions to the combat casualty problems listed in Exhibit 1-2 should be considered a challenge by all military anesthesiologists.

Injury to the CNS was the second-most-common cause of death in combat casualties studied by WDMET. These injuries were almost always so devastating (eg, three or more lobes injured, avulsion of the brain, decapitation, or injury to the brainstem) that they offered little potential for better surgical management to improve outcome. Surprisingly, the most common cause of death at the hospital level was CNS injury. The extent to which better care might be able to decrease this cause of mortality is unclear: one half of these casualties had been triaged into the expectant category because they were considered brain dead. The famous Bougainville study[54] of World War II reached the same conclusion regarding the relative importance of the pathophysiological causes of death: hemorrhage accounted for the largest number of combat fatalities (55%), while those who succumbed to injuries to the CNS composed the second-largest group (26%).

Most of the WDMET casualties in the multiple category had the misfortune to sustain potentially lethal injuries to the head, chest, or abdomen. The most common combinations were head and chest, and chest and abdomen. Some of these casualties sustained what was described as mutilating blast injury, in which the body was essentially disintegrated, but others had combined injuries as a consequence of the propensity of assault rifles and machine guns to cause multiple wounds.

EXHIBIT 1-2

CLINICAL AND ANATOMICAL DIAGNOSES OF 10 CASUALTIES WHO DIED 10 OR MORE MINUTES AFTER BEING WOUNDED

1. Casualty lived 15 minutes; perforating gunshot wound of chest; bullet entered at right anterior axillary line and exited to the left of the spine above the iliac crest; pulmonary laceration, fracture of T12; severed spinal cord; 2,000 mL of blood in right hemithorax.
2. Casualty lived about 10 minutes; through-and-through gunshot wound of abdomen; bullet entered right flank and exited under left costal margin; celiac axis and superior mesenteric vein transected; 1,750 mL of blood in abdominal cavity.
3. Casualty lived less than 1 hour; perforating gunshot wound entered right shoulder and exited lower abdomen; lacerations of right lung, diaphragm, liver, and kidney; a total of 1,600 mL of blood in chest and abdomen.
4. Casualty died 10 to 15 minutes after being wounded: bullet entered laterally on the right side of the abdomen and passed out of the left hip; autopsy showed transection of right internal iliac artery, sigmoid colon, and left femoral artery, multiple perforation of small bowel; 1,750 mL of blood in abdominal cavity.
5. Casualty lived 50 minutes; gunshot wound of chest with fractures of ribs 7, 8, and 9; small hemothorax (250 mL); massive "traumatic atelectasis" of lung [pulmonary contusion?—*RFB*]; casualty became unresponsive 2 minutes after being wounded and after he stated "I think I've got a punctured lung."
6. Casualty lived 15 minutes; 2 gunshot wounds of the upper chest; one bullet, after fracturing T 4-5, lacerated the trachea, esophagus, and one lung; second bullet passed through chest into abdomen, where it injured the liver, kidney, and pancreas; 250 mL of blood in abdomen.
7. Casualty lived for 15 minutes; four gunshot wounds of left lateral hip and lower abdomen; extensive fracture of pelvis; perforation of right common iliac artery; 1,000 mL of blood in abdomen.
8. Casualty may have lived for 15 to 20 minutes; two perforating gunshot wounds of left side of body; one passed through the arm and entered the chest, where it fractured four ribs; no description of hemo- or pneumothorax; second bullet fractured T10 and severed the spinal cord at that location.
9. Casualty lived for 20 to 25 minutes; bullet entered right flank and passed through liver, diaphragm, and all lobes of right lung; several severely fractured ribs at wound of exit; 650 mL of blood in chest and abdomen.
10. Casualty lived 10 to 15 minutes; perforating gunshot wound of abdomen with lacerations of liver, duodenum, and kidney; 1,300 mL of blood in abdomen.

Data source: Wound Data and Munitions Effectiveness Team. *The WDMET Study*. 1970. Original data are in the possession of the Uniformed Services University of the Health Sciences, Bethesda, Maryland 20814-4799. Three summary volumes contain extensive abstracts of the statistical data and can be obtained from Defense Documentation Center, Cameron Station, Alexandria, Virginia 22304-6145.

A minority of the casualties in the multiple category did not have true multiple injuries but had respiratory tract wounds as the cause of death. It is not unusual to find chest X-ray films of WDMET dead that show the presence of a massive tension pneumothorax. In casualties seen alive at the hospital level, about 3.2% were said to be in respiratory distress: about one half had tension pneumothorax and one half had an open chest wound. The importance of injury to the upper airway (face and neck) as a cause of death on the battlefield is unclear; no doubt it is much less important than exsanguination or CNS injury. The WDMET study indicates that of casualties who were alive when they reached a medical treatment facility, about 1.3% required immediate upper airway control.[15(T4-7-9)] However, slightly more than one half of these casualties required airway control because of massive CNS injury; a minority only had direct injury to the upper airway.

About 4% of the fatally wounded soldiers died from what would now be called the systemic inflammatory response syndrome apparent as multiple organ failure and sepsis. The most common manifestations were septic shock (usually caused by severe peritonitis), adult respiratory distress syndrome, and acute renal failure. To put the magnitude of these problems in perspective, about 1 casualty in 1,000 died of renal failure. Assuming that the condition has a mortality of 50%, there would have been about 2 cases of renal failure per 1,000 casualties.

THE ANESTHESIOLOGIST AND COMBAT CASUALTY CARE

Some civilian trauma anesthesiologists, most prominently C. M. Grande,[55] believe that trauma anesthesiologists must go beyond their familiar role in the operating room and become life-support physicians in the broadest sense, involved in all aspects of the casualty's care. In combat casualty care, however, the potential for lifesaving, nonsurgical intervention in the operating room is somewhat limited. In lieu of data from a more recent war, the data contained in Table 1-5 may be taken as evidence for this contention.[37] The table stratifies by phase of treatment the deaths of 1,450 combat casualties, which occurred in hospitals in the Fifth U.S. Army in Italy between January 1944 and May 1945.

Although these data are nearly 50 years old, they suggest that it would be difficult to do much better, because only 6.3% of the total hospital mortality occurred during the anesthetic induction and the operation itself. Where there is room for improvement is in the preoperative, and especially in the postoperative, phases. It is for this reason that the focus of this book goes beyond anesthesia per se and puts strong emphasis on perioperative care. Unfortunately, as has been shown, the battlefield is the site of the great majority (90%) of combat fatalities. For the concept of the trauma anesthesiologist as life-support physician to find its full realization, military anesthesiologists must look beyond the hospital level to the battlefield. The military trauma anesthesiologist must be prepared to assume a leadership role in providing resuscitation at the first and second echelons of care. Because the Advanced Trauma Life Support course (ATLS)[56] of the American College of Surgeons provides the scientific and doctrinal basis for AMEDD's initial care of combat casualties, it is necessary for military trauma anesthesiologists to take a critical look at ATLS as it is presently practiced.

TABLE 1-5

PARTITION OF HOSPITAL DEATHS BY PHASE OF MEDICAL MANAGEMENT

Phase of Management	Deaths (%)
Dead on admission or died shortly after admission	7.8
Died before anesthesia began	23.2
Died during anesthetic induction	1.1
Died during initial surgery	5.2
Died after initial surgery	62.7

Adapted from Snyder HE, Culbertson JW. Studies of Fifth US Army hospitalized casualty deaths. In: Beyer JC, ed. *Wound Ballistics*. Washington, DC: Department of the Army, Medical Department, Office of The Surgeon General; 1962: 473.

Advanced Trauma Life Support Course

The ATLS course is a systematic approach to the initial diagnosis and management of trauma victims. It emphasizes the recognition of immediately life-threatening injuries and provides instruction in the first-aid skills that are necessary to optimize patient survival in the early postinjury period. In the broadest sense, ATLS should be applicable to all trauma victims. However, because it was developed by civilian physicians for managing civilian trauma in a civilian setting, the military anesthesiologist should not be surprised to find that specific aspects of ATLS are not entirely appropriate to combat casualty care. There are significant differences in the epidemiologies of civilian and battlefield trauma. They arise not only from dissimilarities in the mechanisms of injury (eg, blunt trauma is much more common in civilian life than in war), but they also reflect the following characteristics of military medicine:

- Military trauma management is echelon (now also called *level*) based. Each echelon either returns the soldier to duty or evacuates the casualty safely to the next echelon.
- Medical personnel are in much greater physical danger when providing combat casualty care than they are when providing civilian trauma care (about 10% of the soldiers in the WDMET study were wounded while attempting to help a casualty).

- Military trauma care is performed in an austere and resource-limited environment.

It is in the areas of organization and in what can be called the conditions of practice that ATLS in its usual civilian guise may need to be modified when used to care for combat casualties in conventional land warfare.

Military Organization for the Provision of Care

Both civilian and military trauma care depend on an organized system of prehospital treatment. While the civilian prehospital care organization typically consists of ambulances and paramedics, the military prehospital system consists of two levels of deployable medical facilities, ground or air ambulances, and attendant personnel numbering as many as 600 for one division. The extensive nature of the military prehospital system reflects the cost of providing a mobile and self-contained healthcare system for a large number of personnel who are subject to a variety of infectious diseases and environmental hazards and, worse, exposed to a risk of violence that exceeds anything in civilian experience by 1 or 2 orders of magnitude.

The military trauma care organization differs from the civilian model by providing care by echelons, wherein military casualties are either returned to duty or evacuated through successive echelons that are capable of increasingly sophisticated care. Table 1-6 describes the echelons of care and their function. Resuscitative surgery—surgery performed to control bleeding and to eliminate contamination—is carried out at the third echelon (or at lower echelons by a third-echelon forward surgical team [FST]), while restorative surgery—surgery performed to heal wounds and to restore function—is carried out at the fourth echelon or in the continental United States (CONUS). In the civilian system, the emergency department (the site of ATLS) is in the same building as the operating room (the site of resuscitative surgery). In the military system, ATLS is performed at the first and second echelons (where it must be done if acute life-threatening processes are to be reversed), many kilometers (or hours, depending on the mode of evacuation) from the site of resuscitative surgery.

The contents of the preceding paragraph describe the organization as prescribed by army doctrine,[1] but exceptions do exist. During much of the Vietnam War, the first and second echelons of care were frequently so atropic that third-echelon hospitals had a function not too dissimilar from that of a civilian trauma center. Casualties frequently arrived directly from the battlefield without having received any care, which meant that first-aid interventions that ideally should have been performed in the field were commonplace at the hospital level. Still, the analogy with the civilian system was not

TABLE 1-6

LEVELS OF MILITARY MEDICAL CARE AND THEIR USUAL FUNCTION

Echelon/Level	Medical Unit	Trauma Management
First/Unit	Medical platoon, BAS	ATLS
Second/Division	Medical company	ATLS
	Medical battalion	Minor surgery
	FST*	Resuscitative surgery
Third/Corps	MASH†	ATLS
	CSH	Resuscitative surgery
Fourth/COMMZ	Field hospital	Reconstructive surgery
	General hospital	Reconstructive surgery
Fifth/CONUS	Medical center	Reconstructive surgery

*Surgical squads are organic to airborne and air-assault divisions and, in the form of forward surgical teams, may be attached when needed to medical companies of other divisions.
†The MASH is to be deleted; its function will be assumed by the FSTs.
ATLS: Advanced Trauma Life Support; BAS: battalion aid station; COMMZ: communications zone; CONUS: continental United States; CSH: combat support hospital; FST: forward surgical team; MASH: mobile army surgical hospital

total because only resuscitative surgery, and not reconstructive surgery, was normally carried out. In recent years, the U.S. Army's involvement in peacekeeping operations, under the doctrinal guise of operations other than war (OOTW),[1(p1-1)] has raised the possibility that military anesthesiologists will practice in a situation in which the functions of the first three echelons of care are telescoped together into one medical treatment facility. Military anesthesiologists may also have the opportunity to serve in hospitals of the International Committee of the Red Cross. Although typical military wounds are treated in these circumstances, there are no echelons of care and the primitive economic infrastructure, the lack of medical resources, the underlying social chaos, and a perhaps fatalistic acceptance of death by the population being served create conditions that are likely to be new to most medical officers in the U.S. military.[57]

Battlefield Conditions

Four factors—danger, austerity, casualty density, and goals—distinguish the military use of ATLS from its use in the civilian sector.

Danger. Field medical units, especially those of the first and second echelons, are subject to enemy attack. Even necessary defensive measures, such as entrenchment and construction of bunkers, may prevent an optimal flow of casualties. Furthermore, when the possibility of unconventional warfare (chemical or biological) exists, even the individual casualty must be considered a threat to the medical troops, and appropriate steps must be taken to reduce the risk of exposure. These dangerous possibilities may interfere with, or prevent the full application of, ATLS as it is practiced in civilian emergency care.

Austerity. Field medical units lack the pleasant ambience of civilian hospitals. Tents, mud floors, cots, and battery-operated lights are not insurmountable obstacles to the proper application of ATLS, but they can reduce the efficiency of all but the most ardent and most experienced practitioners. The need to employ noise and light discipline complicates battlefield ATLS. The lack of many diagnostic modalities, even such basic ones as X-ray units, seriously impairs the ability of military physicians to apply ATLS as practiced in the civilian sector, especially in first- and second-echelon facilities. Finally, medical supplies such as syringes, intravenous catheters, and even gloves are available in limited amounts; they cannot be expended unless there is good reason to believe that their use will benefit the casualty. Furthermore, the wearing of protective devices against communicable disease (ie, the universal precautions) is not feasible in the field echelons of care.

Casualty Density. Mass casualty situations are not unique to the military, but mass casualty situations among civilians are usually considered atypical, while they are a constant threat in the military. As has been described previously in this chapter, the casualty-generating potential of the modern battlefield is 10- to 100-fold greater than it is in even the most violent urban setting. Although the ATLS primary survey may take only a few seconds to perform, the complete examination is not suited to situations in which only a few minutes per casualty are available for diagnosis and presurgical resuscitation.

Goals. ATLS is designed to assist the physician in recognizing acute, life-threatening, pathophysiological disturbances. The focus is on lethality and the prevention of gross morbidity. The military anesthesiologist cannot forget that the missions of the medical services—conserve fighting strength and maintain the fighting power of the command—can be carried out only if each casualty is assessed in terms of his ability to return rapidly to duty. This is not to say that the demands of military medicine require that the seriously injured be ignored. Rather, the slightly wounded should be accorded higher priority for care than they would be if the military medical treatment system were driven solely by ATLS considerations of lethality.

Specific Aspects of Advanced Trauma Life Support

The following is not to be construed as an attempt to replace ATLS with an alternative approach to managing trauma. Instead, its purpose is to indicate areas in which ATLS should be modified when used in combat casualty care. Perhaps the most important point is that ATLS must be tailored to the echelon of care and to the prevailing tactical posture. For example, in a quiet, third-echelon surgical facility, the military practice of ATLS may not deviate from the civilian standard, but this will certainly not be true at a first-echelon facility that is being shelled while it is receiving several dozen casualties. In general, the more theoretically relevant ATLS may seem to be, the *further forward on the battlefield it must be implemented* to be effective. The realities of the battlefield are, however, that the *further forward the care is needed, the less practical it is to provide.*

Most medical officers, and certainly all military anesthesiologists, will be ATLS trained, so only a brief summary need be given here of the sequence of events and their purposes:

- primary survey (with simultaneous correction of any life-threatening conditions):
  - airway patency with cervical spine control,
  - breathing and ventilation,
  - circulation and hemorrhage control,
  - disability, as determined by neurological status, and
  - exposure;
- triage determination, which may be made as part of the primary survey;
- secondary survey (a detailed examination of the casualty); and
- definitive care.

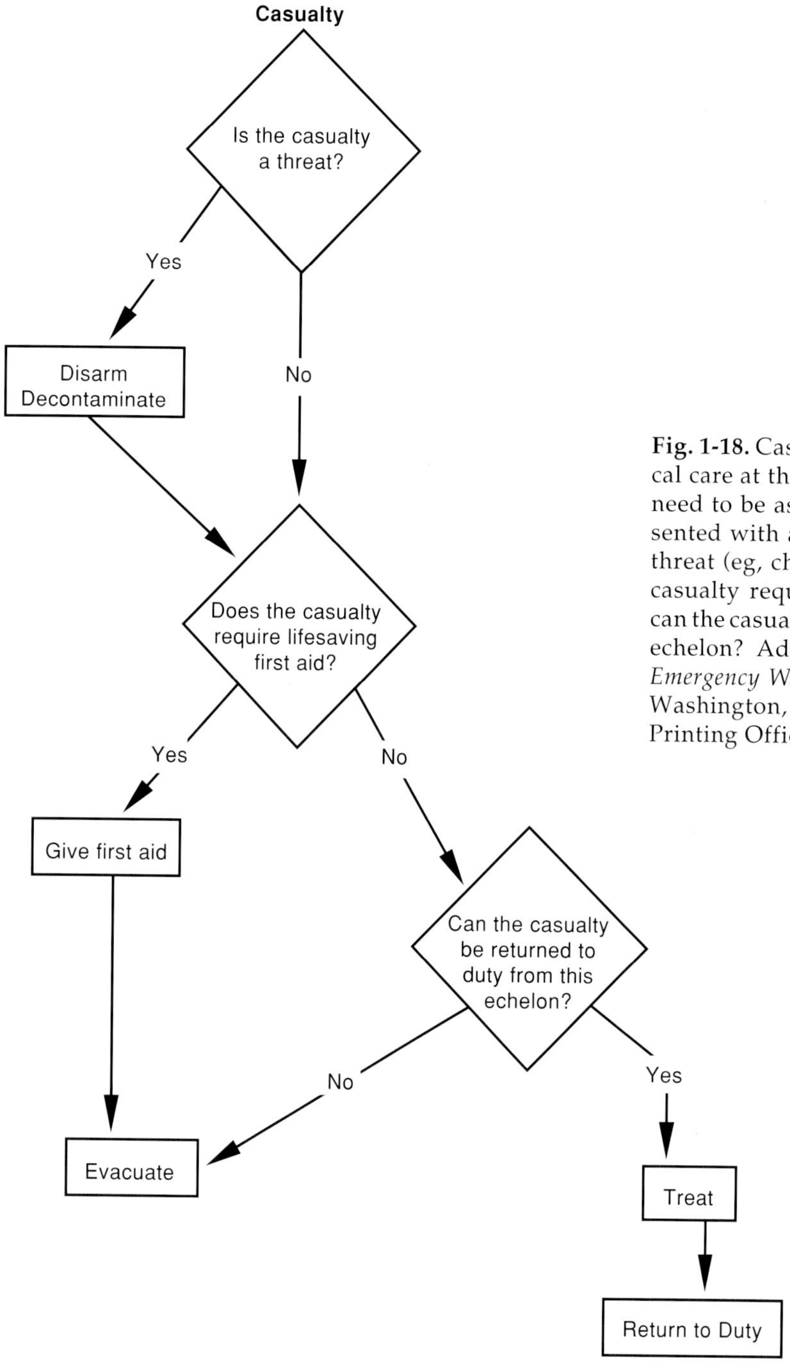

Fig. 1-18. Casualty care decision tree applicable to medical care at the field-echelon level. Three basic questions need to be asked when a field medical provider is presented with a casualty. First, is the casualty a potential threat (eg, chemically contaminated)? Second, does the casualty require immediate lifesaving first aid? Third, can the casualty be treated and returned to duty from this echelon? Adapted from Bowen TE, Bellamy RF, eds. *Emergency War Surgery NATO Handbook*. 2nd rev US ed. Washington, DC: Department of Defense, Government Printing Office; 1988: 204.

The following is a chapter-by-chapter critique of the ATLS manual as it applies to combat casualty care.

Initial Assessment and Management

The triage algorithm from the *Emergency War Surgery NATO Handbook* (Figure 1-18)[58] is applicable to the first and second echelons of care, but it may also be appropriate at facilities that provide surgical care as well.

Medical officers must ask themselves three questions:

1. Is the casualty a threat? The threat comes from casualties who have been contaminated by exposure to chemical or biological agents. Intelligence sources (S-2, G-2) will usually know if the enemy has the capability and the intent to employ unconventional weapons.
2. Does the casualty require emergency lifesaving resuscitation? Medical officers should require no more than a few seconds to determine whether interventions utilizing the ATLS lifesaving skills are needed. As has been indicated previously, the Vietnam War experience showed that about 15% of combat casualties benefited from ATLS airway (1.3%), breathing (3.2%), and shock (10%) interventions.
3. Can the casualty be returned to duty from this echelon? A problem-oriented approach is required: Where is the wound and what is its nature? The medical officer must not waste time preparing a comprehensive list of all the possible diagnoses and *certainly* should not spend time and effort ruling out a large collection of diagnoses that are likely to be important only in the context of ATLS as it is practiced in a civilian emergency department. If the wound will prevent the casualty from performing his duty, and if the treatment capabilities of the echelon cannot reverse the pathophysiology of the injury, then the casualty must safely and expeditiously be evacuated to the next echelon.

Many aspects of the complete ATLS program are not applicable to combat casualty care. For example, it is a mistake to cut off all the casualty's clothing to perform the complete ATLS examination. Not only can climatic conditions make this unwise, but a fresh uniform will not be available as a replacement. Performance of the secondary survey should be left to medical officers at higher echelons. This is especially true because the necessary diagnostic modalities are absent in the battalion aid station, medical company, and even some third-echelon hospitals.

Airway and Ventilatory Management

Combat casualties (exclusive of those with a severe brain injury) who require airway management almost always have such destructive wounds that a surgical airway (tracheostomy or cricothyroidotomy) will be required. The possibility that a casualty whose upper airway problem is the result of a penetrating wound will also have a subtle, unrecognized, coexisting injury to the cervical spine is so remote that it may be ignored. Airway control in combat casualties with facial or neck wounds is a necessary but not a sufficient therapeutic intervention; safe evacuation to the third echelon of care will be impossible unless hemorrhage into the oral cavity can be stopped, or at least free egress of blood from the mouth can be achieved.

Shock

Hemorrhage is the major cause of death in combat casualties. In about 20% of those casualties at risk of exsanguination,[53] bleeding can be controlled by first-aid techniques such as applying pressure at the site of hemorrhage or applying a tourniquet. The latter intervention is especially useful when the site of bleeding is from an amputation stump. There can be little doubt that of the ATLS lifesaving interventions, those associated with the control of bleeding are most important. Nevertheless, the associated intervention—starting two large-bore intravenous lines and infusing 2 L of Ringer's lactate—although having the status of established dogma, has recently been called into question by numerous laboratory studies on experimental animals and human clinical trials.[59,60] It seems well established that infusion of a crystalloid fluid will elevate the systemic blood pressure and thereby potentially increase the rate of hemorrhage from injured vessels. The rationale for administering intravenous fluids in a casualty with ongoing, uncontrolled hemorrhage can only be that a net increase in intravascular volume will take place, and this will occur only if the fluid is infused faster than it can leave the vascular bed. There is an obvious limit to this approach: as was demonstrated during the Vietnam War, massive administration of crystalloid fluid without concomitant rapid control of bleeding may very well result in a degree of hemodilution incompatible with life (ie, the "white blood syndrome").

The value of ATLS in the management of combat casualties in shock will depend on the echelon of care. Clearly, when surgical care is immediately available, the ATLS shock module should be entirely appropriate. Its value at the first and second echelons, where resuscitative surgery is usually not available, is less obvious. It would indeed be ironic if it were to be shown that the importance placed on asanguineous fluid resuscitation in the field of casualties in shock from uncontrolled bleeding did more harm than good. It becomes even more ironic when we are reminded of the World War II experience with fluid resuscitation and combat casualty care:

> When internal hemorrhage persisted...there could be no resuscitation without surgery, and it was wasteful of both time and blood to attempt to raise the patient's blood pressure to normal before operation. The blood or plasma which was administered merely leaked into the traumatized regions and was wasted....[36(p6)]

It is uncertain at this time what should be done about fluid resuscitation in casualties with ongoing hemorrhage, in circumstances in which surgical control of bleeding is not immediately possible. An experimental study published in 1993[61] showed that although infusion of crystalloid fluid during uncontrolled hemorrhage did increase the magnitude of the blood loss, infused animals lived longer than controls that received no fluid. The magnitude of the volume infused is important because both the 1993 study and another one published in 1992[62] found that survival was better when the volume infused did not exceed 40 mL/kg. Some intravenous fluid may be better than none at all, as was appreciated in World War II:

> [Plasma] superbly fulfilled the role of supporting life until transportation could be accomplished to an installation at which whole-blood transfusion was feasible.... By temporarily sustaining a seriously falling blood pressure and increasing the cardiac output, it kept the patient alive long enough for more effective measures to be taken.[36(p22)]

Nevertheless, there are limits to how long such stabilization will be effective. Until asanguineous oxygen-carrying blood substitutes are developed, there is no substitute for immediate surgery in the rapidly exsanguinating casualty; nonsurgical stabilization is an act of futility.

There is an additional area in which the realities of battlefield medicine intrude on the performance of ATLS. Invasive monitoring techniques will not be available in the first three echelons of care; thus, clinical signs will need to be followed during volume replacement. In this regard, the World War II and Vietnam War experiences showed that tachycardia was an unreliable and inappropriate indicator of the degree of shock.[63]

Thoracic Trauma

Casualties with thoracic wounds who survive to be evacuated from the battlefield should be treated following the ATLS algorithm; however, a penetrating chest wound is itself an indication for inserting a chest tube. Reinfusion of shed blood may be possible because autotransfusion devices are being added to the table of organization and equipment (TOE) of third-echelon facilities. Thus, ATLS principles are appropriate, but sepsis remains the main potential source of morbidity. Cardiac tamponade is seen very uncommonly. The decision to perform a pericardiocentesis is usually predicated on the presence of shock that is unresponsive to fluid administration in a casualty who has a wound of the anterior chest wall.

Abdominal Trauma

Casualties with abdominal wounds should be treated by the ATLS algorithm, but the following facts need emphasis:

- Among casualties who have abdominal wounds and who survive to be evacuated from the battlefield, the major threat to life is sepsis from peritoneal contamination rather than shock from hemorrhage. Thus, antibiotic coverage needs to be emphasized.
- Indications for operation are simpler than suggested by ATLS; the presence of a penetrating wound is sufficient justification. Peritoneal lavage as mandated by ATLS has no role in the management of combat casualties with penetrating wounds.

Head Trauma

Casualties with penetrating head wounds who survive to reach a medical treatment facility fall into two main categories: (1) those with tangential gunshot wounds of the skull, with laceration of the brain caused by bony fragments that are driven into the brain parenchyma; and (2) those with penetrating wounds of the brain made by one or two small fragments. Most surviving casualties will be conscious at the time of admission and will have high Glasgow coma scale scores. Thus, the ATLS mini-neurological examination is needed to establish evacuation and treatment priorities. If these casualties fail to receive neurosurgical care within 24 hours, they are at risk of developing potentially fatal cerebral sepsis. A combat casualty who is comatose secondary to penetrating head wounds has a very poor prognosis. In the absence of neurosurgical intervention, the best that can be done is to assure an open airway by inserting an endotracheal tube.

Spine and Spinal Cord Trauma

ATLS and the reality of combat casualty care have their greatest potential conflict with spine and spinal cord trauma. Penetrating missiles that wound the cervical, thoracic, or lumbar spine have a high lethality because the missile has a propensity to also strike contiguous structures (eg, the carotid artery or thoracic aorta). Wounds of the cervical spine may or may not involve the cervical cord, but when they do, the outcome is almost always fatal (98%).[15] There is no evidence that a penetrating missile wound that involves only the cervical spine will predispose the patient to a subsequent cervical *spinal cord* injury when the neck is manipulated. Essentially no combat casualties with *penetrating* neck wounds will benefit from immobilization of the cervical spine, except the rare living casualty who has an existing neurological defect that is thought to be caused by a spinal injury.[64] Given the well-established danger of carrying out care on the battlefield, battlefield immobilization of the neck of a casualty with a penetrating neck wound is therefore unwarranted. However, ATLS principles do apply to casualties with *blunt* trauma to the head and neck.

Extremity Trauma

During the pre-ATLS era, much of field medical training consisted of practicing the application of dressings and splints to casualties with fractures or soft-tissue wounds of the extremities. In fact, these remain the essential skills required to give effective combat casualty care at the first and second echelons. For the military ATLS trainer, the chapter in the ATLS manual on extremity trauma is *the important* chapter. Emphasis should also be placed on the prehospital administration of antibiotics that will decrease the potential for clostridial and streptococcal wound infections.

Third-echelon extremity care will differ from ATLS practice because the radiographic equipment necessary to rule out vascular injury will probably not be available. Although Doppler probes may be available to assist in making the diagnosis of a vascular injury, the diagnosis will usually have to be made by exposing the vessel at the time of soft-tissue wound management.

Burns

Inhalation injury is a major source of mortality and morbidity during naval warfare and will probably become more important in future land warfare because of the prevalence of armored fighting vehicles. Medical officers at field medical facilities should predicate their therapies on the burned casualty's ability to clear the tracheobronchial tree. If secretions cannot be raised, the medical officer will have to decide whether scarce resources should be used for intubation and ventilation. Bronchospasm must be broken and pneumonitis must be prevented or treated. Antibiotic treatment may have to be initiated without the physician's knowing the specific bacterial flora that is growing in the lung, undesirable as this may be. In an important departure from ATLS, topical antimicrobial therapy such as with Sulfamylon (manufactured by Don B. Hickon, Inc., Sugar Land, Tex.) or Silvadene (manufactured by Marion Merrell Dow, Inc., Kansas City, Mo.) burn cream should be started before the casualty is evacuated from the field echelons. The appropriate escharotomies should be performed early when treating a casualty with deep, third-degree extremity burns whose evacuation to a higher echelon is likely to be delayed.

Stabilization and Evacuation

Stabilization and evacuation of casualties are aspects of ATLS that are difficult to implement fully. There is no 911 number to call on the battlefield nor will the referring physician be able to contact the receiving physician. In these respects, the military and civilian trauma-care systems are markedly dissimilar. At the unit and division levels, medical officers will need to know how to contact the supporting ambulance unit for either air or ground evacuation. At the third echelon, the evacuation, which will usually be done by the U.S. Air Force, will be organized by the medical regulating officer.

Regardless of the echelon, the medical officer will be responsible for establishing priorities for evacuation and treatment. ATLS concepts can usefully be combined with existing military criteria for triage at first- and second-echelon medical facilities:

- Priority I—URGENT and Priority IA—URGENT-SURG: the casualty fails to respond or responds transiently to ATLS airway, breathing, and circulation (ABC) skills;
- Priority II—PRIORITY: the casualty responds to ATLS ABC skills and remains stable; and
- Priority III—ROUTINE: ATLS ABC skills are not needed to stabilize the casualty.

Note: casualties with massive injuries to large muscle masses (such as the thigh or the pelvis) and casualties with open comminuted fractures of the femur or the hip should be triaged into the priority category because of the propensity of such wounds to develop anaerobic sepsis.

ATLS concepts can also be used to establish treatment priorities not only at first- and second-echelon facilities but also for third-echelon war surgery:

- Urgent: this triage category includes the uncommon casualty who is at risk of rapid death after an injury that causes airway compromise, respiratory derangement, or shock that is not responsive to ATLS stabilization. Emergency surgery must be performed within minutes for there to be any hope that the casualty will survive.
- Immediate: this triage category includes most casualties with abdominal or chest wounds who responded to ATLS emergency lifesaving skills and those with extensive soft-tissue and bony injuries, especially when a major vascular injury is present. Surgery is needed within 6 hours.
- Delayed: this triage category includes most casualties with fractures or soft-tissue wounds. ATLS ABC skills are not needed, but surgical care must be provided within 12 to 24 hours.
- Minimal or ambulatory: this triage category includes casualties who are carded for record only. These soldiers require outpatient treatment and should not be evacuated to higher echelons.
- Expectant: this triage category includes casualties whose injuries are so severe that they cannot reasonably be expected to survive given the available medical care. Those who are brain dead or who have deep burns over much of their bodies are in this category. These casualties are not evacuated from the echelon that assigns this priority.

The assignment of treatment or evacuation priorities is a dynamic process. The medical officer must continually update priorities. For example, a casualty who is in the delayed category may become immediate. Similarly, a casualty's category will be influenced by the prevailing tactical situation and the availability of medical resources. Given an unfavorable tactical situation, a casualty who might otherwise be classified in the urgent or the immediate category may have to be classified in the expectant. The converse is occasionally true: a casualty who has been classified as expectant may be retriaged into the urgent category because more medical resources have suddenly become available. Furthermore, priorities need to be reassessed for treatment and subsequent evacuation on arrival at the receiving echelon. Triage is ongoing, and no decision should be considered final.

SUMMARY

Although catastrophic attrition from disease or a hostile environment is an ever-present threat in military operations, battle injury is likely to assume an increasing proportion of attrition compared with the historical norm. The magnitude of the attrition depends on the size of the units engaged, their tactical posture, and the intensity of the warfare. Typical battle casualty rates in war are 10- to 100-fold greater than the rate found for civilian trauma. In contrast to civilian trauma, where blunt trauma predominates, combat injuries are overwhelmingly (> 90%) penetrating in origin. Explosive munitions are the most common sources of penetrating missiles in modern warfare. The location of penetrating injuries is, to a first approximation, a function of the size of the body surface over the body regions, except that the head sustains about twice as many injuries as would be expected on the basis of its surface area alone. Surviving casualties usually have injuries to bones or skeletal muscle, while those who are killed most commonly have wounds to the head or trunk.

The mortality of combat trauma is commonly measured by two normalized statistics: the percentage who are killed in action, and the percentage who died of wounds. The former category includes soldiers who expire on the battlefield, while the latter category includes those who expire while receiving treatment at a medical facility. Typical historical data from recent wars indicate that about 20% to 25% of casualties are killed in action and about 3% to 5% die of wounds. Penetrating missile wounds of certain organs have a very high probability of death: wounds of the brain (about 4 of 5); wounds of the chest (about 3 of 4).

Morbidity in combat casualties results in noneffectiveness following a combat injury, which can be measured as man-days lost. The distribution of injury severity in combat casualties has a bimodal appearance with two major subpopulations: the larger consists of soldiers with minor or not–life-threatening (albeit frequently incapacitating) injuries; the smaller subpopulation consists of soldiers with critical and nonsurvivable injuries.

The ATLS course of the American College of Surgeons is the basis for initial assessment and resuscitation of combat casualties. However, modifications in ATLS are necessary to make it compatible with the realities of combat casualty care in three areas: the nature of the injuries, the organization of the military medical system, and the conditions of practice on the battlefield.

REFERENCES

1. US Department of the Army. *Planning for Health Service Support*. Washington, DC: DA; 1994. Field Manual 8-55: 3-1; 4-1–4-3; 5-8–5-15.
2. Hawkins CF. Friendly fire. *Proc USN Instit*. June 1994:54–57.
3. Bodart G. *Losses of Life in Modern Wars*. Oxford, England: Clarendon Press; 1916: 127.
4. Chandler DG. *The Campaigns of Napoleon*. New York, NY: Macmillan; 1966: 853.
5. Clausewitz C. *The Campaign of 1812 in Russia*. Hattiesburg, Miss: Academic International; 1970: 97–98. Reprint of the 1843 London, England, edition.
6. Fischer H. *Der Deutsche Sanitätsdienst 1921–1945*. Vol 3. Osnabrück, Germany: Biblio Verlag; 1983: 1517, 1535.
7. Bellamy RF, Llewellyn CH. Preventable casualties: Rommel's flaw, Slim's edge. *Army*. 1990;40:52–56.
8. Connolly P. *Greece and Rome at War*. Englewood Cliffs, NJ: Prentice-Hall Inc; 1981: 188–189.
9. Fischer H. *Der Deutsche Sanitätsdienst 1921-1945*. Vol 2. Osnabrück, Germany: Biblio Verlag; 1983: 147–149, 633, 705–706.
10. Crew FAE. *Campaigns. North-West Europe*. Vol 4. London, England: The Army Medical Services, Her Majesty's Stationery Office; 1962: 597, 608, 610.
11. Beebe GW, DeBakey ME. *Battle Casualties*. Springfield, Ill: Charles C Thomas; 1952: 21, 92, 125, 186.
12. Dupuy TH. *Understanding War*. New York, NY: Paragon House Publishers; 1987: 73, 188.
13. Baker CC, Oppenheimer L, Stephens B, Lewis FR, Trunkey DD. Epidemiology of trauma deaths. *Am J Surg*. 1980;140:144–148.
14. Ognibene AJ, Barrett O'N. *General Medicine and Infectious Diseases*. Vol 2. In: Ognibene AJ, ed. *Internal Medicine in Vietnam*. Washington DC: US Army, Medical Department, Office of The Surgeon General, Center of Military History; 1982: 64.

15. Wound Data and Munitions Effectiveness Team. *The WDMET Study*. 1970. Original data are in the possession of the Uniformed Services University of the Health Sciences, Bethesda, MD 20814-4799. Three summary volumes contain extensive abstracts of the statistical data and can be obtained from Defense Documentation Center, Cameron Station, Alexandria, VA 22304-6145.

16. US Army Patient Administration Systems and Biostatistics Activity. Battle injury dispositions by causative agent—Active duty Army personnel with initial admission in Vietnam. Fort Sam Houston, Tex: AMEDD Center and School, Department of the Army; 2 June 1981. Unpublished data.

17. Friedman N. *Desert Victory*. Annapolis, Md: Naval Institute Press; 1992: 413.

18. Pirogov NI. *Origins of Military Field Surgery*. St. Petersburg, Russia: 1857. In German: *Grundziige der Allgemeinen Kriegscherurgie*. Leipzig, Germany: 1864. No English translation is available.

19. Dupuy TN, Brinkerhoff JR, Johnson CC, Clark PJ. *Handbook of Ground Forces Attrition in Modern Warfare*. Fairfax, Va: Data Memory Systems, Inc; 1986.

20. Reister FA. *Medical Statistics in World War II*. Washington, DC: Department of the Army, Office of The Surgeon General; 1975: 13; 90, Table 7; 202, Table 17.

21. Reister FA. *Battle Casualties and Medical Statistics: US Army Experience in Korea*. Washington, DC: Department of the Army, The Surgeon General; 1973: 12, 17, 45.

22. Neel S. *Medical Support of the US Army in Vietnam 1965–1970*. Washington, DC: Department of the Army; 1973: 52–54.

23. Phillips YY. Colonel, Medical Corps, US Army. Walter Reed Army Medical Center, Washington, DC. Personal communication, 1992.

24. Bellamy RF. An antitank mine destroys an armored personnel carrier. *Milit Med*. 1987;152:567–570.

25. Wright HB, Harkness RD. *A Survey of Casualties Amongst Armored Units in North West Europe: Survey of Casualties in Tank Crew—21st Army Group, Jan 1946*. Medical Research Council Team. Wright Patterson Air Force Base, Ohio: SURVIAC Co; 1946. Document 1862.

26. Scott R. Major General, Royal Army Medical Corps. Personal communication, 1983.

27. US Army Patient Administration Systems and Biostatistics Activity. *Battle Injury, Active Duty Army Personnel, Vietnam Origin, 1961–1979*. Fort Sam Houston, Tex: AMEDD Center and School, Department of the Army: 28 June 1984. Unpublished data.

28. Blood CG. Analyses of battle casualties by weapon type aboard US Navy warships. *Milit Med*. 1992;157(3):124–130.

29. Every MG, Parker JF. *A Review of Problems Encountered in the Recovery of Navy Aircrewmen Under Combat Conditions*. Wright Patterson Air Force Base, Ohio: SURVIAC Co; 1973. Document 2694.

30. Bellamy RF, Zajtchuk R. Assessing the effectiveness of conventional weapons. In: Bellamy RF, Zajtchuk R, eds. *Conventional Warfare: Ballistic, Blast, and Burn Injuries*. Part l, Vol 5. In: Zajtchuk R, Jenkins DJ, Bellamy RF, eds. *Textbook of Military Medicine*. Washington, DC: Department of the Army, Office of The Surgeon General, Borden Institute; 1991: 53–82.

31. Bellamy RF, Zajtchuk R. The weapons of conventional land warfare. In: Bellamy RF, Zajtchuk R, eds. *Conventional Warfare: Ballistic, Blast, and Burn Injuries*. Part l, Vol 5. In: Zajtchuk R, Jenkins DJ, Bellamy RF, eds. *Textbook of Military Medicine*. Washington, DC: Department of the Army, Office of The Surgeon General, Borden Institute; 1991: 1–52.

32. Ellis J. *The Social History of the Machine Gun*. Baltimore, Md: Johns Hopkins University Press; 1975: 130–141.

33. Palmer A. Survey of battle casualties, Eighth Air Force, June, July, and August 1944. In: Beyer JC, ed. *Wound Ballistics*. Washington, DC: Department of the Army, Medical Department, Office of The Surgeon General; 1962: 573.

34. American Association for Automotive Medicine. *Abbreviated Injury Scale*. 1985 rev. Arlington Heights, Ill: American Association for Automotive Medicine; 1985.

35. Bellamy RF, Vayer JS. Assessment of penetrating injury severity. *Adv Trauma*. 1988;3:163–182.

36. Wolff LH, Giddings WP, Childs SB, Brott CR. Timelag and the multiplicity factor in abdominal injuries. In: DeBakey ME, ed. *General Surgery*. In: Coates JB Jr, ed. *Surgery in World War II*. Vol 2. Washington, DC: Department of the Army, Medical Department, Office of The Surgeon General; 1955: 108.

37. Snyder HE, Culbertson JW. Studies of Fifth U.S. Army hospitalized casualty deaths. In: Beyer JC, ed. *Wound Ballistics*. Washington, DC: Department of the Army, Medical Department, Office of The Surgeon General; 1962: 479, 481.

38. Arnold K, Cutting RT. Causes of death in United States military personnel hospitalized in Vietnam. *Milit Med*. 1978;143:161–164.

39. Trunkey DD. Trauma. *Sci Am*. 1983;249(Aug):28–35.

40. Sauaia A, Moore MD, Moore EE, Moser KS, Read RA, Pons P. Epidemiology of trauma deaths: A reassessment. *J Trauma*. 1993;35:170.

41. Carell P. *Stalingrad*. Atglen, Pa: Schiffler Military History; 1993: 208–209.

42. Laffin J. *Brassey's Battles*. London, England: Brassey's Defence Publishers; 1986: 511.

43. Love AG. *Medical and Casualty Statistics*. Vol 15, Part 2. In: *Statistics*. In: *Medical Department of the United States Army in the World War*. Washington, DC: Government Printing Office; 1925: 1181, 1183.

44. Bellamy RF. Contrasts in combat casualty care. *Milit Med*. 1985;150:405–453.

45. Champion HP, Sacco WJ, Carnazzo AJ, Copes W, Foulty W. Trauma score. *Crit Care Med*. 1981;9:672–676.

46. Wiener L, Barrett J. *Trauma Management*. Philadelphia, Pa: WB Saunders; 1986: 547.

47. Ryan JM, Sibson J, Howell G. Assessing injury severity during general war: Will the military triage system meet future needs? *J R Army Med Corps*. 1990;136:27–35.

48. Baker SP, O'Neill HW Jr, Long WB. The Injury Severity Score: A method for describing patients with multiple injuries and evaluating emergency care. *J Trauma*. 1982;22:187–196.

49. National Transportation Safety Board. Washington, DC. Personal communication, 1987.

50. Rowles JM, Kirsh G, Macey AC, Colton CL. The use of injury scoring in the evaluation of the Kegworth M1 aircrash. *J Trauma*. 1992;32:441–447.

51. Gaddis GM, Gaddis ML. Non-normality of distribution of Glasgow coma scores and revised trauma scores. *Ann Emerg Med*. 1994;23:75–80.

52. Bzik KD, Bellamy RF. A note on combat casualty statistics. *Milit Med*. 1984;149:229–230.

53. Bellamy RF. The causes of death in conventional land warfare: Implications for combat casualty care research. *Milit Med*. 1984;149:55–62.

54. Oughterson AW, Hull HC, Sutherland FA, Greiner DJ. Study on wound ballistics—Bougainville campaign. In: Beyer JC, ed. *Wound Ballistics*. Washington, DC: Department of the Army, Office of The Surgeon General; 1962: 373.

55. Grande CM. The trauma anesthesia/critical care specialist. In: Grande CM, ed. *Textbook of Trauma Anesthesia and Critical Care*. St. Louis, Mo: Mosby–Year Book; 1993: Chap 5: 93–105.

56. Committee on Trauma, American College of Surgeons. *Advanced Trauma Life Support Program for Physicians: Instructor Manual*. 5th ed. Chicago, Ill; 1993.

57. Coupland RM. Epidemiologic approach to surgical management of the casualties of war. *Br Med J*. 1994;308: 1693–1697.

58. Bowen TE, Bellamy RF, eds. *Emergency War Surgery NATO Handbook*. 2nd rev US ed. Washington, DC: Department of Defense, Government Printing Office; 1988: 204.

59. Gross D, Landau EH, Klin B, Krausz MM. Quantitative measurement of bleeding following hypertonic saline therapy in "uncontrolled" hemorrhagic shock. *J Trauma*. 1989;29:79–83.

60. Martin RR, WH Bickell, PE Pepe, JM Burch, KL Mattox. Prospective evaluation of preoperative fluid resuscitation in hypotensive patients with penetrating truncal injury: A preliminary report. *J Trauma*. 1992;33:354–362.

61. Sindlinger JF, Soucy DM, Greene SP, Barber AE, Illner H, Shires GT. The effect of isotonic saline volume resuscitation in uncontrolled hemorrhage. *Surg Gynecol Obstet*. 1993;177:545–550.

62. Kowalenko T, Stern S, Dronen S, Wang X. Improved outcome with hypotensive resuscitation of uncontrolled hemorrhagic shock in a swine model. *J Trauma*. 1992;33:349–353.

63. Vayer JS, Henderson JV, Bellamy RF, Galpen AR. Absence of a tachycardia response to shock in penetrating intraperitoneal injury. *Ann Emerg Med*. 1988;17:227–231.

64. Arishita GI, Vayer JS, Bellamy RF. Cervical spine immobilization of penetrating neck wounds in a hostile environment. *J Trauma*. 1989;29:332–337.

Chapter 2

COMBAT ANESTHESIA OVERVIEW

DENVER E. PERKINS, M.D.*

*Colonel, Medical Corps, U.S. Army; Deputy Commander for Clinical Services, 44th Medical Brigade, Fort Bragg, North Carolina; Assistant Chief, Anesthesia Service, Walter Reed Army Medical Center, Washington, D. C. 20307-5001

THE BATTLEFIELD MEDICAL ENVIRONMENT

As key players in a small unit, the anesthesia providers in deployed hospitals have the ability to influence the most vital aspects of the unit's performance, both directly through their actions and indirectly through the examples they set. Delivering anesthetics for combat casualties is always challenging, frequently difficult, and occasionally dangerous. The patient population overseas will differ from the typical emergency room caseload in hospitals in the continental United States (CONUS). Combat casualties will include a great number of patients with high-velocity wounds and multiple surgical problems. In addition, military hospitals invariably become active in caring for casualties among the indigenous civilian population, who may present with any number of medical challenges. The operating room environment may be quite different from that found in the usual stateside fixed facility. The prospect of working in ISO (International Standards Organization) shelters and TEMPER (*t*ents, *e*xtendable, *m*odular, *per*sonnel) tents with unfamiliar field anesthesia machines (eg, the Ohmeda 885A, manufactured by Ohmeda, Inc., Madison, Wis.) represents a dramatic departure from the norm. The growing emphasis on far-forward surgery introduces the likelihood that anesthetic procedures will be performed in tents or shelters of opportunity with draw-over devices. The pace of operations on the battlefield may also differ significantly from the routine in a civilian hospital. As opposed to carefully managed surgical caseloads planned weeks in advance, there will be unpredictable pulses of emergent patients that will temporarily overwhelm the surgical and evacuation systems. These periods may be followed by weeks or months of waiting—a condition of monotonous inactivity that many medical personnel find almost intolerable. To further complicate matters, all this usually takes place in a remote location at the end of a long and complex chain of logistical and technical support. In any deployment, there will be major problems to be mastered arising from not only the nature of the medical environment but also the support structure and the pace at which casualties are received and evacuated. However, the physicians and nurses of the U.S. Army Medical Department have a long and proud history of adapting to unusual circumstances and meeting difficult challenges. Wounded U.S. soldiers have always received excellent medical care in the past. The continuation of that fine tradition depends in large part on the determination and skill of the people reading this book.

Technological and Logistical Support

The degree of sophistication and permanence of the medical environment may vary greatly from place to place, even at the same time and in the same war. During Operation Desert Storm (the Persian Gulf War, 1991), some hospitals attached to major armored units lived and operated under the most austere field conditions, moving frequently in desperate attempts to keep up with the extremely mobile tactile forces. Other medical units in this same conflict worked without interruption in hospitals in Riyadh, Saudi Arabia, with modern, first-rate equipment at their disposal. The former group had to learn field medicine in its most extreme form; the latter, only to decipher the labels on their machines (which were in French and Arabic). The anesthesia providers working from tents did very few spinal anesthetic procedures for a number of reasons, among them relatively low lighting levels, unstable tables, and ambient dust. The groups in the fixed facilities, however, were free to use whatever techniques they deemed appropriate for their patients.

Complexity of the Medical Network

An equally important consideration is the extent of the theater medical network. In the Persian Gulf War, the U.S. Army had 44 field hospitals and a highly developed evacuation system in place. It was possible, within limits, to transfer patients from one facility to another. This allowed for a certain amount of flexibility. In direct contrast, in Operations Continue Hope and Restore Hope in Somalia (1993–1994), the U.S. Army's task force had one 24-bed combat support hospital that served as the only facility for 3,000 U.S. soldiers and as the principal third-echelon facility for 20,000 other United Nations–coalition peacemaking troops. In this latter instance, there were four functional operating room tables in the theater. The fact that regional anesthetic techniques such as bupivacaine brachial plexus blocks were extremely rare had nothing to do with the nature of the soldiers' wounds. It was a decision based on time, space, and the need to be constantly ready for the next influx of emergent cases.

Nature of the Evacuation Scheme

Operation Just Cause (Panama, December 1989) involved the initial use of forward surgical teams operating as the receiving and stabilization point for an evacuation plan that employed one (albeit one very long) move. After casualties received their surgical treatment in the field hospitals, they were transported by fixed-wing aircraft to CONUS hospitals in San Antonio, Texas, which functioned as the equivalent of third- and fourth-echelon deployed hospitals. The air-transport leg of the move took about 8 hours.

Casualties from the Persian Gulf War faced a 6- to 8-hour, fixed-wing flight from the deployed theater hospitals to fourth-echelon facilities in Germany. Because of the size and complexity of that conflict, there was some variation in the time to transport from the site of injury to the stabilizing hospitals. Additionally, there was some variation in the capabilities of the facilities in the chain proximal to Landstuhl, Germany.

Operations Continue Hope and Restore Hope in Somalia presented another variation on this theme. As in Panama, there was a single receiving and stabilization point, and the flight time to the facility in Landstuhl was quite long: 11 hours. However, casualties of the African conflict were stabilized in a mature field environment prior to transport. The U.S. Army's field medical treatment facilities in Somalia, although based in TEMPER tents, had a computed tomography scanner, sophisticated intensive care units, and other advanced technological support.

The plan for medical support of the operation in Haiti (Operation Restore Democracy, 1994) was quite different. In addition to four surgeons and five anesthesia providers being scheduled to jump in with the 82nd Airborne Division, the USN *Comfort* (an enormous and quite sophisticated hospital ship) was standing just offshore to receive casualties. Had the planned U.S. incursion met significant resistance, a great number of casualties with traumatic injuries would in all likelihood have been stabilized in the field and then evacuated by rotor-wing aircraft directly to the operating rooms of the *Comfort*. That environment would have been an almost exact parallel of a civilian level 1 trauma center in a major urban center in the United States.

Pace of Operations

A mass casualty situation exists when the number of emergent patients exceeds a facility's resources. If there is one operating room table and one surgeon, then it only takes two casualties both triaged in the surgically "immediate" category to throw that facility into a mass casualty situation. On the other hand, if there are 20 operating room tables and 20 surgeons, then 19 simultaneous emergent casualties represent business as usual.

Two examples from recent conflicts illustrate this point. One week *after* the fighting had stopped in the Persian Gulf War, some U.S. Army field hospitals experienced a massive influx of Iraqi soldiers who had sustained serious but nonlethal wounds up to 2 weeks before surrendering. These circumstances created an instant backlog of nonemergent cases. In this unusual situation, the anesthesiologists had the luxury of doing regional techniques if they thought the operating room environment was suitable. There was no compelling need for their hospitals to operate at absolute maximum efficiency in order to be prepared for the next mass casualty situation.

Two years later, anesthesiologists in field hospitals in Somalia found themselves in exactly the opposite situation. During the 5 June and 2 October mass casualty situations in 1993, more than 50 emergency surgeries were performed in about that many hours. Every casualty was assumed to have a full stomach and underwent a rapid-sequence, general, endotracheal anesthetic, regardless of the site of injury. The determining factors in these two situations pertained to

- the limited surgical resources in theater,
- the impracticality of deploying timely medical reinforcements from Germany or CONUS, and
- the uncertainty of the tactical situation.

The foremost consideration was the most efficient way to use operating room time—to get as many cases done in as short a time as possible to free the operating rooms for the following wave of casualties.

Interventions Prior to Surgery

The general *ideas* involved in treating the trauma patient are quite simple. There are, essentially, four things to be done: (1) establish an airway, (2) establish high-capacity venous access, (3) replace volume appropriately, and (4) get the patient to the operating room as soon as possible for definitive treatment. Actually achieving these goals, however, may be difficult or even, at times, impossible.

The first order of business is, as usual, the airway. Many anesthesia providers involved in trauma care have independently arrived at a simple and effective way of determining airway competence: if a patient can talk, the airway is competent. The indications for intubation include coma or shock, as well as the need to protect the airway, relieve obstruction, deliver positive pressure breathing, or perform tracheal toilet. A semiconscious, combative, or otherwise uncontrollable patient may have to be paralyzed and intubated for further diagnosis and treatment to proceed. As a general rule, anesthesia providers should be fairly aggressive in their approach to questionable airways, especially among the many distractions of mass casualty episodes.

Most casualties intubated prior to entering the operating room will be facing one or more life-threatening medical problems. Many will be comatose. The wisest pharmacological approach to these patients is to do as little as possible in terms of depressing their cardiovascular systems while securing an airway. This means doing a lot of intubations with no drugs at all (or with only a muscle relaxant) and accepting a relatively high degree of postevent awareness.

One straightforward approach to the combat casualty with traumatic injuries is diagrammed in Figure 2-1; the following guidance pertains across the spectrum of combat casualty care:

- If the casualties arrive at a measured, controlled pace, if the available medical personnel match the number and kind of casualties, and if the equipment is optimal, then use the same techniques you would apply in your routine practice.
- If the casualties arrive at a controlled pace and do not outnumber the available medical personnel but if the equipment is less than optimal, then do the best you can with what you have.
- If the casualties outnumber the medical personnel required, then a mass casualty situation exists and the casualties must be triaged into the appropriate categories.

All casualties are considered to have full stomachs. Nasotracheal intubation is rarely indicated when dealing with acute trauma. A blind approach in an unconscious casualty is generally unwise due to the high likelihood of vomiting and aspiration. Also, it is possible for a tube passed through the nose to enter the cranial cavity. Casualties who have significant facial trauma or who are unconscious should be treated as if they have unstable cervical spines. Most casualties with acute trauma, then, will be orally intubated using a rapid-sequence technique involving Sellick's maneuver while an assistant holds in-line manual traction.

Safe Anesthetic Induction

Generally, severely injured casualties are intubated before they come to surgery. All patients with severe or multiple injuries should be placed on 100% oxygen. The reasonable assumption is that the casualty's condition is going to improve at some time during the surgery. As the patient's sensorium improves, so may his tendency to move. Therefore, the first drug administered is usually a muscle relaxant. Narcotics or inhaled agents are cautiously added as vital signs, urinary output, and other parameters of cardiovascular stabilization are manifested.

If the casualty reaches the operating room unintubated and conscious, then great care must be taken not to destabilize the situation with induction drugs. *Which* drug is used (ketamine and etomidate are two reasonable choices) is not as important as the *care* taken in its administration. Once again, a certain amount of awareness on the part of the casualty is unavoidable when dealing with trauma—not desirable, just inevitable.

Gaining Venous Access

Venous access is easy to talk about but can be incredibly difficult to achieve, especially in a hypothermic or hypovolemic casualty. Two 16-gauge intravenous lines should be considered the minimum, and some units routinely start three or four. The point is to get some sort of serviceable access quickly. Techniques to enter central veins and surgical cutdowns should be considered very early if initial attempts at peripheral sites are fruitless.

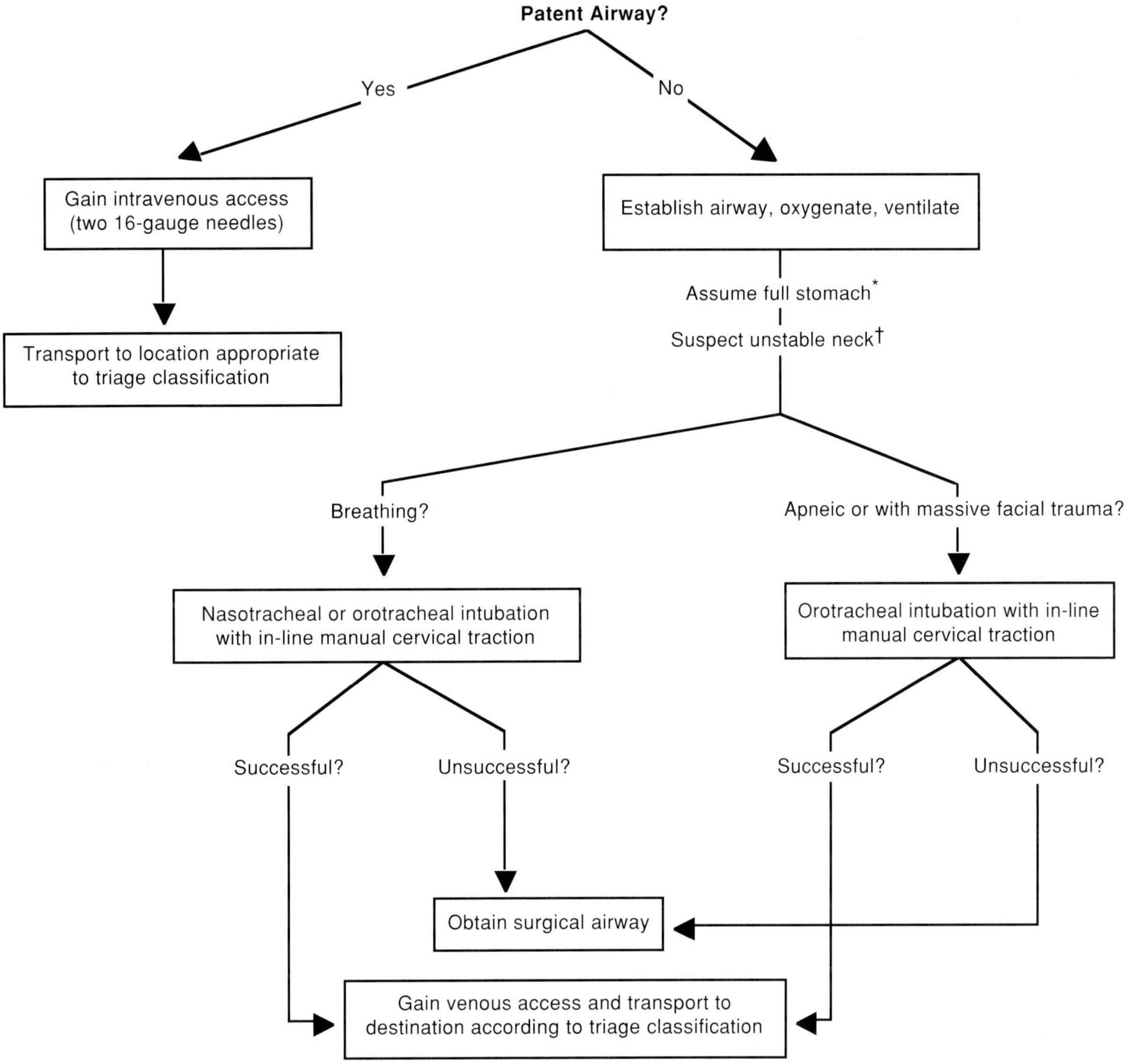

*All casualties with traumatic injuries should be treated as if they had full stomachs.
†In the absence of compelling historical or radiographic evidence to the contrary, unconscious casualties should be treated as if they have unstable cervical spines.

Fig. 2-1. Algorithm for initial treatment of casualties with traumatic injuries.

THE EXPANDED ROLE OF ANESTHESIA PROVIDERS IN BATTLEFIELD HOSPITALS

Education and Training Before Deployment

The familiar maxim holds true: during emergencies and times of crisis, a few people will rise to the occasion and perform unexpected heroics, but most of us will default to the level of our training. Ideally, education in emergency and trauma medicine begins in nursing or medical school and progresses through specialty training. At least some exposure to trauma surgery prior to deployment is highly desirable, not only to reinforce the important anesthetic issues surrounding these cases but also to acclimate anesthesia providers to the pace and stress of this environment. A rotation through a level 1 trauma center during the second or third year of training is highly desirable. Not all U.S. Army anesthesia residency programs and certified registered nurse anesthetist (CRNA) training programs have formal trauma rotations. This issue is currently being addressed and will be changed in the near future.

Because deployed hospitals generally function as more-or less-isolated units and cannot expand their personnel rosters in response to emergencies, certain medical specialists may be forced to expand their professional borders. Anesthesiologists are particularly flexible members of the trauma team. These physicians, with special training in airway management and resuscitation, are capable of moving between the triage/emergency medical treatment/preoperative tent (usually called the emergency tent), the operating room, and the presurgery holding areas to support the most intense resuscitative efforts.

One of the most serious problems in managing protracted mass casualty exercises is the timely detection of significant deterioration in the patients awaiting surgery. When all the surgeons are in the operating rooms, the job of reassessing the casualties in the delayed and immediate triage categories who are awaiting surgery may fall to the anesthesiologist, who has some knowledge of trauma and may be able to leave the operating room, whereas the scrubbed-in surgeon cannot. A casualty with a gunshot wound to the abdomen who has stable vital signs may be triaged in the *delayed* category. However, if this casualty begins to bleed and becomes unstable, his category can change to *immediate* with little or no warning. A system that guarantees relentless, frequent reevaluation of all casualties awaiting surgery is essential to a well-run trauma facility. Clearly, a surgeon is the medical professional most qualified by training to perform this function; an anesthesiologist is perhaps the next best in a crisis.

If new casualties arrive at the facility after all the surgeons are already committed to the operating rooms, it frequently falls to the anesthesiologist (military occupation specialty [MOS] 60N) to participate in the initial triage and to act as an intermediary between the medical officers in the emergency tent and the surgeons in the operating room. Once again this job usually falls to the anesthesiologist because he is a known entity to the surgeon, has some knowledge of trauma and resuscitation, and has some freedom of movement. For this reason, all deployed physicians, not just emergency-treatment specialists and surgeons, should have the training necessary to perform triage and to perform the initial assessment on casualties with multiple trauma and high-velocity missile wounds.

Certified registered nurse anesthetists (MOS 66F) not committed to the operating room may be stationed in the EMT (emergency medical treatment) area to provide immediate airway support for newly arriving casualties, or they may provide the same care to casualties in the intensive care unit whose condition is deteriorating. Certified registered nurse anesthetists have considerable expertise in achieving vascular access and placing intraarterial and intravenous monitoring lines. Physicians and nurses in the EMT, recovery room, and intensive care unit should be made aware of this expertise and be encouraged to ask for assistance from the anesthesia teams.

Because of the diversity of tasks that anesthesia providers may be expected to accomplish, anesthesiologists and nurse anesthetists should be particularly aggressive in seeking relevant experience in the emergency department and intensive care unit—both while they are in training and during their continuing medical education. Even if an anesthesia provider has had formal training in trauma, it is beneficial to direct a reasonable amount of continuing medical education effort in this direction. As a minimum, all providers should have the American College of Surgeons' current Advanced Trauma Life Support (ATLS) training. ATLS is directed toward care of civilians suffering blunt trauma, and it does not cover all aspects of war trauma. However, the ATLS system provides a solid background in casualty assessment, and the effectiveness of that program has been borne out in every conflict since Operation Urgent Fury (Grenada, 1983). If at all possible, reading and conferences should include enough material on high-velocity missile injuries to acquaint the provider with a basic idea of the differences between blunt and penetrating trauma (see Chapter 1, Combat Trauma Overview, in this textbook, and *The Medical Consequences of Conventional Warfare: Ballistic, Blast, and Burn Injuries*, an earlier (1991) volume in the *Textbook of Military Medicine* series). In addition, anesthesia providers should thoroughly review the areas of difficult intubations, hypovolemic shock, hypothermia, muscle relaxants in casualties with burns or traumatic injuries, and massive transfusion procedures.

One specific area of training for the field has been particularly problematic in the past decade: realistic training with field anesthesia machines. Ohmeda's 855A field anesthesia machine (FAM) and its Universal portable anesthesia circuit (PAC), as they are marketed, do not meet all current safety requirements for routine use in CONUS in peacetime. This complex issue has been studied at great length at the highest levels of the U.S. Army Medical Corps' military preparedness community, and a workable solution is now being formulated. Under the guidance of Lieutenant Colonel D. M. Anderson, Consultant in Anesthesiology to The U.S. Army Surgeon General, training sites at Walter Reed Army Medical Center, Washington, D. C., Womack Army Medical Center, Fort Bragg, North Carolina, and Brooke Army Medical Center, San Antonio, Texas, have been established to provide carefully monitored instruction in the use of the draw-over device. Numerous machine monitors are added to the PAC when it is used in this setting. The patients are young and healthy, and their surgery does not involve the thorax, abdomen, or head (ie, they are in American Society of Anesthesiology [ASA] category I). An instructor, designated by the Consultant in Anesthesia to the U.S. Army Surgeon General, is either in the operating room or is immediately available. This augmented "teaching" PAC is always used in conjunction with a standard, modern anesthesia machine, which is positioned for immediate use, plugged in, and turned to the "standby" setting in case any need arises for additional support. As of January 1995, more than 45 operations using this draw-over teaching system had been performed at Walter Reed Army Medical Center and more than 250 at Womack.[1] The Joint Medical Readiness Training Command has developed a curriculum for instruction with the PAC and will implement this program in conjunction with the anesthesia services of Brooke Army Medical Center and Wilford Hall.

A protocol that will allow military anesthesia providers the opportunity to gain experience with the 855A FAM is also being developed. Carefully controlled conditions that involve both upgrading the machine-monitor capabilities, certification of instructors, and presence of standard back-up devices are being worked out to enable teaching the use of the 885A FAM. Two preliminary cycles of 885A FAM training have already occurred at Walter Reed, and an army-wide program should be in place by the end of 1995. With the growing emphasis on readiness, opportunities to train under realistic conditions can be expected to improve steadily in the coming years.

Training the Team After Deployment

Anesthesia providers tend to lead highly specialized, rather isolated, professional lives in peacetime. It is necessary to change this pattern during deployment. To a degree unequaled in any other aspect of medicine, trauma care is a team effort. Members of the anesthesia group must be prepared to shoulder some of the responsibility for planning and training the team to respond to mass casualty events. As a key member of the casualty-receiving, triage, and stabilization teams, as well as of the operating room's main effort, the military anesthesia provider's expertise, training, and problem-solving abilities are among the deployed hospital's most valuable assets. Anesthesia providers tend to become involved at every point in the care of casualties, from the initial assessment on the helipad to the transfer onto C-141s for out-of-theater evacuation. Because of this latitude of involvement, anesthesia providers are ideally placed to understand exactly what does and does not work in their team's efforts. Combat zone hospitals are not the place for a reticent specialist; everyone with the skill and the authority has the responsibility to participate fully in both planning and training.

It is incumbent on anesthesia providers to take a proactive position in the effort to train the nonmedical members of the field hospital. Not only must basic skills be effectively taught, but all members of the unit must understand that their individual efforts are vital to the mission of caring for wounded soldiers. Anesthesia providers have great skill and experience in the areas of transport, intravenous access, monitoring for vital signs, and airway support. These basic skills must be rapidly imparted to personnel without much predeployment day-to-day exposure to patient care. An involved, supportive, leadership/instructor style is well suited to the field environment. By contrast, the more withdrawn, caustic style that is characteristic of many teaching institutions is not effective in this setting and is likely to be misunderstood.

Level 1 trauma centers in CONUS have the luxuries of large ancillary service staffs and a virtually unlimited supply of reinforcements. This is usually not the case with deployed units. When field hospitals go into a crisis-response mode, reinforcements will come from the nonmedical areas of the unit (motor pool, mess hall, laundry and bath, etc).

During overseas mass casualty exercises, for example, patient transport personnel are usually drawn from those sections of the deployed unit that are not involved directly with patient care. During high-volume trauma incidents, the diesel mechanics and cooks assigned as litter bearers will suddenly become key members of the trauma team. It will be up to them to establish and maintain orderly, safe, and efficient patient flow under conditions that are fatiguing, uncomfortable, and sometimes hazardous. The effectiveness of these soldiers in the early phase of a mass casualty situation can set the tone, for better or worse, of an effort that may go on nonstop for days. Their training, no less than that of the medical officers and nurses, must be thorough and inclusive. They must be quite comfortable with the appropriate techniques for safely transferring patients to and from helicopters, fixed-wing aircraft, tracked vehicles, and field ambulances. For example, the off-loading and transport of a litter patient with an unstable cervical spine from a Huey helicopter, at night, under black-out conditions, is not only difficult but is also quite dangerous to all concerned. Litter bearers must also be able to deliver casualties to the minimal care, delayed, and expectant triage category areas without interfering with flow to and from the emergency tent and the operating room. The correct pathways through the tents, ISO shelters, and other structures that make up the maze of a field hospital must be learned thoroughly before the first emergency. Seemingly minor details—such as which entrances must be entered with the litter headfirst and which feetfirst—can take on immense importance in crises where every minute counts.

Not all postdeployment instruction involves taking personnel out of their primary specialties and teaching them new skills. Some of the most important training in this period entails expanding existing capabilities and increasing the breadth and depth of the individual soldier's knowledge. For example, during many of a deployed hospital's most important functions, the unit's radio operators become vital communications links between field medics, evacuation vehicle crews, and members of the emergency and operative services. The radio operators must be taught to understand and accurately record field telephone and radio messages from medics, flight nurses, and medical officers. In addition, these soldiers become an important part of the patient care delivery system, as they are trained to extract accurate information from helicopter crews bringing casualties to your facility. Although there are well-established, detailed, communications formats for medical evacuation, circumstances on the ground or in the air may, understandably, distract the air crews or soldiers at the scene. The initial radio transmission may indicate little more than the fact that casualties are coming to your helipad. Well-trained radio operators can usually overcome the difficulties involved with intermittent or garbled transmissions and at least determine such basic information as the number of wounded, the anatomical sites of injuries, and whether all patients are conscious or at least breathing. Enlisted personnel in the Signal Corps are quite bright; they are well motivated and tend to have excellent judgment. If properly trained and encouraged, they can become great assets to the medical-care efforts. If you conscientiously help them expand their capabilities, they will make your unit's trauma-receiving efforts much more effective.

In times of crisis, almost everyone in your unit will play a direct or immediate support role in the care of casualties. As these two examples have demonstrated, nonmedical members of the field hospital play a key part in achieving a successful outcome during such emergencies. Because these soldiers will be asked to perform vital jobs outside their primary field of expertise with minimal supervision, they must know their jobs inside and out.

To the extent possible, units should train together prior to deployment. At the time of this writing (1995), vast strides are being made in improving the U.S. Army Medical Department's ongoing field training. However, there is no way to anticipate exactly either the environment or the clinical situations you will face. Perhaps more importantly, the inevitable professional isolation and heightened degree of individual responsibility cannot be realistically duplicated in stateside training exercises. For that reason, a planned series of exercises of graduated magnitude, pace, and complexity should begin as soon as possible after arriving in-country. These drills should begin within a few days of arrival at the facility outside CONUS and should continue until the teams have been through more than one real situation. Even if a full-scale mass casualty situation occurs on the first day, you should still go through a measured training cycle during the ensuing weeks, because it is difficult to make on-the-spot corrections or to try new ideas during a real emergency. The training sessions should begin as walk-throughs and proceed to more complex, realistic drills. Moulage is probably not worth the effort in this setting, but drills involving moving soldiers in combat gear on litters all the way through the system—from aircraft and vehicles to the various destinations in the hospital—are essential. There should be no unannounced drills in hostile-fire environments. It should be made abundantly clear to all concerned that everything except announced practice exercises are the real thing and must be responded to without hesitation.

One of the truisms regarding trauma medicine in remote environments is this: if your team members have not worked on live, bleeding patients, they do not *know* whether they can perform effectively or not. U.S. Army field hospitals are sometimes deployed weeks or months before hostilities begin. In this period of quiet before the storm, the worst position to take is one of passive inaction. If the political, tactical, and logistical situations allow, the unit should accept injured coalition soldiers or patients from the indigenous population at a steady, controlled pace. Field hospitals, no less than tactical units, need to perform the equivalent of live-fire exercises. The logistical cost of doing at least one emergent surgical case every other day is small when compared to the dramatic increase in performance that will result from a sustained effort at improving combat casualty care.

Special Problems With Blood and Blood Products

As a part of the surgical team, you will be one of your unit's most important subject-matter experts on blood utilization. As such, you must be aware of the basic problems that face deployed field hospitals and help to develop plans to overcome these difficulties. It is in this area, perhaps more than any other, that the medical environment of the battlefield differs from that of civilian hospitals in the United States. Platelets cannot be stored for more than 48 hours, and it is quite likely that this component of blood therapy will not be available to you in many remote locations. A field plasmapheresis unit is under development but is not currently in distribution. This means that your unit must either be able (*a*) to reliably acquire platelets expeditiously in any emergency, (*b*) to use whole blood as a source of platelets, or (*c*) to accept a certain number of otherwise-preventable lethal exsanguinations. Fresh, whole-blood transfusions from local donors are not commonly performed in CONUS in peacetime, and therefore most physicians have some reservations about the process. Most field hospitals will not be able to screen for hepatitis viruses, human immunodeficiency virus, cytomegalovirus, or malaria in a timely fashion. The use of fresh, whole blood, then, will involve some unavoidable risks.

Fresh frozen plasma may also be difficult to use under some field conditions. During my own deployment to Somalia (1993–1994), the usability of fresh frozen plasma was seriously affected by two technical problems: the field warming unit took 45 minutes to thaw the fresh frozen plasma, and 50% of the bags ruptured during this procedure.

It is crucial that military physicians involved in trauma care overseas understand the essentials of the supply system that delivers packed red blood cells to their facility. A thorough comprehension of the routine delivery schedules and emergency replacement options is necessary so that appropriate stock levels may be maintained. To be able to respond effectively to mass casualty situations, stocks of blood and blood products must be kept at high levels. A single firefight or an incident such as a landmine being detonated by a truck loaded with soldiers can necessitate the expenditure of up to 50 units of blood. Conversely, during conflicts characterized by sporadic fighting, weeks or months may go by with little or no demand for blood or blood products. A high level of resource wastage due to outdating can be anticipated in this setting. Nevertheless, these periods of relative inactivity and the associated waste of a scarce and valuable resource should not lead to a lowering of stock levels. Unless the mission, the number of troops supported, or the essential nature of the conflict change, the deployed field hospital's state of readiness should not be downgraded in response to periodic variations in casualty rates.

It is customary for the chief of the laboratory services to publish a daily accounting of the number and type of units of blood products on hand. It may be beneficial to post this information in the operating room as soon as it is published. One of the most important reasons for the unit to become active in the management of trauma early in the deployment is to allow the medical, laboratory, and logistical elements concerned with blood utilization to learn to function together smoothly. Experience with administering massive transfusions in remote locations will also help medical personnel resist attempts by well-meaning logisticians to reduce blood stockage levels based on temporary declines in usage.

Essentials of Readiness: Equipment, Training, and Attitude

At least one operating room site should be set up for major trauma at all times. This includes an anesthesia machine, airway equipment, a well-stocked cart, a functioning cart top (with resuscitative drugs drawn up and labeled), provisions for rapidly delivering blood and warmed fluids, electronic monitors, and extra supplies. On a broader scale, each hospital unit must establish some method for acquiring and storing the medical supplies necessary to support the dramatic surges experienced during mass casualty situations. The members of the anesthesia service must aggressively identify and solve all problems associated with critical supply items before the emergencies begin. Because the capability for immediate resupply is so limited, the involved medical specialists must take the responsibility of determining both their future needs and their current stock levels. For example, as the medical treatment facility's subject-matter experts on resuscitation, it is incumbent on the anesthesia provider to understand how much crystalloid solution must be readily at hand. In these instances, the training and operations officer (the S-3) is a valuable source of information. For example, if it were learned that an armored brigade had been attached to the division being supported by the field hospital, the training and operations officer should be able to provide a rough estimate of the increase in the number of burned casualties that could be expected in the near future. This information, and a quick inventory of the unit's intravenous fluid stocks, should allow for a reasonable assessment of the hospital's ability to support its expanded mission.

Obviously, key personnel must be in as high a state of readiness as is their equipment. Unless a unit is blessed with an extraordinary level of communication and transportation, at least one anesthesia provider should be in the compound at all times. A routine establishing which member of the anesthesia team will report to the emergency tent and which members will report to the operating room should be set and practiced until responses to incoming trauma are automatic.

Preparing for the Worst Case

Combat-related casualties and fatalities are quite rare among members of the Medical and Nursing Corps, but they do occur. All deployment plans should, at some point, be able to answer this question: Who is going to take care of the hospital's doctors and nurses if they get hurt? Plans should involve both interhospital contingencies and arrangements with other U.S. or coalition medical forces. The advisability of all anesthesia care providers or all surgeons or both traveling together in the same vehicles or aircraft should be carefully considered. Whether or not all members of the operating room team should bunk in the same area is also an issue worth considering in some environments.

Problems of Morale

As numerous afteraction reports have noted, the aspect of preparedness most difficult to maintain is probably the psychological one. The prolonged tedium between emergencies that becomes a part of almost every deployment seems to be especially damaging to the morale of medical department personnel. Physicians and nurses tend to be aggressive and problem-oriented, and they often find the lack of immediate challenge especially hard to bear. This is only one more reason to urge deployed facilities to stay as busy as the tactical and logistical situation will allow. Equipment, skills, attitudes, and systems quickly deteriorate in the vacuum of idleness. If the fighting dies down, consider offering your services to the special forces or civil affairs teams in the theater. An aggressive team of medical personnel can find a patient population in almost any environment. The importance of a smoothly operating trauma response team's maintaining its clinical skills cannot be overemphasized. Anesthesia providers, who always have the rank of at least captain, have a central position in most of the meaningful activities of the team. The influence of the morale of the surgical team on that of the entire hospital is profound; use your influence and authority to help the team stay busy and enthusiastic.

Preparing for the Future

Clearly, it is impossible to identify, in anything more than the most general terms, the nature of the operations the U.S. military's medical services will support in the future. Nor is it possible to predict what new technologies and therapeutic interventions will be introduced into the world of clinical anesthesia in the coming decade. What, then, must we do to prepare for the future?

In all the considerations of wound ballistics, evacuation strategies, plans, training, and logistics, it is possible to forget that what the U.S. Army really expects of its medical officers is that they take the best possible care of soldiers and their families. The single most important element in preparation for treating casualties of war is a strong graduate medical education program. Good residents and students make good doctors and nurses. To be most effective, medical personnel should be made aware of the field hospital environment, the nature of war, and the techniques of care of masses of casualties. However, the drive to educate doctors and nurses to the realities of field medicine must be balanced by the clear understanding that the most important aspect of readiness is the acquisition and sustainment of clinical proficiency. Particular facets of strategy, climate, and geography may force medical personnel to modify their practices to accommodate the realities of any given deployment, but achieving the highest level of care possible under the circumstances should be the deployed hospital's unwavering goal.

REFERENCE

1. Reynolds P. Lieutenant Colonel, Medical Corps, US Army. Personal communication, January 1995.

Chapter 3

AIRWAY MANAGEMENT

RICHARD B. HECKER, D.O.*; AND CHARLES P. KINGSLEY, M.D.†

*Major, Medical Corps, U.S. Army; Anesthesia and Operative Service, Brooke Army Medical Center, Fort Sam Houston, Texas; Clinical Assistant Professor of Anesthesiology, The University of Texas Health Science Center at San Antonio, San Antonio, Texas 78284-7834, and The Uniformed Services University of the Health Sciences, Bethesda, Maryland 20814-4799

†Formerly, Lieutenant Colonel, Medical Corps, U.S. Army; Anesthesia and Operative Service, and Chief, Department of Clinical Investigation, Brooke Army Medical Center, Fort Sam Houston, Texas 78234-6200; currently, Associate Professor of Anesthesia, The Milton S. Hershey Medical Center, The Pennsylvania State University College of Medicine, Hershey, Pennsylvania 17033

INTRODUCTION

Untreated airway obstruction will result in death from cerebral anoxia within several minutes. Fortunately, most causes of airway obstruction can easily be reversed. Although massive exsanguination due to cardiac or aortic injury is not amenable to first-aid measures, the resolution of airway compromise may be lifesaving in the field.

Combat casualties who will require airway interventions can be grouped into four categories:

1. those whose direct trauma to the airway causes obstruction;
2. the severely wounded casualty (eg, with an exsanguinating injury or in a comatose state) who needs a secure airway;
3. those with impending or known respiratory failure due to blast or inhalational injury, exposure to chemical agents, or postinjury or postoperative respiratory insufficiency; and
4. the casualty who needs a controlled airway during the administration of anesthesia for surgery.

In the military, casualties in the last category will certainly constitute the major source of airway interventions, as surgery for most combat injuries will be performed under general anesthesia. Airway management in this setting will be performed by trained anesthesia providers. Most combat casualties arriving at definitive medical facilities will not require immediate operation, and there will be time for a planned approach for airway control.

The number of casualties that comprises the first three categories—those who require emergency airway intervention in the field—is not large. In fact, the data assembled during the Vietnam War by the Wound Data and Munitions Effectiveness Team (WDMET) reveal that only 1.3% of combat casualties who arrived at medical facilities directly from the battlefield required emergency airway management. Only one half of these casualties (0.6% of the total) suffered from a traumatic airway injury.[1] Data collected nearly 30 years later, during the 1991 Persian Gulf War, demonstrated only a 0.4% incidence of airway obstruction due to trauma.[2] On review of the WDMET data, it is impossible to determine the exact number of soldiers who died on the battlefield due to acute airway obstruction prior to medical intervention, although autopsy results suggest that this occurrence was uncommon.[3]

The most gravely wounded casualties—those dying from exsanguination or severe brain injury—will most likely outnumber those seen with direct airway trauma. The major indication for emergency airway management is found in the group with severe head injuries. WDMET data indicate that 0.7% of all casualties who required immediate airway intervention were in this category; these data also show that 10% of casualties treated in medical facilities arrived in a state of hypovolemic shock.[3] Rapid intravenous fluid administration will temporarily reverse shock in most cases, but the treatment of severe hypovolemic shock by rapid fluid resuscitation is facilitated by early airway intubation and mechanical ventilation. These casualties may increase the total percentage of cases in whom immediate airway management is necessary.

Finally, WDMET data indicate that 3.2% of combat casualties arrived alive from the battlefield with difficult breathing due to chest wounds. One half of these casualties had a tension pneumothorax and the remainder had sucking chest wounds.[3] Tension pneumothorax can initially be managed by tube thoracostomy alone, but disruption of the chest wall will usually require tracheal intubation and mechanical ventilation. For the purpose of this discussion, if we exclude (*a*) those casualties who will require ventilatory assistance due to postoperative respiratory insufficiency and (*b*) those suffering from lung damage due to blast overpressure, inhalational injury, or chemical agent exposure, then possibly 5% to 10% of the total combat casualty population entering the military medical system will be candidates for immediate airway management.

In 1980 in the United States alone, 105,000 fatalities and 10 million disabling injuries occurred as a result of accidents.[4–6] In the civilian experience, as in the military, airway management is the *initial* step in resuscitating victims suffering from trauma or sudden cardiac death.[7] Although few data exist regarding the direct impact of appropriate initial airway management on the survival of trauma victims, failure to provide timely emergency airway management in parturient and surgical patients is a leading cause of morbidity and mortality.[8–11] The establishment of trauma centers that foster rapid and appropriate airway management in the prehospital phase of care appears to have a favorable effect on patient outcome.[12,13]

Newcomers to military medicine must appreciate this fundamental fact: the mechanisms of injury are different in civilian and military trauma. Most civilian trauma is caused by blunt injury, while most military battlefield injuries are caused by penetrating missiles. Therefore (owing to the high lethality of penetrating missile wounds of the head, chest, and neck), the percentage of casualties who require lifesaving airway intervention is lower than the percentage seen in civilian accident victims.

FUNDAMENTALS OF AIRWAY MANAGEMENT

The term *airway* is customarily used in two senses: the anatomical (ie, to denote any part of the respiratory tract through which air passes during breathing), and the operational (ie, to denote a device for correcting obstructions to breathing). This semantic imprecision is regrettable because it may confuse the uninitiated, but the usage is well established and we will not attempt to introduce new nomenclature here.

Airway Obstruction

The Medical Service of the Army of the Soviet Union has published data from World War II that help us appreciate the anatomical basis for upper-airway obstruction that is seen in combat casualties (Table 3-1).[14] It appears that almost all classes of injury had a penetrating component as the etiology of the obstruction. Direct airway injury and maxillofacial blunt trauma are also causes. (The nature and detailed management aspects of maxillofacial injury are discussed in Chapter 18, Injuries to the Face and Neck.)

TABLE 3-1

ASPHYXIATION WITH FACIAL AND JAW WOUNDS IN THE RUSSO–GERMAN WAR, 1941–1945

Injury	Frequency (%)
Prolapse of the tongue into the pharynx due to structural damage to the mandible	40
Blockage of upper airway by damaged detached oropharyngeal tissue	29
Compression of the trachea as a result of edema or hematoma in the neck	23
Displacement of the glottis/larynx by surrounding soft tissue	5
Aspiration of blood and vomitus	3

Data source: Rehwald G. *Organization and Tactics of the Medical Service*. Berlin, German Democratic Republic: Military Press, GDR; 1973: Table 3.10.

Many of the battle casualties who require immediate airway intervention will not survive to be evacuated from the site of injury to the field hospital level without first receiving airway control. For these casualties, airway intervention must take place in the first or second echelons of care, where military anesthesia providers are unlikely to be present. Therefore, medics, physician assistants, and physicians providing care at the first and second echelons must be able to provide early airway management. Medical personnel trained in the provision of anesthesia and airway control will be available at the third and fourth echelons of care. The interventions chosen to reverse airway obstruction and to provide definitive airway control will, to some extent, depend on the echelon of care (Table 3-2). Nevertheless, simple maneuvers such as the head tilt and the chin lift, which are discussed later in this chapter, are universally applicable (Figure 3-1). Not only medical officers but also physician assistants within the first and second echelons should be able to use a bag-valve-mask device, place an endotracheal tube, and be familiar with performing an emergency surgical airway intervention such as a cricothyroidotomy. Teaching of these life-saving techniques should be part of any formalized medical training program for these providers.

Goals of Airway Management

The aims of airway management are to (*a*) relieve airway obstruction, (*b*) prevent pulmonary aspiration, and (*c*) serve as an adjunct for therapeutic intervention. The initial and foremost goal of airway management is to ensure relief from obstruction. Obstruction of the upper airway can, in most instances, be dramatically relieved by the simple maneuvers of head tilt and jaw thrust. Cautious sweeping of the oropharynx with the fingers may assist in locating and removing foreign material, teeth, dentures, food, or vomitus. Suctioning of the oropharynx allows for the removal of blood, secretions, and regurgitated gastric contents that may impede spontaneous or assisted ventilation.

TABLE 3-2

AIRWAY MANAGEMENT BY ECHELON

Location	Medical Personnel	Principal Indication for Airway Control
First and second echelons (prehospital levels)	Not anesthesia-trained	Direct upper-airway trauma Exsanguination Comatose state
Third echelon and above (hospital levels)	Anesthesia-trained	Adjunct to general anesthesia and emergency perioperative care

The prevention of pulmonary aspiration of blood, foreign material, or regurgitated gastric contents is the second goal of airway management. The normal protective airway reflexes may be obtunded due to intracranial injury, loss of consciousness, hypoxemia, hypercarbia, or hypovolemia-induced hypotension. Pulmonary aspiration leading to pneumonitis is associated with a very high morbidity, and the mortality rate seen with respiratory insufficiency in these patients may be as high as 50%.[15]

The maintenance of adequate ventilation and gas exchange is the third goal of airway management. Ideally, this is best accomplished by endotracheal intubation. Casualties who present with injury to the central nervous system need not only airway protection but, to maintain a normal acid–base status, may also require mechanical ventilation to assure adequate oxygenation and to eliminate carbon dioxide. Furthermore, control of the airway may allow for hyperventilation to ensure that hypocarbia is used as a temporary therapeutic modality to lower cerebral blood flow and to decrease intracranial pressure in the casualty with acute head injuries. Cervical spine injuries may be associated with spinal cord injury, causing respiratory weakness or paralysis that requires mechanical ventilation. Trauma to the thoracic area, with rib fractures and underlying cardiac or pulmonary contusions, may also require ventilatory assistance. Finally, the pneumonitis resulting from the pulmonary aspiration of gastric contents is best managed by mechanical ventilation and the application of positive end-expiratory pressure (PEEP).

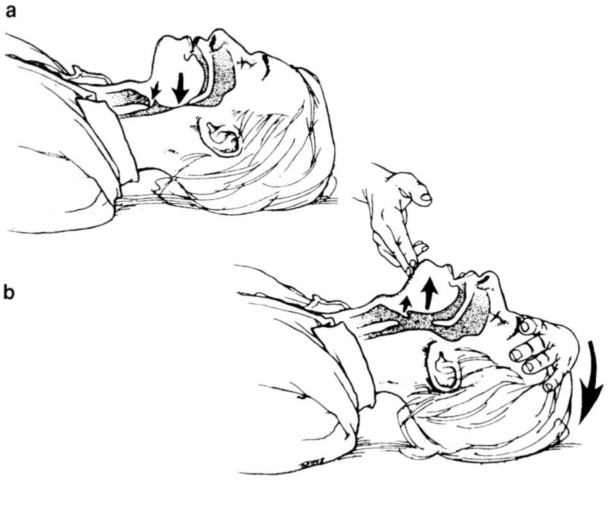

Fig. 3-1. Soft-tissue obstruction (**a**) relieved by head tilt and chin lift (**b**). Reprinted with permission from Cummins RO. *Textbook of Advanced Cardiac Life Support.* Dallas, Tex: American Heart Association; 1994: Chap 2: 2-1.

Patient Evaluation

Assessment of the airway in the combat casualty is an ongoing process. The initial steps in airway management should occur simultaneously with the initial evaluation of the injuries. If supplemental oxygen therapy is available, it should be provided to trauma victims during the initial assessment. Airway patency should be the first priority of the patient evaluation. Signs of airway obstruction include stridor, inability to phonate, nasal flaring, supraclavicular and intercostal muscle retractions, and paradoxical abdominal muscle contractions. If airway obstruction is present, immediate steps must be taken to relieve the obstruction. Once the adequacy of the airway is established, the remainder of the injury evaluation can be completed.

Simple observation and examination of the patient are poor indicators of the adequacy of oxygenation and ventilation. If resources are available, the assessment of arterial or venous oxygen saturation may be helpful in those cases where adequate oxygenation is a concern. A complete physical examination of the patient should be made, in conjunction with other medical personnel, to thoroughly appreciate the extent of the patient's injuries. Examination of the head may reveal scalp lacerations and skull fractures, particularly in the occipital region. These injuries may not be detected during the initial assessment due to their location and may become apparent as the head is manipulated for airway management. If head injuries are found, the technical approach to airway management may have to be altered. Bleeding head wounds may be an unappreciated major cause of hypovolemia. Any casualty who has been unconscious, becomes unconscious, or develops an altered mental status should be assumed to have an intracranial injury and should be treated appropriately. The presence of ocular injuries may also lead to an alteration in airway and anesthetic management.[16]

Although the patency of the airway may have been judged to be adequate during the initial evaluation, continuous and careful patient observation must occur if medical personnel are to recognize changes in mental status or ventilatory ability. These changes can occur in an insidious fashion. All trauma victims who are conscious and complain of cervical pain, those who present with motor or sensory deficits of any extremity, and those who are unconscious must be presumed to have an injury to the cervical spine. These casualties should be treated with cervical immobilization with a rigid collar and back board until radiograph evaluation of the cervical spine, to include visualization of C-7, is performed.[17,18]

Injuries to the airway can be divided anatomically into supraglottic, glottic, and subglottic trauma. Supraglottic injuries (eg, facial fractures) with resultant hemorrhage may be a cause of significant airway obstruction. Glottic injuries may cause stridor and the inability to phonate; casualties with such injuries present with severe respiratory obstruction due to edema or hemorrhage. Subglottic injuries may cause obstruction and can be associated with subcutaneous emphysema that may involve the entire head, thorax, and abdomen, which further complicates airway management. It is paramount that these injuries be detected prior to the insertion of airways, as attempts at endotracheal intubation may be futile, further worsen the airway situation, and delay the establishment of a definitive surgical airway. As most combat casualties have penetrating missile wounds as the mechanism of their injury, an entrance wound in the face or neck will suggest the likelihood for airway compromise that demands surgical intervention.

The presence of a penetrating missile wound to the chest must alert the medical provider to the possibility of lower-airway injury. Lower-airway injury may not be as obvious in the setting of blunt trauma to the chest with possible resultant rib fractures, flail chest, pneumothorax, hemothorax, or pulmonary contusion. The chest should be carefully inspected for asymmetrical motion with ventilation, and for decreased or absent breath sounds. Hypotension seen with distended neck veins is a result of tension pneumothorax compromising venous return to the heart. Needle thoracostomy (with an 18-gauge or larger needle) in the midclavicular second intercostal space can temporarily decompress the tension pneumothorax until a tube thoracostomy can be placed in the T-5 anterior axillary line area. A persistent air leak from a thoracostomy tube may indicate a tracheal or bronchial injury. Chest radiographs should be obtained to detect occult pneumothorax or hemothorax, rib fractures, pulmonary contusion, or to appreciate a widened mediastinum, which suggests injury to the great vessels.

The abdomen, genitourinary system, and extremities must also be examined. Injuries to these areas have only minimal impact on initial airway management. However, it should be appreciated that blood loss in these areas may contribute to profound hypovolemia that necessitates later surgical management requiring airway placement for anesthesia.

BASIC EQUIPMENT FOR AIRWAY MANAGEMENT

The successful approach to airway management requires a thorough understanding of the underlying respiratory pathology, hypoxemia, hypercarbia, or airway obstruction before the selected therapy is applied. To select the correct approach to a particular airway problem, this knowledge must be coordinated with an understanding of the available techniques and airway-management equipment on hand. It is crucial to formulate an individual plan for each casualty and to assemble the proper equipment before attempting to secure an airway. Most importantly, should the original plan prove unsuccessful, all airway-management plans should include several additional approaches.

Standard equipment necessary for emergency airway management is listed in Exhibit 3-1. Depending on the echelon of care that will provide facilities for the management of the airway, addi-

EXHIBIT 3-1

EQUIPMENT NECESSARY FOR EMERGENCY AIRWAY MANAGEMENT

Laryngoscope with blades of various sizes and shapes

Endotracheal tubes of various sizes

Endotracheal tube stylet

Oral and nasal airways

Face masks of various sizes and configurations

Tonsil-tipped suction handle and suction source

Bag-valve-mask device with a self-inflating reservoir and oxygen coupling

Oxygen source and tubing

Nasogastric tubes of various sizes

Emergency drugs

Adapted with permission from Grande CM. Airway management of the trauma patient in the resuscitation area of a trauma center. *Trauma Q*. 1988;5:30-49.

tional equipment and emergency adjuncts may be available.

Oxygen Therapy

The management of hypoxemia is aimed at raising the arterial partial pressure of oxygen (PaO_2). The arterial oxygen content of blood (CaO_2) can be raised by fully saturating hemoglobin and increasing the dissolved oxygen in the blood to maximize its delivery to the tissues. Oxygen therapy allows time for treating the underlying cause of hypoxemia—whether from anemia, hypovolemia, sepsis, pulmonary edema, or cardiac failure. Supplemental oxygen therapy is simple to provide, has minimal short-term risk to the patient, and, because it is so simple, is quite easy for medical personnel to forget to deliver in a crisis.

Oxygen Adjuncts

The simplest method of administering oxygen is via nasal cannulae. The maximal fraction of inspired oxygen (FIO_2) that can be achieved depends on the oxygen flow rate, the patient's minute ventilation, the amount of inspiratory flow, and the volume of the patient's nasopharyngeal anatomical reservoir.[19] The administration of oxygen by this method is effective in mouth breathers because the airflow in the posterior pharynx produces a Bernoulli effect that entrains reservoir oxygen located in the nasopharynx. Each liter of supplemental oxygen that is provided can potentially raise the FIO_2 by 0.03 to 0.04 (3%–4%), although the ceiling flow rate is approximately 6 L. Using nasal prongs, the FIO_2 can therefore be enriched up to 0.45 (45% oxygen).[20] The use of oxygen flow rates greater than 6 L/min wastes resources, serves to be a source of discomfort to the patient, and may dry secretions.

A face mask must be used to achieve further increases in FIO_2. Face masks come in four configurations: simple, partial rebreathing, nonrebreathing, and air-entrainment (eg, Venturi) masks. Simple face masks provide an FIO_2 from 0.35 to 0.60 at a flow rate of 5 to 8 liters of oxygen per minute. In adults, flow rates less than 5 L/min with this type of mask may allow partial rebreathing of exhaled gas. As there is little difference in the maximum FIO_2 that is provided by either nasal cannulae or simple face masks, the choice of using one or the other becomes a matter of patient comfort or preference.[21]

Partial and nonrebreathing masks contain an oxygen reservoir bag and allow for the delivery of an FIO_2 of 0.8 to 1.0, with high flow rates greater than 10 L/min. In the partial rebreathing system, the proper adjustment of oxygen flow allows the oxygen-rich, dead-space portion of the tidal volume to refill the reservoir bag. This constitutes 30% of each tidal-volume breath and, in effect, decreases the required gas flow by one third. Nonrebreathing systems are less efficient but allow for maximum FIO_2 delivery. The rebreathing mask contains one-way valves that prevent rebreathing and entrainment of ambient air into the mask.

Air-entrainment masks employ jet mixing of oxygen with ambient air utilizing the Venturi principle to provide a fixed FIO_2 rate. Oxygen delivery can be specifically selected in an FIO_2 range of 0.24 to 0.50. It is important to appreciate that a specific Venturi setting must be matched to a specific oxygen flow rate to obtain the desired FIO_2. For the application of an FIO_2 in the range of 0.28 to 0.40, a face tent is an alternative to a face mask. In a cooperative patient, a tent is often better tolerated than a mask.

Airway-Management Adjuncts

Casualties suffering from hypoventilation due to airway obstruction may require assistance ranging from simple airway maneuvers to endotracheal intubation and controlled ventilation. The simplest method for airway control entails extending the neck (ie, the head tilt) and elevating the mandible in a forward manner (ie, the chin lift). This maneuver establishes a patent airway by displacing the mass of the tongue away from the posterior pharynx. In the comatose casualty, the loss of muscle tone allows the tongue to fall posteriorly against the pharyngeal tissues and therefore obstruct the airway. This is the most common cause of airway obstruction, and it is easily alleviated. However, cervical extension is contraindicated in patients with known or suspected cervical spine injury, and the chin-lift alone should be attempted with these casualties.

Commonly available airway-management adjuncts may also be used to establish a patent airway. Stiff oropharyngeal airway devices are available in 40- to 100-mm sizes, with the 80- or 90-mm size being acceptable for most adults. The use of these airway devices may cause gagging in awake patients due to stimulation of the pharyngeal structures. Softer nasopharyngeal airway devices are available in French (F) catheter sizes; F28 to F34 are usually placed in adults. They may cause discomfort or epistaxis on insertion, but partially awake patients tolerate them somewhat better than oral airway devices. Nasopharyngeal airway devices can be placed bilaterally if needed (Figures 3-2 and 3-3).

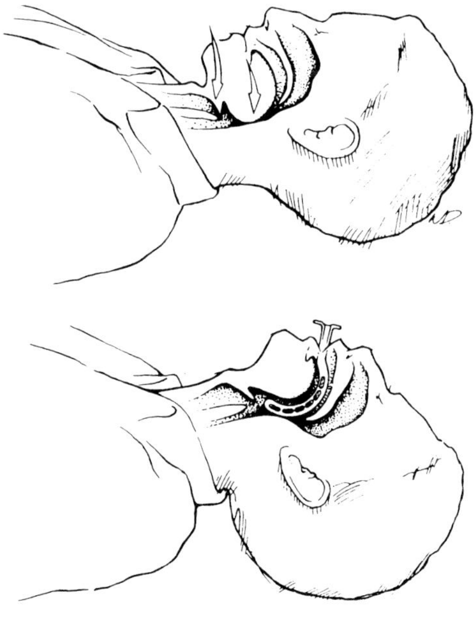

Fig. 3-2. Soft-tissue obstruction relieved by head tilt and placement of an oropharyngeal airway. Reprinted with permission from Cummins RO. *Textbook of Advanced Cardiac Life Support*. Dallas, Tex: American Heart Association; 1994: Chap 2: 2-2.

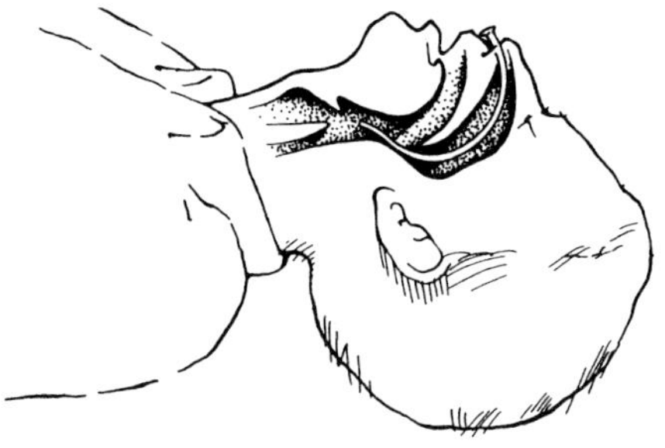

Fig. 3-3. Soft-tissue obstruction relieved by head tilt and the placement of a nasopharyngeal airway. Reprinted with permission from Cummins RO. *Textbook of Advanced Cardiac Life Support*. Dallas, Tex: American Heart Association; 1994: Chap 2: 2-2.

Bag-valve-mask devices may be used to improve oxygenation and ventilation until a more permanent airway can be secured. The face masks that may be fitted to these devices come in a variety of sizes and configurations to better conform to different facial structures. All commercially available bag-valve-mask systems are provided with a standard 22-mm connector that attaches to a standard 15-mm connector fitting, which is found on replaceable masks and endotracheal tubes. The reservoir bags on these devices are either self-inflating or require a flow of oxygen to fill them. The stiffer, self-inflating bag can be used with room air to fill the reservoir, and it comes with an oxygen-inlet port if oxygen supplementation is needed. The use of oxygen allows for an FIO_2 of up to 1.0 with these devices. The bag-valve-mask devices are commonly available in emergency areas and are more easily used by providers who are relatively untrained in airway management. A major disadvantage of this type of device is that little information concerning pulmonary compliance can be obtained by the "feel" of the reservoir bag. These systems have a one-way valve that prevents rebreathing of expired gas. A specialized bag-valve-mask arrangement that is favored by anesthesia-trained personnel is called the Jackson-Rees modification of Ayre's T-Piece, which is essentially a modified Mapleson E circuit.[22,23] This type of bag-valve-mask device has an adjustable exhaust valve that allows for a "feel" of the pulmonary compliance. A disadvantage of this type of device is that a fresh-gas flow is required to inflate the bag, and the exhaust valve must be properly adjusted to prevent the inadvertent application of PEEP. Some degree of rebreathing of exhaled gas may occur at low gas-flow rates.

PLACEMENT OF AIRWAY DEVICES

An appropriate strategy for airway management seeks to accomplish the goals previously described: relief from obstruction, protection from pulmonary aspiration, and treatment of airway injury. The identification of airway injuries in combat casualties requires that immediate attention be instituted to the particular problem. Casualties who are victims of head injury or exposure to chemical agents will need urgent airway control. Casualties with thoracic injuries may need airway control simply to control secretions. Selection of the appropriate airway-management technique requires a knowledge of the injuries received, the availability of airway equipment, and the degree of airway-management skill held by the medical personnel. The goal is to improve the combat casualty's overall status by ensuring safe, effective airway management. It must be understood that there is never a single technique that is most appropriate for a particular patient. Various specialists who will participate in the care of the casualty may have different perceptions regarding the degree to which the injury will influence the problem of airway management. This impression, when combined with another provider's training and experience with airway management, may result in the selection of another technique that is also appropriate for the patient. Suffice it to say that if all providers involved in the care of the battle casualty have a solid understanding of the pathophysiology of injury and select a technique that is compatible with those considerations, then the airway-management plan will be appropriate for that individual patient. Indications for airway and ventilatory management in the postoperative patient are discussed in Chapter 25, Acute Respiratory Failure and Ventilatory Management.

Once the initial airway evaluation has been completed and an adequate airway has been ensured, or at least supported by oxygen therapy and possible airway adjuncts, it is appropriate to complete the assessment of the casualty. It is now possible to consider any anatomical airway limitations and the availability of airway-management equipment to allow for the formulation of primary and alternative plans to formally secure the airway. Suction should be available, and all equipment such as laryngoscopes and endotracheal tubes should be checked. The casualty's level of consciousness will dictate the selection of the technique and the urgency of placing the airway device. It is important to recognize that patients who are alert, oriented to their situation, and who do not demonstrate overt respiratory distress may do well with close observation and supplemental oxygen for a period of time. All too often, these individuals are further traumatized by overly aggressive, hasty attempts to instrument the airway.

Airway Classification

An airway classification system may predict difficult tracheal intubations. The Mallampati airway classification assumes that when the base of the tongue is disproportionately large, the muscular mass of the tongue will encroach upon the larynx and make the laryngoscopic exposure of the glottic opening difficult[24]:

- Class I: Faucial pillars, soft palate, and uvula are visible.
- Class II: Faucial pillars and uvula are visible, but the uvula is masked by the base of the tongue.
- Class III: Only the soft palate is visible; a difficult intubation is predicted.
- Class IV: The soft palate is not visible; a difficult intubation is predicted.

To properly assess the patient according to Mallampati's scheme, the casualty must be able to sit upright with the head in the neutral position, open his mouth as wide as possible, and be able to protrude his tongue. The upper airway is then inspected and graded.[24] Although this classification may not be suitable for all combat casualties due to their inability to sit or perform the required maneuvers, it should be employed on appropriate patients as part of the airway assessment, as Class III and Class IV airways are predicted to be difficult to intubate using standard laryngoscopy (Figure 3-4).[25]

Anesthetizing the Airway

The anatomical areas that will be trespassed during airway management include the nasopharynx, oropharynx, hypopharynx, glottis, and the subglottic areas. The structure that divides the upper and lower airways is the glottis. The upper airway is mainly innervated by the glossopharyngeal (cranial nerve IX) and the superior laryngeal (a branch of cranial nerve X) nerves. The glossopharyngeal nerve supplies the posterior third of the tongue and the oropharynx to its junction with the na-

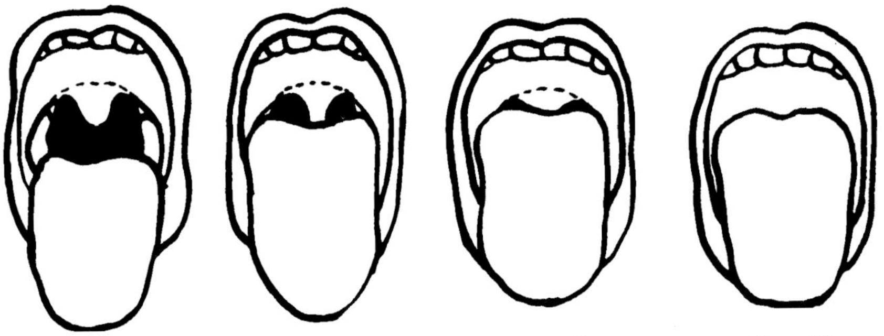

Fig. 3-4. Upper-airway classification is based on visible oral anatomy when the mouth is fully open and the patient is in the sitting position. Class I reveals the soft palate, fauces, uvula, and the anterior and posterior tonsillar pillars. Class II reveals all of the above structures except for the tonsillar pillars. Class III demonstrates that all of the above structures—except the uvula—are obscured. In a class IV airway, all of the pertinent oral structures are obscured by the tongue. Both class III and class IV airways predict a difficult laryngoscopic intubation. Reprinted with permission from Benumof JL. Management of the difficult airway. *Anesthesiology*. 1991;75:1091.

sopharynx. Its distribution includes the pharyngeal surfaces of the soft palate, epiglottis, and the fauces to the junction of the pharynx and esophagus. The superior laryngeal nerve supplies the mucosa from the epiglottis to and including the vocal cords and the motor branch to the cricothyroid muscle. The recurrent laryngeal nerve (a branch of cranial nerve X) supplies the mucosa below the vocal cords and the remainder of the intrinsic muscles of the larynx.

If awake intubation is deemed necessary in a responsive casualty, the application of topical anesthesia to the upper airway and consideration for judicious use of intravenous sedation should be entertained to facilitate airway manipulation. The sensory input for the nasal mucosa is supplied by many named nerve branches that route through the trigeminal (ie, Gasserian) ganglion. Passing a nasotracheal tube can be facilitated by using a local anesthetic agent combined with a topical vasoconstrictor to both anesthetize and shrink the nasal mucosa. Although 4% cocaine can accomplish both purposes, a solution of 1% lidocaine combined with 0.25% neosynephrine or 0.05% oxymetazoline is just as efficacious. Viscous lidocaine or lidocaine, cetacaine, and benzocaine sprays may be used to topically anesthetize the awake patient. Time is required for these agents to penetrate the mucosal tissue to provide adequate anesthesia. Sedation can be accomplished with the judicious use of intravenous benzodiazepines, narcotics, or sedative-hypnotic agents such as sodium thiopental, etomidate, or propofol—in small boluses, if necessary—in arousable patients.

Specific Nerve Blocks

Glossopharyngeal and superior laryngeal nerve blocks augment topical anesthesia applied to the pharynx and upper portion of the larynx. The glossopharyngeal nerve block is performed by injecting 1 to 2 mL of 1% lidocaine behind each tonsillar pillar. Special angled needles and kits are available to perform this block. Caution should be exercised to avoid injecting local anesthetic into the carotid artery: this mishap is associated with seizure activity due to the rapid transport of the anesthetic agent to the brain. The use of a laryngoscope will supply illumination and help to displace the tongue to the side. The superior laryngeal nerve is anesthetized by identifying the superior cornu of the hyoid bone and moving slightly caudally toward the thyrohyoid membrane. The fascia is pierced and 2 to 3 mL of 1% lidocaine is injected bilaterally.

If needed, providing anesthesia to the lower larynx and trachea is best accomplished by the transtracheal instillation of 3 to 4 mL of 4% lidocaine through the cricothyroid membrane to block the recurrent laryngeal branches of the vagus nerve. A note of controversy concerns this maneuver. If we accept the dictum that, by definition, all trauma patients have a "full stomach," then the combat casualty with traumatic wounds is at risk for gastric regurgitation and pulmonary aspiration. Opponents of this practice argue that blocking the recurrent laryngeal nerves removes the last defense the patient has to self-protect against pulmonary aspiration. Proponents argue that the medical provider performs the block to facilitate the process of securing the airway. Regardless of the merits of the argument, however, blocking the recurrent laryngeal nerves allows the anesthesia provider a more rapid and controlled passage of an endotracheal tube whether blindly, under direct vision, or with fiberscope assistance, with less coughing, retching, or vomiting by the casualty.

Nasotracheal Intubation

The awake patient without suspicion of neck injury may tolerate blind nasal endotracheal intubation better than an oral endotracheal tube placed with the use of a laryngoscope. Nasal intubation requires less manipulation of the cervical spine than oral intubation and is not hampered by jaw closing or biting. Slight flexion maneuvers of the neck frequently facilitate blind nasal placement during spontaneous ventilation. The anesthesia provider advances the tube while listening at its end to inspiratory breath sounds. A decrease in sound occurs if the tube passes posterior to the glottic opening. Repositioning and possibly rotating the tube while advancing it toward the open glottis during inspiration is usually successful. Correct placement within the glottis will be associated with an increase in breath sounds heard at the end of the tube, and exhaled vapor that condenses within the tube lumen may be visible during ventilation. Alternatively, the endotracheal tube may be placed nasally and then directly guided into the trachea under laryngoscopic visualization. The tube tip may have to be manipulated into the trachea with Magill forceps. It is important to avoid touching the endotracheal cuff with the Magill forceps, as a tear in the cuff will require that a new endotracheal tube be placed. Nasotracheal intubation is contraindicated in all casualties with midfacial injuries, basilar skull fractures, disorders of hemostasis, foreign bodies in the airway, or airway tumors.

Orotracheal Intubation

Oral intubation is the technique of choice in those casualties who have a contraindication to the nasal route, are obtunded with inadequate ventilation, or are recognized to need the rapid establishment of a secure airway. The goal of laryngoscopy is to align the oral, pharyngeal, and laryngeal axes in such a manner that the glottic opening can be visualized so that an endotracheal tube can be introduced into the trachea (Figure 3-5). The most commonly used blades for laryngoscopy are the straight Miller type and the curved Macintosh type, which are available in various sizes (Figure 3-6).[26] In an obtunded patient, an oral endotracheal intubation can frequently be performed without the use of local anesthetic or supplemental sedative agents.

Since traumatized and obtunded casualties are at risk for pulmonary aspiration, cricoid pressure should be utilized if possible during endotracheal

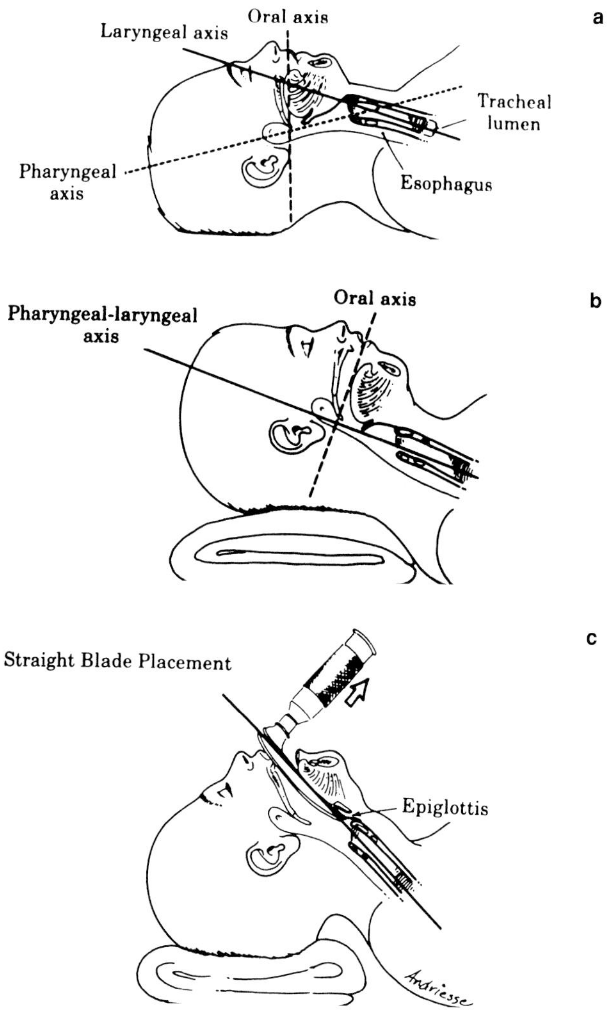

Fig. 3-5. Alignment of the oral–pharyngeal–laryngeal axis to allow for laryngoscopy and endotracheal intubation. (**a**) The long axes of the oral cavity, pharynx, and larynx are not normally aligned when a person is in the supine position. (**b**) Displacing the slightly flexed head forward in relation to the neck aligns the pharyngeal and laryngeal axes. (**c**) Extension of the forward-displaced head will align the oral cavity with the conjoint pharyngeal–laryngeal axis. The blade of the laryngoscope displaces the epiglottis, exposing the glottis. Reprinted with permission from Gaiser R. Airway evaluation and management. In: Davison JK, Eckhardt WF III, Perese DA, eds. *Clinical Anesthesia Procedures of the Massachusetts General Hospital*. 4th ed. Boston, Mass: Little, Brown; 1993: 177.

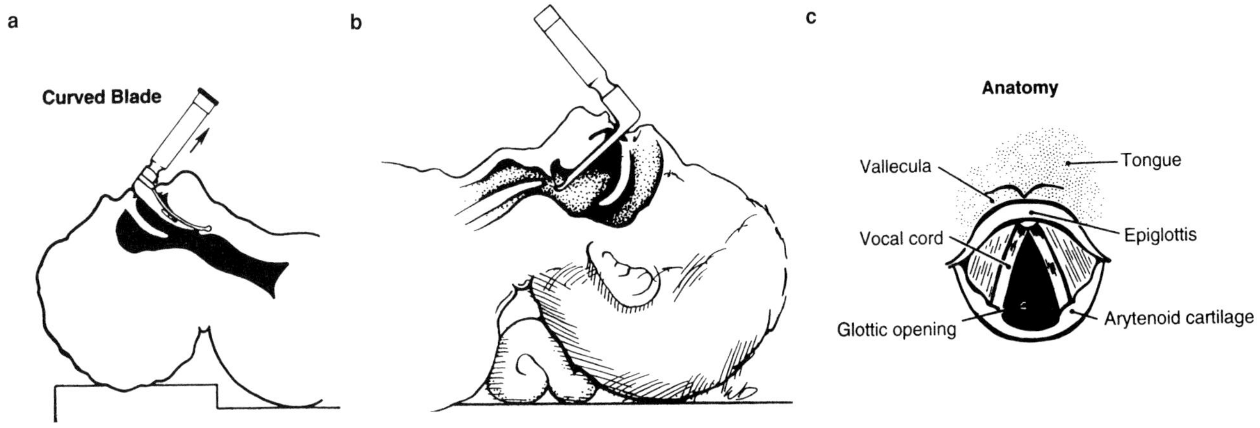

Fig. 3-6. (**a**) The correct placement of the curved blade tip into the vallecula and the use of forward traction allows the epiglottis to be displaced anteriorly to expose the glottic opening. (**b**) The tip of the straight blade is used to lift up the epiglottis to expose the glottic opening. (**c**) The glottic structures visualized during laryngoscopy. Reprinted with permission from Cummins RO. *Textbook of Advanced Cardiac Life Support*. Dallas, Tex: American Heart Association; 1994: 2-4, 2-5.

intubation (Figure 3-7). Firm compression of the cricoid cartilage (*not* the thyroid cartilage) by an assistant is effective in occluding the esophageal lumen and preventing passive gastric regurgitation into the larynx.[27] To avoid esophageal injury, cricoid pressure should be released if the patient retches. The application of cricoid pressure should not displace the cervical spine from the neutral position (the assistant can support the dorsal cervical spine with the other hand).

Cricoid pressure may also facilitate endotracheal intubation by also stabilizing the larynx, thereby helping to guide the tube tip into the glottic opening. The assistant should feel the tube pass through the larynx. Cricoid pressure may be relatively difficult to apply if the casualty is wearing a rigid cervical collar. If the collar can be removed and the cervical spine stabilized in the neutral position during the intubation procedure, the benefits of avoiding pulmonary aspiration will far outweigh the danger of injury to the cervical spinal cord. In many instances, a nasogastric tube will have been placed before the casualty receives endotracheal intubation. The placement of a nasogastric tube relieves increased intragastric pressure and may allow for removal of a portion of the gastric contents. With a nasogastric tube in place, cricoid pressure can be adequately applied without increasing the risk of regurgitation or aspiration.[28] Cricoid pressure should be maintained until successful endotracheal intubation is properly verified.

To complete endotracheal intubation, oxygenation, ventilation if necessary, and oral suctioning are required prior to both induction of general anesthesia and the performance of direct laryngoscopy. Attention to detail regarding laryngoscope and blade selection, patient positioning, and intubating technique is essential, as emergent intubating conditions may be less than optimal. Developing good intubating techniques and adhering to them in these situations are mandatory to provide skillful airway management.

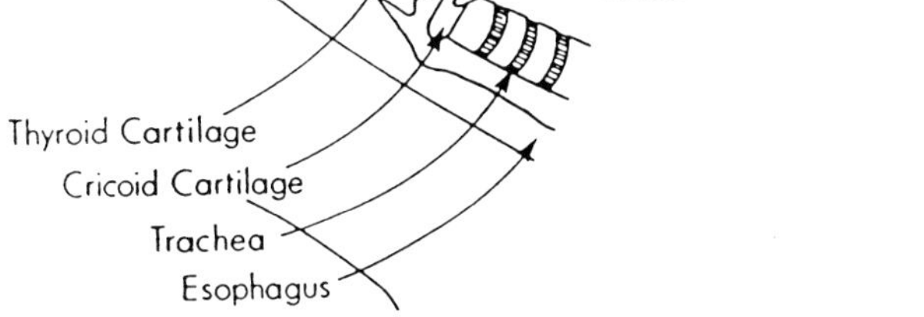

Fig. 3-7. The cricoid cartilage should be firmly compressed with 44 N (10 lb or 4.5 kg) pressure to occlude the esophagus and continue to be held until successful intubation has been verified. Reprinted with permission from Horswell JL, Cobb ML, Owens MD. Anesthetic management of the trauma victim. In: Zuidema GD, Rutherford RB, Ballinger WF, eds. *The Management of Trauma*. 4th ed. Philadelphia, Pa: WB Saunders; 1985: 133.

Rapid-Sequence Induction of Anesthesia

The casualty with a traumatic wound may have neither an airway injury nor difficulty with ventilation yet may require surgical intervention to treat his injury. Again, all casualties are considered to have full stomachs, which puts them at risk for pulmonary aspiration. It is important to realize that it is the time of injury, not the time of last ingestion, that is the most significant. If awake intubation cannot be performed, then a rapid-sequence induction of general anesthesia with cricoid pressure and endotracheal intubation should be performed.

Prior to induction of general anesthesia, it is important to provide an FIO_2 of 1.0 for a few minutes through a tight-fitting mask to denitrogenate the lungs and to ensure maximum alveolar and arterial oxygen saturation. If it is impractical to fully denitrogenate prior to induction, an attempt should be made to maximize oxygen saturation by having the casualty take four deep breaths of pure oxygen prior to induction of anesthesia.

The rapid-sequence induction of anesthesia is a technique of quickly administering a sedative-hypnotic agent in conjunction with a muscle relaxant to cause rapid unconsciousness and tracheal muscle relaxation so that the trachea can be intubated as quickly as possible. It is desirable to accomplish this task within less than 90 seconds if possible. No attempt should be made to ventilate the patient by mask after induction of anesthesia until correct placement of the endotracheal tube has been confirmed. The intravenous induction of general anesthesia can be accomplished with ketamine, etomidate, propofol, or sodium thiopental. Thiopental is the most well-known drug for contributing to myocardial depression and hypotension, but all of the induction agents can be associated with these conditions.[29,30]

To allow for endotracheal intubation, succinylcholine, a depolarizing muscle relaxant agent, remains the most reliable agent for producing rapid relaxation of the airway musculature. It has a short duration of action due to its chemical breakdown by plasma cholinesterase. Newer nondepolarizing agents of the aminosteroid and benzylisoquinoline classes that are administered in large doses have been shown to be acceptable alternatives for rapid tracheal intubation.[31–34] The disadvantage to their use is related to their long duration of action following large doses. The nondepolarizing agents generally require that their action be reversed with a cholinesterase-inhibiting agent such as neostigmine combined with an antimuscarinic agent such as atropine. See Chapter 11, Neuromuscular Blocking Agents, for a more complete discussion of this subject.

COMPLICATIONS OF AIRWAY MANAGEMENT

Casualties with respiratory compromise, in whom an effective airway is not promptly established, can die or suffer irreversible neurological injury. Other complications can be divided into (*a*) an acute group, which includes mechanical trauma to the airway or the sequelae of pulmonary aspiration, and (*b*) a chronic group, which comprises the complications associated with prolonged intubation and mechanical ventilation (Exhibit 3-2). The latter complications are addressed in Chapter 25, Acute Respiratory Failure and Ventilatory Management, and are not discussed further in this chapter.

Traumatic complications include injuries to the nasal septum, dental or labial structures, mucosal tissue disruption, and hemorrhage.[35] Mucosal dissection that is complicated by infection may progress to sinusitis, retropharyngeal abscess formation with possible spread to the mediastinal space, and generalized life-threatening sepsis. Vigorous intubation attempts may disrupt or dislocate arytenoid or other laryngeal cartilages.[36] Although damage to the innervation of the larynx is typically a result of trauma or surgery, paralysis of the vocal cords is occasionally related to endotracheal intubation, especially if the patient is intubated for a prolonged time.[37] This injury is typically unilateral, presents clinically with a complaint of hoarseness, does not cause respiratory obstruction, and resolves with time.

Complications associated with prolonged intubation include pressure necrosis of the nasal alae, lips, and tongue. In a patient with a nasal endotracheal tube in place, unrecognized purulent sinusitis may progress to meningitis or sepsis. Vocal cord granuloma, tracheal ulceration, and subglottic stenosis are known complications of prolonged intubation. Although these complications may be unavoidable, attention to technique and early recognition of complications with appropriate consultation may minimize associated morbidity.

Although a given injury may not directly involve the airway, it may be worsened by delayed, improper, or inadequate airway management. Combat casualties frequently have multiple sites of in-

EXHIBIT 3-2

COMPLICATIONS OF INTUBATIONS IN TRAUMA PATIENTS

Oral Intubation

- Trauma from laryngoscopy
- Excessive cervical spine motion
- Esophageal intubation
- Pneumothorax
- Damage to endotracheal tube
- Vomiting or aspiration or both
- Broken teeth
- Inadvertent extubation
- Laryngeal trauma
- Right main bronchus intubation
- Mouth debris forced down the trachea
- Esophageal perforation
- Laryngotracheal disruption
- Blood clots obstructing the tube

Nasal Intubation

- All complications listed above plus:
- False passage in posterior pharynx
- Air entry from paranasal sinuses into subcutaneous tissues
- Nosebleed
- Prolonged intubation:
  - Sinusitis
  - Necrosis of the nose

Reprinted with permission from Stene JK, Grande CM, Barton CR. Airway management for the trauma patient. In: Stene JK, Grande CM, eds. *Trauma Anesthesia*. Baltimore, Md: Williams & Wilkins; 1991: 80.

jury, which must be prioritized for seriousness of injury and which may require selection of techniques that place one organ system at risk while minimizing damage to another. There are no rigid formulas for selecting a technique for these patients, as each casualty must have an airway-management plan based on individual assessment of the injury and its associated physiological impact. This information, combined with knowledge of the provider skills and the available airway equipment, is used to formulate a prompt, effective approach to airway management.

Regurgitation and Aspiration

All trauma victims and combat casualties are assumed to have gastric atony beginning at the time of their injury and therefore are at risk for gastric regurgitation and pulmonary aspiration due to their having a full stomach. The risk is not minimal, as WDMET autopsy data from soldiers killed on the battlefield confirm that regurgitation and aspiration are common agonal events.[3] Although most endotracheal intubations will be performed by trained anesthesia personnel, an appreciation of the problem must be entertained by all medical personnel who come in contact with the battle casualty.

Manual maneuvers such as the use of cricoid pressure during endotracheal intubation will help to minimize the risk of passive regurgitation and aspiration. A nasogastric tube may help to partially decompress gastric volume and air. If time allows, the intravenous pharmacological manipulation of gastric volume and pH can help to reduce the risk of aspiration. Histamine-2 receptor blocking agents given intravenously (eg, cimetidine 300 mg, ranitidine 50 mg) help both to decrease the rate and volume of acid secretion and to increase the pH of gastric contents.[38–40] Unfortunately, pharmacological treatment for aspiration prophylaxis requires time for the agents to work and may not be helpful in emergency airway-management situations. Metoclopramide 10 mg, administered intravenously, promotes gastric emptying into the small intestine within a few minutes by relaxing the pylorus and increasing peristaltic activity.[41] When time precludes the use of intravenous agents for aspiration prophylaxis, a nonparticulate antacid such as sodium citrate 30 mL, or sodium bicarbonate 8.4% 2.5 to 5.0 mL, administered orally or through a nasogastric tube, will raise the gastric pH for up to 30 minutes.[42] The benefit from the increased gastric pH outweighs any concern over increased volume of stomach contents; in addition, the stomach contents may be less harmful even if aspirated into the airway. Although the acid-buffering power of colloidal antacids is superior to that of nonparticulate solutions, the particulate antacids have been shown to worsen the pneumonitis associated with pulmonary aspiration.[43]

Management of Pulmonary Aspiration

If gastric regurgitation and pulmonary aspiration have occurred, then the oropharynx and trachea should be suctioned immediately, and the pH of the secretions should be determined. The casualty should be intubated if this has not already been accomplished. Bronchoscopy may be indicated if the aspiration of particulate matter has occurred. Casualties with significant aspiration may present with immediate bronchospasm, wheezing on auscultation, and elevated peak airway pressures. A high FIO_2 along with PEEP should be delivered. Serial arterial blood gas measurements will reflect the degree and course of the pulmonary injury. The patient should be observed in an intensive care setting and given supportive therapy. Chest radiography is useful in following the clinical course, but radiographic changes lag behind the clinical course by several hours. Antibiotic therapy is indicated only for proven bacterial infection. Steroids are not indicated for the management of this condition. Pulmonary aspiration progressing to the adult respiratory distress syndrome (ARDS) is associated with mortality as high as 50%.[44]

MANAGEMENT OF THE FAILED INTUBATION

In the general population who present for surgery without evidence of injury to the airway, tracheal intubation or the maintenance of a patent airway will be difficult in an estimated 1% to 3% of patients.[45] The inability to secure a patent airway in a patient who cannot be ventilated is perhaps one of the most serious situations faced in airway management. Consequently, it is imperative that alternative nonsurgical and surgical strategies be considered. Repeated attempts at intubation using the same techniques seldom succeed and increase the potential for iatrogenic airway injury. An algorithmic approach to the difficult airway and failed intubation has been promulgated to help formulate alternative strategies in the management of this problem (Figure 3-8).[25] The key to success is the combination of carefully assessing the airway, formulating and proceeding with a plan that does not limit other options, and having assistance and extra equipment to manage this demanding problem. The decision to place a surgical airway should be considered early if advanced airway equipment or individuals skilled in advanced airway-management techniques are not available.

In the first and second echelons of care, cricothyroidotomy is the accepted approach to securing an emergency surgical airway when it is impossible to ventilate a casualty by nonsurgical means (Figure 3-9). The decision to perform either cricothyroidotomy or tracheostomy at the third or fourth echelons of care will depend on both the availability of surgical personnel trained in tracheostomy and the urgency of airway access. The cricothyroid membrane can be used to gain access to the airway using large-bore catheters, wires, or percutaneous airway devices. If large-bore (12- or 14-gauge) catheters are used, temporary oxygenation and ventilation using a bag-valve-mask or jet-ventilation equipment attached to a high pressure oxygen source can be used. Percutaneous airway devices can be used, if available.[46–49] A guidewire (0.030 in.) or an epidural catheter can be placed through the cricothyroid membrane in a retrograde fashion to pass through the oropharynx or nasopharynx. The guidewire or the catheter can then be retrieved, and an endotracheal tube may then be guided over the device into the laryngeal inlet. The wire or catheter can then be removed and the endotracheal tube advanced into the trachea.[50] Alternatively, at higher echelons of care, if a fiberscope is available, it can be preloaded with an endotracheal tube and then advanced over the retrograde wire and visually directed into the trachea. The wire is then withdrawn and the endotracheal tube is advanced under fiberscope guidance.

Other alternative methods for intubation are available, but these require specialized equipment that may not be available at forward areas of care. These devices, including the laryngeal mask airway (LMA), lightwand, and fiberoptic laryngoscope, all of which may facilitate the management of the difficult or failed intubation, are presently not included in the Department of Defense's Deployable Medical Systems (DEPMEDS) equipment list, although they are available in most fixed hospitals.

The LMA (a new device that is under consideration for the DEPMEDS equipment list) bridges the gap in airway management between a face mask and endotracheal intubation.[45,51] The LMA is designed to be placed blindly into the pharynx, forms a low-pressure seal around the laryngeal inlet, and allows for either spontaneous or low ($\leq$ 20 cm H_2O) positive-pressure ventilation. This device is available in various sizes, is relatively easy to insert, and has a role in the management of the difficult or failed intubation in a casualty who does *not* have trauma to the airway (Figures 3-10 through 3-17). The LMA is not suitable for an awake patient, as it causes as much gagging as an oropharyngeal airway. It is possible to pass a small endotracheal tube through the larger LMAs, either using a fiberscope or blindly through the LMA grate that sits above the glottis.

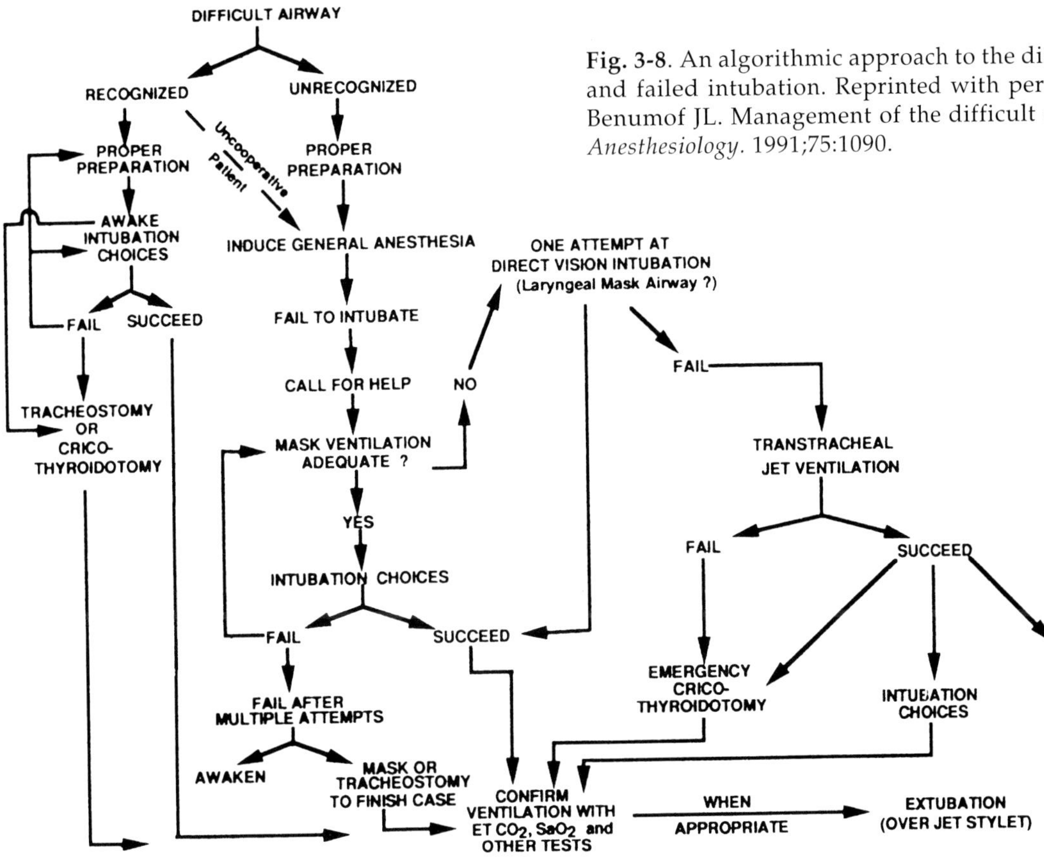

Fig. 3-8. An algorithmic approach to the difficult airway and failed intubation. Reprinted with permission from Benumof JL. Management of the difficult adult airway. *Anesthesiology.* 1991;75:1090.

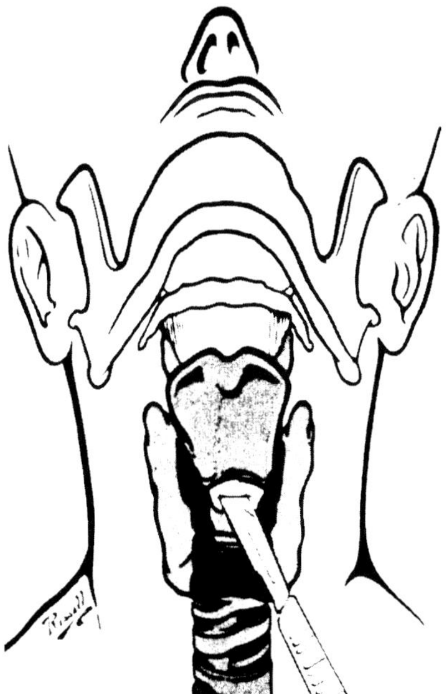

Fig. 3-9. Performance of cricothyroidotomy with a scalpel. Reprinted with permission from Cummins RO. *Textbook of Advanced Cardiac Life Support.* Dallas, Tex: American Heart Association; 1994: Chap 2: 2-13.

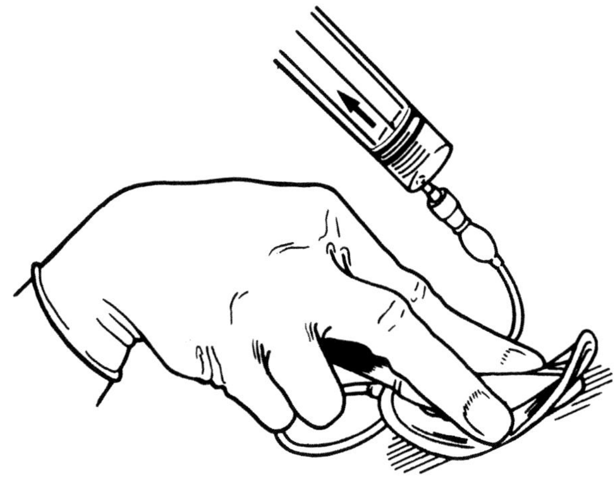

Fig. 3-10. The cuff of the laryngeal mask airway should be tightly deflated to ensure that there are no folds near the tip of the mask. Reprinted with permission from Baskett PJF, Brain AIJ. *The Use of the LMA in Cardiopulmonary Resuscitation Handbook*. 1st ed. Henley-on-Thames, England: Intavent Research Ltd; 1994: 5.

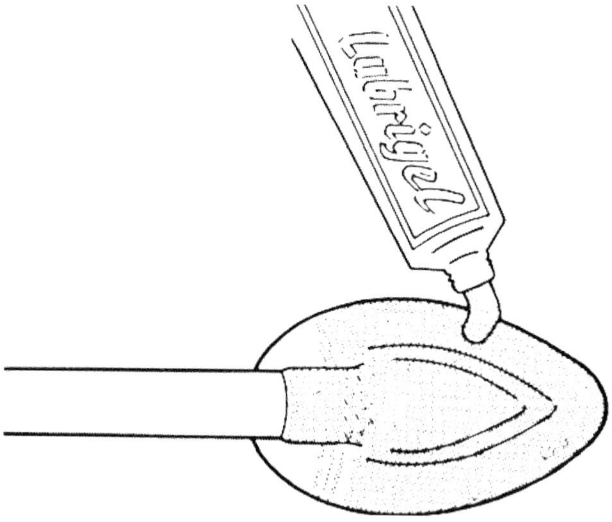

Fig. 3-11. Lubrication should be applied only to the rear of the laryngeal mask airway, *not* to the open bowl of the mask. Reprinted with permission from Baskett PJF, Brain AIJ. *The Use of the LMA in Cardiopulmonary Resuscitation Handbook*. 1st ed. Henley-on-Thames, England: Intavent Research Ltd; 1994: 5.

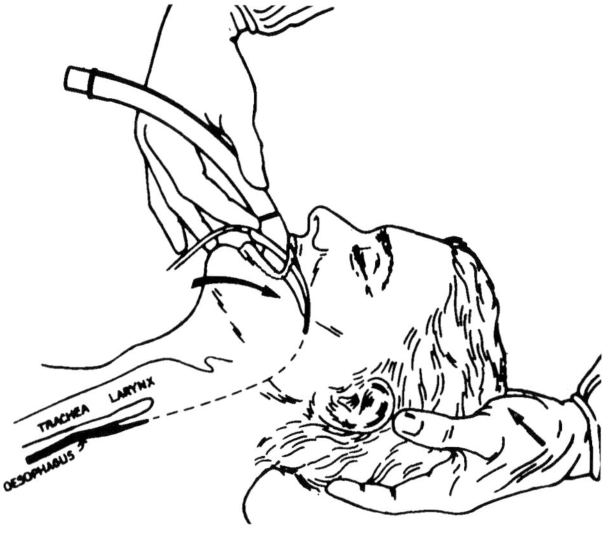

Fig. 3-12. Under direct vision, press the mask tip upward against the inner surface of the patient's upper incisors to flatten the tip. Arrows indicate direction of applied pressure exerted by each hand. Reprinted with permission from Baskett PJF, Brain AIJ. *The Use of the LMA in Cardiopulmonary Resuscitation Handbook*. 1st ed. Henley-on-Thames, England: Intavent Research Ltd; 1994: 7.

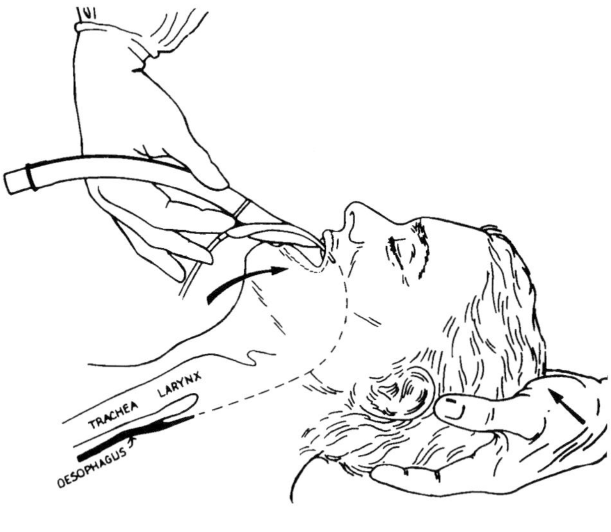

Fig. 3-13. Using the index finger, keep pressing the mask upward as it is advanced into the pharynx, to ensure that the tip of the mask remains flattened and avoids engaging the patient's tongue. Reprinted with permission from Baskett PJF, Brain AIJ. *The Use of the LMA in Cardiopulmonary Resuscitation Handbook*. 1st ed. Henley-on-Thames, England: Intavent Research Ltd; 1994: 8.

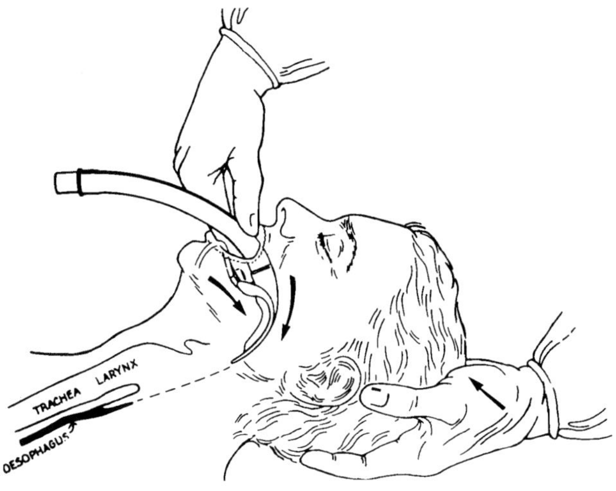

Fig. 3-14. With the patient's neck flexed and head extended, press the mask into the posterior pharyngeal wall using the index finger. The index finger must be directly in line with the mask aperture. Reprinted with permission from Baskett PJF, Brain AIJ. *The Use of the LMA in Cardiopulmonary Resuscitation Handbook.* 1st ed. Henley-on-Thames, England: Intavent Research Ltd; 1994: 8.

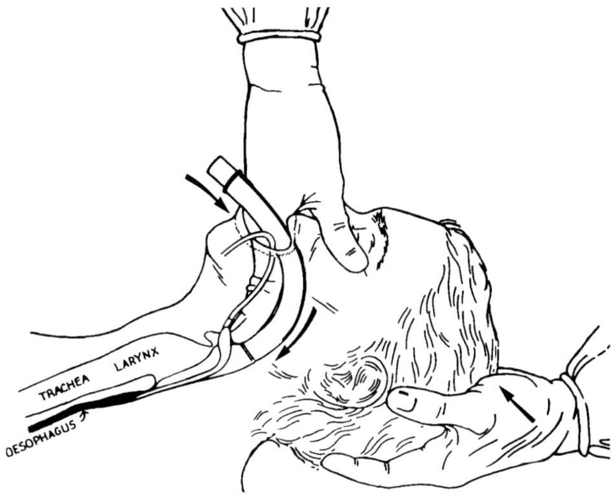

Fig. 3-15. The mask can be seated into position with one fluid motion while the anesthesiologist continues to push the mask with the index finger. Reprinted with permission from Baskett PJF, Brain AIJ. *The Use of the LMA in Cardiopulmonary Resuscitation Handbook.* 1st ed. Henley-on-Thames, England: Intavent Research Ltd; 1994: 9.

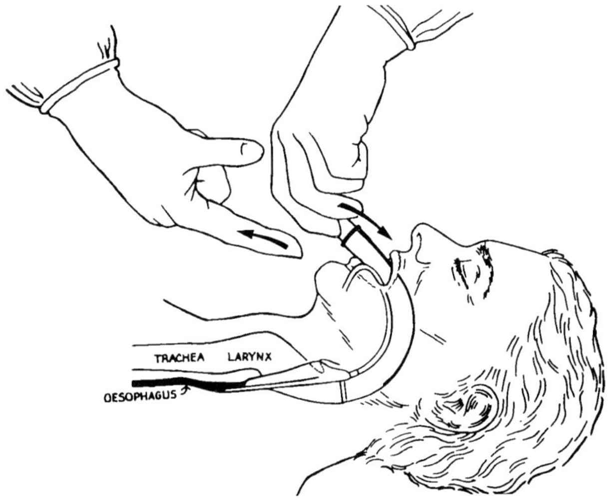

Fig. 3-16. While grasping the tube and continuing to exert downward pressure, remove the index finger from the patient's oral cavity. Reprinted with permission from Baskett PJF, Brain AIJ. *The Use of the LMA in Cardiopulmonary Resuscitation Handbook.* 1st ed. Henley-on-Thames, England: Intavent Research Ltd; 1994: 9.

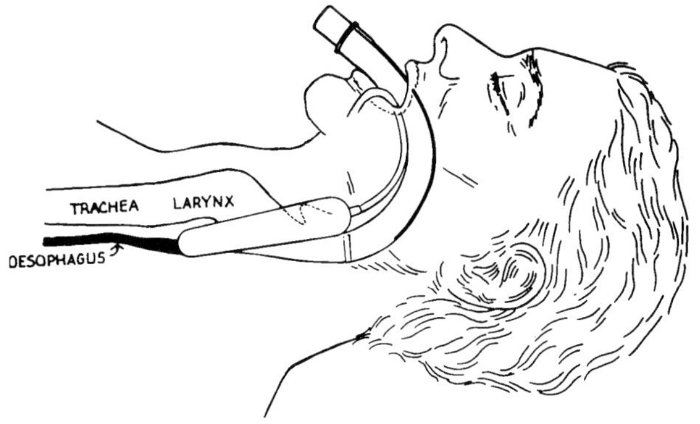

Fig. 3-17. Inflate the mask with the recommended amount of air. The mask should rise slightly as it seats itself in the correct position over the larynx. A slight airleak (< 20 cm H_2O) is acceptable if the chest moves with respiration. Deflate and reseat the mask if there is a large airleak (> 20 cm H_2O). Reprinted with permission from Baskett PJF, Brain AIJ. *The Use of the LMA in Cardiopulmonary Resuscitation Handbook.* 1st ed. Henley-on-Thames, England: Intavent Research Ltd; 1994: 9.

The lightwand is a lighted, flexible stylet over which an anesthesia provider can blindly place an endotracheal tube into the trachea through either the mouth or the nose (Figure 3-18). The lightwand can be positioned easily without manipulating the neck. The instrument should be used in dim ambient light and advanced following the curve of the tongue. A glow seen over the lateral neck indicates that the tip lies in the pyriform fossa. A loss of tip brightness generally indicates that the lightwand has entered the esophagus. A marked glow in the anterior neck with a cone of light pointing caudad indicates its proper position at the glottic opening, and the tube can then be slid off the stylet and passed into the trachea.[52,53]

The fiberoptic laryngoscope is a shortened version of the fiberoptic bronchoscope. It requires a light source and incorporates a suction port (which can also be used to entrain oxygen) and optics into a flexible bundle that fits easily through an endotracheal tube. It allows for direct visualization of the airway structures. These fiberscope devices are expensive, somewhat fragile, and require that anesthesia providers be trained to use them. The devices are likely to be available in only the higher echelons of care. The Patil-Syracuse mask (manufactured by Bay Medical, Clearwater, Fla.) is a face mask modified with an entry port for the introduction of a fiberscope during mask ventilation. Specialized oral airways such as the Williams (manufactured by Bay Medical, Clearwater, Fla.), Berman (manufactured by Sun Medical, Clearwater, Fla.), and Ovassapian (manufactured by Bay Medical, Clearwater, Fla.) intubating airways have been developed to facilitate introduction of the fiberscope tip into the laryngeal orifice.[54–57]

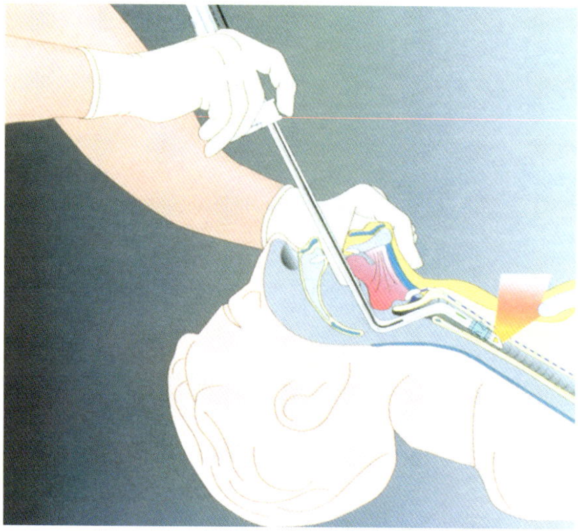

Fig. 3-18. Once the cone of light is seen at the glottic opening, the endotracheal tube is passed from the lighted stylet into the trachea. Photograph: Courtesy of Laerdal California, Inc, Long Beach, Calif.

SPECIAL AIRWAY-MANAGEMENT CONSIDERATIONS

Head Injury

In the civilian setting, where motor-vehicle blunt trauma predominates as the cause for injury,

> a head injury occurs every 15 seconds, and a patient dies of a head injury every 12 minutes, a physician dealing with trauma is confronted with a head-injured patient almost every day. Approximately 50% of all trauma deaths are associated with head injury, and more than 60% of vehicular trauma deaths are due to head injury.[58(p161)]

Both early recognition of intracranial injury and institution of appropriate therapy will minimize secondary neuronal injury and increase the potential for neurological recovery. Airway management for the casualty with head injuries has three goals. The first is to provide adequate ventilation to those whose medullary respiratory centers may have been compromised due to increased intracranial pressure (ICP) from edema or hemorrhage. The second is to reduce the risk for gastric regurgitation and pulmonary aspiration, because a decreased sensorium with possible compromise to cranial nerve function alters the normal protective airway reflexes. The third is to decrease the risk for aspiration and allow for the transient use of hypocapnia ($Paco_2$ 25–30 mm Hg) to prevent or manage increased ICP.[59]

An obtunded state, a deterioration in mental status, or a Glasgow coma scale determination of 8 points or less signals the need for immediate airway management (Exhibit 3-3).[60,61] Ideally, endotracheal intubation should be accomplished rapidly and under deep anesthesia so that the untoward hemodynamic effects of laryngoscopy can be blunted. Hypertension in response to laryngoscopy and endotracheal tube placement may exceed the limits of cerebral autoregulation and contribute to further intracranial hemorrhage, edema, and an increase in ICP with compromise of cerebral perfusion pressure (CPP) and cerebral function. Coughing or bucking in response to intubation efforts elevates not only cerebral-inflow pressure but also central venous pressure, with resultant decreases in CPP.

EXHIBIT 3-3

GLASGOW COMA SCALE

Eye Opening	
Spontaneous	____ 4
To verbal command	____ 3
To pain	____ 2
None	____ 1
Verbal Response	
Oriented and converses	____ 5
Confused and converses	____ 4
Inappropriate words	____ 3
Incomprehensible words	____ 2
None	____ 1
Motor Response	
Obeys command	____ 6
Localizes pain with a purposeful response	____ 5
Flexion withdrawal	____ 4
Abnormal flexion	____ 3
Decerebrate extension	____ 2
None	____ 1

A normal individual would score 15, while a patient in profound coma would score 3. A score of 8 or less is considered indicative of a severe head injury, and endotracheal intubation should be performed to protect the airway.

Painful stimuli should be administered by pressure over the supraorbital notch, or by pressure on a nail bed with a pencil. The best performance score at each time of testing should be reported. Some centers record a score before and after resuscitation has been completed.

Cold caloric testing and tonic neck reflexes provide information regarding the integrity of the brainstem in comatose patients.

While hypertension is poorly tolerated in casualties with brain injuries whose blood–brain barrier is disrupted, hypotension is just as dangerous: inadequate cerebral perfusion may occur in areas of brain injury where cerebral autoregulation of blood flow is compromised or nonexistent.

If a barbiturate such as thiopental is available, its use as an induction agent in the dose range of 3 to 5 mg/kg will provide deep anesthesia, decrease the cerebral metabolic rate of oxygen demand ($CMRO_2$), and not interfere with any cerebral autoregulation that remains intact.[62] Barbiturates can depress cardiovascular function and their use may be limited in a casualty who is hypovolemic and hypotensive. Etomidate 0.1 to 0.3 mg/kg or propofol 1 to 2 mg/kg may be acceptable alternatives. Ketamine should be avoided in the casualty with head injuries. Lidocaine 1.5 to 2.0 mg/kg will blunt the tracheal response to laryngoscopy, augment anesthetic depth, and serve as a cerebral vasoconstrictor.[63] The use of muscle relaxants can provide stable intubating conditions, prevent coughing with resultant elevation of ICP, and minimize the risk for gastric regurgitation and pulmonary aspiration. Succinylcholine has been the muscle relaxant of choice due to its reliable rapid onset and short duration of action, but it has the potential to cause muscle fasciculation–induced increases in ICP, although this issue is controversial.[64–66]

Cervical Spine Injury

Cervical spine injuries with cord compromise at or above the C-3 level mandate immediate airway control and mechanical ventilation. Casualties with cervical injuries may also require intubation due to other areas of trauma.[67] If ventilation is adequate, any conscious casualty presenting with neck pain or neurological deficit, or one who is unconscious, will need radiographic examination of the cervical spine to include visualization of C-7 before cervical-fixation devices are removed or the airway is instrumented. If immediate intubation is required prior to radiographic examination, or if bony or ligamentous cervical instability is diagnosed, then cervical stabilization should be accomplished by the senior surgeon while the most skilled endoscopist manages the airway. If not otherwise indicated, a blind nasal intubation may be accomplished with minimal manipulation of the airway. The application of topical anesthesia may help to minimize coughing or gagging. Direct laryngoscopy can be accomplished with cervical stabilization to avoid flexion, and particularly extension, of the cervical spine. The use of anesthetic agents in any casualty with a high cervical cord injury should be approached with caution, as the casualty may have an altered sympathetic nervous system response to these agents.[68]

Eye Injury

Penetrating (ie, open) ocular injuries are commonly seen in combat casualties who have received multiple fragment wounds. The care of casualties with open globe injuries should minimize any coughing or straining to prevent extrusion of intraocular contents.[16] The potential for ocular salvage and preservation of visual function must be assumed until a complete examination can be performed by an ophthalmic surgeon. Airway management will require deep anesthesia with muscle relaxation to avoid further loss of intraocular contents. Succinylcholine has been considered to be relatively contraindicated in open eye injuries because muscle fasciculations have the potential to increase intraocular pressure. Pretreatment with a small dose of a nondepolarizing muscle relaxant has been shown to minimize but not ablate this problem,[69] although one large study[70] has indicated that the increased intraocular pressure seen with the use of succinylcholine is more a theoretical than a clinical concern.[69] Higher-than-usual intubating doses of nondepolarizing muscle relaxant agents are acceptable alternatives to succinylcholine in appropriate patients.[31–34]

DIRECT INJURY TO THE AIRWAY

Maxillofacial Injury

The combat casualty suffering from multiple traumatic injuries, especially head injures, frequently has associated midfacial and mandibular abnormalities. Medical personnel should determine the presence of these injuries before instrumenting the airway. Casualties with facial lacerations often present with copious bleeding that may contribute to airway obstruction. Relief of obstruction can frequently be obtained with gentle suctioning and, if possible, by allowing the casualty to sit forward rather than lie supine. Gentle, forward traction on an unstable, fractured mandible may also relieve simple obstruction. The nasal approach to endotracheal intubation is contraindicated in the casualty with midfacial fractures. Passage of endotracheal, gastric, or suction tubes via the nares may dislodge bone fragments or introduce infection, or the tube may pass upward into the cranial vault if the cribriform plate has been disrupted.

If endotracheal intubation is required, direct visualization of the larynx is usually possible and can often be performed in an awake patient after the topical application of anesthetic agents to the airway. Fiberoptic intubation can be considered, but secretions and bleeding often obscure the view and make this technique very difficult. A blind oral technique such as using a lightwand may be helpful if direct visualization is difficult. If anesthesia of the larynx and trachea is needed, previously discussed approaches to the airway and aspiration-prevention techniques can be utilized.

It is important to make an early determination if airway instrumentation above the larynx would be very difficult or futile. If this is true, or if multiple intubation approaches fail, then arrangements need to be made for an urgent or emergent surgical approach to the airway.

Laryngeal and Tracheal Injury

Direct trauma to the larynx and trachea is relatively rare, based in part on the anatomical relationship of these to bony structures: the mandible provides a bony shelf that overhangs the larynx and hyoid bone, while the sternum offers protection to the trachea. Injuries to the larynx and trachea can be divided into (*a*) blunt and (*b*) penetrating types.

Airway compromise results either from disruption of laryngotracheal structures or from secondary compression due to hemorrhage or subcutaneous emphysema. Blunt trauma to the anterior neck may cause dislocation or fracture of the thyroid, cricoid, or tracheal cartilages. Alternatively, a blow to the chest may cause a concussive injury to the trachea.[71–73]

Penetrating injuries may also damage the superior or recurrent laryngeal nerves, resulting in partial anesthesia and airway obstruction. A neck wound that causes a divided cervical trachea is best managed by directly intubating the distal portion of the tracheal opening with a tracheostomy or endotracheal tube.

The diagnosis of tracheal injury is based on the history of trauma to the area and finding the signs and symptoms of airway obstruction. Stridor may be the only presenting sign, although some victims may have difficulty with phonation. The inability to vocalize the "E" sound may indicate arytenoid dislocation or injury to the recurrent laryngeal nerve with arytenoid weakness or paralysis. Airway obstruction tends to worsen with deep inspiration and coughing. The proper recognition and care of these patients requires that the examiner have a high index of suspicion for airway injury.

Management of the casualty with a potential airway injury should be predicated on the knowledge that such injuries have the potential to be rapidly fatal. The casualty with obvious signs of obstruction such as hoarseness and dyspnea, especially in the presence of subcutaneous air or a pneumothorax, requires immediate airway control. When the larynx has been separated from the trachea or if the trachea is disrupted, orotracheal intubation—although sometimes possible—can be dangerous. A tracheostomy using local anesthesia is the safest approach in such a casualty. Once the airway is secured, laryngoscopy and bronchoscopy are used to establish the diagnosis. Intubation over a flexible bronchoscope is useful in preparation for operative repair during thoracotomy.

In addition to direct injuries to the airway, the aspiration of foreign bodies can be life threatening. Removal of foreign bodies requires the coordination and planning of anesthesia, surgical, and operating room personnel. The circumstances, location, and description of the foreign body can be obtained from history and physical examination, respiratory symptoms, and radiographic studies. The anesthetic plan should allow for removal of the foreign body without worsening the casualty's respiratory status.

The casualty who has airway obstruction from an expanding infectious site or from aspiration of a foreign body may require an anesthetic approach that deviates from the usual rapid-sequence induction technique. These conditions often require that a mask-inhalational induction of anesthesia be performed to (*a*) preserve spontaneous ventilation and (*b*) allow for intubation under deep inhalational anesthesia. The risk of gastric regurgitation and pulmonary aspiration in these casualties is less than the risk of being unable to ventilate or intubate a patient with an abnormal airway who has received a neuromuscular blocking agent.

Thermal Injury

Injuries to the airway caused by changes in temperature may be purely thermal in nature, due to chemical exposure, or a result of both mechanisms. A history of the events surrounding the inhalational injury and physical evidence of facial burns, charred nasal vibrissae, or carbonaceous sputum may provide an indication for immediate airway management. Although a diagnosis may be suspected, a conclusive diagnosis of airway injury cannot be made without examination of the casualty's upper and lower airways, usually by a surgeon skilled in the management of thermal injuries. Airway edema from the original injury and subsequent airway embarrassment occurs insidiously. Subsequent fluid-resuscitation therapy in the burned casualty may worsen airway edema and cause respiratory obstruction at any time. Therefore, a high index of suspicion of both airway injury and the need for airway management is essential in all thermally injured casualties. During the first 12- to 24-hour period after the burn, succinylcholine may be used to facilitate endotracheal intubation during airway management. After the first day, during the intensive-care phase of treatment, succinylcholine should be avoided. The burn victim's muscles rapidly develop extrajunctional receptors that are associated with an exaggerated release of potassium in response to the administration of succinylcholine, which frequently results in a hyperkalemia-induced cardiac arrest.[74]

SUMMARY

Most combat casualties who survive long enough to be admitted to field hospitals for the treatment of their injuries will require some form of airway management during the course of their treatment. Most of these casualties will have been through triage on arrival at the medical facility and will receive semielective resuscitative or reconstructive surgery. Their airway management will be provided by trained anesthesia providers. In a few casualties (< 5%–10% of the total), emergency, lifesaving airway management may need to be carried out by medical personnel before the casualty reaches a field hospital. Combat casualties who require immediate airway control are usually in extremis due to exsanguination, severe head injury, or destructive injuries to the face or neck. Standard techniques to provide endotracheal intubation should be applied to all casualties except for those with direct airway trauma. Patients with direct airway injuries can be best managed by creating a surgical airway. Other patients may benefit from alternative means to secure an adequate airway with such devices as the laryngeal mask airway or lightwand if standard endotracheal intubation is difficult. Once hypoxia has been averted or treated, gastric regurgitation and pulmonary aspiration remain the greatest threats to the combat casualty who requires airway management. At the hospital level, rapid-sequence induction of anesthesia combined with cricoid pressure to facilitate endotracheal intubation will minimize the risk of pulmonary aspiration. Casualties with potential cervical spine injury due to blunt head or neck trauma need to be approached with special caution, as manipulation of the neck has the potential to cause injury to the cervical spinal cord. Finally, thermally injured patients must be evaluated for airway injury, and appropriate airway management must be instituted as expeditiously as possible.

REFERENCES

1. Wound Data and Munitions Effectiveness Team. *Evaluation of Wound Data and Munitions Effectiveness in Vietnam: Final Report*. Vol 3. Alexandria, Va: Defense Documentation Center, Defense Logistics Agency: 1970: Table 4-7-9.

2. Burkle FM, Newland C, Meister SJ, Blood CG. Emergency medicine in the Persian Gulf War, III: Battle casualties. *Ann Emerg Med*. 1994;23:4755–4760.

3. Bellamy RF. Colonel, Medical Corps, US Army. Personal communication, March 1995. The single most useful database describing combat wounds and the circumstances of wounding is the Wound Data and Munitions Effectiveness Team (WDMET) study prepared by the U.S. Army Materiel Command during the Vietnam War. These data are stored at the National Naval Medical Center, Bethesda, Maryland. Access is controlled by the Uniformed Services University of the Health Sciences, Bethesda, Maryland 20814-4799; telephone (301) 295-6262. Three summary volumes contain extensive abstracts of the statistical data and can be obtained from Defense Documentation Center, Cameron Station, Alexandria, Virginia 22304-6145; telephone (703) 545-6700 and (703) 274-7633.

4. Katz J. Anesthesia for the trauma patient. *Prog Crit Care Med*. 1984:(1):218–230.

5. Weiskopf RB, Fairley HB. Anesthesia for major trauma. *Surg Clin North Am*. 1982;62(1):31–34.

6. Trunkey DD. Trauma. *Sci Am*. 1983;249:28–35.

7. Committee for Cardiopulmonary Resuscitation and Emergency Cardiac Care. Standards and guidelines for cardiopulmonary resuscitation and emergency cardiac care. *JAMA*. 1986;255(21): 2905–2989.

8. Buehler JW, Kaunitz AM, Hogue CJR, et al. Maternal mortality in women aged 35 or older, United States. *JAMA*. 1986;255:53–57.

9. Tomkinson J, Turnbull A, Robson G, et al. *Report on Confidential Enquiries Into Maternal Deaths in England and Wales 1976–1978*. London, England: Her Majesty's Stationery Office; 1982.

10. Kaunitz AM, Hughes JM, Grimes DA, et al. Causes of maternal mortality in the United States. *Obstet Gynecol*. 1985;65:605–612.

11. Utting JE, Gray TC, Shelley FC. Human misadventure in anaesthesia. *Can Anaesth Soc J*. 1979;26:73–79.

12. Stewart RD, Paris PM, Winter PM, et al. Field endotracheal intubation by paramedical personnel: Success rates and complications. *Chest*. 1984;85:341–345.

13. Jacobs LM, Berrizbeitia LD, Bennett B, Madigan C. Endotracheal intubation in the prehospital phase of emergency medical care. *JAMA*. 1983;250:2175–2177.

14. Rehwald G. *Organization and Tactics of the Medical Service*. Berlin, German Democratic Republic: Military Press, GDR; 1973.

15. Mendelson CL. The aspiration of stomach contents into the lungs during obstetric anesthesia. *Am J Obstet Gynecol*. 1946;52:191.

16. Adams AK, Jones RM. Anaesthesia for eye surgery: General considerations. *Br J Anaesth*. 1980;52:663.

17. Desmond J. Paraplegia: Problems confronting the anesthesiologist. *Can Anaesth Soc J*. 1970;17:435.

18. Singer MM, Lee J. Management of thoracic injuries. *Int Anesthesiol Clin*. 1971;9:17.

19. Gibson RL, Comer PB, Beckham RW, McGraw CP. Actual tracheal oxygen concentrations with commonly used oxygen equipment. *Anesthesiology*. 1976;44:71–77.

20. Smith R. Respiratory care: Mechanical. In: Miller R, ed. *Anesthesia*. 2nd ed. New York, NY: Churchill Livingstone; 1986: 2177.

21. Cohen JL, Demers RR, Saklad M. Air-entrainment masks: A performance evaluation. *Respir Care*. 1977;22:277.

22. Ayre P. The T-piece technique. *Br J Anaesth*. 1956;28:520–523.

23. Mapleson WW. The elimination of rebreathing in various semi-closed anaesthetic systems. *Br J Anaesth*. 1954;26:323–332.

24. Mallampati SR, Gatt SP, Gugino LD, et al. A clinical sign to predict difficult tracheal intubations: A prospective study. *Can Anaesth Soc J*. 1985;32:429–434.

25. Benumof JL. Management of the difficult adult airway. *Anesthesiology*. 1991;75:1087–1110.

26. Cummins RO. *Textbook of Advanced Cardiac Life Support*. Dallas, Tex: American Heart Association; 1994: Chap 2.

27. Sellick BA. Cricoid pressure to control regurgitation of stomach contents during induction of anesthesia. *Lancet*. 1961;2:204.

28. Salem MR, Joseph NJ, Heyman HJ, Belani B, Paulissian R, Ferrara TP. Cricoid pressure is effective in obliterating the esophageal lumen in the presence of nasogastric tube. *Anesthesiology*. 1985;63:443–446.

29. Weiskopf RB, Bogetz MS, Roizen MF, et al. Cardiovascular and metabolic sequelae of inducing anesthesia with ketamine or thiopental in hypovolemic swine. *Anesthesiology*. 1984;60:214–219.

30. Bogetz MS, Weiskopf RB, Roizen MF. Ketamine increases catechols, but causes cardiovascular depression and acidosis in hypovolemic swine. *Anesthesiology*. 1982;57:A29.

31. Brown EM, Krishnaprasad D, Smiler BG. Pancuronium for rapid induction technique for tracheal intubation. *Can Anaesth Soc J*. 1979;26:489–491.

32. Waldburger JJ, Nielsen CH, Mulroy MF. Evaluation of atracurium for rapid sequence endotracheal intubation. *Anesthesiology*. 1984;61:A290.

33. Nagashima H, Nguyen HD, Lee S, et al. Facilitation of rapid endotracheal intubation with atracurium. *Anesthesiology*. 1984;61:A289.

34. Foldes FF, Schwarz S, Ilias W, et al. Rapid tracheal intubation with vecuronium: The priming principle. *Anesthesiology*. 1984;61:A294.

35. Blanc VF, Tremblay NAG. The complications of tracheal intubation: A new classification with a review of the literature. *Anesth Analg.* 1974;53:202.

36. Prasertwanitch Y, Schwartz JJH, Vandam LD. Arytenoid cartilage dislocation following prolonged endotracheal intubation. *Anesthesiology.* 1974;41:516.

37. Ellis PDM, Pallister WK. Recurrent laryngeal nerve palsy and endotracheal intubation. *J Laryngol Otol.* 1975;89:823.

38. Strain JD, Moore EE, Markovchick VJ, Van Duzer Moor S. Cimetidine for the prophylaxis of potential gastric acid aspiration pneumonitis in trauma patients. *So J Trauma.* 1981;21(1):49–51.

39. Manchikanti L, Colliver JA, Demeyer RG, et al. Dose response effects of intravenous ranitidine on gastric pH and volume in outpatients. *Anesthesiology.* 1986;65:180–185.

40. Morris RE, Miller GW. Preoperative management of the patient with a full stomach. In: Giesecke AH, ed. *Anesthesia for the Surgery of Trauma.* Philadelphia, Pa: Davis; 1976: Chap 4.

41. Olsson GL, Hallen B. Pharmacological evacuation of the stomach with metoclopramide. *Acta Anaesthesiol Scand.* 1982;26(5):417–420.

42. Gibbs CP, Banner C. Effectiveness of Bicitra as a preoperative antacid. *Anesthesiology.* 1984;61:97–99.

43. Eyler SW, Cullen BF, Murphy ME, et al. Antacid aspiration in rabbits: A comparison of Mylanta and Bicitra. *Anesth Analg.* 1982;61:288–292.

44. Diverte MB. The adult respiratory distress syndrome. *Mayo Clin Proc.* 1982;57:371–378.

45. Pennant JH, White PF. The laryngeal mask airway: Its uses in anesthesiology. *Anesthesiology.* 1993;79:144–163.

46. Bjoraker J, Kumar NB, Brown ACD. Evaluation of an emergency cricothyrotomy instrument. *Crit Care Med.* 1987;5(2):157–160.

47. Weiss S. A new emergency cricothyrotomy instrument. *Trauma.* 1983;23:155.

48. Toye F, Weinstein J. A percutaneous tracheostomy device. *Surgery.* 1969;65:384–389.

49. Ravlo O, Bach V, Lybecke H, Møller JT, Werner M, Nielsen HK. A comparison between the emergency cricothyroidectomy instruments. *Acta Anesthesiologica Scand.* 1987;31:317–319.

50. Powell WF, Ozdil T. A translaryngeal guide for tracheal intubation. *Anesth Analg.* 1967;46:231–234.

51. Brain AIJ. *The Intavent Laryngeal Mask: Instruction Manual.* 2nd ed. Henley-on-Thames, England: Intavent International SA; 1991.

52. Ellis DG, Jakymec A, Kaplan RM, et al. Guided orotracheal intubation in the operating room using a lighted stylet: A comparison with direct laryngoscopic technique. *Anesthesiology.* 1986;64:823.

53. Fox DJ, Castro T, Rastrelli AJ. Comparison of intubation techniques in the awake patient: The Flexi-lum surgical light (lightwand) versus blind nasal approach. *Anesthesiology.* 1986;66:69–71.

54. Messeter KH, Pettersen KI. Endotracheal intubation with the fibre-optic bronchoscope. *Anaesthesia.* 1980; 35(3):294–298.

55. Conyers AB, Wallace DH, Muller DS. Use of fiberoptic bronchoscope for nasotracheal intubation. *Can Anaesth Soc J*. 1972;19:654–656.

56. Raj PP, Forestner J, Watson TD, et al. Techniques for fiberoptic laryngoscopy in anesthesia. *Anesth Analg*. 1974;53:708.

57. Watson CB. Fiberoptic bronchoscopy for anesthesia. *Anesthesiol Rev*. 1982;9:17.

58. American College of Surgeons Committee on Trauma. Head trauma. In: *Advanced Trauma Life Support Program for Physicians*. Chicago, Ill: American College of Surgeons; 1993: Chap 6: 161.

59. Shapiro HM. Intracranial hypertension: Therapeutic and anesthetic considerations. *Anesthesiology*. 1975;43:445.

60. Teasdale G, Jennett B. Assessment of coma and impaired consciousness: A practical scale. *Lancet*. 1974;2:81–84.

61. Wiener SL, Barrett J. *Trauma Management for Civilian and Military Physicians*. Philadelphia, Pa: WB Saunders; 1986: 115.

62. Newfield P. Anesthetic considerations in patients with increased intracranial pressure. *ASA Refresher Courses in Anesthesiology*. 1988;16:157.

63. Hamill J, Bedford R, Weaver D, Colohan A. Lidocaine before endotracheal intubation: Intravenous or intratracheal. *Anesthesiology*. 1981;55:578.

64. Marsh ML, Dunlop BJ, Shapiro HM, et al. Succinylcholine—intracranial pressure effects in neurosurgical patients. *Anesth Analg*. 1980;59:550–551.

65. Contrell JE, Hartung J, Giffin JP, et al. Intracranial and hemodynamic changes after succinylcholine administration in cats. *Anesth Analg*. 1983;62:1006–1009.

66. Minton M, Stirt J, Bedord R. Increased intracranial pressure from succinylcholine: Prevention by prior nondepolarizing blockade. *Anesthesiology*. 1986;63:165.

67. Ciba Foundation. Acute cervical spine injuries. *Ciba Fdn Symp*. 1980;32:1.

68. Milne B, Jenkins MT. Anesthetic considerations in the multiply injured patient. In: Meyer M, ed. *The Multiply Injured Patient with Complex Fractures*. Philadelphia, Pa: Lea & Febiger; 1984: Chap 10: 96–112.

69. Miller RD, Way WL, Hickey RF. Inhibition of succinylcholine-induced increased intraocular pressure by nondepolarizing muscle relaxants. *Anesthesiology*. 1968;29:123–126.

70. Libonati MM, Leahy JJ, Ellison N. The use of succinylcholine in open eye surgery. *Anesthesiology*. 1985;62:637–640.

71. Schaffer S, Anderson R, Carder H. Management of the upper airway in the injured patient. In: Meyer M, ed. *The Multiply Injured Patient with Complex Fractures*. Philadelphia, Pa: Lea & Febiger; 1984: Chap 2: 9–17.

72. Bertz JE. Maxillofacial injuries. *Ciba Clin Symp*. 1981;33:14.

73. Lambert GE Jr, McMurry GT. Laryngotracheal trauma: Recognition and management. *Journal of the American College of Emergency Physicians*. 1976;5:883–887.

74. Haponik EF, Munster AM, Wise RA, et al. Upper airway function in burn patients. *Am Rev Respir Dis*. 1984;129:251–257.

Chapter 4

HEMORRHAGE, SHOCK, AND FLUID RESUSCITATION

FREDERICK W. BURGESS, PH.D, M.D.*; MICHAEL J. SBOROV, M.D.†; AND DEAN E. CALCAGNI, M.D.‡

*Formerly, Major, Medical Corps, U.S. Army Reserve; Director, Anesthesia Research, Madigan Army Medical Center, Tacoma, Washington 98431-5000; currently, Department of Anesthesia, Rhode Island Hospital, 593 Eddy Street, Providence, Rhode Island 02903

†Lieutenant Colonel, Medical Corps, U.S. Army Reserve; Chief, Anesthesia and Operative Services, Madigan Army Medical Center, Tacoma, Washington 98431-5000

‡Lieutenant Colonel, Medical Corps, U.S. Army; Staff Officer, Combat Casualty Care, U.S. Army Medical Research and Materiel Command, Fort Detrick, Frederick, Maryland 21702-5000

INTRODUCTION

Victims of combat-related trauma may present with the classical manifestations of hemorrhagic shock following rapid exsanguination from a major vascular structure. Hemorrhagic shock is the most common cause of death among combat casualties. Early recognition, control of the hemorrhage source by effective first aid, and rapid volume restoration with intravenous fluids are the ideal preparation for definitive surgical repair of the injury. Unfortunately, most combat casualties manifesting evidence of hypovolemia may not be rapidly transported, may not have an obvious bleeding source, may suffer from sleep deprivation, may have occult injuries, and, depending on the climatic conditions, may suffer from hyperthermia, hypothermia, and dehydration. An understanding of the combat environment, the climate, infectious epidemics, and the time of injury are all important factors contributing to the delineation of an appropriate diagnosis and treatment plan. This chapter focuses on the recognition and *initial* treatment of hypovolemic shock in the combat casualty, with an emphasis on associated medical conditions that may accompany and confound the diagnosis and treatment of hypovolemia.

PHYSIOLOGICAL CONSEQUENCES OF HEMORRHAGE

The adverse effects of hemorrhage on young and healthy soldiers are directly related to two primary factors: (1) decreased intravascular volume and (2) inadequate oxygen-carrying capacity. Reductions in intravascular volume and the associated organ hypoperfusion initiate a variety of autonomic and neurohumoral homeostatic responses, which are designed to maintain or restore the circulating plasma volume and organ perfusion. The consequences of inadequate oxygen delivery are organ dysfunction and possible death.

Cardiovascular Response

The response to rapid hemorrhage is complex and time dependent. The sudden fall in venous return to the heart results in an immediate decrease in cardiac stroke volume. Because the aortic arch is less distended by blood, intraluminal pressure will fall. The immediate response to the fall in pressure is a diffuse activation of the sympathetic nervous system caused by reflexes that arise in the aortic and carotid baroreceptors. An additional component of this adrenergic response is caused by the release of catecholamines from the adrenal medulla. The initial physiological effects are (*a*) increased heart rate and myocardial contractility; (*b*) increased systemic vascular resistance, which is due primarily to vasoconstriction of arterioles in the splanchnic viscera and skeletal muscle; and (*c*) decreased vascular capacitance, which arises primarily from constriction of the smaller veins and venules. These responses tend to preserve perfusion of the critically important central organs such as the heart and brain at the expense of the more peripherally situated splanchnic viscera and skeletal muscles.

Augmentation of the immediate vasoconstrictor response to hemorrhage occurs within minutes, with the activation of the renin-angiotensin system (Table 4-1). The formation of angiotensin II, an extremely potent generalized vasoconstrictor, contributes to the restoration of the arterial blood pressure and stimulates sodium conservation via the release of aldosterone. Sodium conservation, together with water conservation mediated via antidiuretic hormone secretion, also tends to restore the missing blood volume. The major mechanism that reestablishes an effective circulating blood volume in the first hours following a major hemorrhage is transcapillary transfer of plasma water from the intracellular fluid space to the intravascular fluid space. Although this process begins within minutes, it requires many hours for completion.

If the hemorrhage continues or if its magnitude overwhelms these compensatory mechanisms, a vicious cycle may begin, arising from the profoundly ischemic splanchnic viscera and skeletal muscle (Figure 4-1). Ultimately, systemic hemostasis fails for the following reasons:

- the ability of ischemic cells to maintain a normal transmembrane ionic gradient is lost,
- precapillary sphincters in the ischemic vascular beds relax,
- intravascular fluid leaves the circulation and collects in the ischemic tissues,
- lactic and inorganic acids as well as possible myocardial depressants enter the circulation, and
- oxygen-derived free radicals are generated—especially at the beginning of resuscitation when the ischemic beds are

TABLE 4-1

COMPENSATORY RESPONSE TO HEMORRHAGIC SHOCK

Response Times	Systemic Response
Few seconds	*Sympathetic nervous system*
	Vasoconstriction
	Tachycardia
Few minutes	*Renin-angiotensin system*
	Vasoconstriction (Angiotensin II)
	Sodium conservation
	Aldosterone secretion
	Glucocorticoid secretion
	Water conservation
	Vasopressin secretion (ADH)
Several minutes	*Fluid compartment shifts*
	Transcapillary refill
	Thirst

reperfused—and add to the cellular damage already caused by ischemia.

As the peripheral component of systemic hemostasis fails, the centrally circulating blood volume falls, leading to cardiac and respiratory dysfunction and further reduction in cardiac output and blood pressure. Respiratory compensation for the increasing metabolic acid load fails as the capacity of respiratory muscles is impaired by hypoperfusion. Acidosis, in conjunction with declining coronary perfusion pressure, impairs cardiac function; this leads to a further fall in cardiac output and blood pressure. Even vigorous resuscitation instituted at this time may not prevent death.

Fluid Compartment Shifts

After an untreated casualty sustains a major hemorrhage, restoration of the intravascular fluid compartment may require many hours as interstitial fluid is drawn into the intravascular compartment through alterations in the normal balance between the transcapillary hydrostatic and oncotic pressures. This phenomenon, *transcapillary refill,* depends on both adequate interstitial fluid reserves and the integrity of the capillary bed. In the average adult male, total body water accounts for approximately

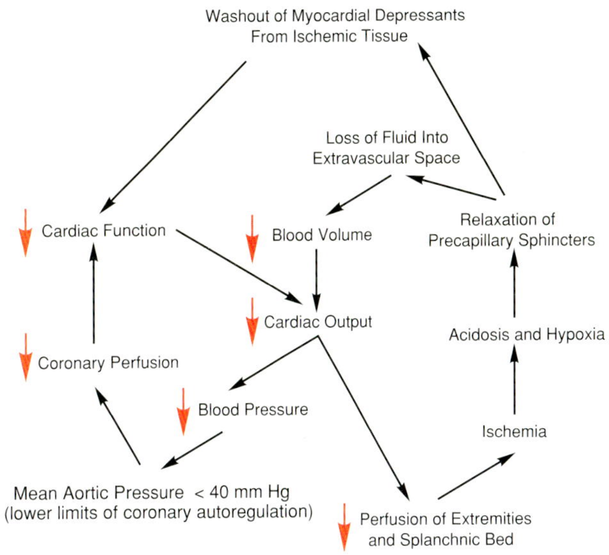

Fig. 4-1. *Positive* feedback loops (a departure from the normal steady state, which induces an ever-increasing departure) that may possibly develop and lead to death following massive hemorrhage can involve either the heart or the peripheral vascular beds of the soft tissues of the extremities and the splanchnic organs. The loops are not independent because the magnitude of cardiac output is a component of both. The central role of cardiac output means that a decline in the heart's pumping action (if of sufficient duration and magnitude) can, by reducing peripheral perfusion, adversely affect myocardial function. This causes a further decline in the heart's pumping action. The importance of myocardial depressants in hemorrhagic shock, in contrast to septic shock, remains controversial. Adapted from Bellamy RF, Pedersen DC, DeGuzman LR. Organ blood flow and the cause of death following massive hemorrhage. *Circ Shock.* 1984;14:115.

60% of total body weight.[1] Two thirds of body water is distributed within the intracellular compartment. The remaining one third is located in the extracellular fluid compartment; 25% to 30% of this compartment comprises the intravascular plasma volume (approximately 5% of the total body water), with the remainder making up the interstitial fluid space. Water freely distributes between each compartment by passive diffusion; however, ionic equilibrium is primarily determined by selective permeability, or ion-selective active transport, or both, within each compartment. Water, ions, and, to a variable extent, proteins, are freely exchanged between the intravascular and much of the interstitial fluid compartments. The transmural exchange of fluid between the intravascular compartment and the interstitium can be described by Starling's equation:

$$\text{fluid flux} = K[(P_c - P_i) - s(\pi_c - \pi_i)]$$

where *K* represents the capillary filtration coefficient; P_c and P_i represent the hydrostatic pressure of the intravascular (capillary) and interstitial compartments, respectively; *s*, which is known as the reflection coefficient, represents the impermeability of the membrane to a given substance; and π_c and π_i represent the oncotic pressure of the intravascular and interstitial fluid compartments, respectively.[2] (See Chapter 25, Acute Respiratory Failure and Ventilatory Management, for further discussion of Starling's equation.)

In hemorrhagic shock, constriction of the precapillary sphincter should decrease the net flow of fluid out of the intravascular space (decreased P_c) and promote the return of interstitial fluid into the intravascular compartment (transcapillary refill). Conversely, the loss of precapillary sphincter tone in late shock is an important factor leading to decompensation and death.

Extracellular Fluid Loss

Combat casualties presenting for care several hours after being injured may suffer from (*a*) hemorrhage-induced intravascular volume depletion and (*b*) preexisting depletion of the extracellular fluid compartment that is caused by concomitant dehydration secondary to environmental or nutritional factors. The importance of restoring the interstitial fluid compartment, in addition to restoring the circulating blood volume, was demonstrated in classic experiments performed during the 1950s.[3] Using a dog hemorrhagic shock model, the researchers found improved survival among the animals that were resuscitated with both lactated Ringer's solution and their shed blood, as opposed to resuscitation with shed blood alone or shed blood and additional plasma. Because the crystalloid fluid is distributed through the body water, it was soon afterwards determined that restoration of the intravascular volume required the infusion of volumes 3- to 4-fold greater than the putative missing volume; that is, after 1 L of lactated Ringer's solution is infused, only 250 mL will remain in the intravascular space.

Trauma and severe hemorrhage frequently lead to a reduction in the functional extracellular fluid compartment. The reduction in extracellular fluid is partly attributable to hemorrhage; transcapillary refill; and the sequestration of interstitial (isotonic) fluid, which represents the third-space loss. Recommendations for replacing the third-space fluid sequestration include administering (*a*) a balanced salt solution at 4, 6, and 8 mL/kg/h for minimal, moderate, and severe trauma, in addition to (*b*) the estimated hourly maintenance fluids.[4]

Oxygen Transport

Hemorrhage interferes with normal tissue oxygenation by two mechanisms: (1) the anemic (ie, inadequate oxygen-carrying capacity) and (2) the hemodynamic (ie, inadequate tissue perfusion). Anemia is rarely appreciated immediately after a hemorrhage. This may be due to inadequate time for equilibration or inadequate interstitial fluid reserves. However, even in the setting of severe hemorrhage, reduced hemoglobin content of the blood is rarely the cause of tissue hypoxia.[5] For example, a healthy, 20-year-old, male soldier (with body surface area of 1.73 m^2) arrives at a combat support hospital within 1 hour of sustaining an extremity wound. Medical personnel there estimate that he has experienced a 40% to 50% hemorrhage from the femoral artery. Fortunately, the bleeding had been controlled at an aid station and he had been resuscitated with 6% hetastarch and lactated Ringer's solution. On arrival at the combat support hospital, his vital signs are stable and the bleeding has stopped. His hemoglobin is determined to be 7 g/dL. Assuming a $Pa{O_2}$ (partial pressure of oxygen in the arteries) of 95 mm Hg, a hemoglobin saturation of 99%, and a normal cardiac output (C.O.) of 5 L/min, the arterial oxygen content ($Ca{O_2}$) and oxygen delivery ($D{O_2}$) of this hypothetical casualty can easily be calculated:

$$CaO_2 = 1.36 \bullet (\text{hemoglobin concentration}) \bullet (\text{hemoglobin saturation}) + 0.003\,(PaO_2)$$

$$CaO_2 = 1.36 \bullet (7\text{ g/dL}) \bullet (.99) + 0.003 \bullet (95) = 9.71\text{ mL }O_2\text{/dL}$$

$$\text{C.O.} \bullet CaO_2 = DO_2$$

$$5\text{ L/min} \bullet 9.71\text{ mL/dL} = 486\text{ mL }O_2\text{/min}$$

Assuming a normal C.O. of 5 L/min, with a CaO_2 of 9.71 mL/dL, this hypothetical patient can deliver 486 mL of O_2/min or 281 mL/m^2. This value exceeds the predicted basal O_2 consumption rate of 250 mL/min. Under stress conditions, the basal oxygen requirement may increase 2- to 3-fold. However, the cardiac output of most young, healthy soldiers can increase 2- to 3-fold to keep up with increased metabolic demand, provided that an adequate cardiac preload has been maintained.

This example demonstrates that (*a*) blood replacement is frequently unnecessary and (*b*) volume restoration with asanguinous plasma expanders is, at least initially, the key element. If the circulating plasma volume is maintained, then the metabolic consequences of severe hemorrhage can be minimized. The critical point to be remembered in this scenario is that the soldier's hemorrhage was not ongoing but had been stopped by appropriate first aid. However, in the setting of unabated hemorrhage and shock (as indicated by hypotension, tachycardia, mental-status changes, and diminished or absent urinary output), the administration of blood is essential and should not be withheld.

When combat casualties who are in shock arrive at a medical treatment facility with surgical capabilities, medical officers should not underestimate the amount of fluid required to reestablish a circulating blood volume compatible with survival. For example, during the Vietnam War, soldiers who required a blood transfusion received, on average, 2.5 L of blood and 2 L of crystalloid fluid during their initial resuscitation and surgery.[6] Even combat casualties who are no longer bleeding—who have normal hemodynamic indices and have received what should be adequate restoration of red blood cell mass on the basis of estimated blood loss—frequently have a deficient red blood cell mass when this is measured several days after the resuscitative surgery.[7]

HYPOVOLEMIA

Vascular and visceral injuries secondary to missile wounds, fractures of the long bones, and crush injuries are frequently accompanied by visible and occult hemorrhage. The amount of blood lost will not always be evident, as blood loss tends to be overestimated with more-visible, superficial injuries and underestimated with abdominal and orthopedic injuries (see Chapter 20, Abdominal Injuries, and Chapter 21, Extremity Injuries). Intervention in the field and mobilization of extracellular fluid stores (transcapillary refill) may serve to confuse the initial estimation of blood loss and result in an underestimation of blood loss. The classic parameters for the estimating the severity of hemorrhage are often a useful starting point for determining the rapidity and types of fluid administered, and for determining the response to resuscitation (Table 4-2). Supine hypotension in all combat casualties should be recognized as hypovolemia that requires rapid and immediate fluid resuscitation.

Trauma victims presenting with a suspected mild hemorrhage (Class I: suspected blood loss in the absence of tachycardia or hypotension) require initial resuscitation with clear solutions, preferably intravenous crystalloids. Resuscitation for moderate hemorrhage (Class II: tachycardia without hypotension) should be initiated with crystalloid or colloid solutions or both; however, in the presence of continued bleeding, early transfusion therapy with packed red blood cells or whole blood should be initiated. The presence of hypotension (Class III or Class IV hemorrhage: tachycardia and hypotension) requires immediate blood-volume replacement with (*a*) packed red blood cells or whole blood and (*b*) crystalloid solutions. Other causes of

TABLE 4-2

ESTIMATION OF HEMORRHAGE

Degree of Hemorrhage	Blood Loss (L)	Blood Vol. Lost (%)	Heart Rate	Blood Pressure	Pulse Pressure	Respiratory Rate	Urinary Flow (mL/h)	Mental Status
Class I	< 1	< 15%	< 100	Normal	Normal or increased	14–20	≥ 30	Slight anxiety
Class II	0.75–1.5	15%–30%	> 100	Normal	Decreased	20–30	20–30	Mild anxiety
Class III	1.5–2.0	30%–40%	> 120	Decreased	Decreased	30–40	< 15	Anxious and confused
Class IV	> 2.0	≥ 40%	≥ 140	Decreased	Decreased	Rapid and shallow	Negligible	Confused and lethargic

Adapted with permission from Committee on Trauma, American College of Surgeons. *Advanced Trauma Life Support Program for Physicians*. Chicago, Ill: American College of Surgeons; 1989: 72.

hypotension (eg, tension pneumothorax, cardiac tamponade) should be sought after fluid resuscitation has begun.

In the combat setting, tachycardia is a useful, but often an insensitive, indicator of hypovolemia. Just how insensitive was one of the more interesting findings of the surgical research unit that worked during World War II. Data on the effects of shock on heart rate were published in the seminal volume, *The Physiologic Effects of Wounds,* published as part of The Surgeon General's official history of the U.S. Army Medical Department in World War II (Table 4-3).[8] The degree of shock in injured soldiers was stratified not only by blood pressure but also by measurement of blood volume. The table demonstrates that the differences between the heart rates in soldiers with varying degrees of shock are so small as to be useless for predictive purposes.

Subsequent studies on combat casualties have confirmed that there may be no simple relation between magnitude of hemorrhage and heart rate.[9] Although the generalized discharge of the sympathetic component of the autonomic nervous system following a precipitous fall in blood pressure leads to tachycardia, the decrease in venous return to the heart by unloading mechanoreceptors in the cardiac chambers, and especially the left ventricle, leads to reflex slowing of the heart through an efferent pathway that involves the parasympathetic nervous system. Thus, hemorrhage activates two different components of the autonomic nervous system, and although tachycardia due to the sympathetic component usually predominates, vagal slowing may also be seen.

In addition, other factors may confound any relation between the observed heart rate and the magnitude of blood loss. For example, atropine administered in the field for chemical exposure, fear, and pain makes the use of heart rate unreliable. Trained athletes and infantry soldiers may tolerate a substantial hemorrhage without manifesting tachycardia or hypotension until they are severely hypovolemic. When possible, performance of a tilt-test will help to distinguish hypovolemia from other causes of tachycardia.

It is important to recognize that heart rate and blood pressure may normalize with initial resuscitation efforts, but this may not be indicative of normal peripheral perfusion. Mixed venous blood oxygen saturation may be the best single index for assessing the adequacy of systemic perfusion.[10] However, this determination requires a blood gas analyzer, a device not usually available in forward surgical hospitals (this subject is discussed more fully in Chapter 5, Physiological Monitoring). Furthermore, a central venous line is required. Unfortunately, invasive arterial and central venous monitoring, although often desirable for fluid management, may not be easily managed in the combat theater.

Traditionally, restoration of urinary output has been used as a monitor of organ perfusion and as a guide to fluid therapy. An indwelling urinary bladder catheter should be considered an essential monitor in all trauma victims. There may be no change in hematocrit immediately following hemorrhage, because only when transcapillary fluid refill occurs (or when fluid resuscitation is initiated) does dilu-

TABLE 4-3

RELATIONSHIP OF DEGREE OF SHOCK TO HEART RATE (106 CASES)

	Degree of Shock			
	None (n=13)	Slight (n=24)	Moderate (n=34)	Severe (n=35)
Reduction of Blood Volume (%)	14.1 ± 4.9	20.7 ± 4.1	34.3 ± 3.1	45.9 ± 4.6
Blood Pressure (m ± SD)				
Systole	126 ± 11.9	109 ± 3.0	95 ± 4.9	49 ± 7.6
Diastole	75 ± 1.5	66 ± 2.7	58 ± 3.5	25 ± 5.8
Heart Rate (m ± SD)	103 ± 7.2	111 ± 3.4	113 ± 3.6	116 ± 3.3
(Range)	(70–140)	(88–150)	(80–160)	(60–144)

Data source: The Board for the Study of the Severely Wounded, North African–Mediterranean Theater of Operations. *The Physiologic Effects of Wounds*. In: Beecher, HK, ed. *Surgery in World War II*. Washington, DC: US Army Medical Department, Office of The Surgeon General; 1952: 34, 35, 56.

tion of the remaining red blood cell mass occur. Thus, acute changes in hematocrit and hemoglobin are not necessarily useful in evaluating ongoing blood loss.

Venous Access

The initial management of all combat trauma casualties must involve a team effort focusing on combined assessment and intervention as indicated by the immediacy of the situation. Casualties presenting with evidence of shock must quickly be inspected for evidence of external hemorrhage. If a site of major bleeding is found, appropriate first-aid maneuvers designed to stop the bleeding (eg, direct pressure) must be instituted immediately. Two or more large-bore (preferably 14-gauge) intravenous fluid cannulae must be established early in all casualties in shock, or those suspected of having injuries that might lead to shock. Venous access can be extremely difficult to obtain in the presence of hypovolemia and dehydration. Additionally, access sites may be limited by the location and nature of the traumatic injuries. Optimal sites for venous cannulation in trauma victims include the antecubital, subclavian, saphenous, and femoral veins.

Surgical access (cutdown) may be required in patients with severe hemorrhagic shock. The saphenous and antecubital vessels are convenient locations for cutdown cannulation. This approach allows the sterile intravenous extension tubing to be inserted directly into the vessel to maximize delivery. A major disadvantage of the surgical approach is the risk of infection.

Central venous access may be obtained via the internal and external jugular veins, the subclavian vein, and the femoral veins. Femoral access eliminates the risk of a pneumothorax (a recognized complication of gaining venous access via the neck and chest); however, the femoral site is remote from the anesthesiologist during most surgical procedures. Also, penetrating intraabdominal injuries may involve the inferior vena cava. In such cases, resuscitation via the femoral vessels may contribute to intraabdominal bleeding or be rendered ineffective by cross-clamping of the femoral vessel. The subclavian vein is a useful site for trauma access; however, this location carries a significant risk of a pneumothorax. Both the subclavian and internal jugular sites carry a significant risk of unintentional arterial injury or cannulation.[11] Major blood loss has occurred following arterial injuries at both sites, and the potential exists for an expanding hematoma in the neck to compromise the airway. Techniques for obtaining peripheral, central, and cutdown venous access are well taught in the American College of Surgeons' Advanced Trauma Life Support course, which should be taken by all medical officers.[12]

Intravenous Fluid-Delivery Systems

Some consideration must be given to ensuring the availability of large-bore, fluid-administration sets. The ideal set contains a large-surface-area combination drip chamber and blood filter (170 µ), dual vessel-access ports, and a hand-operated pumping chamber.

Large-caliber, high-efficiency, blood-warming units are essential for large-volume resuscitation. The Level 1 infusion system (manufactured by Level 1 Technologies, Inc., Rockland, Mass.) is a functional unit that provides rapid warming of intravenous infusions, through a counter-current warming system, at high rates of flow (500 mL/min) (Figure 4-2). This system allows quick and effortless priming, and has an in-line air vent to prevent accidental air emboli when used in conjunction with a pres-

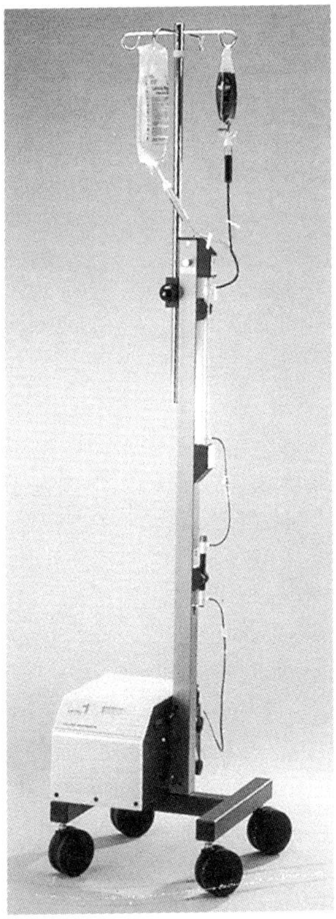

Fig. 4-2. The Level 1 blood warming system is manufactured by Level 1 Technologies, Inc., Rockland, Mass.

sure infuser. These devices are being evaluated by the U.S. Army Medical Department for use in its field hospitals. The space required for the warming unit and the disposable components, and the expense of the disposable components are disadvantages of the Level 1 fluid warmer.

Alternative methods for rapid warming of crystalloid solutions include using microwave ovens or storing the solutions in warming ovens. The use of microwave ovens for blood components is presently not recommended. Under no circumstances should the fluid be infused at a temperature exceeding 40°C.

Pressure-assist, fluid-administration devices (pressure bags) are helpful in speeding fluid delivery. Most of these are manually operated bladder devices. Pneumatic infusers are currently marketed; however, under field conditions, the availability of compressed gas may limit their use. The Biomed Spring Activated Infusion Pressor (manufactured by Migada, Inc., Burbank, Calif.) offers a useful mechanical alternative. This spring-operated system provides a constant pressure and thus a more stable rate of delivery. Complications secondary to pressure-assisted fluid administration can occur (eg, venous air emboli, which may occur with compression of the residual air in an exhausted intravenous fluid bag). Air traps in blood-warming sets and air vents (eg, Level 1 system) can help to minimize this risk. Also, inverting the container and venting the air prior to administration will also reduce this risk. Some concern has been raised over the potential for damage to cellular elements with pressurized delivery systems, but the significance of this concern remains to be clarified.

Blood-Salvage Techniques

Salvaging blood for intraoperative autotransfusion is becoming an increasingly important part of routine anesthetic and surgical practice. Much of the recent emphasis on blood salvage has arisen over concerns about the safety of community autologous blood supplies, predominantly relating to the transmission of the human immunodeficiency virus. Although blood-salvage techniques can reduce the need for homologous transfusion, blood salvage usually does not completely eliminate the need for transfusion of homologous blood products in major trauma. Currently, there are two principal methods for salvaging blood from the operative field. The simplest method involves collecting the blood into sterile vacuum containers containing an anticoagulant (citrate-phosphate-dextrose or heparin) and reinfusing the unwashed filtered blood directly into the patient. The advantages of this technique include low cost, simplicity, and minimal requirements for storage or trained personnel. The disadvantages are that procoagulants, bacteria, and free hemoglobin will also be infused into the patient.[13] This approach appears to be ideally suited for use in field hospitals; unfortunately, the risks and benefits involved with transfusing unwashed blood have not yet been well delineated.

The alternative approach to blood salvage involves the collection of shed blood and processing it through a cell-washing device prior to reinfusion. These cell-washing devices, such as the Cell Saver 4 (manufactured by Haemonetics, Boston, Mass.) have become increasingly efficient and automated (Figure 4-3). The drawbacks include the need for personnel training, equipment expense, the need for expensive disposable plastic ware, and a time delay during processing. Furthermore, the benefits of cell washing, as opposed to the reinfusion of unwashed blood, have not been clearly demonstrated to improve patient outcome. With both techniques, coagulation factors and platelets are lost, and there is a risk of trauma to the cellular elements. Although blood salvage is clearly beneficial in the manage-

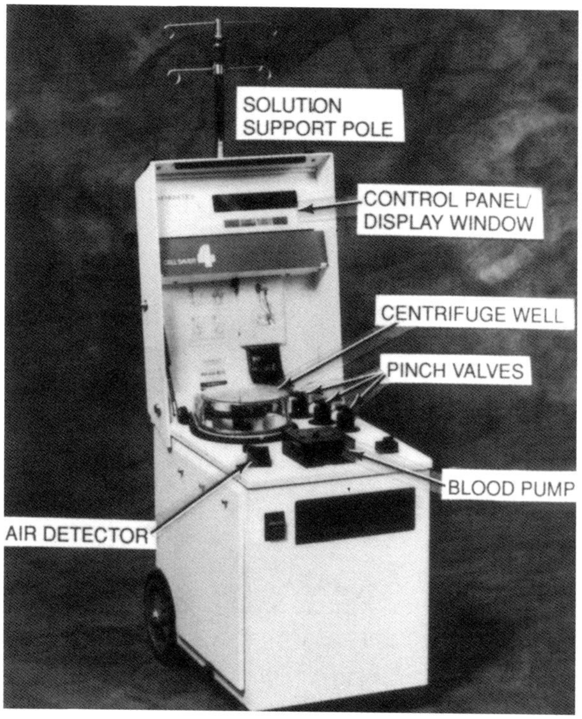

Fig. 4-3. The Cell Saver 4 is manufactured by Haemonetics, Boston, Mass.

ment of elective surgery, the advantages of introducing this methodology into the care of the combat casualty have yet to be demonstrated.

Intraosseous Fluid Infusion

Intraosseous fluid infusion has been advocated in situations in which venous access is difficult or impossible to obtain.[14] This route of delivery is particularly amenable in the pediatric population, and because pediatric casualties always occur in urban warfare, military anesthesiologists need to be familiar with the technique. Intraosseous access in adults is somewhat more difficult to obtain. This is partly related to the replacement of the marrow space by fat and partly related to the density of the overlying bone. Recent experimental animal studies have demonstrated the benefits of intraosseous infusion of a small-volume mixture of hypertonic saline and dextran via the sternum. A sternal infusion device has been developed that could be placed in the field with minimal training of medics, and then utilized for fluid access.[15] This approach is still in the early phase of development and testing.

At present, the intraosseous approach in adults is impractical and inadequately tested. Special needles are required for this technique (bone marrow sets) and the clinical utility in adults is unknown. Typically, the marrow space is entered by inserting a 15- or 18-gauge iliac bone marrow needle into the medial aspect of the proximal tibia. The distal femur, in the midline above the condyles, is an alternative site. The medial malleolus has been used in patients in cardiac arrest, in whom venous access is difficult. This approach may prove useful for the administration of selected drugs. Unfortunately, the distal tibia provides inadequate flow rates for it to prove useful in the management of hypovolemia. Complications with intraosseous infusions are uncommon.[16] The most common complication is that of local extravasation. Local cellulitis and osteomyelitis are fortunately rare (< 1%). Deaths have occurred with the sternal approach secondary to unrecognized penetration of the thoracic cavity.[17]

RESUSCITATION FLUID SELECTION

Hypovolemia and hemorrhagic shock fall along a continuum from mild to profound organ hypoperfusion. As cardiac output falls, oxygen transport to less crucial end-organ cellular elements (eg, skin, muscle) may become progressively inadequate, contributing to anaerobic metabolism and the accumulation of organic acids (eg, lactate). Homeostatic efforts (vasoconstriction) to preserve perfusion to the heart and brain inevitably sacrifice perfusion to the kidneys, muscle, intestine, and skin, leading to the classic manifestations of shock. The eventual lethality of the shock state probably results from the maintenance of this restricted perfusion pattern and progressive tissue hypoxia and acidosis.[18] Some evidence suggests that blockade of the sympathetic nervous system may reverse the vasoconstriction-induced acidosis and improve survival after bleeding has been stopped and blood volume restored.[19–21] However, a more effective and clinically relevant treatment plan is to restore the circulating blood volume and organ perfusion.

A variety of treatment regimens, including colloids, crystalloid solutions, whole blood, and blood components, have been proposed (Table 4-4). Perhaps the best initial approach to the casualty with evidence of a mild-to-moderate hemorrhage (10%–30% of the estimated blood volume) is to rapidly administer an intravenous fluid challenge of a warmed, balanced, salt solution in 10- to 20-mL/kg increments, depending on the severity of symptoms and ongoing blood loss. Repeated fluid challenges are administered until the desired hemodynamic response is obtained. Blood products should be administered to keep pace with concurrent blood loss and to maintain an acceptable hemoglobin level (> 7 g/dL). When uncontrolled bleeding occurs, isovolumic transfusion with fresh whole blood or packed red blood cells, in conjunction with a crystalloid solution, is necessary.

Crystalloid Solutions

Although a variety of crystalloid solutions is available, 0.9% sodium chloride or lactated Ringer's solution are reasonable first choices. Isotonic sodium chloride (0.9%) may be readily mixed with blood products and is an excellent choice for volume resuscitation. However, it has the minor disadvantage of contributing to a hyperchloremic acidosis when large volumes of resuscitation fluid must be used. Lactated Ringer's solution has the advantage of having a somewhat more physiological composition, providing elemental replacement of calcium and potassium, and more physiological concentrations of sodium and chlorine ions. A disadvantage of lactated Ringer's solution is its relative incompatibility with blood products. The

TABLE 4-4

RESUSCITATION FLUIDS

Solution	Advantages	Disadvantages
0.9% NaCl	Inexpensive Compatible with blood Replenishes ECF space Increases GRF	Nonphysiological Na^+ and Cl^- concentrations Contributes to interstitial edema Large volumes required for replacement of blood loss ($\geq$ 3-fold estimated blood loss)
Lactated Ringer's	Inexpensive Physiological electrolyte concentrations Increases GFR Replenishes ECF space	Same as those for NaCl
5% Albumin (MW $6 \bullet 10^4$)	Replaces plasma loss volume for volume Provides rapid expansion of the intravascular space with less volume	Expensive Redistributes into the interstitial fluid space relatively quickly (compared to other colloids) May aggravate edema in leaky capillary states
6% Hetastarch (Hespan, Dupont) (MW 10^4–10^7)	Same as those for 5% albumin Provides a more persistent expansion of the intravascular space, relative to albumin Plasma volume expansion may persist > 24 h	Expensive May interfere with coagulation cascade if > 20 mL/kg is administered
5% Plasma Protein Fraction (83% albumin)	Resembles albumin	Similar to albumin, somewhat less osmotically active Contaminating plasma proteins may produce hypotension with rapid administration
Dextran 40 (average MW $4 \bullet 10^4$)	Provides rapid expansion of the intravascular space with a small volume Reduces incidence of thromboembolism	Risk of anaphylaxis 0.5%–5% May contribute to renal failure Interferes with platelet function and clotting Risk of bleeding with > 1.5 g/kg/d Interferes with blood cross-matching May produce osmotic diuresis
Dextran 70 (average MW $7 \bullet 10^4$)	Same as those for dextran 40 Larger MW confers a greater duration of plasma volume expansion	Same as those for dextran 40
HDS	Very rapid restoration of intravascular volume with a small volume Small volume makes field use easier	Same as those for dextran 40 Brief hypotension with rapid infusion Hypernatremia, especially if used in dehydrated casualties

ECF: extracellular fluid; GRF: glomerular filtration rate; HDS: hypertonic saline (7.5%) and dextran 70 (6%); MW: molecular weight

calcium content of lactated Ringer's solution may activate the coagulation cascade in blood products; however, slight dilution of packed red cells with lactated Ringer's solution has not been shown to cause a problem.[22] The lactate content of lactated Ringer's solution may aggravate the correction of the ongoing metabolic acidosis in individuals suffering from profound acidosis or ketoacidosis. Under most circumstances, however, when organ perfusion has been restored, the liver is quite capable of metabolizing the lactate load; the problem is, therefore, rarely of concern.[23]

Intravenous fluids containing dextrose (glucose) are rarely indicated and are potentially harmful in the management of trauma casualties. The stress response induced by major trauma or surgery frequently contributes to a normal or an elevated blood glucose level. Rapid administration of large volumes of glucose solutions during resuscitation may lead to an osmotic diuresis, confounding efforts to restore the intravascular deficit. Hyperglycemia has also been linked to a poorer neurological outcome among victims of trauma, cardiac arrest, and stroke.[23–25] Glucose may be included in maintenance fluids during the postresuscitation phase.

Colloid Solutions

The use of colloid-containing intravenous solutions in the management of trauma and surgical patients remains a source of controversy and is thoroughly discussed in other textbooks[26,27] and in Chapter 24, The Syndromes of Septic Inflammatory Response and Multiple Organ Dysfunction. Historically, the only colloids that were available in the military for field use were albumin and plasma. More recently, the dextrans and hydroxyethyl starch (Hespan, manufactured by Du Pont Pharmaceuticals, Wilmington, Del.) have become widely available and are used by some civilian paramedic rescue squads for field resuscitation of casualties in hemorrhagic shock. The most significant drawback to these agents is their cost, which is excessive relative to crystalloid solutions. The attractive features of the colloids include

- rapid repletion of the intravascular compartment with a smaller fluid volume,
- a more-prolonged expansion of the plasma volume, and
- less peripheral edema.

Some have suggested a reduced risk of increased intracranial pressure as another attractive feature of colloids. This may be true in comparison to lactated Ringer's solution; however, the effects of isotonic solutions (eg, normal saline) on intracranial pressure appear comparable to those of albumin.[28]

Colloid solutions produce an increase in the intravascular colloid oncotic pressure and may draw interstitial water into the intravascular compartment.[29,30] Thus, the plasma volume expands in excess of the administered fluid volume. Conversely, in "leaky capillary" states (eg, burns, sepsis, the adult respiratory distress syndrome), the colloids can traverse the endothelial barrier and contribute to the formation of pulmonary and peripheral edema. Although abnormal capillary membranes are not likely to be present during the initial treatment of most combat casualties, other disadvantages of colloid solutions that argue against their use include the following:

- the potential for impaired coagulation,
- interference with cross-matching of blood,
- increased viscosity,
- a transient fall in ionized calcium levels (which albumin may produce), and
- the potential for a relative reduction in glomerular filtration.

The reduction in glomerular filtration rate probably reflects (*a*) the depletion of the interstitial fluid compartment through third-space losses and (*b*) the inability of colloids to replace the loss.[30] A relatively hyperoncotic state may result. Crystalloids are better suited to improving glomerular filtration. Patients with compromised glomerular filtration may be placed at increased risk of renal failure if resuscitated with a dextran solution.[31] In hypovolemic patients, renal tubular obstruction may develop due to precipitation of the dextran in the tubules.

In circumstances where blood loss is substantial and continuing, dextran and hetastarch should be used cautiously. Dextran interferes with platelet adhesion and may aggravate blood loss.[32] Hetastarch, when used in large cumulative volumes, has been shown to produce a coagulopathy, probably by interfering with Factor VIII activity.[33] Clinical case reports have linked bleeding catastrophes to the use of hetastarch in quantities greater than 20 mL/kg.[34] Life-threatening anaphylaxis can occur with the dextrans and hetastarch. The overall risk of anaphylaxis appears to be on the order of 0.5% to 5% with the dextrans and 0.08% with hetastarch.[33]

Hypertonic Solutions

Hypertonic saline solutions, alone or in combination with concentrated colloid solutions, have become the focus of intense interest over their possible use as small-volume resuscitation fluids in the field. The primary advantage of hypertonic solutions compared to conventional fluids for field resuscitation is logistical: much less hypertonic fluid is required for an equivalent degree of resuscitation—thus, the load of the combat medic is reduced. The U.S. Army Medical Research and Materiel Command at Fort Detrick, Frederick, Maryland, has had an ongoing research program into the development and clinical application of a hypertonic saline dextran solution (7.5% sodium chloride and 6% high-molecular-weight dextran 70). This solution, when used in animal models for hemorrhagic shock, has effected dramatic improvements in hemodynamic parameters and survival following a hemorrhage that would otherwise have been lethal.[35] Limited field trials using human volunteers have documented the beneficial hemodynamic effects when hypertonic saline dextran is administered by paramedics; however, improved patient outcome has not yet been demonstrated convincingly.[36,37] One reason for this could be the rapidity with which most patients were transported to hospitals and received definitive care.

Hypertonic saline produces a rapid expansion of the intravascular space by drawing extracellular and intracellular water into the vascular compartment. Hypertonic saline alone produces short-lived improvements in hemodynamics, as the sodium tends to redistribute rapidly. The addition of a concentrated colloid solution (eg, dextran, hetastarch) increases the duration of the plasma volume expansion and improves survival in animal models.[35] However, two recent clinical investigation studies involving traumatized humans show no added benefit from dextran compared with 7.5% saline alone.[38,39] Subsequent volume replacement with isotonic, balanced salt solutions is essential to maintain organ perfusion as the effects resolve, and to reverse the relative hypernatremic/hyperoncotic state.[40] Hypertonic saline resuscitation may offer additional advantages in the management of head-injured, hypovolemic casualties by minimizing elevations in intracranial pressure and by improving the cerebral-perfusion pressure.[41] While the benefits are clearly evident in the short term (hours), the long-term benefits or disadvantages of hypertonic solutions on cerebral perfusion and neurological outcome need to be demonstrated.

One important hazard associated with the use of hypertonic-resuscitation measures in the field is the risk of promoting further exsanguination and dehydration. Improvements in blood pressure and cardiac output in casualties with uncontrolled bleeding may increase the rate of blood loss, leading to further loss of oxygen-carrying capacity, progressive acidosis, and increased morbidity. Data from studies[42] with experimental animals appear to support these conclusions. Thus, the administration of hypertonic solutions in the presence of uncontrolled hemorrhage, and in the absence of guaranteed, short-term delivery of definitive supportive and surgical treatment, may be contraindicated. Of course, the same stricture applies to resuscitation with any fluid that raises blood pressure, including lactated Ringer's solution. Further study is needed on this issue.

At present, and under most conditions, crystalloid solutions appear to be the resuscitation fluid of choice. Perhaps some combination of colloid and crystalloid solutions will prove to be the optimal approach. Colloid solutions should probably be avoided during the initial resuscitation (ie, the first 24 h) of victims with extensive burn injuries, casualties suffering from the adult respiratory distress syndrome, and in casualties suffering from preexisting dehydration. Hypertonic solutions may have a role in the immediate resuscitation of hypovolemic trauma casualties, provided continued volume support with isotonic solutions is available. Colloid solutions or hypertonic saline may prove particularly useful prior to the induction of anesthesia in conscious, hypovolemic casualties, or in hypovolemic casualties with head injuries who require immediate surgery. Of course, the development of an oxygen-carrying solution—such as a stroma-free hemoglobin solution—which, in contrast to blood, could be taken into the field by the medic, would be an important step forward in our ability to treat the combat casualty.

SUPPLEMENTAL THERAPEUTIC MEASURES

Although control of bleeding and rapid infusion of crystalloid fluids and blood are the essential steps that must be taken if the combat casualty in shock is to be salvaged, a variety of supplemental therapeutic measures have been suggested in the past; in some instances, they may play an important role. The use of other measures, such as steroid theroid therapy in the management of head trauma, continues to be controversial and unresolved. However, in the absence of Addison's disease, adrenocorticoids are unlikely to be beneficial in the management of hypovolemic shock.

Patient Position

Conventional management of hypotensive trauma victims frequently involves placing the patient in the head-down (Trendelenburg's) position to improve venous return to the heart (Figure 4-4). In otherwise normovolemic subjects experiencing hypotension (ie, those in neurogenic shock), lowering the head or elevating the legs may facilitate venous return. However, studies[43] of subjects with hemorrhagic shock have failed to demonstrate consistent hemodynamic improvement from

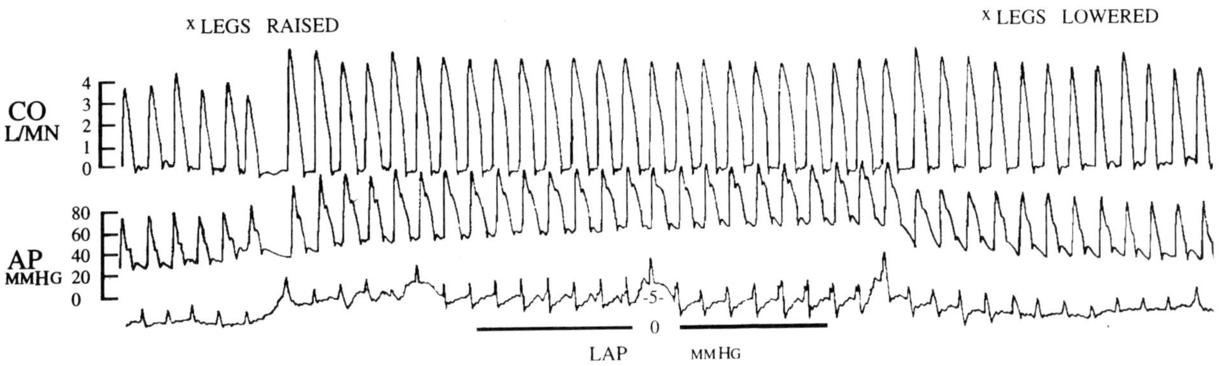

Fig. 4-4. The data shown in this phasic pressure and flow diagram were obtained in an anesthetized swine instrumented with an aortic flow probe for measuring cardiac output (CO) and pressure transducers in the proximal aorta (AP) and left atrium (LAP). When the animal's hind legs were raised abruptly, cardiac output, aortic pressure, and left atrial pressure were transiently elevated. Previously, 50% of the animal's circulating blood volume had been removed. Cardiac output remained elevated when the legs were lowered, suggesting that the blood that transfused into the central circulation when the extremities were raised has not yet been redistributed back to the legs. The fall in aortic pressure caused by lowering the legs may mean that the hydrostatic pressure head above the site of the pressure catheter is itself a factor in determining the magnitude of the measured pressure. If applicable to humans in shock, data such as these suggest that Trendelenburg's position may be hemodynamically beneficial. Source: Medical Audio Visual Aids Division, Letterman Army Institute of Research, Presidio of San Francisco, Calif. File Number 229-82-1, 1983.

Trendelenburg's position, and this position may have an adverse impact on cardiac output and blood pressure.[44] Furthermore, Trendelenburg's position may produce adverse consequences in the hypovolemic, head-injured victim by increasing intracranial pressure and reducing the cerebral perfusion pressure. Most of these problems can be avoided simply by elevating the legs to facilitate venous return, without placing the head in a dependent position.

Pneumatic Antishock Garment

The use of the pneumatic antishock garment (a compression device first known as military antishock trousers [MAST]) was introduced by the U.S. Army during the Vietnam War. Until recently, use of this garment was considered to be a standard of practice but its use in the acute management of hemorrhagic shock has now waned. The pneumatic antishock garment appears to support the blood pressure by a combination of increased systemic vascular resistance and increased venous return.[45]

There seems little doubt that proper use of the pneumatic antishock garment results in an autotransfusion of blood from the compressed tissue in the lower half of the body into the central circulation, but the actual volume is small (2–3 mL/kg) and the augmented cardiac output secondary to the increased venous return is transient (Figure 4-5). Maintenance of blood pressure with this device probably is the result of a mechanical increase in resistance in the compressed tissue and therefore is purchased at the cost of decreased perfusion of already ischemic tissue. Clinical studies[46] have demonstrated significantly reduced survival in patients treated with the pneumatic antishock garment when the site of hemorrhage is in the chest and, therefore, is not compressed by the device. This is not surprising given that any increase in blood pressure will simply increase the rate of hemorrhage. If the pneumatic antishock garment has any utility in combat casualty care, it is in stabilizing fractures of the pelvis and the long bones of the legs. In this setting, the device may help to reduce ongoing blood loss and therefore permit hemodynamic stabilization prior to definitive intervention.

Supplemental Oxygen

The routine administration of supplemental oxygen to trauma casualties may be beneficial in some victims, in that multiple or massive injuries (eg, splinting, flail chest, fat emboli) are often associated with impaired oxygenation. However, expecta-

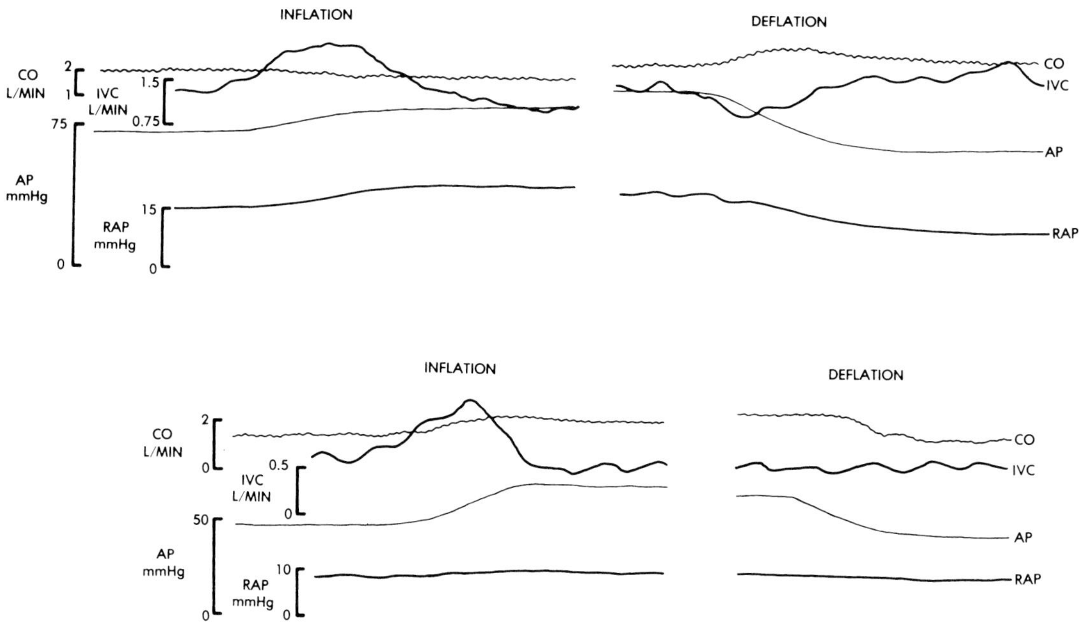

Fig. 4-5. The phasic pressure and flow data shown in this figure were obtained in an anesthetized swine instrumented with an aortic flow probe for measuring cardiac output (C.O.), a flowprobe inserted into the inferior vena cava (IVC), and pressure transducers in the proximal aorta (AP) and right atrium (RAP). A pneumatic antishock garment especially designed for application to a large swine was applied around the animal's lower trunk and hind legs. The upper panel shows pressure and flow transients associated with abrupt inflation and deflation of the pneumatic antishock garment. A bolus of blood is translocated through the inferior vena cava into the heart (equivalent to about 2 mL/kg, or 100 mL total), but cardiac output actually falls. Possibly this is due to an increase in arterial impedance caused by the external compression. The lower panel shows the effects of inflating the pneumatic antishock garment after 50% of the animal's circulating blood volume is removed: both cardiac output and aortic pressure rise. Reprinted with permission from Bellamy RF, DeGuzman LR, Pedersen DC. Immediate hemodynamic consequences of MAST inflation in normo- and hypovolemic anesthetized swine. *J Trauma*. 1984;24:892.

tions of improved tissue oxygenation in the presence of hypovolemic shock are unrealistic: hemoglobin oxygen saturation in the typical young combat casualty—who is usually hyperventilating because of the injury—is already maximal. Furthemore, the added amount of dissolved oxygen in the plasma caused by breathing supplemental oxygen is too small to be of importance. Until the circulating blood volume is restored, supplemental oxygen is unlikely to reverse the anaerobic metabolism in poorly perfused tissues.

Therapeutic Hypothermia

Reductions in body temperature are associated with a reduced metabolic rate: approximately 13% for every 1°C decrease in temperature.[47] In addition, oxygen solubility in plasma increases at reduced temperatures. Thus, hypothermia (< 37°C) may be beneficial in reducing oxygen consumption in individuals with reduced oxygen-carrying capacity if blood transfusion cannot be provided, but this approach to managing the seriously injured combat casualty can only be considered speculative.

Intraarterial Infusion

Intraarterial infusion was advocated during the Korean War because it appeared to provide the potential for more-rapid volume replacement, compared with the intravenous routes then being used. However, clinical evidence failed to show any significant advantage of this route over more conventional intravenous approaches, and its complexity argues against its use today.

Vasopressors

Efforts to support the arterial blood pressure through the administration of vasoconstrictors are mentioned here only to be condemned. Intense vasoconstriction is the typical homeostatic response to hemorrhagic shock and may be primarily responsible for the adverse consequences of hypovolemia (eg, acidosis, tissue hypoxia). Pharmacological support of the blood pressure with vasoconstrictors will only aggravate the reduction in tissue perfusion by decreasing cardiac output, and will contribute to the progressive acidosis. The benefits of transiently supporting the blood pressure with vasoconstrictors, until volume replacement or control of bleeding is possible, have not been carefully evaluated.

Vasodilators

At face value, the administration of vasodilators to a hypovolemic patient would seem to be grossly inappropriate. However, numerous animal studies[19–21]—using fixed-pressure shock models of the Wigger's type, involving the use of epidural anesthesia or the administration of adrenergic antagonists in the presence of hemorrhagic shock—have demonstrated both reductions in the severity of the systemic acidosis and improved survival. The beneficial effects of sympathetic antagonism are related to a reversal of the reflex vasoconstriction associated with hypovolemia. Tissue oxygenation and perfusion, albeit reduced, are maintained at levels adequate to reduce the progression of the acidosis. However, the beneficial application of central neuraxis anesthesia has not rigorously been evaluated in the clinical setting. Case reports have appeared in the literature; however, it is impossible to draw valid conclusions based on a limited number of uncontrolled reports. Conventional wisdom has dictated the avoidance of spinal and epidural anesthesia in hypovolemic and bleeding patients. Further study clearly is needed.

CONDITIONS PECULIAR TO RESUSCITATING COMBAT CASUALTIES

The conditions of the battlefield, which are so unlike those encountered in civilian practice, can create unique problems for military anesthesiologists. Not only are combat injuries quite different from those encountered in civilian practice, but the propensity for environmental hazards to become important sources of comorbidity must also be kept in mind.

Hyperthermia and Dehydration

Military conflicts frequently occur under adverse climatic conditions. Elevated ambient temperatures, physical exertion, and inadequate supplies on the battlefield can combine to contribute to the development of heat injury and dehydration. Coincident trauma and hemorrhage in the setting of preexisting dehydration and volume contraction will adversely influence survival. Elevated body temperature and hypotension will accelerate the progression to renal failure and contribute to the development of rhabdomyolysis. Rapid replacement of the intravascular and extracellular fluid space with isotonic, balanced, salt solutions is key to reversing this life-threatening process. Hyperoncotic colloid or hypertonic saline solutions are relatively contraindicated in casualties suffering from dehydration. The hyperosmotic state will adversely impact on glomerular filtration and further deplete the extracellular and intracellular fluid spaces.

Hypothermia

Hypothermia is a common problem afflicting trauma victims. The pathophysiology of hypothermia affects virtually all organ systems, and is discussed in detail in Chapter 28, Systemic Hypothermia. Profound hypothermia (core temperature < 30°C) is associated with substantial reductions in renal blood flow (75%) and glomerular filtration.[48,49] Despite this, profoundly hypothermic victims become progressively dehydrated due to a cold-induced diuresis secondary to defective tubular reabsorption. The urine produced is usually dilute, contributing to the development of a relatively hyperosmotic serum. Temperatures below 30°C are associated with ventricular fibrillation. Hyperkalemia and hyponatremia frequently occur with hypothermia; however, specific treatment is seldom necessary. Restoration of fluid deficits with warm hypotonic solutions (lactated Ringer's) is generally all that is required. Metabolic acidosis frequently develops as the patient is rewarmed. Fluid resuscitation to restore and maintain perfusion will correct the acidotic state; however, some may choose to treat with intravenous sodium bicarbonate. Colloids and hypertonic solutions are relatively contraindicated in this hyperosmotic state.

Thermal Burns

Fortunately, extensive burns are uncommon combat injuries in land warfare. They are much more common as nonbattle injuries:

> [A]lthough the incidence of combat-related burns has historically been about 3%, in recent wars the incidence is higher because mechanized modern warfare—tanks and other armored vehicles—actually places soldiers at higher risk [than previously] of being burned.... During the Yom Kippur War, burns comprised 10.5% of all injuries; during the Falkland Island Conflict, 18% of British casualties were burned. Furthermore, medical officers should know that in the United States military, burns and inhalation injuries have always been far more important sources of morbidity and mortality in both the navy and the air force than in the army.[50(p350)]

The fluid management of burn victims has been well described elsewhere[51] (also see Chapter 22, Burn Injuries) and will only briefly be discussed here. Ordinarily, burns involving more than 15% of the total body surface area will require intravenous fluid therapy. A number of treatment protocols have been developed to predict fluid requirements in the immediate and delayed phases of injury. However, as with any regimen, any given patient may require more or less fluid. Parameters of adequate organ perfusion (eg, urinary output) provide the most accurate indicators with which to guide fluid therapy.

Most authorities divide the fluid resuscitation of burned patients into two phases: the initial 24 hours and after the initial 24 hours. During the initial 24 hours, burn victims experience a generalized increase in capillary permeability that involves, in addition to the burned areas, normal capillary beds. This increased permeability has led some authorities[52,53] to suggest that colloid solutions be avoided in most patients during the initial 8 to 24 hours; the concern is that protein loss into the extracellular space will accelerate edema formation.[51] This effect is particularly evident during the initial 24-hour period. Isotonic crystalloids will lead to interstitial edema, but they also improve glomerular filtration and allow for replacement of evaporative losses. Hypertonic solutions have been touted to maintain the intravascular compartment with minimal edema.[40] However, careful monitoring of serum sodium is necessary to avoid hypernatremia. In the absence of data demonstrating a clear improvement in survival with any particular solution, it is reasonable to emphasize the use of isotonic crystalloids during the initial 24 hours after the burn. The revised Brooke formula[54] recommends administering 2 mL of lactated Ringer's solution per kilogram of body weight per percentage of total body surface area burned. Of the amount estimated to be required during the first phase, one half should be administered during the initial 8 hours, with the remaining volume dispersed over the next 16 hours. The Rule of Nines[55] is a useful indicator for estimating the percentage of body surface area burned:

- head and neck, 9%;
- anterior and posterior trunk, 18% each;
- upper extremities, 9% each;
- lower extremities, 18% each; and
- perineum, 1%.

After the initial 24 hours, colloid solutions are clearly beneficial for restoring the plasma oncotic pressure. Plasma proteins continue to be lost, not only into the burned areas but also owing to dilution and the patient's general catabolic state. Albumin solutions should be administered to maintain the plasma albumin concentration at 2.0 to 2.5 g/dL to support the plasma oncotic pressure.[51] Evaporative losses may be replaced with hypotonic dextrose solutions during this period. During this second phase, the requirement for sodium replacement generally declines and the risk of hypernatremia arises secondary to free-water loss via evaporation and urine.

Hemorrhagic Shock and Head Injury

Severe head injury coexisting with hypovolemic shock is an ominous combination (this subject is discussed in greater detail in Chapter 16, Neurological Injuries). Cerebral edema or compression by an expanding intracranial hematoma, or both, produce an elevation in intracranial pressure. Hypotension secondary to hemorrhage contributes to further decline in the cerebral perfusion pressure and thereby potentiates ischemic injury. Improvement of the mean arterial pressure with fluid resuscitation may lead to further increases in intracranial pressure, secondary to increased cerebral blood volume and progressive cerebral edema. Resuscitation with hypotonic fluids, especially dextrose solutions, is contraindicated. Unfortunately, lactated Ringer's solution is relatively hypotonic and may contribute to increased cerebral edema. Colloid solutions have been advocated; however, with diffuse injuries, the blood–brain barrier may be damaged, contributing to interstitial leakage of colloid and worsening edema in the area of injury. Because of their adverse interactions with the coagulation system, the dextrans and hetastarch solutions must be used with caution in the setting of intracranial hemorrhage. Isotonic crystalloid solution (0.9% NaCl) does not accelerate brain edema and may be the optimal resuscitation fluid.[28]

The Chemically Contaminated Casualty

Although the anesthetic management of casualties of chemical warfare agents is discussed in detail in Chapter 30, Anesthesia for Casualties of Chemical Warfare Agents, and elsewhere, several brief points on the fluid management of the chemically injured casualty will be outlined here. The risk of exposure to chemical weapons continues to persist throughout the world, particularly in third-world nations, as witnessed by the use of chemical weapons on civilian and military targets during the Iran–Iraq War. Combat casualties in high-risk chemical environments may present a confusing diagnostic picture if chemical protective treatments (atropine, pyridostigmine) have been used. Atropine-induced tachycardia and the associated autonomic effects may present a picture easily confused with hypovolemia. Certain incapacitating agents (eg, quinuclidinyl benzylate) may produce similar effects. Pyridostigmine, an acetylcholinesterase inhibitor, was provided to many troops as a chemical protectant during the Persian Gulf War. Pyridostigmine tends to produce bradycardia and may adversely interact with the compensatory response to hemorrhage.

Fluid replacement is an important component in the management of blister agents (ie, mustard). Casualties exposed to blister agents may present with considerable cutaneous denuding and subsequent fluid loss. Treatment requires aggressive fluid management, similar to the treatment of thermal burns. Choking agents (eg, phosgene, chlorine), which may cause alveolar capillary injury, represent the opposite end of the spectrum, in that strict fluid management is needed to avoid contributing to the development of noncardiac pulmonary edema. Because careful fluid management may not be easily accomplished in patients with multiple trauma who are also exposed to choking agents, supportive therapy, including mechanical ventilation, may be needed in this population.

SUMMARY

Combat injuries associated with hemodynamic instability should be regarded as hypovolemic until proven otherwise. The rapid attainment of large-bore venous access and the initiation of fluid resuscitation should occur simultaneously with evaluation of the casualty's injuries. The administration of fluids—colloid or crystalloid—should be guided by the normalization of hemodynamic indices and especially by evidence of good peripheral perfusion (eg, high urinary output). Coexisting medical concerns peculiar to the battlefield may create confusion in the interpretation of the physiological response to intervention. Military healthcare providers must be aware of the medical implications associated with environmental and chemical concerns of the combat theater.

REFERENCES

1. Gamble JL. *Chemical Anatomy, Physiology, and Pathology of Extracellular Fluid*. 6th ed. Boston, Mass: Harvard University Press; 1954.

2. Starling EH. On the absorption of fluids from the connective tissue spaces. *J Physiol*. 1896;9:312.

3. Shires T, Coln D, Carrico J, et al. Fluid therapy in hemorrhagic shock. *Arch Surg*. 1964;88:688–693.

4. Giesecke AH, Egbert LD. Perioperative fluid therapy. In: Miller R, ed. *Anesthesia*. New York, NY: Churchill Livingstone; 1985: 1313–1328.

5. Lichtenstein A, Eckhart WF, Swanson KJ, et al. Unplanned intraoperative and postoperative hemodilution: Oxygen transport and consumption during severe anemia. *Anesthesiology*. 1988;69:119–122.

6. Mendelson JA. The use of whole blood as blood volume expanders in US military medical facilities in Vietnam 1966–1971. *J Trauma*. 1975;15:1–13.

7. Crosby WH. Acute anemia in the severely wounded battle casualty. *Milit Med.* 1988;153:25–27.

8. Beecher HK, ed. The Board for the Study of the Severely Wounded, North African–Mediterranean Theater of Operations. *The Physiologic Effects of Wounds.* In: *Surgery in World War II.* Washington, DC: US Army Medical Department, Office of The Surgeon General; 1952: 34.

9. Vayer JS, Henderson JV, Bellamy RF, Calper AR. Absence of a tachycardia response to shock in penetrating intraperitoneal injury. *Ann Emerg Med.* 1988;17:227–231.

10. Scolea TM, Holman M, Fuortes M, et al. Central venous blood oxygen saturation: An early, accurate measurement of volume during hemorrhage. *J Trauma.* 1988;28:725–732.

11. Scott WL. Complications associated with central venous catheters. *Chest.* 1988;94:1221–1224.

12. Committee on Trauma, American College of Surgeons. *Advanced Trauma Life Support Program for Physicians: Instructor Manual.* 5th ed. Chicago, Ill: American College of Surgeons; 1993.

13. Glover JL, Broadie TA. Intraoperative autotransfusion. *World J Surg.* 1987;11:60–64.

14. Fiser DH. Intraosseous infusion. *N Engl J Med.* 1990;322:1579–1581.

15. Halvorsen L, Bay BK, Perron PR, Holcroft JW, Blaisdell FW, Kramer, GC. Evaluation of an intraosseous infusion device for the resuscitation of hypovolemic shock. *J Trauma.* 1990;30:652–658.

16. Rosetti VA, Thompson DM, Miller J, et al. Intraosseous infusion: An alternative route of pediatric intravascular access. *Ann Emerg Med.* 1985;14:885–888.

17. Papper EM. Bone marrow route for injecting fluids and drugs into general circulation. *Anesthesiology.* 1942;3:307.

18. Lellehei RC, Longerbeam JK, Bloch JH, et al. The nature of irreversible shock: Experimental and clinical observations. *Ann Surg.* 1964;160:682–710.

19. Shibata K, Yamamoto Y, Murakami S. Effects of epidural anesthesia on cardiovascular response and survival in experimental hemorrhagic shock in dogs. *Anesthesiology.* 1990;71:953–959.

20. Gould L, Ettinger S, Carmichael A, et al. The use of phentolamine in experimental hemorrhagic shock. *Angiology.* 1970;21:330–335.

21. Da Luz PL, Shubin H, Weil MH. Effectiveness of phentolamine for reversal of circulatory failure. *Crit Care Med.* 1973;1:135–140.

22. King WH, Patten ED, Bee DE. An in vitro evaluation of ionized calcium levels and clotting in red blood cells diluted with lactated Ringer's solution. *Anesthesiology.* 1988;68:115–121.

23. Lanier WL, Stangland KJ, Scheithauer BW, et al. The effects of dextrose infusion and head position on neurologic outcome after complete cerebral ischemia in primates: Examination of a model. *Anesthesiology.* 1987;66:39–48.

24. Pulsinelli WA, Levy DE, Sigsbee B, et al. Increased damage after ischemic stroke in patients with hyperglycemia with or without diabetes mellitus. *Am J Med.* 1983;74:540–544.

25. Prough DS, Coker LH, Lee S, et al. Hyperglycemia and neurologic outcome in patients with closed head injury. *Anesthesiology.* 1988;69:A584.

26. Rainey, TG, English JF. Pharmacology of colloids and crystalloids. In: Chernaw B, ed. *The Pharmacologic Approach to the Critically Ill Patient.* 2nd ed. Baltimore, Md: Williams & Wilkins; 1988: Chap 12: 219–240.

27. Haupt MT. The use of crystalloidal and colloidal solutions for volume replacement in hypovolemic shock. *Crit Rev Clin Lab Sci.* 1989;27:1–26.

28. Kaieda R, Todd MM, Warner DS. Prolonged reduction in colloid oncotic pressure does not increase brain edema following cryogenic injury in rabbits. *Anesthesiology*. 1989;71:554–560.

29. Quon CY. Clinical pharmacokinetics and pharmacodynamics of colloidal plasma volume expanders. *J Cardiothoracic Anesth*. 1988;2:13–23.

30. Lamke LO, Liljedahl SO. Plasma volume expansion after infusion of 5%, 20%, and 25% albumin solutions in patients. *Resuscitation*. 1976;5:85–92.

31. Mailoux L, Swartz CD, Capizzi R, et al. Acute renal failure after administration of LMW dextran. *N Engl J Med*. 1967;277:1113–1118.

32. Weiss HJ. The effect of clinical dextran on platelet aggregation, adhesion, and ADP release in man: In vivo and in vitro studies. *J Lab Clin Med*. 1967;69:37–46.

33. Mishler JM. Synthetic plasma volume expanders—Their pharmacology, safety and clinical efficacy. *Clinics in Haematology*. 1984;13:75–92.

34. Cully MD, Larson CP, Silverberg GD. Hetastarch coagulopathy in a neurosurgical patient. *Anesthesiology*. 1987;66:706.

35. Wade CE, Hannon JP, Bossone CA, et al. *Resuscitation of Conscious Pigs Following Hemorrhage: Comparative Efficacy of Small-Volume Resuscitation with Normal Saline, 7.5% NaCl, 6% Dextran 70, and 7.5% NaCl in 6% Dextran 70*. San Francisco, Calif: Letterman Army Institute of Research, US Department of the Army; 1988. Institute Report 305.

36. Holcroft JW, Vassar MJ, Turner GC, et al. 3% NaCl and 7.5% NaCl/dextran 70 in the resuscitation of severely injured patients. *Ann Surg*. 1987;206:279–287.

37. Maningas PA, Mattox KL, Pepe PE, et al. Hypertonic saline–dextran solutions for the prehospital management of traumatic hypotension. *Am J Surg*. 1989;157:528–533.

38. Vassar MJ, Perry CA, Holcroft JW. Prehospital resuscitation of hypotensive trauma patients with 7.5% NaCl versus 7.5% NaCl with added dextran: A controlled trial. *J Trauma*. 1993;34(5):622–633.

39. Vassar MJ, Fischer RP, O'Brien PE, et al. A multicenter trial for resuscitation of injuried patients with 7.5% sodium chloride. *Arch Surg*. 1993;128:1003–1013.

40. Monafo WW, Halverson JD, Schectman K. The role of concentrated sodium solutions in the resuscitation of patients with severe burns. *Surgery*. 1984;95:129–134.

41. Prough DS, Johnson JC, Stump DA, et al. Effects of hypertonic saline versus lactated Ringer's solution on cerebral oxygen transport during resuscitation from hemorrhagic shock. *J Neurosurg*. 1986;64:627–632.

42. Gross D, Landau EH, Klin B, et al. Quantitative measurement of bleeding following hypertonic saline therapy in "uncontrolled" hemorrhagic shock. *J Trauma*. 1989;29:79–83.

43. Taylor J, Weil MH. Failure of the Trendelenburg position to improve circulation during clinical shock. *Surg Gynecol Obstet*. 1967;124:1005–1010.

44. Bivins HG, Knoop R, dos Santos PA. Blood volume distribution in the Trendelenburg position. *Ann Emerg Med*. 1985;14:641–643.

45. Zippe C, Burchard K, Gann D. Trendelenburg versus PASG application in moderate hemorrhagic hypoperfusion. *J Trauma*. 1985;25:923–931.

46. Mattox KL, Bickell W, Pepe PE, et al. Prospective MAST study in 911 patients. *J Trauma*. 1989;29:1104.

47. Michenfelder JD, Uihlein A, Daw EF, et al. Moderate hypothermia in man: Haemodynamic and metabolic effects. *Br J Anaesth*. 1965;37:738–745.

48. Vandam, LD, Burnap, TK. Hypothermia. *N Engl J Med.* 1959;261:546.

49. Hervey GR. Hypothermia. *Proc R Soc Med.* 1973;66:1055.

50. Cioffi WG, Rue LW, Buescher TM, Pruitt BA. The management of burn injury. In: Bellamy RF, Zajtchuk R, eds. *Conventional Warfare: Ballistic, Blast, and Burn Injuries.* Part 1, Vol 5. In: Zajtchuk R, Bellamy RF, eds. *Textbook of Military Medicine.* Washington, DC: US Department of the Army, Office of The Surgeon General, and Borden Institute; 1991: 350.

51. Demling RH. Fluid replacement in burned patients. *Surg Clin North Am.* 1987;67:15–30.

52. Baxter CR. Fluid volume and electrolyte changes in the early post-burn period. *Clin Plast Surg.* 1974;1:693–709.

53. Demling RH, Kramer GC, Gunther R, et al. Effect of non-protein colloid on post-burn edema formation in soft tissues and lung. *Surgery.* 1984;95:593–602.

54. Reiss E, Stirmon JA, Artz CP, Davis JH, Amspacher WH. Fluid and electrolyte balance in burns. *JAMA.* 1953;152:1309.

55. Bowen TE, Bellamy RF, eds. *Emergency War Surgery NATO Handbook.* 2nd rev US ed. Washington, DC: Department of Defense, Government Printing Office; 1988: 37.

Chapter 5

PHYSIOLOGICAL MONITORING

HERMAN V. DeVERA, M.D.*

*Formerly, Lieutenant Colonel, Medical Corps, U.S. Army; Department of Anesthesiology, Walter Reed Army Medical Center, Washington, D. C. 20307-5001; currently, Chief, Anesthesia Services, South Valley Hospital, 9400 No Name Uno, Gilroy, California 95020

INTRODUCTION

Physiological monitoring of combat casualties is often compared unfavorably with monitoring as it is done in civilian trauma situations. However, those who make this comparison are usually not cognizant of the significant differences between the management of trauma in civilian versus military settings. Especially important are the severe constraints that logistics place on the availability of monitoring equipment and the vulnerability of sophisticated monitors to the rough-and-tumble environment of combat zone hospitals. Another important difference is the number of casualties needing care: mass casualties are all too common in wartime.

The type of monitoring for anesthesia and surgery in the field depends on the echelon of care (the casualty flow through the echelons of care is illustrated on page xv in the opening pages of this book). The spectrum extends from the austerity of the battalion aid station (first echelon) and the medical company (second echelon) through the intermediate capability of mobile army surgical and combat support hospitals (third echelon) to the complexity found in general hospitals and in medical centers in the continental United States (fourth echelon).

Another factor determining the sophistication or even the possibility of monitoring will be the number of casualties requiring care. Obviously, the number of casualties is beyond the control of an individual medical unit. In a mass casualty situation, the overriding goal will be to use the available monitoring resources to do the greatest good for the largest number of casualties. The goal of monitoring then becomes one of deciding who needs monitoring and which monitoring devices to use. The standards of care seen in medical centers, or even in small community hospitals, in the continental United States may have to be altered to conform to the reality of the battlefield. Although the standards applied on the battlefield may be unfamiliar to those trained in a modern medical facility equipped with the latest technical devices, this does not mean that medical care in the field is inadequate.

Military trauma anesthesiologists must resist the tendency to become dependent on sophisticated devices such as monitors. Extremes of temperature; delays; and damage to equipment due to transport, dust, or other environmental conditions may all require innovative approaches to monitoring the combat casualty. Flexibility in using more basic (low-tech) monitors is also desirable. The U.S. Army Medical Department should ensure that anesthesia care providers play a role in helping logisticians decide which equipment should be available in field hospitals.

This chapter is divided into two sections. The first deals with the type of monitoring likely to be found in medical treatment facilities from the first through the fourth echelons; the second section deals with the monitors used to evaluate the various body systems. Wherever possible, the principles of monitoring are related to the practical aspects of field anesthesia care.

MONITORS IN THE ECHELONS OF CARE

The monitors that military anesthesia providers can expect to find vary with the level of care from austere through intermediate to complex (Table 5-1). Each unit will, no doubt, modify the list of equipment supplied. Specifically, individual military trauma anesthesiologists will likely go to considerable lengths to obtain (from their colleagues) monitoring equipment not officially included in their units' Table of Organization and Equipment.

First and Second Echelons

Austere conditions prevail at unit- and division-level medical facilities of the first and second echelons as well as forward surgical teams deployed below corps. Although only the most basic devices for monitoring casualties will be found at these levels of care, initial surgery to make the casualty transportable may be necessary. Ideal circumstances would allow monitoring of pulse, ventilation, oxygenation, and blood pressure during monitored anesthesia care or general or regional anesthesia. However, in austere battlefield conditions, general anesthesia will be provided in emergent situations only, and will most likely be provided via the draw-over system and not the portable anesthesia machine. Most monitoring will be for procedures carried out with local or possibly some form of regional anesthesia.

Monitoring at the first and second echelons may consist of recording only vital signs (blood pressure, respirations, and heart rate) and the physical examination. The monitoring equipment available, which needs to be sturdy and transportable, may be

TABLE 5-1

RECOMMENDED EQUIPMENT AVAILABILITY AND MONITORS REQUIRED

Equipment Available	Physiological Parameter	Monitor Required
Austere (First and second echelons)	Hemodynamics	Manual blood pressure cuff Precordial stethoscope
	Temperature	Thermometer
Intermediate (Third echelon)	Hemodynamics	Blood pressure Precordial stethoscope Electrocardiograph
	Temperature	Thermometer
	Urinary output	Foley catheter Specific gravity Sodium concentration
	Respiration	Pulse oximeter
	Blood components	Laboratory analyses (hematocrit, electrolytes, blood urea nitrogen, creatinine, prothrombin time/partial thromboplastin time, whole-blood clotting time, activated clotting time)
	Other	Nerve stimulator Oxygen analyzer Capnography
Complex (Fourth echelon and higher)	Hemodynamics	Blood pressure Precordial stethoscope Electrocardiograph A-line Central venous pressure Pulmonary artery catheter
	Temperature	Thermometer
	Urinary output	Foley catheter Specific gravity Sodium concentration
	Respiration, airway pressure, lung compliance	Pulse oximeter Ventilator pressure gauges
	Blood components	Laboratory analyses (hematocrit, electrolytes, blood urea nitrogen, creatinine, prothrombin time/partial thromboplastin time, whole-blood clotting time, activated clotting time)
	Other	Nerve stimulator Oxygen analyzer Capnography, Doppler

limited to a manual blood pressure cuff and a stethoscope. Whether pulse oximetry can be used will most likely be determined by the availability of electricity to run or charge the equipment. Pulse oximetry would be highly valuable at first- and second-level medical treatment facilities.

If there is a threat that the enemy will use chemical or biological agents, both the providers of care and the casualties are in full mission-oriented protective posture (MOPP) gear. Obviously, any monitoring, other than possibly a cursory mental-status examination, may have to wait until the casualty has been decontaminated. Ambient noise may limit the use of the stethoscope to just determining the presence of heart sounds.

Blood pressure may have to be taken by merely documenting the point at which the systolic pressure becomes palpable or the needle on the aneroid manometer begins to bounce. (Blood pressure can be measured by inflating a manual cuff and slowly letting the cuff deflate while watching for the needle on the manometer to begin to bounce; this correlates with the point at which one can begin to feel the pulse.) This quick, accurate means of monitoring blood pressure may be the only method practicable. The bouncing needle on the sphygmomanometer also allows the observer to form an impression of the patient's heart rate. Heart rate can be counted by either listening with a stethoscope or by taking the pulse. Subtle signs, such as threadiness of pulse and crispness of heart sounds, may provide information about the casualty's volume status.

Third Echelon

The intermediate level of care includes mobile army surgical and combat support hospitals. This setting is more fixed than a medical company clearing station, but third-echelon hospitals must be somewhat mobile also. These hospitals are designed to perform resuscitative surgery. General anesthesia is available and, therefore, more elaborate monitoring equipment will be necessary. The equipment found at this level must be sturdy, able to withstand the multiple moves that may be required of a third-echelon hospital. Much of the equipment used in this setting may arrive by some expedient means (eg, being dropped by parachute from a cargo plane). For these reasons, it is unlikely that sensitive equipment such as mass spectroscopy or other highly sophisticated monitors will be seen at this level of care.

The portable anesthesia machine will probably not contain an automated ventilator with disconnection alarms. The only "monitor" for sensing disconnections of the anesthesia circuit will probably be the individual responsible for providing the manual ventilation. Equipment at this level should include electrocardiograph monitors, blood pressure cuffs, pulse oximetry, temperature-monitoring devices, and perhaps even some form of capnography. The anesthesia machines (Ohio Model 855A Field Anesthesia Machine, manufactured by Ohmeda, Inc., Madison, Wisc.) also should contain an oxygen analyzer.

Pulse oximetry provides such valuable information that it should also be included at this level. Although not standard equipment at this level, the pulse oximeter will often be added as supplementary equipment. The automated blood pressure cuff may or may not be present. It is unlikely that more than one or possibly two will be available—if present at all at this level of care. The manual blood pressure cuff will certainly find use at this level, whether in the operating room or in the recovery areas.

Devices to monitor the casualty's temperature should also be included at this level of care. Adhesive, disposable, skin-temperature monitors will be of little value at the third echelon. A more appropriate device is one able to measure axillary, oral, esophageal, or rectal temperatures. Monitoring of the skin temperature is unlikely to provide useful information in casualties who are either receiving large amounts of fluid or blood or are hypovolemic because of blood loss.

The ability to monitor end-tidal carbon dioxide ($ETCO_2$) can be very useful, not only for verifying endotracheal intubation but also for monitoring carbon dioxide levels in casualties with head trauma. Currently, these monitors are somewhat large and are unlikely to be added as supplementary equipment. With improved technology and as they become more compact, capnographs will no doubt be added even at the third echelon.

One additional method of providing anesthesia that allows significant monitoring of the casualty's respiratory status (including oxygen requirements) is the use of closed-circuit anesthesia. This method of providing anesthesia has many advantages:

- Changes in the patient's oxygen utilization are readily apparent.
- Oxygen waste is minimized (rather than flows of 3–5 L/min, flows of 250–350 mL/min or less are used).
- The use of a sophisticated vaporizer requiring calibration and high oxygen flows to provide accurate delivery of anesthetic agent is omitted; the potent anesthetic agent can be delivered by merely introducing a syringe containing a volatile anesthetic into the breathing circuit.
- The total amount of inhalational anesthetic agent used is decreased. This can be a most significant factor if supplies are short.

The disadvantages of the use of this method of providing anesthesia are few. It behooves providers of anesthesia, particularly those in the military, to become familiar with this technique. Although it may appear to be more time consuming (because recent graduates of anesthesia training programs lack familiarity with this technique), this technique may be safer and more appropriate than the conventional vaporizer technique when supplies of oxygen are short or when vaporizers are broken or uncalibrated. Extremes of ambient temperature (eg, in the desert) may also make the closed-circuit anesthesia delivery technique more desirable (see Chapter 8, Closed-Circuit Anesthesia, for a more complete discussion of this subject).

Fourth Echelon and Higher

Complex levels of equipment are found at fourth and higher echelons of care, including hospital ships and hospitals along the chain of evacuation from the theater of operations. The sophistication of monitoring equipment is more like what anesthesia providers would expect to see at a civilian or military community hospital or small medical center. These are fixed facilities and would be unlikely to move, once set up (the obvious exception being the hospital ship). For this reason, more-elaborate monitoring is likely to be found. At fourth and higher echelons of care, automated blood pressure cuffs, pulse oximeters, automated ventilators with disconnection alarms, capnographs, and invasive hemodynamic monitoring devices (ie, arterial and central lines for measuring central venous and pulmonary artery pressure) will all be found.

The use of these invasive monitoring devices will, of necessity, depend on not only the individual patient's clinical situation but also on the number of casualties requiring treatment. The great majority of casualties will already have received resuscitative surgery at mobile surgical or combat support hospitals; monitoring will be employed either in difficult emergency cases requiring reoperative surgery or, as is more common, in elective reconstructive operations. An inordinate amount of time cannot be spent placing invasive monitors in all casualties; nor is sophisticated monitoring necessary in most operations (eg, delayed primary closure of soft-tissue wounds or reestablishment of gastrointestinal continuity). The intensity of monitoring will have to be tailored to the needs of the casualty. This philosophy, which is inherent in military triage, is likely to be unfamiliar to most civilian personnel, who are accustomed to providing all the care that *can* be done, not just what *must* be done.

SYSTEMIC MONITORING

Anesthesia care providers will be faced with difficult decisions regarding which monitors are practical and necessary at the various echelons of care. The decision regarding what monitoring devices to have available should be based on the level of care to be provided, the expected needs of the casualties, the durability of the equipment, and the storage capability and mobility of the equipment.

Hemostasis and Coagulation

The first step in monitoring for hemostasis is the evaluation of blood loss. This can be done by directly measuring the volume of blood in the suction containers that were used to draw blood from the operative field. Weighing, or estimating the weight of, used surgical sponges is another method of accounting for surgical blood loss. Besides monitoring for vascular integrity, monitoring of the coagulation system is also necessary.

Determining platelet count and function can easily be done at both the intermediate and complex levels of care. A platelet count of 50,000 to 75,000 normal, functioning platelets may be inadequate for intraoperative hemostasis. The Ivy bleeding time test is used to measure platelet function. The test is performed by making a standard, 9-mm–long incision on the volar surface of the forearm while an inflated blood pressure cuff on that arm is maintained at 40 mm Hg. The elapsed time required for bleeding to stop is known as the bleeding time. Normal bleeding times vary between 5 and 8 minutes.[1]

Several methods are available for monitoring coagulation as well as for monitoring the coagulation status of casualties who have received therapeutic anticoagulation drugs. These methods include (1) heparin level measurements; (2) protamine titration; (3) activated clotting times; and (4) other tests such as prothrombin time, thrombin time, fibrinogen levels, and fibrin split product levels.

Heparin, a mucopolysaccharide, acts by stimulating the enzymatic activity of antithrombin III, which inactivates the serine proteases in the coagulation scheme (factors II, VII, IX, and X). Approximately one individual in 2,000 has a physical condition (eg, liver disease, pregnancy, debilitating illness) that depresses the antithrombin III level; therefore, that individual may not respond to heparin. Serum levels of antithrombin III can be depressed by a variety of conditions; such deficiency may be responsible for as many as 2% of clinical cases of venous thrombosis.[2]

Devices used to estimate heparin level include the automated protamine titration system and fluorometric analysis. The automated protamine titration method (Hepcon, manufactured by HemoTec, Inc., Englewood, Colo.) uses protamine titration to estimate heparin levels. Advantages of this method include (1) the rapidity of obtaining results, (2) the ease of use, and (3) the reliability of the results. The disadvantages are (1) the cartridges expire in a short time (60 d) and (2) the reagents require refrigeration.

The Hemochron system (manufactured by Technidyne Corp, Edison, N.J.)—a simple, reliable, automated activated clotting time test—was introduced during the mid-1970s; (unfortunately, however, it is not available in field hospitals). A normal baseline activated clotting time is 110 to 130 seconds. A low baseline should alert the anesthesia provider to a hypercoagulable state. Activated clotting times between 300 and 600 seconds are acceptable for cardiopulmonary bypass to be initiated. There is a linear relationship between the activated clotting time and the milligram per kilogram heparin dose for any given patient.[3] Determining the adequacy of protamine reversal is one area in which heparin-level tests may be more useful. Although plotting the heparin dose against the activated clotting time can be used to determine the protamine-reversal dose, the difficulty arises when the clotting time remains elevated after the protamine has been given. The reasons for this can be (1) continued excess heparin or (2) a derangement of the coagulation system. The usual clinical response is to give an additional dose of protamine. If the activated clotting time remains the same or is elevated further, then a coagulopathy should be suspected.

Physiological monitoring of the hematological system in the first echelon of care will be very basic. Accuracy in the evaluation of the nonmechanical bleeding can be obtained with a whole-blood clotting time. Decreased clotting factors should be suspected if whole blood does not clot within 15 minutes. Measurements of prothrombin, partial prothrombin, and bleeding time should be available at the third or fourth echelons. The ability to measure activated clotting time intraoperatively would also be useful. This approach should be considered when logisticians are determining which monitoring devices to include for each unit that provides complex care.

Cardiovascular System

Physical examination will remain a mainstay in the evaluation of the casualty's cardiovascular system. Assessment should include mental status examination, presence of nausea or vomiting, capillary refill, vital signs, coolness of extremities, and so forth. Other, more-direct monitors of the cardiovascular system include methods to monitor blood pressure and central venous pressure, and monitors of the heart for rhythm and ischemia.

Blood Pressure

Noninvasive Monitoring. Depending on the equipment available, blood pressure can be monitored by several noninvasive methods:

- Doppler technique,
- oscillations of an aneroid manometer during deflation of a manual cuff,
- return of tactile pulses during deflation of a manual cuff,
- auscultatory method using Korotkoff's sounds, and
- automated blood pressure devices.

Of these, the first three monitor only systolic pressures; the others, in addition, monitor diastolic and mean pressures.

The simplest way to detect systolic blood pressure is to palpate the pulse while an occluding cuff is deflating. A modification of this technique involves watching for oscillations of the aneroid manometer during deflation of the occluding cuff.

Once, the most common technique for indirect manual measurement of blood pressure employed by anesthesia care providers in hospitals in the continental United States was the auscultatory method of using Korotkoff's sounds.[4] A stethoscope or an automatic blood pressure–monitoring device placed over an artery serves as a detector. Slightly more sophisticated detectors include a Doppler or other sound-amplifying device as a signal detector. By placing the ultrasonic Doppler device over the radial artery, the anesthesia provider detects blood flow by listening for the characteristic "swishing" sounds. The Doppler method utilizes a 10-Hz ultrasonic device coupled to a transducer/receiver assembly. This device detects the difference in frequency between transmitted and reflected sound in response to deflation of an occluding cuff. The Doppler signal is detected when blood flow causes movement of the arterial wall during systole. There is good correlation between measurement of systolic blood pressure via Doppler and direct arterial monitoring.[5] Ultrasonic gel (if available) will provide a helpful medium for transmitting sound. The blood pressure cuff on the patient's arm is inflated as above. As the cuff is slowly deflated, the point at which sounds are again heard correspond to the systolic pressure. The Doppler device may be useful

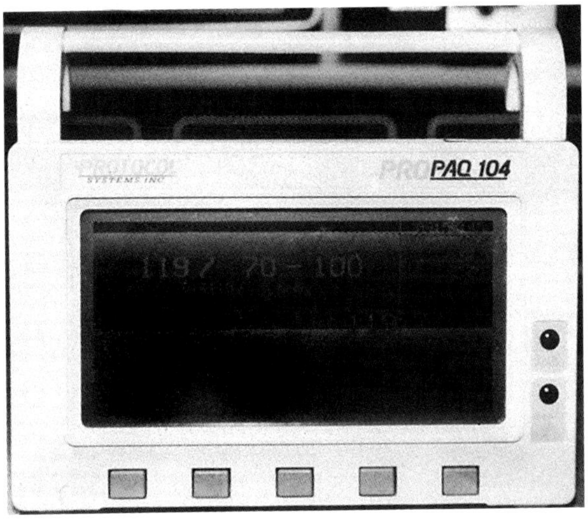

Fig. 5-1. This patient monitor, the PROPAC 104 (portable anesthesia circuit, manufactured by Protocol Systems, Inc., Beaverton, Ore.), has ports for noninvasive measurement of arterial blood pressure, electrical activity of the heart, and temperature, and has two additional pressure ports.

and should be considered as supplementary equipment for the intermediate and complex levels of care.

The automated oscillometric method for measuring blood pressure has become the most common method used by anesthesia care providers for noninvasive blood pressure monitoring. Its advantages over the techniques discussed above are its greater accuracy and ability to measure mean blood pressure. The devices manufactured currently employ an electric pump to generate the pressure required to inflate the occluding cuff. A microprocessor controls the cuff inflations and deflations. A solenoid valve allows incremental deflation of the cuff. The cuff also acts as the signal sensor that responds to oscillations in the limb. A pressure-sensing function is performed by a pressure transducer, and digital readout of the systolic, diastolic, and mean blood pressure is provided. Under ideal circumstances, the accuracy of these units compared with direct arterial measurements is usually within 10 mm Hg.[6] Problems in obtaining measurements occur when the patient moves, when there is substantial beat-to-beat variability in the blood pressure (eg, atrial fibrillation), and with very slow heart rates. Originally, automated oscillometric units were somewhat bulky and required electricity to operate. Newer units have backlit liquid crystal displays. In addition to their ability to monitor blood pressure noninvasively, many units currently manufactured are also capable of monitoring pulse oximetry and the heart's electrocardiographic status, and have transduced pressure-monitoring capability (Figure 5-1). These new units can run on alternating or direct current. They are compact, weighing just a few pounds, and are currently used in tertiary-care centers as transport monitors. In the future, we are likely to find these units at third, fourth, and higher echelons of combat casualty care.

Invasive Monitoring. The medical officer's ability to evaluate a casualty's arterial waveform is a major advantage of direct monitoring of arterial blood pressure in the trauma setting. The arterial waveform allows a qualitative assessment of the patient's blood volume status to be made. The area beneath the arterial waveform is affected by myocardial performance, systemic vascular resistance, and circulatory volume status. The more common sites of arterial cannulation are listed in Exhibit 5-1. Most studies reporting the complications of direct arterial cannulation involve the radial artery. Complications include decreased circulation, infection, vasospasm, thrombosis, embolism, aneurysm formation, and hematomas.

The necessity of performing an Allen's test before cannulation of the radial artery has been questioned.[7] The incidence of thrombosis of the radial artery relates to the size of the catheter used. One study[8] found a 34% incidence of thrombosis when a 18-gauge catheter was used, compared to an 8% prevalence when a 20-gauge catheter was used. The incidence of catheter thrombosis also increases with the duration of cannulation. The safety of brachial-

EXHIBIT 5-1

SITES OF ARTERIAL CANNULATION

End Arteries
- Brachial
- Femoral

Other Arteries
- Radial*
- Ulnar*
- Dorsalis pedis
- Axillary

* Cannulation of both arteries of the same arm is not recommended because of the risk of significant occlusion of blood flow to the hand.

and femoral-artery cannulations is established; they serve as other sites of direct arterial monitoring.[9,10]

The common way of measuring direct arterial pressure is to connect the indwelling arterial catheter to a transducer that converts hydrostatic pressure into movement of a thin diaphragm. Ultimately, this energy is converted into an electrical signal, which is amplified and converted to analog or digital signals or both. Digital readouts and analogue displays of waveforms can be viewed on small monitors. A useful invasive means of measuring mean blood pressure is to use a manometer connected to the arterial tubing (formerly connected to a transducer) (Figure 5-2). This method provides a means of monitoring the patient's mean blood pressure, which may be particularly useful during transport or when transducers become unavailable for whatever reason. This type of monitor has the disadvantages of only giving an analog display of the mean blood pressure. The arterial waveform cannot be viewed.

Central Venous and Pulmonary Artery Pressures. Central venous lines are used for several reasons,

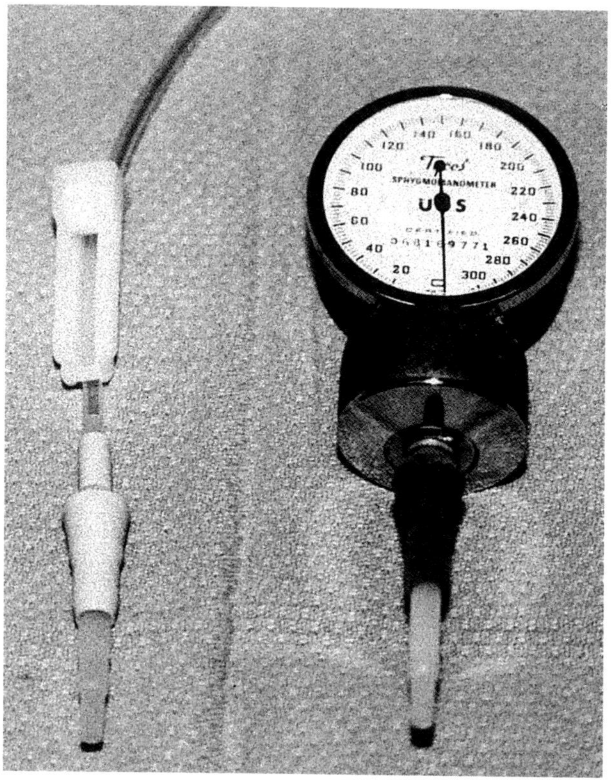

Fig. 5-2. A sphygmomanometer can be used as an ad hoc field blood pressure monitor, but only the mean pressure can be measured.

including perioperative administration and management of fluids in the critically ill patient, administration of vasoactive drugs, and obtaining blood samples. Central venous pressures can be monitored by using either pressure transducers or a water manometer.

Normal central venous pressure is between 0 and 5 mm Hg or 0 and 7 cm H_2O. Although it is unlikely, it is possible that central venous pressure monitoring will be used at the third echelon of care. At this level, saline-filled manometers may be used because pressure transducers will be in short supply. The saline-filled manometers are measured in centimeters of water (1 mm Hg is equal to 1.36 cm H_2O). Measurements are made at the level of the right atrium (the midaxillary line). This is considered the zero point (the point at which the zero on the manometer is positioned). In fixed facilities, where more-complex monitoring is available, central venous pressure can be monitored using a pressure transducer. This allows both an analog display of the central venous waveform and a digital readout of the pressures. One advantage of having the waveform displayed is that the right ventricular wave pattern can be differentiated from the right atrial wave pattern. This would be particularly useful in verifying correct location of the catheter tip.

The four most accessible sites available for the insertion of central venous pressure–monitoring lines are the internal or external jugular, subclavian, antecubital, and femoral veins. The right internal jugular approach is the one most commonly used for central vein catheterization. This is because it (*a*) provides a straight path to the right atrium; (*b*) provides a clean site (the incidence of thrombophlebitis is low); and, perhaps most importantly, it (*c*) is easily accessible to the anesthesia provider during the operative procedure. The external jugular approach requires the use of a guide wire with a J-tip to allow it to be maneuvered into the central circulation.

Although the pulmonary artery catheter is used in medical centers in the continental United States, it has not yet been *hardened* (miniaturized and/or made sufficiently sturdy) for battlefield use; therefore, this device is seen only infrequently at third-echelon hospitals. Pulmonary artery catheters require that pressure transducers be used to confirm placement. The same approaches that are used for placement of a central venous pressure line can be used for pulmonary artery catheter placement. The insertion and management of this device require experience with its use.

The uses of pulmonary artery catheters include

the following:

- hemodynamic monitoring of both central venous pressure and pulmonary artery pressures;
- monitoring of cardiac output via the thermodilution technique;
- evaluation of changes in compliance of the left ventricle and, thus, evaluation of myocardial ischemia;
- measurement of mixed venous saturation;
- central infusion of cardiotonic drugs; and
- insertion of intravenous pacing wires through pacing ports added to the catheter.

The use of these catheters would most likely be restricted to the complex level of care provided by the evacuation hospital or specialized hospital ship.

Electrocardiography

The electrocardiograph is used for monitoring heart rhythm and ischemia. Hospitals throughout the United States use either three-lead or five-lead systems. The standard limb leads in general use monitor cardiac rhythm. Precordial leads are better for evaluation of ischemia. It is possible that only a three-lead system may be available in field hospitals. When using only three leads, the heart can still be evaluated for rhythm and ischemia: place the reference lead on the patient's left shoulder and the positive lead over the lateral precordial surface (V_5 position). By switching between lead I and lead II on the electrocardiograph, we can then view a limb lead and a modified precordial lead (modified V_5). The capability to monitor the electrical activity of the heart should be found at both the intermediate and complex levels of care.

Transesophageal Echocardiography

At present, evaluation of the cardiovascular system primarily involves hemodynamic monitoring. The introduction of transesophageal echocardiography has presented a new tool that provides useful information to the physician in highly sophisticated centers. The uses of transesophageal echocardiography include both monitoring for air embolism and monitoring of cardiac function.

Echocardiography uses sound waves emitted by sound transducers in a narrow beam. The sound waves travel through tissues and are reflected. The intensity of the reflected echoes is a function of the density of the reflecting tissue. Sound waves emitted by an esophageal transducer have to pass through only the esophageal wall and pericardium before reaching the heart. Thus, there is less likelihood of image distortion. Other advantages of transesophageal echocardiography include both the stability of the position of the transducer and the potential of continuous intraoperative recording.[11]

This monitor is very unlikely to be present during the operative care of the combat casualty. Currently, these monitors require excessive space and specialized training for their use. Although transesophageal echocardiography might provide useful information in specific instances, it remains a monitor that most likely will not be seen in hospitals that receive battlefield casualties.

Respiratory System

The respiratory system can be monitored by physical exam (presence or absence of labored breathing), stethoscopy, the casualty's color (presence or absence of cyanosis), pulse oximetry, arterial blood gases, and various sophisticated monitors such as capnography or mass spectrometry.

Pulse Oximetry

The pulse oximeter continuously measures the oxygen saturation of the arterial blood ($Sa{O_2}$, which is expressed as a percentage). Of more importance, however, is the oxygen content of the arterial blood ($Ca{O_2}$, which is expressed as grams of oxygen per 100 mL of blood), which is defined as $Sa{O_2}$ multiplied by the oxygen capacity (1.36 mL of oxygen per gram of hemoglobin [Hb]), multiplied by the concentration of Hb (grams per 100 mL of blood) divided by 100. The definition of Hb saturation (also called oxyhemoglobin, O_2Hb) does not include that fraction of Hb that may be either methemoglobin (MetHb) or carboxyhemoglobin (COHb). Therefore, the saturation percentage of Hb can be expressed as

$$\%\ \text{saturation}\ (Sa{O_2}) = (Ca{O_2}\ /\ \text{total Hb content}) \bullet 100$$

where total Hg is equal to O_2Hb + Hb + COHb + MetHb. Under normal circumstances, this correction is of little importance. However, in the casualty who is suffering from smoke inhalation (with the associated potential for carbon monoxide poisoning, in which 10%–20% of the total Hg content may be in the form of COHb), use of the complete formula to estimate saturation becomes mandatory.

The oximeter estimates Sao_2 by transilluminating the ear or other appendage with light of two different wavelengths (one in the red range, the other in the infrared). The transmitted light is then measured with a photodetector. The pulsatile component of the transmitted light is related to the absorbances of the Sao_2. All pulse oximeters assume that the only pulsatile absorbance between the light source and the photodetector is due to arterial blood. The baseline absorbance represents the light that is absorbed by tissue, venous blood, or the capillary bed. Thus, the oximeter is able to differentiate Sao_2 from venous or tissue saturation. The pulse oximeter further assumes that there are only two absorbing Hb types in the blood (ie, O_2Hb and Hb). If MetHb or COHb or both are present, they contribute to the pulse absorbance signal and, therefore, alter the Sao_2. Other limitations include any substance that absorbs light at the red and infrared pulse oximeter wavelengths used. Examples would be the use of methylene blue, indigo carmine, and indocyanine green dyes, which decrease the Sao_2. Colored nail polish also can adversely effect the measurement of Sao_2.

Pulse oximetry is an extremely useful noninvasive monitor of the respiratory system and has quickly become a standard of practice in operating rooms throughout the continental United States. Although it provides much information, however, pulse oximetry is not without pitfalls. Oxygen saturations greater than 90% indicate an arterial oxygen tension (Pao_2) greater than 60 torr. Patients who are given supplemental oxygen can have a significant shunt (causing decreases in Pao_2) before alterations in Sao_2 are noted. For example, if a casualty with lung contusions were placed on supplemental O_2, his initial arterial blood gas could show a Pao_2 of 300 torr. Oxygen saturation would show 100%. The casualty's condition could worsen such that the arterial blood gas might show a Pao_2 of 100 torr and the Sao_2 would still be 99% to 100%. Thus, a significant decrease in Pao_2 might not be noted by the pulse oximeter. Another pitfall could occur in the casualty who has been exposed to cyanide. In this instance, Sao_2 may remain high, despite the need for high concentrations of oxygen and treatment of cyanide toxicity.

The pulse oximeter may not be part of the standard equipment found at the second or third echelons of care, but it should be added as additional equipment. It should also be considered in the austere first-echelon setting when it is anticipated that anesthesia will be provided if electricity and space for equipment are available and maintenance can be provided.

Arterial Blood Gases

The ability to measure arterial blood gases serves as the standard in evaluating oxygenation. Modern measurement devices depend on selectively permeable membranes and the electrochemical activity of the gases present; besides measuring oxygen tension, modern electrodes also measure pH and pCO_2. The platinum electrode (Blood Gas System, manufactured by CIBA Corning Diagnostics, Medfield, Mass.) is used for measuring oxygen tension. The devices that monitor arterial blood gases are small, precise, and very sturdy. Arterial blood gas monitors will most likely be found at the more complex level of care (general hospitals); they may also be found at the intermediate level but certainly not in the austere setting.

Equipment able to continuously monitor oxygen tension is currently under development. The primary problem has been with miniaturization of the electrode. Another technology uses fiberoptic sensors, which can be miniaturized more easily. A continuous oxygen-tension monitor has recently been approved for clinical use, and this technology may soon be available for combat casualty care. At present, however, oxygen tension is measured only intermittently and only at the fourth echelon of medical care and higher.

Capnography

The analysis of end-tidal carbon dioxide ($ETco_2$) has only recently become commonplace in operating suites, but it has rapidly become a standard of practice in many community hospitals. This type of monitoring

- provides useful information regarding mechanical and gas-exchange functions of the patient's lungs,
- detects changes in the patient's metabolic and cardiovascular function, and
- helps identify malfunctions of breathing circuits that are used while patients are under anesthesia.

The systems most commonly available use infrared light absorption by carbon dioxide. The expired carbon dioxide absorbs light in proportion to its concentration. The sensors are placed in line with the expired gases, and a continuous waveform provides the capnograph. This type of in-line system for measuring $ETco_2$ is relatively fragile and the equipment is bulky. Capnography can also use a gas-withdrawal system (ie, mass spectrometry) as a way of measuring $ETco_2$; however, this requires very sophisticated instrumentation. The gas-withdrawal system to transport the gas to be measured to the measuring device causes a delay in measurement of the capnogram. Also, the moisture that develops within the gas-transport tubing often will obstruct the flow of the gases to the measuring device. $ETco_2$-measuring devices are not likely to be seen except at the more complex levels of combat casualty care.

Pulmonary Function

Lung compliance (the change in volume for a given change in transpulmonary pressure) is another monitor for evaluating the respiratory system in patients who require intubation, but we should bear in mind that the word "lung" is something of a misnomer: what is actually measured is the total compliance of the pulmonary tissue and the chest wall. Furthermore, two different compliances—dynamic and static—can be measured, depending on whether air is in motion when the measurements are made. Most mechanical ventilators have a pressure gauge that can be used to determine airway pressure on a moment-by-moment basis and, therefore, can be used to measure dynamic compliance. Dynamic compliance (DC) for a patient on a ventilator is defined as tidal volume (TV) divided by the peak airway pressure (PAP) minus the pressure at end expiration (PEEP):

$$DC = TV / (PAP - PEEP)$$

Normal lung compliance is approximately 100 mL/cm H_2O. A compliance of 25 mL/cm H_2O) is significantly decreased. Decreased dynamic compliance (increased peak airway pressure) may mean an obstructed endotracheal tube, bronchospasm, or a pneumothorax. Static compliance (SC) is calculated:

$$SC = TV / (\text{plateau pressure} - PEEP)$$

where *plateau pressure* is the pressure during the period in which there is no airflow. This is commonly estimated during the period of inspiratory pause. Decreased static compliance may signify atelectasis or increased lung water. Static compliance is a useful monitor for casualties with adult respiratory distress syndrome (ARDS).

Renal System

Monitoring the renal system serves as a means of measuring not only renal function but also the casualty's intravascular volume status. Useful monitors include urinary output, sodium concentration, and specific gravity. The patient should be able to maintain a urinary output of at least 0.5 mL/kg/h. Urinary specific gravity and sodium concentration help the medical officer determine whether the kidneys are attempting to conserve water (an indicator of the casualty's volume status). In nonhypovolemic patients who are not taking diuretics, urinary sodium concentration should be higher than 20 mEq/L and specific gravity lower than 1.020.

Above the second echelon of care, Foley catheters will be the primary device for monitoring renal function. Laboratory methods capable of measuring blood urea nitrogen or creatinine or urinary sodium concentration are not likely to be found at other than fourth-echelon medical treatment facilities.

Nervous System

Monitoring the nervous system involves both physical examination and the use of sophisticated equipment. Due to equipment limitations of durability and size, anesthesia care providers currently have limited ability to monitor the nervous system.

Central Nervous System

Monitoring the central nervous system is discussed in detail in Chapter 16, Neurological Injuries. The equipment used in this monitoring is often highly sensitive, fragile, and bulky; it is found only at the highest echelons of care. However, as technology improves and miniaturization of equipment then becomes practicable, these monitors will likely be used in the field.

Intracranial Pressure. For the most part, monitoring of the central nervous system will consist of mental-status checks and the physical examination. Intracranial pressure can be monitored at the fourth echelon of care and higher: specialized equipment is required and the monitors are generally inserted by neurosurgeons. The normal value for intracranial pressure is less than 10 cm H_2O.

Devices for monitoring intracranial pressure can be classified according to (*a*) the anatomical location at which the device is placed and (*b*) the method by which intracranial pressure is measured. Anatomically, these monitors can be placed in the lumbar spine, cervical spine, posterior fossa, or supratentorial area of the cranium. The supratentorial area is the preferred location for placement of the monitor, because insertion of a catheter into the subarachnoid space below the tentorium cerebri can cause a potentially fatal decrease in pressure there and subsequent herniation of the uncus of the temporal lobe or the cerebellar tonsils.

Devices in current use can be fluid-coupled (ie, the pressure-monitoring device is connected to a transducer by a column of fluid). The transducer should be at the level of the external auditory meatus while the intracranial pressure is being measured. Routine pressure tubing and transducers used for arterial and central venous pressure monitoring are *not* used to monitor intracranial pressure. The flow through the standard tubing (approximately 2 mL/h) could harm a patient with increased intracranial pressure. Flushing the monitor tubing would also be harmful. Care must be taken not to inject any fluid into this system. Newer devices now use fiberoptics instead of a fluid-coupled system to transmit pressure waves to the pressure-measuring device.

The intraventricular catheter is a simple device used for measuring intracranial pressure. It can be used both as a monitor and as part of a therapeutic regimen. The device is coupled directly to the cerebrospinal fluid and the transducer. In the event of increased intracranial pressure, fluid can be drawn off as needed. Iatrogenic infection can be introduced because this technique requires that the catheter be inserted through brain tissue; the incidence of such infection is estimated to be less than 6.3%.[12] Other devices used to monitor intracranial pressure include the subarachnoid bolt and epidural devices. These devices allow for monitoring without invading brain tissue.

Encephalography. The conventional, multichannel electroencephalograph is the standard against which all other types of monitors of the electrical activity of the brain are compared. The electroencephalograph and its electrodes are large and cumbersome. In addition, conditions within the operating room make it a hostile environment for electroencephalography (eg, electrocautery interference). The difficulty in using the conventional, multichannel electroencephalograph is largely overcome by monitoring a processed electroencephalogram (eg, the cerebral function monitor, which is a single-channel processed electroencephalogram). The use of the cerebral function monitor during carotid endarterectomy,[13] deliberate hypotension,[14] and cardiopulmonary bypass[15] is well documented. However, the inability to examine the behavior of different frequencies within the electroencephalograph is a major drawback. The Lifescan Monitor (manufactured by Neurometrics Inc., San Diego, Calif.) displays a processed electroencephalogram in which brain waves can be viewed as three-dimensional vertical spikes. The height of the spike represents the amplitude of the wave, its horizontal position represents its frequency, and time is represented on the Z axis. This device also can monitor sensory evoked potentials. The processed electroencephalogram is useful in monitoring cerebral ischemia and the effects of anesthetic drugs.[16–18]

There are many types of electroencephalographs that have differing processing techniques. Clinically, all the processing techniques show frequency changes when the raw electroencephalogram slows, and amplitude changes when it flattens. The difficulty lies in comparing two differing processing techniques. Qualitatively, the processed electroencephalogram may be quite useful. However, this monitor is unlikely to be seen at any echelon of care except in hospitals within the continental United States.

Sensory Evoked Potentials. The intraoperative use of sensory evoked potentials is labor intensive. Because many anesthesia care providers lack the time or skill to monitor and interpret sensory evoked potentials, their use has often been limited to large medical centers where neurologists or electrophysiologists are available. Some facilities have a specialized technician who assists in the technical aspects of the monitoring.

Sensory evoked potentials have been used in neurosurgery,[19,20] orthopedic spinal surgery,[21] and during positioning of the patient where brachial plexus injuries may occur.[22] Its usefulness as a monitor during care of combat casualties is doubtful, because even the most basic machines are so labor intensive and bulky. This monitor will most likely be found only at the larger medical centers in the continental United States.

Peripheral Nerve Stimulators

Peripheral nerve–stimulator devices allow muscle relaxation to be monitored while potent muscle relaxants are administered. They can also be useful when regional anesthesia is performed using a nerve-stimulation technique (see Chapter 11, Neuromuscular Blocking Agents, Figure 11-2). Those who select the nerve stimulator that will be used at the third and fourth echelons of care should take this dual use into consideration. A nerve stimulator with the ability to adjust the amount of output in milliamps (0–10.0 mA and 0–100 mA) will be more versatile. The ability to identify nerve structures by direct stimulation of nerves or muscles or both during the surgical procedure would be an additional benefit to the surgeon.

Temperature

The ability to monitor temperature will no doubt be found at both the third and fourth echelons of care. Thermocoupled liquid crystal display devices that paste onto the skin will have little value in the field. Nondisposable devices that allow temperature monitoring at various sites will be most helpful. Monitoring core body temperature—via esophageal or rectal temperature probes—will provide the most useful information regarding the casualty's temperature.

COMPUTERS IN ANESTHESIA

In anesthesia, computers can be used as microprocessor-based drug and anesthesia delivery systems or as a means of patient-data management. Currently, there are no well-established systems in which physiological data are processed by computer and which subsequently permit the delivery of anesthesia drugs to be modified based on the data received by the microprocessor. More commonly, computers receive physiological data and record it on the anesthesia record. The ability to detect detrimental changes in the casualty's status and trigger the appropriate alarms are what separates simple data collection from computerized monitoring. Improvements in the technology of artificial intelligence will be required before useful microprocessor-based anesthesia drug delivery systems are seen either outside the research area or on the battlefield. The computers required for such elaborate tasks require processing in parallel with data received from monitors measuring cardiovascular, respiratory, and other physiological parameters. The enormous amount of data will then require processing so that appropriate responses (mimicking those of a human expert) will be made.

Computerized data recording is a much more manageable task. The objective is to make record keeping easy and complete: to free the anesthesia provider to monitor the casualty, not to institute time-consuming tasks. Accurate, detailed records of data from various physiological monitors can be stored and printed. The medical officer's ability to distinguish between artifact and real data, and a user-friendly computer program's processing of human input are essential to the practicability of any computerized record system.

SUMMARY

Monitoring of the combat casualty can be both adequate and austere. Levels of care practiced in fixed medical facilities such as combat support or general hospitals differ from those practiced closer to the battlefield. Strategies for obtaining data from various physiological systems for use in management of the medical care of the combat casualty need to be decided in advance, as do the types of monitors that can be expected at each echelon of care.

As technological advances make sophisticated equipment smaller, simpler, and sturdier for transport, the kinds of monitoring devices that are available at each echelon will undoubtedly change, making more-sophisticated monitoring available closer to the battlefront. The pulse oximeter is one example; capnography will most likely follow.

REFERENCES

1. Harken LA, Slichter SJ. The bleeding time as a screening test for evaluation of platelet function and perioperative blood loss. *N Engl J Med*. 1972;287:155–159.

2. Rosenberg RD. Actions and interactions of antithrombin and heparin. *N Engl J Med*. 1975;292:146–151.

3. Bull BS, Brauer FS, Korpman RA. Heparin therapy during extracorporeal circulation, II: The use of a dose-response curve to individualize heparin and protamine dosage. *J Thorac Cardiovasc Surg*. 1975;69:685–689.

4. Korotkoff N. On the subject of methods of determining blood pressure. *Bull Imperial Med Acad*. 1905;1:365.

5. Stegall HF, Kardon MB, Kemmerer WT. Indirect measurement of arterial blood pressure by Doppler ultrasonic sphygmomanometry. *J Appl Physiol*. 1968;25:793–798.

6. Ramsey MI. Noninvasive automatic determination of mean arterial pressure. *Med Biol Eng Comput*. 1979;17:11–18.

7. Slogoff S, Keats AS, Arlund C. On the safety of radial artery cannulation. *Anesthesiology*. 1983;59:42–47.

8. Bedford RF. Radial arterial function following percutaneous cannulation with 18- and 20-gauge catheters. *Anesthesiology*. 1977;47:37–39.

9. Barnes RW, Foster EJ, Janssen GA, Boutros AR. Safety of brachial arterial catheters as monitors in the intensive care unit: Prospective evaluation with Doppler ultrasonic velocity detector. *Anesthesiology*. 1976;44:260–264.

10. Glenski JA, Beynen FM, Brady J. A prospective evaluation of femoral artery monitoring in pediatric patients. *Anesthesiology*. 1987;66:227–229.

11. Thys DM, Konstadt S, Hillel Z. Intraoperative echocardiography. In: Lake C, ed. *Clinical Monitoring*. Philadelphia, Pa: WB Saunders; 1990: 197–235.

12. Rosner JJ, Becker DP. ICP monitoring: Complications and associated factors. *Clin Neurosurg*. 1976;23:494–519.

13. Cucchiara RF, Sharbrough FW, Messick JM, Tinker JH. An electroencephalographic filter-processor as an indicator of cerebral ischemia during carotid endarterectomy. *Anesthesiology*. 1979;51:77–5179.

14. Patel H. Experience with the cerebral function monitor during deliberate hypotension. *Br J Anaesth*. 1981;53:639–644.

15. Kritikou PE, Branthwaite MA. Significant changes in cerebral electrical activity at onset of cardiopulmonary bypass. *Thorax*. 1977;32:534–538.

16. Spackman TN, Faust RJ, Cucchiara RF, Sharbrough FW. The comparison of the Lifescan EEG monitor with EEG and cerebral blood flow for detection of cerebral ischemia. *Anesthesiology*. 1985;63:A187. Abstract.

17. Smith NT, Demetrescu M. The EEG during high-dose fentanyl anesthesia. *Anesthesiology*. 1980;53:S7.

18. Demetrescu M, Kavan E, Smith NT. Monitoring the brain condition by advanced EEG. *Anesthesiology*. 1981;53:A130. Abstract.

19. Grundy BL, Lina A, Porocopio PT, Jannetta PJ. Reversible evoked potential changes with retraction of the eighth cranial nerve. *Anesth Analg*. 1981;60:835–838.

20. Symon L, Wang AD, Costa e Silva IE, Gentili F. Perioperative use of somatosensory evoked potentials in aneurysm surgery. *J Neurosurg*. 1984;70:269–275.

21. McPherson RW, North RB, Udvarhelyi GB, Rosenbaum AE. Migrating disc complicating spinal decompression in an achondroplastic dwarf: Intraoperative demonstration of spinal cord compression by somatosensory evoked potentials. *Anesthesiology*. 1984;61:764–767.

22. Mahla M, Long DM, McKennett J, Green C, McPherson R. Detection of brachial plexus dysfunction by somatosensory evoked potential monitoring—A report of two cases. *Anesthesiology*. 1984;60:248–252.

Chapter 6

DEPLOYABLE HOSPITALS

WILLIAM JAMES PHILLIPS, M.D.*; MARC A. PARADIS, M.D.†; AND RONALD F. BELLAMY, M.D.‡

*Major, Medical Corps, U.S. Army Reserve; formerly, Anesthesiologist, 528th Special Operations Support Battalion (Airborne), U.S. Army Special Operations Command, Fort Bragg; Staff Anesthesiologist, Womack Army Medical Center, Fort Bragg, North Carolina 28307; currently, Staff Anesthesiologist, Mayo Clinic, Rochester, Minnesota

†Formerly, Lieutenant Colonel, Medical Corps, U.S. Army; Staff Anesthesiologist, Walter Reed Army Medical Center, Washington, D. C. 20307-5001; currently, Chief, Cardiac Anesthesiology Section, Hartford Hospital, Hartford, Connecticut 06106

‡Colonel, Medical Corps, U.S. Army; Managing Editor and Officer in Charge, Textbook of Military Medicine, Borden Institute, Walter Reed Army Medical Center, Washington, D. C. 20307-5001

INTRODUCTION

No modern general will go into battle without taking with him at least a rudimentary hospital system. When the tempo of warfare was governed by the speed of marching men and horses, existing deployable hospitals were usually able to keep pace with combat units. The primitive nature of medicine and surgery minimized the logistical and transportation needs of such hospitals, which were frequently nothing more than tents with cots. The imperatives of modern medicine and surgery, together with the advent of mechanized warfare, have vastly increased the challenge of providing medical support—especially surgical care for combat casualties. The problems implicit in designing mobile hospitals were not especially apparent during the positional warfare that characterized much of World War I, but they became obvious during World War II. Medical commanders soon recognized that unless hospitals capable of providing surgical care for combat casualties were able to accompany rapidly moving armored units, casualties would necessarily be subjected to a lengthy evacuation. For many, this was incompatible with survival. Furthermore, the lifesaving potential of modern surgery could be realized only if operations were carried out shortly after wounding had occurred. To wait for the combat casualty to reach a communications zone hospital, as was done in World War I, was to minimize the value of modern surgery.

The need for hospitals that had the tactical mobility of combat units became apparent to the U.S. Army during the campaigns in North Africa and Italy in 1943. It was recognized that a small fraction of those wounded in action (perhaps 10%) were "nontransportable": they could not survive evacuation from the battlefield to the corps-level hospitals. The major achievement of military surgery by the U.S. Army in World War II was forward surgical care for such casualties. Small ad hoc surgical hospitals (30–60 beds) were created and attached to, and could move with, division-level medical units. The basic hospital module was a platoon-sized unit, three of which constituted an existing Table of Organization and Equipment (TOE) unit: the field hospital. Teams of surgeons and anesthesia providers were attached to the field hospital platoons from army level medical replacement units known as auxiliary surgery groups. Mobility for the combined surgical team–field hospital platoon was provided by its own *organic* (ie, intrinsic; included in the TOE) vehicles (Figure 6-1). Simplicity to the point of austerity was their dominant feature; for example, operating rooms were tents or buildings of convenience (Figures 6-2 and 6-3). The equipment believed to be essential by World War II surgical teams is listed in Exhibit 6-1. The field hospital platoon supplied the tentage, cots, and ancillary equipment for the casualties, while logistical and administrative support was provided by the supported division.

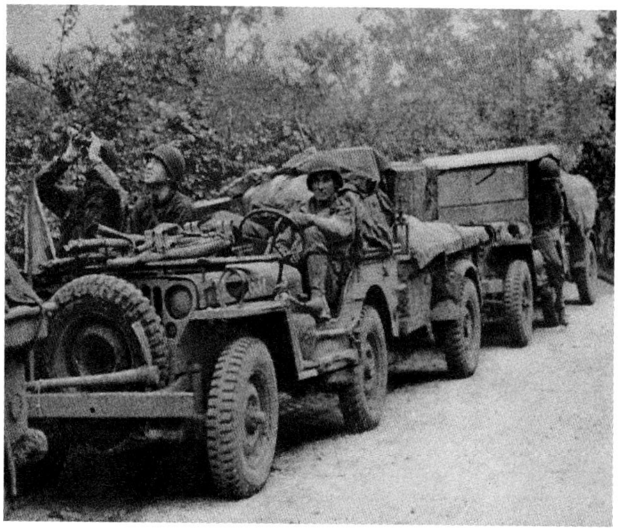

Fig. 6-1. The mobility and simplicity of World War II–vintage surgical teams are apparent in this photograph taken in Italy in 1944. Several jeeps with trailers and a small truck were found to be sufficient to transport the surgical personnel and specialty equipment. Tents, cots, and other equipment were provided by the unit being supported. Note that several members are watching the sky, possibly for enemy aircraft. Their actions emphasize how far forward surgical teams were deployed. Reprinted from Brewer LA III, Burford TH. Administrative considerations in the Mediterranean (formerly North African) Theater of Operations. In: Berry FB, ed. *Thoracic Surgery*. Vol 1. In: Coates JB Jr, ed. *Surgery in World War II*. Washington, DC: US Department of the Army, Medical Department, Office of The Surgeon General; 1963: 88.

Only casualties who were considered to be likely to die or to develop life-threatening complications during evacuation to a corps-level evacuation hospital were treated by the surgical team–field hospital platoon. In general, the following categories were treated in forward surgical hospitals[1]:

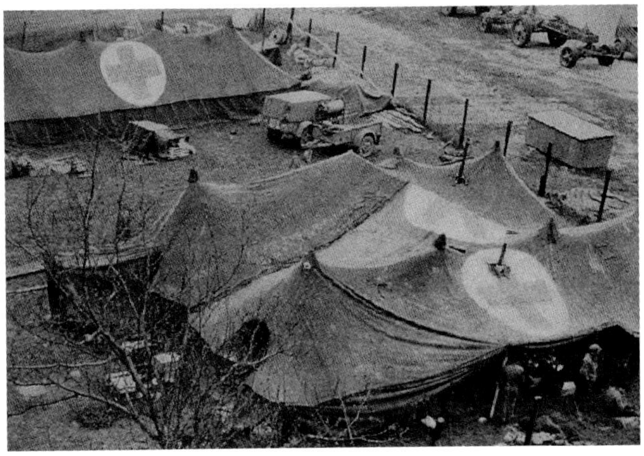

Fig. 6-2. A forward surgical unit set up somewhere in France in 1944. Several tents house the operating room, the shock or resuscitation ward, and the postoperative/recovery ward. Environmental control was obviously not optimal by today's standards, nor was there much protection against enemy action. Reprinted from Odom CB. Third US Army. In: Carter BN, ed. *Activities of Surgical Consultants*. Vol 1. In: Coates JB Jr. *Surgery in World War II*. Washington DC: US Department of the Army, Medical Department, Office of The Surgeon General; 1962: 305.

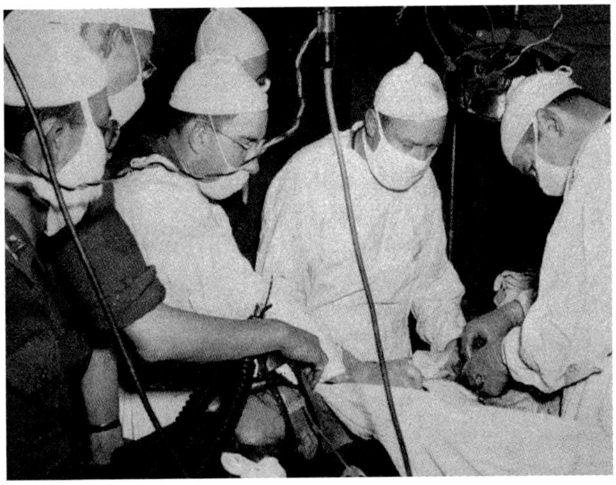

Fig. 6-3. A World War II surgical team performing an operation. The notable austerity is in marked contrast to what is found in today's DEPMEDS (Department of Defense's Deployable Medical Systems)-equipped hospitals. Yet all the components required to perform lifesaving surgery are present. Reprinted from Odom CB. Third US Army. In: Carter BN, ed. *Activities of Surgical Consultants*. Vol 1. In: Coates JB Jr. *Surgery in World War II*. Washington DC: US Department of the Army, Medical Department, Office of The Surgeon General; 1962: 309.

EXHIBIT 6-1

ESSENTIAL EQUIPMENT FOR WORLD WAR II SURGICAL TEAMS

1. Adequate transportation assigned permanently to the team
2. Adequate lighting: at least 200 W candlepower for each operating table
3. A portable oxygen apparatus, with a large-cylinder reducing valve
4. A simple transfusion set for giving whole blood with citrate as the anticoagulant
5. A large autoclave for sterilizing towels, gowns, and sheets
6. Two covered metal sterilizers for boiling instruments
7. Two stoves for sterilizing
8. Three large, 30-gal galvanized cans for washing, waste, and soaking dirty and bloody linen
9. Linen, including 200 towels, 20 gowns, and 40 sheets; drapes for the surgical tents to keep out dirt and dust
10. A positive-pressure anesthesia machine and a portable suction apparatus
11. Basic surgical instruments as well as specialty instruments needed for such operations as a thoracotomy
12. A walled or pyramidal tent to furnish living quarters for the surgical team

Adapted from: Brewer LA III, Burford TH. Administrative considerations in the Mediterranean (formerly North African) Theater of Operations. In: Berry FB, ed. *Thoracic Surgery*. Vol 1. In: Coates JB Jr, ed. *Surgery in World War II*. Washington, DC: US Department of the Army, Medical Department, Office of The Surgeon General; 1963: 88–89.

- casualties with multiple wounds, who remained in shock despite intensive therapy;
- casualties with abdominal wounds, particularly those with possible concealed hemorrhage;
- casualties with large, sucking chest wounds or massive intrathoracic hemorrhage;
- casualties with thoracoabdominal wounds; and
- casualties with wounds about the face and neck that caused mechanical interference with respiration.

Most casualties—those with orthopedic, soft-tissue, and head injuries—were sent to evacuation hospitals in the rear after being given initial care by the division-level medical unit with which the surgical hospital was collocated. The decision as to whether a casualty would be sent to the forward surgical hospital was made by the triage officer of the host division-level medical unit. The latter unit was also responsible for evacuation of treated casualties. Strangely enough, although professional relationships were clearly defined, formal command-and-control relationships among the three units—the surgical team (army level), the field-hospital platoon (corps level), and the supported division—were ill defined. In all, about 100,000 operations were performed in the European theater by auxiliary surgery group surgical teams. Probably one half were carried out in forward surgical hospitals, of which there may have been several hundred.[2]

Given the great success of the surgical team–field hospital approach to providing forward surgical care, it is not surprising that after World War II, it was decided to develop a formal TOE surgical hospital. From this decision came the famous mobile army surgical hospital (MASH) of the Korean War. Ironically, the conditions that gave rise to the forward surgical hospital during World War II were absent in Korea: after the first 9 months, a static battlefield reminiscent of World War I had developed. The MASHs remained immobile and, in fact, became functionally identical to other hospitals (ie, they no longer were dedicated to the treatment of only the most severely wounded casualties).

The MASH concept underwent considerable refinement during the period between the end of the Korean War in 1953 and the United States' intervention in Vietnam in the 1960s. One obvious defect in the MASH and its World War II predecessor was that the use of canvas tents precluded environmental control: a clean operating room was not possible. Furthermore, not only was there a potential for pollution from the environment but the tents offered no protection against chemical and biological warfare agents. To correct this, an advanced-technology approach was undertaken, with the goal of creating an environmentally controlled hospital with both strategic and tactical mobility. By 1963, this program had led to the development of the medical unit, self-contained, transportable (MUST) hospital.

The MUST hospital consisted of hard-walled, expandable shelters for certain parts of the facility (eg, the operating room), and inflatable shelters for other areas (eg, patient wards) (Figure 6-4). The facility was transportable using special transporter vehicles; electricity, air conditioning, and water were supplied via utility packs. The utility packs were large units powered by a gas turbine that burned jet engine fuel (JP4), and they provided heating and cooling to all the inflatable and hard-walled shelters (Figure 6-5). The utility packs worked well but consumed large amounts of fuel. In 1966, the first MUST hospital was deployed to Vietnam. Four more were deployed before the war ended.

In retrospect, the MUST cannot be judged a success. Part of the reason for its relative failure arose from the nature of the Vietnam War. Small U.S.

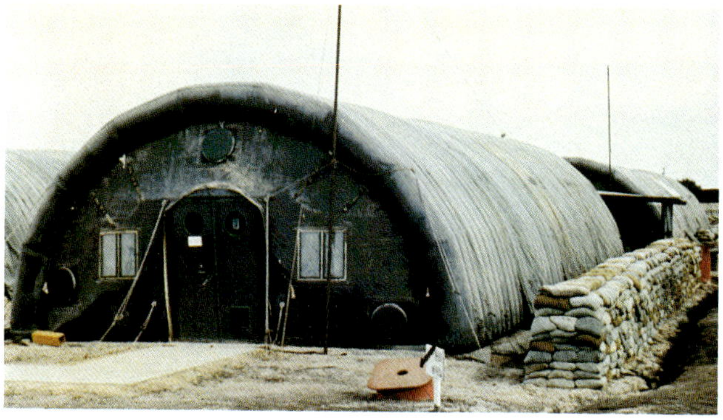

Fig. 6-4. An inflatable shelter in use in Vietnam, 1967. The MUST (medical unit, self-contained, transportable) surgical hospital used two characteristic structures: hard-walled, expandable shelters that contained the operating rooms and supporting services; and inflatable shelters that served as patient wards. Although representing an advanced-technology approach to providing a deployable surgical facility, inflatable shelters were probably not worth the effort. Setting them up was not easy and the equipment required to keep them inflated was labor-intensive. The inflatable shelters were also notably sensitive to battle damage.

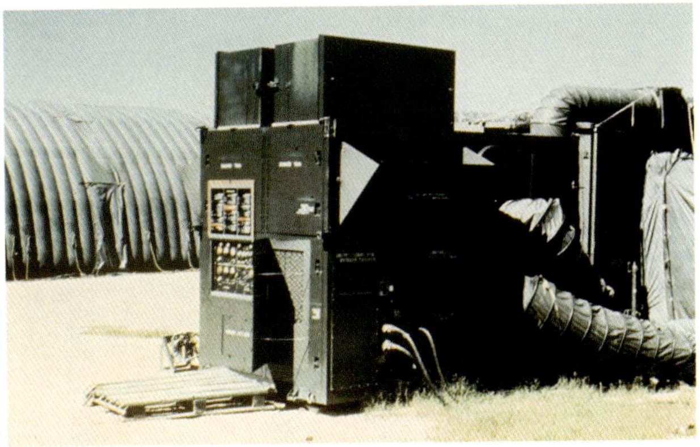

Fig. 6-5. The mechanical equipment used to operate a MUST (medical unit, self-contained, transportable) hospital consisted of a gas turbine, a generator, and an air-cooling unit, which together constituted a utility pack. Large tubes acted as conduits to provide cooled or heated air to the treatment areas.

Army units deployed from base camps into the surrounding enemy-held territory. By World War II standards, distances in Vietnam were small, control of the air complete, and the number of casualties slight. It was, therefore, much more reasonable to fly casualties into hospitals established in the base camps than to move the hospitals with the combat units. Given the nature of the Vietnam War, MUST hospitals were never used the way they were envisioned: as mobile hospitals to provide resuscitative surgery only to the most seriously injured. Thus, MUST hospitals became immobile and increasingly lost their primary function. For example, it was not unusual for the prototype MUST—the 45th Surgical Hospital—to function as a station hospital and hold daily sick call for other units assigned to the Tay Ninh base camp.

The major deficiencies of the MUST facilities were as follows:

- They were not as adaptable to changing mission requirements nor as deployable as originally intended.
- The inflatable shelters were easily damaged by enemy action and difficult to maintain.
- Fuel consumption and the cost of supplying power to the utility packs were unacceptably high.
- MUST-equipped hospitals lacked commonality among the army, navy, and air force.

Consequently, the U.S. Congress ended the MUST program in 1979, and mandated in 1981 that all future North Atlantic Treaty Organization (NATO) third- and fourth-echelon hospitals would be standardized among the military services. This standardization program led to what is now known as the Department of Defense's Deployable Medical Systems (DEPMEDS).

HISTORY OF DEPLOYABLE MEDICAL SYSTEMS

In June 1982, the Department of Defense established the Military Field Medical Systems Standardization Steering Group, which consisted of general and flag officers of the U.S. Army, Navy, Air Force, and Marine Corps, and was responsible for directing the development of DEPMEDS.[3] Their mission was to standardize DEPMEDS to the degree that would still allow the four services to accomplish their distinct missions. DEPMEDS would (*a*) improve on the MUST's modular design and reassembly and (*b*) be more flexible and easier to deploy. To this end, the Military Field Medical Systems Standardization Steering Group established that DEPMEDS equipment sets be adequate, affordable, austere, maintainable, modular, transportable, usable in multiple service-specific configurations, usable by all four services, and suitable for transportation by strategic airlift. Other requirements came from the Health Service Support Tenets, which stress (*a*) providing healthcare as far forward as possible and (*b*) maximizing the number of soldiers who return to duty. DEPMEDS was designed for use only in the third and fourth echelons of medical care.

The most important task for the Military Field Medical Systems Standardization Steering Group was to select medical and nonmedical equipment and supplies that were not only acceptable to all four services but would also adhere to their individual requirements. To do this, the steering group convened 21 panels of medical experts from all four services. The panels selected the medical equipment after reviewing and studying the Combat Zone Assessment and Requirements (CZAR) model.

The original DEPMEDS database contained 316 patient conditions, which encompassed most of the workload expected to be seen if war were to occur in the NATO theater of combat. These 316 patient conditions were accompanied by brief descriptions of the conditions and their treatment. The treatment briefs, developed in late 1985, summarized the procedures recommended for each hypothetical patient. Because each hypothetical patient repre-

EXHIBIT 6-2

SELECTED DEPMEDS TREATMENT BRIEFS AND DEFINITIONS OF PATIENT CONDITIONS

No.	Injury	Description	Degree of Severity
1.	Cerebral concussion	Closed, with or without nondepressed linear skull fracture	Severe; loss of consciousness 2–12 h
3.	Cerebral contusion	Closed, with or without nondepressed linear skull fracture	Severe; loss of consciousness > 24 h, with focal neurological deficit
4.	Cerebral contusion	Closed, with or without nondepressed linear skull fracture	Moderate; loss of consciousness 12–24 h, without focal neurological deficit
5.	Cerebral contusion	Closed, with intracranial hematoma, with or without nondepressed linear skull fracture	Severe; large hematoma (including hematoma) with rapidly deteriorating, comatose patient
7.	Cerebral contusion	Closed, with depressed skull fracture	Severe; with associated intracerebral hematoma and/or massive depression
9.	Cerebral contusion	Open skull fracture	Severe; with intracranial fragments and/or depressed skull fracture
10.	Cerebral contusion	Open skull fracture	Moderate; without intracranial fragments and/or depressed skull fracture
45.	Wound: upper arm	Open, penetrating, lacerated, without fracture, with nerve and/or vascular injury	Severe
46.	Wound: upper arm	Open, penetrating, lacerated, without fracture, without nerve or vascular injury	Moderate
47.	Wound: upper arm	Open, with fractures and nerve and vascular injury	Arm not salvageable
48.	Wound: upper arm	Open with fractures and nerve injury, without vascular injury	Arm salvageable
83.	Injury: lung	Closed (blast, crush) with pneumo-hemothorax	Severe, one lung with pulmonary contusion and acute, severe respiratory distress
85.	Wound: thorax (anterior or posterior)	Open, superficial, lacerated, contused, abraded, avulsed	Requires major debridement
87.	Wound: thorax (anterior or posterior)	Open, penetrating, with associated rib fractures and pneumohemothorax	Acute, severe respiratory distress
94.	Thermal burn: trunk	> 20% but < 30% of TBSA	Full thickness
95.	Thermal burn: trunk	> 10% but < 20% of TBSA	Full thickness
96.	Wound: abdominal wall (anterior or posterior)	Lacerated, abraded, contused, avulsed without entering the abdominal cavity	Severe, requiring major debridement
130.	Wound: lower leg	Open, lacerated, penetrating, perforating, with fracture and nerve/vascular injury	Limb not salvageable
131.	Wound: lower leg	Open, lacerated, penetrating, perforating, with fracture and nerve/vascular damage	Limb salvageable
134.	Wound: ankle, foot, toes	Open, lacerated, contused, without fractures	Requiring major debridement
135.	Wound: ankle, foot, toes	Open, lacerated, contused, without fractures	Not requiring major debridement
136.	Wound: ankle, foot, toes	Open, penetrating, perforating, with fractures and nerve/vascular injury	Limb not salvageable

Adapted from Scotti MJ, chairman. Defense Medical Standardization Board. *DEPMEDS Policies/Guidelines: Treatment Briefs*. Fort Detrick, Frederick, Md: 1990: E-1, E-2, E-4.

Exhibit 6-2 *continues*

EXHIBIT 6-2: PATIENT CONDITIONS *(continued)*

PATIENT CONDITION 9:

CEREBRAL CONTUSION WITH OPEN SKULL FRACTURE, SEVERE—WITH INTRACRANIAL FRAGMENTS OR DEPRESSED SKULL FRACTURE OR BOTH

LENGTH-OF-STAY MATRIX

	Echelon			
	3	4	5	Total Days
ICU	3	3	7	13
ICW	0	5	143	148
MCW	0	0	0	0
Total days	**3**	**8**	**150**	**161**

BLOOD USAGE

	Blood	Hemorrhage Class
Echelon 3	2	II
Echelon 4	0	

NATO Echelon 2

Assumptions: Litter, unconscious; moderate neuro deficits; responds to painful stimuli only; vital signs—moderate tachycardia; rapid shallow resp; some require assisted ventilation; blood pressure normal; minimal-to-moderate hemorrhage; 4% die at this echelon.

Treatment: Stabilize head and C-spine; start IV; intubate 80%; dress and bandage open head wound. Transport on litter, head-up 15°–30° position.

NATO Echelon 3

Assumptions: Litter; neuro status unchanged; Class II hemorrhage; vital signs same as Echelon 2; X ray shows depressed skull fracture with intracranial frag; requires craniotomy; (50% died in hospital).

Treatment: *Emergency Medical Treatment area*: Place endotracheal tube in 20%; assist ventilation 100%; cardiac monitor in 100%; IV to keep open 1 L Ringer's lactate; inspect and dress head wound; nasogastric tube; Foley cath; neurosurg meds; antibiotics; protect neck; X ray: skull, cervical spine; 100% portable chest; Lab: complete blood count, electrolytes, type and crossmatch 3 units

Operating Room: 100% have craniotomies; central venous pressure monitor; 2 units blood; endotracheal tube; antibiotics; 2 L Ringer's lactate; operating room table time 150 min.

Wards: *Intensive Care Unit*: hyperventilate via endotracheal tube with 40% O_2; Ringer's lactate 3 L 1st day; change head dressing; insert tube feeding; abdomen X ray; 100% tube feeding 2nd day; steroids; Foley; IV to keep open after tube feeding begun; may require mannitol; IV antibiotic; cardiac monitor while on ventilator, possible 5% cardiac arrest; complete blood count, electrolytes every other day; transcutaneous O_2 for 3 days. Remove central venous pressure monitor on day 3.

NATO Echelon 4

Assumptions: Litter; 50% conscious/50% unchanged; all require assisted ventilation x 2 days; all on tube feeding; vital signs stable.

Treatment: *Emergency Medical Treatment area*: Check vitals, check IV, suction: ventilate; transport to ward; complete blood count and electrolytes in emergency treatment area on 20%.

Operating Room: 100% have tracheostomies (30 min); operating room table time 60 min.

Wards: *Intensive Care Unit*: control ventilation with tracheostomy; continue IV; continue tube feeding; continue monitoring; continue antibiotics; steroids; disconnect ventilator at day 2; complete blood count & electrolytes every other day; continue Foley; transcutaneous O_2 monitor 2 day; *Intermediate Care Ward*: vital signs; heparin lock to continue IV antibiotics and steroids; tube feeding to continental United States; continue Foley to continental United States; parenteral pain meds; prepare to transfer to Veterans Administration hospital Echelon 5.*

Ancillary Support: occupational therapy/physical therapy evaluation.

*Echelon 5 hospitals are within the continental United States, not in the theater

Reprinted from Scotti MJ, chairman. Defense Medical Standardization Board. *DEPMEDS Policies/Guidelines: Treatment Briefs.* Defense Medical Standardization Board, Fort Detrick, Frederick, Md: 1990: Rev 7/90.

sents the *average* in the spectrum of a particular injury or disease, each treatment brief described (*a*) the average amount of time and equipment needed and (*b*) the average number of personnel and procedures required to treat a given injury.

The lists of equipment the panel had selected were reviewed by a group of senior physicians representing each service—the Joint Services Clinical Review Group—which, along with Logistics, Dental, Nursing, and Pharmacy Quad-Service Review Groups, continues to review DEPMEDS equipment and supplies to ensure that the items are reliable, compatible, complete, and ready to use. There have been numerous annual revisions; major changes were made in 1987 and 1990, and a major update and revision occurred in March 1992.

Once the Joint Services Clinical Review Group review was completed, the Medical Assemblage Design Branch of the Academy of Health Sciences, Fort Sam Houston, San Antonio, Texas, organized the items into functional modules known as medical material sets (MMSs). It is these sets that allow the armed services to deploy medical facilities with markedly different capabilities and still maintain the mandate for standardization. Three types of sets were created[4(p8)]:

- the basic MMS, which contains all the equipment, durable goods and a 3-day supply of consumable equipment for a specific module in the hospital (eg, the Operating Room MMS D301);
- the special-module MMS, which contains equipment for additional capability (eg, the Orthopedic Cast Clinic MMS D314); and
- the resupply MMS, which contains expendable and some durable goods, and can be configured as needed for each individual hospital.

In June 1984, the standardization mission of the Military Field Medical Systems Standardization Steering Group was given to the Defense Medical Material Board, which was renamed the Defense Medical Standardization Board. The Defense Medical Standardization Board continues to direct the development of DEPMEDS and to standardize all medical equipment to the extent consistent with the missions of the individual military services.

The DEPMEDS MMSs were initially tested in November 1984 at Fort Hood, Texas. In November 1985, the DEPMEDS database was again reviewed by a quad-service panel of medical experts. Based on the panel's review, final changes to the MMSs were made, and in March 1987, the Assistant Secretary of Defense for Health Affairs approved the sets as the Department of Defense DEPMEDS sets. DEPMEDS was further evaluated and tested by the U.S. Navy during Operation Safe Haven (1987), the U.S. Army with Joint Task Force Bravo in Honduras during the 1980s, and the U.S. Air Force during REFORGER exercises (1984–1988). Changes based on these experiences resulted in the 1990 version of DEPMEDS, which was more streamlined and fully capable of meeting the quad-service field medical requirements. Based on the experience gained from the Persian Gulf War, DEPMEDS was again updated in March 1992.

The Defense Medical Standardization Board, located at Fort Detrick, Frederick, Maryland, publishes *DEPMEDS Policies/Guidelines Treatment Briefs*, most recently in July 1990.[4] This manual is neither a set of orders nor standing operating procedures for the care of *individual* patients but is the doctrinal basis for medical care in a theater of combat. It contains the concept of operation for DEPMEDS and treatment briefs for the 339 patient conditions used currently in the development of DEPMEDS (examples are shown in Exhibit 6-2). It must be emphasized that these patient conditions were designed to facilitate planning for manpower, equipment, and supply needs; they were never intended to predict every wartime injury nor were they intended to dictate therapy. The patient conditions, which are based on a combination of historical data, computer modeling, experience, and enlightened speculation, provide planning parameters for medical treatment facilities. Of note is the changing number of patient conditions, which occur as patient conditions are added, deleted, or coalesced depending on the threat and changing medical modeling requirements:

> The treatment briefs should be viewed as a living document that will require continual review for currency. At periodic intervals particular types of diseases or injuries will have to be modified due to the advent of new treatment modalities or the change in the medical threat.[4(p92)]

The patient conditions did not change substantially after the Persian Gulf War.

The DEPMEDS manual also contains specific policies for specialties (including anesthesiology), and guidelines for emergency medical treatment, fluid resuscitation, laboratory tests, the use of cell savers, and the use of blood. Anesthesiologists and nurse anesthetists who are deploying with a DEPMEDS-equipped unit should review the manual and note the following policies[4(p49)]:

- Pulse oximetry is available intraoperatively and postoperatively.
- Halothane and isoflurane are the only inhalational anesthetics currently available.
- Nitrous oxide is not available.
- Patients recover in an intensive care unit adapted for that purpose.
- The care of postoperative patients is one of the most important responsibilities of anesthesia personnel.
- In-line oxygen monitoring is available (end-tidal carbon dioxide monitoring currently is not available but was recommended as a part of the monitoring package at the March 1992 update).
- Regional anesthesia kits are supplied for spinal and axillary blocks only (an epidural kit has been requested).
- Draw-over vaporizers are available for use when other methods are unavailable in extremely austere environments.

DEPLOYABLE ANESTHESIA EQUIPMENT

Most of the equipment used by anesthesiologists is currently contained in Operating Room MMS D301. The March 1992 revision strongly recommended that a *separate* anesthesia MMS be created to facilitate accountability, periodic review, maintenance, and rapid accessibility. The only significant piece of equipment not included in the Operating Room MMS for which anesthesia providers have expressed a desire is for a 5-mm flexible, fiberoptic bronchoscope. This instrument is contained in Central Material Supply Special Augmentation Set D342.

Physiological Monitors

The physiological monitors that are part of DEPMEDS include electrocardiographs, automated blood pressure machines, several types of thermometry (including glass oral and rectal thermometers), electronic esophageal stethoscopes, central venous manometers, transcutaneous peripheral nerve stimulators, and pulse oximeters. Monitoring of arterial blood gases is considered vital: DEPMEDS purchased a GEM-STAT blood-gas analyzer (manufactured by Mallinckrodt Sensor Systems, Ann Arbor, Mich.) for the Persian Gulf War and it was included in the 1990 database. Active duty TOE units have this monitor.

Resuscitative Equipment

Resuscitative equipment available includes one defibrillator for each operating room; one external, noninvasive pacemaker in each Emergency Medical Treatment module; and two invasive, external pacemakers, all of which are included in each Medical Services Augmentation set (D413) at the fourth echelon. Gas-powered volume ventilators (the Ohmeda 7000, manufactured by Ohmeda, Inc., Madison, Wis.) and the Ohmeda PAC (portable anesthesia circuit, manufactured by Ohmeda, Inc., Madison, Wis.) unit have been added to the armamentarium. Pressure transducers are not part of the DEPMEDS equipment, but were recommended and requested at the March 1992 update. The Uni-Vent 750 ventilator (manufactured by Impact Medical Corp., West Caldwell, N.J.), a compact, portable ventilator used to provide short-term ventilatory support for an intensive-care-unit patient population, was first made available to the U.S. Army Medical Department (AMEDD) during the Persian Gulf War. Approximately 1,900 units are currently in the DEPMEDS inventory.[5]

Medical Gases

Medical gases are supplied in the operating room MMS. Oxygen tanks include the D cylinder for use as back-up on the Ohmeda 885 Field Anesthesia Machine (manufactured by Ohmeda, Inc., Madison, Wis.) and the M cylinder for use as the central source. H cylinders (6,900 L) are also available. The D cylinder contains approximately 360 L of oxygen and the M cylinder contains 2,835 L at standard temperature and pressure. Medical Supply, a part of Medical Logistics, is responsible for receiving, storing, and issuing all necessary supplies consumed during an operation, including delivery of and exchanging of medical gas cylinders in the operating room. Oxygen tanks are changed on a regular basis and the potential for errors related to the oxygen supply exists, making the in-line oxygen monitor a valuable device. Preventive and corrective maintenance is very limited. An anesthesiologist assigned to a DEPMEDS unit should check with Medical Logistics once the hospital is set up to determine not only what replacement equipment is available but also the extent of the biomedical repair staff's repair capability.

Blood-Recovery Equipment

Blood-recovery equipment is contained in the Blood Recovery/Delivery System Augmentation set (D343) and currently consists of one Haemonetics Cell Saver 4 (manufactured by Haemonics Corp., Braintree, Mass.) machine and the equipment necessary to perform 100 cases (including harnesses, bags, tubing, sterile fluids, and heparin). The blood-recovery system is expected to be used in the preoperative and intraoperative periods in cases of massive hemorrhage. The system is also approved for use in cases of gross blood contamination.

Setup and cleaning are the responsibility of the operating room technicians, and intraoperative use is the responsibility of anesthesia personnel. Efficient intraoperative use of the blood-recovery system requires a second person besides the primary anesthesia provider.

A Level 1 blood-warming infusion device (manufactured by Level 1 Technologies, Inc., Rockland, Mass.) is currently available in DEPMEDS (one Level 1 for every two operating room beds).

Anesthetic Drugs

The pharmacological armamentarium of anesthetics and anesthetic adjuvants available in the operating room set was revised in March 1992 (Table 6-1). At the onset of Operation Desert Shield (ie, the build-up phase of the Persian Gulf War) in August 1990, the primary induction agents were pentothal, ketamine, and diazepam. Maintenance agents were fentanyl and halothane. Muscle relaxants were succinylcholine and pancuronium. The local anesthetic agents were lidocaine, bupivacaine, mepivacaine, and tetracaine. Anesthetics that were deleted at the 1992 update include diazepam, pancuronium, Demerol (meperidine; manufactured by Sanofi Winthrop Pharmaceuticals, New York, N. Y.), and curare. Drugs that had not been available in the basic Operating Room MMS but were added at the March 1992 update include phenylephrine, vecuronium, esmolol, labetalol, nitroglycerin (intravenous preparation), isoflurane, propofol, preservative-free morphine, sufentanil, midazolam, sodium citrate, metoclopramide, 7.5% bupivacaine in dextrose, dexamethasone, albuterol inhalers, and verapamil.

Miscellaneous Equipment

Miscellaneous equipment items that were added at the March 1992 update include epidural kits, hygroscopic humidifiers, Y-type blood-administration sets, and 8.5 French central venous catheter kits. Also added were 3.0- to 6.0-mm (internal diameter) uncuffed pediatric endotracheal tubes, 22-gauge intravenous catheters, and mini-drip intravenous-infusion sets. At the March 1992 update, it was also recommended that a discrete monitoring package be adopted for DEPMEDS. The prototype for this would be the PROPAQ 106 monitor (manufactured by Propaq Systems, Beaverton, Ore.) and ideally would include the ability to monitor the electrical activity of the heart, oxygen saturation, blood pressure (noninvasive), end-tidal carbon dioxide, and to measure two invasive pressures (ie, arterial and central venous pressure).

Essential characteristics for a new field anesthesia machine to replace the Ohio 885 were also submitted by anesthesia representatives to the March 1992 update. Shortcomings of the Ohio 885 include obsolete technology and heavy reliance on compressed gas. Most importantly, because the machine does not meet American Society for Testing and Materials (ASTM) standards, it cannot be used during peacetime for training or patient care. Ideally, the new machine would

- be a small, compact, durable, closed-circuit system;
- be powered by compressed gas (45 psi), an oxygen concentrator, or an air compressor;
- be a multiagent (isoflurane and halothane) vaporizer; and
- meet all ASTM standards.

Work on the development of and procurement for this machine is in progress. Market and industry surveys, development, field testing, and procurement will probably take 3 to 5 years.

The anesthesia drugs and equipment were selected to provide general anesthesia via mask or endotracheal tube, with either controlled or spontaneous ventilation; and regional anesthesia including Bier, axillary, spinal, epidural, and peripheral

TABLE 6-1

ANESTHESIA-RELATED DRUGS CONTAINED IN THE BASIC OPERATING ROOM MEDICAL MATERIAL SETS*

Drug	Concentration or Amount	Quantity or Size Dispensed
Albumin	25 %	100 mL
Albuterol inhaler†	—	17 g
Atropine	0.4 mg/mL	20 mL
Benzoin	—	1 pint
Bupivacaine	0.5%	30 mL
Bupivacaine HCl in dextrose†	7.5 mg/mL	2-mL ampule
$CaCl_2$	100 mg/mL	10-mL syringe
Dyphenhydramine HCl	50 mg/mL	1 mL
Dantrolene sodium	—	20-mg vial
Dextrose in H_2O	5%	50-mL bag
Droperidol inj†	2.5 mg/mL	2-mL ampule
Dexamethasone sodium phosphate inj†	4 mg/mL	5-mL vial
Epinephrine inj USP†	1 mg/mL	1-mL ampule
Epinephrine inj	0.1 mg/mL	10-mL syringe
Esmolol HCl†	10 mg/mL	10-mL vial
Ephedrine sulfate	25 mg/mL	1-mL ampule
Fentanyl citrate inj USP	25 µg/mL	2-mL ampule
Glycopyrrolate inj†	0.2 mg/mL	20-mL vial
Halothane	—	250 mL
Heparin sodium	1,000 units/mL	10 mL
Hetastarch in NaCl	500-mL bag	—
Hydralazine†	20 mg/mL	1-mL vial
Isoflurane USP†	—	100-mL bottle
Isopropyl alcohol USP	—	1 quart
Ketamine HCl inj	50 mg/mL	10-mL vial
Lidocaine	40 mg/mL	25 mL, for infusion
Lidocaine	1%	50 mL
Lidocaine	2%	20-mL vial
Lidocaine HCl + dextrose†	5%	2-mL vial
Lidocaine ointment	5%	35 g
Lidocaine and USP epinephrine inj	1%	20 mL
Lidocaine HCl	1% inj	10-mL syringe
Labetolol HCl inj USP†	5 mg/mL	20 mL
Lubricant, ophthalmic	—	—
Mepivacaine HCl inj†	20mg/mL	50 mL
Midazolam HCl†	5 mg/mL	1-mL vial
Morphine sulfate inj	10 mg/mL	1-mL ampule
Morphine sulfate inj, preservative-free†	—	5-mg vial
Naloxone	0.4 mg/mL	1 mL
Nitroglycerine	5 mg/mL	10-mL vial
Neostigmine	1 mg/mL	10 mL
Nitroprusside†	5 mg/mL	10 mL
Povidone-iodine topical solution	—	3.8 L
Phenylephrine HCl†	1%	1-mL vial
Propofol inj†	10 mg/mL	20-mL ampule
Ringer's lactate	—	1,000-mL bag
Soda lime cartridge	—	—
Sodium bicarbonate	8.4% syringe	50 mL
Sodium chloride inj USP	—	1,000-mL bag
Sodium citrate and citric acid†	oral solution	—
Succinylcholine	20 mg/mL	10-mL vial
Succinylcholine	—	1 g powder
Tetracaine	—	20-mg ampule
Thiopental sodium inj	—	5-g bottle
Vecuronium bromide†	—	10 mg powder, vial
Verapamil†	2.5 mg/mL	2-mL vial
Water for inj, sterile	—	5-mL vial

inj: injection
*As of March 1992
†Recommended additions from the March 1992 DEPMEDS update. These drugs will have to be approved and then purchased before they are placed in DEPMEDS hospitals.
Adapted from Scotti MJ, chairman. Defense Medical Standardization Board. *DEPMEDS Policies/Guidelines: Treatment Briefs*. Fort Detrick, Frederick, Md: 1990: App D.

nerve blocks. Anesthetic drugs and equipment may be available for other techniques to be performed, depending on the experience and innovation of the anesthesiologist or nurse anesthetist.

Fluid Resuscitation

Fluid resuscitation has been stressed appropriately in the outfitting of DEPMEDS facilities. Lactated Ringer's solution and normal saline are the primary crystalloid resuscitative solutions. Hetastarch and albumin are the colloid solutions available and are supplied for use in patients whose estimated blood losses exceed 1,500 mL. Blood products including packed red blood cells, fresh frozen plasma, and platelets (which are typically provided as 200- to 300-mL "six-packs") are also available.

DEPMEDS-EQUIPPED HOSPITALS

DEPMEDS-equipped hospitals are designed to be used in all situations by all four armed services of the U.S. military. By 1990, the army had decided on fielding six types of DEPMEDS-equipped hospitals: general, station, field, evacuation, combat support, and MASH, which have differing mobility, missions, numbers of operating rooms, numbers and types of beds, and types of patients. Physically, DEPMEDS-configured hospitals consist of expandable metal boxes, which, although they are somewhat similar to the hard-walled expandable shelters of the MUST, are really quite different; and TEMPER (*t*ents, *e*xtendable, *m*odular, *per*sonnel) tents, which replaced the MUST program's inflatable shelters. The equipment needed to make the International Standards Organization (ISO) shelters and TEMPER tents functional in their various configurations is contained within MMSs. Electricity is provided by 100-kW, diesel-powered generators.

The expandable shelters were made to conform to the dimensions established for cargo containers by the ISO, and for this reason they are known as ISO shelters. An ISO shelter is, however, not simply a box. Its walls are composed of several layers that, when folded out, can be reconfigured into one or two additional boxes. Thus, the internal volume of a single ISO shelter can be doubled (2:1) or tripled (3:1) (Figure 6-6).

TEMPER tents are the second major component of DEPMEDS hospitals. They differ from standard army tents by having a magnesium-alloy frame instead of wooden poles and a covering that is made of vinyl-covered fabric rather than canvas. In contrast to standard-issue tents, TEMPER tents have fabric floors, a feature that not only limits dust and mud within the patient treatment areas but also makes possible more-efficient cooling and heating of the enclosed space. Individual modules are 8 ft long x 20 ft wide and are extended into either two- or eight-section tents (Figure 6-7). The triage/emergency medical treatment/preoperative module and the postoperative/intensive care units are both composed of eight-module TEMPER tents.

Each DEPMEDS hospital is composed of the same integral components, including (*a*) the patient treatment areas: operating room, emergency medical treatment area, intensive care unit, intensive care ward, and minimal care ward; and (*b*) the ancillary support areas: the clinical laboratory and blood bank, the radiology area, and the pharmacy, among others. The exact configuration of these various areas can be changed depending on the tactical situation and patient flow. These functional areas are not likely to change with Medical Force 2000 (MF2K, which is discussed later in this chapter); the

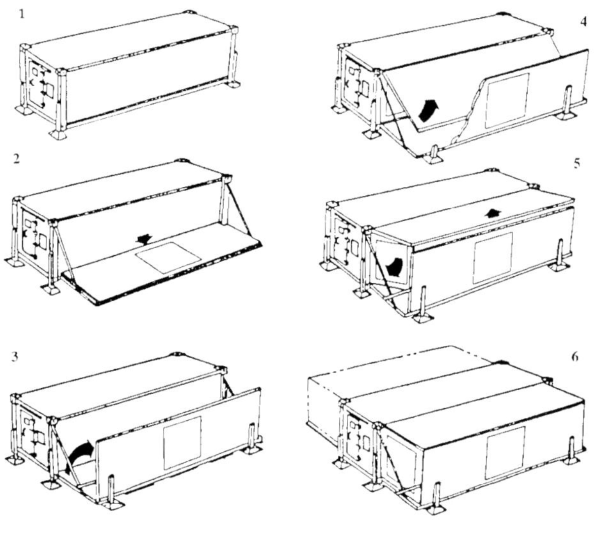

Fig. 6-6. The construction of a 2:1 ISO (International Standards Organization) shelter (**1–5**). The side wall of the original box consists of three individual walls that are folded out to enclose the additional space. A 3:1 ISO shelter can be formed by a similar process performed on the opposite wall (**6**). Adapted from Department of the Army. *Deployable Medical Systems*. Washington, DC: Headquarters, DA; 1990. TC 8-13: 3-21–3-26.

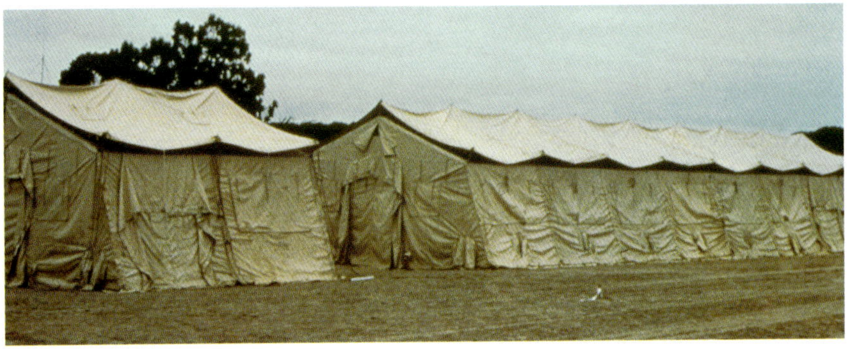

Fig. 6-7. Two TEMPER tent modules have been combined to form the tent on the left, while eight modules have been combined to form the tent shown in the rear. TEMPER: *t*ents, *e*xtendable, *m*odular, *per*sonnel.

equipment contained in them, though, will continue to change as technological advancements are made.

Patient Care Areas

The operating room in a DEPMEDS facility is a 3:1 ISO shelter, which houses two operating tables and the necessary equipment to perform two operations simultaneously (Figure 6-8). The layout of the operating room specifies that both operating room tables face in the same direction, which allows the anesthesia provider more flexibility in monitoring patients. The anesthesiologist is equipped with an Ohmeda 885 Field Anesthesia Machine, Ohmeda 7000 volume ventilator, anesthesia cart, intravenous infusion pole, and suction from an operating room suction machine. The main oxygen supply (two M cylinders per operating room table) and both a fluid and a blanket warmer are all located within the operating room. The operating room layout is schematic and can be changed depending on the type of surgery. Having two operating room tables in one room allows personnel to be used more efficiently and creates a mutual back-up system for equipment and supplies. An associated operating room preparation MMS was supposed to be available, but this appears not to have been deployed.

The emergency medical treatment area is set up to provide initial medical evaluation and treatment, triage, and resuscitation, and to serve as a preoperative holding area when no surgical delay is anticipated (Figure 6-9). Each emergency medical treatment area has space for 12 litter patients and is capable of monitoring vital signs including oxygen saturation and the electrical activity of the heart in a limited number of patients. It is equipped to provide Advanced Trauma Life Support (ATLS; discussed in Chapter 1, Combat Trauma Overview) care to all patients, and mechanical ventilation to a very limited number (but only to two patients at a time). Depending on the size of the hospital, two or more emergency medical treatment sets were designed into the new MF2K structure to accommodate the hypothetical number of incoming casualties.

The intensive care unit is designed to provide care to the most seriously injured and to sick patients of all types (Figure 6-10). Each intensive care unit has 12 beds and can mechanically ventilate six patients using volume ventilators. The unit is capable of monitoring the patients' electrocardiographic status and oxygen saturation but, as is the case throughout DEPMEDS, does not currently have the capability for any type of invasive blood pressure monitoring except central venous pressure via manometry. The intensive care unit may also be used as a postanesthetic recovery area.

The intermediate care ward is designed to provide care to acutely injured or sick patients of all types. The ward does not normally care for patients who require continuous monitoring or life-support devices, but the level of acuity can vary greatly depending on the type of conflict or catastrophe. The intermediate care ward can also serve as a specialty area (ie, a burn ward). It has the capacity for 20 patients.

The minimal care ward provides care to medical and surgical patients who are ambulatory and partially self-sufficient. No intravenous fluids or parenteral medications are administered on this ward. The primary focus on the ward is the physical and psychological conditioning of soldiers expected to return to duty. The ward has a capacity of 40 patients housed in two general purpose, large (GPL) tents.

The relative mix of anesthesia-relevant MMSs, ISO shelters, and TEMPER tents depends on the type of hospital. The authorization matrix for the 1990 version of DEPMEDS is shown in Table 6-2. Updating of the matrix is continuous, however, and this information has already been changed by MF2K.

a

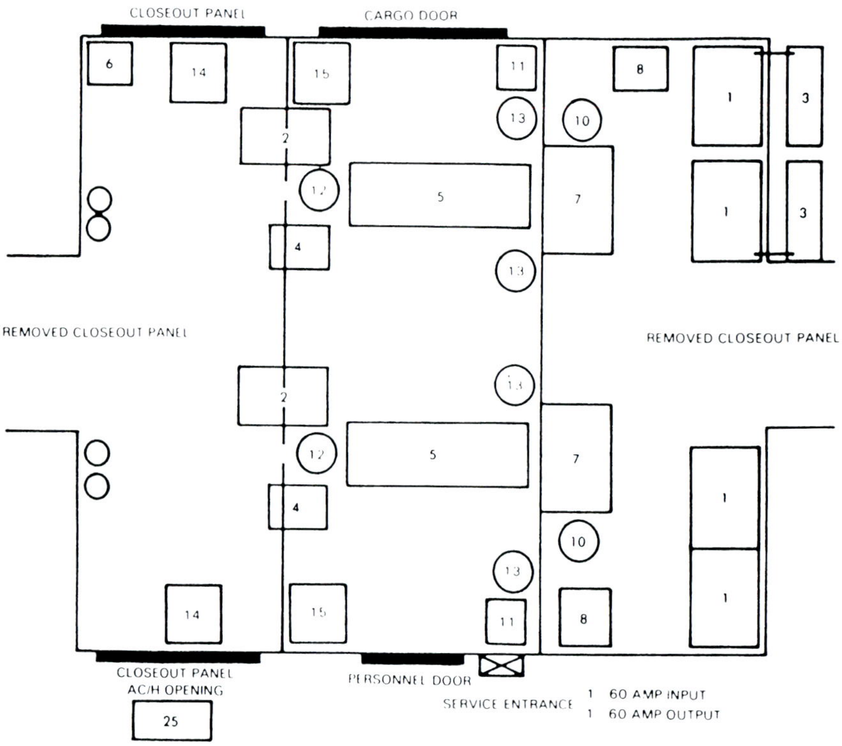

1: Cabinet, pharmacy, base
2: Cart, anesthetic equipment
3: Cabinet, pharmacy, upper
4: Apparatus, anesthetic
5: Table, operating, field
6: Regulator, thermo
7: Table, surgical instrument
8: Table, surgical instrument and dressing
10: Stand, basin, folding
11: Apparatus, electrosurgical
12: Stool, revolving
13: Pail
14: Cloth, frame
15: Apparatus, suction
25: Air conditioner/heater

b

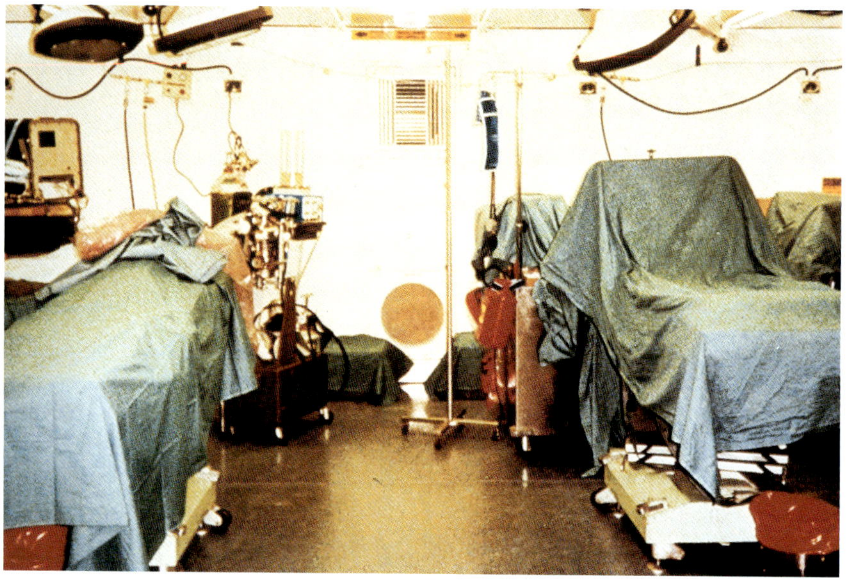

Fig. 6-8. (**a**) The recommended arrangement of the DEPMEDS operating room medical material set in a 3:1 ISO shelter. (**b**) The two operating tables in a 3:1 ISO face in the same direction, which allows the anesthesia provider more flexibility in monitoring patients. DEPMEDS: Department of Defense's Deployable Medical Systems; ISO: International Standards Organization. Diagram (a) : Reprinted from Department of the Army. Deployable Medical Systems. Washington, DC: Headquarters, DA; 1990. TC 8-13: 2-2.

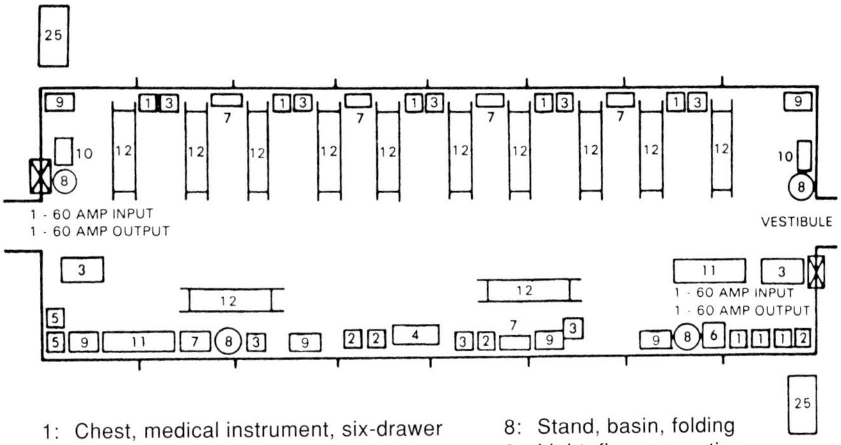

1: Chest, medical instrument, six-drawer
2: Chest, medical instrument, #3 field
3: Chest, medical instrument, two-shelf
4: Cart, resuscitation, mobile
5: Chest, medical instrument (utility)
6: Refrigerator-freezer, mechanical
7: Stand, surgical instrument
8: Stand, basin, folding
9: Light, floor, operating
10: Sink unit, surgical
11: Table, folding legs, laboratory
12: Litter
25: Air conditioner/heater

Fig. 6-9. The recommended arrangement of the DEPMEDS triage/emergency medical treatment area/preoperative room medical material set in an eight-module TEMPER tent. This facility may or may not be connected to the operating room by an interposed operating room preparation area medical material set. DEPMEDS: Department of Defense's Deployable Medical Systems; TEMPER: *t*ents, *e*xtendable, *m*odular, *per*sonnel. Reprinted from Department of the Army. *Deployable Medical Systems.* Washington, DC: Headquarters, DA; 1990. TC 8-13: 2-36.

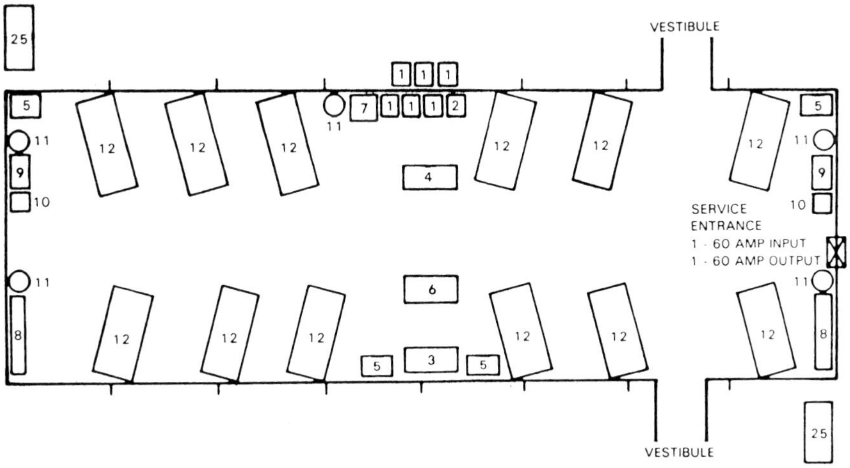

1: Chest, medical instrument, two-shelf
2: Chest, medical instrument with 22-drawer insert
3: Cart, resuscitation
4: Desk, field with folding chairs
5: Light, floor, operating and exam
6: Cart, surgical dressing
7: Refrigerator-freezer
8: Shelf, chrome, 1848
9: Sink unit, surgical
10: Frame, cloth basket, folding
11: Stand, basin, folding
12: Bed, adjustable, hospital
25: Air conditioner/heater

Fig. 6-10. The recommended arrangement of the DEPMEDS postoperative/intensive care unit medical material set in an eight-module TEMPER tent. This facility would be connected to the end of the operating room medical material set opposite the triage/emergency medical treatment area/preoperative room medical material set. DEPMEDS: Department of Defense's Deployable Medical Systems; TEMPER: *t*ents, *e*xtendable, *m*odular, *per*sonnel. Reprinted from Department of the Army.*Deployable Medical Systems.* Washington, DC : Headquarters, DA; 1990. TC 8-13: 2-32.

TABLE 6-2

DEPLOYABLE MEDICAL SYSTEMS–MEDICAL MATERIAL SET AUTHORIZATION MATRIX

Medical Material Set	DEPMEDS-Equipped Hospitals (Number of Sets)						
	MASH	CSH	EVAC	STA 300	STA 500	FH	GH
Operating room	2	2	3	1	2	3	3
Triage area	1	1	1	1	1	3	1
Intensive care unit	5	4	4	2	4	3	8
Intermediate care	0	4	8	9	15	9	30
Minimal care	0	4	10	5	8	9	15

MASH: Mobile Army Surgical Hospital; CSH: Combat Support Hospital; EVAC: Evacuation Hospital; STA 300: Station Hospital, 300 beds; STA 500: Station Hospital, 500 beds; FH: Field Hospital; GH: General Hospital
Adapted from US Department of the Army. *Deployable Medical Systems: Tactics, Techniques, and Procedures*. Washington, DC: Headquarters, DA; 7 Dec 1990. Training Circular 8-13, Table 2-1, p 2-24.

Ancillary Support Areas

The laboratory section of a DEPMEDS-equipped facility consists of two parts: the clinical laboratory and the blood bank. The clinical laboratory provides basic hematology, chemistry, urinalysis, microbiology, and serology; cytology and pathology can be performed only if an augmentation team with equipment is added to the hospital. The complete list of tests provided is contained in the *DEPMEDS Policies/Treatment Briefs*; Table 6-3 includes only tests of particular interest to anesthesiologists.

There are two types of blood bank sections: the Liquid Blood Bank MMS D304 and the Liquid/Frozen Blood Bank MMS D404. The liquid blood bank can store 500 units of packed red blood cells and can issue 250 units for transfusion in a 24-hour period. Each patient's blood is ABO grouped and Rh typed. A single-tube (major-side saline, immediate spin) cross-match is performed on each patient. The liquid blood bank can draw and type 180 units of fresh whole blood for extreme emergencies. The liquid/frozen blood bank can store 500 units of packed red blood cells, 485 units of frozen red blood cells, 10 units of fresh frozen plasma, and 5 packs of platelets, and is capable of reconstituting 180 units of frozen red blood cells per 24 hours. It can issue up to 250 units of blood for transfusion in a 24-hour period. It has the same emergency blood-drawing capabilities as the liquid blood bank. The storage and transfusion shelf life of the different blood products was established in accordance with the Military Blood Program 2004 Study (which is available from U.S. Army Medical Department [AMEDD] Center and School, Fort Sam Houston, San Antonio, Tex.).

Several assumptions and planning factors are used in calculating blood usage:

- Only blood that is actually to be transfused is ordered.
- Patients with hematocrits of 0.21 or lower will frequently require blood transfusions.
- Single units of blood will not be requested.
- Fresh frozen plasma is transfused at a ratio no greater than 1 unit per 10 units of red blood cells infused into the same patient.
- Platelets are transfused at a ratio no greater than 1 unit per 20 units of red blood cells infused into the same patient.
- Each platelet transfusion is expected to raise the platelet count in a 70-kg man by 30,000 to 80,000 platelets/mm^3.

Both platelets and fresh frozen plasma supplies are extremely limited in the theater of action, and the current recommendation is that they be used only for documented thrombocytopenia or coagulopathy. The transfusion ratios were established using accepted standards of transfusion medicine in trauma settings. However, these are guidelines, and the decision to administer any blood products is a clinical one that is the medical officer's responsibility. A more detailed discussion can be found in Chapter 15, Military Transfusion Practice.

Radiographic support is provided by a fixed, high-capacity, combination X-ray and fluoroscopy unit, and by portable machines. The radiographic capabilities include plain X-ray examinations

TABLE 6-3

LABORATORY PROCEDURES PERFORMED AT THE THIRD AND FOURTH ECHELONS

Test	Task No.	Description	Third Echelon	Fourth Echelon
Chemistry	E001	Blood gas estimation	+	+
	E002	Electrolyte levels (Na^+, K^+, Cl^-, HCO_3)	+	+
	E003	Total serum protein level	+	+
	E004	Urinary protein level	+	+
	E005	Serum creatinine level	+	+
	E007	Serum amalyse level	+	+
	E008	SGPT level	+	+
	E009	CK level	+	+
	E010	Blood glucose	+	+
	E011	BUN level	+	+
	E012	Serum bilirubin	+	+
	E013	Spinal-fluid sugar	+	+
	E014	Spinal-fluid protein	+	+
	E015	SGOT level	—	+
	E017	Calcium level	+	+
Hematology/Urinalysis	E020	CBC (WBC, Hgb, Hct)	+	+
	E021	White cell count	+	+
	E022	Hematocrit level	+	+
	E024	White cell differential count	+	+
	E025	Prothrombin time	+	+
	E026	PTT	+	+
	E028	Spinal fluid cell count and differential	+	+
	E029	Urinalysis with specific gravity	+	+
	E030	Microscopic urinalysis	+	+
	E031	Platelet estimate	+	+
	E032	Platelet count	+	+
	E033	Fibrinogen level and fibrin split products	—	+

SGPT: serum glutamic-pyruvic transaminase (alanine aminotransferase); CK: creatine kinase; BUN: blood urea nitrogen; SGOT: serum glutamic-oxaloacetic transaminase (aspartate aminotransferase); CBC: complete blood count; WBC: white blood cell; Hgb: hemoglobin; Hct: hematocrit; PTT: partial thromboplastin time

Adapted from Scotti MJ, chairman. Defense Medical Standardization Board. *DEPMEDS Policies/Guidelines: Treatment Briefs.* Fort Detrick, Frederick, Md: 1990: 82.

and some special studies (eg, upper gastrointestinal series, intravenous pyelogram, and single-shot angiography). Although only the portable X-ray unit is available in the operating room, the unit can be taken throughout the hospital. A refined C-arm module is in the process of approval and was suggested for procurement and fielding by the year 2000.

The pharmacy stocks a number of drugs that are not part of the operating room MMS. Once the hospital has deployed, the actual placement and distribution of drugs may vary depending on the standing operating procedures of the hospital. The handling of controlled substances will likewise vary depending on the situation and the guidance of the hospital commander.

DEPLOYABLE HOSPITALS IN THE PERSIAN GULF WAR

Forty-four DEPMEDS-equipped hospitals were deployed to Saudi Arabia in support of the Persian Gulf War (Table 6-4).[6] The enormous size and complexity of a typical DEPMEDS-equipped hospital is apparent in Figure 6-11, which shows two evacuation hospitals collocated in the same base camp in the Arabian desert during the Persian Gulf War. Ad hoc forward surgical teams (FSTs) were also deployed and were used in support of combat arms units far forward in the combat zone. These elements were not DEPMEDS-equipped owing to mobility constraints; important components of DEPMEDS equipment (eg, ISO shelters, TEMPER tents, C-arms, laundry units, and other bulky equipment items) were found to be incompatible with high mobility. The ISO shelters require specially designed dolly sets for their movement; they are not designed to be transported by truck, a significant drawback in a war characterized by movement. The DEPMEDS equipment is too heavy and too complex, and the reassembly is too time-consuming for modern maneuver warfare. The afteraction reports from Operation Desert Storm are replete with statements that hospital equipment cannot be moved rapidly enough to support the needs of a highly mobile army:

> There were strong feelings in regard to the mobility of DEPMEDS equipment, especially in this conflict when hospitals had to move long distances in short periods of time, and then rapidly prepare to receive casualties.[7(p8–24)]
>
> . . . .
>
> A hospital following the forward maneuver units and providing surgical care should be capable of establishing the Emergency Medical Treatment (EMT) section and one to two operating rooms (OR) in 1 to 2 hours, and the entire hospital in 6 to 8 hours. The hospital should be able to break down and be prepared to move in less than 12 hours. The hospital should be capable of moving in sandy and rough terrain.
>
> In Operation Desert Storm, most forward hospitals took 3 to 4 hours to have an operating room set up, 6 to 8 hours to set up the EMT section, and almost 24 hours to establish the entire hospital. Thirty-six to 48 hours were required to break down and pack the hospital. Thirty 5-ton trucks were required to move the hospital, with only approximately 10 contained in the unit TOE. Each truck also had an attached dolly set. Each dolly set required 8 to 12 people a half hour (or more at night) to attach. The dolly set had only a 12-inch clearance, causing it to be easily hung up, in the front, in rough terrain (offroad).[7(p1–11)]

TABLE 6-4

HOSPITALS DEPLOYED TO SAUDI ARABIA (1990)

Hospital	Number Deployed
Mobile Army Surgical Hospital	8
Combat Support Hospital	9
Evacuation Hospital	22
Station Hospital	1
Field Hospital	3
General Hospital	1
Total	**44**

Hospitals deployed during the Persian Gulf War included both active duty and reserve or National Guard units. By August 1990, very few active duty units had converted to DEPMEDS. Those that had invariably suffered from shortages of equipment and pharmaceuticals. The training sets that reserve and National Guard hospitals were issued contained only minimal essential equipment, while the complete hospital sets were placed in storage as prepositioned material configured in units and sets (POMCUS) or primary mobilization stations (PRIMOB). Shortages were attributed to the newness of the system, delays in purchase from the industrial base, and sometimes delayed decisions from clinical groups that reviewed equipment and drug selection. The following priority sequence was used in fielding DEPMEDS:

1. unequipped reserve and National Guard units,
2. active duty, rapid-deployment units,
3. regional training sites, and
4. active duty TOE hospitals.

At the time of deployment, the decision was made to modernize in theater. Therefore, equipment sets that had been packed for long-term storage were lacking (ie, short) some equipment and were not functionally operational when they arrived in country. These equipment shortages led to the ship-short concept: the package of missing equip-

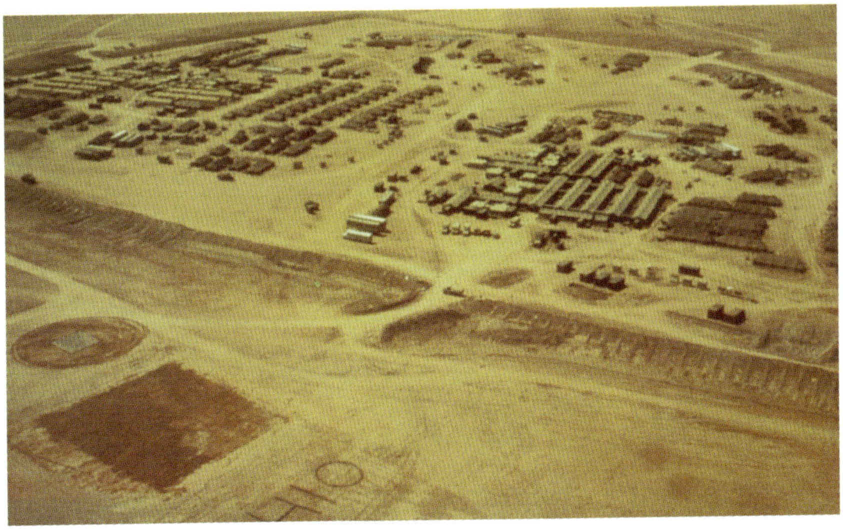

Fig. 6-11. Two evacuation hospitals, the 148th in the distance on the left and the 410th in the near right, deployed in the Kuwaiti Theater of Operations during the Persian Gulf War. TEMPER tents form much of the central portion of the 410th. ISO shelters can be identified by their lighter color. Hospital personnel are billeted in the complex of canvas tents that occupy the right side of the hospital. TEMPER: *t*ents, *e*xtendable, *m*odular, *per*sonnel; ISO: International Standards Organization. Photograph: Courtesy of Public Affairs, Office of The Surgeon General, US Army.

ment (ie, the push packet) would be sent to the units in theater as soon as it could be procured. Correction of shortages was actually a complex process; it involved six independent, functional areas that procured equipment and supplies. Delivery to specific hospitals in theater then required the coordinated efforts of the Medical Supply, Optical, and Maintenance (MEDSOM) Battalion (which is now called the Medical Logistics Battalion).

Communication—both between hospitals and between air force and army evacuation assets—was frequently a problem. Deployed personnel cited premobilization instruction in theater communications networks and standing operating procedures as critical information to help avoid future problems.

Afteraction reports by anesthesiologists (60N) and nurse anesthetists (66F) expressed concerns about the following missing equipment:

- noninvasive blood pressure machines,
- pulse oximeters,
- electrocardiographs,
- adequate suction devices,
- regional anesthesia kits and needles,
- oxygen tubing, and
- medications (eg, isoflurane, vecuronium, midazolam, reversal agents, and pentothal).

It must be emphasized, however, that many of the items and drugs (including isoflurane, vecuronium, and even nitrous oxide) that deployed personnel expected to have, were *never* on the TOE for DEPMEDS hospitals, and therefore should not have been expected. However, the Office of The Surgeon General decided to attempt to provide non-TOE pharmaceuticals if such were requested by deployed physicians. In addition to standard U.S. Army channels, sources for equipment procurement included local purchase, Air Force logistics, and even personal mail from hospitals in the continental United States. All hospitals were operational by the onset of the ground war.

Work load, patient type, and frequency of movement varied widely among the 44 DEPMEDS hospitals deployed to Saudi Arabia. Patient categories included U.S. and allied military battle injury and nonbattle injury, civilian disease and injury, and Iraqi prisoners. The variety of patient conditions encountered emphasized the need for the DEPMEDS system to be able to support all aspects of clinical anesthesia: emergency and elective (neurosurgical, thoracic, abdominal, vascular, etc), and regional, obstetrical, and even pediatric anesthesia. The percentages of multiple-trauma cases varied widely in the afteraction reports.[7]

The most frequently used anesthetic agents included isoflurane, succinylcholine, vecuronium, thiopental, ketamine, local anesthetics, and fentanyl. By far the most commonly used general anesthetic technique was a rapid-sequence induction with tracheal intubation, followed by a balanced anesthetic. Packed red blood cells were frequently used, but the use and availability of fresh frozen plasma or platelets was minimal to nonexistent. Oxygen supplies, particularly for refilling tanks, were frequently inadequate. Sterile water was supplied in plastic bottles.

The Persian Gulf War provided the first true test of the DEPMEDS system. As with any new system, problems were encountered and weaknesses uncovered; nevertheless, the conversion to DEPMEDS was completed in theater and all hospitals were ready by the time the ground offensive commenced. Overall, the system worked well under often adverse conditions, although the limited number of casualties makes an assessment of DEPMEDS' true value difficult to make. The Defense Medical Standardization Board will continue to conduct a review of equipment and drugs approximately every 2 years; changes will be made as necessary. The system will always be in transition so that it can keep up with changes in warfare, medical doctrine, and new developments in medical technology. The structure of the medical force will continue to evolve. Changes in war-fighting doctrine, changes in the nature and sophistication of threat forces, and the increasing requirement for AMEDD to be involved in peacetime missions will necessitate constant changes and force modifications.

MEDICAL FORCE 2000

While DEPMEDS is essentially a system describing the characteristics of hardware, Medical Force 2000 (MF2K) deals not only with equipment but also with personnel and organization. Four types of hospitals—MASH, combat support, field, and general—and a medical holding company were initially envisioned by MF2K. Under MF2K, station and evacuation hospitals will be deleted from the system, and the MASH configuration will change dramatically. These changes will largely be made to prevent duplication in the system and to streamline the patient-evacuation flow. The original concept calls for the MASH to be changed from a 60-bed, DEPMEDS-configured facility to a more-mobile, 30-bed, non-DEPMEDS unit. The MASH remains a surgical unit only, with minimal medical-treatment or patient-holding capability. Likewise, for mobility considerations, the MASH will not use ISO shelters. The combat support, field, and general hospitals will remain DEPMEDS equipped. The numbers of anesthesiologists and nurse anesthetists proposed for each type of hospital are found in Table 6-5. The third echelon includes the MASH, combat support hospital, and medical holding company; the fourth echelon includes field and general hospitals. Like DEPMEDS, MF2K is subject to revision, the process being known as the medical reengineering initiative (MRI).

The MF2K designs for the combat support, field, and general hospitals are built using a four-module concept:

- Hospital Unit, Base (HUB)
- Hospital Unit, Surgical (HUS)
- Hospital Unit, Medical (HUM)
- Hospital Unit, Holding (HUH)

The HUB, a base, can operate independently and is located in each hospital as the initial building block. The exact composition of the base may vary among the different hospitals. The other modules contain the necessary equipment, supplies, and assigned personnel to accomplish the particular mission (eg, to provide an operating room capability for a certain number of operating tables, in the case of the HUS). Future AMEDD force-structure doctrine, as expressed in MF2K and MRI, will emphasize the tailoring of medical assets for the proposed mission, an undertaking less easily accomplished with previous DEPMEDS-configured hospitals designed for a high-intensity war.

Mobile Army Surgical Hospital

The original MF2K design for the MASH converted the existing 60-bed hospital to a highly mobile 30-bed facility designed to function in the rear area of the division or the forward area of the corps. Surgical capability was based on three operating room tables for general, orthopedic, and thoracic surgery. Preoperative and postoperative acute nursing care for up to 30 patients was provided in three wards. The following services were planned: pharmacy, clinical laboratory, liquid-blood bank, radi-

TABLE 6-5

MEDICAL FORCE 2000 ANESTHESIA STAFFING

Hospital	Anesthesiologists* (Number)	CRNAs† (Number)
MASH	1	4
Combat Support Hospital	3	15
Field Hospital	1	2
General Hospital	3	15

*60N
†66F
MASH: Mobile Army Surgical Hospital; CRNA: Certified Registered Nurse Anesthetist
Source: Perkins DE. Colonel, Medical Corps, US Army. Washington, DC: Walter Reed Army Medical Center. Personal communication, June 1995.

ology, and food services. Unfortunately, it soon became apparent that the reduction in weight and volume was less than desired: in 1992, a MASH weighed 240,500 lb and occupied 17,514 ft^3, and the MF2K MASH weighed 184,331 lb and occupied 15,498 ft^3.[8] In the future, neither the 30- nor the 60-bed MASH will be fielded.

The configuration of the army's forward surgical hospitals has undergone a great deal of study, analysis, and field testing during the last half century and an entirely satisfactory design is not yet available. In no other type of hospital is the tension between the perceived need for ever-increasing medical sophistication and complexity and the military logistical requirements for a high degree of strategic and tactical mobility more apparent. One of the implicit assumptions behind DEPMEDS was to match the standards of civilian hospitals while also being able to care for the massive casualty load expected to be generated by a high-intensity war in Europe. Planners tacitly assumed that transportation capability would appear when needed. In essence, bed capacity and sophistication of care were favored over mobility and sustainment. The MASH, which has long been criticized as being too heavy and bulky to have the needed degree of strategic or tactical mobility, was more affected by this design philosophy than was any other DEPMEDS hospital. The commander of the 5th MASH during the Persian Gulf War has written of the need to reverse the DEPMEDS approach to the design of deployable hospitals by first defining weight and volume limits compatible with strategic and tactical mobility. Weight and volume limits should then be used to determine the number of beds, surgical capability, and staffing.[9]

Forward Surgical Team

The MASH is to be replaced by a TOE unit to be known as the FST. This unit, of which at least 30 are planned, will have 2 operating tables and 8 beds. It will be staffed by 3 general surgeons and 1 orthopedic surgeon; 2 nurse anesthetists; 1 each operating room nurse, intensive care nurse, medical-surgical nurse; and 11 medics. The FST will be housed in lightweight collective protective equipment developed by the U.S. army and known as chemical biological protective shelters (CBPS). The tents are made of synthetic materials, and will be moved in six high-mobility, multipurpose, wheeled vehicles (HMMWVs) (Figure 6-12). The CBPS, which looks superficially like the Vietnam War–era MUST shelter (see Figure 6-4), has a rib structure and is inflated by a compressor integral to the HMMWV. The inflated, insulated CBPS has airlocks for both litter and ambulatory access.[10]

An FST is eminently air-transportable and can, with its organic vehicles, be moved by two C-141 missions (or possibly only one). By way of contrast, the 1990 version of the MASH required no less than 32 C-141 missions for its deployment.[9] Standard DEPMEDS MMSs will not be used. Supplies will be available for 72 hours of continuous operations, during which period 30 major operations can be performed. Supplies include 60 units of Group O, Rh-negative blood.

The original plan called for the FST to be collocated with a brigade- or division-level medical company, with the patient flow being through the medical company. The critically injured casualties were to be sent directly to the FST, with the remainder of the casualties to be evacuated after resuscitation to third-echelon hospitals. Because a medical company may not always be available, or because logistical and personnel constraints may have reduced the capability of the medical company, an additional option has been formulated: the FST can be deployed with both a holding and a treatment squad, the combined unit being called a Medical Readiness Task Force.

Command and control of the FST was to have been from the combat support hospital to which the FST was originally attached (but not part of) when not deployed, but it is now likely that the FST will be controlled by the corps-level medical brigade. Regardless of the resolution of the command-and-control issues, today's FST is nearly identical in form and function to the forward battlefield surgical team of World War II (see Figures 6-1 through 6-3).

The effect of advanced technology has been more incremental than revolutionary on AMEDD's ability to care for gravely wounded, nontransportable casualties. Numerous incremental changes, however, can have a significant total impact. Compare the following points with the list of essential equipment that was compiled by World War II surgeons (see Exhibit 6-1):

1. Transportation is now accomplished on HMMWVs, which are much more mobile and capacious than jeeps.
2. Modern lighting, including the use of headlights by the surgeons, is a fundamental improvement on previous equipment. This is an example of a seemingly minor change that is, in fact, extremely beneficial to surgeons and therefore to combat casualty care.
3. Heavy oxygen cylinders and other equipment need no longer be transported to

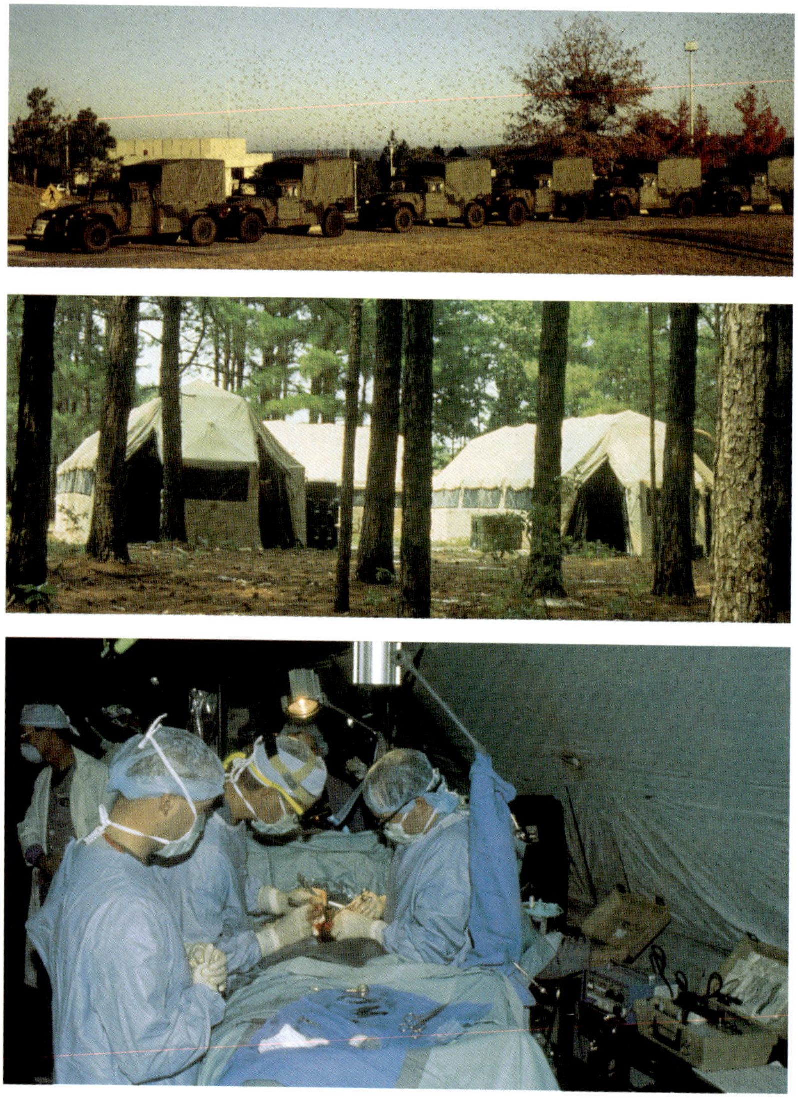

Fig. 6-12. The *d*eployable *r*apid *a*ssembly *sh*elter (DRASH) was used in early prototype forward surgical teams (FSTs), before the decision was made to use the chemical biological protective shelter (CBPS). These photographs of DRASHs were taken during a field exercise carried out by the 274th Forward Surgical Team of the 44th Medical Brigade, Fort Bragg, North Carolina, in November 1995. They illustrate some of the similarities to and changes from forward surgery during World War II (see Figures 6-1 through 6-3). (**a**) The entire team and its equipment are deployed in six high-mobility, multipurpose, wheeled vehicles (HMMWVs). (**b**) The FST works in three interconnected shelters. The first tent is for receiving and resuscitating casualties; the second contains two operating tables, draw-over anesthesia equipment, and surgical instruments; and the third, which has eight beds, is the intensive care and recovery area. The DRASH could be set up and made fully functioning within 1 hour; an individual CBPS, using only three men, in 15 minutes.[1] (**c**) An actual operation is seen in progress in the operating tent. (1) Gander TJ. *Jane's NBC Protection Equipment*. 5th ed. Surry, United Kingdom: Jane's Information Group Limited; 1992: 203. Photographs: Courtesy of Major Thomas E. Knuth, MD, MPH, Medical Corps, US Army; Eisenhower Army Medical Center, Fort Gordon, Ga.

forward hospitals. Oxygen concentrators are part of DEPMEDS equipment, and oxygen can be manufactured in situ.

4. The vagaries and possible complications of using fresh blood donations have been obviated by the availability of the hospital's own blood bank and the blood transfusion program.
5. Autoclaving is not used in FSTs; surgical instruments are chemically sterilized. This improvement has relieved the logistical demands of transporting heavy autoclaving equipment.
6. The laundry function of the hospital has been supplanted by the use of disposable towels, gowns, sheets, and other linen.
7. CBPS tents are made of a high-performance fluoropolymer/aramid laminate, in contrast to the heavy canvas that has been used since at least World War I. The lightweight synthetic material can be decontaminated easily and protects personnel inside against chemical and biological warfare agents (liquid and vapor). In addition, individual CBPS units can be connected to make complex collective protection modules.[10] These improvements may provide a more pleasant, climate-controlled environment for casualties and medical personnel, but they do not necessarily translate directly into lower mortality in combat casualty care.

Anesthesiologists in command-and-control positions need to assure the proper use of the FST. In a conventional war, in which the casualty load may fluctuate in a widely unpredictable manner, the FST should be used to care for *only* the critically wounded, the transportable casualties being evacuated to the combat support hospital. If this is not done, the meager resources of the FST may be exhausted just when they are needed to care for an influx of gravely wounded soldiers. Members of the FST and commanders of medical companies in a position to refer casualties *must* understand the role of the FST in the overall context of field medical support. By way of contrast, in operations other than war (OOTW), such as when an FST is deployed to support a small unit not engaged in combat operations, the FST will probably assume treatment functions going beyond the exclusive care of the critically wounded.

Combat Support, Field, and General Hospitals

The mission of the combat support hospital is to stabilize patients for further evacuation and to return to duty those soldiers who fall within the corps evacuation policy. This hospital is capable of handling all types of patients and will be employed in the corps area. Surgical capability is based on eight operating room tables (each used for 18 h/d), for a surgical capacity of 144 operating room–table hours per day. Hospitalization for up to 296 patients includes 96 intensive care beds. The combat support hospital has, organic to its TOE, 35% of the vehicles needed for a tactical move; it is DEPMEDS configured.

The field hospital provides hospitalization for general classes of patients and reconditioning or rehabilitating services for those who can return to duty within the theater evacuation policy. Most patients at this facility will be there for rehabilitation. The field hospital will usually be located in the communication zone. Hospitalization for up to 504 patients includes 36 intensive care beds. Surgical capability is based on two operating room tables, for a capacity of 24 operating room–table hours per day. All movement requirements are the responsibility of theater transportation units. This hospital is DEPMEDS configured.

The general hospital, a 476-bed facility, serves as the main conduit for patient evacuation to the continental United States. It provides stabilization and hospitalization for general classes of patients. Surgical capability is based on eight operating room tables for a capacity of 144 operating room–table hours per day. Intensive nursing care is available for up to 96 patients. The general hospital relies on theater transportation units for movement and is DEPMEDS configured.

MEDICAL REENGINEERING INITIATIVE

The characteristics of U.S. Army deployable hospitals continue to change. The need for change arises from the design of MF2K deployable hospitals, which was based on a high-intensity NATO war-fighting scenario that anticipated vast numbers of combat casualties. The recent U.S. Army experience in the Middle East, Somalia, Haiti, and Bosnia suggests a less apocalyptic battlefield. To meet the multiple deployment contingencies in the early 21st century, the MRI envisions one basic hospital design (not the seven of the original DEPMEDS or the four of MF2K), composed of small but self-sufficient modules. The MRI hospital size and the mix of its beds (eg, intensive care, minimal care) will differ from that of DEPMEDS hospitals. The basic hospital will consist of 248 beds: 48 in intensive care and 200 in intermediate care. Minimal care beds will be provided by a separate medical detachment that will be added to the basic hospital as needed. The basic hospital design calls for five operating tables disposed in three operating room modules. Two of these modules will have two tables each; the third will have one table plus a C-arm for radiographic studies and an operating microscope. The major component of the basic hospital, an 84-bed module, is fully deployable forward with one of the two-table operating room modules.

The new MRI hospital will be able to provide general, orthopedic, thoracic, and oral maxillofacial surgical care. Neurosurgery and eye, ear, nose, and throat surgical capabilities can be added to the basic hospital by attaching a Hospital Augmentation Team–Head and Neck, which will include computed tomography capability. Additional Hospital Augmentation Teams are proposed, including those for Renal Dialysis, Infectious Disease Pathology, and OOTW. Typically civilian medical and public health problems are likely to be encountered in OOTW, and that team will include a pediatrician, pediatric nurse practitioner, community health nurse, obstetrician–gynecologist, midwife, preventive medicine physician, and primary care physician. DEPMEDS equipment, including shelters, will be used in the basic MRI hospital. Lighterweight shelters, based on the recently fielded CBPS system, may become available in the near future.

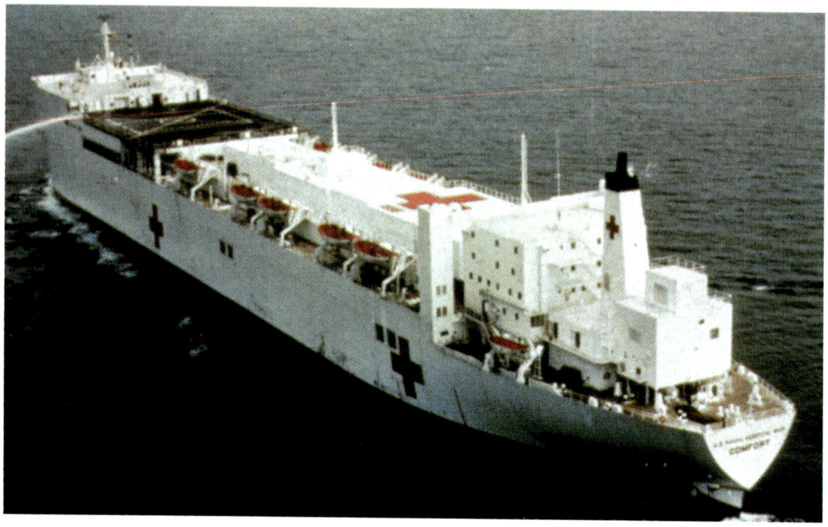

Fig. 6-13. The USNS *Comfort* as viewed from the stern. The helicopter flight deck, designated by the cross, is forward. In addition to having access by two elevators, one next to the helicopter flight deck and one forward, casualties can enter the ship through two water-level loading portals. The *Comfort* and her sister, the *Mercy*, each have an overall length of 894 ft, a beam of 105 ft 9 in., a draft of 32 ft 9 in., a displacement of 69,360 tons, a maximum sustained speed of 17.5 knots, and an endurance of 13,420 nautical miles. Photograph: Courtesy of Colonel James Collins, MD, Medical Corps, US Army, Commandant, Uniformed Services University of the Health Sciences, Bethesda, Md.

A major difference between the MRI hospital and its DEPMEDS/MF2K predecessors is the heavy emphasis in the former on telemedicine and hospital information and communications systems. At present the order of priority will be to develop (1) intrahospital communication with telephones, either wired or cellular; (2) local and wide-area networks for interhospital communications; (3) digital radiology; and ultimately, (4) full-motion video teleconsultation.

The proposed MRI hospital will be deployed to both the corps and the echelon above corps, differing only in that the latter may have fewer organic transportation assets and therefore will be less mobile. Far forward resuscitative surgery will be provided by FSTs as proposed in MF2K.

HOSPITAL SHIPS

The U.S. Navy's hospital ships are the ultimate deployable hospitals. Although the ships are obviously not AMEDD assets, U.S. Army anesthesia providers need to know about their capabilities because of the increasing interdependence of the nation's military medical services. The U.S.N.S. *Mercy* (T-AH 19) and *Comfort* (T-AH 20) were originally 80,000-ton supertankers. During the mid 1980s they were converted into hospital ships with a 50-bed casualty receiving area, 12 operating rooms, 500 acute care beds (20 recovery room, 80 intensive care, and 400 intermediate care beds), and 500 minimal care beds (Figure 6-13). Staffing consisted of 77 physicians, 160 nurses, and 250 enlisted personnel.

During the Persian Gulf War, the ships were given the resources to receive 200 casualties per day for 30 days. The internal organization of the ship's medical treatment facilities and the casualty flow plan, from the helicopter flight deck through the treatment areas to the patient wards, was designed to be simple and rational (Figure 6-14). Although a hospital ship is a remarkable facility with extraordinary treatment capabilities, medical officers should remember that like any hospital, it is useful only if it can be reached by casualties. For the casualty who requires resuscitative surgery, a hospital ship is useful only if the combat occurs near a coastline.[11]

SUMMARY

A modern army must take a hospital system with it. To be useful, the deployed hospitals must have some degree of strategic and tactical mobility. Tactical mobility is essential for hospitals that are to care for combat casualties since, to be optimally effective, surgical care must be rendered far forward on the battlefield. During World War II, this was achieved by attaching small teams of surgeons and anesthesia providers to platoon-sized units from field hospitals. Austere surgical hospitals in tents were set up in the division rear area, where they were collocated with medical units organic to the division. The MASH, a TOE version of the World War II surgical team–field hospital platoon, was

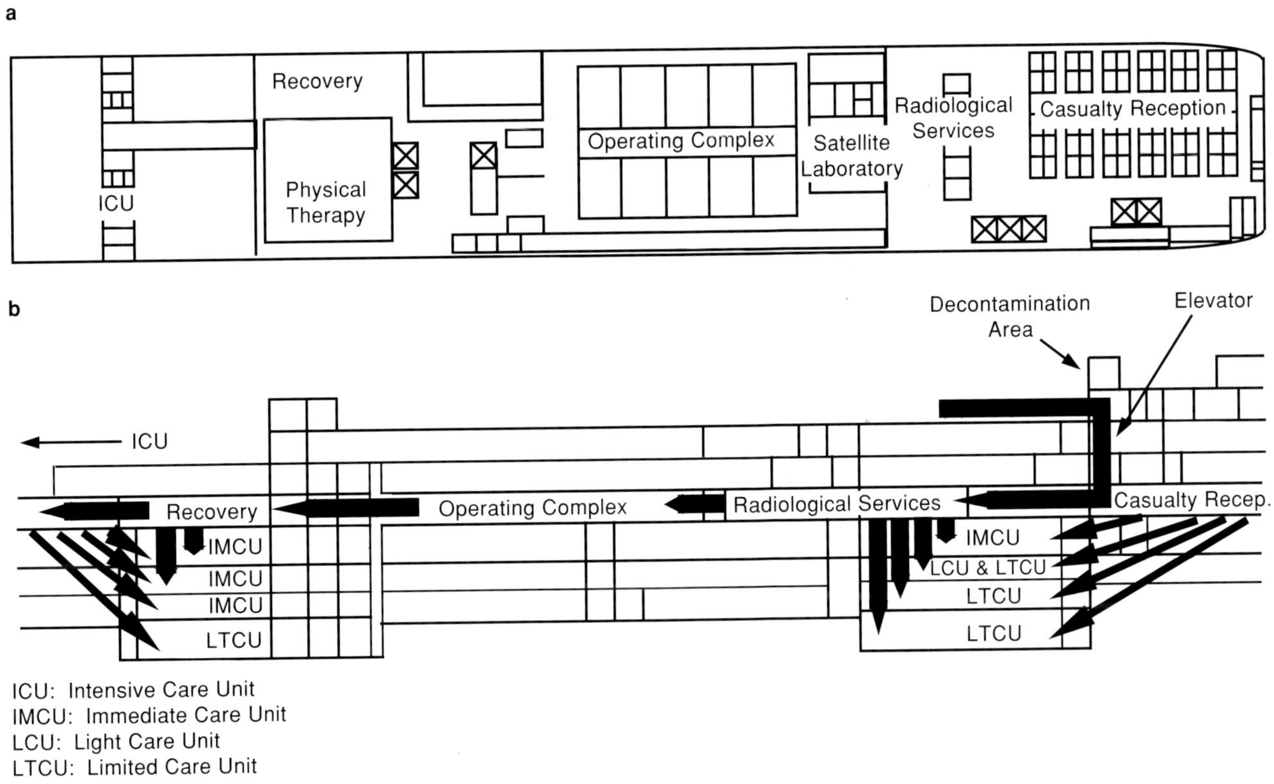

Fig. 6-14. Casualty flow in the USNS *Comfort* as it was originally configured prior to its service in the Persian Gulf War; (**a**) the arrangement of the main deck of the ship and (**b**) a cross-section of the ship with arrows indicating the casualty flow. The most important medical treatment facilities—the casualty receiving area, the operating rooms, and the intensive care wards—are all amidship on the main deck. This location ensures minimal rocking and rolling in a seaway and provides maximal protection from enemy action. Reprinted from Auxiliary and Special Mission Ship Acquisition Project Office. *FY 83 Shipbuilding Program*. Naval Sea Systems Command, Washington, DC; February 1984. T-AH 19 Hospital Ship. Diagram: Courtesy of Captain T.G. Patel, Medical Corps, US Navy, Bureau of Medicine and Surgery, Washington, DC.

used in the Korean War. During the Vietnam War, the MUST, an advanced-technology approach, replaced the tented MASH with an environmentally controlled facility. The MUST's complexity and cost detracted from its value. During the 1980s, DEPMEDS, another advanced-technology approach, was begun. DEPMEDS was based on an extensive systems analysis of field medical needs, and a variety of modular hospitals housed in special tents and metal boxes were fielded. Although DEPMEDS both improved the level of medical care in deployed hospitals and simplified equipment procurement, excessive weight and volume gravely compromised deployability.

Analysis of afteraction reports from the Persian Gulf War raised questions regarding the appropriateness of DEPMEDS equipment and the lack of mobility of deployable hospitals. Owing to the fluidity of the deployment, and particularly of the ground offensive itself, deployed hospitals were frequently required to relocate on short notice. Distances traveled and the degree of mobility varied widely. Transportation assigned to the unit was sometimes inadequate. The time required to become fully operational varied from several hours to 2 weeks. All personnel assigned to the hospital were required to help pack and unpack equipment for movements. Logistical supply lines were usually able to keep pace with this often-rapid forward deployment, however, and few chronic shortages of supplies and equipment were experienced by the onset of the ground war.

MF2K and MRI are refinements of DEPMEDS. These systems will decrease the number and types of hospitals and make it possible to tailor medical assets by mission. Perhaps the two most important changes are the deletion of the MASH and its replacement by the FST, and the design of one single hospital type to replace the present multiple hospital types.

REFERENCES

1. Odom CB. Third US Army. In: Carter BN, ed. *Activities of Surgical Consultants.* Vol 1. In: Coates JB Jr. *Surgery in World War II.* Washington DC: US Department of the Army, Medical Department, Office of The Surgeon General; 1962: 315.

2. Brewer LA III, Burford TH. Administrative considerations in the Mediterranean (formerly North African) Theater of Operations. In: Berry FB, ed. *Thoracic Surgery.* Vol 1. In: Coates JB Jr, ed. *Surgery in World War II.* Washington, DC: US Department of the Army, Medical Department, Office of The Surgeon General; 1963: 129–131.

3. Department of Defense Instruction 6430.1, dated 21 June 1982. Washington, DC: DoD. In: Scotti MJ, chairman. Defense Medical Standardization Board. *DEPMEDS Policies/Guidelines: Treatment Briefs.* Fort Detrick, Frederick, Md: Defense Medical Standardization Board; 1990: 1.

4. Scotti MJ, chairman. Defense Medical Standardization Board. *DEPMEDS Policies/Guidelines: Treatment Briefs.* Fort Detrick, Frederick, Md: Defense Medical Standardization Board; 1990.

5. Johannigman JA, Putnam AT. Clinical evaluation of the Impact Uni-Vent 750. *Milit Med.* 1994;159(5):403–408.

6. Perkins DE. Colonel, Medical Corps, US Army. Personal communication, June 1995.

7. US Army Office of The Surgeon General, Professional Services Directorate. *Operation Desert Storm: Professional Afteraction Review.* Phoenix, Ariz: US Army Office of The Surgeon General; June–July 1991.

8. Dorsey DA. Military and emergency medicine. Paper prepared for Military Studies 1, Uniformed Services University of the Health Sciences, Bethesda, Md; 1992.

9. Steinweg KK. Mobile surgical hospital design: Lessons from 5th MASH surgical packages for Operations Desert Shield/Storm. *Milit Med.* 1993;158:733–739.

10. Gander TJ. *Jane's NBC Protection Equipment.* 5th ed. Surry, United Kingdom: Jane's Information Group Limited; 1992: 203.

11. Oschner MG, Harviel JD, Stafford PW, et al. Development and organization for casualty management on a 1,000 bed hospital ship in the Persian Gulf. *J Trauma.* 1993;32:501–513.

Chapter 7

MILITARY ANESTHESIA MACHINES

W. CLAYTON PETTY, M.D.*

*Captain, Medical Corps, U.S. Navy; formerly, Professor and Vice Chairman, Department of Anesthesiology, Uniformed Services University of the Health Sciences, 4301 Jones Bridge Road, Bethesda, Maryland 20814-4799; currently, Professor and Chairman, Department of Anesthesiology, Madigan Army Medical Center, Tacoma, Washington 98431-5000

INTRODUCTION

Anesthesia machines designed and manufactured for the U. S. military have had unique features since their inception during World War II. Prior to World War II, physicians, nurses, and dentists usually administered ether by an open-drop technique, which consisted of dripping it onto a face mask covered with two to four thin layers of cotton mesh (Figure 7-1). Until the Persian Gulf War, anesthesia machines in the field of combat were very similar to those used in civilian hospitals in the United States. During and after World War II, the first militarily specific anesthesia machines were sold. Chapter 31, A Brief History of Military Anesthesia, describes the milestones in the development of anesthesia machine Models 675 (manufactured by the former McKesson Appliance Co.), 685A, 685B, and 785 (manufactured by Ohio Chemical and Manufacturing Co., which is now owned by Ohmeda, Inc., Madison, Wis.), and the present Field Anesthesia Machine (FAM) Model 885A (manufactured by Ohmeda).

One of the major problems in the development of anesthesia machines for the military has been the lag time between the concept and the delivery of the product. Since the Korean War, not one anesthesia machine designed for civilian use has met the immediate needs of the U. S. military in combat. At the beginning of the Vietnam War, U.S. military hospitals in Vietnam delivered ether with the "pig" (Ohio 685A) anesthesia machine, which was designed immediately after World War II and used in the Korean War. In the Vietnam War, the FAM Model 785 was introduced but was immediately outmoded because halothane had been introduced while the 785 Model was being developed. The FAM Model 785 had a cyclopropane flowmeter (which rapidly became obsolete), and a large, in-circuit vaporizer for ether, but was unsafe for the delivery of halothane. Anesthesia providers overcame this problem by attaching a halothane single-agent, temperature-compensated vaporizer to the FAM 785; they buried all the cyclopropane tanks and used halothane as the major inhalational anesthetic (with the addition of nitrous oxide) for the remainder of the war. The FAM Model 885 was developed in the hiatus between the Vietnam War and the Persian Gulf War. An additional oxygen flowmeter was mounted in place of the cyclopropane flowmeter, and a universal vaporizer replaced the in-circuit ether vaporizer. A Model 885-Conversion superseded the Model 885 and was eventually replaced

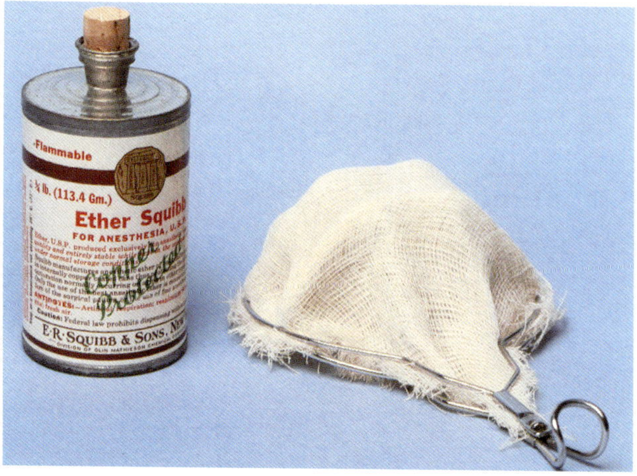

Fig. 7-1. Most anesthetics given during the American Civil War, World War I, and World War II were administered by dripping ether onto a gauze-covered face mask.

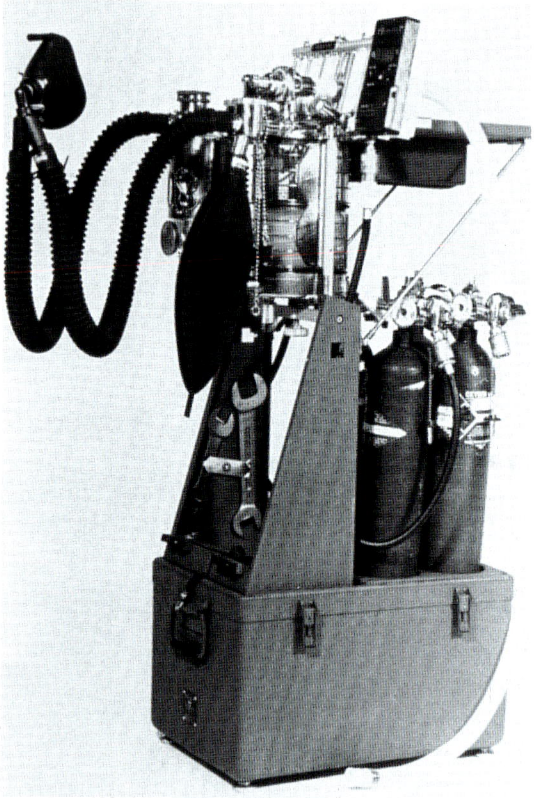

Fig. 7-2. Field Anesthesia Machine (FAM) Model 885A with an oxygen analyzer. The circle-system machine has a vaporizer, carbon dioxide absorber, flowmeters, and an adult patient breathing circuit. Compressed medical gases are required. Photograph: Permission granted by Ohmeda, Inc, Madison, Wis.

by Model 885A. Hospitals mobilized for Operation Desert Shield (the build-up phase of the Persian Gulf War) were initially supplied with the FAM Model 885A and later with the Ohmeda Universal Portable Anesthesia Circuit (PAC) (Figures 7-2 and 7-3). Military anesthesia providers (especially those who were members of the reserves) realized that both anesthesia machines were not compatible with the techniques and standards of practice used in civilian and military hospitals in the United States. Most of the anesthesia providers in Operation Desert Storm (the fighting phase of the Persian Gulf War) considered the FAM and the PAC to be of historical importance only. Training with the machines was extremely limited, and the majority of anesthesia providers had been exposed only superficially to the principles of operation of a universal vaporizer. Many were hesitant to use the FAM and the PAC because they were unfamiliar with the machines and they were genuinely concerned about the standard of care and medicoliability issues.

Military anesthesia providers require a small, lightweight, versatile, easily transportable anesthesia machine for use in a frontline aid station and in a rear, full-service field hospital. Historically, anesthesia providers in the United States have leaned heavily toward circle breathing systems; thus, this was a major determining factor in the development of anesthesia machines for the military. Two anesthesia machines are stocked by the Department of Defense's Deployable Medical Systems (DEPMEDS): the FAM and the PAC. The FAM is geared for use in field hospitals and in conflicts lasting longer than 2 weeks. The PAC fits inside a briefcase and is suitable for use in the battalion aid station and for fast-in and fast-out conflicts. Our discussion will focus on detailed descriptions of the FAM Model 885A and the PAC, and on concepts that might influence evolutionary changes for a new FAM.

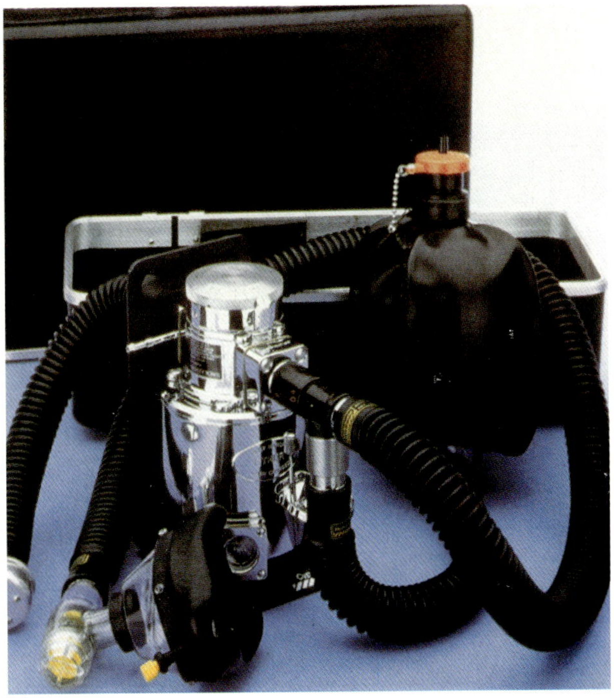

Fig. 7-3. Ohmeda Portable Anesthesia Circuit (PAC). A draw-over vaporizer is the heart of this nonrebreathing lightweight anesthesia machine. Photograph: Permission granted by Ohmeda, Inc, Madison, Wis.

FIELD ANESTHESIA MACHINE MODEL 885A

Military anesthesia providers should familiarize themselves with the manufacturer's *Instruction and Service Manual With Illustrated Parts List*,[1] on which much of the following information is based. A distinctive carrying container, 13 in. wide x 20 in. long x 18 in. high, holds the entire FAM (Figure 7-4). All that is needed to put the machine into service is a cylinder of oxygen, carbon dioxide–absorbent granules, and a bottle of liquid anesthetic agent. The FAM and its container have a combined weight of 115 lb and can be lifted by grasping two handles on the lower case. During shipment, four glides are inserted into sprockets on the bottom of the container and these glides are replaced with four casters when the machine is assembled (Figure 7-5).

A pressure-release valve keeps dust from entering the container. The pressure-relief device must be pushed in to relieve the pressure inside the case before the lower and upper cases can be separated. Releasing four drawbolt fasteners separates the container into upper and lower cases (Figures 7-6 and 7-7).

Lower Case

The lower case contains the anesthesia machine, accessories, and spare parts (Exhibit 7-1). As the absorber head is pulled upward, the support arms are held in vertical position by a spring-loaded snap bar at the base. A hinged thumb bolt is tightened into a slot on one support arm to keep the absorber head vertical (Figures 7-8 and 7-9). Between the two support arms are an open and a latched compartment (Figure 7-10). The open compartment has spring holders that secure adult- and child-sized

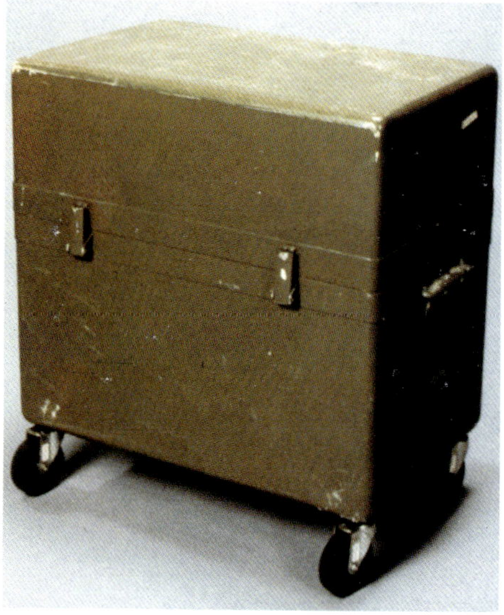

Fig. 7-4. Carrying case for the Field Anesthesia Machine (FAM) Model 885A. The upper and lower cases are held together by two drawbolts on each side of the case. Shipping glides have been replaced by four casters. Note one of the carrying handles on the end of the case.

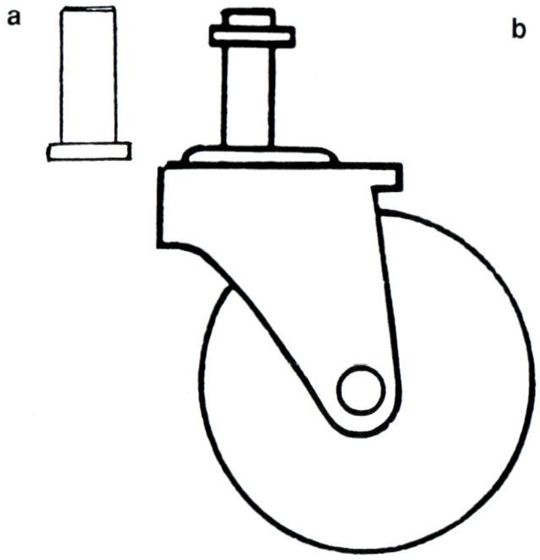

Fig. 7-5. Four glides (**a**) are placed in sprockets on the bottom of the lower case for shipment and storage. Four casters (**b**), stored inside the bottom case, replace the glides when the Field Anesthesia Machine Model (FAM) 885A is in use. Redrawn with permission from Ohmeda, Inc, Madison, Wis.

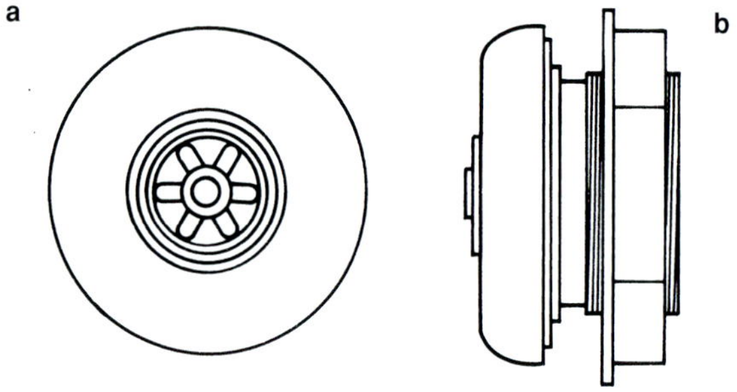

Fig. 7-6. A pressure-release valve keeps dust and other materials from entering the case. Prior to opening the case, the center button (**a**, front view) is pushed to return pressure within the case to atmospheric conditions. A groove (**b**, side view) fits in a hole cut in the case wall and a flat bolt secures the device from the inside. Redrawn with permission from Ohmeda, Inc, Madison, Wis.

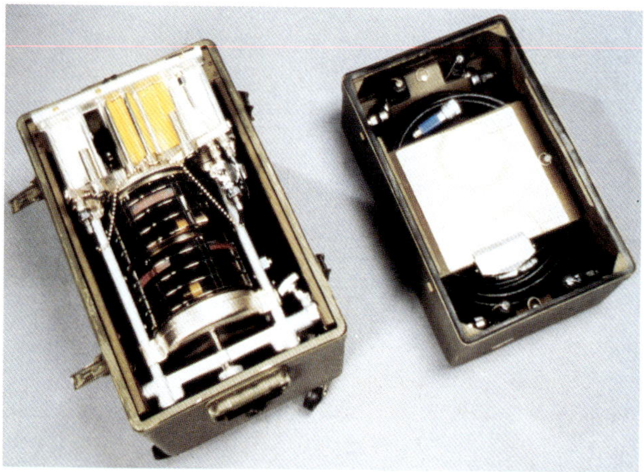

Fig. 7-7. Field Anesthesia Machine (FAM) Model 885A carrying case, opened. Bottom case (left) showing the FAM canister and rear of the flowmeter manifold. Upper case (right) with the medical gas hoses, a clipboard, and compressed gas regulators (one at each corner).

EXHIBIT 7-1

ITEMS IN LOWER CASE, FIELD ANESTHESIA MACHINE MODEL 885A

$1^5/_{16}$- and $1^1/_8$-in. open-end wrench
$^7/_8$- and $^3/_4$-in. open-end wrench
Tee-valve wrench
Flow calculator
$^3/_{16}$-in. hex Allen wrench
Y-inhaler
Mask elbow
Large and medium adult masks
Child and infant masks
Extra check valve disks
Extra cylinder gaskets
Extra funnel plug with chain
Four wheels
Large cylinder adapters for oxygen and nitrous oxide
Protective closure devices for cylinder adapters
Extra absorber gaskets
Instrument tray
Cylinder holder
Gas evacuation tubing
19-mm connector
Instrument tray with oxygen monitor case
Oxygen sensor tee, probe, and cable
Sight level

Adapted with permission from Ohmeda, Inc. *Instruction and Service Manual With Illustrated Parts List. Model 885A. Anesthesia Apparatus, Gas, Nitrous Oxide, Oxygen and Volatile Liquid Anesthetics, Portable 4-Cylinder Capacity.* Ohmeda, Madison, Wis: 1990: 14.

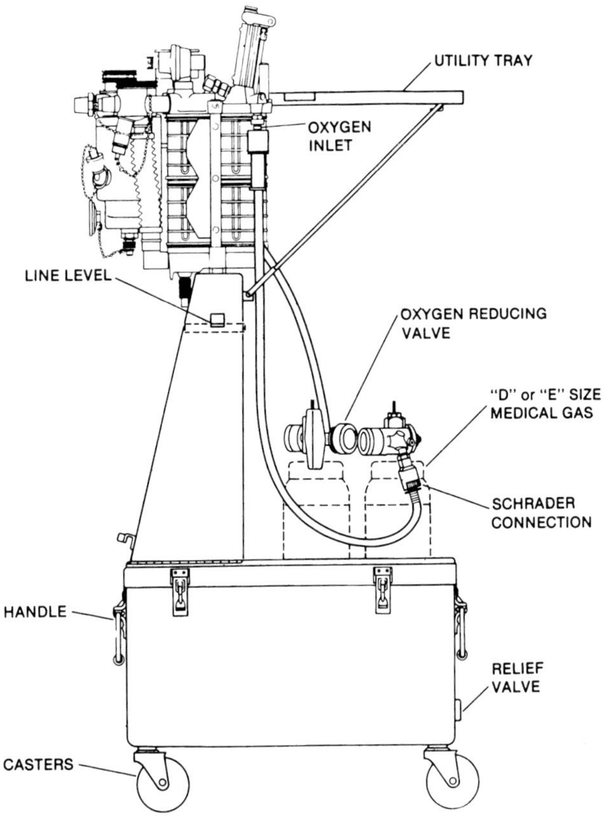

Fig. 7-8. Field Anesthesia Machine (FAM) Model 885A in the upright position. Side arms support the vaporizer and flowmeter manifold. One end of the utility tray is supported by a brace connected to the support arms. A line level on the inside of the support arm is used to level the machine prior to use. Casters have replaced the shipping glides. A gas-specific noninterchangeable male Schrader valve is attached to the female outlet of the pin-indexed reducing valve on the compressed oxygen cylinder. The opposite end of the oxygen hose has a female Schrader valve that is attached to the male oxygen inlet of the FAM. A carrying handle, two drawbolts, and the pressure-relief valve can be seen. A spring-latched bar (not seen) secures the bottom end of the support arms. Redrawn with permission from Ohmeda, Inc, Madison, Wis.

masks. Adjacent to the masks, in FAM models with an oxygen monitor, is an unsecured box containing the oxygen sensor cartridge. The latched compartment contains the elbow connector, the Y-connector for the breathing circuit, a box with three vials of extra parts, and the tee-valve wrench (which is used to turn the E-cylinder to the ON position). Replacement parts in the three vials include vaporizer replacement parts, cylinder yoke gaskets, and disks for the inhalation and exhalation check valves. If the FAM has an oxygen monitor, the cable assembly and sensor tee will be stored in the box.

Corrugated scavenger hoses are stored inside the absorber chamber. Lifting the absorber head reveals the utility tray, which is held in place by a hook-and-loop strap and four casters snapped into spring holders (Figure 7-11). The front end of the tray has two round brackets that slide onto two mounting studs behind the flowmeter manifold (Figure 7-12). A tray brace is permanently attached to the top of the support arms and fits snugly

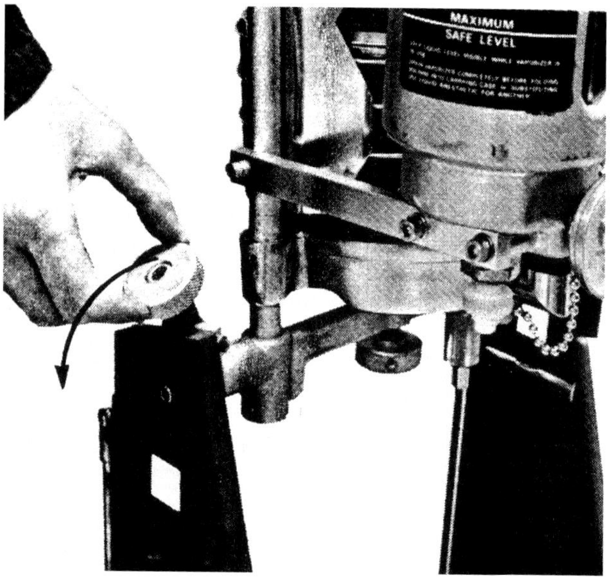

Fig. 7-9. Field Anesthesia Machine (FAM) Model 885A. A hinged thumb bolt secures the absorber head in the vertical position. Photograph: Printed with permission from Ohmeda, Inc, Madison, Wis.

Fig. 7-10. Field Anesthesia Machine (FAM) Model 885A. The space between the support arms contains two compartments. An open compartment has two posts holding oronasal masks. A lid (shown removed) for the closed compartment protects the Y breathing-circuit connector, the elbow adapter, spare parts containers, and the tee valve wrench for E-cylinders. Models with an oxygen sensor have the sensor cartridge stored next to the masks and the sensing cable and sensing tee inside the closed compartment. Redrawn with permission from Ohmeda, Inc, Madison, Wis.

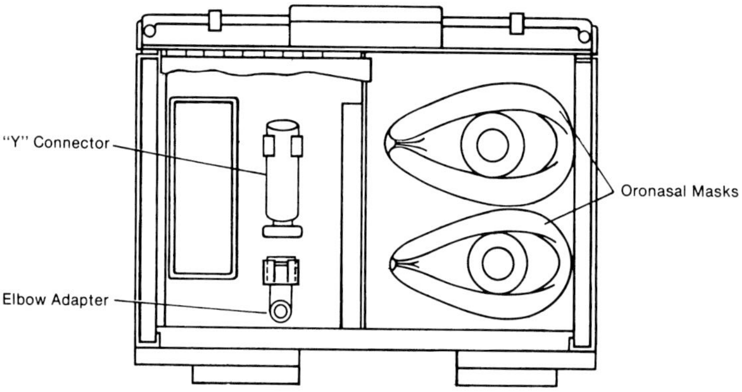

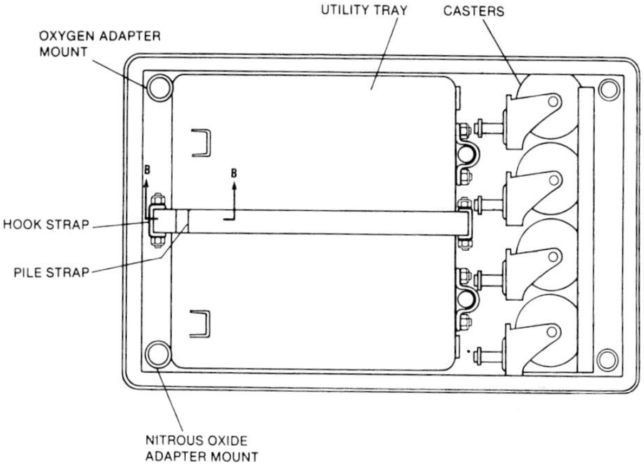

Fig. 7-11. Field Anesthesia Machine (FAM) Model 885A. After the absorber head is in the vertical position, the utility tray, casters, and mounts for the oxygen and nitrous oxide H-cylinder adapter can be seen. Spring-loaded clamps in the end of the case secure either the casters or glides. A strap holds the utility tray in place. Redrawn with permission from Ohmeda, Inc, Madison, Wis.

against the edge of the support arms when not in use. The tray brace slides into two brackets on the underside of the utility tray to support the opposite end of the tray (see Figure 7-8).

The mounting bracket for the oxygen monitor is attached by a set screw to the utility mounting stud on the side of the metabolic oxygen flowmeter (Figure 7-13). During assembly, the set screw is loosened and the bracket is moved parallel to the flowmeter manifold, and the oxygen monitor is then mounted to the bracket. The oxygen sensor probe is inserted in the sensor tee placed between

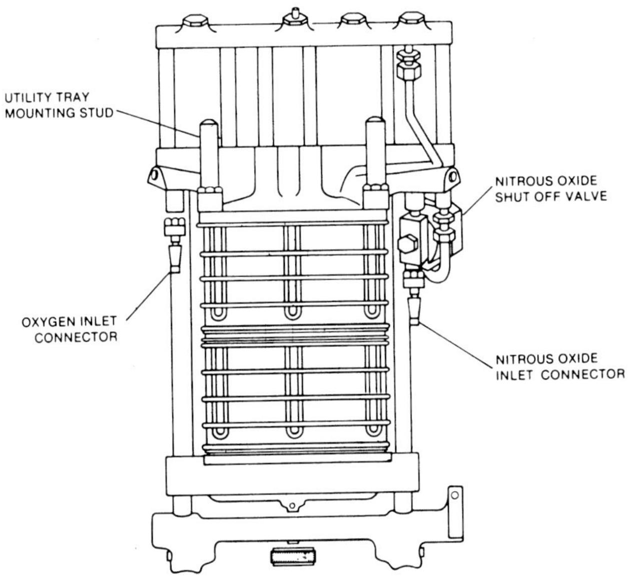

Fig. 7-12. Field Anesthesia Machine (FAM) Model 885A. Rear view of the absorber head. Two mounting studs hold one end of the utility tray. Inlet male noninterchangeable Schrader connectors for oxygen and nitrous oxide are shown. The nitrous oxide pressure-sensor shutoff valve blocks the flow of nitrous oxide to the flowmeter when the pressure of oxygen in the pipeline is less than 20 psig. Reprinted with permission from Ohmeda, Inc, Madison, Wis.

Fig. 7-13. Field Anesthesia Machine (FAM) Model 885A. The oxygen mounting bracket is attached to one of the utility mounting studs during shipment (left). Releasing the set screw allows the bracket to be moved approximately 180°. The oxygen monitor is mounted on the bolt pictured at the end of the bracket (right). Redrawn with permission from Ohmeda, Inc, Madison, Wis.

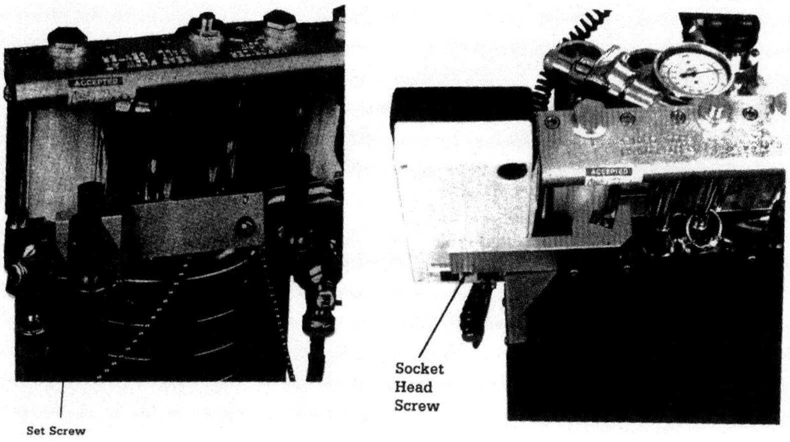

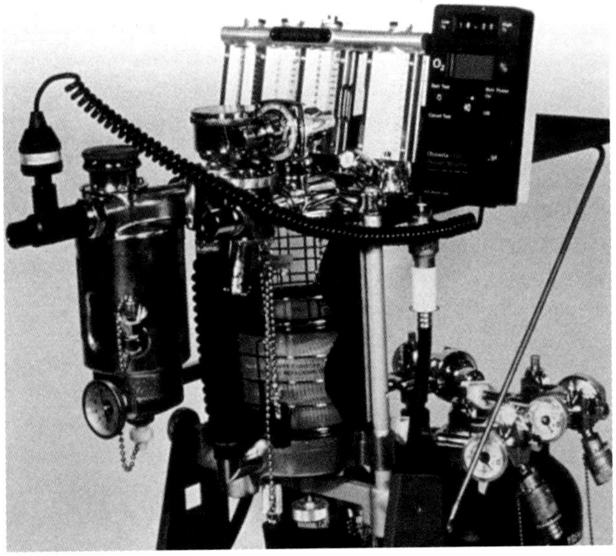

Fig. 7-14. Field Anesthesia Machine (FAM) Model 885A. The oxygen monitor is mounted to the bracket of the absorber head. A sensor cable connects the oxygen sensor in the sensor tee of the fresh-gas outlet of the breathing circuit to the monitor. The inspiratory limb of the breathing circuit will be attached to the open end of the sensor tee. Photograph: Printed with permission from Ohmeda, Inc, Madison, Wis.

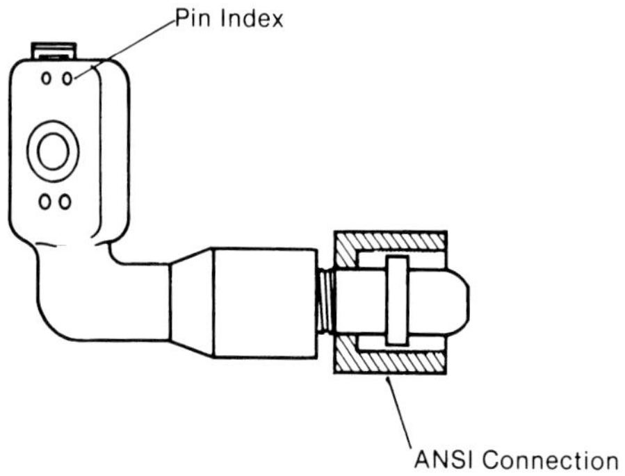

Fig. 7-15. Field Anesthesia Machine (FAM) Model 885A, large-cylinder adapter. An American National Standards Institute (ANSI) nut-and-gland medical gas–coded thread attaches to a matching threaded cylinder outlet. The opposite end of the adapter has a pin-index safety system (PISS) that is gas-specific (a PISS regulator is attached to the PISS fitting). Redrawn with permission from Ohmeda, Inc, Madison, Wis.

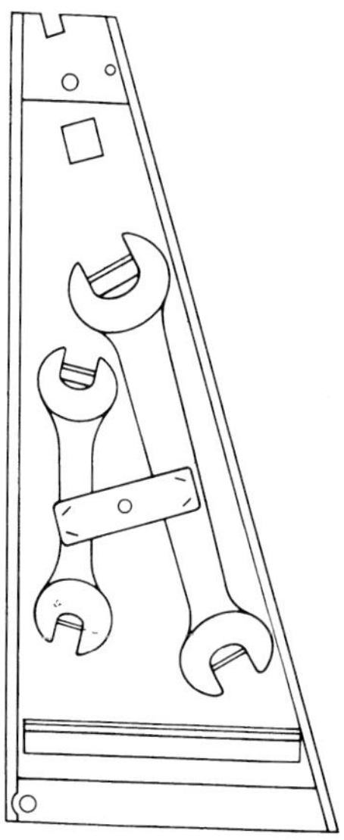

Fig. 7-17. Field Anesthesia Machine (FAM) Model 885A. Two wrenches for connecting cylinder adapters are mounted on the inside of one support arm. Redrawn with permission from Ohmeda, Inc, Madison, Wis.

the common gas outlet and the inspiratory limb of the patient breathing circuit (Figure 7-14).

Large cylinder connectors for oxygen and nitrous oxide are stored on threaded mounts (see Figure 7-11) adjacent to the end of the utility tray. These connectors attach to cylinders, which do not have the pin index safety system (PISS) holes drilled in the cylinder valve. An American National Standards Institute (ANSI) nut-and-gland medical-gas–coded thread of the connector attaches to the threaded cylinder outlet; the other end of the connector has the appropriate PISS for the gas-specific cylinder regulator gauge (Figure 7-15). Beneath the utility tray is a four-holed cylinder holder that mounts on the top of the lower case and keeps the E-cylinders in place during use (Figure 7-16). Mounted on one side of the lower case wall is the flow calculator, which is used to determine anesthetic concentrations delivered by the universal vaporizer.

On the inside of one support arm are extra absorber gaskets and a small sight level for leveling the machine during assembly (see Figure 7-8). On the inside of the other support arm are two open-end wrenches, which are used for connecting connectors to cylinders, and for other purposes (Figure 7-17).

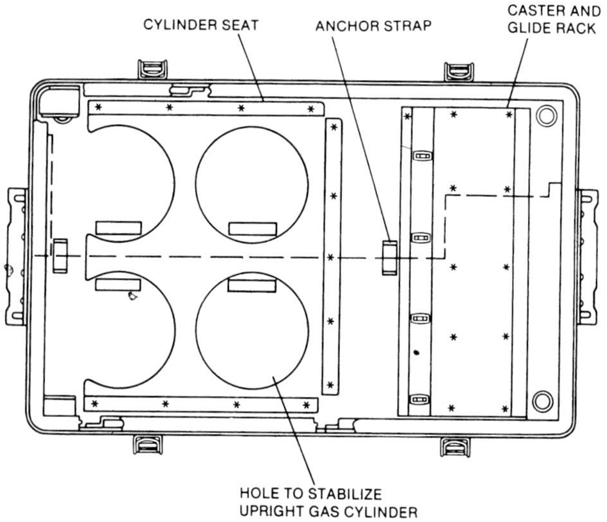

Fig. 7-16. Field Anesthesia Machine (FAM) Model 885A. After the utility tray is removed, the four-holed cylinder holder can be taken out and fitted to the cylinder seat on top of the lower case to help secure the E-cylinders in the upright position. The weight of the cylinders contributes to the stability of the FAM. Redrawn with permission from Ohmeda, Inc, Madison, Wis.

Upper Case

Additional equipment and accessories for assembling the completed anesthesia machine are contained in the upper case (Exhibit 7-2). Figure 7-18 shows the fastener holding the clipboard in place. A compartment secured by a fastener is on each end of the upper case. When the clipboard is removed and the compartments are opened, the rebreathing bags, head harness, oxygen and nitrous oxide PISS regulators, long and short gas-supply hoses, corrugated breathing tubes, and equipment for a pediatric nonrebreathing system are revealed (Figure 7-19).

EXHIBIT 7-2

ITEMS IN UPPER CASE, FIELD ANESTHESIA MACHINE MODEL 885A

Long and short gas-supply hoses for oxygen and nitrous oxide

Regulator assemblies for oxygen and nitrous oxide

Head strap

Long and short corrugated breathing tubes

Clipboard

Pediatric supply hose

1-L Breathing bag with scavenging valve

3-L Breathing bag

Adapted with permission from Ohmeda, Inc. *Instruction and Service Manual With Illustrated Parts List. Model 885A. Anesthesia Apparatus, Gas, Nitrous Oxide, Oxygen and Volatile Liquid Anesthetics, Portable 4-Cylinder Capacity.* Ohmeda, Madison, Wis: 1990: 14.

Attaching the Medical Gas Supply

Cylinders containing oxygen and nitrous oxide are connected to the anesthesia machine by using the PISS regulator for E-cylinders or the large-cylinder PISS adapters. E- or D-cylinders will fit inside the four-holed holder in the lower case (see Figures 7-8 and 7-16). It is important to briefly review the differences in physical characteristics between the storage and the delivery of oxygen and nitrous oxide. E-cylinders (internal volume 4.8 L) at 21.1°C (70°F) contain either 660 L of compressed oxygen at a pressure of 1,900 psig or 2.92 kg of liquid nitrous oxide (which evaporates to provide 1,590 L) at a pressure of 750 psig.[2] Oxygen boils at –183.0°C at 1 atm and has a *critical temperature* (ie, the temperature above which a substance cannot be liquefied regardless of the pressure applied) of –118.6°C.[3] Oxygen can only be stored as a gas at room temperature, and the amount of oxygen in the cylinder is proportional to the cylinder pressure (Figure 7-20). Nitrous oxide at room temperature is below its critical temperature and is stored as a liquid under pressure

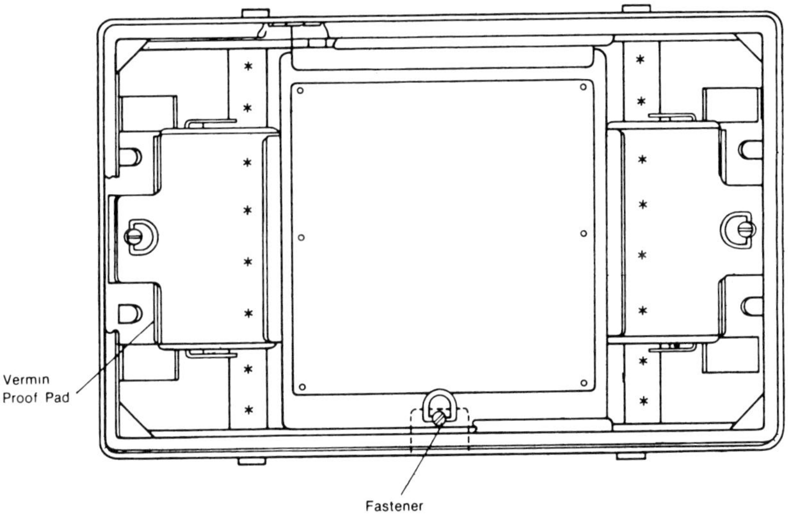

Fig. 7-18. Field Anesthesia Machine (FAM) Model 885A. Upper case. A fastener is holding the clipboard in place. Fastened compartments are shown at opposite ends of the case. Redrawn with permission from Ohmeda, Inc, Madison, Wis.

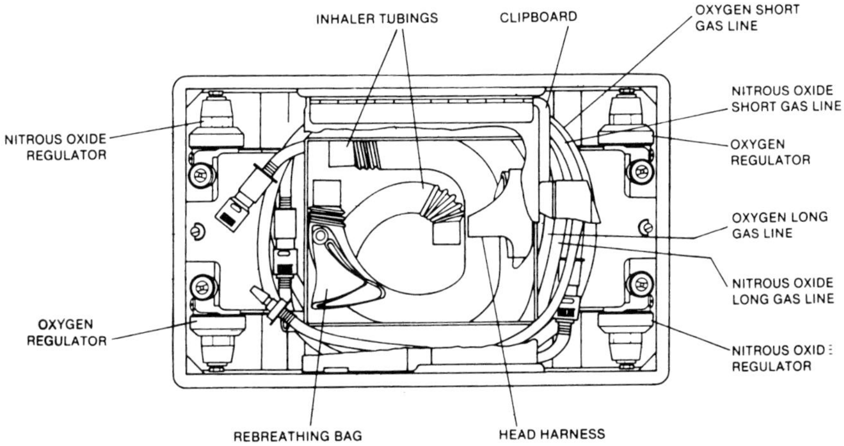

Fig. 7-19. Field Anesthesia Machine (FAM) Model 885A. Breathing tubes, a head harness, rebreathing bags, a pediatric nonrebreathing circuit, and gas hoses are stored beneath the clipboard in the upper case. A pin index safety system (PISS) gas regulator is secured at each corner of the case. Redrawn with permission from Ohmeda, Inc, Madison, Wis.

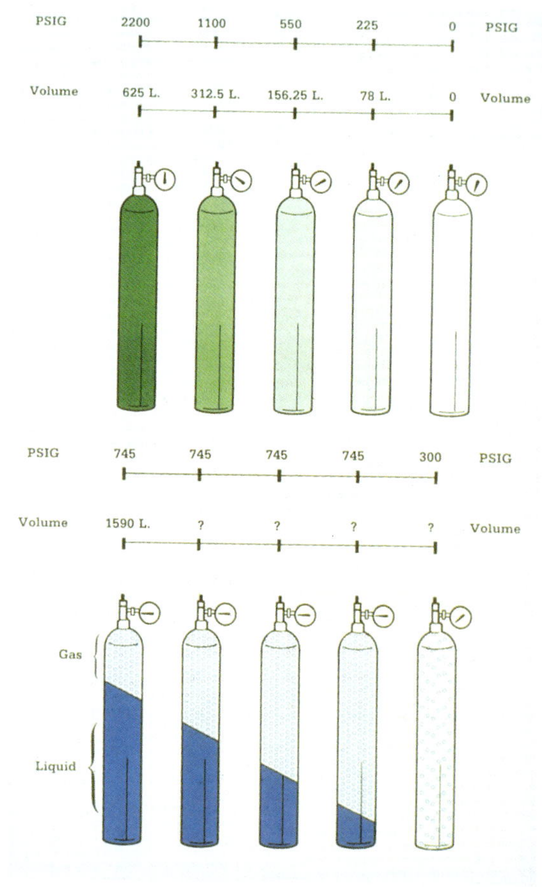

Fig. 7-20. Oxygen and nitrous oxide compressed-gas cylinders. Oxygen (green) is stored as a compressed gas because it is above its critical temperature at room temperature. The amount of oxygen in the cylinder is proportional to the cylinder pressure. Nitrous oxide (blue) is stored as a liquid under pressure. As the tank empties, the amount of nitrous oxide in the cylinder is *not* proportional to the pressure in the cylinder. When the last drop of liquid nitrous oxide is evaporated, the cylinder contains *only* gas, and *then* the amount of nitrous oxide in the cylinder is proportional to the amount of gaseous nitrous oxide. Photograph: Printed with permission granted by Medical Systems Division, Ohmeda, Inc, Madison, Wis.

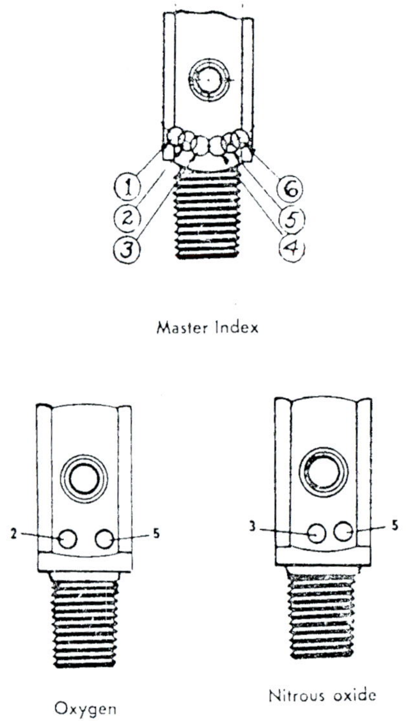

Fig. 7-21. The pin index safety system (PISS), which is designed for medical gases compressed in cylinders. Each medical gas is assigned two holes of the six-holed main index (upper figure). Oxygen is assigned positions 2 and 5 and nitrous oxide positions 3 and 5. Above the two holes is the cylinder-gas outlet.

in the cylinder. The content of the nitrous oxide cylinder is *not* proportional to the cylinder pressure *until* the liquid nitrous oxide has completely evaporated.

An E-cylinder valve in the United States must comply with the PISS. Three holes are drilled in the cylinder valve: one is the gas outlet and the other two are limited-depth holes that are positioned to correspond with the assigned PISS for oxygen (numbers 2 and 5) or nitrous oxide (numbers 3 and 5) (Figure 7-21). Both FAM oxygen and nitrous oxide regulators have two pins that mate with the paired holes in the cylinder valve (Figure 7-22). The oxygen regulator is marked with the chemical symbol O_2 and is painted white (the international color code for oxygen) on the pressure gauge dial face and the tee-securement handle. The nitrous oxide regulator is marked with the chemical symbol N_2O and painted blue (the international color code for nitrous oxide) on the pressure gauge dial face and the tee-securement handle. After a regulator is attached to either an E-cylinder valve or a large-cylinder PISS connector, a male Schrader noninterchangeable connector (Figure 7-23) on the

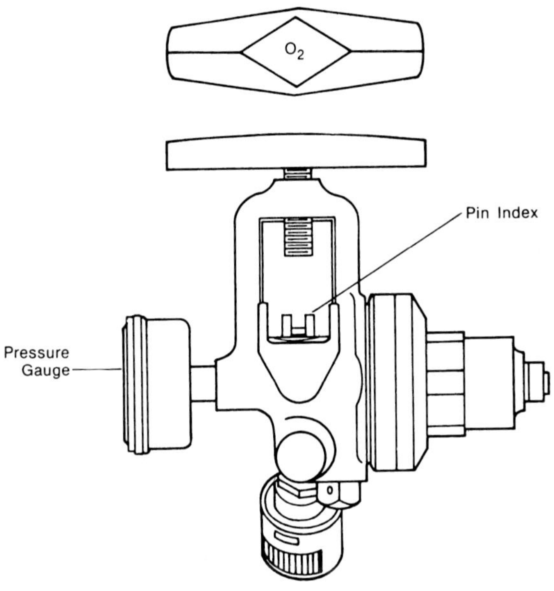

Fig. 7-22. Oxygen regulator. Two pins are positioned to fit the 2,5 pin index safety system (PISS) of the oxygen cylinder valve. The handle is painted white (international color assigned to oxygen) and is labeled with the chemical symbol for oxygen. A pressure gauge reflects the cylinder pressure in psig and kg/cm^2, is painted white, and labeled O_2. A male Schrader noninterchangable connector can be seen at the bottom of the regulator. Redrawn with permission from Ohmeda, Inc, Madison, Wis.

Fig. 7-23. Schrader noninterchangeable connectors at the ends of the gas hoses. Each medical gas has a specific connector assigned to avoid cross-connection of gases. One end of the gas hose has a male connector (left) that fits the gas-specific female connector (right) on the pin index safety system (PISS) regulator, and the other end has a female connector that fits the male inlet connection on the Field Anesthesia Machine (FAM) Model 885A. Schrader adapters allow rapid connections and disconnections without the use of special tools. Photograph: Printed with permission of Ohmeda, Inc, Madison, Wis.

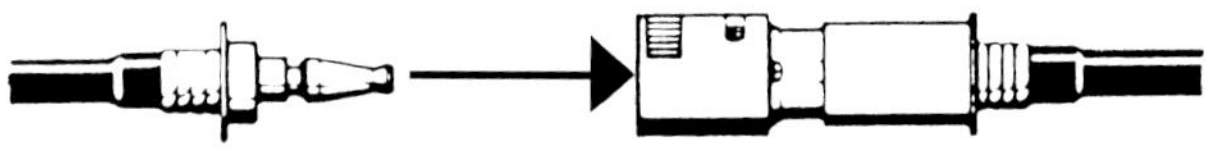

medical gas–supply hose is inserted into the gas-specific female Schrader connector on the regulator. Gas-supply hoses come in two lengths, 114 and 40 in. A color-coded identification disk is found on each end of the supply hose. The female Schrader connection on the opposite end of the medical gas–supply hose is then connected to the male Schrader inlet connector on the control head. Figure 7-8 shows the connection of an E-cylinder containing oxygen to the FAM.

Cylinders larger than E-cylinders are sometimes supplied to combat hospitals to improve the efficiency of the medical gas supply (Figures 7-24 and 7-25). A large cylinder connector (see Figure 7-15), which is nut-and-gland coded for either oxygen or nitrous oxide, is attached to the threaded cylinder outlet, and a PISS oxygen or nitrous oxide regulator is attached to the PISS-connector outlet.

When an oxygen-powered ventilator is required, it is necessary to use either (*a*) the second oxygen regulator, attached to an E-cylinder or large-cylinder connector, or (*b*) an oxygen regulator equipped with two male Schrader connectors (Figure 7-26).

Pipeline Circuits

Gases from the oxygen and nitrous oxide cylinders enter the FAM through the two male Schrader noninterchangeable inlets on the rear of the control head (see Figure 7-12). Before the gases enter the FAM circuit, the regulator has reduced the pressure to approximately 40 psig. Nitrous oxide must flow through the pressure-sensor shutoff valve before it can enter the nitrous oxide flowmeter (see Figure 7-12 and Figures 7-27 and 7-28). The pressure-sensor shutoff valve will block the flow of nitrous oxide to the flowmeter if the oxygen pressure on its diaphragm is less than 20 psig.

Oxygen is distributed to four areas after it enters the FAM: (1) the metabolic oxygen flowmeter control valve, (2) the diaphragm of the nitrous oxide pressure-sensor shutoff valve, (3) the oxygen

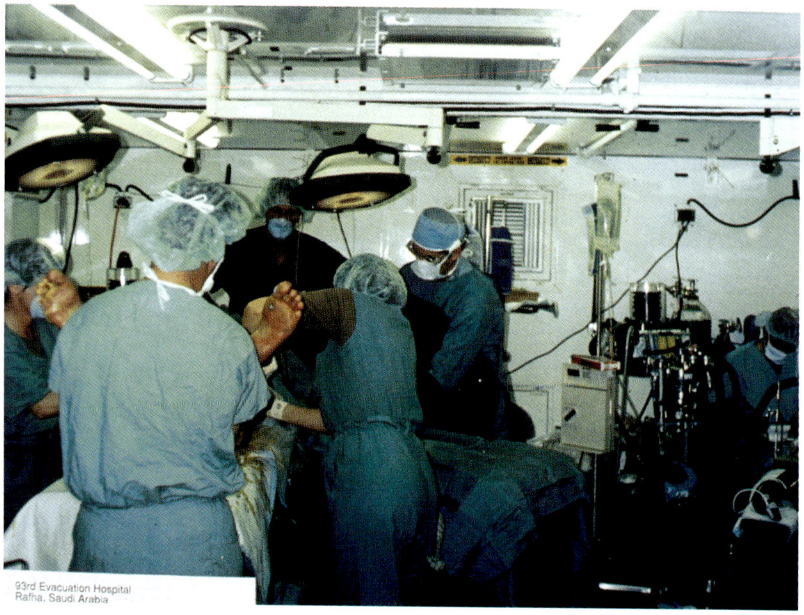

Fig. 7-24. Field Anesthesia Machine (FAM) Model 885A at the 93rd Evacuation Hospital, Rafha, Saudi Arabia, during the Persian Gulf War. Two operations are under way in the same operating room. The FAM can be seen on the right. Photograph: Courtesy of Captain DJ Rutkowski, CRNA, US Army Nurse Corps.

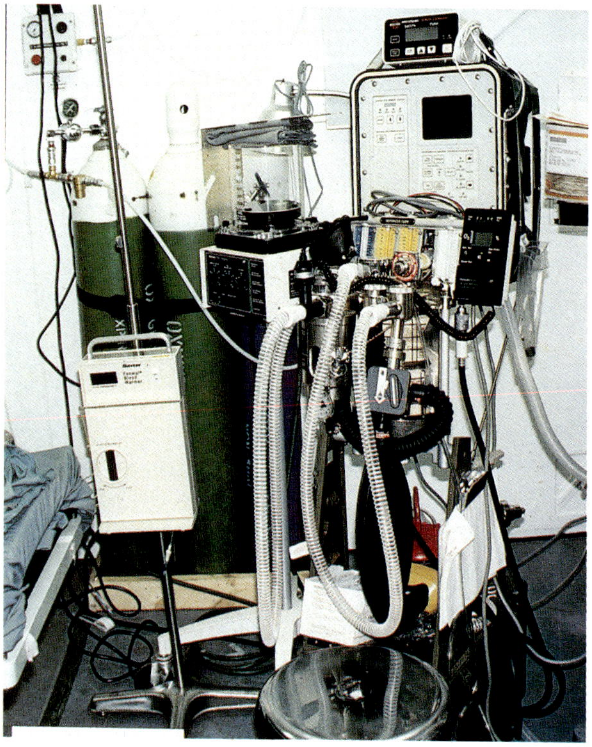

Fig. 7-25. Anesthesia equipment at the 12th Evacuation Hospital in Saudi Arabia during the Persian Gulf War. Patient monitors, a Field Anesthesia Machine (FAM) Model 885A with an oxygen monitor, a ventilator, and a blood warmer are shown. The rebreathing bag is attached to a switch-over valve that simplifies the adaptation of the ventilator to the breathing circuit. Against the wall (left) are two H-cylinders of compressed oxygen. These cylinders are painted two colors: green (US designation for oxygen) and white (international color assigned to oxygen), and are stamped OXYGEN in white letters on the green section of the cylinder. One oxygen H-cylinder is being used to power the ventilator, and the adapter and pin index safety system (PISS) regulator provided with the FAM are not being used. Nonstandard breathing tubes are connected to the FAM. Photograph: Courtesy of Captain D J Rutkowski, CRNA, US Army Nurse Corps.

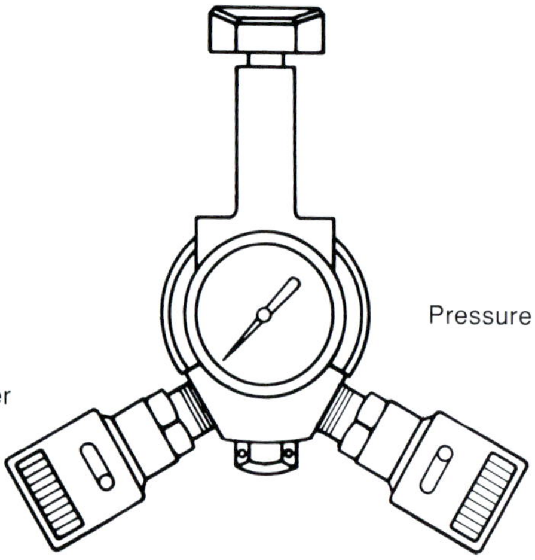

Fig. 7-26. A pin index safety system (PISS) oxygen regulator fitted with two Schrader couplers. One supplies oxygen to the Field Anesthesia Machine (FAM) Model 885A, and the other is a power outlet for the ventilator. Redrawn with permission from Ohmeda, Inc, Madison, Wis.

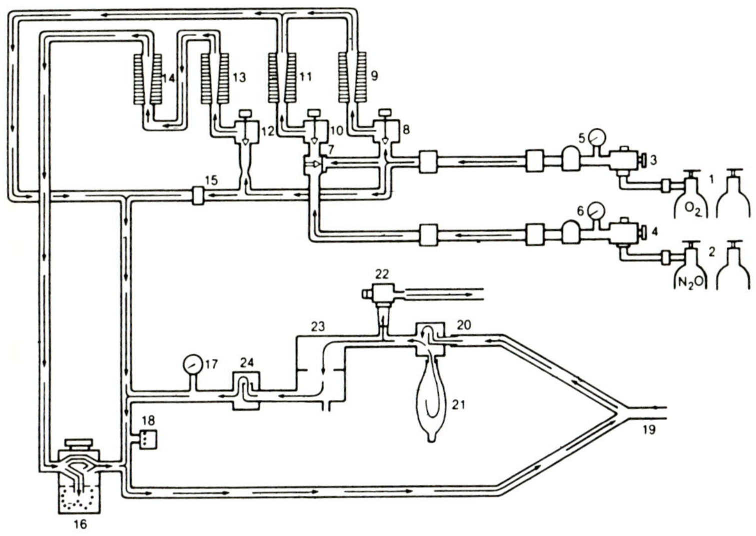

Fig. 7-27. Field Anesthesia Machine (FAM) Model 885A pipeline schematic for oxygen and nitrous oxide. Oxygen from the compressed medical oxygen cylinder (**1**) is reduced (**3**) to a pressure of 40 psig (**5**) before entering the FAM. Oxygen is distributed to metabolic oxygen flowmeter control valve (**8**), diaphragm of the nitrous oxide pressure sensor shutoff valve (**7**), oxygen flush valve (**15**), and the oxygen-for-vaporizer flowmeter control valve (**12**). Nitrous oxide in cylinders (**2**) is reduced (**4**) to 40 psig (**6**) before it enters the FAM. Nitrous oxide passes through the nitrous oxide pressure-sensor shutoff valve (**7**) to the nitrous oxide flowmeter control valve (**10**). Metabolic oxygen (**9**) and nitrous oxide (**11**) mix in a common pipeline and then combine with the oxygen-for-vaporizer (**13**, **14**) and anesthetic agent emitting from the vaporizer (**16**). Mixed gases are carried by the inspiration limb of the breathing circuit to the Y piece (**19**) and then to the patient. Exhaled gases enter the expiratory limb and flow through the exhalation check valve (**20**), some of the gases go into the rebreathing bag (**21**), and some exit through the adjustable pressure-limiting valve (**22**), if it is open, into the scavenging system; the remaining gases pass through the carbon dioxide absorber (**23**), through the inspiration check valve (**24**), and begin the cycle again. A pressure gauge (**17**) monitors breathing-circuit pressure. An emergency nonadjustable pressure-relief valve (**18**) releases gases into the atmosphere when the circuit pressure exceeds 60 to 80 mmHg. Photograph: Printed with permission from Ohmeda, Inc, Madison, Wis.

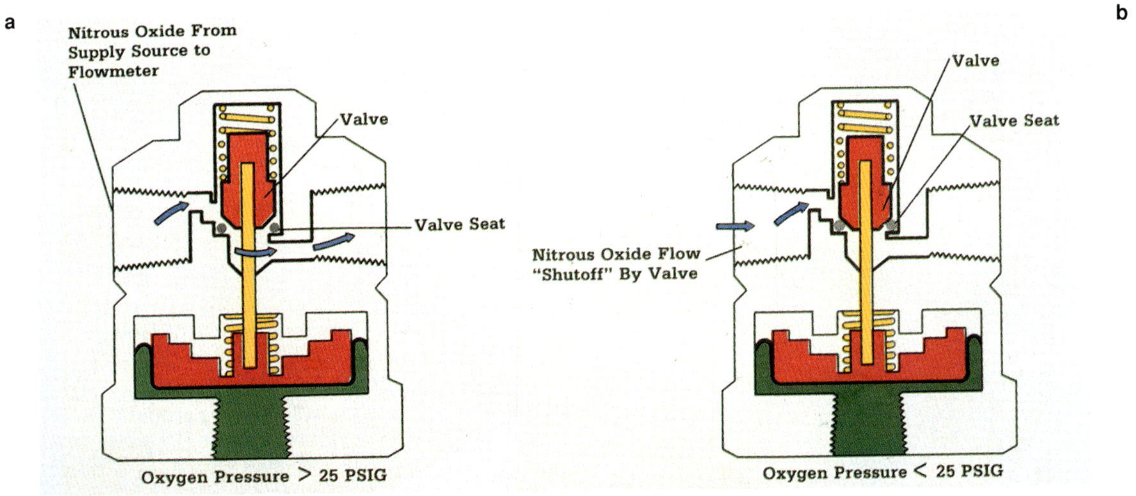

Fig. 7-28. This diagram shows how the nitrous oxide pressure-sensor shutoff valve works. (**a**) When the oxygen line pressure exceeds 25 psig, a large diaphragm counteracts the force applied by a valve-return spring on the valve. In this position, nitrous oxide flows through the shutoff valve. (**b**) Oxygen pressure drops below 25 psig and the valve-return spring forces the valve to seat, closing the shutoff orifice. Nitrous oxide still flows to the pressure-sensor shutoff valve but cannot flow through the valve to the nitrous oxide flowmeter. Photograph: Printed with permission granted by Medical Systems Division, Ohmeda, Inc, Madison, Wis.

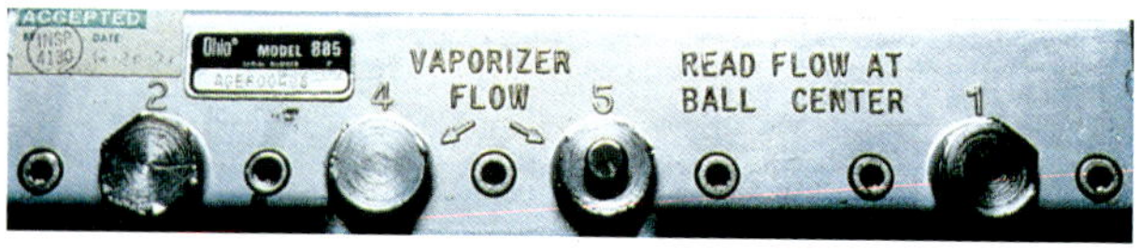

Fig. 7-29. Top of the flowmeter manifold, showing the assigned numbers imprinted for each medical gas. The numbers above the bolt holding the flow tube in place must match the number on the bottom of the flow tube. From the left, number 2 is for nitrous oxide, 4 is for low-flow oxygen-for-vaporizer, 5 is for high-flow oxygen-for-vaporizer, and 1 is for metabolic oxygen. Switching flow tubes can be disastrous because the output of the flowmeter is determined by the specific viscosity and density of the medical gas flowing through the flow tube.

flush valve, and (4) the oxygen-for-vaporizer flowmeter.

Flowmeters

Flowmeters are provided for metabolic oxygen, oxygen for the vaporizer, and nitrous oxide. The range for the flowmeters is, for metabolic oxygen, 200 mL/min to 7 L/min; for low-flow oxygen for the vaporizer, 20 to 180 mL/min; for high-flow oxygen for the vaporizer, 100 mL/min to 1 L/min; and for nitrous oxide, 200 mL/min to 8 L/min. Accuracy for all flowmeters is ±20% up to flows of 1,000 mL/min; above flows of 1,000 mL/min, the accuracy is ±10% (eg, at a setting of 5 L/min, the output would be 4.5–5.5 L/min). Each flowmeter tube, float, and scale are a matched set and must be replaced as a unit. Each flow tube is gas-specific, and a numbering system on the flowmeter manifold and each matching flow tube enhances the correct placement of the flow tubes if they are removed for maintenance or replacement. Numbers on the top of the flowmeter manifold are placed above the bolt that holds the flowmeter in place (Figure 7-29). Metabolic oxygen is number 1; oxygen-for-vaporizer, high flow, is 5; oxygen-for-vaporizer, low flow, is 4; and nitrous oxide is 2. The corresponding number is printed on the bottom of the flow tube. Switching flow tubes can be disastrous. One of the two documented deaths attributed to the FAM occurred when someone switched the nitrous oxide flow tube with the high-flow oxygen-for-vaporizer flow tube.[4] This switch resulted in a delivery of 6.2% isoflurane instead of the expected 1.5% setting, and the overdosing and eventual death of the patient.

Flowmeter scales and control knobs are color coded: metabolic oxygen is white, oxygen-for-va-

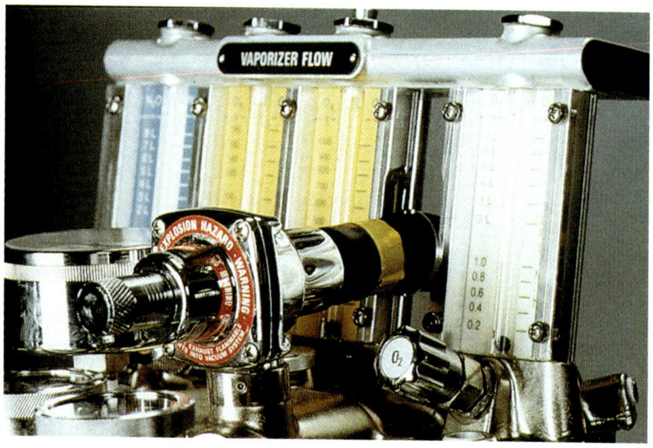

Fig. 7-30. The metabolic oxygen flowmeter control knob is fluted, labeled O_2, painted white (international color assigned to oxygen), and is positioned on the far right. The flow-tube scale is labeled O_2, ranges from 0.2 to 7 L/min, is also white, and is protected by a plastic shield. The adjustable pressure-limiting (pop-off) valve can be seen, with the proximal end of the scavenger hose attached.

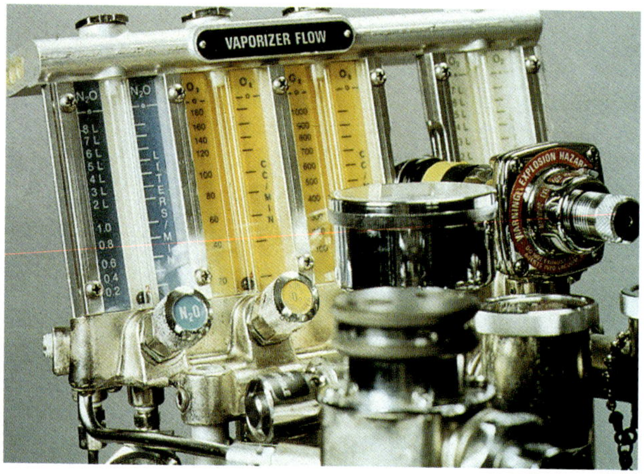

Fig. 7-31. Nitrous oxide and oxygen-for-vaporizer flowmeter control knobs and flow tubes. Nitrous oxide is labeled N_2O and is painted blue (international and US color assigned to nitrous oxide). The nitrous oxide–flow-tube scale is labeled N_2O, ranges from 0.2 to 8 L/min, is painted blue, and is protected by a plastic shield. The oxygen-for-vaporizer control knob is painted yellow (manufacturer's choice), and is labeled O_2 FOR VAPORIZER. The single oxygen-for-vaporizer flowmeter control knob meters both low- and high-flow oxygen. The flow-tube scales are labeled O_2, painted yellow, and protected by a plastic shield; the low-flow tube ranges from 20 to 180 cc/min, and the high-flow tube ranges from 100 to 1,000 cc/min. The nitrous oxide pressure-sensor shutoff valve can be seen below the nitrous oxide flowmeter housing.

porizer is yellow, and nitrous oxide is blue (Figures 7-30 and 7-31). Flowmeters and scales are protected by a transparent plastic shield. Metabolic oxygen and nitrous oxide flow into a common pipeline circuit at the top of the flowmeter manifold. The high and low flowmeters for oxygen-for-vaporizer are controlled by a single knob. The flow first enters the bottom of the low-flow tube, exits the top and enters the bottom of the high-flow tube, and finally exits the top of the high-flow tube to enter the common gas pipeline (Figure 7-32). Oxygen-for-vaporizer bubbles through the anesthetic liquid and carries anesthetic vapor into the common gas outlet *if* the vaporizer control dial is in the ON position; otherwise, the oxygen bypasses the vaporizer and enters directly into the common gas outlet. The metabolic oxygen flowmeter control knob is fluted (see Figure 7-30) to enhance identification.

Vaporizer

The FAM 250 mL vaporizer will deliver accurate, metered concentrations of isoflurane, halothane,

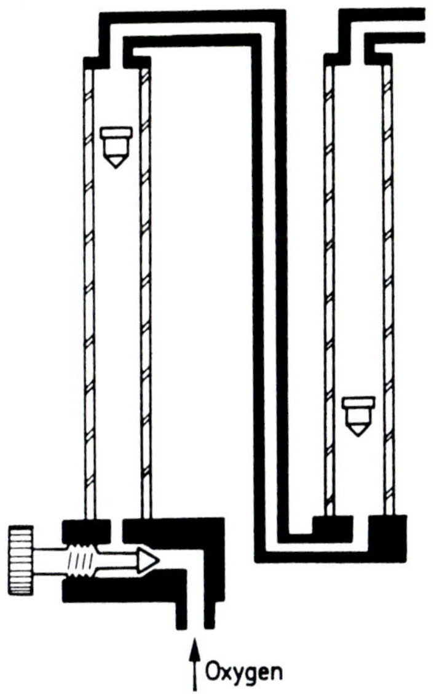

Fig. 7-32. The single-control flowmeter knob controls flow through the low- and high-flow tubes. Oxygen flow rate is metered by the position of the control knob in the cone-shaped orifice. Oxygen passes into the low-flow tube, causing the float to rise. Increasing the flow of oxygen causes the float in the low-flow tube to stay at the top, as oxygen passes into the high-flow tube and begins to lift the float in the high-flow tube. All oxygen eventually exits from the top of the high-flow tube on its way to the vaporizer. Photograph: Reprinted with permission from Schreiber P. *Safety Guidelines for Anesthesia Systems.* Telford, Pa: North American Dräger; 1985: 17.

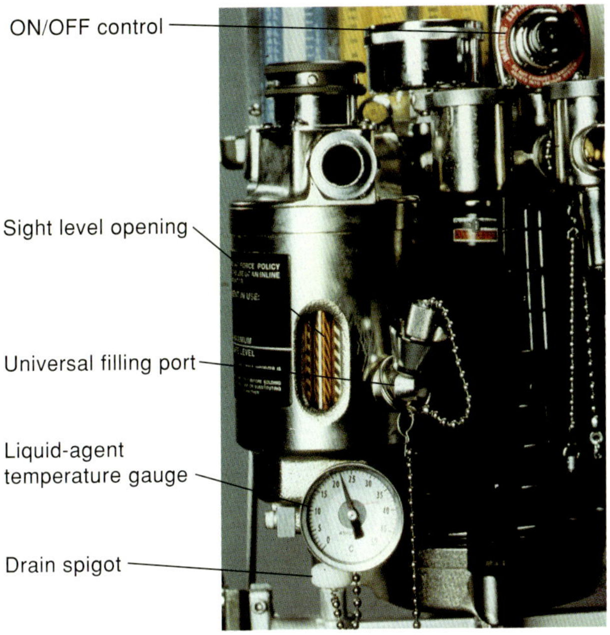

Fig. 7-33. Field Anesthesia Machine (FAM) Model 885A vaporizer, showing the ON/OFF control, the sight level opening, the universal filling port, the liquid-agent temperature gauge, the drain spigot, and the common gas-outlet port.

enflurane, ether, and chloroform (Figure 7-33). Desflurane cannot be used in the vaporizer because of its unique vapor pressure. The vaporizer is a brass container filled with a liquid anesthetic. Brass is a reasonably priced metal with acceptable thermal conductivity and specific heat characteristics. A dedicated oxygen-for-vaporizer flowmeter bubbles oxygen through the liquid in the vaporizer when the ON/OFF control is in the ON position. Agent output is determined by the same principles that govern the copper kettle (Figure 7-34). Each bubble of oxygen is saturated with the vapor of the liquid anesthetic. The large surface area of the oxygen bubble allows ample time for the liquid anesthetic agent to evaporate inside the bubble and to fully saturate the oxygen flowing through the vaporizer. Eventually, the oxygen entering the liquid anesthetic plus the anesthetic vapor exit the top of the vaporizer and are diluted by the metabolic oxygen and nitrous oxide in the common gas outlet. At least 50 mL of anesthetic liquid must be in the vaporizer for the anesthesia provider to be certain that the desired vapor concentration is delivered.

Many formulas can be used to calculate the final output of anesthetic agent concentration in the inspiratory limb of the breathing circuit. Approxi-

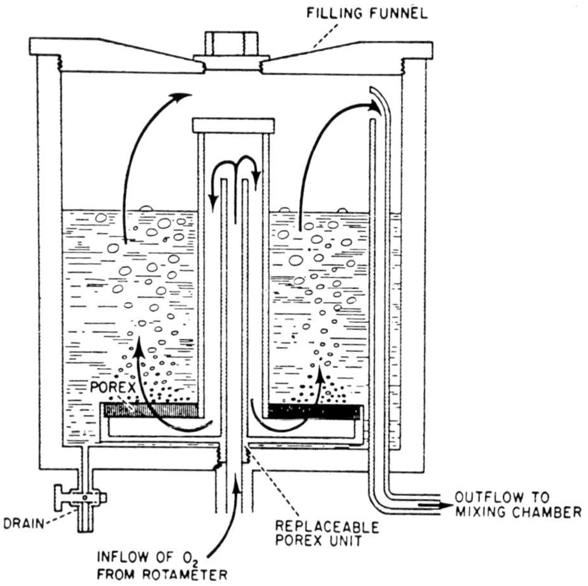

Fig. 7-34. Copper kettle bubble-through vaporizer. Output is determined by the temperature of the liquid anesthetic, the vapor pressure of the liquid anesthetic, the rate of oxygen bubbling through the liquid, and the barometric pressure. The Field Anesthesia Machine (FAM) Model 885A is a bubble-through vaporizer that can accept the majority of inhalational anesthetic agents. Photograph: Reprinted with permission from Morris LE. A new vaporizer for liquid anesthetic agents. *Anesthesiology.* 1952;13:587.

mate calculations of output are accurate enough for clinical application, of which the following is one method[5]:

- Derivation:

$$\% = \frac{\text{VF [mL/min]} \bullet [P_a / \{P_b - P_a\}] \bullet 100}{\text{TF [L/min]} \bullet 1{,}000}$$

where % represents the percentage concentration of anesthetic in the inspiratory limb of the breathing circuit, *VF* represents the flow of oxygen through the vaporizer (in mL/min), *TF* represents the total gas flow (in L/min), P_a represents the vapor pressure of volatile agent (in mm Hg), and P_b represents barometric pressure (in mm Hg).

- Simplification:
  - Vapor pressure of halothane is 243 mm Hg at 20°C and 760 mm Hg barometric pressure
  - Therefore, by substitution:

$$\% = \frac{\text{VF} \bullet [243/\{760 - 243\}] \bullet 100}{\text{TF} \bullet 1{,}000}$$

$$\% = \frac{0.47\ \text{VF}}{10\ \text{TF}} \quad \text{or} \quad \% \sim \frac{0.5\ \text{VF}}{10\ \text{TF}}$$

  - Therefore, VF ~ TF • 20 • %.
- Practical applications:
  1. An induction concentration of 3% halothane is desired.

     Temperature 20°C, barometric pressure 760 mm Hg, fresh-gas flow of 5 L/min:

     VF ~ 5 • 20 • 3%

     VF = 300 mL/min

     - Set vaporizer control to the ON position.
     - Set metabolic oxygen and nitrous oxide flowmeters to deliver a combined flow of 5 L/min.
     - Set oxygen-for-vaporizer flowmeter at 300 mL/min.
  2. To obtain a maintenance of 1% halothane in the inspiratory limb of the breathing circuit at 20°C, barometric pressure of 760 mm Hg, and a fresh-gas flow of 2 L/min:

     VF ~ 2 • 20 • 1%

     VF = 40 mL/min

     - Leave vaporizer control at ON position.
     - Set metabolic oxygen and nitrous oxide flowmeters to give a combined flow of 2 L/min.
     - Set oxygen-for-vaporizer flowmeter at 40 mL/min.

To simplify the calculation of vaporizer output concentration, a Verni-Trol (manufactured by Ohmeda, Inc., Madison, Wis.) anesthetic vaporizer-flow calculator is included in the lower case of the FAM (Figure 7-35). This calculator is a miniature slide rule designed for one task: to determine the final concentration of anesthetic agent in the inspiratory limb of the breathing circuit. The anesthesia provider first finds the desired concentration of the anesthetic agent vapor on the outermost scale of the calculator (labeled % CONCENTRATION). Then the desired total flow rate on the TOTAL FLOW scale is aligned with the anesthetic agent concentration value. Set the hairline LIQUID TEMPERATURE scale value for the agent in the vaporizer to correspond to the temperature of the liquid in the vaporizer. Finally, read the required oxygen-for-vaporizer flowmeter setting where the hairline crosses the Flow Thru Verni-Trol scale. These steps are illustrated in the following example:

1. The desired total flow rate is 5 L/min.
   - Desired concentration of *halothane* is 1%.
   - Vaporizer thermometer reading is 25°C.
2. Find 1% on the CONCENTRATION scale.
   - Align 5 L/min value on the TOTAL FLOW scale with the 1% value.
   - Find 25°C on the halothane LIQUID TEMPERATURE scale and set the hairline.
   - The hairline will cross Flow Thru Verni-Trol scale at 100 mL/min value.
3. Set metabolic oxygen and nitrous oxide flowmeters to give a combined 5 L/min flow.
   - Set vaporizer control on vaporizer to the ON position.
   - Set oxygen-for-vaporizer flowmeter at 100 mL/min.

Temperature has a profound effect on vapor pressure and must always be factored in when using the vaporizer in field conditions. Total flow rates have major effects on concentration. During induction, high flow rates are used; when switching to lower flows for maintenance, the anesthesia provider must recalculate the flow required through the vaporizer for maintenance levels of anesthetic.

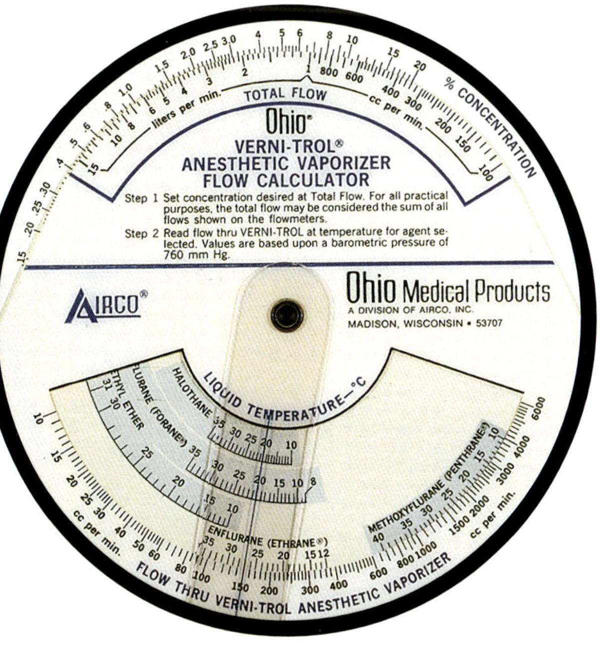

Most anesthesia providers are not familiar with the calculations or the Verni-Trol calculator because single-agent temperature- and pressure-compensated vaporizers have replaced Verni-Trol–type vaporizers. During the Persian Gulf War, many anesthesia providers believed that the FAM Model 885 vaporizer was outmoded, dangerous, and should have been replaced immediately. Not many took the time to learn the technology of a past era, and only a few felt comfortable administering an anesthetic with the FAM. A new anesthesia machine for the field will have agent-specific vaporizers available for at least halothane and isoflurane.

A common funnel port is provided on the side of the vaporizer with a liquid level sight tube. Under the vaporizer are found a drain, a spigot, and a plug (see Figure 7-33). The manufacturer recommends rinsing the vaporizer, first with hot water and then with ethyl alcohol, after one agent has been drained and a different agent is to be added. Gas from the metabolic oxygen and nitrous oxide flowmeters mix prior to entering the vaporizer housing and do not enter the vaporizer at any time. The oxygen from the oxygen-for-vaporizer flowmeter bubbles through the liquid anesthetic, and both the oxygen and anesthetic vapor mix with the metabolic oxy-

Fig. 7-35. The Ohio Verni-Trol anesthetic vaporizer-flow calculator is attached to the inside of the wall of the bottom case of the Field Anesthesia Machine (FAM) Model 885A. The calculator is positioned to calculate the parameters to deliver approximately 1.3% halothane to the breathing circuit at a liquid anesthetic temperature of 20°C, a barometric pressure of 760 mm Hg, an oxygen-for-vaporizer flowmeter setting of 150 cc/min, and a metabolic oxygen flowmeter setting of 5 L/min. Find the bar for HALOTHANE; note that the center of the hairline crosses the 20°C mark (all agent markings are in °C) and that the outer end of the hairline crosses the 150 cc/min mark. Next, read the desired concentration (1.3%, in this case) and the total flow immediately below the concentration (5 L/min). At the same setting, you could give 1% halothane by increasing the total flow to 6.5 L/min or 3% halothane by decreasing the total flow to 2.2 L/min. If you wanted to induce anesthesia in a patient, using 3% halothane at a total flow of 5 L/min and the halothane in the vaporizer was at a temperature of 20°C (barometric pressure 760 mm Hg), you would have to set the oxygen-for-vaporizer flow rate to 320 cc/min. Instructions for use are printed on the calculator. The accuracy of output is reasonable for clinical anesthesia. Remember: each time the metabolic oxygen flows change (eg, induction to maintenance) or the anesthetic liquid temperature changes, an adjustment must be made in the flow rate of oxygen through the vaporizer.

gen and nitrous oxide in the common gas outlet (see Figure 7-27). An oxygen sensor tee is connected to the vaporizer port (see Figure 7-14), and the inspiratory breathing circuit is attached to one limb of the tee and the oxygen sensor housing is attached to the other limb.

The FAM Model 885 vaporizer is well designed, versatile, functional, and safe in the hands of anesthesia providers who are familiar with how it works.

Breathing Circuit

The circuit has a breathing-circuit pressure gauge, an oxygen monitor, an oxygen flush valve, and a nonadjustable pressure-relief valve (which releases gases to the atmosphere if the circuit pressure exceeds 60–80 mm Hg) (see Figures 7-27 and 7-31). The adult circuit has, in addition, an adjustable pressure-limiting valve (ie, the pop-off valve), a 3-L rebreathing bag, two one-way valves, two corrugated breathing tubes, a scavenger, a carbon dioxide absorber, a Y-piece, an elbow, and an adult's face mask (see Figure 7-27 and Figure 7-36). The pediatric partial nonrebreathing circuit is attached to the vaporizer port and has a tee connector, a breathing tube, a 1-L rebreathing bag, a one-way scavenger valve, and a child's face mask (Figures 7-37 and 7-38). When using the pediatric circuit, it is essential to close the pop-off valve to prevent the loss of gases to the atmosphere.

Oxygen Flush Valve

The oxygen flush valve is mounted in front of the flowmeter manifold, behind the breathing pressure gauge, and between the flowmeter control knobs for metabolic oxygen and oxygen-for-vaporizer (Figure 7-39). The valve is identified by a white semicircular label with the words OXYGEN FLUSH printed in black letters. When the anesthesia provider presses down on the oxygen flush valve, the spring pressure holding a ball valve against a valve seat is counteracted, and oxygen is allowed to flow into the breathing circuit at a flow rate of approximately 40 L/min (Figure 7-40). Releasing the pressure on the button allows the spring to reseat the ball valve.

Carbon Dioxide Absorber

A standard two-chamber carbon dioxide absorber is positioned beneath the control head (see Figure 7-12 and Figure 7-41). Once the chambers are filled with carbon dioxide–absorbent granules, the unit is secured with a clamping knob. If the clamping knob is tightened excessively, the chamber wall can be warped, causing leaks. An absorber drain plug is located on the bottom of the unit.

Carbon dioxide–absorbent granules react irreversibly with carbon dioxide. Sodasorb (manufactured by W. R. Grace, Lexington, Mass.), a mixture of hydrated lime, sodium hydroxide, potassium hydroxide, and inert materials, reacts with carbon dioxide according to the following equations:

1. $CO_2 + H_2O \rightleftharpoons H_2CO_3$
2. $2H_2CO_3 + 2NaOH + 2KOH \longrightarrow Na_2CO_3 + K_2CO_3 + 4H_2O + \text{Heat}$
3. $2Na_2CO_3 + 2Ca(OH)_2 + K_2CO_3 \longrightarrow 2CaCO_3 + 2NaOH + 2KOH + \text{Heat}$

The net reaction can be expressed as follows:

4. $Ca(OH)_2 + CO_2 \longrightarrow CaCO_3 + H_2O + \text{Heat}$

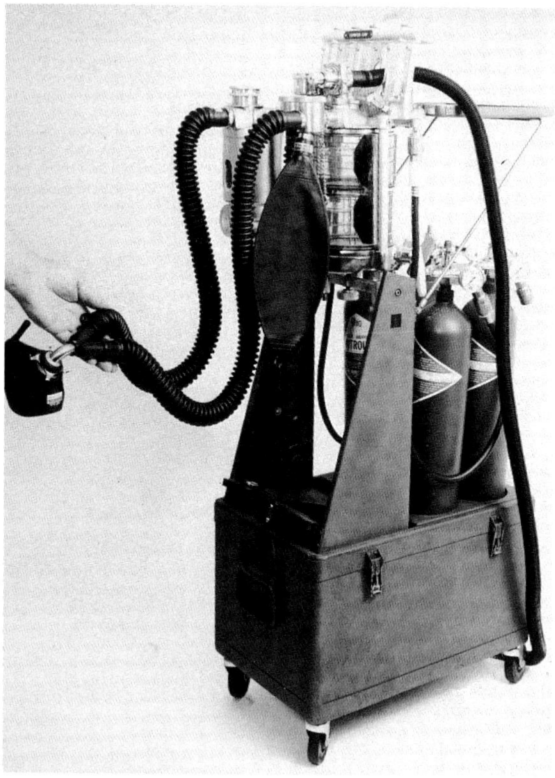

Fig. 7-36. The Field Anesthesia Machine (FAM) Model 885A is configured with an adult breathing circuit. A corrugated hose is attached to the scavenger port of the pop-off valve. The inspiratory limb of the breathing circuit is attached to the outlet port near the vaporizer, and the expiratory limb is attached to the inlet port near the exhalation valve. Photograph: Printed with permission from Ohmeda, Inc, Madison, Wis.

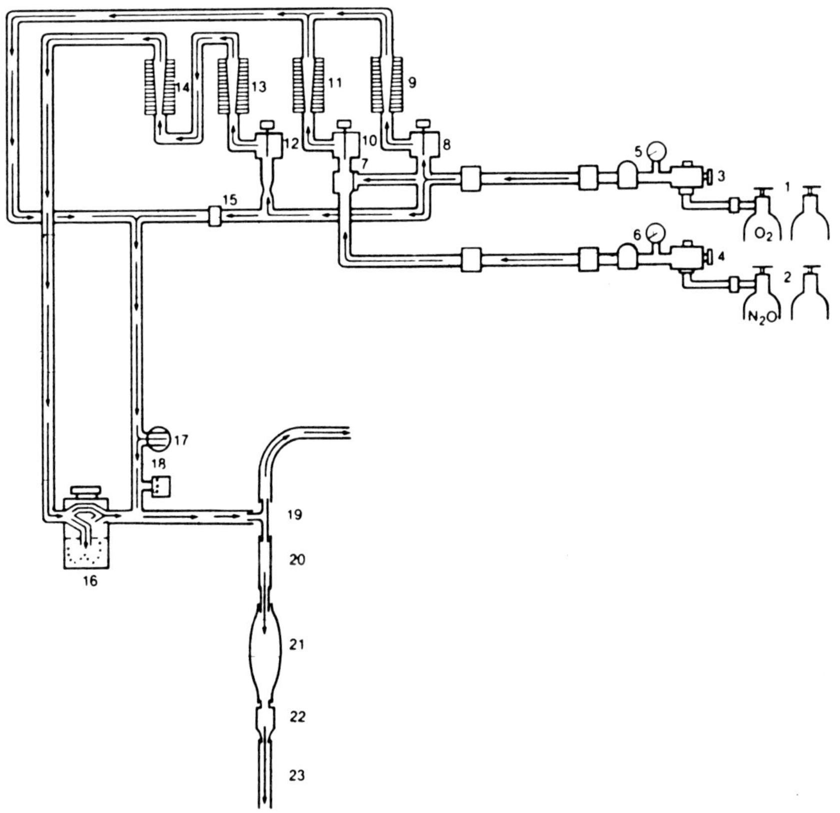

Fig. 7-37. A schematic drawing of the pediatric nonrebreathing circuit. The circuit is the same as the adult system in Fig. 7-14 except that the mixed gases do not recirculate. Mixed gases enter the tee connector (19) and flow through a short tube (20) into the rebreathing bag (21). Squeezing the rebreathing bag forces the mixed gases into the patient. Exhaled gases pass through the rebreathing bag, the scavenger valve (22), and out the gas-evacuation tubing. Low-flow rates are associated with partial rebreathing. The pop-off valve must be closed when using the pediatric circuit to prevent significant loss of gases to the atmosphere. Drawing: Printed with permission from Ohmeda, Inc, Madison, Wis.

The granules most frequently used in the United States have been Sodasorb, SODALIME USP/NF (manufactured in England by Molecular Products, Ltd.; distributed in the United States by Puritan-Bennett, Lenexa, Kan.), and Baralyme (manufactured by Allied Healthcare Products, Inc., St. Louis, Mo.). Table 7-1 compares some of the basic characteristics of the three granules. Figures 7-42 and 7-43 illustrate the differences in the three granules' absorption of carbon dioxide. Granules are provided in different kinds of packaging (Figure 7-44).

Carbon dioxide–absorbent granules are imbedded with ethyl violet, an indicator dye, which changes from white to purple at pH 10.3. Absorp-

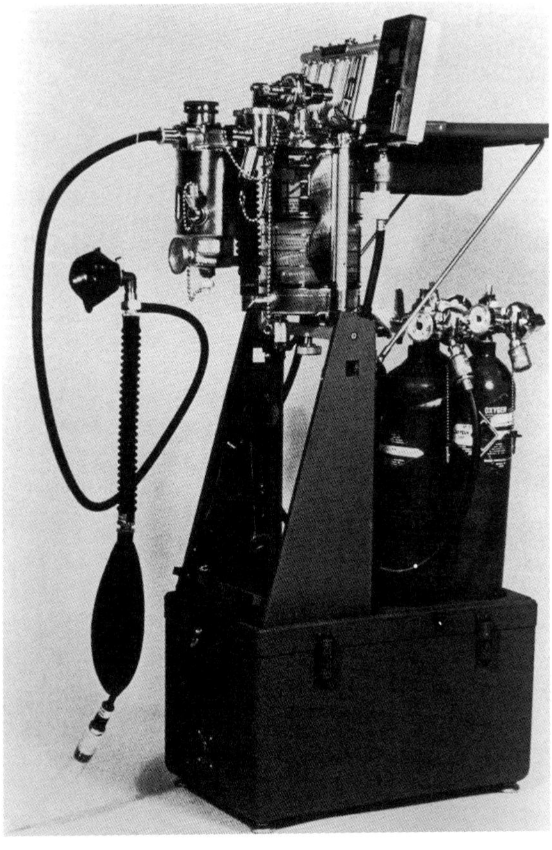

Fig. 7-38. Field Anesthesia Machine (FAM) Model 885A configured with a pediatric nonrebreathing circuit. Fresh gases flow from the outlet port near the vaporizer to the tee of the pediatric nonbreathing circuit. The pop-off valve of the FAM is closed to prevent gas escaping to the atmosphere. Scavenged gases leave the tip of the rebreathing bag and flow into a corrugated hose. Photograph: Printed with permission from Ohmeda, Inc, Madison, Wis.

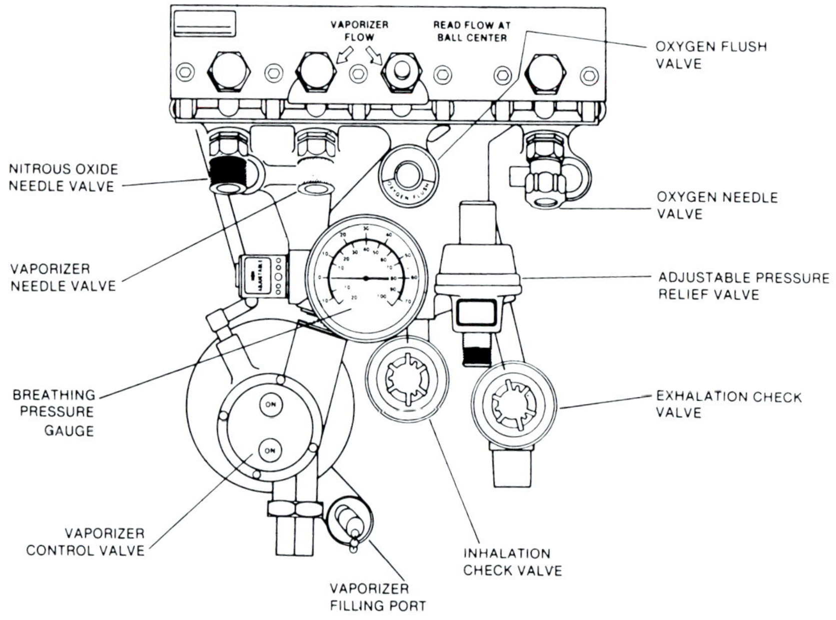

Fig. 7-39. Diagram of the top view of the Field Anesthesia Machine (FAM) Model 885A showing the position of the oxygen flush valve. Note the fluted oxygen needle valve, the adjustable pressure-limiting (pop-off) valve, and the two breathing-circuit check valves. The breathing-pressure gauge is in the horizontal position, making it somewhat difficult to read. Two orifices in the vaporizer control valve read ON. The nonadjustable pressure-relief valve can be seen immediately adjacent to and to the left of the breathing-pressure gauge. Redrawn with permission from Ohmeda, Inc, Madison, Wis.

tion of carbon dioxide is not the same throughout the canister. Figure 7-45 depicts the zones of absorption; the granules immediately adjacent to and along the top encounter carbon dioxide first. Once the granules are purple, their structures are permanently changed and they should be discarded (Figure 7-46).

Oxygen Monitor

An oxygen monitor is assembled for use with the following parts: oxygen monitor, tee, cable, oxygen sensor cartridge, mounting bracket, and batteries. The heart of the oxygen monitor is the galvanic cell sensor cartridge (Figure 7-47). Oxygen molecules

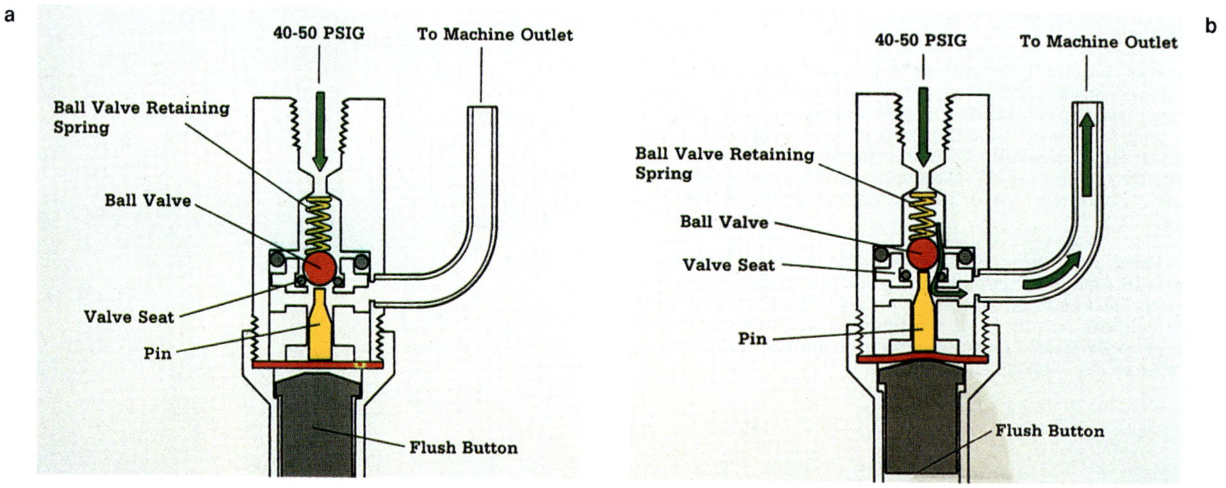

Fig. 7-40. How the oxygen flush valve works in the Field Anesthesia Machine (FAM) Model 885A. (**a**) A ball-valve retaining spring is holding the ball valve against the valve seat, preventing oxygen from escaping into the machine outlet. (**b**) The flush button has been pushed in, counteracting the pressure from the ball-valve retaining spring. As the pin moves, the ball valve is lifted off the valve seat, and oxygen at a pressure of 40 psig escapes into the machine outlet at 40 to 60 L/min. Photograph: Printed with permission granted by Medical Systems Division, Ohmeda, Inc, Madison, Wis.

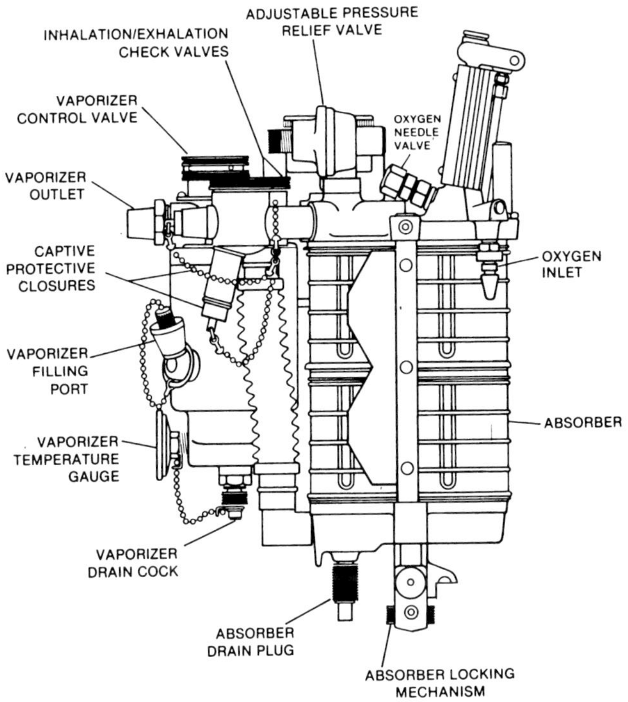

Fig. 7-41. Right side of the absorber head of the Field Anesthesia Machine (FAM) Model 885A. A two-canister carbon dioxide absorber is positioned directly below the flowmeter manifold. After the absorption granules have been placed in the absorber, the absorber's locking mechanism is gently tightened to avoid leaks between the two chambers and around the gaskets. Overtightening the locking mechanism will warp the canister walls, causing permanent leaks. Protective devices used during storage are shown in place. The vaporizer's filling port, temperature gauge, and drain cock are shown. Fluid accumulating in the absorber can be drained by opening the drain plug. Redrawn with permission from Ohmeda, Inc, Madison, Wis.

TABLE 7-1

COMPARISON OF COMMERCIALLY AVAILABLE CARBON DIOXIDE–ABSORBENT GRANULES

Attribute	SODALIME USP/NF* (4–8 mesh w/v granules)	Sodasorb† (4–8 mesh w/v granules)	Baralyme‡ (4–8 mesh w/v agglomerates)
Moisture (%)	16.3	14.7	14.4
NaOH content (%)	3.01	0.82	0.3
KOH content (%)	0.01	2.1	3.3
Bulk density (g/mL)	0.82	0.83	0.97
Attrition (%)	92.7	95.2	94.1
Crush strength (%)	91.9	94.1	90.5
Hardness (%)	96.2	90.1	89.0
Mesh analysis:			
> 8 mm	0	0	0
4.75–8 mm	0.9	1.7	5.9
2.36–4.75 mm	89.1	89.9	87.9
0.42–2.36 mm	9.4	7.3	5.2
< 0.42 mm	0.6	1.1	1.0

*Manufactured by Molecular Products, Ltd (England); distributed in the US by Puritan-Bennett, Lenexa, Kan
†Manufactured by WR Grace, Lexington, Mass
‡Manufactured by Allied Healthcare, St Louis, Mo
Information provided by Puritan-Bennett Corporation, Lenexa, Kan, distributors of SODALIME USP/NF.

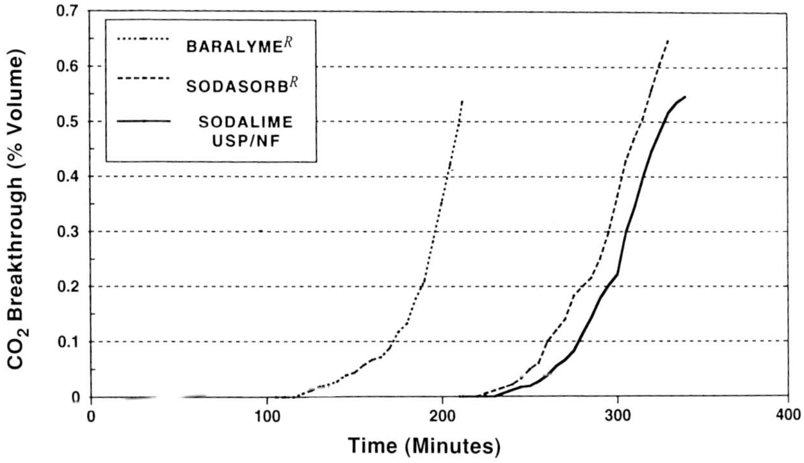

Fig. 7-42. Length-of-life comparison of carbon dioxide–absorbent granules. A closed-circuit test was done with 5% CO_2 at 500 mL • 20 breaths per minute. Carbon dioxide breakthrough occurred first with Baralyme (manufactured by Allied Healthcare, St Louis, Mo). Sodasorb (manufactured by WR Grace, Lexington, Mass) and SODALIME USP/NF (manufactured by Molecular Products, Ltd (England); distributed in the United States by Puritan-Bennett, Lenexa, Kan) absorbed more carbon dioxide than Baralyme. Information provided by Puritan-Bennett Corporation, Lenexa, Kan, distributors of SODALIME USP/NF.

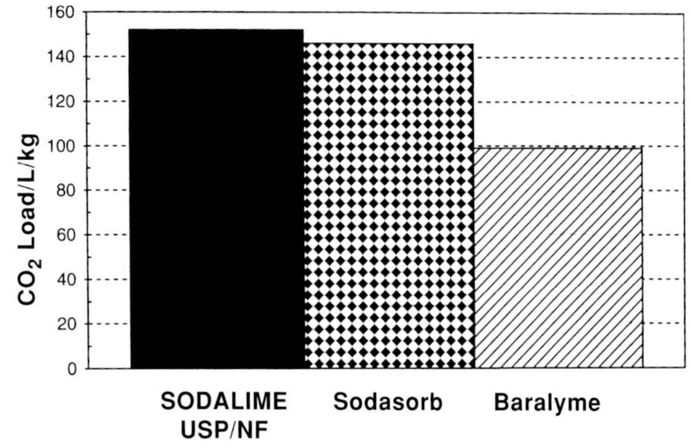

Fig. 7-43. Comparison of carbon dioxide loading by three absorbent granules. A closed-circuit test was done with 5% CO_2 at 500 mL • 20 breaths per minute. Carbon dioxide load was complete when 0.5% CO_2 appeared in the exit gas from the absorber. Baralyme (manufactured by Allied Healthcare, St Louis, Mo) absorbed less carbon dioxide than Sodasorb (manufactured by WR Grace, Lexington, Mass) or SODALIME USP/NF (manufactured by Molecular Products, Ltd; distributed in the US by Puritan-Bennett, Lenexa, Kans). Information provided by Puritan-Bennett Corporation, Lenexa, Kans, distributors of SODALIME USP/NF.

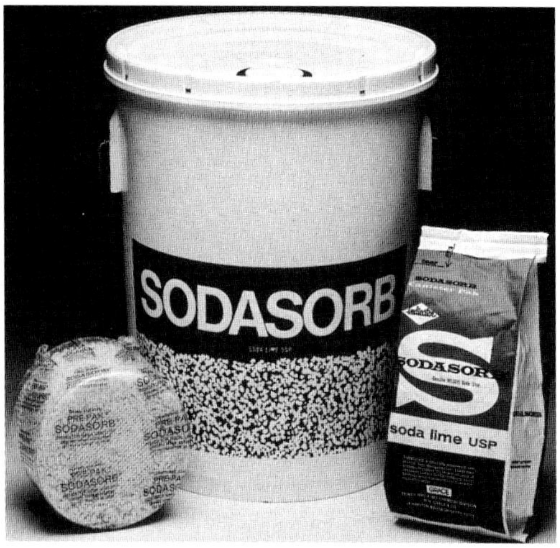

Fig. 7-44. Carbon dioxide–absorption granules can be purchased in a variety of packages. Sodasorb is available in large buckets, small sacks, and prefilled canisters. Photograph: Printed with permission of WR Grace & Co, Lexington, Mass.

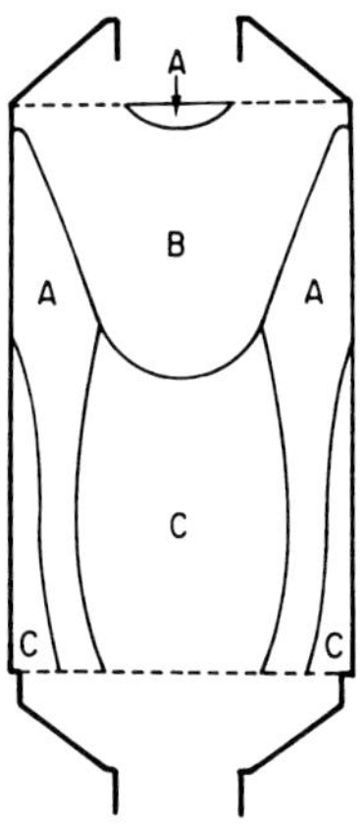

Fig. 7-45. Zones of absorption in the carbon dioxide–absorber head. Exhaled gases enter the top of the carbon dioxide–absorber head. Granules in the **A** areas are rapidly depleted and change from white to purple very early. Granules in the **B** and **C** zones change slowly. Photograph: Reprinted with permission from Conry WA, Seevers MH. Studies in carbon dioxide absorption. *Anesthesiology*. 1943;4:160.

a b

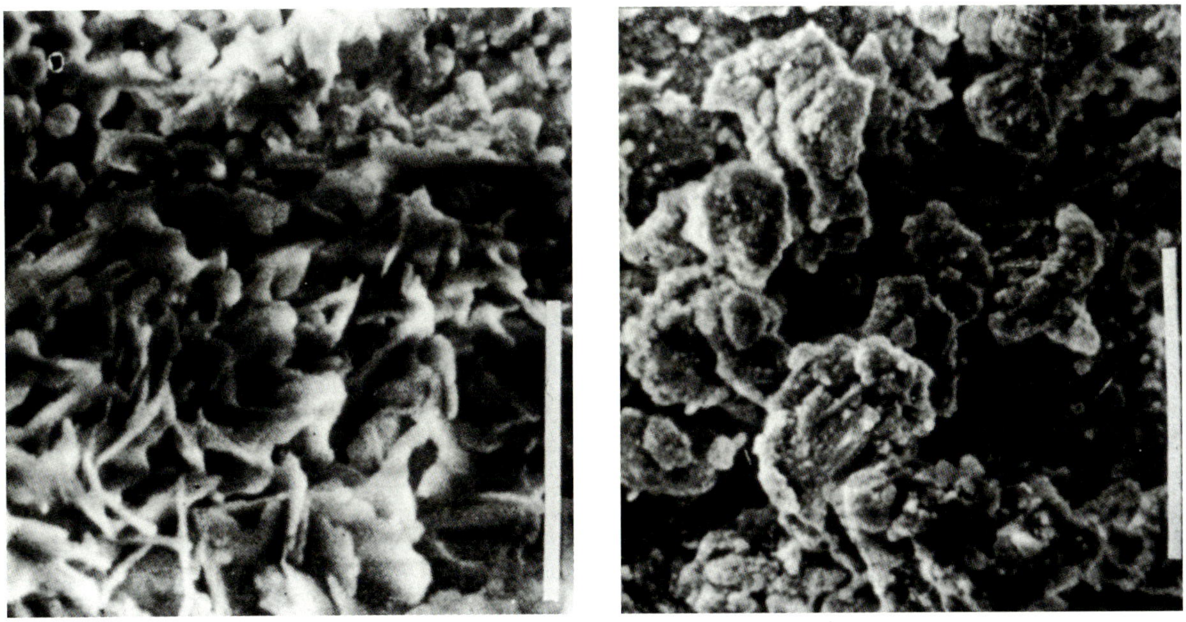

Fig. 7-46. (**a**) Normal structure of carbon dioxide–absorption granules before exposure to carbon dioxide (scanning electron micrograph, original magnification x 3,000). (**b**) Carbon dioxide–absorbent granules undergo irreversible structural changes after absorbing carbon dioxide. Soda lime granules become less defined and look cokelike (scanning electron micrograph, original magnification x 3,000). Reprinted with permission from Sato T, Hori T, Yusa T, Fujii A. The surface structure of carbon dioxide absorbents observed with scanning electron microscopy. *Jap J Anes*. 1970;19(1):26. In Japanese.

selectively pass through a Teflon (polytetrafluoroethylene, manufactured by Du Pont Polymers, Wilmington, Del.) membrane and react with gold to produce hydroxyl ions (Figure 7-48). Hydroxyl ions then react with lead to release electrons, which create a voltage output across an external load resistor. Computer chips allow the electron flow to be displayed as the percentage of oxygen (Figure 7-49). High– and low–percentage-of-oxygen alarms are included. Sensor life is exposure-dependent. Each sensor is initially packed in an inert gas and if stored under refrigeration at 6°C ± 3°C (CAUTION: do not freeze), can be expected to last a long time. Refrigeration is not always available in the field, so the replacement sensors should be stored (when possible) between 18°C and 22°C and between 50% and 60% relative humidity. Lifespan in use (approximately 438,000 percent hours) is determined by the time of exposure (in hours) and the concentration of oxygen (as a percentage). For example, the sensor would last 1 year if exposed to 50% oxygen but only 6 months if exposed to 100% oxygen.

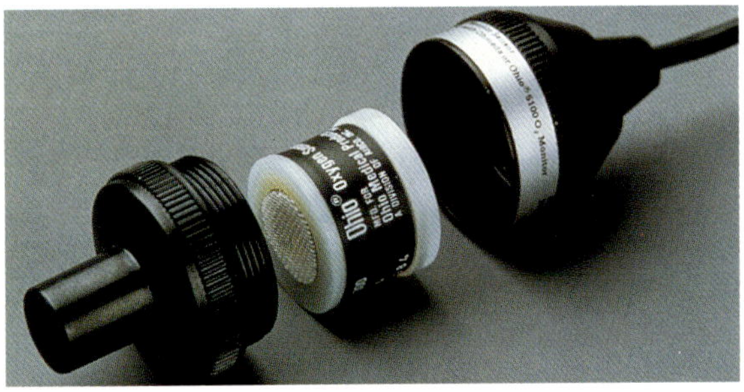

Fig. 7-47. An oxygen sensor housing showing the galvanic cell sensor cartridge. A cable from the housing connects the cartridge to the processor in the monitor, and the opposite end is placed in the tee of the inspiratory limb of the breathing circuit. Photograph: Printed with permission of Ohmeda, Inc, Madison, Wis.

After the tee is inserted in the breathing circuit between the vaporizer outlet port and the inspiratory limb of the breathing circuit, the oxygen sensor is inserted in the remaining open port of the tee. A cable connects the sensor to the monitor mounted on the bracket of the absorber head (see Figures 7-13 and 7-14).

Checkout and Maintenance

Each FAM's *Instruction and Service Manual*[1] outlines in detail how to set up the machine, contains a checklist to complete prior to use, and describes how to maintain and repair the machine. In the

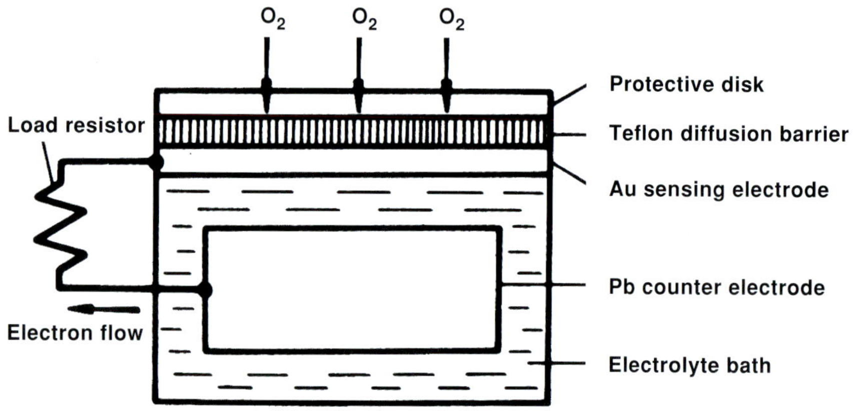

Fig. 7-48. How an oxygen galvanic cell sensor works. Oxygen molecules selectively pass through a Teflon (polytetrafluoroethylene, manufactured by Du Pont Polymers, Wilmington, Del) membrane and immediately react with gold (Au, the cathode), producing hydroxyl ions. The hydroxyl ions pass into the electrolyte bath and react with lead (Pb, the anode) to form lead oxide and release electrons. These electrons produce a current proportional to the number of oxygen molecules that are reduced at the gold cathode. An external load resistor connects the anode and the cathode. Reprinted with permission from Schreiber P. *Anesthesia Equipment, Performance, Classification and Safety.* New York, NY: Springer-Verlag; 1972: 130.

back of the manual are blow-up illustrations of the parts, and numbers for ordering parts. A videotape, *Set Up and Use of the Military Field Anesthesia Machine*,[6] is also available to assist the first-time user in how to give an anesthetic with the FAM.

Once the machine has been set up, it is important to perform a checkout of the machine prior to the administration of anesthesia. The FAM will not require the same checkout as an anesthesia machine meeting the *Standard Specification for Minimum Performance and Safety Requirements for Components and Systems of Anesthesia Gas Machines*[7] defined by the American Society for Testing and Materials (ASTM) because it was manufactured prior to the standards. The FAM instruction manual outlines a specific checkout list covering the following areas[1]:

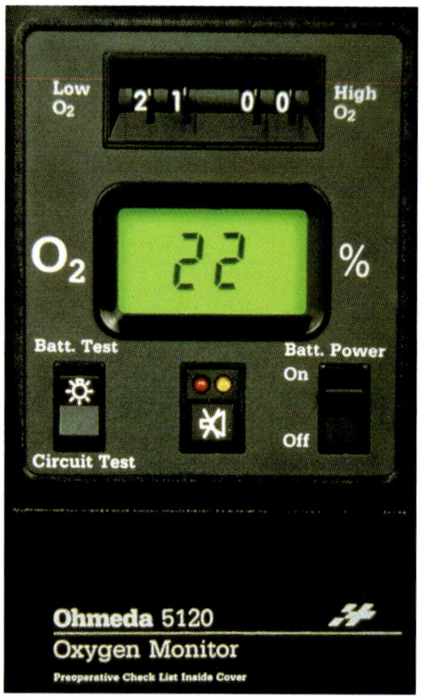

Fig. 7-49. An oxygen display of the percentage of oxygen in the gas mixture. Low-concentration and high-concentration alarms can be used by the anesthesia provider as conditions warrant. Photograph: Printed with permission of Ohmeda, Inc, Madison, Wis.

- visual inspection,
- high-pressure gas circuit check,
- low-pressure gas circuit check,
- adult breathing circuit check,
- pediatric breathing circuit check,
- the oxygen monitor,
- the gas-ratio output of metabolic oxygen and nitrous oxide,
- zeroing the breathing-circuit pressure gauge, and
- the nonadjustable pressure relief valve.

In three different places in the instruction manual, the manufacturer warns in boldface type:

> "CAUTION: **No repair should ever be undertaken or attempted by anyone not having experience repairing devices of this nature.**"[1(p35)]

Internal repairs should not be performed in the field.

Simple procedures can be done by anesthesia personnel or anesthesia technicians. Soda lime should be changed when the top portion of the bottom canister begins to turn purple (exhaled gases pass into the top of the absorber and the top container is the first to be depleted). Check valves must be kept clean to avoid sticking. The pop-off valve can be dismantled easily and then inspected, washed, dried, and reassembled. Surface areas need to be wiped regularly with a damp cloth to keep dirt and grime from collecting. Special attention must be paid to the absorber and the rubber goods. Cloudiness on the inside of the canisters can be removed by buffing with Bon Ami (feldspar and calcite abrasive cleanser, manufactured by Faultless Starch/Bon Ami Co., Kansas City, Mo.). Anesthesia agents and oxygen take their toll on the rubber goods; rubber gaskets and so forth should routinely be inspected and worn parts replaced. Preventive maintenance should be done at least every 4 months when the FAM is in service.

Sterilization is sometimes difficult to perform in field conditions, owing to the limited access to equipment and materials. Most of the components of the FAM can be washed with a mild alkali detergent and sterilized in a cold germicidal solution. Steam sterilization and ethylene oxide sterilization can be used, but with caution.

FAMs in storage with oxygen monitor sensors should be inspected at least once a year. FAMs without sensors should be inspected every 30 months. Records should be kept of all inspections, part replacements, and performance of preoperative checks.

OHMEDA UNIVERSAL PORTABLE ANESTHESIA CIRCUIT

Before the discovery of anesthesia, surgery usually lasted less than 5 minutes because patients could not tolerate the pain. On October 16, 1846, William Morton performed the first public demonstration of anesthesia by using a draw-over vaporizer to administer ether to Gilbert Abbott.[8] Ether was poured onto a sponge in a glass container, later called the Morton inhaler (see Figure 31-5, in Chapter 31, Military Anesthesia From Open-Drop Ether to Critical Care). A wooden tube was placed in the patient's mouth and as the patient inhaled, a valve was opened, air that was pulled through the glass container picked up the ether vapor, and the induction of anesthesia began. The Morton inhaler proved to be cumbersome, inaccurate, and was soon replaced by the simplest form of draw-over vaporizer: a gauze-covered mask (see Figure 7-1).

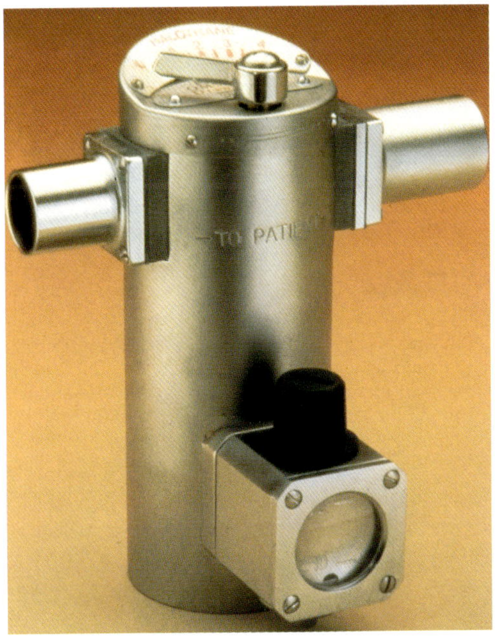

Fig. 7-50. The Tri-Service draw-over vaporizer (manufactured by Penlon, Ltd, Abingdon, England) is used by the British armed forces. Atmospheric air is the primary carrying gas. The unit can be used with a mechanical ventilator, supplemental oxygen, and a self-inflating bag. Photograph: Printed with permission of Penlon Ltd, Abingdon, England.

Ether dripped onto a gauze-covered mask was widely used in the U.S. military from 1846 to the end of World War II. After World War II, anesthesia providers adopted circle systems in civilian hospitals and the use of draw-over vaporizers ended. In the Vietnam War, a few U.S. military anesthesia providers used draw-over vaporizers, loaned by the Australian Armed Forces, as a novelty. During the Falklands War, the British armed forces used the Tri-Service draw-over vaporizer (manufactured by Penlon, Ltd., Abingdon, England) with great success (Figure 7-50). This war was especially suited for a draw-over vaporizer: it was short, featured highly mobile forces, and long-standing field hospitals were not required. British anesthetists continued to praise the draw-over vaporizer via such vehicles as journal publications and medical meetings. Members of the U.S. military anesthesia community eventually became interested in the draw-over vaporizer. Basic research was done on the machine in the United States, and some military anesthesia provid-

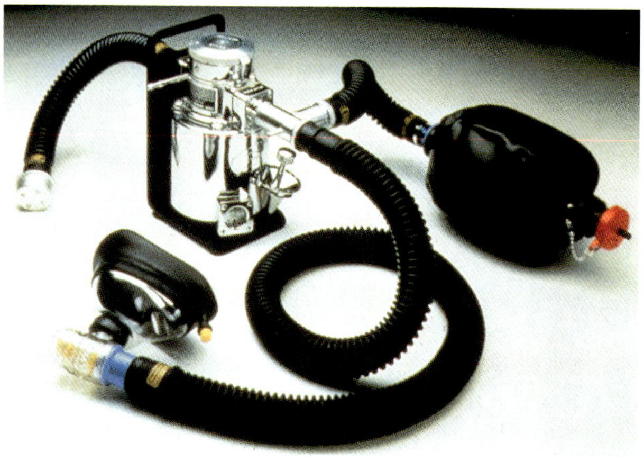

Fig. 7-51. The Ohmeda Universal Portable Anesthesia Circuit (PAC) is shown assembled and ready for use. Photograph: Printed with permission of Ohmeda, Inc, Madison, Wis.

ers took draw-over vaporizers with them on volunteer humanitarian missions to the Third World.

Once Operation Desert Shield was mobilized, military anesthesia providers requested draw-over vaporizers as backup to the FAMs. The Ohmeda Universal PAC was chosen as the draw-over vaporizer for the U.S. military (Figure 7-51). Appropriate paperwork and PAC units were sent to the U.S. Food and Drug Administration (FDA) for its 510(k) approval for sale. The FDA was attuned to the needs of the military and was able to give its approval before the onset of Operation Desert Storm. This approval allowed the PAC to be sold to the military but restricted its use to wartime conditions. The manufacturer was requested to include the following statement in the PAC *Operation and Maintenance Manual*:

> WARNING: The Ohmeda Universal PAC system is intended for use only in military battlefield situations where conventional closed, semi-closed continuous low flow or other more sophisticated anesthesia systems are not available. Failure to utilize a conventional anesthesia system when available significantly increases the risk of patient injury.[9(p3)]

PAC units were taken to Saudi Arabia and became an inventory item in the DEPMEDS system. The majority of anesthesia providers in the United States have not seen a draw-over vaporizer, are only vaguely familiar with its operating principles, and do not know how to use one safely. Learning to use a draw-over vaporizer is not complicated, but it was extremely difficult to train our military personnel during the Persian Gulf War. Anesthesia standards of care, anesthesia machine standards,[7] and medicolegal pressures would not allow the routine use of draw-over vaporizers in civilian hospitals and stateside military hospitals. Efforts have recently been begun to establish training sites at stateside military hospitals to provide instruction.

Specifications and Operation

The PAC fits into a small container about the size of a small briefcase (see Figure 7-3). Figure 7-52 is a labeled diagram of the components and Figure 7-53 shows the PAC assembled. The PAC unit weighs about 5 lb and measures $7\frac{1}{2}$ in. x $5\frac{1}{8}$ in. x $3\frac{3}{4}$ in; the vaporizer holds 85 mL of liquid anesthetic and has

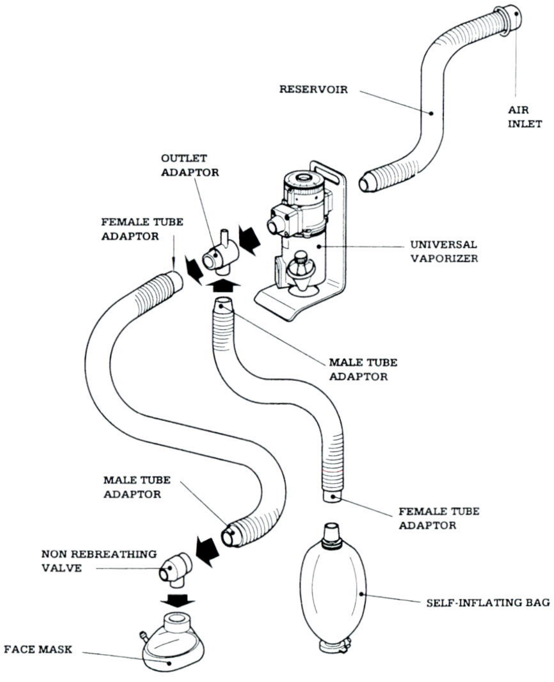

Fig. 7-52. Break-out view of the Ohmeda Universal Portable Anesthesia Circuit (PAC). Atmospheric air is pulled through the air inlet and the vaporizer by the recoil inflation of the self-inflating bag. The reservoir hose is a catchment area for supplemental oxygen to accumulate during the respiratory cycle. A nonrebreathing valve at the face mask keeps the air/anesthetic mixture flowing in one direction. As the self-inflating bag is squeezed, the patient's lungs are ventilated. Elastic recoil of the patient's lungs empties the exhaled gases into the room via a scavenger hose. During inflation of the self-inflating bag, air is drawn through the vaporizer, picking up anesthetic vapor and filling the self-inflating bag and connecting tube with air/anesthetic mixture. Photograph: Printed with permission of Ohmeda, Inc, Steeton, West Yorkshire, England.

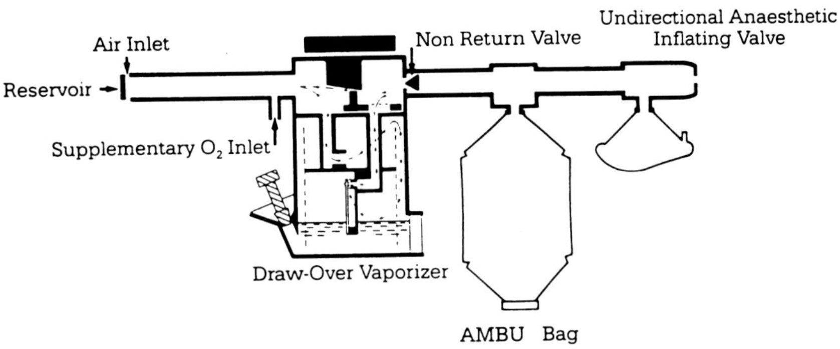

Fig. 7-53. Schematic of the Portable Anesthesia Circuit (PAC). Air is drawn through the air inlet into the vaporizer. A portion of the air enters the vaporizer chamber to pick up the anesthetic vapor and combine with the portion of air that bypassed the vaporizing chamber. Note the nonreturn valve at the vaporizer outlet and the nonrebreathing valve at the face mask. Both function to ensure one-way airflow. A supplementary oxygen inlet is present between the air inlet and the vaporizer inlet. Oxygen can accumulate in the reservoir hose to provide enrichment of the carrier gas. Photograph: Printed with permission of Ohmeda, Inc, Steeton, West Yorkshire, England.

a nominal working temperature range of 18°C to 35°C (65°F–95°F).[9]

A one-way valve at the face mask, combined with the nonreturn valve at the vaporizer outlet, ensures the one-way movement of air from the air inlet to the face mask (Figure 7-53). Air is drawn through the PAC by the recoil negative pressure created by filling of the deflated self-inflating bag. Air flow within the vaporizer is governed by a rotary valve, which is controlled by adjusting the concentration setting dial (Figure 7-54). Two calibrated concentration dial disks are available: isoflurane/halothane and diethyl ether/enflurane (Figure 7-55). The reversible dial disk, graduated from 0.5% to 5%, is provided as a convenient concentration dial for isoflurane/halothane. The main dial, which is attached to the vaporizer, is graduated alphabetically from A to F, and a label permanently affixed to the vaporizer gives the output for diethyl ether, enflurane, halothane, and isoflurane at each setting. As air enters the vaporizer, the vertical rotary valve divides the stream; some en-

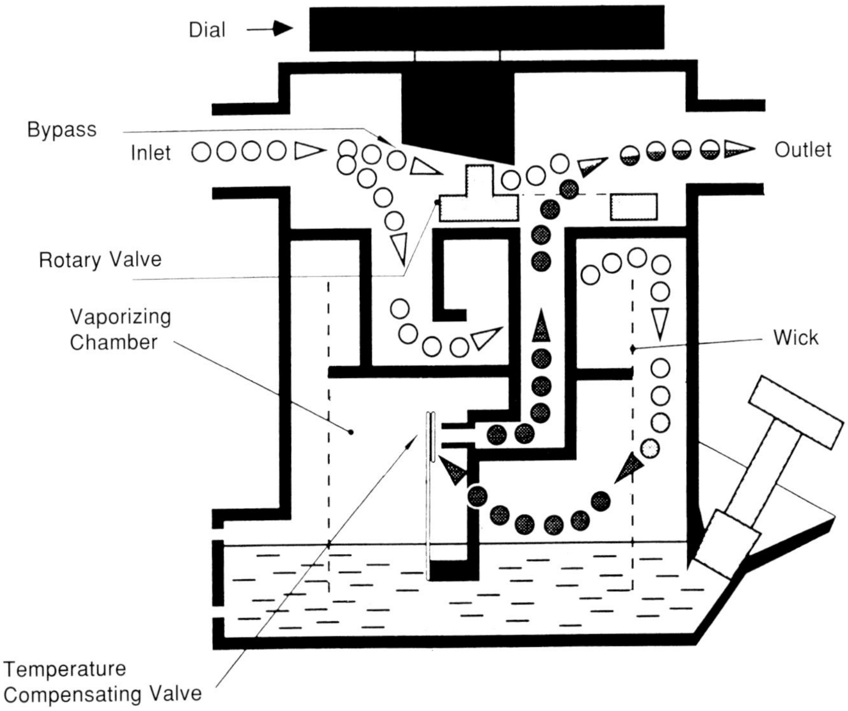

Fig. 7-54. Cross section of the Portable Anesthesia Circuit (PAC) Universal vaporizer. A rotary valve is connected to the concentration dial. Changing the concentration dial setting changes both the amount of air bypassing the vaporizing chamber and the amount entering the vaporizing chamber. The vaporizer chamber holds 85 mL of anesthetic liquid; 13 mL is retained in the wick. A bimetallic strip (see Fig. 7-58) serves as a temperature-compensation valve. Photograph: Printed with permission of Ohmeda, Inc, Steeton, West Yorkshire, England.

a

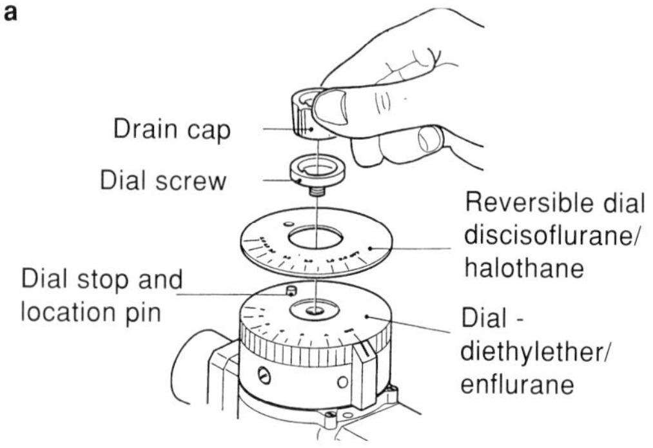

b

Drug Type / Dial Setting	Nominal Calibrations			
	% v/v Diethylether	% v/v Enflurane	% v/v Halothane	% v/v Isoflurane
A	1.55	0.50	0.50	0.60
B	2.70	0.90	1.00	1.20
C	4.80	1.70	2.00	2.15
D	6.65	2.40	3.00	3.10
E	8.20	3.10	4.00	4.00
F	10.10	3.85	5.00	5.00

Fig. 7-55. The diagram (**a**) shows the agent-concentration dials of the Portable Anesthesia Circuit (PAC). The reversible dial disk has halothane on one side and isoflurane on the other. Gradations of concentration from 0.5% to 5% are present for both agents. The main agent-concentration dial is divided alphabetically from A to F. The tabular information (**b**) is affixed to the vaporizer for interpreting the concentration output for each agent. The concentration output of the main dial is graduated from A to F for diethyl ether, enflurane, halothane, and isoflurane. Filling the vaporizer with isoflurane and setting the main concententration dial at C will deliver 2.15% isoflurane at a flow rate of 4 to 6 L/min and a temperature of 20°C to 22°C. Photographs: Printed with permission of Ohmeda, Inc, Madison, Wis.

ters the vaporizer chamber and some bypasses the vaporizer. In the Tri-Service draw-over vaporizer, a sliding valve opens and closes the vapor chamber (Figure 7-56).[10]

As the PAC bypass gap is reduced, greater proportions of air enter the vaporizing chamber. A wick in the vaporizing chamber increases the surface area for evaporation. Heat is required for evaporation of the liquid anesthetic. A temperature compensation valve controls the orifice where the mixture of air and anesthetic exits the vaporizing chamber to mix with the air bypassing the vaporizing chamber.

Output from the vaporizer is dependent on flow rate (tidal volume and respiratory rate), inspiratory/expiratory rate, and temperature.[11] High flow rates do not allow enough time for temperature compensation, so the liquid cools rapidly and out-

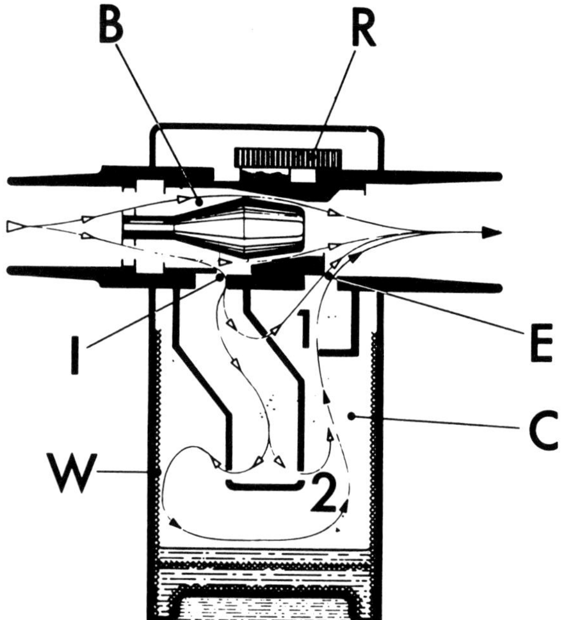

Fig. 7-56. Cross section of the Tri-Service draw-over vaporizer, which is used by the British armed forces. Air enters the vaporizer and a portion of the stream goes into the vaporizing chamber (**C**) through the inlet of the vapor chamber opening controlled by a sliding valve (**R**). The remainder of the air stream enters the bypass passage (**B**). Wicks (**W**) of stainless steel mesh increase the evaporation surface area inside the vaporizing chamber. A heat reservoir (**H**) filled with antifreeze liquid compensates for temperature changes. Air and anesthetic vapor pass out the vaporizing chamber outlet (**E**) to mix with the air coming through the bypass passage. Two different paths (**1** and **2**) through the vaporizing chamber provide a method of temperature and flow compensation. Photograph: Printed with permission of Penlon, Ltd, Abingdon, England.

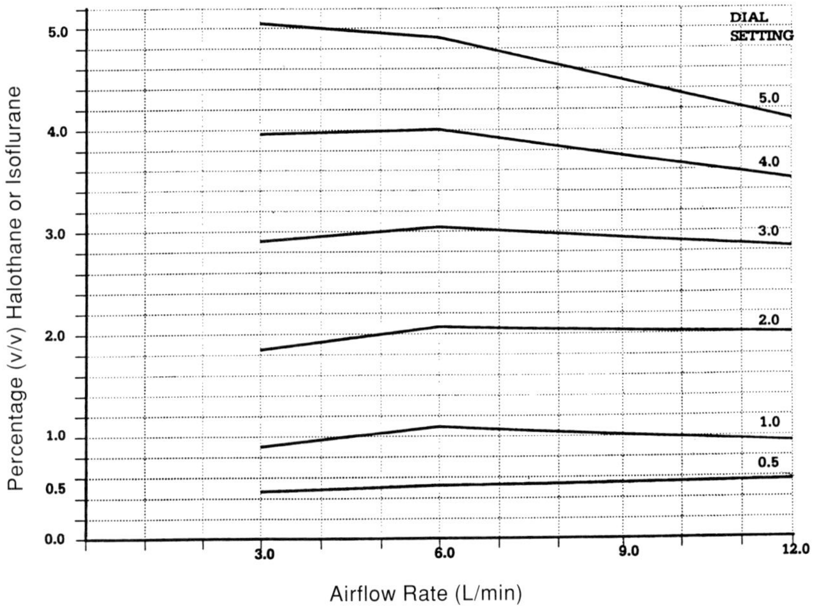

Fig. 7-57. The effect of flow rate on output concentration for halothane and isoflurane from the Portable Anesthesia Circuit (PAC). Lower concentrations are seen at higher levels of flow. The most accurate outputs are between 3 and 6 L/min. Photograph: Printed with permission of Ohmeda, Inc, Steeton, West Yorkshire, England.

put falls (Figure 7-57). Temperature compensation in the PAC is accomplished by a bimetallic strip that controls the vaporizing chamber outlet orifice (Figure 7-58). Flow rates between 4 and 6 L/min for halothane, isoflurane, and enflurane deliver concentrations close to the dial settings. If the flow rate is kept constant and the temperature of the liquid anesthetic is raised or lowered during ambient temperature changes, the output of the agent will become temperature dependent (Figure 7-59). At about 22°C, the output concentration is approximately equal to the dial setting. Vapor pressure is determined by temperature; thus, the amount of evaporated anesthetic is reduced at low temperatures and increased at high temperatures. The manufacturer warns that "potentially hazardous excessive concentrations of anesthetic agent may occur at temperatures above 35°C (95°F)."[9(p11)] Tipping the vaporizer can result in unpredictable output concentrations.

An estimated hourly drug usage can be calculated by using the following formula[12]:

3 • % • flow (L/min) = agent usage (mL/h)

For example, if the vaporizer is set to deliver 1% halothane at 5 L/min, then

3 • 1% • 5 L/min = 15 mL/h

of halothane will be used.

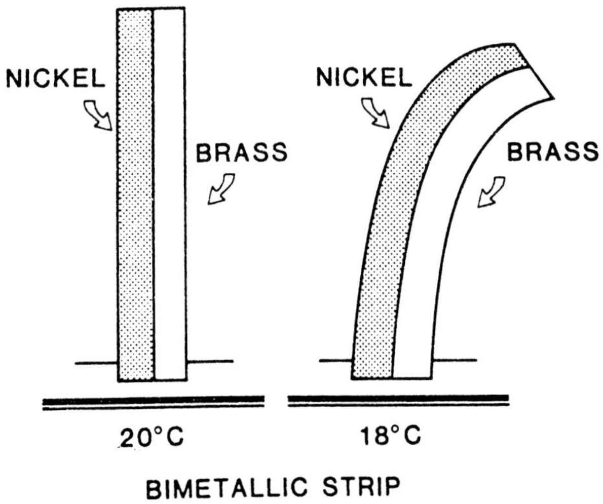

Fig. 7-58. In this bimetallic strip, brass has been welded to nickel. The strip's bending depends on the temperature and the difference in the linear expansion coefficient of brass and nickel. Temperature compensation for the Portable Anesthesia Circuit (PAC, manufactured by Ohmeda, Inc, Steeton, West Yorkshire, England) is controlled by a similar bimetallic strip at the vaporizing chamber exit (see Fig. 7-54).

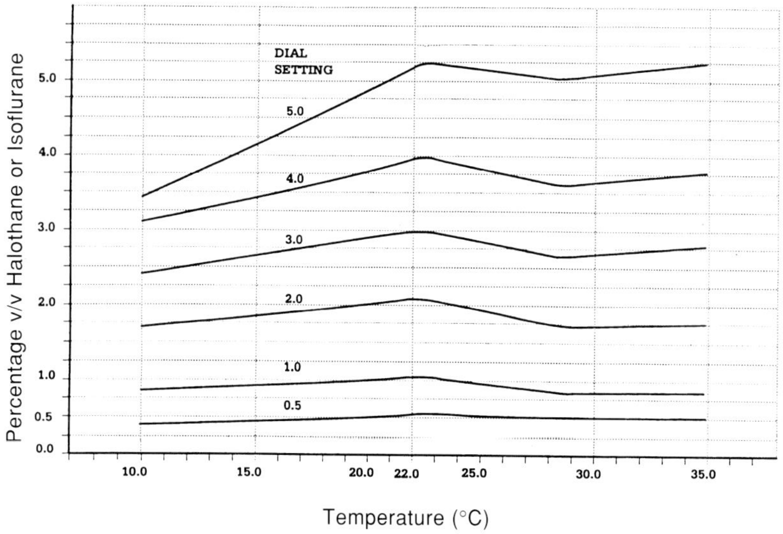

Fig. 7-59. Effect of temperature on the output concentration of halothane and isoflurane from the Portable Anesthesia Circuit (PAC). The most stable output is found between 21°C and 27°C. Photograph: Printed with permission of Ohmeda, Inc, Steeton, West Yorkshire, England.

A nipple is provided at the vaporizer inlet for connecting supplementary oxygen. Oxygen improves the safety margin for the patient and should be added whenever available. Availability of oxygen concentrators in combat areas will greatly enhance the safety of draw-over vaporizers. A ventilator and scavenger apparatus can be used with the PAC.[9] A training film is also available on how to use the PAC.[13]

Checkout and Maintenance

A visual inspection must be made of the vaporizer, hoses, self-inflating bag, nonrebreathing valve, and any other attachments. Make sure the concentration dial on the vaporizer is the one for the liquid anesthetic agent in the vaporizer. Internal leaks can be tested by squeezing the self-inflating bag with the vaporizer in the ON position, capping the air inlet and oxygen nipple, and releasing the self-inflating bag. The bag should not reinflate. External leaks can be detected by capping the face mask and expiratory valve ports and by squeezing the self-inflating bag. The bag should not deflate.

Clean the exterior with a damp cloth. Be sure to completely drain the vaporizer of anesthetic agent and dry the wicks before filling with a different agent. Dry the wicks by passing air through the vaporizer (minimum rate of 750 mL at 24 cycles per minute), until no vapor can be smelled at the vaporizer outlet. This drying process may take 15 to 20 minutes for isoflurane or halothane. Make sure that the vaporizer wicks are dried thoroughly when storing the vaporizer.

The manufacturer recommends yearly service if the vaporizer is used daily, servicing every 2 to 3 years with intermittent use, and every 5 years with occasional use if the vaporizer is stored dry.

IDEAS FOR FUTURE MILITARY ANESTHESIA MACHINES

Comparison of the FAM Model 885A and the PAC with conventional anesthesia machines in stateside civilian and military hospitals finds them sorely deficient in safety features. Patient monitoring in combat areas can easily be brought up to standard with excellent portable monitors now available as off-the-shelf items (Figure 7-60). Elevating the FAM and PAC to the level expected of anesthesia machines in the United States is not possible in combat. The central problem, in the opinion of this writer, is: How do we train anesthesia providers to use the two available anesthesia machines when these machines do not meet current standards? For training purposes, many military hospitals are putting the FAM Model 885A in the operating room with a standard anesthesia machine and transferring the machine's monitors to the FAM. Some military hospitals are even transferring the standard machine monitors to a PAC, denying that the PAC is an anesthesia machine (calling it an "apparatus"), using the PAC without the consent of the patient, and ignoring the warning in the instruction manual.[14]

Training for the FAM and the PAC is difficult to provide in military hospitals, since they are expected to meet the same patient-care standards as civilian hospitals. Anesthesia providers in civilian hospitals would be aghast to see a FAM 885A or a PAC in one of their operating rooms. Neither machine

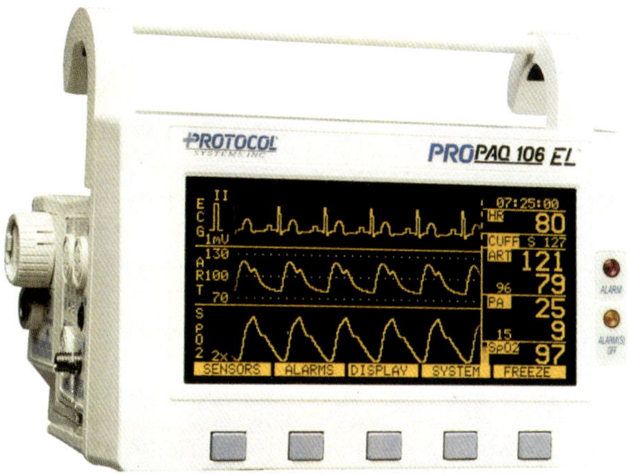

Fig. 7-60. PROPAC portable patient monitor. A unit this size can be fitted to monitor temperature, the electrical activity of the heart, pulse oximetry, blood pressure (direct and indirect methods), end-tidal carbon dioxide, venous pressure, and pressure from a pulmonary catheter. Photograph: Printed with permission of Protocol Systems, Inc., Beaverton, Ore.

meets the ASTM standards for anesthesia machines and the medicolegal implications of using either machine "as is" would be unthinkable. The FAM 885A, with state-of-the-art machine monitoring transferred from an anesthesia machine that meets all ASTM standards, can be used safely in the operating room if rigid protocols are established and if approval is given by the patient. Such programs are being or have been established at Naval Hospital, San Diego, California; Brooke Army Medical Center, San Antonio, Texas; and Walter Reed Army Medical Center, Washington, D. C. Exposure to FAM 885A training for anesthesia personnel in the reserves is still rather limited, but formalizing the present programs and instituting some manner of required certification may widen the scope of available training sites.

Adaptation of the PAC to present ASTM standards is not possible because the standards do not address such outdated technology. There are those within the military who have used the PAC in training programs in military hospitals in the United States in recent years by stating that the PAC is not an anesthesia machine and then using such logic to remove the medicolegal implications from the use of the machine. However, in the view of this author, *the PAC is a draw-over vaporizer anesthesia machine*, and, as such, must meet the same standards of patient care as those used in *any* hospital in the United States. A carefully prepared teaching program could allow the PAC to be used in military hospitals. The first step would be for participants to become familiar with the PAC by reading the instruction manual, watching the videotape, listening to a didactic program, and then administering an anesthetic to animals. The second step would be to obtain permission from the risk-management department of the hospital to use the PAC in the operating room. Transferring the monitors from an ASTM-qualified anesthesia machine to the PAC and using state-of-the-art patient monitors would be essential. The third and final step would be to obtain permission from the patient. A carefully designed plan would allow the PAC to be used safely in the operating room and would allow us to train military personnel in a formalized program with some kind of certification or record of training. Some military centers are designing programs to allow restricted use of the PAC in the operating room. To push forward and use the PAC without a formalized protocol (including patient permission) is to flout the manufacturer's warning, which explicitly states that such use will significantly increase the risk to the patient. Plans are under way at the U.S. Army Medical Materiel Development Activity, Fort Detrick, Frederick, Maryland, to (*a*) upgrade a few of the FAM Model 885As with machine monitors and single-agent vaporizers to more closely approximate ASTM standards,[7] and (*b*) design a new FAM that will be more versatile, weigh less, and meet all the ASTM standards. A Joint Services Working Group has reviewed the characteristics of both the upgrade and a new machine. Anesthesia machine manufacturers have submitted designs for the upgrade. Money has been allocated for a military–industry cooperative effort to develop a new FAM.

The PAC might be improved by adopting some of the features of the ULCO Field Anaesthesia Apparatus (manufactured by ULCO Engineering Pty. Ltd., Marrickville, NSW, Australia) that has been developed for the Australian Armed Forces (Figure 7-61).[15] Its total weight is 55 lb. Versatility is the keynote feature of the apparatus. Different breathing circuits and multiple gas sources (eg, compressed-gas cylinders, pipeline gases, oxygen concentrators) can be used. Two Oxford Miniature Vaporizers (OMV, manufactured by Penlon, Ltd., Abingdon, England) connected to Tri-Service draw-over vaporizers are the heart of the apparatus (Figure 7-62) The machine can be used as a circle system or as a nonrebreathing system. In the circle-system mode, a carbon dioxide absorber, and either compressed-cylinder or pipeline oxygen and / or nitrous oxide are required. When the self-inflating bag is used, the oxygen in atmospheric air is sufficient or supplemented oxygen can be added.

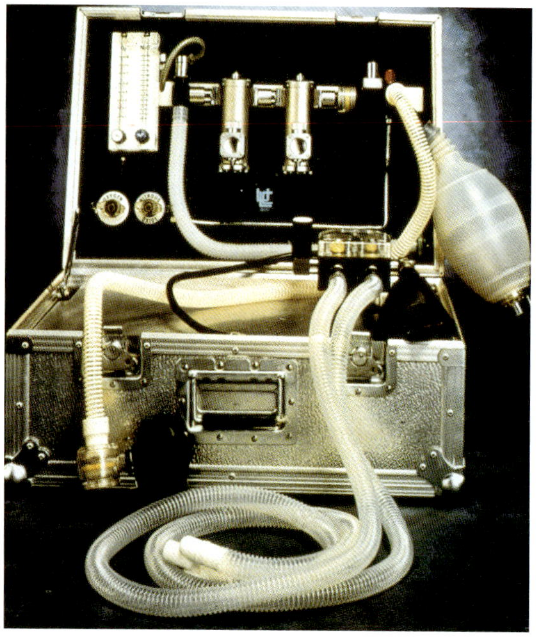

Fig. 7-61. The ULCO Anaesthesia Apparatus is used by the Australian Armed Forces. Two agent-specific Oxford Miniature Vaporizer (OMV) Tri-Service draw-over vaporizers (manufactured by Penlon, Ltd, Abingdon, England) are connected in series. Flowmeters are used for compressed or piped oxygen and nitrous oxide when available. A self-inflating bag converts the apparatus to a nonrebreathing circuit and can be used with atmospheric air and supplemental oxygen. A small carrying case houses the 55-lb unit. A mechanical ventilator and a carbon dioxide absorber can be used with the apparatus. Photograph: Printed with permission of ULCO Engineering Pty, Ltd, Marrickville, NSW 2204, Australia.

a

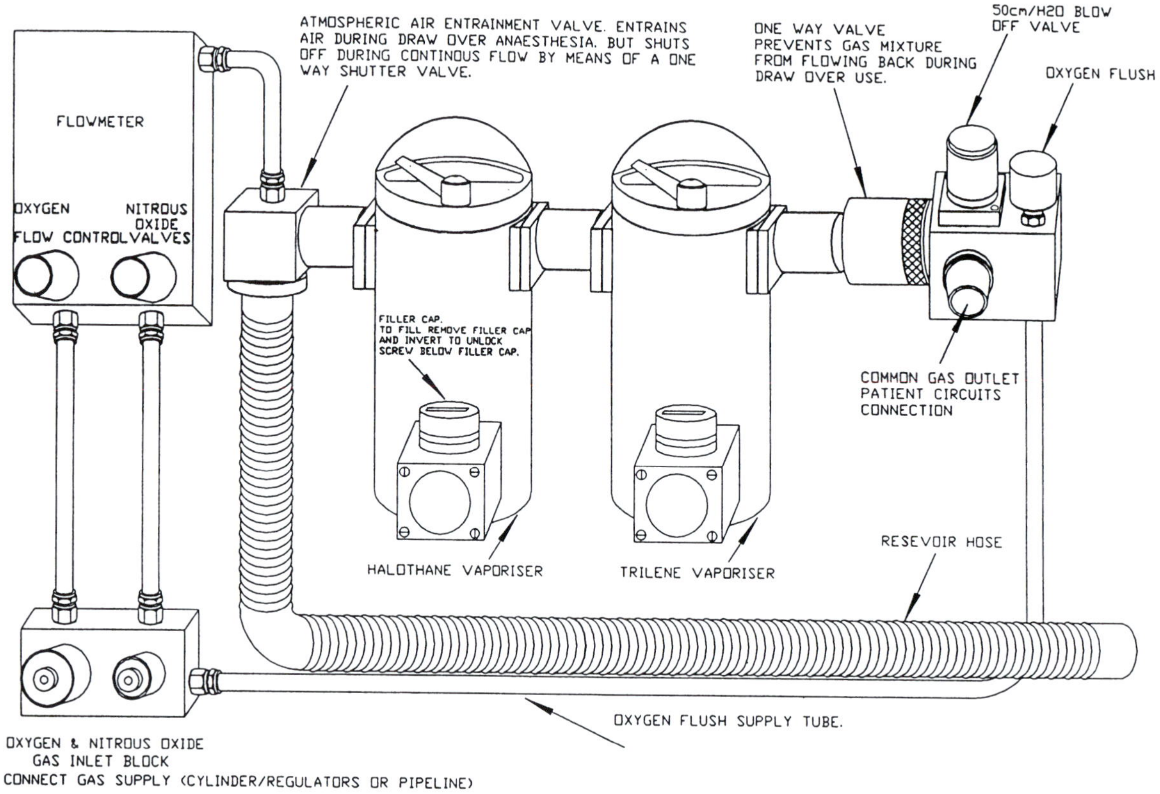

Fig. 7-62 In the basic configuration of the ULCO Field Anaesthesia Apparatus (**a**), flowmeters for oxygen and nitrous oxide are used with compressed or pipeline gases when available. Two single-agent (halothane and trilene) Oxford Miniature Vaporizer (OMV) Tri-Service draw-over vaporizers (manufactured by Penlon, Ltd, Abingdon, England) are connected in series (see Figure 7-61). Atmospheric air enters the circuit when the unit is used with the self-inflating bag. A one-way valve prevents reverse flow in the circuit. An oxygen flush valve is activated when oxygen under pressure is attached. The common gas outlet is where the various circuit configurations are connected. When configured as a closed-circuit system (**b**), the circuit's fresh-gas connector is attached to the common gas outlet of the anesthesia apparatus. A carbon dioxide absorber with one-way valves, exhaust valve, patient breathing hoses, and connections for a ventilator or rebreathing bag are present. When configured as a non- **(continued on p 173)**

b

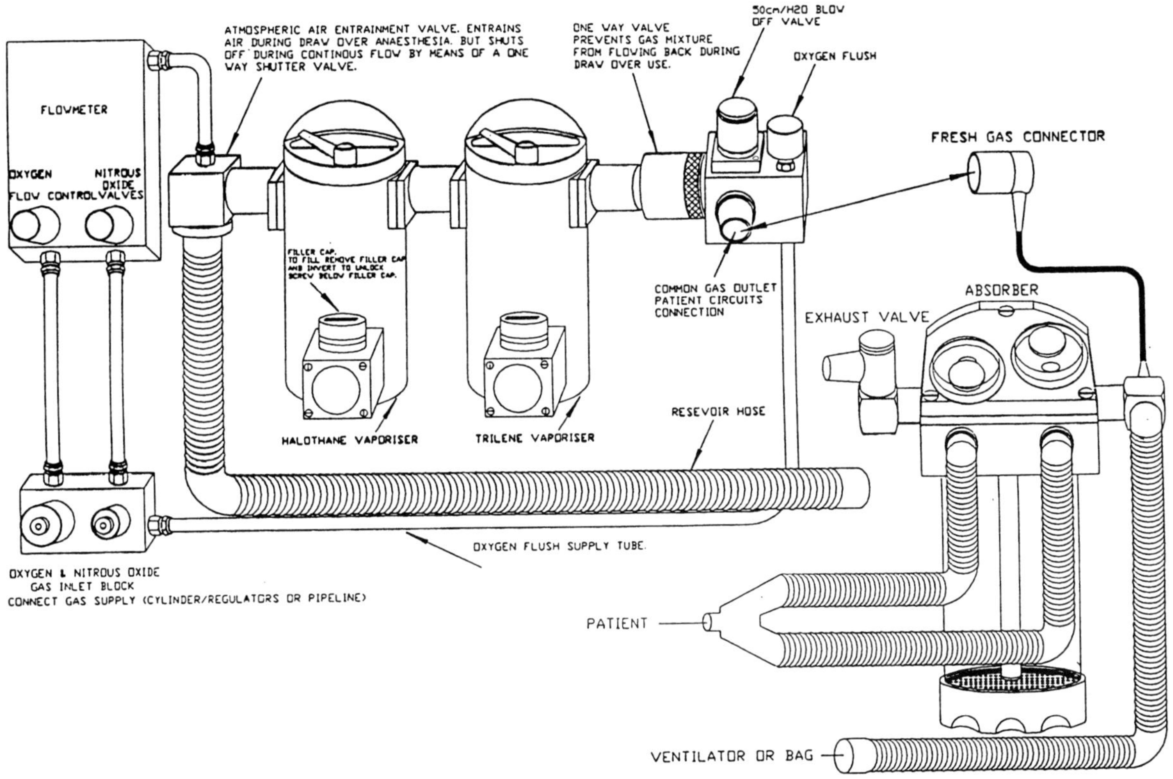

c

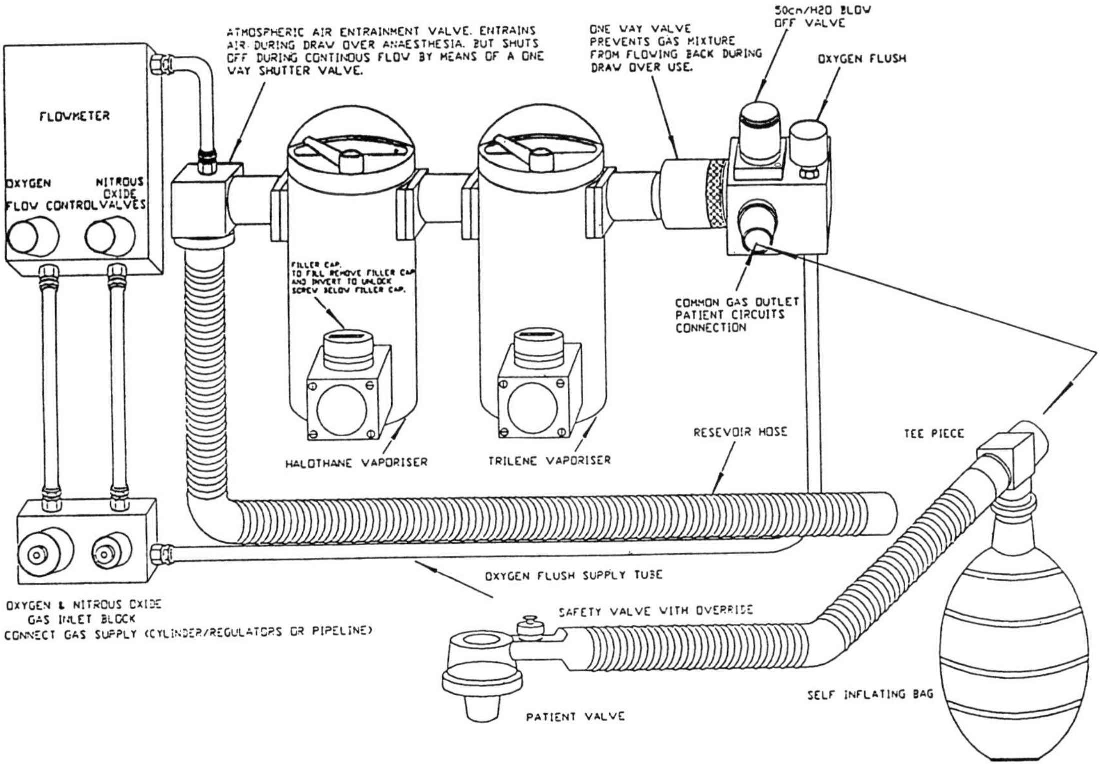

rebreathing circuit (**c**), a tee piece is attached to the common gas outlet of the anesthesia apparatus. A self-inflating bag is connected to one arm of the tee, and the patient breathing hose is attached to the other arm of the tee. A nonrebreathing valve at the connection of the face mask allows fresh gas to enter the patient's lungs and exhaled gases to exit into the room. Photographs: Printed with permission of ULCO Engineering Pty, Ltd, Marrickville, NSW 2204, Australia.

SUMMARY

Military anesthesia machines have been essential for the care of the wounded since the discovery of anesthesia in 1846. Each war and humanitarian effort has required military anesthesia providers to adapt to the equipment provided. At present, the military has in inventory the FAM Model 885A and the PAC anesthesia machines. Both machines are adequate for their designed task. The PAC has a limited application for rapid deployment and a short battle. Anesthesia providers and standards have outpaced the FAM Model 885A. Expectations of anesthesia providers and standards can only be met by a stop-gap measure of a FAM upgrade and an eventual replacement with a new FAM.

REFERENCES

1. Ohmeda. *Instruction and Service Manual With Illustrated Parts List. Model 885A. Anesthesia Apparatus, Gas, Nitrous Oxide, Oxygen and Volatile Liquid Anesthetics, Portable 4-Cylinder Capacity.* Stock Number 0178-1683-000. Madison, Wis: Ohmeda; Sept 1990. National Stock Number 6515-01-185-8446, Defense Personnel Support Center.

2. Compressed Gas Association. *Characteristics and Safe Handling of Medical Gases.* Manual P-2. 7th ed. Arlington, Va: Compressed Gas Association, Inc; 1989.

3. Parbrook GD, Davis PD, Parbrook EO. *Basic Physics and Measurements in Anaesthesia.* 2nd ed. Norwalk, Conn: Appleton-Century-Crofts; 1986.

4. Food and Drug Administration. Medical Device Report 372985. Product: 10-134 Anesthesia Units. Common Device Name: Military Anesthesia Machine. Washington, DC: FDA; 25 March 1993.

5. DesMarteau JK. Flow through the copper kettle flowmeter. *Anesthesiology.* 1984;61:789.

6. Department of Anesthesiology, Uniformed Services University of the Health Sciences. *Set Up and Use of the Military Field Anesthesia Machine.* March 1991. Videotape; Beta, VHS, Umatic formats. Production Identification Number 503005. Bethesda, Md: Dept of Anesthesiology, USUHS; Military Medicine Education Institute. Requests, US Army, Navy, Marine Corps: Chief, Joint Visual Information Activity, ATTN; ASQNV-OJVT-ID, Tobyhanna Army Depot, Pennsylvania 18466-5100; Air Force: Commander, 1352 AVS/DOL, Bldg. 248, Norton Air Force Base, California 92409-5996.

7. American Society for Testing and Materials. *Standard Specification for Minimum Performance and Safety Requirements for Components and Systems of Anesthesia Gas Machines.* Philadelphia, Pa: ASTM; March 1989. F 1161-88.

8. William TG Morton (1819–1868), demonstrator of ether anesthesia. *JAMA.* 1965;194:190. Editorial.

9. Ohmeda. *Operation and Maintenance Manual: Ohmeda Universal PAC.* West Yorkshire, England: Ohmeda. Dec 1990. Part No. 1101-0001-000.

10. Penlon, Ltd. *User's Instruction Manual: OMV Fifty Vaporizer.* Abingdon, England: Penlon, Ltd; Oct 1989. Catalog No 51216.

11. Kingsley CP, Petty C, Olson K. Anesthesia equipment for austere conditions. In: Grande CM, ed. *Textbook of Trauma Anesthesia and Critical Care.* St. Louis, Mo: Mosby–Year Book; 1993: Chap 97.

12. Ohmeda. *PAC Range.* West Yorkshire, England: Ohmeda; 1985.

13. *Draw-over Anesthesia.* Videotape. Production No. A1908-94-002. Washington, DC: Department of Motion Picture Production, Division of Medical Audio-Visual Services, Walter Reed Army Institute of Research; 1994.

14. Casinelli PE, Reynolds PC. Adapting the Ohmeda UPAC draw-over vaporizer for use in the modern operating room. *Milit Med.* 1994;159:600–602.

15. ULCO Engineering Pty, Ltd. *Manual for ULCO Portable Anaesthesia Apparatus.* Marrickville, NSW, 2204, Australia: ULCO Engineering Pty Ltd; ca 1993.

Chapter 8

CLOSED-CIRCUIT ANESTHESIA

RICHARD K. BAUMGARTEN, M.D.*

*Lieutenant Colonel, Medical Corps, U.S. Army (ret); formerly, Associate Clinical Professor of Anesthesiology, Uniformed Services University of the Health Sciences, Bethesda, Maryland 20814-4799; currently, Senior Staff Physician, Department of Anesthesia and Pain Management, Henry Ford Hospital, 2799 West Grand Boulevard, Detroit, Michigan 48202

INTRODUCTION

The military anesthesia provider may be required to provide many hours of care in battlefield medical treatment facilities while working under restrictions that make the usual peacetime practice of anesthesiology infeasible:

- Supplies of compressed gas may be very limited in the field.
- Most ventilators in the inventory are oxygen powered.
- Nitrous oxide, the most commonly used anesthetic during peacetime and in civilian hospitals, has been removed from the U.S. military field inventory.

With oxygen at a premium, the anesthesia provider may need to "squeeze the bag," (ie, to provide manual positive-pressure ventilation) sometimes for many hours, when controlled ventilation is required.

Two anesthetic options may aid the anesthesia provider in these circumstances: (1) regional anesthesia and (2) spontaneous ventilation under general anesthesia. Where appropriate to the injury, regional anesthetic techniques, such as brachial plexus blockade and spinal anesthesia, which use a minimum of supplies, can be used. With certain caveats, draw-over vaporizers can provide anesthesia with no compressed gas at all.[1] Because ether is a respiratory stimulant, its use with spontaneous ventilation in a draw-over system does not require oxygen supplementation. Potent volatile agents, such as halothane and isoflurane, are respiratory depressants; therefore, supplementation with at least 1 L/min of oxygen is required during spontaneous ventilation. If these agents are utilized with only air, ventilation should be controlled. The anesthetist must squeeze the bag constantly, because on room air the patient has little reserve during even short periods of apnea. Providing manual ventilation for many hours with a draw-over system's self-inflating reservoir bag can be very uncomfortable.[2] Intravenous anesthetics, such as ketamine, opioids, benzodiazepines, and muscle relaxants can be utilized; however, their use often mandates controlled ventilation.

Two field anesthesia machines are available for deployment with the U.S. Army Medical Department: the Field Anesthesia Machine (FAM) Model 885A and the Ohmeda Universal Portable Anesthesia Circuit (PAC, both manufactured by Ohmeda, Inc., Madison, Wis.) draw-over system (see Chapter 2, Combat Anesthesia Overview and Chapter 7, Military Anesthesia Machines). The FAM 885A is a circle system; the PAC is a nonrebreathing system. A circle system is a closed circuit of gases from which the patient is breathing. These gases consist of oxygen, water vapor, carbon dioxide, sometimes nitrogen, and anesthetic agents, and are confined within breathing tubes with one-way valves, a reservoir bag, a fresh-gas inlet, a pop-off device (ie, an adjustable positive-pressure relief valve), and a carbon dioxide absorption canister, which permits rebreathing of some or all of the exhaled gases. In a closed circuit, the inflow of gases is set to replace only those gases taken up by the patient, in order to maintain the set percentages and volume within the system. A nonrebreathing system, on the other hand, contains only an inspiratory limb of tubing, a reservoir bag, a fresh-gas inflow, and a single nonrebreathing valve between the patient and the system. A nonrebreathing system must supply all of the tidal volume delivered to the patient as fresh gas inflow with each breath. This inflow must contain the appropriate mixture of gases required for anesthesia, as there will be no equilibration between patient and system. The closed-circle system efficiently conserves patient heat, water vapor, anesthetic agent, and oxygen; the nonrebreathing system is smaller and simpler but conserves nothing, as the patient's entire tidal volume is lost to the room or scavenging device.

In its usual semiclosed configuration, the FAM 885A is profligate in its use of compressed gas. However, when low flows are utilized, it can provide a high fraction of inspired oxygen (F_{IO_2}) with very modest expenditure (0.3–0.5 L/min) of compressed oxygen. The compliant reservoir bag is comfortable and controlled ventilation can be provided for many hours without undue fatigue. Additionally, the high F_{IO_2} provides a reserve so that the patient can tolerate short periods of apnea while the anesthetist performs other tasks (eg, hanging a unit of blood for transfusion).

During deployment, with compressed gas at a premium, controlled ventilation will be provided manually. The closed-circuit technique can be used advantageously in two ways: (1) to provide controlled ventilation with a high F_{IO_2} for intravenous techniques and (2) to deliver potent volatile agents by liquid injection for techniques utilizing spontaneous or controlled ventilation. Anesthesia personnel deployed with the U.S. Marines during the Persian Gulf War used closed circuit anesthesia with liquid injection of halothane. With high ambient temperatures and limited logistical reserves, the method proved both workable and useful.[3]

OXYGEN AND POSITIVE-PRESSURE VENTILATION

The circle system can be used to provide a high FIO_2 and positive-pressure ventilation while conserving oxygen supplies. This is a very effective adjunct to total intravenous anesthesia techniques, especially when a muscle relaxant is used.

To understand low-flow anesthesia with oxygen, we must consider the various contributions to the volume of gas in the anesthesia system. The anesthesia system consists of the tubing, reservoir bag, gas in the carbon dioxide absorber, and the patient's functional residual capacity (FRC) (Figure 8-1). For an adult, the volume of gas in this system is approximately 10 L.[4] Several potential positive and negative contributions to this system occur during the anesthetic-delivery period. The patient consumes oxygen from the anesthesia system. Normal adult oxygen consumption (VO_2) is approximately 200 mL/min.[5] Carbon dioxide produced by the patient is removed by the carbon dioxide absorber. During closed-circuit anesthesia, the anesthesia provider closes the relief valve and adjusts the oxygen flow to maintain a *constant volume* in the anesthesia system. Changes in system volume are assessed at end-expiration. When a rising-bellows ventilator is used, system volume is constant when the bellows returns to the same height with each breath. The same principle applies when a reservoir bag is used; however, the extent to which the bag is filled is assessed relative to the anesthesia provider's hand. If the anesthesia system is leak-free, only enough fresh oxygen to replace the patient's consumption is required.

Inward and Outward Leaks

In practice, some leaks usually occur, especially around the face mask or endotracheal tube. Leaks can be either into or out of the circuit (Figure 8-2). A leak into the system can occur when negative pressure develops in the circuit, the most common source being a hanging bellows ventilator. Negative pressure and a potential inward leak can also arise during spontaneous ventilation. An inward leak introduces room air (nitrogen and oxygen) into the circuit. Outward leaks arise when the circuit pressure is positive. During controlled ventilation (ei-

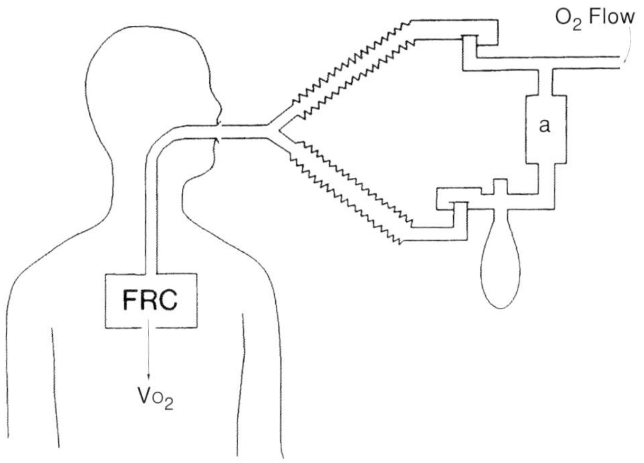

Fig. 8-1. The closed anesthesia system consists of the circuit, reservoir bag, and the patient's functional residual capacity. The total volume of the anesthesia system for an adult is approximately 10 L. If the circuit is free of leaks and the system volume is held constant, oxygen flow will equal oxygen consumption. FRC: functional residual capacity; O_2: oxygen; VO_2: normal adult consumption of oxygen; a: carbon dioxide absorbant.

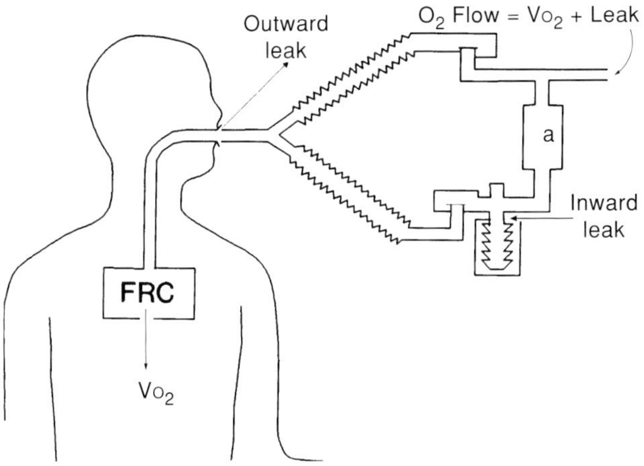

Fig. 8-2. Leaks usually occur in a closed-circuit anesthesia system, including those that incorporate a hanging bellows ventilator. When the system volume is held constant, oxygen flow equals oxygen consumption plus the leak. This is an algebraic sum. An inward leak lowers the oxygen flow required to maintain system volume, while an outward leak increases the required flow. FRC: functional residual capacity; O_2: oxygen; VO_2: normal adult consumption of oxygen; a: carbon dioxide absorbant.

ther manually controlled or using a rising-bellows ventilator), circuit pressure will be positive and any leak will be out of the anesthesia system. A substantial outward leak can also arise when a gas analyzer or mass spectrometer is used (unless the sampled gas is returned to the circuit). In common peacetime practice, gas analysis produces the most substantial leak.

The distinction between inward and outward leaks is important. An inward leak introduces nitrogen into the circuit, which will tend to lower the FIO_2 in the system. When the circuit is closed soon after induction, the initial FIO_2 is usually 0.5 to 0.6. To understand the effect of an inward leak, consider a patient with a VO_2 of 200 mL/min, an initial system FIO_2 of 0.5 and an inward leak of 10 mL/min. With an inward leak of 10 mL/min, a fresh-gas oxygen flow of 190 mL/min will maintain the system volume. During each minute, the inward leak introduces 8 mL of nitrogen and 2 mL of oxygen. Each minute, the patient consumes 200 mL of oxygen while 192 mL of oxygen is added to the system. Therefore, the FIO_2 will decrease with time. After 1 hour, 480 mL (60 min • 8 mL/min) of nitrogen will be introduced into the system. The circuit initially contained 5,000 mL of nitrogen and 5,000 mL of oxygen, so after an hour it will contain 4,520 mL of oxygen and 5,480 mL nitrogen (FIO_2 = 0.452). The FIO_2 has decreased by 0.048.

In contrast, outward leaks increase the FIO_2 in the system because the leak removes oxygen and nitrogen, which are replaced with oxygen only. Let us again consider a patient whose VO_2 is 200 mL/min, and a system with an outward leak of 50 mL/min. To maintain circuit volume, 250 mL of oxygen per minute must be added via the fresh-gas flow. During the first minute, the FIO_2 is 0.5; therefore, the leak removes approximately 25 mL of nitrogen, which is replaced with oxygen. After a minute, the circuit will contain 5,025 mL of oxygen and 4,975 mL of nitrogen. The FIO_2 will have increased slightly. During the second minute, the leak removes approximately 25 mL [(4,975 ÷ 10,000) • 50 mL = 24.95 mL] of nitrogen. As the system FIO_2 increases, less nitrogen is removed in the leak. This change in FIO_2 is actually a continuous process that can be summarized by an exponential expression of the form:

$$1 - e^{-t/T_c}$$

where t represents time and T_c represents the time constant, which equals the volume divided by the flow.[6] In this example,

$$T_c = \frac{10,000 \text{ mL}}{50 \text{ mL/min}} = 200 \text{ min}$$

The initial FIO_2 was 50% and the FIO_2 of the fresh-gas flow entering the circuit is 100%; after one time constant (ie, 200 min), the FIO_2 will be 0.835 (ie, 67% of the difference between 50% and 100%); after two time constants (400 min), it will be 0.935 (87% of the difference between 50% and 100%); and after three time constants, it will be 0.975 (95% of the difference between 50% and 100%). Note that with leaks of 50 to 100 mL/min, the FIO_2 increase is quite slow. Therefore, when FIO_2 is measured during closed-circuit anesthesia, it is quite common to see values of 0.5 to 0.7 despite the fact that the fresh gas is 100% oxygen.

There are two additional sources of nitrogen in the closed anesthesia system. First, nitrogen can enter the closed system from the release of dissolved nitrogen by body tissues. The total nitrogen dissolved in the body is approximately 1 L. Because the volume of the closed system is 10 L, dissolved nitrogen could potentially lower the FIO_2 by one tenth (1 L÷10 L). Second, nitrogen remains in the FRC when the circuit is closed. This nitrogen distributes throughout the entire system. As an example, consider an adult patient who is intubated awake with no preoxygenation. The anesthesia circuit contains pure oxygen and the circuit is closed immediately after intubation. The adult patient's FRC is approximately 2 L. Because the patient was breathing room air prior to awake intubation, the FIO_2 in the FRC is 21%. Therefore, the FRC contains 1,580 mL of nitrogen (2,000 mL • 0.79). This nitrogen will be distributed throughout the anesthesia system, producing an initial FIO_2 of 0.84 [(10,000 – 1580) ÷ 10,000 = 0.84]. In this example, the circuit contained oxygen and the patient's FRC was the source of the nitrogen. If the patient is preoxygenated for several minutes with a tight-fitting face mask, a semiclosed circuit, and high flows of oxygen (4–5 L/min), then the FRC nitrogen can largely be removed, and when the circuit is closed the initial FIO_2 will be high (0.7–1.0). If, however, a loose-fitting face mask is utilized, nitrogen will enter around the mask and be distributed throughout the system. The initial FIO_2 may then be as low as 0.30 to 0.40.

Conserving Oxygen

With this understanding of the sources and losses of oxygen and nitrogen in the closed circuit, oxygen can be conserved to a large extent. The following checks are required before using the closed circuit:

1. The circuit should be tested for leaks. The circuit should hold 40 cm H_2O with an inflow of less than 200 mL/min.
2. The carbon dioxide absorbent should be checked. With a double-canister system, the absorbent should not be changed until the indicator has begun to change color in the lower canister. At this point, the bottom canister should be moved to the top and a fresh canister placed in the bottom. Changing canisters when the indicator has changed in only the upper canister will waste substantial amounts of soda lime.[7]
3. The function of the one-way valves should be confirmed since incompetent valves may allow rebreathing of carbon dioxide.
4. The oxygen analyzer, if available, should be calibrated and the low-F_{IO_2} alarm set.

During low-flow anesthesia, we wish to produce a slight outward leak so that the F_{IO_2} will not fall during the case. A hanging bellows ventilator should not be used. If ventilation is controlled, it should be done either manually or with a rising-bellows ventilator. Any leaks will be outward so long as the flows are adjusted to fill the bag or bellows at the end of expiration. Flows of 250 to 350 mL/min should be adequate. If the anesthesia provider finds that larger flows are required to maintain system volume, a search should be made for leaks. Common sources of leaks include around the face mask, around the endotracheal tube, and loose fittings.

Most discussions of closed-circuit anesthesia have emphasized the delivery of nitrous oxide.[8,9] Several of the steps required for the delivery of this relatively impotent anesthetic are no longer required when it is eliminated. Thorough denitrogenation is required if nitrous oxide is used, as any residual nitrogen limits the amount of nitrous oxide that can be given. When only oxygen is being administered, the circuit can be closed after partial denitrogenation (F_{IO_2} of 0.4–0.5). With only outward leaks, the F_{IO_2} will slowly increase during the case. An oxygen analyzer is mandatory when nitrous oxide is a component of the anesthetic. When only oxygen is used, continuous F_{IO_2} monitoring is no longer essential. In the field, oxygen analyzers may not be available or may be in short supply. If available, the analyzers should probably be utilized intermittently to conserve their function. A top priority for their use is confirmation of the contents of newly opened oxygen cylinders. Additionally, they may be helpful to check the initial F_{IO_2} and at intervals during the case to assure that an inward leak has not developed.

POTENT VOLATILE ANESTHETIC AGENTS

Although intravenous agents will probably be the mainstay in field anesthesia, occasions will arise when supplementation with low doses of a potent volatile agent would be desirable. The closed circuit can be used to deliver potent volatile agents while conserving precious oxygen supplies. Closed-circuit administration of potent volatile agents requires a special pharmacokinetic conceptualization.

The intravenous line and the closed anesthetic circuit are both extensions of the patient's vasculature (Figure 8-3). When a drug is injected into the intravenous line, it flows to the vasculature and is distributed to body tissues. For purposes of this chapter, *dosage* is defined as the amount of drug that reaches the vasculature. Because little of the drug is lost in the line, the dose is equivalent to the amount injected. Strictly speaking, dosage should be expressed in moles; however, it is usually expressed as mass (grams, milligrams, or micrograms), which is the amount in moles multiplied by the molecular weight.

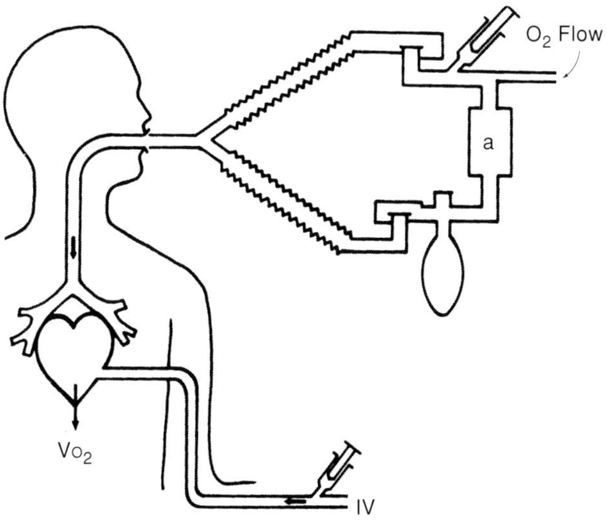

Fig. 8-3. Like the intravenous (IV) line, the closed circuit is an extension of the patient's vasculature. O_2: oxygen; V_{O_2}: normal adult consumption of oxygen; a: carbon dioxide absorbant.

Dosage is defined similarly for volatile anesthetics. Provided that the anesthetic circuit is closed, the fate of volatile agents is straightforward. After it is injected into the circuit, the volatile anesthetic vaporizes, enters the vasculature via the alveolar capillary membrane, and is distributed to body tissues. Except for the amount that primes the circuit, all volatile agent injected into the circuit reaches the patient's vasculature. Therefore, dosage is clearly defined: it is the amount injected into the circuit. Strictly, dosage of a volatile anesthetic should also be expressed in moles; however, because each agent is a pure liquid with a constant molarity, it is more convenient to express dosage as milliliters of liquid, which is equal to the dosage in moles multiplied by the molecular weight and divided by the density. Please note that the various anesthetics vary in potency, molecular weight, and density, so that liquid dosage requirements differ between agents (ie, 1 mL of halothane is not the same as 1 mL of isoflurane, just as 1 mg of fentanyl is not the same as 1 mg of morphine).

If the circuit is not closed, the dosage is still the amount of anesthetic that reaches the patient's vasculature; however, this can no longer be conveniently measured because a large, unpredictable amount escapes via the relief valve. Please note that the concentration of volatile agent in the circuit is *not* the dosage, just as the concentration of an intravenous anesthetic in the intravenous line is not the dosage. In other words, when liquid volatile anesthetics are injected into a closed circuit, the dosage the patient receives is the amount of liquid injected into the closed circuit, just as the dosage of an intravenous agent is the amount injected into the intravenous line.

Pharmacokinetics

With dosage defined, the next question is: How much volatile anesthetic should we give? Inhaled anesthetics display square-root-of-time (SQRT) kinetics.[10,11] When the cumulative dose (in milliliters of liquid) of a potent inhalational anesthetic is plotted against time required to maintain a constant blood concentration, a constant amount of anesthetic (unit dose) is seen to be absorbed in each SQRT interval (0–1 min, 1–4 min, 4–9 min, 9–16 min, etc) (Figure 8-4). These intervals increase in length throughout the case. In the graph, the curve does not pass through the origin because one additional unit dose is required to prime the circuit. When the

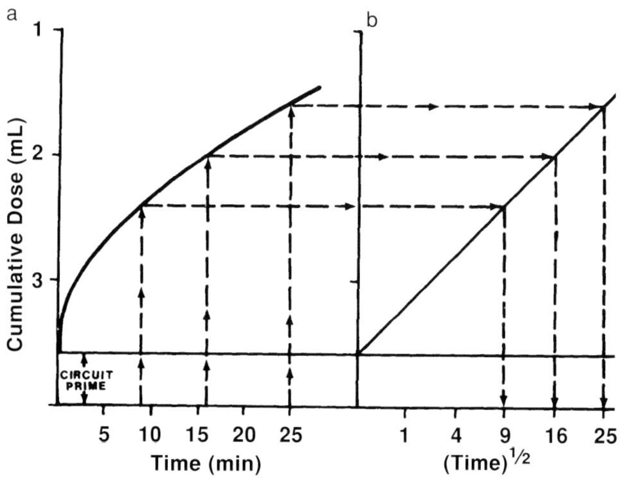

Fig. 8-4. To maintain a constant blood concentration of volatile liquid anesthetic, (**a**) cumulative dose of volatile liquid anesthetic (in milliliters) is plotted against the time required to maintain a constant blood concentration. (**b**) Cumulative dose vs. square root of time (SQRT) yields a straight line.

time axis is transformed to SQRT, the plot becomes linear with a slope equal to the unit dose (UD):

$$\text{UD} = \frac{\text{TD}}{1 + \sqrt{t}} \quad (1)$$

where t represents elapsed time in minutes and *TD* represents the cumulative (total) dose in milliliters of liquid. The 1 added in the denominator accounts for the circuit prime.

It is possible to utilize rigid dosage regimens based on the model in which the patient receives a predetermined unit dose at each SQRT interval (0 min, 1 min, 4 min, 9 min, 16 min, etc.). This would be comparable to giving the same predetermined dose of an intravenous agent, such as sodium nitroprusside, fentanyl, or atracurium, to every patient: dosage requirements vary among individual patients; so, while a single infusion regimen treats the average patient, it underdoses some and overdoses others. Dosage requirements for volatile anesthetics also vary among patients. Therefore, except in some experimental situations, it is prudent to adjust administration based on patient response.

SQRT kinetics can be used to assess dosage requirements during anesthesia and to assist the anesthesia provider in adjusting the dose, based on patient response. Figure 8-5 shows the curves obtained when cumulative dosage is plotted against time for two individuals with different dosage re-

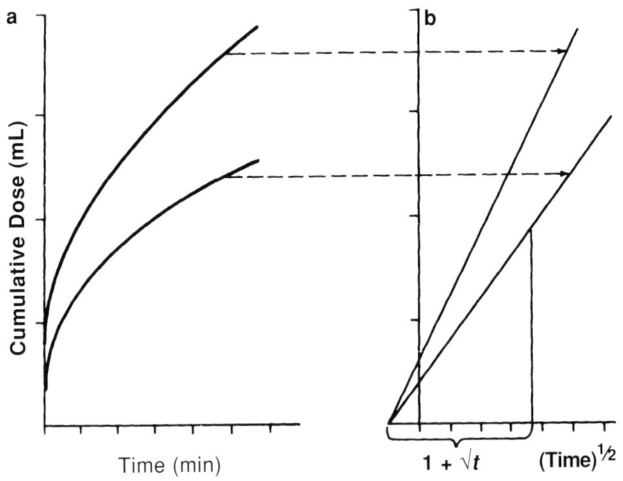

Fig. 8-5. (**a**) Cumulative dose is plotted against time for two individuals with different dosage requirements. (**b**) When cumulative dose is plotted against the square root of time (SQRT), two lines with different slopes are obtained. The slope equals the unit dose.

quirements; when concentration is plotted against SQRT, lines with different slopes are obtained. The slopes of these lines are the respective unit doses for the two patients.

In many areas of pharmacology, it is customary to index dosage based on patient size. Weight and body surface area (BSA) are two common measures. Although BSA is usually derived from a nomogram or formula involving height and weight, some physiologists believe that the weight expressed in kilograms, raised to the three-fourths power ($kg^{3/4}$), is a more precise parameter.[12] In closed-circuit anesthesia, it has become customary to index dosage based on this physiological BSA–weight relation. The dosage index f represents the unit dose from equation 1 indexed for patient size using equations 2 and 3:

$$(2) \qquad f = \frac{UD}{UD_1} = \frac{TD}{UD_1(1 + \sqrt{t})}$$

$$(3) \qquad UD_1 = m \bullet kg^{3/4}$$

The multiplier m in equation 3 accounts for differences in density, molecular weight, and potency among the volatile anesthetics and is different for each agent (Table 8-1). In an individual patient, a given dosage index should provide the same depth of anesthesia no matter which inhalational agent is used.

TABLE 8-1

MULTIPLIERS FOR CALCULATING UD_1

Anesthetic	Multiplier
Halothane	0.029
Isoflurane	0.038
Enflurane	0.062
Diethylether	0.24

The dosage index f can be used to compare dosage requirements between patients. Additionally, since the dosage requirement for an individual patient remains fairly constant, the index guides administration while the patient is receiving the anesthetic. In theory, during a pure inhalational anesthetic procedure, a dosage index of 1 should prevent movement to skin incision in one half of patients, and an index of 1.3 should prevent movement in 95% of patients.[4] In practice, however, various intravenous agents (eg, opioids, benzodiazepines, and muscle relaxants) are utilized, so the required dosage index is much less.

Figure 8-6 shows a frequency distribution of the dosage index f during a fentanyl/isoflurane/pancuronium/oxygen anesthetic administered for elective surgery in healthy adults.[13] Note that the mean dosage index was 0.42, with 46 of 52 (88%) patients requiring a dosage index between 0.32 and 0.52. The required dosage index may be lower in patients whose physical status is poor, or when large amounts of intravenous medications are utilized. The dosage requirement is also usually lower during surgical preparation when little stimulus is provided and the effect of induction agents is still present.

Concentration and Dosage

The foregoing discussion of closed-circuit pharmacokinetics was prefaced by a careful definition of dosage. Most anesthesia providers are more accustomed to thinking in terms of *concentration* of volatile anesthetics with semiclosed anesthesia systems. A concentration-response curve (ie, a minimal alveolar concentration [MAC] assay) has become widely used in conceptualizing inhalational anesthetic pharmacology.[14] Because blood concentrations of volatile agents are difficult to measure, the end-tidal concentration is utilized instead.[15] As

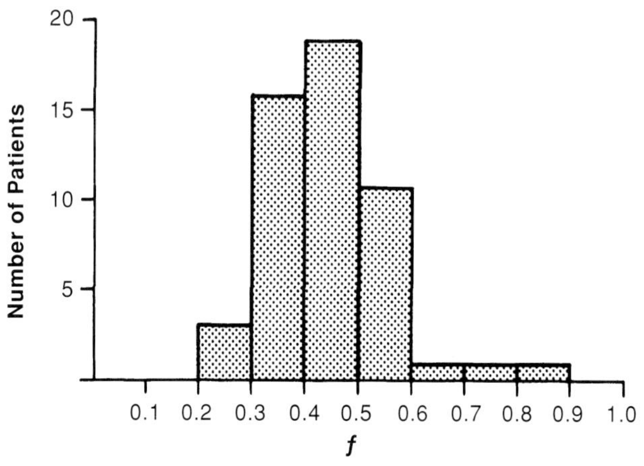

Fig. 8-6. Frequency distribution of dosage index *f*. Data were extracted retrospectively from 52 anesthesia records in which closed-circuit isoflurane/fentanyl/pancuronium/oxygen technique was utilized. All patients were American Society of Anesthesia categories I and II and were scheduled for elective orthopedic or gynecologic surgery. Anesthesia was induced with thiopental (3–5 mg/kg). Tracheal intubation was facilitated with succinylcholine or pancuronium. Maintenance muscle relaxation was provided with pancuronium. The patients received fentanyl (150–250 µg) during the first hour of anesthesia. After intubation, the circuit was closed and isoflurane was administered by liquid injection, guided by clinical signs of anesthesia. The dosage index was recorded every 10 to 15 minutes on the anesthesia records. The mean dosage index during the first hour of surgical stimulation was extracted from each record; these values were used to construct the frequency distribution. Reprinted with permission from Baumgarten RK, Elms MK. Dosage requirements for closed circuit anesthesia. In: Bergmann H, Kramar H, *Beiträge zur Anaesthesiologie und Intensivmedizin*. Vol 7. In: *European Congress of Anaesthesiology*. Vienna, Austria: Verlag Wilhelm Maudrich; 1986: 55. Abstract 107.

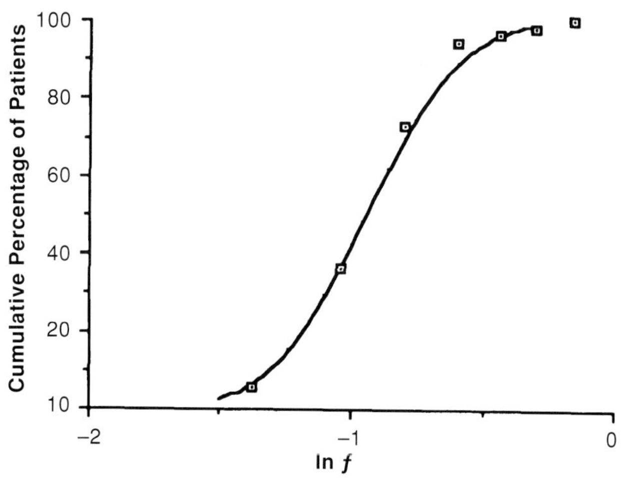

Fig. 8-7. The data from Fig. 8-6 were used to construct this dose-response curve for isoflurane. The frequency histogram is reexpressed as cumulative percentage versus the natural logarithm of *f* (ln *f*).

would be expected, the dose-response curve (Figure 8-7) for volatile anesthetics is very similar to the MAC assay.

The Pharmacological Uncertainty Principle

With the proliferation of mass spectrometers now being used in clinical anesthesia, many anesthesia providers are now accustomed to adjusting the end-tidal concentration to achieve the desired depth of anesthesia. It might be attractive to measure both dosage and end-tidal concentration during closed-circuit anesthesia; however, this is very difficult with current equipment. Because one of the largest leaks in anesthesia equipment is the gas removed by a mass spectrometer, it is no longer possible to assess dosage accurately. Therefore, we can either know the dosage or the concentration but not both. This is analogous to Heisenberg's principle: one can precisely measure the position or the momentum of a subatomic particle, but not both. The advent of stand-alone monitors that can return sampled gas to the circuit should make it possible to measure concentration and dosage simultaneously. This may be very useful for teaching closed-circuit anesthesia.

With adult patients, leaks of 50 to 100 mL/min are tolerable because the amount of agent lost in the leak is small relative to the amount absorbed by the patient. This is important, as small leaks are useful to assure that any leak is outward. (With pediatric patients, leaks are more serious because the amount lost in even a small leak is significant compared with the patient's smaller dosage requirement. When closed-circuit anesthesia is used with small children, a tight-fitting face mask is necessary to prevent leaks, and a tuberculin syringe is used to deliver small, incremental doses of anesthetic agent to the circuit.[16]

Equipment for Administering Volatile Agents

We have emphasized the importance of knowing

the dosage of volatile agent administered to the patient. Although vaporizers can be used for closed-circuit anesthesia, they can also introduce some complexity. When a vaporizer is used, molar dosage rate will depend on the vaporizer setting. To obtain the cumulative dose, the anesthesia provider must add all the various settings that have been used and multiply by the time that each was used—a cumbersome task. Liquid injection eliminates these difficulties.[11] The cumulative dose is readily apparent by subtracting from the amount remaining in the syringe. Additionally, the molar dose is the same at any ambient temperature and pressure, as this only depends on the molecular weight and the density of the liquid, which are constant. Molar dosage does not depend on vapor pressure. This is important because vapor pressure varies dramatically over the range of ambient pressures and temperatures in which field anesthesia may be practiced. The molar output of many vaporizers, especially the copper kettle, increases substantially with increasing temperature.[17]

In the case of in-circuit vaporizers, dosage rate will also depend on the oxygen flow rate (see Figure 8-3). It may be difficult to assure the accuracy of flowmeters in field medical treatment facilities. With liquid injection, the dose does not depend on the oxygen flow rate, just as the dose of an intravenous agent will not depend on the intravenous flow rate.

It is vitally important to prevent accidental intravenous injection of liquid volatile anesthetic agents. Prominent labeling is crucial. At one time, injection ports were commercially available and the syringe could be left in the port throughout the case[18]; however, the port was interchangeable with intravenous fitting so the potential for intravenous injection still existed. An injection port can also be fabricated from a metal T-piece.[9] An expedient injector is pictured in Figure 8-8. A disposable syringe is used with a long needle, either an 18-gauge spinal needle or the introducer from a 16-gauge intravenous cannula. The long needle facilitates drawing up the liquid anesthetic from the bottle. The injector is inserted into the tubing, in either the inspiratory or the expiratory limb, and left in place. Therefore, it is very unlikely that it will be interchanged with other syringes. The needle never leaves the syringe and its length draws attention—the contents of this syringe are unusual and not for intravenous injection. With disposable syringes, the plunger swells slightly on contact with volatile agent so that it will not release agent into the circuit without the plunger's being purposefully pushed.

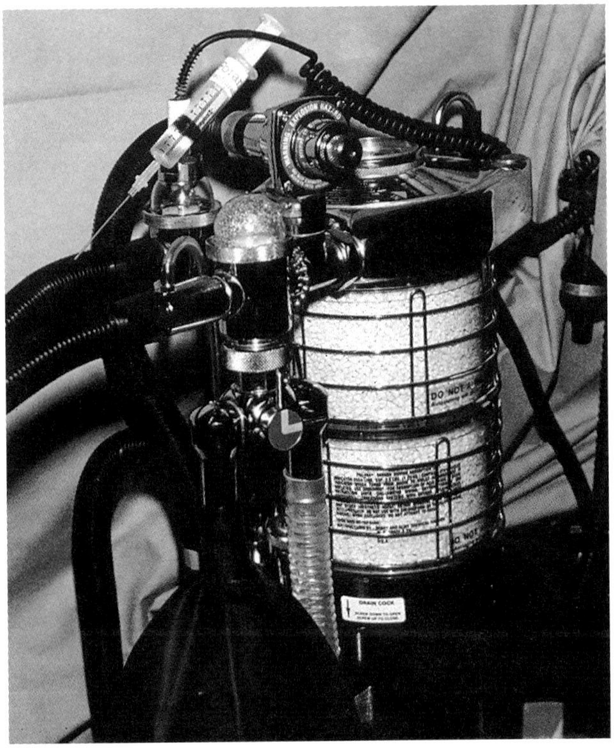

Fig. 8-8. Note the prominent label on this expedient liquid injector. The large needle facilitates filling the syringe and advertises that this is not a syringe intended for intravenous injection. The syringe remains in the circuit and is not placed with other syringes. If the syringe requires refilling, a new location in the tubing can be used for reinsertion.

Square-Root-of-Time Kinetics for Intravenous Agents

Because the dosage concept (see Figure 8-3) applies to both closed-circuit and intravenous administration, it is quite possible that the pharmacokinetics of volatile and intravenous anesthetics are quite similar. Intravenous agents are usually described with linear multicompartmental models; infusion schemes that produce constant blood levels in these models have been described.[19,20] These schemes consist of an initial bolus followed by an exponentially decreasing infusion. Using these equations, the cumulative dose was plotted against time for two typical intravenous agents, lidocaine[21] and fentanyl[22,23] (Figures 8-9 and 8-10). When these curves are transformed to SQRT, an excellent

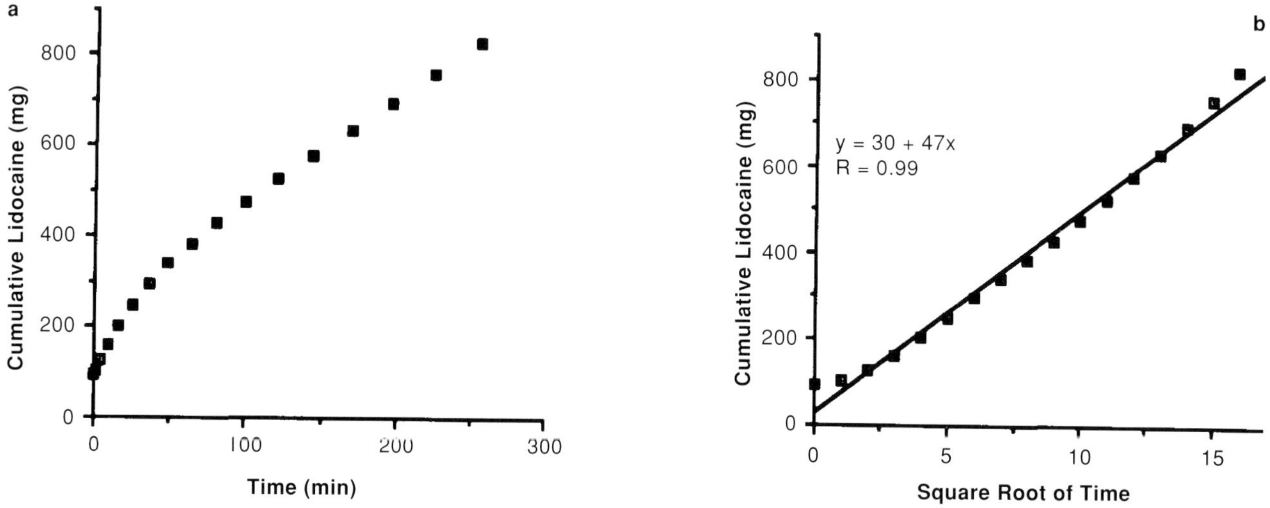

Fig. 8-9. (**a**) Cumulative dose of lidocaine is plotted against time, from a pharmacokinetic simulation with a target concentration of 3 µg/mL. A two-compartment open model was used with an initial bolus followed by an exponentially decreasing infusion. (**b**) Cumulative dose of lidocaine plotted against the square root of time (SQRT). Note that the slope of the line (ie, the unit dose) is 46 mg. Data source: Riddel JG, McCallister GB, Wilkinson GR. A new method for constant plasma drug concentrations: Application to lidocaine. *Ann Int Med.* 1984;100:25–28.

linear fit is achieved over the first 3 to 4 hours of administration. Thus, the SQRT model may also apply to intravenous agents. As anesthesia providers become more comfortable with intravenous anesthesia based on adjusting dosage to patient response, the generalization to dosage-based administration of volatile anesthetics may become easier.

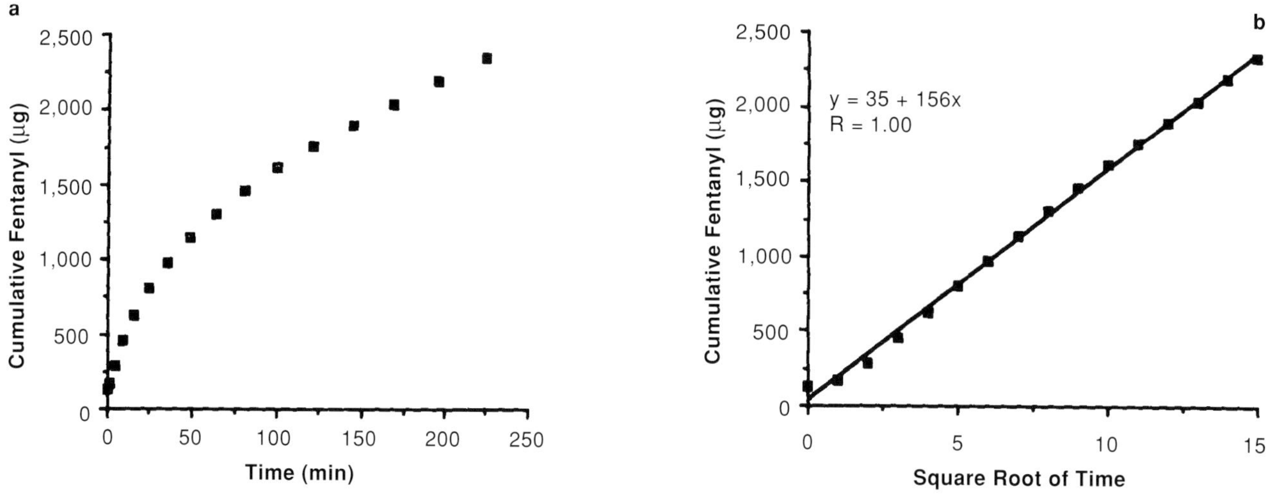

Fig. 8-10. (**a**) Cumulative dose of fentanyl plotted against time, from a pharmacokinetic simulation for a 70-kg subject with a target concentration of 5 ng/mL. A three-compartment open model was used. (**b**) Cumulative dose of fentanyl plotted against the square root of time (SQRT). The unit dose equals 156 µg. Data sources: (1) Alvis JM, Reves JG, Govier AV. Computer assisted continuous infusions of fentanyl during cardiac anesthesia: comparison with a manual method. *Anesthesiology.* 1985;63:41. (2) McClain DA, Hug CC. Intravenous fentanyl kinetics. *Clin Pharmacol Ther.* 1980;28:106–114.

SUMMARY

Compressed oxygen will probably be in short supply in many deployment situations. Nitrous oxide will not be available at all. Simplicity and ease of use are also important in difficult settings. Therefore, the use of the closed circuit to provide a high F_{IO_2} during anesthesia is a valid and practical approach to the management of casualties in field medical treatment facilities. Closed-circuit delivery of anesthetic agents can be used as an adjunct to intravenous techniques with which the anesthesia provider is already familiar. This approach can conserve limited supplies of compressed gas. Additionally, the pharmacokinetic analogy between intravenous and potent volatile anesthetics may be used to balance intravenous techniques with moderate doses of inhalational anesthetics.

REFERENCES

1. King M. *Primary Anaesthesia*. Oxford, England: Oxford University Press; 1986: 82.

2. Jowitt MD, Knight RJ. Anesthesia during the Falklands campaign: The land battles. *Anaesthesia*. 1983;38:776–783.

3. Waters, J. Commander, US Navy. Personal communication, October 1991.

4. Lowe HJ, Ernst EA. Uptake and distribution: Model development. In: *The Quantitative Practice of Anesthesia: Use of the Closed Circuit*. Baltimore, Md: Williams & Wilkins; 1981: Chap 4: 58–60.

5. Nunn JF. *Applied Respiratory Physiology*. London, England: Butterworths; 1987: 366.

6. Lowe HJ, Ernst EA. Basic anesthetic concepts. In: *The Quantitative Practice of Anesthesia: Use of the Closed Circuit*. Baltimore, Md: Williams & Wilkins; 1981: Chap 3: 47–50.

7. Dorsch JA, Dorsch SE. The Breathing System. IV. The Circle System. *Understanding Anesthesia Equipment. Construction, Care and Complications*. Baltimore, Md: Williams & Wilkins; 1984: 210–246.

8. Lowe HJ, Ernst EA. *The Quantitative Practice of Anesthesia: Use of the Closed Circuit*. Baltimore, Md: Williams & Wilkins; 1981: Chap 9: 153–173.

9. Kofke W, Andrew L, William B. Closed circuit anesthesia. In: Firestone LL, ed. *Clinical Anesthesia Procedures of the Massachusetts General Hospital*. New York, NY: Little, Brown; 1988: Chap 14: 226–243.

10. Severinghouse JW. The rate of uptake of nitrous oxide in man. *J Clin Invest*. 1954;33:1183.

11. Lowe HJ, Ernst EA. Uptake and distribution: Square root of time model. In: *The Quantitative Practice of Anesthesia: Use of the Closed Circuit*. Baltimore, Md: Williams & Wilkins; 1981: Chap 5: 67–97.

12. Brody S. *Bioenergetics and Growth*. New York, NY: Reinhold; 1945.

13. Baumgarten RK, Elms MK. Dosage requirements for closed circuit anesthesia. In: Bergmann H, Kramar H, *Beiträge zur Anaesthesiologie und Intensivmedizin*. Vol 7. In: *European Congress of Anaesthesiology*. Vienna, Austria: Verlag Wilhelm Maudrich; 1986: 55. Abstract 107.

14. Eger EI, II, Saidman LJ, Brandstater B. Minimum alveolar anesthetic concentration: A standard of anesthetic potency. *Anesthesiology* 1965;26:756–763.

15. Eger EI, II, Bahlman SH. Is end-tidal anesthetic partial pressure an accurate measure of the arterial anesthetic partial pressure? *Anesthesiology*. 1971;35:301–303.

16. Couta da Silva JM, Tubino PJ, Vieira ZEG. Closed circuit anesthesia in infants and children. *Anesth Analg*. 1984;63:765–769.

17. Dorsch JA, Dorsch SE. Vaporizers. *Understanding Anesthesia Equipment. Construction, Care and Com;ications.* Baltimore, Md: Williams & Wilkins; 1984: 77–135.

18. Lowe HJ, Ernst EA. Using volatile agents. In: *The Quantitative Practice of Anesthesia: Use of the Closed Circuit.* Baltimore, Md: Williams & Wilkins; 1981: Chap 11: 183.

19. Krueger-Thiemer E. Continuous intravenous infusion and multi-compartment accumulation. *Eur J Clin Pharmacol.* 1968;4:317.

20. Schwilden H. A general method for calculating the dosage scheme in linear pharmacokinetics. *Eur J Clin Pharmacol.* 1981;20:379.

21. Riddel JG, McCallister GB, Wilkinson GR. A new method for constant plasma drug concentrations: Application to lidocaine. *Ann Int Med.* 1984;100:25–28.

22. Alvis JM, Reves JG, Govier AV. Computer assisted continuous infusions of fentanyl during cardiac anesthesia: Comparison with a manual method. *Anesthesiology.* 1985;63:41.

23. McClain DA, Hug CC. Intravenous fentanyl kinetics. *Clin Pharmacol Ther.* 1980;28:106–114.

Chapter 9

INHALATIONAL ANESTHESIA

RICHARD B. HECKER, D.O.*

*Major, Medical Corps, U.S. Army; Anesthesia and Operative Service, Brooke Army Medical Center, Fort Sam Houston, Texas; Clinical Assistant Professor of Anesthesiology, The University of Texas Health Science Center at San Antonio, San Antonio, Texas 78284-7834, and The Uniformed Services University of the Health Sciences, Bethesda, Maryland 20814-4799

INTRODUCTION

A variety of anesthetic agents may be administered by different routes to produce both unconsciousness and the absence of sensation to allow for surgical procedures. Typically, general anesthesia is accomplished by the inhalation of anesthetic gases, and although drug administration by inhalation may appear to be unusual, complicated, and awkward to most physicians, it is a familiar route of drug delivery to all anesthesiologists. The pulmonary bed provides an excellent interface for controlling the delivery or removal of inhaled anesthetic agents, oxygen, or carbon dioxide, and measuring the alveolar partial pressure of gases allows for precise control of the depth of anesthesia.

With the exception of nitrous oxide, the modern inhalational anesthetic agents are volatile liquids that are vaporized for administration. These agents are potent, stable, storable for extended periods of time, nonflammable, and useful in almost any surgical setting. Military anesthesia providers deployed with the U.S. Department of Defense's Deployable Medical Systems (DEPMEDS)–equipped forward hospitals may find that the inhalational anesthetic technique, not regional or other methods that are commonly used in civilian hospitals, is the one most often used.

OBSERVATIONS ON MECHANISMS OF ACTION

Although general inhalational anesthetics have been employed for almost 150 years, an understanding of their interaction with organ systems and structures to produce the anesthetic state has not been well delineated. Modern research has been focusing on structural changes in biological membranes on exposure to anesthetic molecules, but any theory of anesthetic action must take into account the following observations that are related to a state of narcosis[1]:

- An extensive array of unrelated chemical structures produce general anesthesia. They do not share any common structure–activity relationship.
- During narcosis, alterations of function occur in all body systems. Physiological, metabolic, and structural changes occur that must be rationalized and explained by an organized system.
- The lipid solubility of anesthetics seems to be important, as the wide range of effective concentrations of agents is reduced to a small range when lipid solubility is calculated and taken into account.
- The phenomenon of pressure reversal that is observed in general anesthesia must be explained by any mechanistic theory of anesthesia.

To expand on the above observations, a major point in the study of the action of general anesthetics is that all the proposed theories have been based on observations of anesthetic agents in living organisms. Based on these observations, and after careful determinations of an anesthetic's potency, four specific pharmacological characteristics have been described for an agent to be considered to have the qualities of a true general anesthetic: (1) lack of structural specificity, (2) cutoff effect of anesthetic potency, (3) lack of stereoselectivity, and (4) demonstration of pressure reversal.

Lack of Structural Specificity

An amazing number of chemically different molecules cause general anesthesia. The implication of this observation is that there is no single specific receptor that mediates general anesthesia. Early in this century, Hans H. Meyer and Charles E. Overton each independently observed that anesthetic potency correlates well with an agent's solubility in the simple organic solvent, olive oil.[2,3] This correlation of anesthetic potency with lipid solubility has been termed the Meyer-Overton rule and is easily demonstrated (Figure 9-1).[4] The Meyer-Overton rule can be interpreted to mean that the product of an index of anesthetic potency and the agent's solubility in a lipid is a constant, which, in theory, should be the same for all inhalational agents. The Meyer-Overton rule is usually taken to mean that inhalational agents have their site of action in the lipid component of cells. However, it is more correct to say that the site is nonpolar.

J. Ferguson proposed in 1939 that an anesthetic's potency can be expressed in terms of thermodynamic activity: whatever the concentration of a given anesthetic agent required to produce a given level of anesthesia, the thermodynamic activity would be

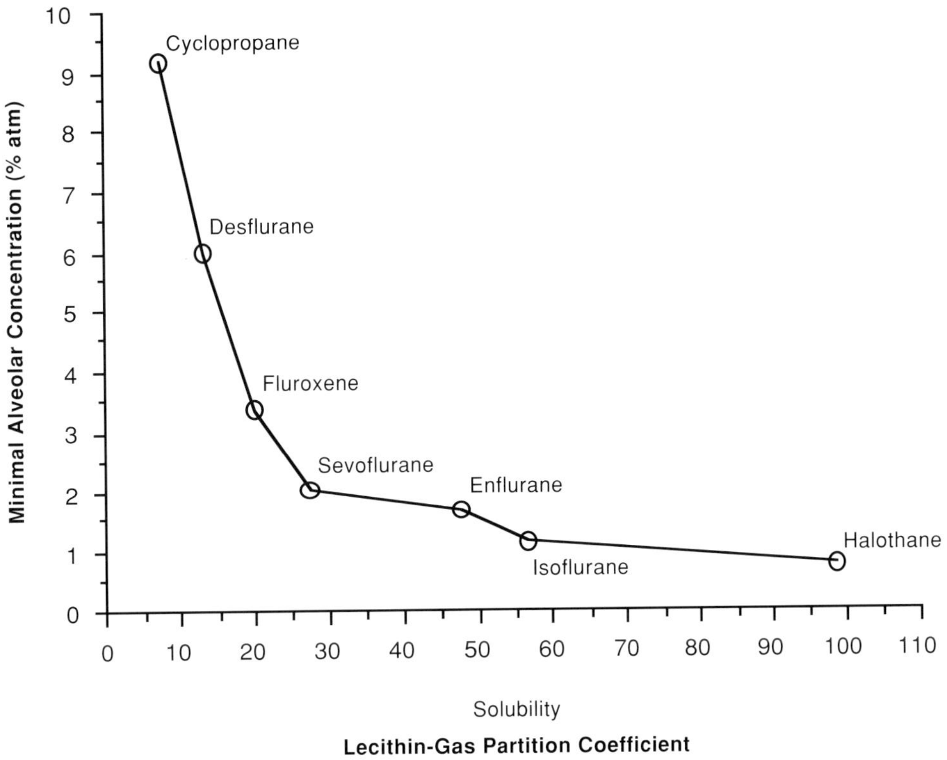

Fig. 9-1. These data, in which an inhalational anesthetic's minimal alveolar concentration is plotted as a function of its solubility in lecithin, are shown in a modern representation of the observations that led Meyer and Overton individually to propose that anesthetic potency is related to lipid solubility. The curve has the mathematical form: constant = XY. A straight line with a negative slope is obtained when the data are plotted using log-log coordinates. Data source: Taheri S, Halsey MJ, Liu J, Eger EI II, Koblin DD, Laster MJ. What solvent best represents the site of action of inhaled anesthetics in humans, rats, and dogs? *Anesth Analg*. 1991;72:Table 1, p 631; Table 4, p 632.

the same.[5] The thermodynamic activity of a volatile agent (which, for purposes of this chapter, can be considered its vapor pressure) is a property of the anesthetic molecule. Ferguson's rule can be interpreted to mean that the quotient of (*a*) the partial pressure of an anesthetic agent at which one half of the subjects are anesthetized, and (*b*) the vapor pressure of the agent at the appropriate temperature is a constant that, in theory, should be the same for all inhalational agents. Ferguson's rule is silent as to the anesthetic's site of action.

The rules of Meyer-Overton and Ferguson both have notable exceptions that provide insight into the mechanisms by which inhalational anesthetics act. Both exaggerate the potency of hydrogen and certain inert gases such as helium and neon, while the Ferguson rule also underestimates the anesthetic potency of short-chained fluorocarbons. The failure to predict the anesthetic potential of low-molecular-weight gases is now recognized to be a consequence of the phenomenon of pressure reversal.[6]

Cutoff Effect

In 1939, when he was studying homologous series of primary alcohols, Ferguson noted that carbon chained compounds demonstrate an anesthetic cutoff effect.[5] Beginning with methanol (C_N=1), anesthetic potency increases logarithmically with the addition of carbon atoms until the effect abruptly stops, and further addition of carbon moieties not only does not enhance potency, but such molecules are devoid of anesthetic potential. In the first series studied, potency ended at C_N=12. This was termed the *cutoff* effect. When other homologous series were studied, both the type of bonds in the compound and the addition of other radicals attached to the first carbon were found to alter the absolute number of carbon atoms required for anesthetic cutoff. Interestingly, the fully fluorinated alkanes demonstrate cutoff at a very short carbon length: at octafluropropane (C_3F_8).[7] The cutoff effect may have implications regarding the molecular binding site of anesthetics.

It has generally been assumed that the cutoff effect results from the failure of anesthetic agents with large molecular dimensions to dissolve at the site of action in a concentration sufficient to cause an effect. This explanation is now known to be untenable, at least for highly lipophilic alcohols with more than 12 carbon atoms.[6]

Stereoselectivity

In general, anesthetics do not exhibit stereoselective effects. For example, both D-halothane and L-halothane, when inhaled, inhibit synaptic transmission and cause a disordered spin-labeling of the bilipid membrane.[8] Interestingly, the optical isomers of isoflurane have markedly different effects on the nicotinic acetylcholine receptors of isolated neurons, even though their bulk lipid solubilities are identical.[9] Although such findings suggest that an agonist–receptor interaction could mediate the effects of certain inhalational agents, the lack of stereospecificity for inhalational agents, when assessed as general anesthetics, speaks against such a phenomenon's importance.

Pressure Reversal

The phenomenon of an anesthetic action's being reversed by the application of high pressure was described in 1951 in tadpoles and confirmed later in other species.[10,11] One possible explanation for pressure reversal is that it is an artifact caused by the helium gas that is used to raise atmospheric pressure in these studies. Helium itself is now known to be an anesthetic agent but has such limited lipid solubility that anesthesia is seen only at the very high pressures that are associated with pressure reversal.[12] It is now accepted that pressure reversal is caused by ambient pressure acting on specific anesthetic sites of action in the lipid bilayer that constitutes the membrane of excitable cells. The mechanism is unclear but was originally thought to be due to the direct hydrostatic compression of the dissolved anesthetic agent; this smaller volume lessens the perturbation of the lipid bilayer in proximity to ion channels. Not all ion channels show pressure reversal—the nicotinic acetylcholine receptor, for example, does not[13]—and even more interestingly, pressure reversal is seen only in species in which the amino acid glycine functions as a neurotransmitter.[14] The latter observations strongly suggest that pressure acts on specific receptors rather than causing a generalized effect (eg, the compression of dissolved gas to a critical volume that is unable to affect the structure of ionic channels).

HYPOTHESES OF INHALATIONAL ANESTHETIC ACTION

Determining the mechanisms of action of inhalational anesthetic agents is one of the most difficult problems facing neuropharmacology. Based on the aforementioned observations, prevailing hypotheses as to the modes of action fall into the categories of lipid, protein, and lipid–protein interaction (Figure 9-2).

Lipid Hypotheses

Both Meyer and Overton pursued their lipid hypotheses of anesthetic action without the benefit of our current understanding of the phospholipid bilayer structure of cell membranes. They used olive oil as a surrogate for a biological lipid, although, interestingly, Meyer proposed that *the* biologically important lipid in which inhalational anesthetics exert their effect is the phosphocholine lecithin, which we now know is an important constituent of myelin sheaths. The simple dissolving of the anesthetic agent throughout the lipid-containing portion of the cell can no longer be viewed as a tenable hypothesis: there is no obvious mechanism through which the bulk presence of the agent can alter the function of ionic channels, which mediate the excitability of cells. Although it might seem possible that the presence of dissolved inhalational agent, by swelling or expanding the membrane (Figure 9-2a), might sufficiently distort the function of ionic channels, measured changes in the thickness of cell membranes due to the presence of an inhalational agent are surprisingly small: from 0.15% to 0.36%.[15–17]

Attempts have been made to refine the lipid membrane–expansion hypothesis by assuming that the action of the inhalational agents is actually localized to discrete sites within the cell membrane, where a local change in the physical properties of the phospholipid bilayer affects ionic channels responsible for anesthesia. The "lipid–phase-transition"[14] and "membrane-disordering"[18] hypotheses are the best-known formulations that employ this approach.

The lipid–phase-transition hypothesis proposes that the lipid moiety of the lipid bilayer that is in proximity to ionic channels exists in two phases: the first consisting of liquid, low-density crystals; the

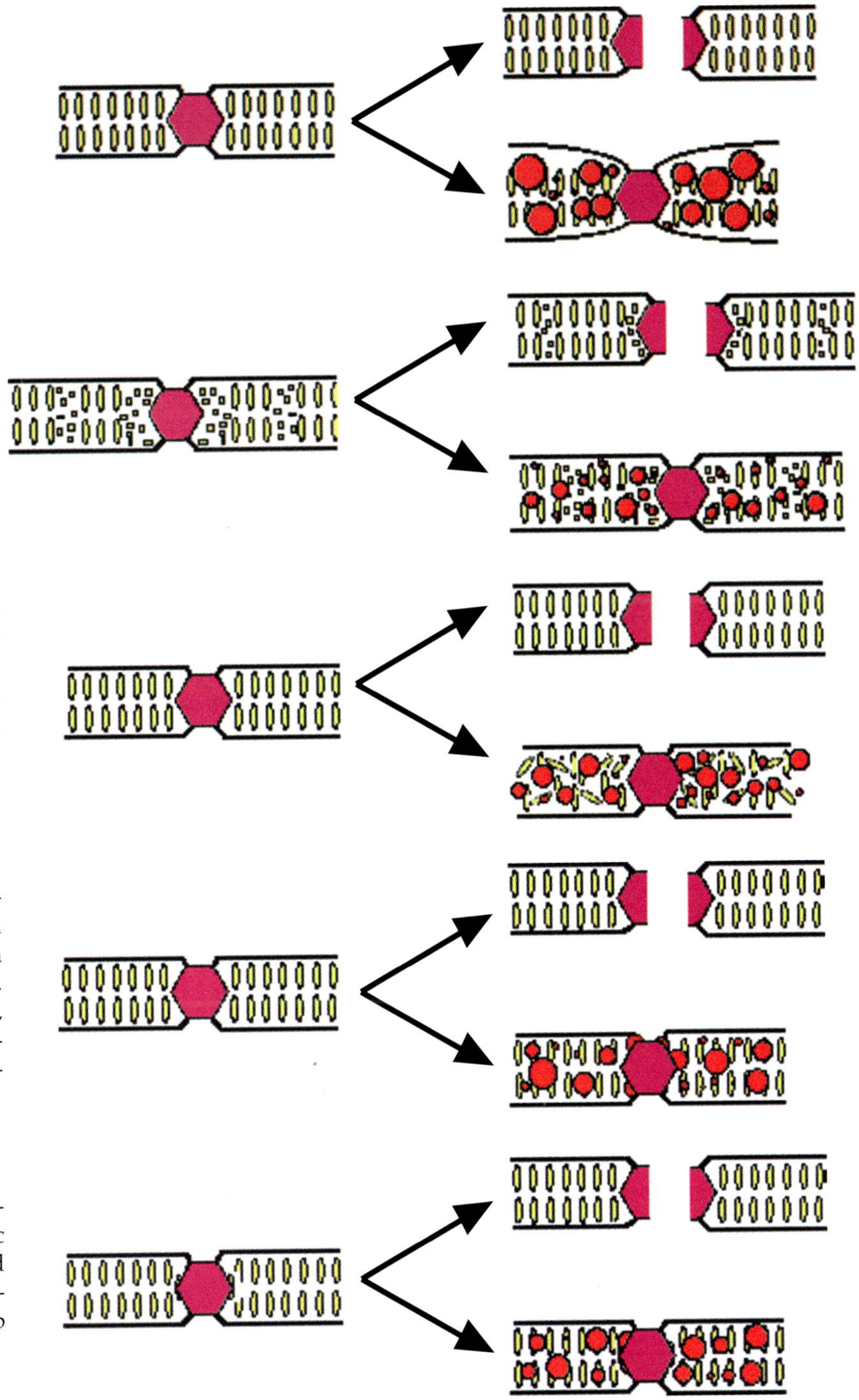

a
The membrane-expansion hypothesis. The inhalational agent so distorts the membrane that the ionic channel cannot open.

b
The phase-separation hypothesis. The lipid within the cell membrane is assumed to exist in two physical states: as a tightly packed gel and as loosely packed liquid crystals. When the ionic channel opens, neighboring liquid crystals are converted to gel. The presence of an inhalational agent prevents this phase transition, thereby inhibiting the opening of the channel.

c
The membrane-disordering hypothesis. The presence of an inhalational agent breaks up the normally parallel arrangement of lipid molecules. In an unknown manner, this perturbation prevents the ionic channel from opening.

d
The protein hypothesis. The inhalational agent activates a receptor on a protein which is a constituent of an ionic channel causing it to open. Viewed in terms of this hypothesis, the correlation between lipid solubility and anesthetic potency is epiphenomenal.

e
The lipid–protein interaction hypothesis. Normal functioning of an ionic channel depends on contact with lipid molecules. The inhalational agent affects the lipid so that this relationship is broken.

Fig. 9-2. A highly schematic and speculative rendering of hypotheses that purport to show possible mechanisms by which inhalational anesthetic agents might cause anesthesia. The crucial assumption is that the agent interferes with the normal function of neuroexcitatory cells. In each of the five sets of diagrams, membrane lipid is shown in yellow; ionic channels in cell membranes are shown in blue; and inhalational agent is shown in red. Each figure shows the ionic channel's resting state (left); the bifurcating arrows indicate the transition to the active state (right), with the ionic channel open (upper) and the state caused by the anesthetic agent (lower).

second, a solid, high-density gel. Opening of the ionic channel pushes aside the neighboring liquid crystals, which then undergo a transition to the more tightly packed gel phase (Figure 9-2b). The presence of the dissolved inhalational agent is thought to prevent this transition. This hypothesis, however, finds little experimental support.

The membrane-disordering hypothesis is derived from spectroscopic evidence that the normal parallel orientation of fatty acid chains of lipid molecules in the cell membrane is disordered by the presence of an inhalational agent (Figure 9-2c). The disordering effect of inhalational agents is seen only when the membrane contains cholesterol in an amount equal to the phospholipid component—an important observation.[19] The membrane-disordering hypothesis assumes that the disorder introduced into the membrane in some unknown way interferes with the function of ionic channels. How and why this happens remain to be determined, but two of the phenomena that must be understood for a putative theory of inhalational agents to have face validity find explanation in the membrane-disordering hypothesis:

1. Pressure reversal is seen to result from the pressure-induced decrease in the random molecular motion of the fatty acid chains that comprise the central portion of the membrane lipids. This ordering of the membrane components reverses the disordering caused by the dissolved inhalational agent.[20]
2. The cutoff phenomenon may be related not to the inability of high-molecular-weight agents to dissolve in the lipid membranes in a concentration that would cause anesthesia, but from their failure to disrupt or disorder the architecture of the lipid bilayer.[6]

Protein Hypothesis

Although the affinity of inhalational anesthetic agents for lipids is commonly used as evidence that their site of action must be in lipids, the term "lipid solubility" actually refers to their solubility in nonpolar or hydrophobic media. Many proteins have nonpolar regions that could serve as sites for the dissolving of inhalational agents.[21] However, these regions are usually centrally located within the protein and, therefore, are effectively shielded from the action of all but pharmacological concentrations of inhalational agents. Such unlikely, nonspecific interactions of proteins and inhalational agents are to be distinguished from interactions of great specificity (eg, those that occur between receptor and agonist). There is no question that inhalational anesthetic agents are capable of specific interactions with proteins[22] (Figure 9-2d):

- Nicotinic acetylcholine receptors are inhibited by halothane, isoflurane, and methoxyflurane at minimal alveolar concentrations (MAC, which is discussed later in this chapter), the end-alveolar concentration of an inhalational anesthetic agent that prevents somatic response to a painful stimulus in 50% of individuals.
- γ-Aminobutyric acid (GABA) receptors are activated by halothane and isoflurane at MAC concentrations.
- The calcium-release channel of the sarcoplasmic reticulum in skeletal muscle is activated by halothane.[23]
- Chemoluminescence liberated by the action of the firefly enzyme D-luciferase is inhibited by inhalational agents.[24]

The question is not so much *whether* inhalational agents can affect proteins—they can—but whether these effects are *necessary* for the induction of general anesthesia. Much needs to be known before this question can be answered. For example, is either (*a*) the inhibition of the nicotinic acetylcholine receptor or (*b*) the activation of the GABA receptor a necessary concomitant for anesthesia? In genetically predetermined individuals, intracellular calcium release by halothane is a profoundly important clinical problem but in normal people is trivial. The inhibition of chemoluminescence by inhalational agents is well described, but there is no evidence that a mammalian equivalent exists. It is perhaps best to defer judgment as to the importance of the protein hypothesis until more data have been collected and reviewed.

Lipid–Protein Interaction Hypothesis

The evidence supporting the protein hypothesis was derived from lipid-free systems. Since biomembranes are aggregates of lipoproteins, it is appropriate to ask whether inhalational agents produce anesthesia by affecting lipoproteins or those lipids in direct contact with proteins of the ionic channel (Figure 9-2e). The lipids that are in direct association with the transmembrane-receptor proteins are known as the *boundary* lipids.[25]

Current research is centered on trying to establish whether inhalational anesthetic–induced perturbation of boundary lipids can be coupled selectively to ionic channels, causing protein conformational changes.[26]

Knowledge of the mechanism of action of inhalational anesthetics has practical importance, because it furthers the process of designing new agents. Nevertheless, it is apparent that a given agent may have a multitude of effects, some of which may be unrelated to the induction of a state of general anesthesia. Even the induction of general anesthesia can be mediated by several mechanisms. For example, inhalational anesthetics fall into two broad classes: alkanes and ethers. Cyclopropane and halothane are alkanes; diethyl ether, enflurane, isoflurane, desflurane, and sevoflurane are ethers. The alkanes are purely lipophilic and therefore dissolve primarily in the lipid portion of the cell membrane, where they exert a nonspecific effect. The halogenated ethers, being more polar, both dissolve in the lipid membrane and form hydrogen bonds with protein moieties of ionic channels. Thus, the ether anesthetics are capable of both specific and nonspecific interactions. It is likely that the stereospecificity of the optical isomers of isoflurane arises from the ability of only one isomer to form hydrogen bonds with receptor proteins.

SITE OF ACTION

A large body of work has been directed toward locating the major areas of interaction within the central nervous system (CNS) that are influenced by the anesthetic agents. It is now obvious that anesthetics do not exert their action through one specific effect in any one particular region of the CNS. Based on this information, more recent work has been directed at the cellular rather than the regional level of the CNS. One early and consistent observation has been that general anesthetic agents block neural transmission at the synapse at much lower concentrations than the concentrations required to block conductance within the axon. Based on this information, the synapse has been the focus of most recent studies. Because synapses are either excitatory or inhibitory in nature, general anesthetic agents should have a depressant effect on excitatory postsynaptic potentials (EPSPs), an augmentation of inhibitory postsynaptic potentials (IPSPs), or both. It should be appreciated, however, that synaptic transmission can be subdivided into four areas for further study:

1. axonal conductance along the afferent axon,
2. neurotransmitter release into the synaptic cleft,
3. binding of the neurotransmitter by specific receptors in the postjunctional area, and
4. changes in conductance, leading to propagation of the action potential.

When both the CNS and the peripheral nervous system have been studied, the general anesthetic agents do have a depressant effect on EPSPs, although the magnitude of effect on EPSPs is diverse within the area of the hippocampus. These findings suggest that either (*a*) EPSPs do not play a major role in the action of anesthetic agents or (*b*) the hippocampus is not relevant to general anesthetic action.[27]

The principal inhibitory neurotransmitter within the CNS is GABA. The data regarding general anesthetic action on IPSPs are conflicting, especially information suggesting that halothane and isoflurane cause a reduction in IPSPs. This phenomenon has been explained as an indirect action due to a depression of excitatory synapses acting on GABA-ergic inhibitory cells.[28] More work is necessary to elucidate the role of inhibitory monosynapses in the absence of excitatory synapse transmission.

To summarize, the synapse is probably the cellular site of action of the general anesthetic agents, based on the low concentrations needed to affect transmission. What is not understood is exactly how these agents work at this level, as there is not an anesthetic effect that is common to all synapses or, indeed, to all anesthetic agents that have been studied. Based on all available information, two main theories have been promulgated to explain anesthetic action at the synaptic level. The unitary theory holds that all general anesthetic agents work by a common mechanism. A more robust, conflicting theory called the degenerate theory holds that different general anesthetic agents have different mechanisms of actions at possibly different sites of action. Two strategies attempt to elucidate information surrounding the degenerate theory: the pharmacological approach studies relative potencies of anesthetic agents in animals, while the mechanistic approach looks at well-defined molecular models in an attempt to discover a yet-unknown site of action in the CNS.

OVERVIEW: MODERN INHALATIONAL ANESTHETIC AGENTS

During the 1920s, the frustrations encountered in clinical practice (eg, difficulties with the older inhalational agents in delivery, side effects, and flammability) coupled with an understanding of the expanding scientific basis for anesthesia and surgery mandated that newer anesthetic agents be developed to replace ether and chloroform. A variety of carbon-chain–based agents were studied and marketed, and cyclopropane became the most important new inhaled anesthetic introduced in the 1930s. Prior to the 1950s, all inhalational anesthetic agents possessed one or both of these two defects: they were explosive, and they were toxic to biological tissues. Fortuitously, research in other fields made possible the development and production of fluorinated carbon-based anesthetic agents, which are both biologically safe and nonexplosive.

A vast increase in our knowledge of the chemistry of elemental fluorine occurred during World War II as a byproduct of the Manhattan Project. A crucial step in the fabrication of the first atomic bombs was the separation of the naturally fissionable isotope of uranium, ^{235}U, from the much more common ^{238}U. The separation depended on the availability of uranium hexafluoride, and the ability to synthesize and manipulate this unusual substance safely led to a better understanding of fluorine chemistry. The mass manufacturing of fluorinated carbon-based compounds could then follow. The addition of a fluorine molecule to carbon was associated with decreased flammability. The fluorine–carbon bond was more stable than the carbon–carbon bond, tended to undergo less biological metabolism, and was therefore associated with less organ toxicity. The fluorinated anesthetic compound first marketed was fluroxene, which was introduced in 1954 and used until 1975. Although fluroxene had the desirable qualities of low solubility in blood and minimal tendency to depress cardiovascular function, it was associated with nausea and vomiting and was flammable at higher concentrations. After a large experience with fluroxene had been collected, this compound was found to be rarely associated with hepatotoxicity and possible carcinogenesis. Fluroxene was an important bridging compound in inhalational anesthetic practice until the development and clinical introduction of safer and more desirable agents.

Fluorinated compounds are today's anesthetic agents of choice (Table 9-1). The ones most commonly used are halothane, enflurane, isoflurane, and desflurane; sevoflurane was added to the armamentarium in 1995. Nitrous oxide is neither fluorinated nor available in DEPMEDS-equipped hospitals but is included for the sake of completeness.

Halothane

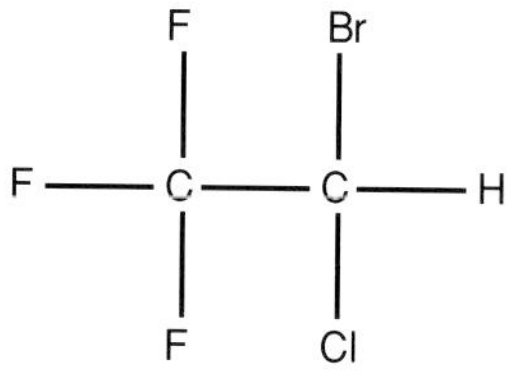

Halothane (1,1,1-trifluoro-2-bromo-2-chloroethane) is an aliphatic hydrocarbon of the alkane series (specifically, a halogenated ethane) that was introduced into the clinical practice of anesthesia in 1956. This important compound was a tremendous improvement over the earlier alkanes and ethers and still has a role in civilian and military anesthesia. The agent is somewhat unstable in the presence of physical factors associated with the delivery of anesthesia, and due to its spontaneous oxidation and affinity for breakdown by ultraviolet light must be stabilized with 0.01% thymol and stored in dark brown bottles. In current practice, halothane's main drawbacks are its propensity to sensitize the myocardium to the effects of epinephrine and its association with a metabolic-related hepatotoxicity.

Halothane is well known to conventionally trained anesthesiologists and continues to be a very useful inhalational anesthetic agent—although its use in the United States is much less than that of the inhalational ethers. Halothane enjoys a greater potency and has less airway irritability than the newer halogenated ether agents and, therefore, is better tolerated when a straight inhalational induction technique is employed. Owing to its association with a metabolic-related hepatotoxicity, halothane has been used as an induction agent in adults and then discontinued and replaced by one of the halogenated ether agents. A main disadvantage of halothane is its effect on the myocardium—from both a dose-related myocardial depression, which causes hypotension, and the enhanced sensitizing effect it has with circulating and administered catecholamines. Cerebral blood flow (CBF) increases with halothane (due to its

TABLE 9-1

GENERAL PROPERTIES OF INHALATIONAL ANESTHETICS

Property	N_2O	ISO	ENF	HAL	DES	SEV
Molecular weight	44	184.5	184.5	197.4	168	218
Boiling point (°C)	–88.5	48.5	56.5	50.2	23.5	58.5
Specific gravity (25°C)*	1.53	1.5	1.52	1.86	1.45	1.50
Vapor pressure (20°C) (mm Hg)	38,770 (gas)	238	172	243	664	160
MAC (in O_2) (%)	105	1.28	1.58	0.75	4.6–6	1.71
MAC (in 70% N_2O) (%)	—	0.56	0.57	0.29		0.66
AD_{95}	—	1.68	1.88	0.90		2.07
MAC-awake (multiple)	0.6–0.8			0.52	0.53	
MAC as partial pressure (mm Hg)	800	9.7	12.0	5.7	34.9–45.6	13.0
Partition coefficients (37°C)						
Blood–gas	0.47	1.4	1.8	2.3	0.42	0.59
Brain–blood	1.1	2.6	1.4	2.9	1.3	1.7
Muscle–blood	1.2	4.0	1.7	3.5	2.0	3.1
Fat–blood	2.3	45	36	60	27	48
Rubber–gas	1.2	62	74	120	20	30
Flammability (in 70% N_2O/ 30%O_2) (%)		7	5.8	4.8	17	10
Stability						
Alkali	Stable	Stable	Stable	Some instability	Stable	Very unstable
Ultraviolet	Stable	Stable	Stable	Unstable		
Metal	Stable	Stable	Stable	Corrodes	Stable	Stable
Preservative	None	None	None	Thymol	None	None
Recovered as metabolites (%)	0.0	0.2	2.4	20		

N_2O: Nitrous oxide; ISO: Isoflurane; ENF: Enflurane; HAL: Halothane; DES: Desflurane; SEV: Sevoflurane; MAC: minimal alveolar concentration; AD_{95}: anesthetic depth (the dose that prevents movement in 95% of subjects in response to standard surgical incision)
*Specific gravity for N_2O is for the gas relative to air, but for the other anesthetics is for the liquid relative to water
Reprinted with permission from Longnecker DE, Miller FL. Pharmacology of inhalational anesthetics. In: Rogers MC, Tinker JH, Covino BG, Longnecker DE. *Principles and Practice of Anesthesiology*. St. Louis, Mo: Mosby–Year Book; 1993: 1054.

vasodilating properties), and the potential exists for an increase in intracranial pressure (ICP) that may only be partially responsive to the elimination of carbon dioxide via hyperventilation. Halothane also causes an important decrease in splanchnic circulation and decreased total hepatic circulation, with portal venous and hepatic arterial blood-flow decrements that may place the patient at risk for hepatic ischemia and hepatocellular tissue hypoxia. The major route of elimination is via the pulmonary bed, but up to 20% of halothane may be biotransformed in the liver. A combination of decreased hepatic blood flow, major hepatic biotransformation, and a possible immunologically mediated tissue injury may contribute to the hepatotoxicity seen in a small number (1:10,000) of adult patients exposed to halothane. This incidence is even lower in children. All the potent volatile agents are associated with a dose-related, muscle-relaxation effect.

Enflurane and Isoflurane

The ethers enflurane (1,1,2-trifluoro-2-chloroethyl difluoromethyl ether) and isoflurane (1-chloro-2,2,2-trifluoroethyl difluoromethyl ether) are isomers. They share the same chemical formulae and molecular weight but differ in their physical and pharmacological properties owing to the position of the carbon atom to which hydrogen and chlorine are attached. These methyl-ethyl ethers are synthesized when bromine is removed from the halothane molecule and an ether link, with a difluoromethyl group attached, is created. The substitution of fluorine for chlorine and bromine increases molecular stability while reducing potency and solubility. The alkanes (eg, halothane) appear to be associated with cardiac toxicity, due to their ability to sensitize the myocardium to catecholamines. The interposition of oxygen in an ether linkage within an anesthetic molecule reduces this myocardial irritability.

Enflurane

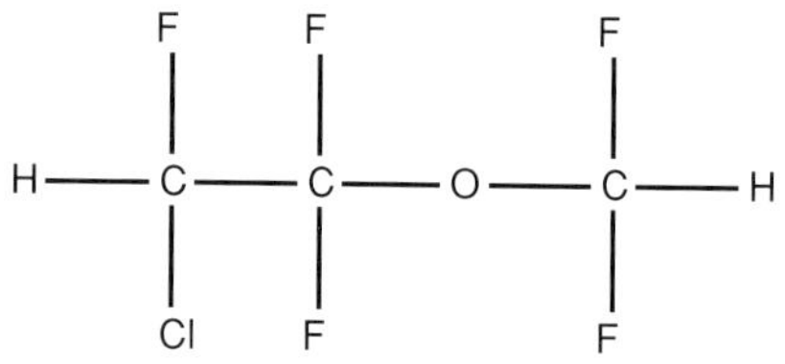

Enflurane was the first of the modern halogenated ether inhalational agents to be released for clinical use (in 1972). Its principal advantage over halothane is its reduced association with hepatotoxicity and catecholamine-induced myocardial irritability. Enflurane is approximately one half as potent as halothane but can still provide prompt induction of anesthesia. Like halothane, enflurane causes a dose-related decrease in blood pressure that makes this drug difficult to titrate between adequate depth of anesthesia and unacceptable hypotension.[29] The dose-related hypotension is due to a combination of myocardial depression and peripheral vasodilation with decreased systemic vascular resistance (SVR). As does halothane, enflurane causes increased CBF and the potential exists for increased ICP and cerebral hypoxia. Although total hepatic blood flow is decreased during enflurane anesthesia, the relation between hepatic arterial and portal blood flow remains preserved.[30] Enflurane produces a dose-dependent respiratory depression, hypercarbia, and an increased alveolar–arterial gradient that is greater than that seen with halothane.[31,32] Enflurane has been associated with tonic-clonic muscle activity and confirmed electroencephalographic (EEG) evidence of seizure activity at higher doses, especially in the setting of hypocarbia, although at lower doses it does not appear to predispose patients with epilepsy to further seizure activity.[33] The major route of elimination is via the lungs, with 2% to 3% being biotransformed in the liver. Major metabolic by-products of concern include fluoride ions and difluoromethoxydifluoroacetic acid.[34] Because nephrotoxicity has been associated with the fluoride ion by-product during very prolonged use, many anesthesiologists prefer to avoid enflurane in patients with renal compromise. The level of fluoride ion that is required to produce nephrotoxicity (40–50 µmol/L) is rarely exceeded except during dramatically prolonged enflurane anesthesia.[27]

Isoflurane

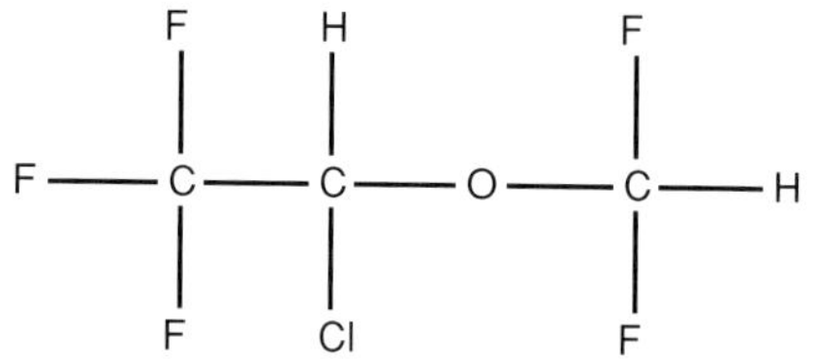

Isoflurane, released for clinical use in 1981, is probably the most popular potent volatile anesthetic agent currently administered in the United States. Its major advantages include its ease of administration, lack of serious hepatotoxicity, and minimal biotransformation with fluoride ion production. As with all of the volatile vapors, it is a potent respiratory depressant and, although isoflurane can be used to induce anesthesia, some patients have complained of respiratory discomfort on inhalational induction. Isoflurane preserves cardiac output throughout all levels of anesthesia better than either halothane or enflurane (Figure 9-3).

Isoflurane is associated with a dose-dependent hypotension without myocardial depression that is solely mediated by a decrease in SVR. This vasodilating effect can actually be exploited when a relatively hypotensive anesthetic technique is desirable. Tachycardia is a commonly seen event with isoflurane and appears more frequently with younger patients.[35] There does not appear to be any appreciable myocardial irritability with circulating catecholamines during the use of isoflurane,

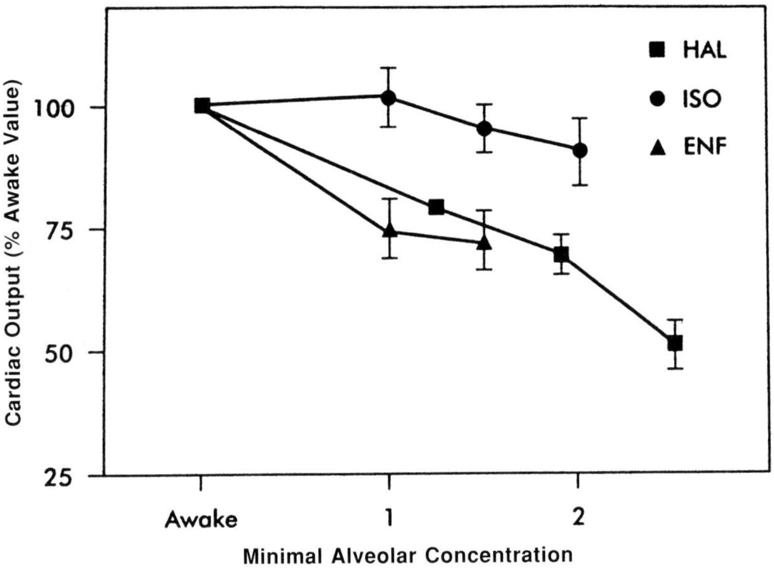

Fig. 9-3. Cardiac output is best preserved in humans by isoflurane, compared with halothane and enflurane. HAL: halothane; ISO: isoflurane; ENF: enflurane. Reprinted with permission from Longnecker DE, Miller FL. Pharmacology of inhalational anesthetics. In: Rogers MC, Tinker JH, Covino BG, Longnecker DE. *Principles and Practice of Anesthesiology*. St. Louis, Mo: Mosby–Year Book; 1993: 1073.

and although the phenomenon of coronary steal is theoretically possible, it is infrequently observed. Again, as with halothane, CBF increases. Although isoflurane may cause an increase in ICP, this effect can be totally abolished with hypocarbia.[36] Previously, isoflurane had been thought to have less effect on cerebral circulation than halothane, but the effect may, in fact, be the same.[30,37] Evidence from studies with animals indicates that isoflurane offers better cerebral protection from ischemia or hypoxia when compared with the other volatile agents, and anesthesiologists who provide care for neurosurgical procedures may therefore consider isoflurane to be the potent volatile agent of choice.[38] There is a reduction of total hepatic blood flow seen with isoflurane; however, total flow, hepatic oxygen transport, hepatic oxygenation, and arterial compensation for reduced portal flow are all better maintained with isoflurane than with either halothane or enflurane.[30,39,40] Hepatic injury has not been associated with isoflurane, and this may be related to the protective mechanisms mentioned above. Renal blood flow is decreased under isoflurane administration, but this appears to be a function of decreased total perfusion rather than changes in regional vascular resistance.[41] Isoflurane is excreted via the lungs, and only 0.2% of the agent undergoes biotransformation. The biotransformation of isoflurane is only 1% of that of halothane and 10% of that of enflurane, with the fluoride and trifluoroacetic acid metabolites being insufficient to be associated with significant cellular injury or toxicity.[42] The major complications associated with isoflurane are related to the spectrum of its pharmacological activity (eg, hypotension, tachycardia, hypercarbia) rather than to any specific organ toxicity per se. Indeed, the major advantage of isoflurane is its rather remarkable lack of significant complications or evidence of associated hepatic toxicity. Isoflurane is a major inhalational agent available to the military anesthesiologist in the field.

Desflurane

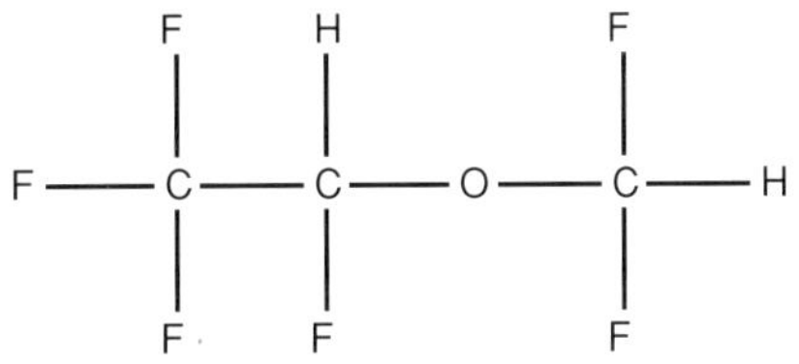

Desflurane (1-fluoro-2,2,2-trifluoroethyl difluoromethyl ether) is a fluorinated methyl-ethyl ether in which the chlorine has been totally removed from the molecule. The lower solubility and chemical stability afforded by this fluorine substitution is at the cost of lower potency and a very high vapor pressure: 664 mm Hg at 20°C. A special vaporizer is required to deliver this agent. Although desflurane may prove to be a valuable agent in the civilian setting because it allows for rapid emergence from anesthesia, the need for a special vaporizer makes it highly unlikely that this agent will be used in the military field setting.

Introduced into clinical practice in 1992, desflurane has the lowest solubility in blood of any of the inhalational agents. Owing to its physical property of a low blood–gas partition coefficient (0.42), its main clinical advantage appears to be a rapid emergence from anesthesia. Its main disadvantages are airway irritation, which limits its use as an induction agent, and its physical property of a high vapor pressure (desflurane boils at room temperature), which requires a specially constructed vaporizer to allow for its delivery in ordinary operating room settings. The circulatory and cerebral effects of desflurane are identical to those seen with isoflurane.[43,44] The route of excretion is via the lungs, and the biotransformation of desflurane is trivial. Trifluoroacetic acid production is slight (0.17 µmol/L), and is 10% of that seen with isoflurane.[27] The desflurane molecule is extremely stable.

Sevoflurane

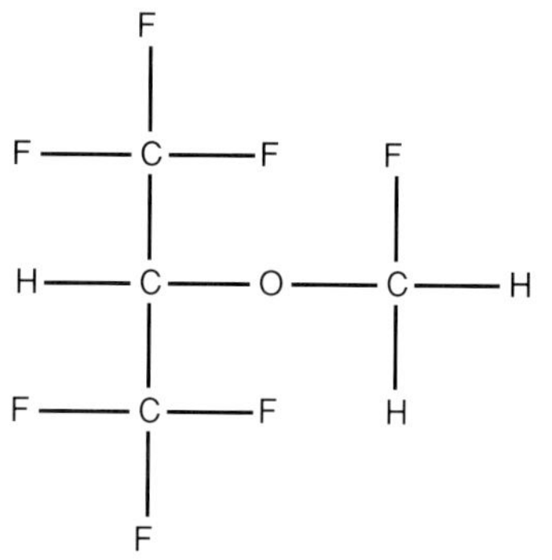

Sevoflurane (1,1,1,3,3,3-hexafluoro-2-propyl fluoroethyl ether) is another highly fluorine-substituted structural modification of the ether link. In this situation, the oxygen is located between an ethyl and a propyl group, which allows for low solubility. The addition of the propyl side chain increases the agent's potency.

Sevoflurane is the newest halogenated ether anesthetic agent and was released for clinical use in the United States in 1995. Due to its low blood–gas partition coefficient (0.59), sevoflurane has the advantage of rapid induction and emergence from anesthesia. The cardiovascular effects of sevoflurane appear to be similar to those of isoflurane.[45,46] The respiratory depression seen with sevoflurane is significant but less than that seen with halothane. Changes in tidal volume and respiratory excursion are greater with sevoflurane than with isoflurane, and this suggests a neural control response to sevoflurane different from that seen with isoflurane.[47] The route of excretion is via the lungs but the biotransformation of sevoflurane is very significant: up to 10% of patients undergoing sevoflurane anesthesia have plasma fluoride levels that exceed 50 µmol/L, which is considered to be the threshold for renal toxicity.[48] Thus, a major disadvantage of sevoflurane is that it may be limited to use for short procedures to avoid potential renal damage, although prolonged sevoflurane anesthesia (9.5 MAC-hours) has been reported not to impair renal concentrating function on days 1 and 5 after anesthesia.[49] Finally, sevoflurane is very unstable in alkali and may not be suitable in situations where low fresh-gas-flow states are needed, such as the military setting, where gas supplies must be conserved and strict economy of available resources preserved.

Nitrous Oxide

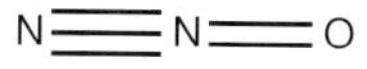

In passing, it should be noted that the old standby inhalational agent of the past—nitrous oxide—is not fielded with DEPMEDS equipment and will only be available in fixed military medical treatment facilities. Although nitrous oxide can successfully be coadministered with other inhalational anesthetic agents, it must be stored in bulky gas cylinders, it supports combustion almost as well as oxygen, and it is subject to contamination from other oxides of nitrogen that may be toxic, owing to the production of free radicals. Because of weight and storage constraints, and especially because it expands in closed spaces, nitrous oxide will probably not be available to military anesthesia providers in the field.

Although nitrous oxide can be used by itself as an analgesic agent for minor surgical procedures, it is rarely used as a sole agent in modern anesthetic practice: its lack of potency and its MAC of 105% make it impossible to use as a total anesthetic agent. Nitrous oxide is employed mainly to minimize the total dose of other potent volatile anesthetic agents by taking advantage of the additive property of MAC. Owing to its physical properties, nitrous oxide exhibits both the *second-gas* and the *concentration* effects, which are discussed later in this chapter. Nitrous oxide demonstrates a mild increase in sympathetic nervous system activity that may be matched by a mild myocardial depressant effect. By itself, nitrous oxide exerts little effect on carbon dioxide response but is associated with respiratory depression when combined with other potent agents.[50] Elimination of nitrous oxide is via the pulmonary system, with minimal biotransformation. The main complications associated with the use of nitrous oxide center on its association with the diffusion anoxia experienced on anesthetic emergence; its ability to expand in closed, gas-containing spaces; and a dose-related bone marrow depression caused by the inhibition of methionine synthetase, which is a cofactor in amino acid and vitamin metabolism.

UPTAKE AND DISTRIBUTION

Biophysical Properties

The amount of inhalational anesthetic agent that is delivered to a patient can be expressed as a percentage of the total gas volume delivered (vol %) or as a partial pressure of the total gas pressure (mm Hg). The convention in the United States is to use the expression "volume percent delivered," but an understanding of partial atmospheric pressure is essential to appreciate how anesthetic agents reach equilibrium. For example, a 2% concentration of isoflurane delivered at sea level at standard temperature with a standard barometric pressure (P_{bar}) of 760 mm Hg (ie, 1 atm) would contain a partial pressure of 15.2 mm Hg (0.02 • 760 = 15.2) isoflurane. However, if 2% isoflurane were to be delivered at an elevation of 6,000 ft above sea level (a slightly higher elevation than that seen in Denver, Colo.), where the P_{bar} is 609 mm Hg, the calculated delivered partial pressure would be 12.2 mm Hg. To further complicate the issue, if a modern temperature-compensated variable-bypass vaporizer were used, the vaporizer constants would be (*a*) the gas dilution ratio of the vaporizer (21:1 diluent gas to gas flow at 2% flow) and (*b*) the saturated vapor pressure of isoflurane (238 mm Hg), both of which are independent of P_{bar}. The actual delivery of isoflurane set at 2% on the dial at an altitude just higher than that of Denver, Colorado, would be 17.1 mm Hg (or 2.8% isoflurane) instead of the calculated 15.2 mm Hg. Therefore, it may be more prudent to consider anesthetic delivery in terms of partial pressure rather than volume percent (Figure 9-4).[27]

Although the inhalational anesthetic agents are delivered via the pulmonary alveolar bed, and the desired inhaled and exhaled anesthetic concentrations are measured as alveolar gas concentrations, the primary intent is to deliver these agents to the brain. The main determinant of anesthetic delivery to target tissues is the biophysical property of solubility, which is also related to anesthetic potency. As the brain is an organ that is extraordinarily well perfused, the partial pressure of anesthetic agent in the blood and that of the brain approach equilibrium very quickly. The exchange of anesthetic gases across the alveolar membrane is quite efficient, and the partial pressure of agent in the pulmonary circulation is very close to that found in the alveolar gas; therefore, the brain partial pressure closely follows alveolar partial pressure. The reason that patients do not fall asleep immediately on exposure to an anesthetic gas, or wake up immedi-

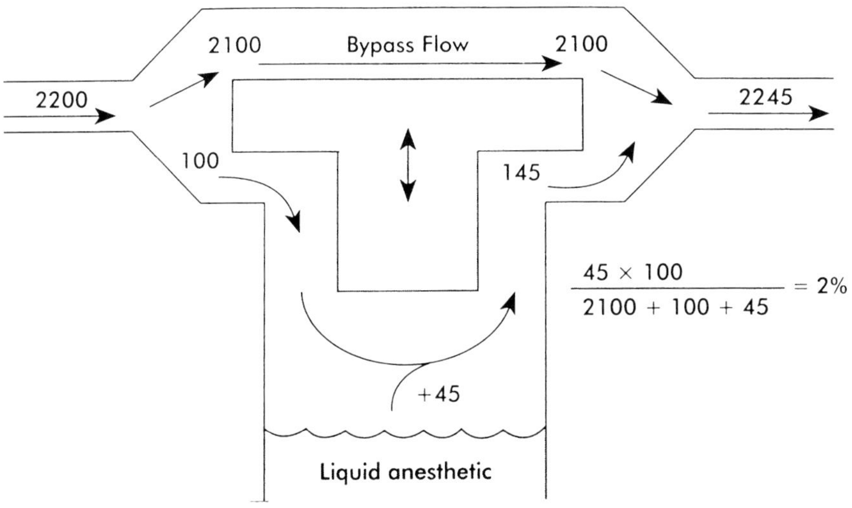

Fig. 9-4. The numbers represent gas flows in milliliters per minute for a 2% isoflurane gas mixture by passing through a vaporizer with a 21:1 splitting ratio at a constant temperature of 20°C. Reprinted with permission from Longnecker DE, Miller FL. Pharmacology of inhalational anesthetics. In: Rogers MC, Tinker JH, Covino BG, Longnecker DE. *Principles and Practice of Anesthesiology*. St. Louis, Mo: Mosby–Year Book; 1993: 1057.

ately on discontinuation, is mainly due to the solubility of the anesthetic agent in the blood. It may be helpful to understand that the uptake of anesthetic agent occurs in three stages of delivery:

1. vaporization and delivery into the airways,
2. transfer across the alveolar membrane with uptake into the blood, and
3. transfer from the blood across a tissue membrane, with uptake into target tissue.

There may be factors that influence any of these stages of anesthetic delivery.

The solubility of an anesthetic agent can be expressed as a partition coefficient, which is essentially the ratio of the solubilities for two media. Partition coefficients are independent of partial pressure and are critical in describing uptake and distribution properties of each agent. An example would be the brain–blood partition coefficient, which quantitates the ratio of solubility for blood compared with that of the brain. The solubility of anesthetic agents in the blood and tissues determines how much drug uptake is required across the alveolar membrane to increase anesthetic partial pressure in the brain, the ultimate target organ for anesthetic agents. Drug uptake ultimately influences the time of induction or emergence from anesthesia. A low blood–gas partition coefficient is desirable for a potent anesthetic agent.

Three points need to be appreciated regarding the practical use of inhalational agents. First, to reach equilibrium, the direction that gas molecules move will always be from the higher partial-pressure phase to the lower. Second, when partial pressures are expressed for media in both gaseous and nongaseous phases, the ultimate reference is to the gaseous phase. Third, the actual amount of vapor contained in a nongaseous phase (eg, within tissues) depends on the partial pressure and its solubility in that particular tissue. This is important, as different body tissues such as brain, muscle, and fat have different partition coefficients, which are expressed as the brain–blood, muscle–blood, and fat–blood coefficients. Prior to achieving equilibrium, an inhalational agent moves from alveolar gas to blood, then to brain, to muscle, and finally to fat. Well-perfused tissues such as the brain are called the vessel-rich group, whereas poorly perfused tissues such as fat are called the vessel-poor group. The brain may reach an anesthetic partial pressure concentration that is adequate for anesthesia, while the partial pressure lags behind in the vessel-poor tissues. On termination of inhalational anesthetic agents, the order is reversed, but ultimate excretion of anesthetic gas is limited to these pressure gradients (Figure 9-5).

The blood–gas coefficient of nitrous oxide at 37°C is 0.47 and is one of the lowest of the available inhalational agents. However, this coefficient is still approximately 31-fold greater than the blood–gas coefficient for gaseous nitrogen. When nitrous

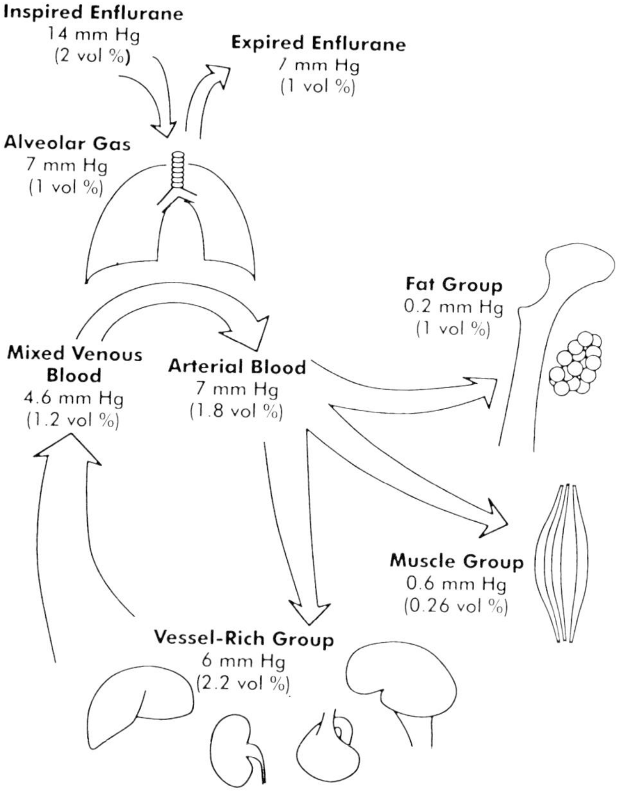

Fig. 9-5. A representation of the distribution of partial pressures (mm Hg) and concentration (vol %) of 2% enflurane into body tissues 10 minutes after induction of anesthesia. At this time, alveolar partial pressure is approximately half of inspired pressure. The anesthetic flow is in the direction of decreasing partial pressure, and is quantitatively represented by the magnitude and direction of the arrows. Note that the vessel-rich groups are close to equilibrium with blood and that the muscle and fat groups are not. The concentration of enflurane depends on partition coefficients, and anesthetic uptake continues into vessel-rich and fat groups. If the anesthetic were terminated at this point, the fat group would continue to take up anesthetic while the vessel-rich groups would begin to release agent back into the blood for ultimate elimination through the lungs. Reprinted with permission from Longnecker DE, Miller FL. Pharmacology of inhalational anesthetics. In: Rogers MC, Tinker JH, Covino BG, Longnecker DE. *Principles and Practice of Anesthesiology*. St. Louis, Mo: Mosby–Year Book; 1993: 1059.

oxide is administered, it will exchange for nitrogen and occupy a volume 30-fold greater than that occupied by nitrogen. At equilibrium using an inhalational gas mixture that contains 70% nitrous oxide, any gas-filled cavity—whether caused by a pathological or a therapeutic process—will expand in size up to 4-fold. Therefore, the use of nitrous oxide is contraindicated in those situations (eg, bowel obstruction, thoracic injury). Although the same exchange phenomenon occurs with the potent inhalational agents, their partial pressures are small (eg, 2% isoflurane vs 70% nitrous oxide) and they occupy less volume in gas-filled spaces.

Factors Affecting Uptake and Distribution

When an anesthetic mixture is selected for administration, three variables must be taken into account for the intended alveolar partial pressure of the desired agent to be achieved. First, the gas circuit itself must be washed out with the fresh gas mixture to achieve a circuit concentration equal to that selected on the vaporizer. This can be accomplished by elapsed time, high gas flows, and the overpressure effect (ie, selecting an initial higher inspired concentration than is ultimately intended). Second, the inhalational agent will move into rubber and plastic parts of the anesthesia circuit (as predicted by the rubber–gas partition coefficient) and the soda lime absorbent will also absorb agent to some degree. The third and most important factor is the concept of alveolar gas uptake (FA_X) in relation to the inspired fractional concentration (FI_X) and the ultimate uptake by the blood (X). This has been expressed as FA_X/FI_X (Figure 9-6). The major factors that can delay anesthetic uptake to the brain include

- highly soluble anesthetic agents,
- a state of increased cardiac output, and
- a large gradient between the partial pressures of alveolar and mixed-venous blood.

Increasing the speed of delivery of the inhaled agents to the brain can be simply accomplished by increasing the inspired partial pressure of the anesthetic or by increasing alveolar ventilation. Figure 9-7 demonstrates how partition coefficients for various tissue groups affect drug delivery to these sites.

Two other phenomena that can affect anesthetic uptake are known as the concentration effect and the second-gas effect. When high concentrations (ie, overpressures) of gas are delivered, large volumes of gas are removed by alveolar uptake and a large gradient is established. Returning expired gases are enriched and concentrated by the high inspired concentration, therefore maintaining a high inspired fraction. The second-gas effect is stated,

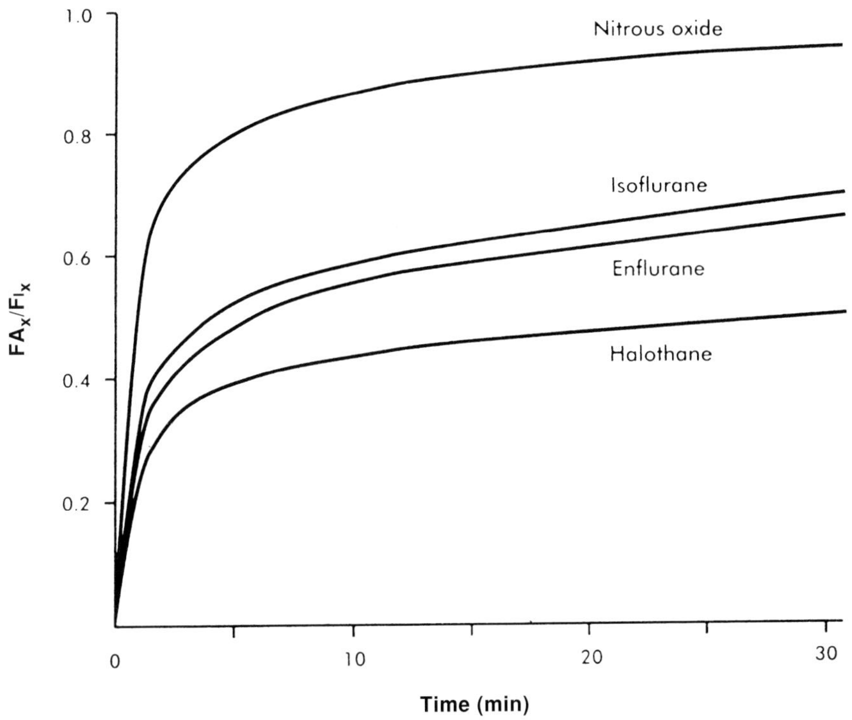

Fig. 9-6. A comparison of different agents regarding the increase of alveolar fractional concentration (FA_X) toward that of inspired concentration (FI_X) over time. Agents that are less soluble in blood rise more rapidly. Reprinted with permission from Longnecker DE, Miller FL. Pharmacology of inhalational anesthetics. In: Rogers MC, Tinker JH, Covino BG, Longnecker DE. *Principles and Practice of Anesthesiology*. St. Louis, Mo: Mosby–Year Book; 1993: 1062.

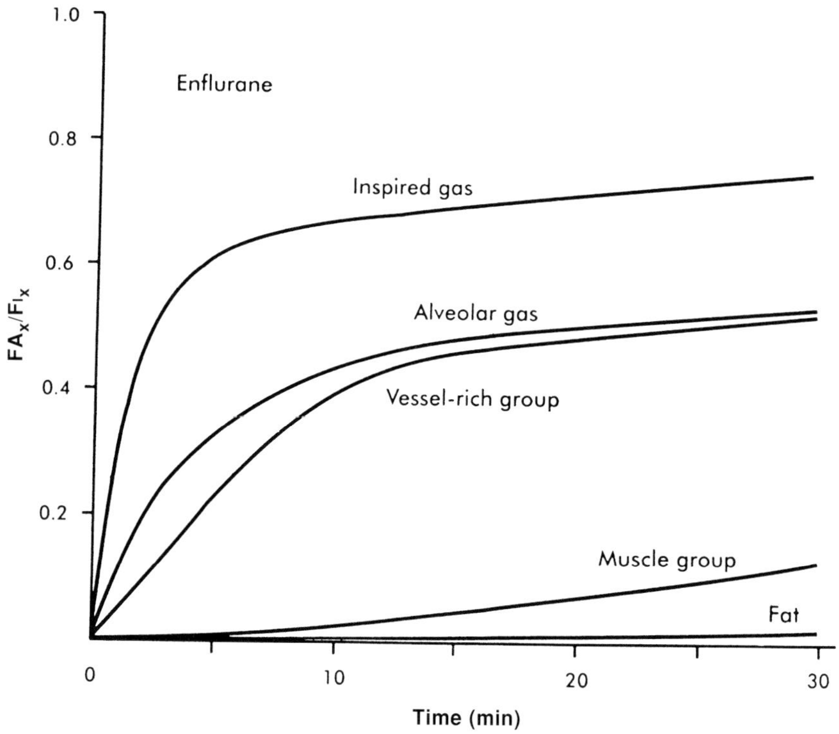

Fig. 9-7. A comparison of anesthetic partial pressures in body compartments for enflurane over time. The vessel-rich group lags behind alveolar concentration for about the first 10 minutes of administration. The muscle group lags behind substantially more, and does not reach even 10% of the fresh gas concentration of enflurane until about 30 minutes after induction. Reprinted with permission from Longnecker DE, Miller FL. Pharmacology of inhalational anesthetics. In: Rogers MC, Tinker JH, Covino BG, Longnecker DE. *Principles and Practice of Anesthesiology*. St. Louis, Mo: Mosby–Year Book; 1993: 1063.

essentially, as follows: if one gas is taken up in high concentrations by the blood, then any other gas associated with the first gas may be similarly affected. This has implications regarding alveolar oxygen, which can be increased when high concentrations of nitrous oxide are administered. The phenomenon may also be seen in reverse, especially with nitrous oxide, if a diffusion anoxia occurs at the termination of anesthesia. If nitrous oxide has been used, hypoxia can be avoided by providing the patient with oxygen for several minutes at the conclusion of the operation.

Minimal Alveolar Concentration

The understanding of the potency of the inhaled anesthetic agents during their clinical administration was made conceptually simpler by the introduction of the term MAC in 1965.[51] MAC was defined as the minimal alveolar concentration (in volume percent of atmosphere) of an anesthetic that prevented movement in 50% of subjects in response to a noxious stimulus. Although it was originally defined in terms of volume percent, the relevant unit for MAC is actually partial pressure. This unit is most important when anesthetics are administered under hyperbaric or hypobaric conditions and has been introduced earlier in this chapter. The MAC for each agent is not static and may vary with the age of the patient, extremes of physiology, the environment (eg, temperature), and the effects of drugs or alcohol. The addition of drugs such as narcotics or sedatives lowers inhalational MAC requirements to prevent patients from responding to the noxious stimulus of a surgical incision. Conceptually, MAC parallels the median effective dose (ED_{50}) that has been described for other pharmacological agents. Since most clinicians would prefer that fewer than 50% of patients respond to a surgical stimulus, the term anesthetic depth (AD_{95}) is used to describe the MAC of an anesthetic agent at which 95% of patients do not respond. A total dose of approximately 1.3 MAC prevents movement in nearly all patients during surgery.[52] The MAC and AD_{95} for each of the inhalational agents are found in Table 9-1. In addition, other values such as MAC-awake (the concentration at which awareness returns) have been described. A very useful and important concept of MAC is that MACs are additive and may also be proportionally substituted. In other words, inhalational agents may be added to one another, and their combined MACs are equal to that of a single agent. This concept is commonly used clinically when 70% nitrous oxide (0.66 MAC) is combined with another potent inhalational agent such as 0.74% isoflurane (0.64 MAC) in oxygen to administer a total dose of 1.3 MAC (0.66 MAC + 0.64 MAC = 1.3 MAC).

MAJOR ORGAN SYSTEM EFFECTS OF THE POTENT INHALED AGENTS

Although there is no one perfect anesthetic agent, an ideal one would have the characteristics listed in Exhibit 9-1. Until the perfect anesthetic agent can be produced, the potent inhalational agents—halothane, enflurane, isoflurane, desflurane, and sevoflurane—provide the major components needed in a single, complete anesthetic agent: analgesia, amnesia, hypnosis, and relaxation of skeletal muscles. Unfortunately, all the potent inhaled agents alter normal organ-system physiology. For the sake of simplicity, only the effects of the first three potent agents on major organ systems will be discussed, and those briefly.

The Respiratory System and the Carbon Dioxide–Response Curve

Control of respiration is mediated by the medulla and the pons. Inspiration and expiration are modulated within the medulla at the dorsal respiratory group and the ventral respiratory group, respectively. In the pons, the pneumotaxic center regulates the rate and pattern of respiration and the apneustic center theoretically has a feedback loop to the dorsal respiratory group to affect maximal inspiration. The physiological goal is to maintain oxygen, carbon dioxide, and hydrogen ion concentration (clinically represented as blood pH) in normal ranges, and the feedback for these parameters is accomplished by chemoreceptors within the medulla that are in close relationship with the cerebral spinal fluid. The inspiratory centers are sensitive to changes in pH and concentrations of carbon dioxide. If the alveolar ventilatory response is plotted against carbon dioxide concentration and pH, a response curve can then be constructed (Figure 9-8). A decrease in the PO_2 will increase the slope of the curve, while a state of acidosis will shift the curve to the left without a change in slope.

The administration of halothane, enflurane, or isoflurane will cause a dose-dependent decrease in the ventilatory response to carbon dioxide, with enflurane tending to be the most potent in this regard. This is graphically expressed by a decreased slope of the carbon dioxide–response curve without a shift to either the left or the right. Clinically, in the patient who is spontaneously breathing a potent inhalational agent at a surgical plane, the $PaCO_2$ should be in the range of 50 to 55 mm Hg. A reaction to surgical stimulation may lower this response by 4 to 5 mm Hg. The addition of a narcotic to a potent inhalational anesthetic technique will further depress and shift to the right the slope of the carbon dioxide–response curve.

EXHIBIT 9-1

CHARACTERISTICS OF AN IDEAL INHALATIONAL ANESTHETIC AGENT

Absence of flammability

Easily vaporized at ambient temperature

Low blood solubility (rapid induction and recovery from anesthesia)

Minimal metabolism

Compatible with epinephrine

Produces skeletal muscle relaxation

Suppresses excessive sympathetic nervous system response

Not irritating to airways

Absent or minimal myocardial depression

Absence of cerebrovascular dilation

Absence of hepatic and renal toxicity

The Central Nervous System

The clinical endpoint of the potent inhalational anesthetic agents is a dose-related, reversible depression or excitation of brain function that results in the anesthetized state. This change in CNS function is associated with alterations in cerebral metabolic rate for oxygen ($CMRO_2$), CBF, EEG changes, and somatosensory (SSEP) and motor evoked potentials (MEP). In the normal brain, CBF and $CMRO_2$ enjoy a proportionally coupled relation that does not usually change independently. Under inhalational anesthesia with the potent volatile agents, there appears to be an uncoupling of the normal CBF:$CMRO_2$ ratio with increasing anesthetic doses. It is important to realize that this effect is seen only when cerebral vascular autoregulation is intact and normal intracranial blood pressure ranges (50–150 mm Hg) are maintained. An increase in cerebral vasodilation with increased CBF results in a decrease in $CMRO_2$. This effect is diminished or abolished with decreasing blood pressure. The effect is

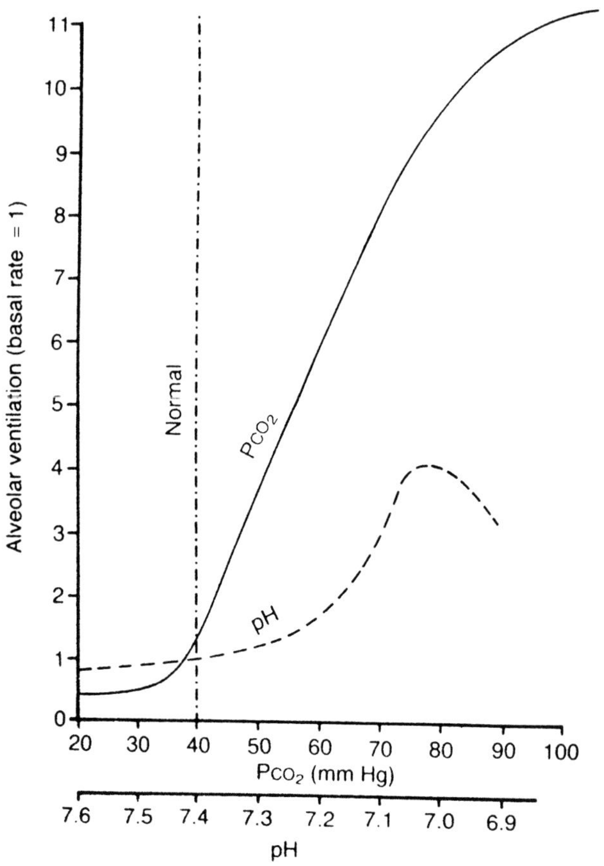

Fig. 9-8. The effects of increased arterial P_{CO_2} and decreased arterial pH on the rate of alveolar ventilation. Reprinted with permission from Guyton AC. *Textbook of Medical Physiology*. 8th ed. Philadelphia, Pa: WB Saunders; 1991: 447

also blunted by an increase in the amount of hypocapnia produced. Therefore, the cerebral vasodilation caused by the volatile anesthetic agents can be attenuated by hypocapnia, although these responses may not be operative in the injured brain. Of the three inhalational agents under discussion, halothane is the most potent cerebral vasodilator, followed by enflurane and isoflurane. The main problem associated with increased CBF is that the cerebral volume is increased, with a resultant increase in ICP. Critical CBF (cCBF) has been defined as the flow at which ipsilateral EEG changes indicative of cerebral ischemia are seen.[53] In the presence of halothane, the cCBF is 18 to 20 mL/100 g/min; for enflurane, it is 15 mL/100 g/min; and for isoflurane, 10 mL/100 g/min.

At clinically useful concentrations, halothane cannot cause an isoelectric EEG. While decreasing CMR_{O_2} may be beneficial, especially in the setting of an isoelectric EEG, halothane has been associated with dangerously low levels of CMR_{O_2} that may reflect cerebral toxicity. Enflurane has been associated with seizure activity at 1.5 to 2 MAC concentrations, with a resultant 50% increased CMR_{O_2}. On the other hand, isoflurane can cause an isoelectric EEG that is associated with a 50% reduction in CMR_{O_2}. The effective recording of SSEPs is not abolished by concentrations of 0.5 to 0.75 MAC with any of the volatile agents. Data concerning the recording of MEPs during inhalational anesthesia are sparse, although MEPs appear to be hindered at clinical doses. Recent work concerning the successful recording of spinal evoked potentials (SpEP) in animals during 1.3 to 2.0 MAC halothane has entered the literature.[54]

The Cardiovascular System

All of the potent, volatile anesthetic agents depress the cardiovascular system, but their hemodynamic effects differ. The clinical endpoint of cardiovascular depression is hypotension. Halothane's effect is due mainly to a decrease in myocardial contractility and rate, with minimal decrement in SVR. Enflurane causes both myocardial depression and decreased SVR, while isoflurane's effect is due mainly to its action on SVR. The newer agents can be expected to have an effect on the cardiovascular system similar to that of isoflurane. This depressive effect is dose related, and for any potent volatile anesthetic, the arterial blood pressure can be decreased by approximately 50% of baseline by the administration of 2 MAC of agent. Although halothane is associated with negative chronotropic effects, both enflurane and isoflurane may cause an increase in heart rate. This chronotropic effect may be related to halothane's impairing the baroreceptor function to a greater degree than enflurane or isoflurane, but studies with animals[55] indicate that while isoflurane may depress both vagal and sympathetic function, vagal depression predominates, leading to a noticeably increased heart rate. This positive chronotropic effect with isoflurane is seen especially in younger patients but tapers off after age 40. Cardiac output is decreased—due mainly to a decreased stroke volume—by halothane and enflurane (minimally by isoflurane). All of the aliphatic hydrocarbon anesthetic agents sensitize the myocardium to circulating catecholamines; this effect is greatest for halothane and least for isoflurane. Because of its vasodilating effects, isoflurane has been implicated theoretically in the phenomenon of coronary steal in dogs, but this effect has not been proven clinically in human subjects.[56]

The Hepatic System

Because of its high metabolic rate, the liver is a highly vascular organ; it receives 25% of the cardiac output. The blood supply consists of two parallel circulations: the hepatic artery supplies fully oxygenated blood at high pressure, and the low-pressure portal vein supplies partially desaturated blood from the splanchnic bed. Owing to this unique anatomical arrangement, the hepatic cells adjacent to the hepatic venules are very susceptible to hypoxia, and centrilobular necrosis can occur. Although autoregulation of total hepatic blood flow can be demonstrated during the metabolically active fed state in dogs, its presence in humans is controversial. Hepatic blood flow is subject to the effects of multiple hormones. The main determinants of hepatic compromise during inhalational anesthesia are related to diminished total hepatic blood flow, which is primarily due to decreases in cardiac output and mean arterial blood pressure. Halothane is more closely associated with these decrements in total hepatic blood flow, cardiac output, and blood pressure than is isoflurane, and although the data are limited, enflurane appears to be similar to halothane.[57] Hepatic oxygen supply–demand ratios are better preserved by isoflurane than by halothane.[58] Other factors that may compromise total hepatic blood flow include (*a*) an operative site near the liver and (*b*) the use of controlled ventilation with high peak pressures and positive end-expiratory pressures, which causes an increase in hepatic venous pressure. The metabolism of drugs with a high extraction ratio is affected by decreased total hepatic blood flow. Finally, transient elevations of liver function tests sometimes occur following anesthesia, but owing to the enormous reserve of the liver, the significance of these elevations is not known and possibly may be related to a surgical site close to the hepatic bed.

The Renal System

The potent inhalational anesthetic agents usually have an adverse impact on renal function due to the secondary effects of the altered cardiovascular, endocrine, and sympathetic nervous systems. The main determinants of an adverse renal outcome are decreased cardiac output and blood pressure. These effects on the renal system are typically transient in nature and resolve spontaneously once the anesthetic action has been terminated. The main key to preventing these altered physiological effects is the maintenance of an adequate preoperative state of hydration. All the potent inhalational agents in use today are fluorinated to some degree, and there is some concern that inorganic fluoride released during their oxidative dehalogenation during hepatic metabolism can cause a primary renal injury. Renal injury from this cause is rarely seen clinically. Owing to the way it is metabolized, enflurane can theoretically place the kidney at the most risk for fluoride toxicity, although a recent clinical study[59] did not support this contention. Interestingly, the metabolism of sevoflurane, the newest halogenated agent, is associated with increased serum fluoride levels and may again open this issue to further discussion and investigation.

ANESTHESIA IN THE FIELD

It is impossible to predict the nature of deployments. The most reasonable assumption is that most military anesthesia in the future will take place in the DEPMEDS environment of ISO (International Standards Organization) shelters and TEMPER (***t***ents, ***e***xtendable, ***m***odular, ***per***sonnel) tents. However, reasonable alternative possibilities range from the marked austerity of draw-over devices in shelters of opportunity to the sophistication of servo-mechanism ventilators in modern, host-nation, fixed facilities. Most anesthesiologists routinely use a balanced anesthetic technique in their peacetime practice, and it should be possible to use this same method in the vast majority of field environments.

Currently, the U.S. Army stocks two devices for delivering inhaled anesthetic agents, the Ohmeda Portable Anesthesia Circuit (PAC) and the Ohmeda Model 885A field anesthesia machine (both manufactured by Ohmeda, Inc., Madison, Wis.), in its DEPMEDS inventory. The Ohmeda PAC is a draw-over device, and the 885A is an anesthesia machine based on flow-over technology. Neither apparatus is supplied with a ventilator, although many field hospitals do carry small ventilators as separate items of operating room equipment. Until recently, little or no training was provided on either apparatus. However, the teaching protocol for the draw-over device is now being implemented at selected medical centers, and a protocol for the 885A is being developed (see also Chapter 2, Combat Anesthesia Overview, and Chapter 7, Military Anesthesia Machines). Military anesthesia providers should at least read about these two devices before they deploy. The draw-over device is simple, but its unfamiliarity may cause the inexperienced anesthesiologist some concern. The 885A is an actual anesthesia machine and may appear more familiar than the PAC to the unpracticed eye, but it, too, has dangers associated with its operation. The 885A is capable of delivering hypoxic mixtures of nitrous oxide and oxygen, and the ambient temperature in the operating room can drastically affect the output of the vaporizer. These two design problems can lead to lethal hypoxic mixtures.[60]

Both halothane and isoflurane are available through the medical logistics system. As a general rule, if the logistical support necessary for surgery is available, the support will also be sufficient to perform the usual anesthetic methods. More than anything else, the condition of the patient will dictate the anesthetic technique. For example, if routine surgery is being done on children as part of a civil action program, an inhalational technique might be selected. On the other hand, some casualties with traumatic injuries will be severely hypovolemic and will not be able to tolerate any anesthetic at all until the hemorrhage is controlled and volume and red blood cell mass restored. A common practice in these latter cases is to begin the procedure with oxygen, a muscle relaxant, and scopolamine (as an amnestic agent), and then carefully titrate small increments of inhaled agents as the casualty's vital signs begin to improve. In other words, anesthetic practice in the field will usually closely resemble the balanced techniques prevalent in peacetime practice.

SUMMARY

Inhalational anesthetic agents are the most important drugs in the pharmacopoeia of both military anesthesia providers and civilian practitioners. It is, therefore, not a little odd that their mechanism of action remains imperfectly understood. Although there is clear evidence that anesthetic potency correlates with lipid solubility, the physical basis for this observation is unknown. It is unlikely to be due to a generalized expansion of the lipid membrane that is caused by the presence of a large volume of the inhalational agent, which thereby prevents normal function of ionic channels. More likely explanations are that inhalational agents either (*a*) perturb the normal, ordered structure of the bilipid membrane or (*b*) reversibly alter lipids in contact with proteins in ionic channels; both changes interfere with membrane excitability. There is less doubt about the *site* of action of inhalational anesthetics: this is at the neural synapse rather than at the axon.

Presently used inhalational agents fall into two categories: the alkanes, such as halothane, and the ethers, such as enflurane and isoflurane. Halothane is more potent and less irritating to the airway than more recently developed inhalational agents, has the propensity to sensitize the myocardium to epinephrine, and may cause severe hepatotoxicity (in isolated instances). Enflurane, although less potent than halothane, has fewer of the potential side effects of the latter. Isoflurane is notable for its ease of administration, lack of serious hepatotoxicity, and minimal biotransformation with fluoride-ion production. Isoflurane is associated with dose-dependent hypotension that is solely mediated by a decrease in systemic vascular resistance and not by myocardial depression.

The amount of inhalational anesthetic agent that is delivered to a patient can be expressed as a percentage of the total gas volume delivered or as a partial pressure of the total gas pressure. The solubility of an anesthetic agent can be expressed as a partition coefficient, which is essentially the ratio of the solubilities for two media. The solubility of anesthetic agents in the blood and tissues determines how much drug uptake is required across the alveolar membrane to increase the partial pressure of the anesthetic agent in the brain, the ultimate target organ for anesthetic agents. Major factors can delay anesthetic uptake to the brain, including the use of an agent with a high solubility, a state of increased cardiac output, and a large gradient between the partial pressures of alveolar and mixed-venous blood. The amount of inhalational agent required is quantitated as the MAC, and is measured as the partial pressure.

Inhalational agents have the potential to cause major organ dysfunction outside the CNS. Depression of the respiratory and cardiovascular systems is to be expected. The liver and kidneys are at risk from decreased blood flow and, in rare instances, devastating agent-induced toxicity.

The administration of inhalational agents in deployed hospitals requires a special understanding of the characteristics of the agents because they will be administered by draw-over and flow-over technologies. Halothane and isoflurane are available in DEPMEDS-equipped hospitals.

REFERENCES

1. Dripps RD, Eckenhoff JE, Vandam LD. *Introduction to Anesthesia: The Principles of Safe Practice.* 6th ed. Philadelphia, Pa: WB Saunders; 1982: 101–115.
2. Meyer HH. The theory of narcosis. *Harvey Lect.* 1906;99:11.
3. Overton CE; Lipnick RL, trans-ed. *Studies of Narcosis.* New York, NY: Chapman and Hall, and Park Ridge, Ill: Wood Library-Museum of Anesthesiology; 1991.
4. Taheri S, Halsey MJ, Liu J, Eger EI II, Koblin DD, Laster MJ. What solvent best represents the site of action of inhaled anesthetics in humans, rats, and dogs. *Anesth Analg.* 1991;72:627–634.
5. Ferguson J. The use of chemical potentials as indices of toxicity. *Proc R Soc Lond Biol.* 1939;127:387–404.
6. Miller KW, Firestone LL, Alifimoff JK, Streicher P. Nonanesthetic alcohols dissolve in synaptic membranes without perturbing their lipids. *Proc Natl Acad Sci USA.* 1989;86:1084–1087.
7. Miller KW, Paton WD, Smith EB, Smith RA. Physiochemical approaches to the mode of action of general anesthetics. *Anesthesiology.* 1972;36:339–351.
8. Kendig JJ, Trudell JR, Cohen EN. Halothane stereoisomers: Lack of stereospecificity in two model systems. *Anesthesiology.* 1973;39:518–524.
9. Franks NP, Lieb WR. Stereospecific effects of inhalational general anesthetics optical isomers on nerve ion channels. *Science.* 1991;254:427–430.
10. Johnson FH, Flagler EA. Hydrostatic pressure reversal of narcosis in tadpoles. *Science.* 1951;112:91.
11. Lever MJ, Miller KW, Paton WD, Smith EB. Pressure reversal of anesthesia. *Nature.* 1971;231:368–371.
12. Dobson BA, Furmaniuk ZW, Miller KW. The physiological effects of hydrostatic pressures are not equivalent to those of helium pressure on *Rana pipiens. J Physiol (Lond).* 1985;362:233–238.
13. Kendig JJ. Anesthetics and pressure in nerve cells. In: Fink BR, ed. *Molecular Mechanisms of Anesthesia.* Vol 2. In: *Progress in Anesthesiology.* New York, NY: Raven Press; 1982.
14. Trudell JR. A unitary hypothesis of anesthesia based on lateral phase separations in nerve membranes. *Anesthesiology.* 1977;46:5–14.
15. Kita Y, Bennett L, Miller KW. The partial molar volumes of anesthetics in lipid bilayers. *Biochim Biophys Acta.* 1981;647:131–139. Cited by: Miller KW. The nature of the site of general anesthesia. *Int Rev Neurobiol.* 1985;27;51.
16. Kita Y, Miller KW. Partial molar volumes of some 1-alkanols in erythrocyte ghosts and lipid layers. *Biochemistry.* 1982;21:2840–2847. Cited by: Miller KW. The nature of the site of general anesthesia. *Int Rev Neurobiol.* 1985;27;51.
17. Franks NP, Lieb WR. Is membrane expansion relevant to anaesthesia? *Nature.* 1981;292:248–251. Cited by: Miller KW. The nature of the site of general anesthesia. *Int Rev Neurobiol.* 1985;27;51.

18. Trudell JR, Hubbell WL, Cohen EN, Kendig JJ. Pressure reversal of anesthesia: The extent of small-molecule exclusion from spin-labeled phospholipid model membranes. *Anesthesiology*. 1973;38(3)207–211.

19. Pang KYY, Miller KW. Cholesterol modulates the effect of membrane perturbers in phospholipid vesicles and biomembranes. *Biochim Biophys Acta*. 1978;511:1–14.

20. Chin JH, Trudell JR, Cohen EN. The compression-ordering and solubility-disordering effects of high pressure gases on phospholipid bilayers. *Life Sciences*. 1977;18:489–498.

21. Miller KW. The nature of the site of general anesthesia. *Int Rev Neurobiol*. 1985;27:1–61.

22. Franks NP, Lieb WR. Selective actions of volatile general anaesthetics at molecular and cellular levels. *Br J Anaesth*. 1993;71:65–76.

23. Terrar DA. Structure and function of calcium channels and the actions of anaesthetics. *Br J Anaesth*. 1993;71:31–46.

24. Franks NP, Lieb WR. Do general anaesthetics act by competitive binding to specific receptors? *Nature*. 1984;310:599–601.

25. Alifimoff JK, Miller KW. Mechanism of action of general anesthetic agents. In: Rogers MC, Tinker JH, Covino BG, Longnecker DE. *Principles and Practice of Anesthesiology*. St. Louis, Mo: Mosby–Year Book; 1993: 1034–1052.

26. Fraser DM, Louro SR, Horvath LI, Miller KW, Watts A. A study of the effect of general anesthetics on lipid-protein interactions in acetylcholine receptor enriched membranes from *Torpedo nobiliana* using nitroxide spin-labels. *Biochemistry*. 1990;29:2664–2669.

27. Longnecker DE, Miller FL. Pharmacology of inhalational anesthetics. In: Rogers MC, Tinker JH, Covino BG, Longnecker DE. *Principles and Practice of Anesthesiology*. St Louis, Mo: Mosby–Year Book; 1993: 1053–1086.

28. Krnjevic K. Cellular mechanisms of anesthesia. *Ann N Y Acad Sci*. 1991;625:1–16.

29. Calverley RK, Smith NT, Prys-Roberts C, Eger EI II, Jones CW. Cardiovascular effects of enflurane anesthesia during controlled ventilation in man. *Anesth Analg*. 1978;57:619–628.

30. Seyde WC, Longnecker DE. Anesthetic influences on regional hemodynamics in normal and hemorrhaged rats. *Anesthesiology*. 1984;61:686698.

31. Eger EI II. Isoflurane: A review. *Anesthesiology*. 1981;55:559–576.

32. Hirshman CA, McCullough RE, Cohen PJ, Weil JV. Depression of hypoxic ventilatory response by halothane, enflurane and isoflurane in dogs. *Br J Anaesth*. 1977;49:957–963.

33. Clark DL, Rosner BD. Neurophysiologic effects of general anesthetics, I: The electroencephalogram and sensory evoked responses in man. *Anesthesiology*. 1986;38:564.

34. Sakai T, Takaori M. Biodegradation of halothane, enflurane, and methoxyflurane. *Br J Anaesth*. 1978;50:785–791.

35. Stevens WC, Cromwell TH, Halsey MJ, Eger EI II, Shakespeare TF. The cardiovascular effects of a new inhalational anesthetic, Forane, in human volunteers at constant arterial carbon dioxide tension. *Anesthesiology*. 1971;35:8–16.

36. McPherson RW, Briar JE, Traystman RJ. Cerebrovascular responsiveness to carbon dioxide in dogs with 1.4% and 2.8% isoflurane. *Anesthesiology*. 1989;70:843–850.

37. Eintrei C, Lezniewski W, Carlsson C. Local application of ^{133}Xenon for measurement of regional blood flow (rCBF) during halothane, enflurane, and isoflurane anesthesia in humans. *Anesthesiology*. 1985;63:391–394.

38. Newberg LA, Michenfelder JD. Cerebral protection by isoflurane during hypoxemia or ischemia. *Anesthesiology*. 1983;59:29–35.

39. Conzen PF, Hobbhahn J, Goetz AE, et al. Splanchnic oxygen consumption and hepatic surface oxygen tensions during isoflurane anesthesia. *Anesthesiology*. 1988;69:643–651.

40. Gelman S. General anesthesia and hepatic circulation. *Can J Physiol Pharmacol*. 1987;65:1762–1779.

41. Mazze RI, Cousins MJ, Barr GA. Renal effects and metabolism of isoflurane in man. *Anesthesiology*. 1974;40:536–542.

42. Holaday DA, Fiserova-Bergerova V, Latto IP, Zumbiel MA. Resistance of isoflurane to biotransformation in man. *Anesthesiology*. 1975;43:325–332.

43. Pagel PS, Kampine JP, Schmeling WT, Warltier DC. Comparison of the systemic and coronary hemodynamic actions of desflurane, isoflurane, halothane, and enflurane in the chronically instrumented dog. *Anesthesiology*. 1991;74:539–551.

44. Lutz LJ, Milde JH, Milde LN. The cerebral functional, metabolic, and hemodynamic effects of desflurane in dogs. *Anesthesiology*. 1990;73:125–131.

45. Bernard JM, Wouters PF, Doursout MJ, Florence B, Chelly JE, Merlin RJ. Effects of sevoflurane and isoflurane on cardiac and coronary dynamics in chronically instrumented dogs. *Anesthesiology*. 1990;72:659–662.

46. Conzen PF, Vollmar B, Habazettl H, Frink EJ, Peter K, Messmer K. Systemic and regional hemodynamics of isoflurane and sevoflurane in rats. *Anesth Analg*. 1992;74:79–88.

47. Kochi T, Izumu Y, Isono S, Ide T, Mizuguchi T. Breathing pattern and occlusion pressure waveform in humans anesthetized with halothane or sevoflurane. *Anesth Analg*. 1991;73:327–332.

48. Frink EJ Jr, Ghantous H, Malan TP, et al. Plasma inorganic fluoride with sevoflurane anesthesia: Correlation with indices of hepatic and renal function. *Anesth Analg*. 1992;74:231–235.

49. Frink EJ, Malan TP, Isner RJ, Brown EA, Morgan SE, Brown BR. Renal concentrating function with prolonged sevoflurane or enflurane anesthesia in volunteers. *Anesthesiology*. 1994:80:1019–1025.

50. Hornbein TF, Martin WE, Bonica JJ, Freund FG, Parmentier P. Nitrous oxide effects on the circulatory and ventilatory responses to halothane. *Anesthesiology*. 1969;31:250–260.

51. Eger EI II, Saidman LJ, Brandstater B. Minimum alveolar anesthetic concentration: A standard of anesthetic potency. *Anesthesiology*. 1965;26:756–763.

52. Stoelting RK, Miller RD. *Basics of Anesthesia*. 2nd ed. New York, NY: Churchill Livingstone; 1989: 17.

53. Michenfelder JD. *Anesthesia and the Brain*. New York, NY: Churchill Livingstone; 1988.

54. Mongan PD, Peterson RE, Williams D. Spinal evoked potentials are predictive of neurologic function in a porcine model of aortic occlusion. *Anesth Analg*. 1994;78:257–266.

55. Skovsted P, Sapthavichaikul S. The effects of isoflurane on arterial pressure, pulse rate, and autonomic nervous activity and barostatic reflexes. *Can Anaesth Soc J*. 1977;24:304–314.

56. Sill JC, Bove AA, Nugent M, Blaise GA, Dewwy JD, Grabau C. Effects of isoflurane on coronary arteries and coronary arterioles in the intact dog. *Anesthesiology*. 1987;66:273–279.

57. Gelman S, Dillard E, Bradley EL Jr. Hepatic circulation during surgical stress and anesthesia with halothane, isoflurane, or fentanyl. *Anesth Analg*. 1987;66:936–943.

58. Gelman S, Fowler KC, Smith LR. Liver circulation and function during isoflurane and halothane anesthesia. *Anesthesiology*. 1984;61:726–730.

59. Mazze RI. Anesthesia and the renal and genitourinary systems. In: Miller RD, ed. *Anesthesia*. 3rd ed. New York, NY: Churchill Livingstone; 1990: 1791.

60. Perkins DE. Colonel, Medical Corps, US Army. Personal communication, April 1995.

Chapter 10

INTRAVENOUS ANESTHESIA

DONALD J. FOX, M.D.*; LISA D. SAUNDERS, M.D.†; EMIL J. MENK, M.D.‡; AND ROBERT MIDDAUGH, M.D.§

*Formerly, Major, Medical Corps, U.S. Army; Anesthesia and Operative Service, Department of Surgery, Brooke Army Medical Center, Fort Sam Houston, Texas 78234-6200; currently, Chief, Department of Anesthesia, Mercy Medical Center, 1512 12th Avenue Road, Nampa, Idaho 83686

†Formerly, Major, Medical Corps, U.S. Army; Anesthesia and Operative Service, Department of Surgery, Letterman Army Medical Center, Presidio of San Francisco, California 94129-6700; currently, Staff Anesthesiologist, Stanford Medical Center, 300 Pasteur Drive, Stanford, California 94305

‡Formerly, Lieutenant Colonel, Medical Corps, U.S. Army; Chief, Anesthesia and Operative Service, Department of Surgery, Brooke Army Medical Center, Fort Sam Houston, Texas 78234-6200; currently, Staff Anesthesiologist, Presbyterian Hospital, 200 Hawthorne Lane, Charlotte, North Carolina 28204

§Formerly, Major, Medical Corps, U.S. Army Reserve; Anesthesia and Operative Service, Department of Surgery, Brooke Army Medical Center, Fort Sam Houston, Texas 78234-6200; currently, Staff Anesthesiologist, St. Vincent Infirmary Medical Center, 2 St. Vincent Circle, Little Rock, Arkansas 72205

INTRODUCTION

Delivering safe and effective anesthesia to casualties with combat injuries presents unique challenges to military trauma anesthesiologists. These casualties may have sustained severe injuries involving significant blood loss and varying degrees of shock. They will be in pain and emotional distress, and possibly suffering from sequelae of prolonged transport such as inadequate ventilation, hypothermia, uncorrected hypovolemia, in any combination. They may have full stomachs, which places them at risk for pulmonary aspiration during general anesthesia.

Certain other conditions in the field further complicate the anesthetic management of these difficult patients. For one, casualties may arrive en masse, exceeding the ability of a small medical staff to provide scrupulous individual monitoring. In these situations, relatively untrained personnel may be required to achieve airway patency and hemodynamic stabilization in the perioperative period. Likewise, recovery care after anesthesia may be marginal. As for the course of the anesthetic itself, bulky and elaborate anesthesia equipment may not be available or practical at the site of combat casualty surgery. In particular, apparatus for the delivery of compressed gases such as oxygen may pose logistical problems.

Ideally, then, an anesthetic approach for combat casualty care should have the following characteristics: preservation of airway reflexes with minimal hemodynamic effects; ease of delivery, which would allow for management by relatively unskilled practitioners; and a minimal requirement for unwieldy or complex anesthetic delivery systems. Unfortunately, no anesthetic technique meets all of these requirements, although many approaches have been used with varying degrees of success in the battlefield setting. Among these are general anesthesia using simple gas-delivery systems, regional techniques, and intravenous anesthesia with or without supplementary inhaled agents. A full discussion of the first two methods is presented in Chapter 8, Closed-Circuit Anesthesia; Chapter 9, Inhalational Anesthesia; and Chapter 12, Regional Anesthesia. In general, their use dictates a significant level of skill on the part of the practitioner, particularly in dealing with hypotension, which is a sequela of both regional and general anesthesia, and from the loss of airway reflexes that ensue from general anesthesia with volatile agents.

Intravenous anesthetic agents are advantageous in the field for many reasons. Transportability and technical ease of administration are excellent. Many of these drugs are able to rapidly induce a state of surgical anesthesia. This is particularly important in traumatized soldiers, as experience has shown most to have full stomachs at the time of injury.[1] To prevent the aspiration of regurgitated material into the lungs, a rapidly induced state of unconsciousness is necessary to facilitate endotracheal intubation and airway protection. With careful use, these drugs will also allow early awakening and extubation of the trachea, shortening stays in the recovery area. Residual analgesia is a benefit with some intravenous agents. These drugs can also be used to supplement inhalational anesthetic agents, providing balanced anesthesia. Some intravenous anesthetic agents can be used as the sole or primary agents for the maintenance of surgical anesthesia by means of an initial bolus followed by continuous infusion. This technique adds a degree of controllability to the duration of action of the anesthetic and reduces the total amount of drug administered, allowing the anesthesia provider to have an awake patient at the end of the case. Such a patient will be easier for recovery area personnel to deal with than an overly sedated or unconscious patient. Indeed, recovery room personnel may be in very short supply or extremely busy. As the patient may receive relatively little attention during this period, recovery time is best kept to a minimum.[2]

INTRAVENOUS ANESTHETIC AGENTS FOR BATTLEFIELD ANESTHESIA

Complete surgical anesthesia, when properly administered, provides amnesia, analgesia, unconsciousness, and muscle relaxation. The ideal anesthetic drug would induce such a state of surgical anesthesia rapidly, be quickly reversible, maintain hemodynamic stability, and be nontoxic to the patient. There is no drug available today that, when used alone, satisfies all of these criteria. However, the intravenous drugs we will discuss in this chapter each provide one or more component parts of the ideal (ie, complete) anesthetic regimen.

Much of the initial anesthetic care of combat casualties consists of the vigorous resuscitation of hemorrhagic shock. It is likely that many of these injured soldiers would not survive the physiological effects of the sudden imposition of a complete anesthetic, which could compound the hemodynamic instability seen with hypovolemic shock states. Careful selection and meticulous titration of anesthetic agents, whether inhalational or intravenous, usually become feasible only as resuscitative efforts progress. Failure to recognize and adequately treat hypovolemic shock before the induction of anesthesia can convert a casualty to a fatality. Indeed, the careless use of thiopental in hypovolemic patients after the Japanese attack at Pearl Harbor on 7 December 1941 caused a large number of intraoperative deaths and led some anesthesiologists to criticize its use in war casualties.[3] It is clear in retrospect that many of the anesthesia providers involved were unfamiliar with the proper use of this agent. It is also clear that volume resuscitation was inadequate in these cases. Thiopental was subsequently used with good success throughout the remainder of World War II,[4–8] the Korean and Vietnam wars,[1] the Falklands War,[9] and remains a valuable anesthetic drug today when properly administered. The intravenous anesthetic and adjuvant drugs currently available have a broad spectrum of effects, indications, and contraindications (Table 10-1). Each of the agents described in this chapter has unique advantages and disadvantages for the anesthetic management of wartime casualties. The anesthesia provider must be able to assess the clinical situation in each case and select the best anesthetic technique and agents for the casualty.

For some short surgical procedures, one or two intravenous bolus injections of anesthetic agent may be all that is required for patient comfort. For very minor procedures, a subanesthetic dose may be sufficient for analgesia, sedation, and anxiolysis. Subanesthetic doses are also useful for supplementing regional anesthetic techniques. Disadvantages of many of the intravenous anesthetic agents include the possibility of overdosage, with resultant respiratory depression or arrest. Mechanical ventilators may not be available at battlefield hospitals.[2] Because the patient's metabolism of the drug is required for these drugs' termination of action, anesthesia-recovery personnel may be forced to commit themselves to one-on-one care for such patients until they are once again breathing on their own. Intravenous

TABLE 10-1

PHARMACOLOGICAL EFFECTS OF VARIOUS INTRAVENOUS ANESTHETIC AGENTS

Agent	Onset	Duration	Loss of Consciousness	Analgesia	Amnesia
Barbiturates					
Thiopental	Rapid	Ultra-short	Yes	Anti*	Yes
Methohexital	Rapid	Ultra-short	Yes	Anti	Yes
Benzodiazepines					
Diazepam	Slow	Long	High-dose	None	Yes
Midazolam	Intermediate	Intermediate	High-dose	None	Yes
Narcotics					
Morphine	Slow	Long	High-dose	Yes	+/–†
Meperidine	Slow	Long	High-dose	Yes	+/–
Fentanyl	Intermediate	Intermediate	High-dose	Yes	+/–
Sufentanil	Intermediate	Intermediate	High-dose	Yes	+/–
Alfentanil	Rapid	Short	Yes	Yes	+/–
Ketamine	Rapid	Short	Yes	Yes	Yes
Etomidate	Rapid	Short	Yes	No	Yes
Propofol	Rapid	Ultra-short	Yes	No	Yes
Scopolamine	Rapid	Long	No	No	Yes

*Pain perception is increased
†The effect may or may not be present

anesthetic techniques, while technically simple, tend to be less forgiving of error than inhalational techniques. Constant vigilance and attention to detail are mandatory when these drugs are used.

Military medical planners have noted that the limiting factor in performing surgery in the field may be the number of personnel who are trained to administer anesthesia.[2] It is recognized that many military physicians and nurses who have had minimal exposure to anesthesiology as a specialty will have to be trained on the job to deliver a safe anesthetic. Simplicity, technical ease of administration, and the relatively high margins of safety of many of the intravenous anesthetic drugs will permit such personnel to deliver safe anesthesia to combat casualties.

USEFUL DRUGS FOR THE INDUCTION OF ANESTHESIA

When induction of general anesthesia is necessary in casualties with traumatic injuries, two properties of an anesthetic drug are of primary importance. The first is whether the selected drug can be expected to cause serious depression of the patient's cardiovascular system. The patient may be severely hypovolemic from blood loss, exposure, or other causes. The choice of an induction agent must therefore take into account the victim's volume status and degree of hemodynamic compromise. The second important factor in the choice of an induction agent is the rapidity of onset of unconsciousness following intravenous injection. Because soldiers injured on the battlefield nearly always present for treatment with a full stomach,[1] the airway must be rapidly protected with an endotracheal tube to prevent aspiration of gastric contents into the bronchopulmonary tree. A drug with a long onset time will therefore expose the patient to greater anesthetic risk.

Agents that are useful for induction of anesthesia are presented below, grouped by drug type.

Barbiturates

Intravenous barbiturates produce central nervous system depression ranging from mild sedation to coma, depending on the dosage given. The two barbiturates most commonly used to induce anesthesia are sodium thiopental (Pentothal, manufactured by Abbott Laboratories, North Chicago, Ill.) and methohexital (Brevital, manufactured by Eli Lilly and Co., Indianapolis, Ind.). These agents rapidly produce a state of unconsciousness and amnesia without significant analgesia.

Pharmacology

Thiopental is usually prepared as a 2.5% mixture (25 mg/mL), while methohexital is made up as a 1% solution (10 mg/mL). Unconsciousness occurs within seconds following intravenous bolus and lasts for approximately 3 to 5 minutes. Clinical recovery from methohexital is slightly faster than from thiopental.

The brief clinical effect seen after intravenous bolus of these drugs is not due to metabolism, but rather to redistribution of agent from the brain and other vessel-rich organs to less metabolically active compartments. However, multiple doses or continuous infusions may result in slow recovery, owing to protein binding and the slow release of drug from muscle and fatty tissues.[10]

Physiological Effects

Central Nervous System. The barbiturate anesthetic agents induce a state of hypnosis and amnesia. However, they tend to reduce the patient's pain threshold (ie, the *antalgesic* effect), with a resultant significant increase in heart rate and blood pressure during painful or stimulating procedures.[11]

Cerebral metabolic rate is markedly reduced following a dose of a barbiturate drug, which, in turn, causes cerebral vasoconstriction. This effect, in turn, results in decreased cerebral blood volume and reduced intracranial pressure. Cerebral perfusion may improve, as intracranial pressure falls to a greater extent than the mean arterial pressure in normovolemic patients.[11] These effects are very beneficial in the patient with a closed head injury. In addition, the barbiturates are potent anticonvulsant agents.

Cardiovascular System. The principal hemodynamic effects of the barbiturates are a decrease in contractility and an associated increase in heart rate. Dose-dependent decreases in arterial blood pressure, stroke volume, and cardiac output are seen. The mechanisms for the decrease in cardiac output include (1) direct negative inotropic effect on the myocardium, (2) decreased ventricular filling owing to increased venous capacitance, and (3) transiently decreased sympathetic outflow from the central nervous system.[11]

Respiratory System. The barbiturates are potent central nervous system depressants. As a consequence of these effects, they produce profound respiratory depression. This is first seen as a decrease in tidal volume, followed by apnea. Positive-pressure ventilation will be necessary following the usual induction doses of both thiopental and methohexital.

Clinical Use and Contraindications

Both sodium thiopental and methohexital are safe induction agents in the normovolemic casualty whose cardiac function is not compromised. Usual induction doses are 4 mg/mL for thiopental or 1 mg/mL for methohexital (Table 10-2). Although these agents are not the drugs of first choice in trauma patients, experience has shown that they may also be used safely in such cases, provided that the dosages are adjusted downward.[4–6] Easy intubating conditions are generally obtained within 60 seconds when given with succinylcholine for rapid-sequence induction (which is discussed later in this chapter). Thiopental (or methohexital) may also be administered as a continuous infusion following an initial bolus (Table 10-3). This allows a state of surgical anesthesia to be maintained for extended periods. However, these agents accumulate in the tissues when used in this manner, and recovery from anesthesia may be prolonged.

Extreme caution should be used in the hypovolemic casualty or one with cardiac compromise such as tamponade. In general, barbiturates should be avoided as induction agents in these casualties until the hypovolemic state or the cardiac tamponade is corrected.

TABLE 10-2

SUGGESTED DOSE RANGES FOR INTRAVENOUS INDUCTION OF ANESTHESIA

	Casualty's Resuscitation Status	
Agent	Normovolemic (Dose)	Hypovolemic (Dose)
Sodium Thiopental	2–4 mg/kg	1–2 mg/kg
Ketamine	1–2 mg/kg	0.5–1.0 mg/kg
Etomidate	0.2–0.4 mg/kg	0.1–0.2 mg/kg
Methohexital*	0.5–1.0 mg/kg	0.25 mg/kg
Midazolam*	0.15–0.3 mg/kg	0.075–0.15 mg/kg
Alfentanil	100–200 µg/kg	not known

*Will cause prolonged sedation and respiratory depression

TABLE 10-3

DRUG DOSES FOR CONTINUOUS INTRAVENOUS INFUSION TECHNIQUES

Agent	Loading Dose	Infusion Rate
Ketamine	1.0–2.0 mg/kg	20–50 µg/kg/min
Etomidate	0.2–0.4 mg/kg	40–100 µg/kg/min for 10 min, then 10–40 µg/kg/min
Thiopental	2.0–4.0 mg/kg	0.1 mg/kg/min
Propofol	2.0–2.5 mg/kg	0.1–0.2 mg/kg/min
Alfentanil	100–200 µg/kg*	0.5–2.5 µg/kg/min

*30–40 µg/kg when combined with thiopental

Etomidate

Etomidate (Amidate, manufactured by Abbott Laboratories, North Chicago, Ill.) is an imidazole compound that is chemically unrelated to any other intravenous anesthetic agent. It is a potent sedative and hypnotic agent with rapid onset and recovery, and its use is associated with excellent cardiovascular and respiratory stability in the normovolemic patient.[12]

Pharmacology

As with the barbiturates, etomidate is rapidly distributed to the brain and other vessel-rich groups following intravenous injection. Termination of clinical action occurs as the agent is redistributed away from these highly perfused organs.[13] Etomidate's distribution half-life is in the 2- to 4-minute range. The drug is cleared from plasma 5-fold faster than is thiopental. Etomidate is prepared as a 2% solution (20 mg/mL).

Physiological Effects

Central Nervous System. Intravenous injection causes a rapid, dose-dependent depression of the central nervous system. As with the barbiturates, etomidate is a potent anticonvulsant agent. This anticonvulsant effect lasts significantly longer than its hypnotic and anesthetic effects. In common with the barbiturates, etomidate also causes a significant reduction in the cerebral metabolic rate, with associated cerebral vasoconstriction[14] and decreased intracranial pressure. Cerebral perfusion pressure is not altered appreciably.

Cardiovascular System. In normovolemic patients, etomidate causes no significant changes in heart rate or cardiac output.[12] A slight fall in systemic blood pressure may be noted, secondary to a mild decrease in peripheral vascular resistance. However, in the trauma patient suffering from hypovolemic shock, serious hypotension may result from usual induction doses of etomidate due to suppression of sympathetic nervous system outflow.

Respiratory System. Etomidate is a potent central nervous system depressant. As a consequence of these effects, it produces dose-related respiratory depression. Respiratory rate and tidal volume are affected, although the magnitude is less than that produced by the barbiturate anesthetic agents.[11] Positive-pressure ventilation will be necessary either after an induction dose or during continuous infusions for maintenance of general anesthesia.

Clinical Use and Contraindications

The usual dose range for induction is 0.2 to 0.4 mg/kg (see Table 10-2). The clinical duration of a single bolus injection is 3 to 12 minutes.

Psychomotor recovery is intermediate between that of thiopental and methohexital. Short surgical procedures may be done using etomidate, maintaining anesthesia with repeated, small boluses or continuous infusion (see Table 10-3). Following a bolus injection of 0.2 to 0.4 mg/kg, a continuous infusion can be set up to flow at a rate of 40 to 100 µg/kg/min (20–40 µg/kg/min if nitrous oxide is being used, although nitrous oxide is not available in deployable hospitals). After the initial 10 minutes of infusion, the rate should be reduced to 10 to 40 µg/kg/min. (Many anesthesiologists would supplement this infusion technique with a potent opioid such as fentanyl, since etomidate is an incomplete anesthetic, ie, it provides no analgesia).

Prudence would dictate a reduction in drug dose for induction of anesthesia during the resuscitative phase of shock (ie, in the acutely traumatized battlefield casualty). A good starting dose would be 0.1 mg/kg, titrating more agent as the patient's condition allows.

Two characteristics of etomidate make it useful for anesthesia in the traumatized patient[11]:

- Relative hemodynamic stability; this is most important when the casualty is hypovolemic (eg, in hemorrhagic shock).
- Its effect on the central nervous system; by decreasing intracranial pressure and cerebral metabolic rate while preserving stable hemodynamic parameters, etomidate may prove to be the agent of choice for anesthetic induction in the hemodynamically unstable trauma patient with a head injury.

Relatively minor drawbacks to the use of etomidate include the following[11]:

- Venous irritation; etomidate is dissolved in propylene glycol, giving rise to pain or irritation or both on intravenous injection in some patients. This side effect can be reduced somewhat by prior administration of an opioid drug such as fentanyl.
- Myoclonus; this centrally mediated effect is frequently observed. It is not indicative of awareness, and is not harmful to the patient, per se. Once again, these movements may be reduced by pretreating the patient with an opioid drug.
- Postanesthetic nausea and vomiting; this side effect may be seen in up to 40% of patients on emergence from anesthesia with etomidate, is probably centrally mediated, and may be reduced in incidence if an antiemetic drug such as droperidol is given.
- Adrenocortical suppression; this effect lasts from 6 to 8 hours and is probably not clinically significant unless prolonged or large total doses are administered. Suppression of adrenal steroid production may predispose critically ill patients to sepsis.

Propofol

Pharmacology

Propofol (Diprivan, manufactured by Stuart Pharmaceuticals, Wilmington, Del.) is a recently introduced intravenous anesthetic agent. It rapidly produces unconsciousness following bolus injection, with a time course on onset and recovery very similar to that of thiopental and methohexital. Propofol is completely insoluble in aqueous solution and is therefore administered in a lecithin-based emulsion. Because this emulsion is a very favorable medium for bacteria, strict aseptic technique should accompany its use. The drug is extremely lipid soluble, a property that allows it to cross the blood–brain barrier very quickly. Clinical experience has shown that less residual postoperative sedation and psychomotor impairment follow administration of propofol, and side effects such as nausea and vomiting are uncommon.[15]

Physiological Effects

As do the barbiturates, propofol causes dose-dependent cardiac and respiratory depression.[11,12,15] The magnitude of these effects is similar to those seen with thiopental. Propofol has no analgesic properties but, in contrast to thiopental, neither does it appear to have an antalgesic effect.

Clinical Usage and Contraindications

Induction of anesthesia is achieved with a propofol dose of 1.5 to 3.0 mg/kg (see Table 10-2). Unconsciousness occurs less than 1 minute following an intravenous bolus, and lasts from 4 to 8 minutes. The drug is redistributed and eliminated very rapidly. A continuous infusion or repeated, small-bolus injections may be used to maintain a surgical plane of anesthesia. The drug does not accumulate in the tissues to a clinically significant degree and thus is better suited to continuous-infusion techniques than the barbiturates or etomidate. Recovery is characterized by rapid emergence from anesthesia and minimal postoperative confusion.[15] A continuous infusion may be used following an induction dose of 2.0 mg/kg (see Table 10-3). The infusion rate is titrated to the desired effect, with a usual dose range of 0.1 to 0.2 mg/kg/min (6.0–12.0 mg/kg/h); in critically ill or debilitated patients, the dosage regimen may be halved. This technique is enhanced by the addition of an opioid drug or nitrous oxide for analgesia.

Propofol's greatest advantage over other intravenous anesthetic agents is its relatively rapid elimination from the body. This may diminish the degree of hangover seen after continuous infusions or repeated boluses of the barbiturates and etomidate, and could potentially shorten time spent in the recovery area.[16]

Ketamine

Pharmacology

In the field, the aim of the military anesthesia provider is to deliver the minimum level of anesthesia necessary to provide adequate surgical depth, thereby assuring a rapidly resolving anesthetic state. Ketamine was developed through investigation of phencyclidine (PCP) and cyclohexamine, both of which provide profound anesthesia accompanied by intolerable psychotomimetic effects.[17] Ketamine resembles these drugs structurally, but it delivers sedation, analgesia, and surgical anesthesia with much milder psychic side effects.

The administration of ketamine produces an unusual clinical state called *dissociative* anesthesia (ie, the patient does not move specifically in response to noxious stimuli[18]). Some researchers[19] have postulated that ketamine depresses central nervous system centers that are crucial to the transmission of the emotional component of pain signals from the spinal cord to the higher centers. Others[20,21] believe that ketamine may work through direct suppression of spinal cord activity or by an action on opiate receptors throughout the central nervous system.

Ketamine has a rapid onset of action attributable to its high lipid solubility, and a short duration of action owing to redistribution out of the central nervous system. These features make it very similar to the barbiturate induction agents such as sodium thiopental. When ketamine is administered intravenously, peak plasma levels are achieved in 1 minute, while peak plasma levels following an intramuscular dose are reached by 15 minutes after the injection. Anesthetic effects last approximately 10 to 15 minutes, and analgesia may last as long as 4 hours. The elimination half-life of ketamine from the peripheral tissues is 2 to 3 hours. Therefore, despite the swift termination of its hypnotic effects after an initial injection, prolonged sedation may ensue from repeated doses or infusions. The development of tolerance to ketamine may occur following repeated exposures.

Does ketamine meet the requirements for combat casualty anesthesia? Certainly, it is an extremely useful agent in this setting. Among its many valuable attributes, ketamine

- is nonlabile in solution and easily transported in powdered form, and can be delivered intravenously or intramuscularly;
- provides a rapid, smooth induction to surgical depth anesthesia, as well as an acceptably brief interval to termination of its sedative effects;
- is a profound analgesic, unlike other nonnarcotic intravenous anesthetic agents; and
- allows the patient's stable cardiovascular and respiratory physiology to be maintained, with consequent preservation of blood pressure and airway reflexes.

This last point is probably the most significant. However, this is not meant to imply that a patient under ketamine anesthesia can be left unattended, since apnea, airway obstruction, aspiration of gastric contents, and hypotension may still be seen. Rather, the use of ketamine allows the administration of general anesthesia by relatively unskilled personnel with an increased margin of safety when compared to other, more conventional methods. While not an ideal situation, this may be unavoidable in times of war. On the negative side, ketamine anesthesia has two major drawbacks in the battlefield setting:

- Time to full recovery is prolonged when the drug is used as a maintenance agent, compared with the inhaled anesthetics and many other intravenous drugs.
- The psychic phenomena accompanying emergence may be severe in young soldiers.

Nonetheless, it is clear that ketamine's unique characteristics make it an important tool for use in combat surgery.

Physiological Effects

Central Nervous System. Ketamine has potent analgesic actions. However, because of its unique nervous system effects, the administration of ketamine produces an anesthetic state unlike that of more traditional agents such as thiopental or the opioid narcotics. Thus, it can be difficult to assess anesthetic depth. When surgical anesthesia is achieved with ketamine, the patient's eyes may remain open and exhibit nystagmus as well as intact corneal and light reflexes. Myoclonus is observed frequently, as are actual purposeful movements that are not necessarily in response to painful stimuli. Even with very small doses of ketamine, patients may lose a sense of contact with their environment and an ability to think coherently. Nonetheless, with appropriate dosing, a trancelike state accompanied by profound anesthesia can be achieved, which allows surgery to proceed. A good approach to assessing the adequacy of anesthesia under ketamine is to aim for suppression of reaction to surgical stimulation.[22] In other words, the goal should not necessarily be a completely motionless patient but rather the dissociative state.[18]

An unfortunate aspect of ketamine's central nervous system effects is a phenomenon known as the *emergence* reaction. This refers to an altered mental state experienced by many patients on awakening from the drug, and is characterized by vivid dreams, floating or "out-of-body" sensations, disorientation, and hallucinations. Although these feelings usually end on full awakening, some patients may experience flashbacklike sensations as late as several weeks after receiving ketamine.[17] Frequently they are very disturbing to the patient. The incidence of emergence reactions is on the order of 5% to 30%.[17,23] Predisposing factors include age older than 16 years, female gender, a history of emotional problems, and a history of an active dream life. This phenomenon also occurs more commonly when ketamine is given rapidly, in relatively large intravenous doses, and when atropine or droperidol are given as premedicants. Finally, many anesthesiologists believe that psychic disturbances are exacerbated by a noisy or otherwise stimulating environment.

The most effective prophylaxis against emergence reactions appears to be the concomitant use of a benzodiazepine drug.[24,25] These drugs are useful either as premedicants or when administered during the course of an operation. When ketamine is used solely as an induction agent, followed by maintenance of anesthesia with other drugs, emergence reactions are virtually unheard of in cases lasting longer than 45 minutes.[23] Some investigators[17] suggest preoperative and postoperative counseling regarding possible psychic phenomena as a very effective means for reducing their incidence.

Cardiovascular System. Ketamine causes dose-related increases in arterial blood pressure and heart rate. These effects are believed to derive from direct sympathetic stimulation. Heart rate, blood pressure, and cardiac output are increased, with variable effects on stroke volume and systemic vascular resistance. These effects make ketamine a very valuable drug for the induction of anesthesia in patients who are suffering from hypovolemic shock.[17]

In addition to sympathetically mediated cardiac stimulation and vasoconstriction, ketamine has been shown to dilate vascular smooth muscle and to depress myocardial function by direct actions.[26] If the sympathetic nervous system is depressed by anesthetic or other drugs, or if the patient is critically ill, a bolus injection of ketamine may cause profound cardiovascular collapse. Ketamine-induced direct myocardial depression and peripheral vasodilation are usually effectively masked by its sympathomimetic actions. In the absence of a fully functioning autonomic nervous system, the predominant cardiovascular effect of ketamine is to depress cardiac function.[11] At least one authority[26] has observed decreases in cardiac performance following the use of ketamine in the setting of acute trauma, but most investigations of the cardiostimulatory effects of ketamine in the presence of hemorrhagic shock have shown a significant increase in both systolic and diastolic blood pressure.[26–28] Cardiovascular stimulation may be attenuated by inhaled anesthetic agents, sodium thiopental, or premedication with a benzodiazepine.[17,29]

Respiratory System. In contrast to the narcotics and barbiturates, ketamine preserves the respiratory response to carbon dioxide.[17] Decreases in the partial pressures of oxygen in arterial blood (Pa_{O_2}) are modest and transient at commonly used doses. Significant respiratory depression occurs when ketamine is given rapidly in high doses.

Ketamine is known to produce bronchial smooth-muscle relaxation, which increases pulmonary compliance in patients with bronchoconstriction.[17] Tracheopharyngeal reflexes are maintained to a greater extent than with other commonly used induction agents, but pulmonary aspiration of gastric contents may occur at even relatively low doses. Finally, salivation is markedly increased on administration of the drug.[30,31]

Relative to other intravenous agents, the effects of ketamine on the respiratory system increase its margin of safety in the field setting. It maintains respiratory drive in the spontaneously ventilating patient, minimizes airway reactivity, and preserves airway-protective reflexes, at least in part. However, this in no way obviates the need for skilled airway management, as respiratory depression or tracheal soiling or both are still possible, particularly when the casualty is not only acutely traumatized but also in a chaotic setting.

Contraindications

Based on the physiological effects just presented, several clinical conditions constitute contraindications to the use of ketamine. As mentioned, since postanesthetic emergence reactions are a troublesome side effect, ketamine probably should not be used when there is preexisting psychopathology.

Ketamine raises intracranial pressure by increasing cerebral blood flow and systemic blood pressure.[11] Likewise, intraocular pressure is increased. Ketamine is therefore contraindicated in casualties who have closed head or penetrating eye injuries, and in all other situations where intracranial or intraocular pressure is raised.

Clinical Use

Ketamine is available in a variety of strengths, most commonly 10 mg/mL, 50 mg/mL, and 100 mg/mL. The usual intravenous induction dose is 1 to 2 mg/kg. (The intramuscular dose for induction of anesthesia is 5–10 mg/kg). Following an intravenous induction dose, ketamine is rapidly distributed to the brain and other vessel-rich groups in a manner analogous to that of thiopental. For short surgical cases, repeated boluses of one half the induction dose may be administered at appropriate intervals as needed. As an alternative to this technique, a solution of 0.1% ketamine may be prepared (1 mg/mL) and a continuous infusion maintained at a rate of 25 to 50 µg/kg/min.

Termination of ketamine's action is due to redistribution (the distribution half-life is 7–11 min) and hepatic metabolism. The elimination half-life is 2 to 3 hours. Effective analgesia is possible with subanesthetic bolus doses of ketamine (0.25 to 0.5 mg/kg).

Initial enthusiasm for ketamine as a possible single-agent, total, intravenous anesthetic has waned somewhat as actual field trials have demonstrated its inadequacies. For example, experiences with ketamine in the Falkland Islands and Southeast Asia have yielded mixed results. In Cambodia, British anesthetists have used ketamine as a sole agent for superficial procedures and brief minor surgeries, but they reported prolonged recovery times, particularly when benzodiazepines were used as a prophylaxis against emergence reactions. In addition, they noted rare laryngospasm and other airway compromise.[32] During the Falklands War, total intravenous anesthesia was employed with success in operations of short duration not involving the body cavity. For more major surgeries in patients in hypovolemic shock, ketamine was recommended as an induction agent and adjunct to maintenance with halothane. In the cases described using this technique, recovery time was not appreciably prolonged despite the routine administration of diazepam at the end of the procedures. Emergence phenomena were not an issue.[33] The consensus drawn from these two experiences is that ketamine delivers adequate anesthesia only for peripheral procedures and when used with a benzodiazepine to prevent postoperative delirium.

In the large majority of cases, airway reflexes were preserved. While supplemental inhaled agents were deemed necessary for casualties who required intraabdominal surgery, total intravenous anesthesia was used successfully for over one half of the casualties who presented to this group of anesthesia providers, owing to the superficial nature of the surgeries involved. Therefore, with a few provisos, it would appear that ketamine as a sole agent is a feasible anesthetic for many situations encountered in wartime.

A marked improvement in outcome was achieved through the introduction of an infusion technique, which reduces the total administered ketamine dose. Two large series[25,34] describing both minor and major abdominal procedures under continuous ketamine infusion report minimal prolongation of recovery time, with favorable respiratory and cardiovascular effects. Nitrous oxide and muscle relaxants were used, as was diazepam. Very encouraging work has been done by anesthetists in South Africa who have used a ketamine infusion with only muscle relaxation and oxygen-enriched room air for major abdominal cases.[35] A critical feature of their work was the use of a benzodiazepine as the induction agent, which served to prevent emergence phenomena but also prolonged the recovery phase. The clear advantage of such a technique to field anesthesia is that the need to transport compressed gas could be reduced or eliminated by maintaining anesthetized casualties on room air.

Minor Procedures and Transport. Ketamine can be used in a wide range of situations encountered in a field hospital. It probably is most effective in providing anesthesia for peripheral or surface procedures. For minor operations such as debridement, incision and drainage, and delayed primary closure, ketamine may be delivered as a bolus of 0.25 to 1.0 mg/kg, administered intravenously, or 1 to 4 mg/kg, administered intramuscularly. These doses are also appropriate for analgesia during transport. Airway reflexes and respiratory drive generally remain intact in this dose range. Repeat doses may be required at 5- to 15-minute intervals. Another approach is to administer a continuous infusion of 5 to 20 µg/kg/min throughout the procedure. A similar dosage schedule is appropriate for analgesia during transport. Benzodiazepines in small doses will attenuate psychic disturbances, although these are seldom significant with low-dose ketamine.[17,33,36]

For minor surgery such as superficial soft-tissue debridement or brief genitourinary or general surgery, general anesthesia can be accomplished using ketamine 2 mg/kg intravenously or up to 10 mg/kg intramuscularly. Repeat doses may be titrated to abolish purposeful movements or nystagmus. Care must be taken to monitor airway adequacy at these doses, and supplemental oxygen is prudent. However, this technique still represents a relatively safe approach to general anesthesia in a setting where skilled personnel and elaborate equipment or compressed gases may not be available. Emergence reactions will pose a problem at these doses, and administration of a benzodiazepine will necessitate more expert and vigilant care of the airway. Recovery time may take up to 45 minutes or longer, especially if other anesthetic agents are used. Recovery from low-dose ketamine should be well under 30 minutes.[25,37]

Major Procedures. In patients suffering from hypovolemia, severe anemia, or cardiovascular compromise, ketamine is an excellent choice for an induction agent.[23,28] While most intravenous induction agents cause hypotension, ketamine generally will preserve blood pressure and cardiac output in casualties in hypovolemic shock. Doses for induction of anesthesia are in the range of 1 to 2 mg/kg intravenously or 4 to 6 mg/kg intramuscularly, with decreased doses as appropriate when the patient is severely ill or in profound shock. Ketamine is suitable for use in patients with full stomachs, with the usual precautionary measures such as application of cricoid pressure and preoxygenation. In the previously healthy, normovolemic patient, ketamine induction may result in undesired blood pressure elevation.

Ketamine can be used to maintain surgical anesthesia for major intraabdominal or intrathoracic cases in combination with inhaled agents, particularly when hypotension limits the dosage of the latter. Following induction, ketamine may be administered intravenously at 15- to 30-minute intervals, as needed, in boluses of 0.5 to 2.0 mg/kg. The patient breathes a low dose of a volatile agent delivered via a field anesthesia machine or similar equipment, or the agent is given via positive-pressure ventilation as necessary. If available, nitrous oxide may be used to supplement ketamine maintenance. A benzodiazepine administered during the operation will reduce the incidence of postoperative delirium.[17]

Alternatively, a continuous ketamine infusion will maintain surgical anesthesia.[38–40] Use in combination with another agent will minimize the total ketamine dose. Usually, 10 to 30 µg/kg/min with 50% to 70% nitrous oxide or a background volatile agent will be sufficient. Again, a benzodiazepine is recommended. An antisialagogue such as atropine or glycopyrrolate will minimize salivation and upper-airway secretions.

Total Intravenous Anesthesia With Ketamine. Finally, when compressed gases are not available, ketamine can act as the primary agent in a total intravenous anesthetic for major operations. The best results have been obtained using a benzodiazepine for induction, followed by intubation using a muscle relaxant, and then initiation of a ketamine infusion (see Table 10-3) in the range of 20 to 40 µg/kg/min, with controlled ventilation on air or oxygen-enriched air, as available. Although this technique has been used successfully for abdominal surgery with little postoperative psychic disturbance, recovery time is likely to be prolonged.[35] In the injured casualty in hypovolemic shock, induction is probably more safely achieved using ketamine rather than a benzodiazepine.

Ketamine for Pediatric Anesthesia. The treatment of combat casualties includes the care of civilians, among whom may be injured children. Ketamine has long been a mainstay in pediatric anesthesia, and it adapts well for use in the field. In a child, an intramuscular dose of 5 to 10 mg/kg will provide surgical anesthesia that will last from 10 to 30 minutes. Lower doses may provide adequate sedation for brief, minor procedures. A sedating intravenous dose would be 0.25 to 0.5 mg/kg. Production of significant upper-airway secretions accompanies the use of this agent in children and necessitates the use of an anticholinergic drug (eg, atropine or glycopyrrolate). Although airway reflexes and respiratory drive are generally well preserved, close attention must be paid to adequacy of ventilation, as is done in any case of general anesthesia or deep sedation. The incidence of postoperative psychic disturbances in children is thought to be lower than that in adults.[17,23]

ANXIOLYTIC AND AMNESTIC AGENTS

Anxiety and fear are very common in the preoperative patient, and even more so in wounded soldiers. Severe anxiety may cause significant tachycardia, hypertension, and increased respiratory rate. Oxygen consumption and carbon dioxide production are increased. Such patients may also be uncooperative, irrational, or combative. Finally, serious psychic trauma may occur in some patients due to their recall of events in the operating room—during resuscitative efforts or surgery or both. In addition to the humane considerations, physiological benefits can be attained if the casualty's fear and anxiety are reduced. The agents discussed in the following section have proven useful for producing amnesia to both preoperative and intraoperative events, and some are potent anxiolytics as well. In high doses, some of these agents have a hypnotic effect and may be used to induce an anesthetic state.

Benzodiazepines

The drugs of this class that are most likely to see clinical use during wartime are diazepam (Valium, manufactured by Roche Products, Inc., Manati, Puerto Rico) and midazolam (Versed, manufactured by Roche Laboratories, Nutley, N.J.).

Pharmacology

All the benzodiazepine drugs possess similar anxiolytic, sedative, hypnotic, amnestic, anticonvulsant, and muscle-relaxant properties.[11] While the pharmacodynamics (ie, what the drug does to the body) of diazepam and midazolam are very similar, their pharmacokinetics (ie, what the body does to the drug) are quite different.

Diazepam has a distribution half-life of 30 to 60 minutes and an elimination half-life of 20 hours or more. Its primary metabolite is active and has an elimination half-life of 41 to 139 hours. The clinical effects of an intravenous diazepam dose are seen within 1 to 2 minutes and last from 1 to 3 hours, with widely variable individual responses.

Midazolam is water soluble, more potent than diazepam, and has no active metabolites.[41] Distribution half-life is 7 to 15 minutes, and elimination half-life is 2 to 4 hours. Its higher potency and shorter duration of clinical action make midazolam particularly attractive in situations where a benzodiazepine drug is indicated.

Physiological Effects

Central Nervous System. Diazepam and midazolam are potent anxiolytics, acting on the centers in the central nervous system that generate fear, anxiety, and aggression. In addition to reducing anxiety, these drugs provide excellent amnesia. In high doses, either drug can be used as an anesthetic induction agent (see Table 10-2), although their primary usefulness is as sedative or anxiolytic agents or both. Recovery from an induction dose of midazolam or diazepam is likely to take longer than is practical in a field hospital.

The benzodiazepines raise the seizure threshold. Thus they confer central nervous system protective effects to the patient who receives large (and potentially toxic) amounts of local anesthetic agent during regional anesthetic techniques, as well as to the patient with brain injury from head trauma.

Cardiovascular System. In otherwise healthy patients, minimal cardiovascular effects are seen with diazepam or midazolam.[11,41] Mean arterial pressure is typically decreased from 0% to 15%, and moderate increases in heart rate are seen when midazolam is used (0.15 mg/kg administered intravenously over 15 s) for induction of anesthesia. This is considerably less hypotension than is routinely seen when sodium thiopental is used as an induction agent. When midazolam is given in a dose of 0.3 mg/kg, hemodynamic changes are similar to those seen with thiopental at a dose of 4.0 mg/kg. Compared with diazepam, midazolam produces a greater decrease in blood pressure, and a slightly greater decrease in systemic vascular resistance.[42]

Combining other anesthetic drugs with diazepam or midazolam in a healthy patient may cause more hemodynamic depression than either agent used alone. In patients with no preexisting heart disease, combining benzodiazepines with narcotics is necessary to prevent hemodynamic changes associated with laryngoscopy and intubation.[41]

Respiratory System. An induction dose of midazolam significantly reduces the ventilatory response to carbon dioxide and produces respiratory depression. This effect has a slower onset and lasts longer than that obtained with thiopental.[43]

Continual vigilance and monitoring will be required in the trauma patient who has received a benzodiazepine drug, particularly when other potent anesthetic drugs have been administered. Postoperative respiratory depression in such a patient is a very real danger. Death secondary to respiratory arrest is a preventable event when the patient is adequately monitored.

Clinical Use

Although diazepam may be used for induction of anesthesia (at a dose range of 0.5–1.0 mg/kg), its relatively prolonged clinical effects limit its clinical usefulness as a primary anesthetic agent. The drug is poorly soluble in aqueous solution and is supplied in an ethylene glycol carrier solution. This causes a troublesome stinging or burning sensation on injection, particularly with the relatively large doses needed for induction of anesthesia. The true usefulness of diazepam in wartime surgery is as an adjunct to other anesthetic agents and techniques, and in allaying anxiety in the perioperative period. Sedation and anxiolysis are achieved with diazepam by titrating to desired effect, with a typical total dose range of 5 to 10 mg.

Because of its rapid onset of action and relatively short duration of action (60–90 min following an induction dose), midazolam can be used as an alternative to the barbiturates for induction of anesthesia for surgery that is expected to last 2 hours or longer. The dose is 0.15 to 0.3 mg/kg when used for this purpose. When surgery lasts less than 60 to 90 minutes, the anesthesia provider can expect to see significant postoperative respiratory depression with this induction regimen. When titrated to effect with 0.5 to 1.0 mg intravenous boluses, midazolam is an excellent anxiolytic and produces profound amnesia, making it a useful agent in the patient receiving a regional anesthetic technique.

As has already been mentioned, ketamine frequently causes vivid dreaming, nightmares, hallucinations and other emergence phenomena. The incidence of these undesirable effects is significantly reduced when a benzodiazepine is administered concomitantly. A useful regimen is diazepam 0.15 mg/kg administered intravenously 5 minutes prior to induction with ketamine. Midazolam 0.075 mg administered intravenously may be used in place of diazepam. Since ketamine has proven to be a very popular field anesthetic agent during recent conflicts, the benzodiazepine drugs will no doubt be useful adjuncts to its use.

Scopolamine

Scopolamine is a naturally occurring drug, obtained from plants of the belladonna family. Other drugs in this class include atropine and glycopyrrolate (Robinul, manufactured by A. H. Robins Co., Richmond, Va.). All of these agents will reduce salivation and upper airway secretions. Scopolamine possesses unique features that make it useful in trauma anesthesia.

Physiological Effects

Central Nervous System. Scopolamine crosses the blood–brain barrier and depresses the central nervous system. In therapeutic doses (0.4 mg administered intravenously), it causes drowsiness, euphoria, amnesia, fatigue, and dreamless sleep. Scopolamine is 9-fold more potent than atropine as an amnestic agent. (Another antimuscarinic agent, glycopyrrolate, does not cross the blood–brain barrier. This makes it useful when parasympathetic inhibition is desirable but the potential central nervous system effects of scopolamine are not).

Cardiovascular System. Drugs with antimuscarinic effects inhibit the actions of acetylcholine on the postganglionic cholinergic nerves of the parasympathetic nervous system, and thus reduce or inhibit parasympathetic tone. This is seen clinically as an increase in heart rate (usually lasting less than 30 min).

Clinical Use and Contraindications

The severely traumatized battlefield casualty is likely to be suffering from hemorrhagic shock. The nature of the wounds may dictate immediate surgery, even as the anesthesia team is resuscitating with airway management and intravenous fluid therapy. Because of adverse hemodynamic effects, it is unlikely that such a casualty would tolerate the administration of most of the intravenous anesthetic agents we have discussed in this chapter. Scopolamine (0.4 mg administered intravenously), with its minimal cardiovascular effects and its desirable amnestic qualities, may be the only safe anesthetic drug in this circumstance. As resuscitative efforts proceed and the patient's hemodynamic status stabilizes, additional anesthetic agents may be judiciously titrated.

The central nervous system effects of scopolamine are not absolutely reliable, and fully conscious patients may find them unpleasant. For this reason, use of this drug should be reserved for the severely traumatized and unstable patient, or in those cases where drying of upper airway secretions is desirable (eg, if the casualty requires nasal and oral surgical procedures). If they are available, atropine or glycopyrrolate are better choices for the latter indication.

Droperidol

Droperidol is a major tranquilizer of the butyrophenone class with antipsychotic activity and potent antiemetic effects.

Physiological Effects

Central Nervous System. Droperidol may be used in combination with an opioid narcotic to induce a state of neuroleptanalgesia or neuroleptanesthesia. Such states are characterized by altered awareness, sedation, and, ultimately, unconsciousness. During the state of neuroleptanalgesia, the patient remains conscious but may tolerate short, painful surgical procedures. Droperidol is also an excellent centrally acting antiemetic drug.

Cardiovascular System. Droperidol produces mild α-adrenergic blockade with peripheral vascular dilation. The resultant decrease in systemic vascular resistance is seen clinically as a fall in blood pressure. This effect may be very significant in the hypovolemic patient.

Clinical Use and Contraindications

The onset of action of droperidol occurs in 3 to 10 minutes following intravenous (75 µg/kg) or intramuscular (150 µg/kg) injection. The full effect may not be apparent for 30 minutes. With therapeutic doses, the duration of sedative effect is 2 to 4 hours, although alteration of consciousness may persist up to 12 hours. Additionally, intravenous doses greater than 100 µg/kg may result in prolonged postoperative somnolence.

When a neuroleptic technique is chosen, the opioid agent most commonly used with droperidol is fentanyl, generally in a ratio of 50 µg fentanyl per 2.5 mg droperidol. This combination is available premixed and is called Innovar (manufactured by Janssen Pharmaceutica Inc., Piscataway, N.J.). Nitrous oxide is frequently added to the neuroleptanalgesia regimen to induce unconsciousness and neuroleptanesthesia. The effects of droperidol last longer than the analgesic properties of fentanyl. The result may be a patient who is outwardly calm, yet is experiencing pain and mental agitation. A therapeutic dose for sedation (when used alone for this purpose) is 5 to 10 mg for a 70-kg individual.

Droperidol's undesirable effects on blood pressure in therapeutic doses, as well as its unpleasant and prolonged psychic effects, limit its usefulness as an anesthetic agent. However, the drug is a potent antiemetic in doses that cause minimal sedation (0.625–1.25 mg administered intravenously, which is 0.25–0.5 mL of the standard preparation). The awake patient with minimal postoperative anesthetic side effects (such as nausea and vomiting) will be the easiest to care for with the limited resources of the field hospital recovery room.

ANESTHETIC AGENTS THAT PRODUCE ANALGESIA

Analgesia is a very desirable attribute of an anesthetic agent. However, many of the commonly used intravenous anesthetic agents (including the barbiturates, etomidate, and propofol) have no analgesic properties. Analgesic drugs may be used in combination with agents that produce unconsciousness. The benefits of such combined regimens include maintenance of surgical anesthesia with reduced dosages of each drug, and residual postoperative pain relief. This chapter deals primarily with the opioid narcotic agents. However, it should be noted that ketamine, which is an extremely useful anesthetic-induction agent, provides very potent analgesia in small intravenous bolus doses (5–10 mg). Opioid narcotic agents are the most commonly used analgesics. The term *opioid* refers to compounds that bind to one or more subpopulations of opiate receptors in the central nervous system. Most anesthesiologists classify the opioid drugs on the basis of their primary effects at the opiate receptor site. This classification scheme results in three primary drug groups: the opioid agonists, the agonist–antagonists, and the antagonists. See Chapter 13, Perioperative Pain Management, for a discussion of the use of these agents purely for analgesia.

Opioid Agonist Drugs

The opioid agonist drugs commonly used intraoperatively (either to supplement or to provide the primary anesthetic) include morphine, meperidine, and the relatively recently discovered phenylpiperidine derivatives, namely, fentanyl, sufentanil, and alfentanil. While these agents differ in potency and pharmacokinetics, they share the important properties of dose-related analgesia as well as respiratory depression.[44]

Because the combat medical corpsman may be supplied with prefilled morphine syringes for prehospital field use, it is imperative that the preanesthetic evaluation of the patient should include whether the patient was medicated during or prior to transport to the field medical facility. Failure to ascertain the dose given may lead to the need for prolonged postoperative ventilatory support if additional morphine or other opioid agonists are given intraoperatively.

Physiological Effects

Central Nervous System. The opioid agonists produce analgesia, sedation, euphoria, and a feeling of body warmth. In the absence of pain, dysphoria rather than euphoria may be produced. Analgesia is most effective when administered prior to onset of the painful stimulus. Continuous, dull pain is relieved more effectively than sharp, intermittent pain. These effects are a result of drug interaction with opioid receptors in the brain and spinal cord. Another important effect of the opioids is stimulation of the central nervous system chemoreceptor trigger zone, producing nausea or emesis in many patients.[44]

Cardiovascular System. Direct stimulation of the medullary vagal nucleus may cause bradycardia following a dose of an opioid agonist.[44] Compensatory sympathetic nervous system responses are blunted, producing or contributing to orthostatic hypotension. Hypotension may also be seen secondary to morphine-induced histamine release.[45] This effect is widely variable, and can be mitigated somewhat by slow administration, supporting intravascular volume, slight head-down position, and prior administration of antihistaminic drugs. Meperidine also causes histamine release, but fentanyl and sufentanil do not.[45]

Meperidine is the only opioid drug with a direct myocardial depressant effect (when given in large doses). Also in contrast with the other opioid agonists, meperidine rarely causes bradycardia and may, in fact, be associated with tachycardia. This property probably reflects its structural similarity to atropine. Like morphine, meperidine may interfere with compensatory sympathetic nervous system reflexes. In analgesic doses, meperidine is associated with hypotension more commonly than is morphine.

The principal advantages of fentanyl (and its more recent analogs) are its maintenance of stable hemodynamics due to the absence of histamine release, the relative lack of direct myocardial depressant effects, and the suppression of the stress responses to surgery.

Respiratory System. All opioid agonists depress ventilation. This initially manifests clinically as a decreased rate of breathing with maintenance of tidal volume. With higher doses, tidal volume diminishes as well. Thus, a dose-related increase in the partial pressure of carbon dioxide in arterial blood ($Paco_2$) is seen. It is important to note, however, that morphine and other opioid agonists may actually lower $Paco_2$ values postoperatively in some patients who have been breathing with small tidal volumes because of pain. Pain is a natural antagonist to the respiratory depressant action of opioids.[44]

Respiratory depression in a casualty who has a closed head injury is particularly dangerous. Because opioid narcotic agents depress the ventilatory response to carbon dioxide, increased $Paco_2$ in the spontaneously breathing combat trauma victim will cause increased intracranial pressure with potentially lethal consequences when head injuries are present. Extreme caution must attend the use of opioid narcotics in such patients.

Respiratory depression is also a problem when these drugs are given in dosage ranges high enough to produce unconsciousness or surgical anesthesia. Because prolonged mechanical ventilatory support will generally be impossible in the austere environment of the combat support hospital, pure narcotic anesthetic techniques will not be useful. The utility of the narcotic drugs will be as adjuncts to inhalational or intravenous anesthetic techniques, using shorter-acting drugs that depress the respiratory system less as the primary anesthetic agents.

Morphine

Morphine is the classic opioid agonist. Intravenous administration of morphine produces a peak effect in about 20 minutes. This relatively slow onset reflects prolonged penetration of the blood–brain barrier by morphine, owing to its poor lipid solubility. The elimination half-life is approximately 2 hours and is largely dependent on excretion by the kidney following conjugation in the liver. A typical intraoperative dose, when morphine is used as an adjuvant agent for general anesthesia, is 0.1 to 0.2 mg/kg. The ideal dose will vary with the duration of the operation. Excellent and relatively prolonged postoperative analgesia generally results when this regimen is used. When morphine is used as the primary anesthetic agent, a dose of 1.0 to 2.0 mg/kg is necessary. The inability to provide adequate postoperative ventilatory support in the field medical environment severely limits the usefulness of the latter technique. Side effects include nausea, pruritus, and depressed ventilatory response to carbon dioxide. When morphine is used with other anesthetic agents, its respiratory depressant effects are augmented. This necessitates careful titration and monitoring in the operating room.

Meperidine

Meperidine (Demerol, manufactured by Sanofi Winthrop Pharmaceuticals, New York, N.Y.) is an older synthetic opioid agonist with one tenth the potency of morphine. Although it has been supplanted by newer and better synthetic drugs for intraoperative use in the United States, meperidine may prove to be readily available in third-world nations, and is still commonly used for analgesia outside the operating room. A typical intramuscular dose for postoperative pain is 1 to 2 mg/kg. If given via the intravenous route, this dose should be reduced by half. Precautions for intraoperative and postoperative meperidine use are similar to those for morphine.

Fentanyl

Fentanyl (Sublimaze, manufactured by Janssen Pharmaceutica Inc., Piscataway, N.J.) is a synthetic opioid agonist that is 100-fold more potent than morphine. It is supplied in a preparation of 50 µg/mL. Fentanyl has a faster onset and shorter duration of action than morphine. Potency and onset are related to the drug's high lipid solubility, and the shorter half-life reflects redistribution.[44] Like thiopental, repeated doses or continuous infusions saturate inactive tissue sites, interfering with the ability of redistribution to lower serum concentrations of the drug. The elimination half-life of fentanyl is 200 minutes, which is actually longer than that of morphine. This apparent contradiction is explained by both redistribution of drug from the active site and the greater volume of distribution of fentanyl. Serum concentration is partially maintained by slow re-uptake from inactive tissue sites.

Clinically, fentanyl has been popular in a wide range of doses. One to two micrograms per kilogram is a useful analgesic dose; 3 to 10 µg/kg is a useful dose range as an adjunct to other anesthetic drugs for induction or maintenance of anesthesia. Once again, prolonged postoperative respiratory depression severely limits the utility of this latter technique in most combat-support medical settings. If intraoperative mechanical ventilation is available, fentanyl may be administered with a continuous-infusion technique. Following a loading dose of 5 to 10 µg/kg (depending on the predicted length of the surgery), a continuous infusion is begun and maintained at 1 to 2 µg/kg/h. If the infusion is stopped 20 to 30 minutes prior to the completion of surgery, the patient will generally awaken promptly with excellent residual analgesia. Used in this manner, fentanyl augments the effects of the volatile anesthetic drugs, allowing the use of lower inspired concentrations of these agents. This technique should not be used unless the patient's respirations are controlled in the operating room.

The shorter duration of action of fentanyl (relative to morphine) allows greater ease of titration in the clinical setting. The absence of histamine release in clinically relevant doses results in less dilation of the venous capacitance vessels, producing less hypotension and a decreased need for temporary fluid supplementation.

Potential problems include persistent or recurrent respiratory depression. Fentanyl circulating in the plasma may be secreted into and sequestered by acidic gastric fluid, with subsequent reabsorption.

This reabsorbed fentanyl will once again act on the central nervous system. Fentanyl may also become trapped in poorly perfused areas of the lung during general anesthesia. Washout of these areas as perfusion improves would also tend to increase the plasma fentanyl level. Other potential problems are bradycardia, which may become hemodynamically significant in the traumatized patient, and truncal rigidity. The latter can make controlled ventilation of the patient quite difficult, necessitating the use of a neuromuscular blocking agent to relax the chest wall. The incidence and severity of both bradycardia and truncal rigidity appear to be related to the rate of administration, and each is readily managed with the appropriate pharmacological intervention.

Sufentanil

Sufentanil (Sufenta, manufactured by Janssen Pharmaceutica Inc., Piscataway, N.J.) is an analog of fentanyl, with an elimination half-life of approximately 156 minutes. Its anesthetic potency is estimated to be 5- to 10-fold greater that of fentanyl. This increased potency is a result of sufentanil's greater affinity for the opioid receptor.[46] The greater potency and more rapid onset of sufentanil make it a more titratable drug than fentanyl. This reduces the incidence and likelihood of tachycardia and hypertension in response to painful stimuli. Side effects and potential problems are the same as those seen with fentanyl.

Like fentanyl, sufentanil is supplied in a strength of 50 µg/mL. For analgesia, 5 to 10 µg administered intravenously may be sufficient. Note that this is 0.1 to 0.2 mL of undiluted drug. Obviously, great care is required when sufentanil is used in this way. This dose may be repeated as necessary to achieve adequate analgesia.

As an adjunct to general anesthesia, sufentanil possesses all the advantages of fentanyl with respect to hemodynamic stability and suppression of the stress response to surgery. It appears to be even better than fentanyl in preventing or reducing the hemodynamic response to endotracheal intubation. When used as part of a balanced anesthetic technique, a useful starting dose of sufentanil is 0.5 to 1.0 µg/kg. As with fentanyl, a continuous infusion may be established at a rate of 0.1 to 0.2 µg/kg/h.

Alfentanil

In contrast to sufentanil, alfentanil (Alfenta, manufactured by Janssen Pharmaceutica Inc., Piscataway, N.J.), the fentanyl analog, is much less potent than its parent compound. Alfentanil is supplied in a strength of 500 µg/mL. It has one tenth to one fifth the potency, one fourth the time to onset of action, and about one third the duration of action of fentanyl. The relatively fast onset and short duration of alfentanil allow for excellent titratability and make it very useful for shorter surgical procedures and continuous infusions.

Alfentanil rapidly crosses the blood–brain barrier because it is almost entirely un-ionized at physiological pH.[46] After an intravenous bolus, plasma levels fall rapidly owing to both redistribution and metabolism. Unlike most other drugs, alfentanil in a continuous infusion does not produce a significant cumulative effect in the length of time that most surgery requires. The elimination half-life is about one half that of fentanyl. The clinical duration of action of this agent may be as little as 15 minutes following an intravenous bolus injection.

When used as part of a balanced anesthetic technique, a continuous infusion is recommended because of its short duration of action. Alfentanil, in a dose of 150 to 300 µg/kg, will induce anesthesia in less than 1 minute. An infusion rate of 25 to 150 µg/kg/h, when combined with another amnestic sedative (such as a low-dose potent inhalational agent), is effective for the maintenance of anesthesia and will produce minimal cumulative drug effect. Such a technique may prove to be very useful in the combat medical facility.

Alfentanil shares with all of the fentanyl analogs the potential for problems with respiratory depression and bradycardia.

Opioid Agonist–Antagonist Drugs

As the name implies, opioid drugs in this group have both excitatory and inhibitory effects at opiate receptor sites in the central nervous system. The mixture of agonist and antagonist properties limits somewhat their clinical usefulness when used as the sole narcotic agents during general anesthesia. A theoretical advantage of these drugs is that their partial antagonist action may reduce the incidence or degree of respiratory depression that is seen with equivalent doses of pure opioid agonist agents. However, this same mechanism limits the achievable degree of analgesia when agonist–antagonist drugs are administered.

Clinical experience has shown that significant respiratory depression remains a potentially serious side effect with these agents, despite their partial antagonist properties. They are most useful as analgesic adjuncts to regional anesthetic procedures, and in the recovery room. Another potential problem is triggering of the withdrawal syndrome in the opioid-narcotic addicted patient.

Nalbuphine

The analgesic potency of nalbuphine (Nubain, manufactured by Du Pont Multi-Source Products, Garden City, N.Y.) is approximately the same (milligram for milligram) as that of morphine. Onset of action is within 2 to 3 minutes following intravenous injection, with a duration of effect in the range of 3 to 6 hours.

Respiratory depression may occur within the usual dose range (generally 10–15 mg) for preoperative sedation or analgesia. The degree of respiratory depression is similar to that of an equianalgesic dose of morphine. There is a ceiling effect to the magnitude of respiratory compromise; that is, depressed respiration does not become more pronounced as the dose of nalbuphine is increased. However, there also appears to be a ceiling effect to the degree of analgesia achieved with increasing doses of nalbuphine. What this means clinically is that doses in excess of 0.15 mg/kg will confer no greater respiratory depression or analgesia than lower doses.[44]

Butorphanol

Butorphanol (Stadol, manufactured by Bristol Laboratories, Evansville, Ind.) resembles nalbuphine in its clinical usage and effects. It is approximately 5-fold more potent than morphine on a weight basis. Butorphanol may be given intramuscularly (1–4 mg) or intravenously (0.5–2.0 mg). Duration of analgesia is 3 to 4 hours. As with nalbuphine, an analgesic and respiratory depressant ceiling effect is seen.

Opioid Antagonist Drugs

Naloxone (Narcan, manufactured by Du Pont Multi-Source Products, Garden City, N.Y.) is the prototypical narcotic antagonist, with strong affinity for opiate receptors and almost no agonist effect. In cases of opiate-induced respiratory depression (such as might be seen following a relative overdose of narcotic agent during general anesthesia), respiratory rate and tidal volume are promptly increased following an intravenous dose of naloxone. However, the analgesic and sedative effects of these drugs will also be antagonized. Thus, the dose of naloxone should be carefully titrated in 0.1- to 0.2-mg doses (for children, 0.01 mg/kg) at 2- to 3-minute intervals until the desired effect is achieved. The onset of action is rapid (within 2 min) following intravenous injection and is only slightly longer via the intramuscular route.

The clinical effects of naloxone last from 1 to 4 hours, depending on the dose given. The plasma half-life is about 1 hour. Since the respiratory depressant effects of some opioid narcotics may persist longer than the naloxone dose administered, personnel in the recovery room must be informed whenever this drug is used in the operating room prior to transport. Such a patient will require more than usual vigilance in the recovery area to prevent hypoventilation or apnea should the narcotic effect outlast that of naloxone.

Naloxone possesses some undesirable side effects. The most serious potential problems include increased intracranial pressure in the patient with a head injury, hypertension, pulmonary edema, dysrhythmias, and cardiac arrest.[47]

Naloxone (as well as the agonist–antagonist drugs) may precipitate a moderate to severe withdrawal syndrome. The symptoms and signs of acute narcotic withdrawal include irritability, nervousness, mental confusion, generalized pain, diaphoresis, abdominal cramping with diarrhea, nausea, and vomiting. This syndrome appears within 2 minutes of the administration of naloxone to a patient with narcotic dependency, and is self-limiting owing to its short plasma half-life of approximately 60 minutes. Soldiers are not entirely exempt from narcotic abuse, and this history must be obtained preoperatively, if possible.

TECHNIQUES FOR USING INTRAVENOUS ANESTHETICS

Rapid-Sequence Intravenous Induction

Experience with battlefield casualties in Vietnam showed that the majority of wounded soldiers have undigested material in their stomachs at the time of emergency surgery.[1] Regurgitation and aspiration of gastric contents into the tracheobronchial tree causes severe pulmonary dysfunction and is potentially fatal. At the very least, such complications require the allocation of scarce recovery and critical care resources to treat what is nearly always a preventable complication of general anesthesia. The risk of regurgitation and aspiration is markedly reduced when the trachea is intubated with a cuffed endotracheal tube. This must be accomplished quickly, following the administration of (1) an intravenous anesthetic agent that causes a rapid loss of consciousness and (2) a muscle relaxant with a similar rapid onset of clinical action. Rapid-sequence induction of anesthesia is performed in a definite sequence (Exhibit 10-1).

The intravenous agents that are most useful for rapid-sequence induction of anesthesia include sodium thiopental, ketamine, and etomidate (see Table 10-2). The reader is encouraged to review the specific advantages and disadvantages of these agents. The only currently available neuromuscular blocking agent with a fast-enough clinical onset time for use in a rapid-sequence induction technique is succinylcholine. The following are suggested dose regimens for rapid-sequence induction of anesthesia in combat casualties:

- ketamine (1–2 mg/kg) immediately followed by succinylcholine (1–2 mg/kg);
- etomidate (0.2–0.4 mg/kg) immediately followed by succinylcholine, as above; and
- sodium thiopental (1–4 mg/kg) immediately followed by succinylcholine, as above.

Each of these drug regimens will typically provide good intubating conditions within 45 to 60 seconds. Dosages should be adjusted downward in the hemodynamically unstable patient, particularly when thiopental is being used.

Not uncommonly, a combat casualty may already be unconscious and in a hypovolemic shock state. In such cases, any of the above agents may cause further deterioration of the patient's condition. A rapid-sequence technique using succinylcholine alone may be the safest alternative in such situations. In the worst case, even succinylcholine may be dispensed with and the patient intubated through cricoid pressure. Scopolamine 0.4 mg administered intravenously may provide amnesia during the initial period of resuscitation.

Adjuvants to Inhalational Anesthesia

Following induction of anesthesia with an intravenous drug, surgical anesthesia must be maintained. Most commonly this will be accomplished with a volatile anesthetic agent delivered by drawover vaporizer or a field anesthesia machine. If the patient is to breathe spontaneously during the procedure, adjuvant drugs such as opioid narcotic agents must be used with extreme caution to prevent respiratory arrest.

When inhalational anesthesia is being used as the primary technique, the addition of a narcotic drug is part of a balanced anesthetic, with the advantages of lower total overall doses of individual anesthetic drugs as well as residual postoperative analgesia (Exhibit 10-2). Because of the respiratory depression that accompanies a balanced anesthetic technique, it is most useful in the field environment in those cases during which the casualty's respirations are to be manually controlled. Such instances would include those there the casualties were undergoing thoracotomies, craniotomies, and major intraabdominal procedures. A muscle relaxant drug is an important component of the technique.

EXHIBIT 10-1

RAPID-SEQUENCE INDUCTION OF ANESTHESIA

1. The patient is given four to five large breaths of 100% oxygen by anesthesia mask.
2. Firm pressure is applied by an assistant with thumb and finger over the patient's cricoid cartilage in the anterior neck. (This compresses the esophagus between the vertebral column and cricoid ring to minimize the risk of passive regurgitation of gastric contents into the posterior pharynx.)
3. The chosen anesthetic agent and muscle relaxant are administered.
4. When the patient is unresponsive and has lost his lid reflex, the larynx is visualized and the endotracheal tube is passed into the trachea. The cuff is inflated. (During the interval prior to intubation, the patient must *not* be ventilated by bag and mask, as air may be forced into the stomach, increasing the risk of regurgitation.)
5. The presence of bilateral equal breath sounds is confirmed. Only after this fifth step is completed should the assistant release the cricoid pressure.

EXHIBIT 10-2

OPIOID NARCOTICS AS ADJUVANTS TO INHALATIONAL ANESTHESIA

- ***Morphine*** 0.1 to 0.2 mg/kg.
- ***Meperidine*** 0.5 to 1.0 mg/kg.
- ***Fentanyl*** 3 to 5 µg/kg on induction of anesthesia. Additional bolus doses of 50 µg/h or a continuous infusion at 1 to 2 µg/kg/h are used for maintenance. Continuous infusions should be stopped 15 to 30 minutes before the end of surgery. An alternative technique is to estimate the time of the proposed surgical procedure. The projected time (in minutes) is divided by 10 and 15. The resulting values represent the fentanyl dose in µg/kg to be administered prior to skin incision, after which no more is given.[1] For example, during a 60-minute procedure, 4 to 6 µg/kg of fentanyl may be given prior to skin incision.
- ***Sufentanil*** 0.5 to 1.0 µg/kg on induction. Additional bolus doses of 5 to 10 µg may be given every 20 to 30 minutes as necessary. If a continuous infusion is to be used, the dosage rate should be 0.1 to 0.2 µg/kg/h following the loading dose. Stop the infusion approximately 30 minutes before the end of surgery.
- ***Alfentanil*** 20 to 60 µg/kg following 2 mg/kg thiopental provides good surgical anesthesia. Larger doses of alfentanil (150–300 µg/kg) will induce anesthesia in less than 1 minute when used alone. Alfentanil's duration of action is quite short (as little as 15 min following a bolus injection). For longer cases, a continuous infusion is necessary to maintain anesthesia. The infusion rate should be set at 25 to 150 µg/kg/h, and can be continued until the end of surgery. The patient can be expected to awaken promptly, but residual analgesia will be relatively short-lived.

1. Ross, AL. How to give an anaesthetic using intravenous analgesics: An alternative from California. *Can Anaesth Soc J*. 1983;30:259-260.

When spontaneous ventilation is to be maintained during general anesthesia for surgery outside the major body cavities, narcotic agents may be administered cautiously as the case is nearing completion. A useful regimen is to reduce slightly the percentage of inspired concentration of the inhalational anesthetic agent. Morphine 0.5 to 1.0 mg is then administered. This is repeated at about 10-minute intervals, to a total morphine dose of 0.1 to 0.2 mg/kg. Respiratory rate and other vital signs must be carefully monitored. Ideally, the last morphine dose is given and the inhalational agent completely turned off 10 to 15 minutes before the end of the procedure. The result is a patient who is spontaneously ventilating with excellent analgesia. This technique works best when the patient is breathing 50% to 60% nitrous oxide, which is shut off as the last skin sutures are in place. Fentanyl may be substituted for morphine and used in a similar fashion, to a final dose of 3 to 5 µg/kg.

Total Intravenous Anesthesia

In contrast to regional techniques and general anesthesia using inhaled gases, total intravenous anesthesia using a single agent seems suited to battlefield use, owing to its relative simplicity (see Table 10-3). Since its introduction in 1970, ketamine has been touted as such an agent. Although ketamine has some untoward side effects, its tendency to preserve blood pressure and airway reflexes make it a very useful drug in the field (see the foregoing section on ketamine in this chapter). It remains the only available intravenous medication that can serve as the sole agent in a general anesthetic.[17] Its use in this manner is described below.

It is conceivable that shortages of various anesthetic agents may occur in forward medical units during wartime. If inhalational anesthetic agents become scarce or unavailable, alternative techniques will become necessary for maintenance of surgical anesthesia. Even in the absence of such shortages, total intravenous anesthesia may occasionally be the technique of choice for brief surgical procedures. Total intravenous anesthesia is possible using a variety of techniques (Exhibit 10-3).

Adjuvants for Regional and Local Anesthesia

For brief, minor surgical procedures, profound anesthetic depth and complicated techniques are not always necessary. If the procedure can be per-

EXHIBIT 10-3

TECHNIQUES FOR TOTAL INTRAVENOUS ANESTHETICS

- ***Ketamine***. An induction dose of ketamine 1.0 to 2.0 mg/kg is preceded by midazolam 1 to 2 mg (or diazepam 5–10 mg). Following induction, a continuous infusion is maintained at 20 to 50 µg/kg/min (2–4 mg/min for a 70-kg soldier). At the lower end of the dosage spectrum, spontaneous ventilation is possible. However, regurgitation and aspiration are still risks. Therefore, in acutely injured patients, the airway should be protected with an endotracheal tube. Midazolam or diazepam will reduce or eliminate emergence phenomena such as unpleasant dreams and hallucinations. When a neuromuscular blocking agent is used, the maintenance dose of ketamine may be reduced somewhat.
- ***Etomidate***. An induction dose of etomidate 0.2 to 0.4 mg/kg is given, followed by a maintenance dose of 40 to 100 µg/kg/min. After 10 minutes, this is reduced to 10 to 40 µg/kg/min. Since etomidate has no analgesic properties, a narcotic (such as fentanyl 3 to 5 µg/kg) may be added to the regimen. For a 70-kg patient, these maintenance doses are 170 to 400 mg/h for the first 10 minutes, followed by a rate of 40 to 170 mg/h. The combination of etomidate, a narcotic agent, and a neuromuscular blocking agent can produce acceptable surgical anesthesia. The infusion should be discontinued 15 to 30 minutes before the end of surgery.
- ***Sodium Thiopental***. Incremental doses of sodium thiopental (1–2 mg/kg) may be titrated to onset of unconsciousness. In this way, spontaneous ventilation may be preserved. This technique is useful for very short procedures and to "smooth" the patient's emergence from inhalational anesthesia. Due to its cumulative central nervous system– and cardiopulmonary-depressant effects, however, thiopental must be administered judiciously. For a surgical case that will last longer than 20 to 30 minutes, a continuous infusion may be prepared by putting 1 to 2 g of thiopental in 250 mL of 5% dextrose in water. Following an induction dose of 2 to 4 mg/kg, a continuous infusion is maintained at 0.1 mg/kg/min. This infusion should be supplemented with an intravenous narcotic and is not recommended unless the patient's respirations are controlled.
- ***Propofol***. Following an induction dose of propofol 2.0 to 3.0 mg/kg, a continuous infusion of 0.1 to 0.2 mg/kg/min (6–12 mg/kg/h) is started. This dose may be reduced by one half or more for critically ill or debilitated patients.
- ***Alfentanil***. An induction dose of alfentanil 150 to 300 µg/kg will induce general anesthesia. A continuous infusion should be set to run at 25 to 150 µg/kg/h for maintenance. Because alfentanil may produce chest-wall rigidity and will definitely cause respiratory depression, the patient should be ventilated mechanically when this technique is used.

formed under local anesthesia, intravenous agents such as the benzodiazepines may be useful in allaying anxiety. Small, intravenous bolus doses of thiopental (1–2 mg/kg) or etomidate (0.1 mg/kg) will not provide analgesia, but may alter consciousness sufficiently to allow a short, painful procedure. If the patient has had no oral intake for at least 6 hours, aspiration risk with these techniques should be minimal. If he has eaten recently, any drug-induced blunting of the airway and gag reflexes should be avoided unless the trachea is protected with an endotracheal tube.

Ketamine is very useful for short procedures in which deep general anesthesia is not required. Incremental bolus doses of 5 to 10 mg provide intense analgesia and altered consciousness. The opioid narcotic agents can also be used in these types of cases. They are most effective if given *before* the painful stimulus. Because they cause more blunting of spontaneous respiration, they allow somewhat less flexibility in dosing than ketamine.

Small-bolus injections of an opioid narcotic drug may be useful in this setting for producing sedation and supplying additional analgesia.

SUMMARY

An impressive number of intravenous anesthetic drugs are available to the anesthesiologist in civilian practice. The wartime anesthesia provider, however, may have to make do with a more limited drug repertoire. It is possible that many physicians and nurses who have little or no training in the field of anesthesiology will be called on to assist in providing this service in battlefield hospitals.

While the combat anesthesia provider may not have access to all of the anesthetic agents described in this chapter, at least one or two agents for each anesthetic indication will almost certainly be available. Thus, only thiopental and ketamine may be available for induction of anesthesia. For analgesia, morphine or fentanyl may be the only drugs in the pharmacy. Perhaps one of the benzodiazepines will be available as well. Whatever the contents of the drug locker, the wartime anesthesia provider must have a rational plan of action for each casualty, and should know how to use safely the intravenous anesthetic agents available in the medical treatment facility.

REFERENCES

1. Noble MJ, Bryant T, Ing FYW. Casualty anesthesia experiences in Vietnam. *Anesth Analg*. 1968;47:5–11.
2. Courington FW. Anesthesia at the battlefield: The present and the future. *Sem Anesth*. 1988;7:26–32.
3. Halford FJ. A critique of intravenous anesthesia in war surgery. *Anesthesiology*. 1943;4:67–69.
4. Adams RC, Gray HK. Intravenous anesthesia with pentothal sodium in the case of gunshot wound associated with accompanying severe traumatic shock and loss of blood: Report of a case. *Anesthesiology*. 1943;4:70–73.
5. The question of intravenous anesthesia in war surgery. *Anesthesiology*. 1943;4:74–77. Editorial.
6. Rose AT. Sodium pentothal: Actual experience in the combat zone. *Anesthesiology*. 1943;4:534–539.
7. Papper EM, Sheehan WC. Anesthesiology in military medicine. *Anesthesiology*. 1943;4:619–624.
8. Lieberman SL. Experiences with pentothal sodium anesthesia on war casualties. *Anesthesiology*. 1944;5: 517–519.
9. Bull PT, Merrill SB, Moody RA, et al. Anaesthesia during the Falklands campaign: The experience of the Royal Navy. *Anaesthesia*. 1983;38:770–775.
10. Turcant A, Delhumeau A, Premel-Cabic A, et al. Thiopental pharmacokinetics under conditions of long-term infusion. *Anesthesiology*. 1985;63:50–54.
11. White PF. What's new in intravenous anesthetics. *Anesth Clin N Am*. 1988;6:297–318.
12. Brussel T, Theissen JL, Vigfusson G, Lunkenheimer PP, Van Aken H, Lawin P. Hemodynamic and cardiodynamic effects of propofol and etomidate: Negative inotropic properties of propofol. *Anesth Analg*. 1989;69:35–40.
13. Giese JL, Stanley TH. Etomidate—a new intravenous anesthetic induction agent. *Pharmacotherapy*. 1983;3:251–258.
14. Milde LM, Milde JH, Michenfelder JD. Cerebral functional, metabolic, and hemodynamic effects of etomidate in dogs. *Anesthesiology*. 1985;63:371–377.
15. Sebel PS, Lowdon, JD. Propofol: A new intravenous anesthetic. *Anesthesiology*. 1989;71:260–277.
16. Doze VA, Westphal LM, White PF. Comparison of propofol with methohexital for outpatient anesthesia. *Anesth Analg*. 1986;65:1189–1195.
17. White PF, Way WL, Trevor AJ. Ketamine—its pharmacology and uses. *Anesthesiology*. 1982;56:119–136.
18. Corssen G, Domino E. Further pharmacologic studies and first clinical experience with phencyclidine derivative Cl-581 (ketamine). *Anesth Analg*. 1966;45:29–39.
19. Ontani M, Kikuchi H, Kitahata LM. Effects of ketamine on nociceptive cells in the medial medullary reticular formation of the cat. *Anesthesiology*. 1979;51:414–417.

20. Kitahata LM, Taub A, Kosaka Y. Lamina-specific suppression of dorsal-horn unit activity by ketamine hydrochloride. *Anesthesiology*. 1973;38:4–11.

21. Vincent JP, Corey D. Kamenka JM. Interaction of phencyclidines with the muscarinic and opiate receptors of the central nervous system. *Brain Res*. 1972;152:176–182.

22. Morgan M, Loh L, Singer L, Moore PH. Ketamine as the sole anesthetic agent for minor surgical procedures. *Anaesthesia*. 1971;26:158–165.

23. Boulton TB. Twenty years of dissociative anesthesia with ketamine (Cl-581): Its origin and present significance. *Surv Anesth*. 1987;5:62–67.

24. Kothary SP, Zsigmond EK. A double-blind study of the effective antihallucinatory doses of diazepam prior to ketamine anesthesia. *Clin Pharm Ther*. 1977;21:108–109.

25. Hatano S, Nishiwada M, Matsumaura M. Ketamine–diazepam anaesthesia for abdominal surgery: A review of 1000 cases with continuous "micro-mini" drip administration technique. *Anaesthesia*. 1978;27:172–182.

26. Waxman K, Shoemaker WC, Lippman M. Cardiovascular effects of anesthetic induction with ketamine. *Anesth Analg*. 1980;59:355–358.

27. Bond AC, Davies CK. Ketamine and pancuronium for the shocked patient. *Anaesthesia*. 1974;29:59–62.

28. Longnecker DE, Sturgill BC. Influence of anesthetic agent on survival following hemorrhage. *Anesthesiology*. 1976;45:516–521.

29. Zsigmond EK, Kothary SP, Martinez OA. Diazepam for prevention of the rise in plasma catecholamines caused by ketamine. *Clin Pharm Ther*. 1974;15:223–224.

30. Way WL, Trevor AJ. Pharmacology of intravenous nonnarcotic anesthetics. In: Miller RD, ed. *Anesthesia*. New York, NY: Churchill-Livingstone; 1986: 813–817.

31. Lundy PM, Gowdy CW, Colhoun FH. Tracheal smooth muscle relaxant effects of ketamine. *Br J Anaesth*. 1974;46:333.

32. Carmichael GLM. Anaesthesia under civil war conditions. *Anaesthesia*. 1981;36:1077–1088.

33. Jowitt MD, Knight RJ. Anaesthesia during the Falklands campaign: The land battles. *Anaesthesia*. 1983;38:776–783.

34. Idvall J, Ahlgren I, Aronsen KF, Stenberg P. Ketamine infusions: Pharmacokinetics and clinical effects. *Br J Anaesth*. 1979;51:1167–1172.

35. Barclay A, Houlton PC, Downing JW. Total intravenous anaesthesia: A technique using flunitrazepam, ketamine, muscle relaxants and controlled ventilation of the lung. *Anaesthesia*. 1980;35:287–290.

36. Bion JF. An anaesthetist in a camp for Cambodian refugees. *Anaesthesia*. 1983;38:798–801.

37. White PF, Dworsky WA, Horai Y, Trevor AJ. Comparison of continuous infusion fentanyl or ketamine versus thiopental: Determining the mean effective serum concentrations for outpatient surgery. *Anesthesiology*. 1983;59:564–569.

38. Bion JF. Infusion analgesia for acute war injuries: A comparison of pentazocine and ketamine. *Anaesthesia*. 1984;39:560–564.

39. Kamm GD, Bewes PC. Ketamine anaesthesia by continuous intravenous drip. *Trop Doct*. 1978;8:68–72.

40. Lilburn JK, Dundee JW, Moore J. Ketamine infusions: Observations on technique, dosage and cardiovascular effects. *Anaesthesia*. 1978;33:315–321.

41. Reves JG, Fragen RJ, Vinik HR, Greenblatt DJ. Midazolam: Pharmacology and uses. *Anesthesiology*. 1985;62:310–324.

42. Samuelson PN, Reves JG, Kouchoukos NT, Smith LR, Dole KM. Hemodynamic responses to anesthetic induction with midazolam or diazepam in patients with ischemic heart disease. *Anesth Analg*. 1981;60:802–809.

43. Gross JB, Zebrowski ME, Carel WD, Gardner S, Smith TC. Time course of ventilatory depression after thiopental and midazolam in normal subjects and in patients with chronic obstructive pulmonary disease. *Anesthesiology*. 1983;58:540–544.

44. Murphy MR. Opioids. In: Barash PG, Cullen BF, Stoelting RK. *Clinical Anesthesia*. Philadelphia, Pa: JB Lippincott; 1989: 255–279.

45. Flacke JW, Flacke WE, Bloor BC, Van Etten AP, Kripke BJ. Histamine release by four narcotics: A double-blind study in humans. *Anesth Analg*. 1987;66:723–730.

46. Rosow C. Newer opioid analgesics and antagonists. *Anesth Clin N Am*. 1988;6:319–333.

47. Smith G, Pinnock C. Naloxone—paradox or panacea. *Br J Anaesth*. 1985;57:547.

Chapter 11

NEUROMUSCULAR BLOCKING AGENTS

RICHARD B. HECKER, D.O.*; JAMES B. STEVENS, M.D.†; AND GERARD F. MELANSON, M.D.‡

**Major, Medical Corps, U.S. Army; Anesthesia and Operative Service, Brooke Army Medical Center, Fort Sam Houston, Texas 78234-6200; Clinical Assistant Professor of Anesthesiology, The University of Texas Health Science Center at San Antonio, San Antonio, Texas 78284-7834, and The Uniformed Services University of the Health Sciences, Bethesda, Maryland 20814-4799*

†*Major, Medical Corps, U.S. Army; Anesthesia and Operative Service, Brooke Army Medical Center, Fort Sam Houston, Texas 78234-6200; Clinical Assistant Professor of Anesthesiology, The University of Texas Health Science Center at San Antonio, Texas 78284-7834*

‡*Major, Medical Corps, U.S. Army; Fellow in Multidisciplinary Critical Care Medicine, Brooke Army Medical Center, Fort Sam Houston, Texas 78234-6200*

INTRODUCTION

The primary reason for administering neuromuscular blocking agents to casualties with traumatic injuries is to permit the airway to be secured with endotracheal intubation and mechanical ventilation. Because battlefield injuries can cause inadequate ventilation and oxygenation, intubation is often required. Many casualties with traumatic injuries have an altered level of consciousness and are at risk for aspiration of stomach contents because they are unable to protect the airway. On occasion, the casualty may simply be so confused and uncooperative that intubation with sedation and muscle relaxation may be required to care for him.

The first description of the clinical use of neuromuscular blockade was reported in 1932, when *d*-Tubocurarine was administered to control the muscle spasms of tetanus.[1] Since then, the pharmacology and clinical use of neuromuscular blocking agents, commonly referred to as muscle relaxants, have been greatly expanded. Today, these drugs are frequently used in surgery, the intensive care unit, and the emergency department. This chapter discusses the mechanisms of action, pharmacodynamics, uses, and complications of the most common neuromuscular blocking agents.

Classically, neuromuscular transmission is viewed as the release of the neurotransmitter substance *acetylcholine* at the motor nerve terminal in response to the neural action potential (Figure 11-1). A cationic channel protein on the postjunctional membrane possesses nicotinic cholinergic receptor sites. When these sites are occupied by acetylcholine or a suitable agonist, the receptor channel protein undergoes conformational change. This causes an influx of sodium ions and a corresponding efflux (although of lesser magnitude) of potassium ions. A smaller number of calcium ions then pass inward with the sodium, with a change in the endplate potential. Simultaneous opening of approximately 200,000 nicotinic receptor channels in response to the evoked release of acetylcholine generates a motor endplate potential. If this change in potential is of sufficient magnitude, the voltage-gated sodium ion channels of the adjacent muscle membrane open, and a large number of sodium ions pass into the interior of the cell, which depolarizes the cell. In some manner, this process is coupled to the activation of the contractile mechanism.[2] In addition to this mechanism, another population of cholinergic receptors appears to exist on the motor nerve terminal itself. Their physiological role is obscure, but their inactivation reduces the amount of acetylcholine that is released in response to a nerve impulse.

Through a combination of acetylcholine reuptake and local degradation within the synaptic cleft by the enzyme acetylcholinesterase, muscle repolarization occurs and the opportunity for contraction is restored. A second nonspecific plasma enzyme, pseudocholinesterase (ie, plasma cholinesterase), is also involved in the breakdown of acetylcholine and acetylcholine-like molecules.

It is customary to consider neuromuscular blocking agents in two groups: the *depolarizing* and the *nondepolarizing* agents. Depolarizing agents, of which succinylcholine is by far the best known, resemble acetylcholine stereochemically and mimic its action at the neuromuscular junction, causing depolarization of the endplate and adjacent muscle membrane, with clinically evident muscle fasciculations. The neuromuscular junction remains depolarized until succinylcholine diffuses away from the receptor site. Breakdown of succinylcholine occurs in a two-stage process away from the receptor site:

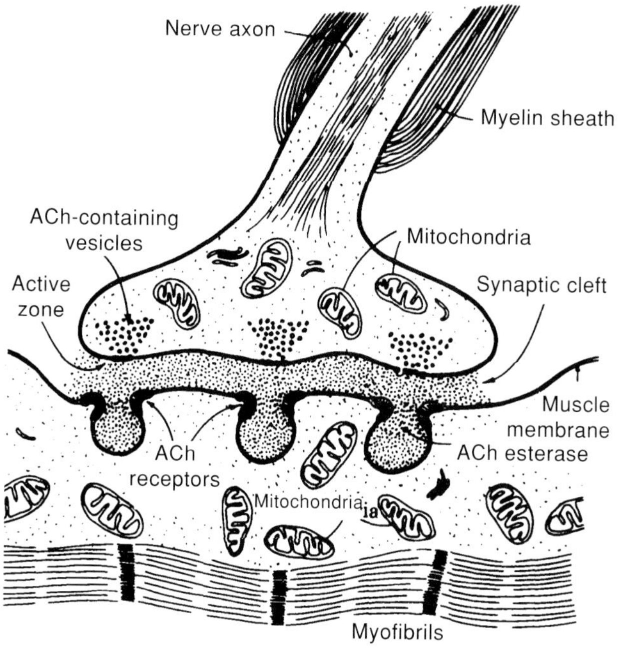

Fig. 11-1. The neuromuscular junction. Reprinted with permission from Shorten G. Neuromuscular blockade. In: Davison JK, Eckhardt WF III, Perese DA, eds. *Clinical Anesthesia Procedures of the Massachusetts General Hospital*. 4th ed. Boston, Mass: Little, Brown; 1993: 152.

1. pseudocholinesterase hydrolyzes succinylcholine to choline and succinylmonocholine (which has weak depolarizing relaxant activity), and
2. succinylmonocholine slowly breaks down to choline and succinic acid by the actions of both acetylcholinesterase and pseudocholinesterase.

Low pseudocholinesterase levels, drug-induced inhibition of cholinesterase activity, or the possession of a genetically atypical enzyme may be associated with prolonged neuromuscular blockade following the use of succinylcholine.

Nondepolarizing agents, on the other hand, act by passively binding acetylcholine receptor sites and thereby prevent their occupancy by acetylcholine. Because nondepolarizing agents act by blocking at the neuromuscular junction, muscle endplate depolarization and clinical fasciculations are not seen. The nondepolarizing agents are quaternary ammonium compounds that include two major categories: the steroid-based derivatives and the benzylisoquinoline series. Recovery from neuromuscular junction blockade occurs spontaneously but can be accelerated by the use of pharmacological agents that inhibit acetylcholinesterase, which therefore increases the availability of acetylcholine to compete for the binding site. Theoretically, experimental research drugs such as 4-aminopyridine can presynaptically increase the amount of acetylcholine and thereby competitively reverse the blockade caused by nondepolarizing agents. Currently, however, only the anticholinesterase agents are used clinically to antagonize neuromuscular junction blockade.

NEUROMUSCULAR MONITORING TECHNIQUES

It is important to emphasize that monitoring of neuromuscular function should be employed whenever neuromuscular blocking agents are used. The military anesthesiologist should consider four main questions when using neuromuscular blocking agents:

1. Is the blockade adequate?
2. Is the blockade excessive?
3. Can the blockade be reversed?
4. Is the blockade fully reversed?

Although there are many ways to stimulate a peripheral nerve, a typical commercially available hand-held peripheral nerve stimulator should provide the ability to choose stimulation by the single twitch, train-of-four (TOF), tetanic, and double-burst methods (Figure 11-2). The most commonly recommended method to monitor neuromuscular function is to observe the contraction of the fingers (adductor pollicis and flexor digitorum muscles) in response to electrical stimulation of the ulnar nerve at the wrist or elbow (Figure 11-3). Other areas may be stimulated, such as the facial nerve or the peroneal or posterior tibial nerves of the lower extremity (Figures 11-4 and 11-5). The magnitude of the muscle contraction response can be a rough gauge to monitor neuromuscular blockade. It is important to emphasize that direct muscle stimulation should be avoided, as this can be mistaken for the responses seen with nerve stimulation.

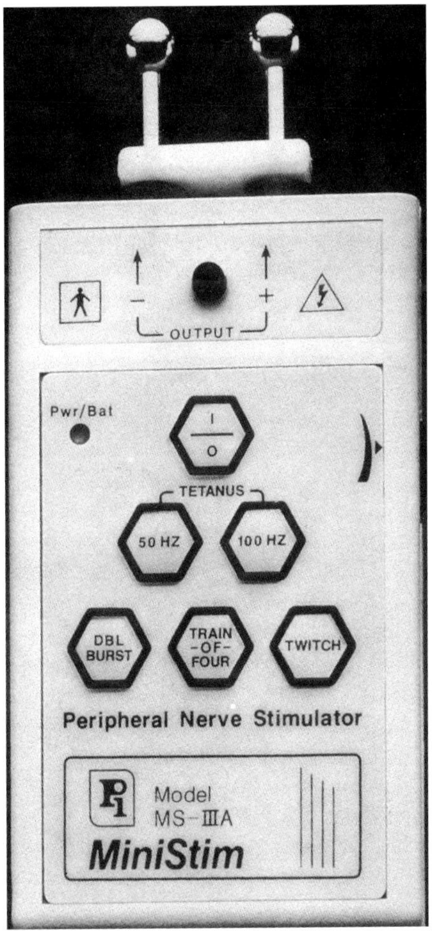

Fig. 11-2. The MiniStim is a portable, battery-operated, adjustable-amplitude, hand-held peripheral nerve stimulator. Photograph: Courtesy of Life-Tech, Inc, Houston, Tex.

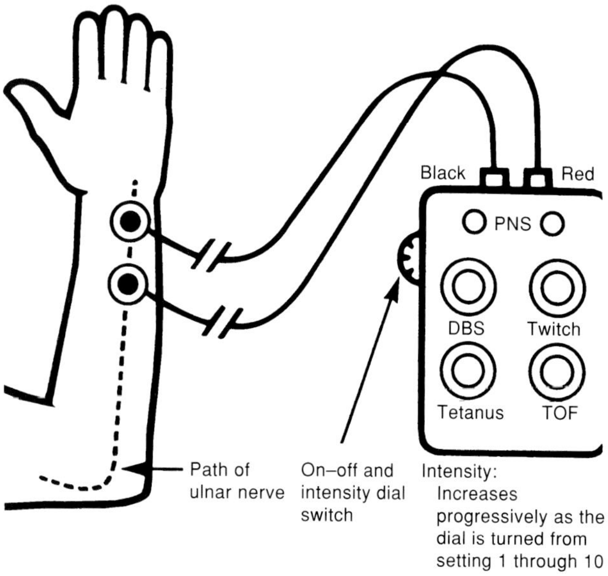

Fig. 11-3. Placement of nerve-stimulator electrodes over the ulnar nerve. Photograph: Courtesy of Organon, Inc, West Orange, NJ.

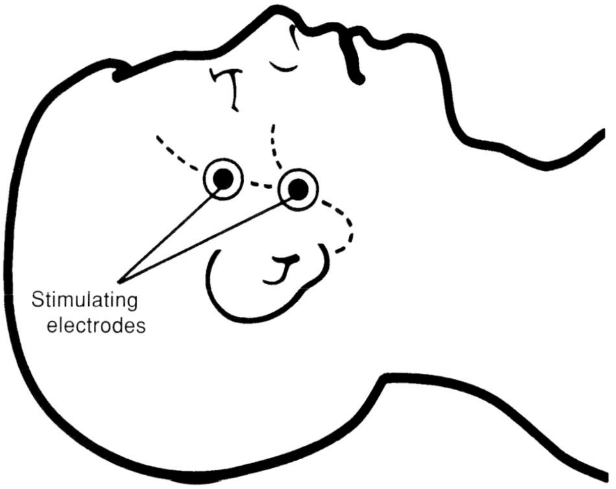

Fig. 11-4. Placement of nerve-stimulator electrodes over the facial nerve. Photograph: Courtesy of Organon, Inc, West Orange, NJ.

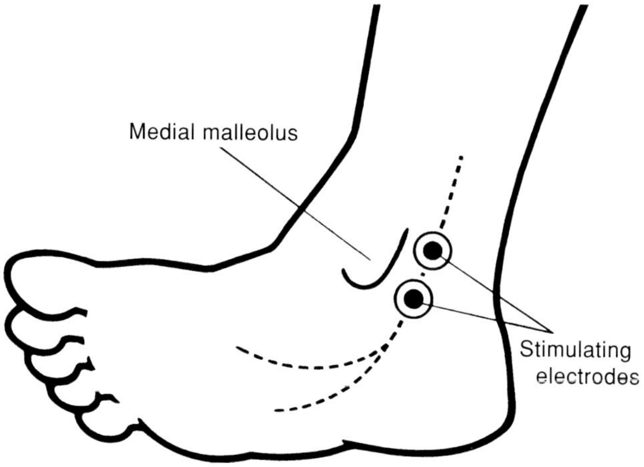

Fig. 11-5. Placement of nerve-stimulator electrodes over the posterior tibial nerve. Photograph: Courtesy of Organon, Inc, West Orange, NJ.

Single Twitch

A single supramaximal stimulus lasting less than 0.2 ms at a frequency of 0.1 Hz is employed to determine control muscle-contraction response before the neuromuscular blocking agent is administered. Subsequent single-twitch stimuli are then employed to assess the diminution of the twitch response so that the depth of muscle blockade can be gauged. This type of monitoring is only a crude measure unless a sophisticated recording device (eg, a force transducer) can be attached to the patient. Quantifying the loss of twitch height is crucial to assess the blockade accurately. For example, a 90% suppression of the twitch height is adequate for endotracheal intubation. Furthermore, 75% to 90% suppression is adequate for surgical relaxation in the presence of anesthetic agents, while a 25% suppression is only clinically associated with a decreased vital capacity. Unfortunately, 75% of receptors must be occupied with the neuromuscular blocking before there is a loss of twitch height. Given its minimal sensitivity, the single-twitch testing method is not recommended.

Train-of-Four

Four supramaximal stimuli at a frequency of 2 Hz are repeated at intervals longer than 10 seconds apart. The number of muscle-twitch responses corresponds to the degree of suppression of the initial twitch response. Loss of the fourth twitch (ie, only three twitches are seen) corresponds to a 75% suppression of the twitch height, compared to the control. Loss of the third, second, and first twitch responses corresponds to 80%, 90%, and 100% of the twitch height, respectively (Table 11-1). Monitoring the TOF is a very useful method of determining neuromuscular blockade because it does not re-

TABLE 11-1

CLINICAL EVALUATION OF NEUROMUSCULAR BLOCKADE

Train-of-Four Response (Twitches)	% Block (Approximate)	Clinical Implication of Neuromuscular Blockade
0	> 95	Response indicates clinical overdose of neuromuscular blockade
1	90	Blockade is adequate for intubation
2	80–90	Blockade is adequate for surgery or long-term ventilation
3	75–80	Additional dosing may be required for surgery or long-term ventilation
3–4	75	Patient is susceptible to reversal of neuromuscular blockade with anticholinesterase agents
4	≤ 75	Patient is recovering from neuromuscular blockade

quire a control height. Loss of more than three twitches signifies good intubating conditions, and maintenance of one to two twitches during continuous neuromuscular blockade confirms adequate relaxation and preserves the ability to reverse the neuromuscular blocking agents. Total loss of the four twitches during incremental-bolus or continuous-infusion therapy signifies excessive blockade. A return of the TOF twitch response suggests recovery from neuromuscular blockade (Figure 11-6).

Tetanic Stimulation

Tetanic nerve stimulation varies in frequency from 50 to 200 Hz, with 50 Hz or 100 Hz being more commonly employed. Tetanic stimulation at 50 Hz for 5 seconds is clinically useful to estimate peak muscle tension. Stimulation at this frequency corresponds to what may be seen with maximum voluntary muscular effort. Peak muscle tension in response to tetanic stimulation is reduced in the presence of both depolarizing and nondepolarizing blockade, but fade to tetanic stimulation is only seen with the latter. This fade to tetanus is a pre-neuromuscular junction phenomenon. It is due to curare-like drugs acting on acetylcholine mobilization during high-frequency stimulation. Evidence of fade with tetanus suggests incomplete recovery from the neuromuscular blocking agents (Figure 11-7). Fade is termed *recurarization* if it is seen after clinical recovery has been determined. Tetanic stimulation is painful and should only be employed with this consideration in mind.

Double-Burst Stimulation

Double-burst stimulation is two, short, 50-Hz tetanic stimuli delivered 750 ms apart. If the response to the second stimulation is less than the first, then residual curarization can be suspected. This method is more sensitive in detecting residual curarization than other methods. As with tetanic stimulation, double-burst stimulation is also painful to apply.

Clinical Assessment

Although the use of a nerve stimulator is strongly recommended when neuromuscular blocking agents are being employed, this type of monitor may be unavailable to the anesthesiologist in the field setting. The clinician must then gauge the degree of muscle strength that has returned so that the casualty's readiness for extubation can be assessed. The casualty's ability to sustain a head lift for 5 seconds, demonstrate a vital capacity of 15 to 20 mL/kg, or generate an inspiratory force of –25 cm H_2O pressure corresponds clinically to a TOF ratio greater than 0.75 or sustained tetanus at 50 Hz for 5 seconds. The ability to cough effectively may also indicate adequate respiratory muscle strength for extubation. Finally, the demonstration of a normal expiratory flow rate, vital capacity, and inspiratory force greater than 40 cm H_2O pressure can be equated with a TOF ratio of 1.0, indicating full recovery from neuromuscular blockade.

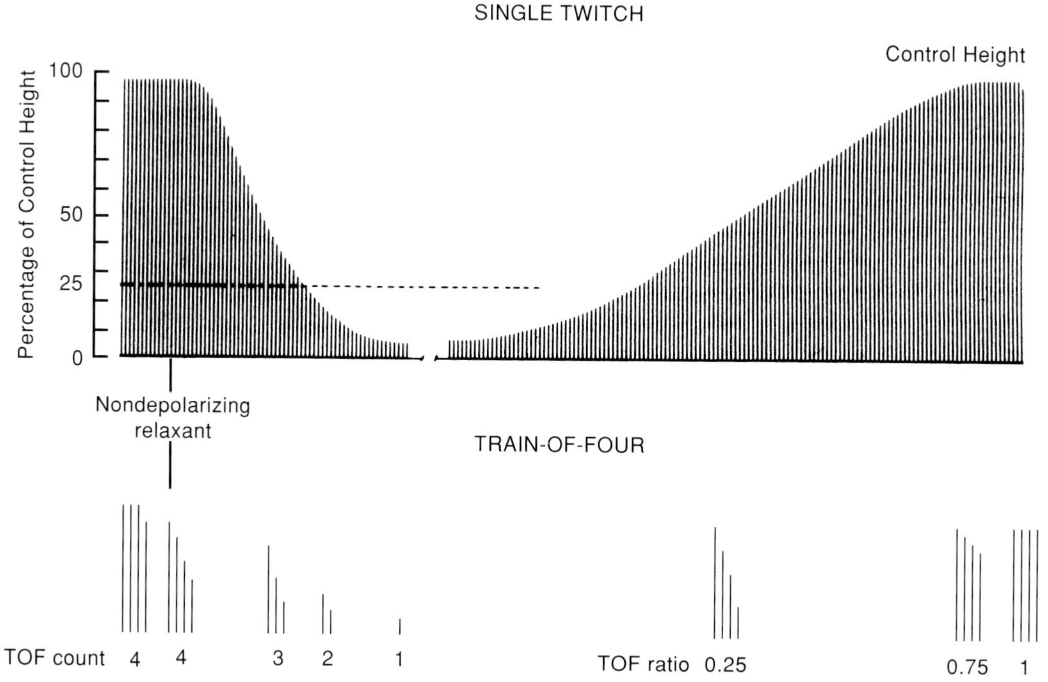

Fig. 11-6. Graphic demonstrations of single-twitch (above) and train-of-four response (below) during onset of and recovery from nondepolarizing neuromuscular blockade. Reprinted with permission from Shorten G. Neuromuscular blockade. In: Davison JK, Eckhardt WF III, Perese DA, eds. *Clinical Anesthesia Procedures of the Massachusetts General Hospital*. 4th ed. Boston: Mass: Little, Brown; 1993: 167.

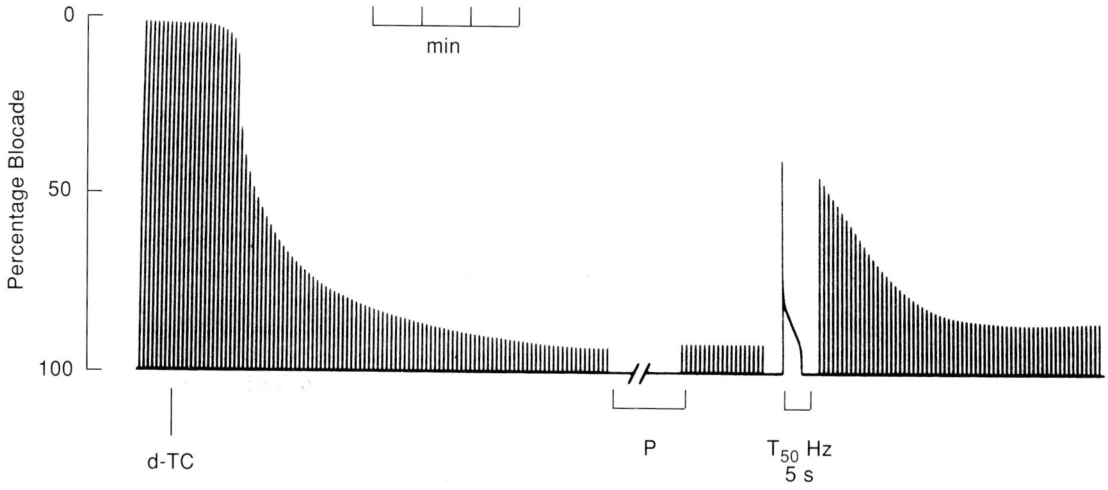

Fig. 11-7. Loss of response to 0.1 Hz after *d*-Tubocurarine (left). Decrease in peak muscle tension followed by fade (no sustained response) after 50-Hz tetanic stimulation (right). Reprinted with permission from Shorten G. Neuromuscular blockade. In: Davison JK, Eckhardt WF III, Perese DA, eds. *Clinical Anesthesia Procedures of the Massachusetts General Hospital*. 4th ed. Boston, Mass: Little, Brown; 1993: 158.

INDICATIONS FOR NEUROMUSCULAR BLOCKADE

Neuromuscular blocking agents are routinely used as adjuncts for general anesthesia. Their most common use is in the facilitation of endotracheal intubation. For elective surgery, general anesthesia is typically induced with a hypnotic agent such as thiopental sodium and a narcotic. Once the patient is asleep and the ability to ventilate the patient with a bag-valve-mask system is confirmed, a muscle relaxant is administered to relax the jaw, larynx, and diaphragm, and thus to facilitate smooth endotracheal intubation. Without a neuromuscular blocking agent, a deeper plane of anesthesia is required to achieve the best possible intubating conditions, which may cause significant hypotension and other detrimental side effects in some patients.

During the maintenance of general anesthesia, supplemental doses of neuromuscular blocking agents are often given to provide optimal operating conditions for the surgeon. This is especially important in abdominal surgery because the anesthetic agents alone do not provide adequate muscle relaxation for these procedures unless very high doses are used.

There is currently great controversy surrounding the use of muscle relaxant agents outside the operating room, particularly in the intensive care unit. Muscle relaxation to facilitate endotracheal intubation by eliminating biting, gagging, combativeness, and laryngospasm is probably the most common clinical indication for their use outside the operating room. Caution in using neuromuscular blocking agents for this purpose must be exercised, particularly in those patients who may be identified as difficult to intubate. The need for a possible surgical airway should be understood, and trained personnel should be available. Physicians who prescribe neuromuscular blockade should be trained experts in airway-management techniques. It is important to realize that once muscle relaxants are given, the patient will be totally dependent on controlled ventilation until the drug is eliminated or antagonized. If the airway cannot be controlled, the patient will asphyxiate.

Many clinicians contend that there is no role for these drugs in appropriately sedated patients in the intensive care unit.[3] It is important to stress that muscle relaxation should never be used without concomitantly administering sedation in doses adequate to produce amnesia or unconsciousness. Furthermore, the use of neuromuscular blocking agents should be limited to the shortest possible time. Generally accepted clinical applications include those listed in Exhibit 11-1.

Rarely, neuromuscular blockade can aid in the treatment of medical conditions such as tetanus, where muscular contraction is itself harmful.[4] Likewise, patients suffering from cardiovascular or metabolic instability due to intractable convulsive activity may transiently benefit from neuromuscular blockade. Because muscle relaxant agents do nothing to protect the brain or terminate intracerebral seizure activity, continuous electroencephalographic monitoring is recommended when the clinical signs of seizure activity are abolished by their use.[5]

The use of a muscle relaxant may occasionally be a useful adjunct to sedative agents when obtaining diagnostic procedures or studies.[6] There are rare patients (eg, those with alcohol withdrawal) whose combativeness may endanger themselves despite large amounts of sedative agents. In situations of this type, muscle relaxants may be necessary temporarily to avoid injury. In addition, these agents have been used to prevent muscle-activity–induced increases in intracranial pressure in patients with head injury.

Neuromuscular blocking agents are useful in facilitating mechanical ventilation in the intensive care unit.[7,8] Certain modes of mechanical ventila-

EXHIBIT 11-1

RATIONALES FOR NEUROMUSCULAR BLOCKADE IN THE INTENSIVE CARE UNIT

Facilitate endotracheal intubation

Minimize increased oxygen consumption associated with muscular activity

Abolish ventilator–patient discoordination

Establish pharmacological restraint

Adjunct to treat septic shock complicated by acute respiratory failure

Rest fatigued respiratory musculature

Adapted with permission from Hall JB, Schmidt GA, Wood LDH. *Principles of Critical Care*. New York, NY: McGraw Hill; 1992: 976.

tion that use prolonged inspiratory times may be actively opposed by the patient. Allowing permissive hypercapnia and using high levels of positive end-expiratory pressure may be uncomfortable to the patient, thus requiring muscle relaxation. Although the use of sedation alone is usually sufficient, some patients demonstrate a respiratory pattern that is discordant with settings chosen for the mechanical ventilator. The resulting bucking and straining against the ventilator may provoke pulmonary barotrauma and bronchospasm. Most often, this discordancy signals that ventilator settings are not suited to the patient's requirements. Adjustment of the ventilator settings must be considered prior to the institution of muscle-relaxant therapy.

Theoretically, muscle relaxation can be used to reduce oxygen consumption in patients with marginal oxygenation. Oxygen consumption by ventilatory muscles is normally 1% to 3% of the available supply. In acute respiratory distress, the oxygen cost of breathing can increase to 24% of the supply.[9] This increased oxygen consumption and perfusion of the stressed respiratory muscles that accompanies the adult respiratory distress syndrome may potentially deprive the body of desperately needed energy supplies when oxygen transport is impaired by a reduction in cardiac output, hypoxemia, or anemia.[10] Neuromuscular blockade has been shown to improve arterial oxygenation and decrease oxygen consumption in patients suffering from respiratory failure, although it has not yet been shown to improve patient outcome.[7,11]

TYPES OF MUSCLE RELAXANTS

Muscle relaxants are classified as depolarizing or nondepolarizing. The only depolarizing agent in clinical use in the United States is succinylcholine chloride. All other muscle relaxants in clinical use are nondepolarizing in their mechanism of action.

Succinylcholine Chloride

Succinylcholine, consisting of two linked acetylcholine molecules, is a potent acetylcholine agonist with a rapid onset of action (< 1 min) and brief duration at clinically used doses (5–10 min). Because of these characteristics, it is an ideal agent in situations where expedient endotracheal intubation is required. The intravenous dose used for intubation is 1 to 1.5 mg/kg in adults and 2 to 2.5 mg/kg in children younger than 2 years of age.[12] In emergency situations where intravenous access is unavailable, succinylcholine can be administered intramuscularly in a dose of 4 mg/kg, with a rapid onset of activity. Great caution should be exercised when using succinylcholine in children, especially boys under the age of 8 years. There have been isolated reports of a succinylcholine-induced hyperkalemic cardiac arrest in this cohort that may be related to an undiagnosed muscular dystrophy, typically of the Duchenne type.

Succinylcholine is rapidly degraded by pseudocholinesterase. Its duration of action may be increased owing to deficiencies in the amount of enzyme (eg, as is seen in patients with liver disease, pregnancy, cytotoxic agents, and malnutrition).[13,14] In addition, genetic abnormalities exist: abnormal isozymes are estimated to occur in 1 per 3,000 in the general population.[15] Even in situations such as these, the duration of muscle relaxation is rarely longer than 20 to 30 minutes.[13–15] If it is necessary to antagonize the prolonged neuromuscular blockade caused by succinylcholine, then administering fresh frozen plasma to provide pseudocholinesterase is effective.[16]

The administration of succinylcholine has been associated with many adverse effects. The serum potassium level is expected to rise from 0.5 to 1.0 mEq/L because potassium leaks from the muscle cell during depolarization. High serum-potassium concentrations have been specifically reported after administration of succinylcholine in patients with spinal cord transection, nerve damage, burns, major central nervous system injuries, and prolonged periods of immobility.[17,18] The common factor that appears to link these conditions and the potential for succinylcholine-induced hyperkalemia is a proliferation of nicotinic cholenergic receptors on myocytes located *away* from the neuromuscular junctions. Such nonjunctional, or extrajunctional, receptors, when stimulated, remain open 4-fold longer than normal junctional receptors, a difference that greatly increases the time for potassium flux.[19] It is therefore unwise to administer succinylcholine to such patients after the first 24 hours from injury, although this effect can be delayed up to 1 week from injury. Succinylcholine may safely be administered during the first hours after a traumatic injury. The risk of ventricular fibrillation or cardiac arrest due to hyperkalemia may persist for 6 months or longer after initial injury in these patients.[20] Life-threatening hyperkalemic events can be treated in the usual fashion with insulin, calcium, and sodium bicarbonate.

Succinylcholine can cause an increase in intraocular pressure and should therefore be used cautiously in patients who have penetrating injuries of the globe and some types of glaucoma. Controversy exists as to whether succinylcholine should be used in patients who may have increased intracranial pressure. After succinylcholine has been administered, small increases in intracranial pressure have been detected in patients whose pressure previously was normal.[21] On the other hand, the advantage of using succinylcholine in patients who require tracheal intubation is that it produces a rapid and profound neuromuscular blockade, which attenuates any substantial increase in intracranial pressure due to coughing or bucking during the intubation process.

Another potential adverse effect of succinylcholine is the rare malignant hyperthermia syndrome. This hypermetabolic syndrome manifests with severe metabolic acidosis and carries a high mortality if not aggressively treated. The key to treatment is early administration of dantrolene sodium and supportive therapy until the acidosis and its sequelae resolve. (For a more complete discussion, see Chapter 29, Malignant Hyperthermia: Military Implications.)

Repeated bolus dosing of succinylcholine should be avoided: it may cause profound bradycardia due to repeated stimulation of the muscarinic receptors. Although this drug is available as a continuous infusion, its use by this method is not recommended. Long-term administration of succinylcholine with doses higher than 5 mg/kg alters the character of the blockade to that of a nondepolarizing muscular blockade. This is termed a Phase II blockade and has the clinical and electromyographic characteristics of a nondepolarizing neuromuscular blockade.

Given its many side effects, the clinical trend has been to avoid the routine use of succinylcholine for intubation and general anesthesia in elective surgery. However, when rapid control of the airway is required, succinylcholine remains the drug of choice for most clinicians.

Nondepolarizing Agents

Nondepolarizing agents act as competitive inhibitors at the motor endplate, preventing acetylcholine from binding at receptor sites and therefore interrupting neuromuscular transmission. Neuromuscular blockade is the result. Because of their competitive mechanisms of action, the effects of these drugs can be antagonized (ie, reversed) with acetylcholinesterase inhibitors such as neostigmine, pyridostigmine, or edrophonium. The reversal agent will also increase acetylcholine at both the nicotinic and muscarinic cholinergic receptors, with resultant bradycardia and other unpleasant muscarinic effects. Therefore, anticholinergic drugs such as atropine or glycopyrrolate should accompany the use of acetylcholinesterase inhibitors when antagonizing neuromuscular blockade. The nondepolarizing neuromuscular blocking agents and their characteristics are found in Table 11-2.[22] The recommended dosages for the acetylcholinesterase inhibitor drugs and the antimuscarinic agents used for reversal of nondepolarizing neuromuscular blockade are found in Table 11-3.

Pancuronium Bromide

Pancuronium is an aminosteroid neuromuscular blocking agent with a long-acting duration of action. Following a dose of 0.08 to 0.12 mg/kg, administered intravenously, pancuronium will produce adequate relaxation for intubation in 90 to 120 seconds, with a duration of approximately 60 minutes.[23] Pancuronium undergoes substantial hepatic metabolism; however, its metabolites are partially active and depend on renal excretion.[8] Owing to these metabolites, this drug is a poor choice for patients with renal failure, and hemodialysis is ineffective for its elimination.[24] Increases in the half-life of pancuronium also occur with liver failure. Thus, any patient with compromised hepatic or renal function is at risk for prolonged neuromuscular blockade during pancuronium administration. Pancuronium also demonstrates vagolytic effects that cause tachycardia.[25] Generally, the use of pancuronium in all settings has decreased in the last several years as newer nondepolarizing drugs with fewer side effects, faster onset, and shorter duration have become available.

Vecuronium Bromide

Vecuronium is the 2-desmethyl analog of pancuronium. It has an intermediate duration of action, with an onset of dense neuromuscular blockade in 2 to 3 minutes following a dose of 0.1 mg/kg. The drug is in large part removed via hepatic metabolism and biliary excretion, and is therefore a poor choice for patients with liver disease.[26] Vecuronium has an active 3-desacetyl metabolite. Renal clearance accounts for up to 25% of the parent compound and its metabolite's excretion. Drug accumulation may account for prolonged recovery in patients with renal failure. Vecuronium has no autonomic or vagal blocking activities, and its use

TABLE 11-2

NONDEPOLARIZING NEUROMUSCULAR BLOCKING DRUGS

Drug	Intubating Dose (mg/kg)	25% Recovery of Control Height (min)	Infusion Rate (µg/kg/min)
Pancuronium bromide (LA)	0.08–0.12	60–120	0.3–0.8
Vecuronium bromide (IA)	0.1–0.2	45–90	0.8–2.0
Atracurium besylate (IA)	0.5–0.6	30–45	4–12
Mivacurium chloride (SA)	0.2–0.25	15–20	3–15
Rocuronium bromide (SO-IA)	0.6–1.0	45–75	8–12
Pipecuronium bromide (LA)	0.8–0.12	60–120	NA
Doxacurium chloride (LA)	0.05–0.08	90–150	NA
51W89 (atracurium stereoisomer)* (Mfg: Burroughs Wellcome, Research Triangle Park, NJ)	0.15–0.2	40–75	1–2
ORG 9487 (steroid based)* (Mfg: Organon, West Orange, NJ)	1.5	24	NA

*Investigational drug
LA: long acting; IA: intermediate acting; SA: short acting; SO-IA: short onset and intermediate acting; NA: information not available

offers hemodynamic stability.[27] In addition, the absence of histamine release during its administration makes it attractive for use in patients with reactive airway disease. Its shorter duration of action makes this drug more titratable than pancuronium. Vecuronium has one advantage of considerable military medical importance, which it shares only with succinylcholine: it is available as a lyophilized powder and can be stored without refrigeration.

Atracurium Besylate

Atracurium is an intermediate-acting neuromuscular blocking agent with onset characteristics approximately equal to vecuronium at an equivalent

TABLE 11-3

NEUROMUSCULAR BLOCKADE REVERSAL AGENTS

Neuromuscular Blocking Agent	Dose (mg/kg)	Time to Peak Antagonism (min)	Duration of Antagonism (min)	Antimuscarinic Agent	Dose (µg/kg)
Edrophonium	0.5–1.0	1	40–65	Atropine	7–10
Neostigmine	0.03–0.06	7	55–75	Atropine	15–30
				Glycopyrrolate	10–15
Pyridostigmine	0.25	10–13	80–130	Atropine	15–20
				Glycopyrrolate	10–15

Adapted with permission from Shorten G. Neuromuscular blockade. In: Davison JK, Eckhardt WF III, Perese DA, eds. *Clinical Anesthesia Procedures of the Massachusetts General Hospital*. 4th ed. Boston, Mass: Little, Brown; 1993: 163.

dosage that produces skeletal muscle relaxation in 95% of subjects (ED_{95}). Atracurium has potential advantages in patients who have hepatic or renal failure, because it undergoes extensive plasma degradation.[28] Additionally, atracurium is metabolized via the Hofmann elimination pathway. Hofmann elimination[29] is the spontaneous degradation of atracurium at physiological pH and temperature into laudanosine and a monoquaternary acrylate. Since Hofmann degradation does not require complete organ function or enzymes for its metabolism, there is no significant prolongation of its action in patients with renal or hepatic dysfunction.[30,31] Although the clinical importance of laudanosine in humans is uncertain, this metabolite causes seizures when high doses are given to animals.[32] However, this association with seizures has not been demonstrated in humans.

Atracurium has minimal cardiovascular effects following single- or incremental-dose administration sufficient to cause adequate relaxation for intubation and surgical procedures. In susceptible individuals, large-bolus doses of atracurium administered over a short time may induce bronchospasm or hypotension due to histamine release.

Mivacurium Chloride

Mivacurium chloride is the newest benzisoquinolinium nondepolarizing muscle relaxant. Its onset characteristics are similar to those of atracurium and vecuronium, but it has a shorter duration of action. Its short duration, like succinylcholine's, results from its rapid metabolism by pseudocholinesterases. At clinically used doses, mivacurium releases significant amounts of histamine, with a resultant potential for inducing hypotension and bronchospasm. Like patients who have received succinylcholine, those with deficient or atypical pseudocholinesterase may have greatly prolonged neuromuscular blockade. The primary use of mivacurium is in surgery of short duration, especially if there is a contraindication for the use of succinylcholine.

Rocuronium Bromide

Rocuronium is the latest muscle relaxant to be introduced into clinical practice in the United States. While structurally analogous to vecuronium and pancuronium, it has much faster onset characteristics.[33,34] Given in appropriate doses (3- to 4-fold > ED_{95}), its profile of clinical onset after administration is comparable to that of succinylcholine.[34] Like vecuronium, rocuronium depends primarily on the liver for metabolism and is excreted by the biliary system.[35,36] The duration of rocuronium is comparable to that of vecuronium (2- to 4-fold > ED_{95}).[34]

The onset characteristics of this drug are a major advance in muscle-relaxant pharmacology, allowing clinicians to perform reliable, rapid endotracheal intubations with excellent intubating conditions in 60 to 90 seconds without succinylcholine. Like other currently available nondepolarizing muscle relaxants, rocuronium's duration of effect is much longer than succinylcholine's, which may limit its use in some situations. However, given circumstances where a muscle relaxant is indicated for rapid intubation and succinylcholine is contraindicated, rocuronium is the best alternative currently available.

Because all patients requiring emergency intubation are considered to be at risk for aspiration of stomach contents during the intubation sequence, a rapid-sequence intubation with cricoid pressure is commonly performed. If muscle relaxants are to be used to facilitate intubation, a fast-acting agent should be selected so that the trachea can be intubated promptly and the airway protected. Succinylcholine is most commonly used in this scenario. The list of contraindications and risks with the use of succinylcholine should be considered. Most patients with acute (< 24 h) trauma can safely be given succinylcholine, and the risks of using this agent should not be overstated. The most reasonable alternative is rocuronium, which has a similarly fast onset at a dose of 0.9 to 1.2 mg/kg (3- to 4-fold > ED_{95}) but much longer duration (50–90 min). Rocuronium should be substituted in the patient with a normal airway who has trauma (including burns) greater than 24 hours old, increased intracranial pressure, history of neurologic disease, significantly increased serum potassium (renal failure), penetrating eye injury, or a family history of malignant hyperthermia. The primary disadvantage of rocuronium at this dosage is the duration of neuromuscular blockade: 1 hour or longer.

Other Agents

Newer neuromuscular blocking agents currently available for use in the operating room or the intensive care unit include the long-acting drugs benzylisoquinoline doxacurium chloride and aminosteroid pipecuronium bromide. Many other investigational agents are currently being studied. These newer agents have minimal cardiovascular effects, but their usefulness in the clinical setting remains to be determined.

COMPLICATIONS OF NEUROMUSCULAR BLOCKADE

As with all interventions, the use of neuromuscular blocking agents has associated risks and complications. It is important to realize that when a muscle relaxant is administered, the patient will be unable to ventilate on his own. Therefore, some method of ventilation must be supplied externally. Neuromuscular blocking agents should never be administered unless the necessary equipment is available to supply this need. In a patient who is not already intubated or who does not have a tracheostomy, at a minimum there should be a laryngoscope with different types of blades, endotracheal tubes, suction, an oxygen supply, and a method to deliver positive-pressure ventilation (eg, bag-valve-mask system, mechanical ventilator). The possibility of difficult intubation should be considered. This cannot be emphasized strongly enough: if the airway is not secured in some manner after the muscle relaxant is administered, the patient will suffocate.

Once intubated, the most serious risk to the patient is accidental disconnection from the mechanical ventilator. Another risk is that the patient will fail to cough during tracheal suction, which can lead to retention of secretions. In addition to these, an increased risk of pulmonary embolism has been described.[37] Patients under neuromuscular blockade are also prone to develop decubitus ulcers and nerve-compression syndromes. In addition, owing to these concerns, the nursing workload increases appreciably when patients are treated with neuromuscular blocking agents.

Recently, numerous reports[38–41] have implicated muscle relaxants as causing generalized weakness or myopathy following their long-term administration, with recovery periods lasting as long as 6 months. These reports have implicated the aminosteroid-based agents primarily, although a later report[42] suggests that any of the neuromuscular blocking agents may be involved. However, it is not yet clear whether muscle relaxants are the precipitating factor. Other possible contributing factors have been identified, including polyneuropathy and polymyopathy of critical illness, disuse atrophy, aminoglycoside use, and, in particular, steroid administration.[43–45] Particularly noteworthy are the numerous reports describing otherwise healthy patients suffering from asthma who were simultaneously treated with corticosteroids and muscle relaxants for acute respiratory failure.[46,47] Patients who have muscle weakness or difficulty in weaning from ventilatory management may need electromyographic or histological studies to delineate their basic neuromuscular problems. Drug interactions may affect the degree and duration of neuromuscular blockade. The aminoglycosides can prolong the action of nondepolarizing agents. The mechanisms of action include inhibition of presynaptic acetylcholine release and stabilization of postjunctional membranes.[48] Patients on anticonvulsants or aminophylline may be more resistant to depolarizing agents.[49]

The soldier on the battlefield where unconventional weapons have been or might be used may present for anesthesia and surgery after having been exposed to a variety of agents that impact on the management of neuromuscular blocking agents and anesthesia. These agents include not only chemical warfare agents but also pyridostigmine, which would have been given to the soldiers for nerve agent prophylaxis, and atropine and cholinesterase reactivators such as 2-pyridine aldoxime methyl chloride (2-PAM Cl), with which soldiers are expected to treat themselves immediately after exposure. Medical officers who are performing triage on chemical casualties who also need surgery may not be able to ascertain exactly how much nerve agent, prophylactic agent, and early treatment drugs the casualty has received. This topic is discussed more fully in Chapter 30, Anesthesia for Casualties of Chemical Warfare Agents.

SUMMARY

Muscle relaxants have four important adjunctive roles in the management of combat casualties: (1) to assist in airway intubation; (2) to optimize operative exposure, especially during laparotomy; (3) to assure a quiet operating field; and (4) to assure adequate mechanical ventilation to patients in the intensive care ward. Muscle relaxants such as succinylcholine, which depolarizes motor endplates, have a rapid onset and a short duration of action. Unfortunately, the use of succinylcholine in certain types of casualties (eg, those with chronic burns or injuries to the spinal cord, or who are recovering from massive injury) has been associated with fatal cardiac dysrhythmias due to hyperkalemia. Succinylcholine should not be used in such casualties, nor in casualties in whom the initial increase in local muscle tension caused by depolarization is undesirable. An example of the latter contraindication is the casualty with a penetrating wound of the eye, in whom prolapse of the intraocular contents is possible.

Nondepolarizing muscle relaxants block the acetylcholine receptor without causing depolarization. They typically have a slower onset of action than does succinylcholine, but their duration of action is more prolonged. Nondepolarizing neuromuscular blocking agents may be used when succinylcholine is contraindicated or when the casualty has impaired cardiovascular function. When quantitative assessments of neuromuscular function using a nerve stimulator cannot be made, extubation of a casualty who has received a muscle relaxant should be considered only after return of muscle function is assessed by the patient's ability to sustain a 5-second head lift and to generate an inspiratory force of –25 cm H_2O pressure. Some of the newer nondepolarizing muscle relaxants such as atracurium, vecuronium, and rocuronium are not dependent on renal metabolism and should be considered safe to administer to patients in acute renal failure.

The use of neuromuscular blocking agents in casualties who have been exposed to nerve agents, and in those who have been given nerve agent prophylaxis in the form of pyridostigmine, can cause special treatment problems for military anesthesia providers. Soldiers who have received pyridostigmine may be especially sensitive to succinylcholine, while simultaneously being relatively refractory to the effects of nondepolarizing agents.

REFERENCES

1. West R. Curare in man. *Proc R Soc Med.* 1932;25:1107–1116.
2. Torda TA. The neuromuscular blocking drugs. *Med J Aust.* 1988;149:316–319.
3. Wheeler AP. Sedation, analgesia and paralysis in the ICU. *Chest.* 1993;104:566–577.
4. Peat SJ, Potter DR, Hunter JM. The prolonged use of atracurium in a patient with tetanus. *Anaesthesia.* 1988;43:962–963.
5. Delgado-Escueta AV, Wasterlain C. Management of status epilepticus. *N Engl J Med.* 1982;306:1337–1340.
6. Roberts DJ, Clinton JE, Ruiz E. Neuromuscular blockade for critical patients in the emergency department. *Ann Emerg Med.* 1986;15:152–156.
7. Coggeshall JW, Marini JJ, Newman JH. Improved oxygenation after muscle relaxation in adult respiratory distress syndrome. *Arch Int Med.* 1985;145:1718–1720.
8. Buck ML, Reed MD. Use of nondepolarizing neuromuscular blocking agents in mechanically ventilated patients. *Clin Pharm.* 1991;10:32–48.
9. Hubmayr RD, Abel MD, Rehder K. Physiologic approach to mechanical ventilation. *Crit Care Med.* 1990;18:103–113.
10. Roussos C, Macklem PT. The respiratory muscle. *N Engl J Med.* 1982;307:786–797.
11. Bishop MJ. Hemodynamic and gas exchange effects of pancuronium bromide in sedated patients with respiratory failure. *Anesthesiology.* 1984;60:369–371.
12. Durbin CG Jr. Neuromuscular blocking agents and sedative drugs: Clinical uses and toxic effects in the critical care unit. *Crit Care Clin.* 1991;7:489–506.
13. Whittaker M. Plasma cholinesterase variants and the anaesthetist. *Anaesthesia.* 1980;35:174–197.
14. Evans RT, Wroe JM. Plasma cholinesterase changes during pregnancy: Their interpretations as a cause of suxamethonium-induced apnoea. *Anaesthesia.* 1980;35:651–654.
15. Viby-Mogensen J. Correlation of succinylcholine duration of action with plasma cholinesterase activity in subjects with genotypically normal enzyme. *Anesthesiology.* 1980;53:517–520.

16. Epstein HM, Jarzemsky D, Zuckerman L, Vagher P. Plasma cholinesterase activity in the blood bank. *Anesth Analg*. 1980;59:211–214.

17. Isenstein DA, Venner DS, Duggan J. Neuromuscular blockade in the intensive care unit. *Chest*. 1992;102:1258–1266.

18. Gronert GA, Theye RA. Pathophysiology of hyperkalemia induced by succinylcholine. *Anesthesiology*. 1975;43:83–99.

19. Brenner HR, Samann B. Neurotrophic control of channel properties at neuromusclar synapses of rat muscle. *J Physiol* (Lond). 1983;337:159–166.

20. Sharpe MD. The use of muscle relaxants in the intensive care unit. *Can J Anesth*. 1992;39:949–962.

21. Minton MD, Grosslight K, Stirt JA, Bedford RF. Increases in intracranial pressure from succinylcholine: Prevention by prior nondepolarizing blockade. *Anesthesiology*. 1986;65:165–169.

22. Savarese JJ, Miller RD, Lien CA, Caldwell JE. Pharmacology of muscle relaxants and their antagonists. In: Miller RD, ed. *Anesthesia*. 4th ed. New York, NY: Churchill Livingstone; 1994: 417–487.

23. Hilgenberg JC. Comparison of the pharmacology of vecuronium and atracurium with that of other currently available muscle relaxants. *Anesth Analg*. 1983;62:524–531.

24. Sangala W, Dixon J. Pancuronium and renal failure. *Anaesthesia*. 1987;42:1236. Letter.

25. Kelman GR, Kennedy BR. Cardiovascular effects of pancuronium in man. *Br J Anaesth*. 1971;43:335–338.

26. Lebrault C, Berger JL, D'Hollander AA, Gomeni R, Henzel D, Duvaldestin P. Pharmacokinetics and pharmacodynamics of vecuronium (ORG NC 45) in patients with cirrhosis. *Anesthesiology*. 1985; 62:601–605.

27. Robertson EN, Booij LH, Fragen RJ, Crul JF. Clinical comparison of atracurium and vecuronium (ORG NC 45). *Br J Anaesth*. 1983; 55:125–129.

28. Fisher DM, Canfell PC, Fahey MR, et al. Elimination of atracurium in humans: Contribution of Hofman elimination and ester hydrolysis versus organ based elimination. *Anesthesiology*. 1986;65:6–12.

29. Hofmann AW. Beitrages zur Kenntriss der fluchtragen organischen Basen. *Ann Chem*. 1851;78:253–259.

30. Nigrovic V, Fox JL. Atracurium decay and the formation of laudanosine in humans. *Anesthesiology*. 1991;74:446–454.

31. Fahey MR, Rupp SM, Fisher DM, et al. The pharmacokinetics and pharmacodynamics of atracurium in patients with and without renal failure. *Anesthesiology*. 1984; 61;699–702.

32. Chapple DJ, Miller AA, Ward JB, Wheatley PL. Cardiovascular and neurological effects of laudanosine: Studies in mice and rats, and in conscious and anesthetized dogs. *Brit J Anaesth*. 1987; 59:218–225.

33. Bowman WC, Rodger IW, Houston J, Marshall RJ, McIndewar I. Structure:action relationships among some desacetoxy analogues of pancuronium and vecuronium in the anesthetized cat. *Anesthesiology*. 1988;69:57–62.

34. Magorian T, Flannery KB, Miller RD. Comparison of rocuronium, succinylcholine, and vecuronium for rapid-sequence induction of anesthesia in adult patients. *Anesthesiology*. 1993; 79:913–918.

35. Khuenl-Brady K, Castagnoli KP, Canfell PC, Caldwell JE, Agoston S, Miller RD. The neuromuscular blocking effects and pharmacokinetics of ORG 9426 and ORG 9616 in the cat. *Anesthesiology*. 1990;72:669–674.

36. Magorian T, Wood P, Caldwell J, et al. The pharmacokinetics and neuromuscular effects of rocuronium bromide in patients with liver disease. *Anesth Analg*. 1995;80:754–759.

37. Miller-Jones CM, Williams JH. Sedation for ventilation: A retrospective study of fifty patients. *Anaesthesia*. 1980; 35:1104–1106.

38. Gooch JL, Suchyta MR, Balbierz JM, Pentajan JH, Clemmer TP. Prolonged paralysis after treatment with neuromuscular blocking agents. *Crit Care Med.* 1991;19:1125–1131.

39. Vanderheyden BA, Reynolds HN, Gerold KB, Emanuele T. Prolonged paralysis after long-term vecuronium infusion. *Crit Care Med.* 1992; 20:304–307.

40. Margolis B, Khachikeon M, Friedmen Y, Gorrad C. Prolonged reversible quadriparesis in mechanically ventilated patients who received long-term infusions of vecuronium. *Chest.* 1991; 100:877–878.

41. Segredo V, Caldwell JE, Matthay MA, Sharma ML, Gruenke LD, Miller RD. Persistent paralysis in critically ill patients after long term administration of vecuronium. *N Engl J Med.* 1992;327:524–528.

42. Manthous CA, Chatila W. Prolonged weakness after the withdrawal of atracurium. *Am J Respir Crit Care Med.* 1994;150:1441–1443.

43. Zochodne DW, Bolton CF, Wells GA, et al. Critical illness polyneuropathy: A complication of sepsis and multiple organ failure. *Brain.* 1987;110:819–841.

44. Danon MJ, Carpenter S. Myopathy with thick filament (myosin) loss following prolonged paralysis with vecuronium during steroid treatment. *Muscle Nerve.* 991;14:1131–1139.

45. Vital Brazil O, Prado-Franceschi J. The nature of neuromuscular block produced by neomycin and gentamicin. *Arch Int Pharmacodyn Ther.* 1969;179;78–85.

46. Douglass JA, Tuxen DV, Horne M, et al. Myopathy in severe asthma. *Am Rev Respir Dis.* 1992;146:517–519.

47. Williams TJ, O'Hehir RE, Czarny D, Horne M, Bowes G. Acute myopathy in severe asthma treated with intracavernously administered corticosteroids. *Am Rev Respir Dis.* 1988;137:460–463.

48. Sokoll MD, Gergis SD. Antibiotics and neuromuscular function. *Anesthesiology.* 1981;55:148–159.

49. Doll DC, Rosenberg H. Antagonism of neuromuscular blockage by theophylline. *Anesth Analg.* 1979;58:139–140.

CHAPTER 12

REGIONAL ANESTHESIA

BEN H. BOEDEKER, D.V.M., M.D., PH.D.*; AND GEORGE W. RUNG, M.D.†

*Major, Medical Corps, U.S. Army; Assistant Professor, Department of Anesthesiology, Uniformed Services University of the Health Sciences, Bethesda, Maryland 20814-4799; Assistant Clinical Professor, Pennsylvania State University, College of Medicine, Department of Anesthesia, Hershey Medical Center, Hershey, Pennsylvania 17033
†Associate Professor and Director, Acute Pain Management Service, Pennsylvania State University, College of Medicine, Department of Anesthesia, Hershey Medical Center, Hershey, Pennsylvania 17033

INTRODUCTION

Regional anesthesia has its greatest use in the surgical repair of extremity wounds, and during wartime, extremity wounds occur more frequently (see Figure 1-6, Chapter 1, Combat Trauma Overview) than any others. A regional anesthetic procedure can be done for (*a*) almost any isolated wound that does not cross the midline of the body, and (*b*) multiple wounds of a single extremity or both legs. A craniotomy can be done under local infiltration, although penetrating head wounds are rarely managed without general anesthesia. Intrathoracic and intraabdominal pain may be relieved quite well by regional block, and this technique should be a major part of preoperative and postoperative management. Surgery in these areas is best accomplished under general anesthesia owing to the need, in many cases, for control of the airway and ventilation. Not more than 10%[1] of all combat casualties will arrive in a state of shock at a medical treatment facility with surgical capabilities, thereby assuming hypovolemia and a significant risk for major conduction nerve block anesthesia.

Nerve blocks may be useful to provide preoperative analgesia, intraoperative anesthesia as the sole anesthetic or as a supplement to general anesthesia, or postoperative analgesia. Some nerve blocks are suited for all three of these uses, while others provide good analgesia but may not be acceptable for intraoperative anesthesia.

The physiological benefits of regional anesthesia are numerous (Exhibit 12-1), but *the most important advantage of regional anesthesia is that general anesthesia is avoided,* with its associated loss of airway reflexes, cardiac and respiratory depression, need for endotracheal intubation and mechanical ventilation, loss of patient cooperation, and residual anesthetic effects. Regional anesthesia is not without risk; however, nerve blocks are usually less invasive and affect fewer vital body systems than general anesthesia (Table 12-1).

EXHIBIT 12-1

PHYSIOLOGICAL BENEFITS OF REGIONAL ANESTHESIA

- Analgesia
- Clear sensorium
- Deafferentation
- Improved respiratory mechanics
- Unimpaired ventilatory control
- Hemodynamic stability
- Improved regional blood flow
- Blunted neurohumoral response to injury
- Reduced metabolic effects of injury
- Reduced urinary retention
- Improved bowel function
- Improved immune function
- Reduced muscle spasm

BENEFITS OF NEURAL BLOCKADE

Any new therapy or new indication for an older technique must be evaluated in terms of the potential benefits to be gained versus the possible risks. The risks of these procedures include immediate and long-term complications arising from (*a*) needle and catheter placement, (*b*) toxicity from the local anesthetic agent itself, and (*c*) side effects of neural blockade (eg, hypotension). The risks associated with individual blocks are discussed in the sections describing each technique and the section on local anesthetic pharmacology.

The quality of analgesia provided by neural blockade is superior to that provided by other forms of pain relief, because local anesthetics may completely block the transmission of afferent and efferent nerve impulses.[2] Other forms of analgesia only modify the perception of pain by various mechanisms in the central nervous system (CNS) and the periphery. For example, salicylates and other nonsteroidal antiinflammatory drugs (NSAIDs) decrease afferent nerve activity after a noxious stimulus by desensitizing peripheral pain receptors (ie, nociceptors) and decreasing local inflammation.[3] Inflammatory mediators cause increased blood flow and capillary permeability (ie, the wheal and flare reaction) around the point of injury, which leads to edema and an increased perception of pain (ie, hyperalgesia).[4] Afferent impulses are subject to

TABLE 12-1

REGIONAL VERSUS GENERAL ANESTHESIA

Clinical Criteria	Regional	General
Sensorium	Lucid	Unconscious
Patient Positioning	Self-assist	Dead weight
Airway Reflexes	Intact	Lost
Respiratory Drive	Intact	Impaired
Circulatory Effects	Sympathectomy	Cardiac depression
Medications Administered	Few	Many
Postoperative Analgesia	Yes	No

modulation at the level of the spinal cord prior to transmission to higher centers. One site of modulation by several systems is the dorsal horn of the spinal cord. Endogenous and exogenous opioids, α-adrenergic agonists, serotonin, substance P, and descending inhibitory nerves have been shown[5] to affect neural activity in the dorsal horn. Inhibitory systems may be stimulated by administering epidural or intrathecal opioids, systemic opioids (increases descending inhibitory impulses), or α-adrenergic agents (clonidine).[5] (Also see Chapter 13, Perioperative Pain Management, and Figure 13-1.) None of these treatments are as effective as local anesthetics applied to peripheral nerves or injected into the epidural or intrathecal space because nerve impulses are completely blocked by local anesthetics and may provide surgical anesthesia. Studies[2,6,7] that compare nerve blocks using local anesthetics to systemic, epidural, or intrathecal opioids uniformly reveal that the analgesia provided by neural blockade is superior to that of the other forms.

Owing to their close proximity, somatic neural blockade with local anesthetics will often also block sympathetic afferent and efferent nerves. Selective sympathetic nerve block may also be accomplished, usually at a paravertebral location, in which a ganglion of the sympathetic chain is blocked. A transient condition equivalent in effect to a sympathectomy by either mechanism has several potentially beneficial effects. Decreased sympathetic outflow causes vasodilation and increased regional blood flow to the area innervated, which may decrease ischemic pain, promote healing, improve plastic surgical graft survival, and retard vascular graft thrombosis.[8,9] Blockade of sympathetic afferent fibers inhibits segmental spinal reflexes that may increase pain perception by local secretion of norepinephrine, substance P, and bradykinin, which increases nociceptor sensitivity. The vasodilation caused by sympathectomy may also decrease systemic blood pressure if an adequate intravascular volume is not maintained. A mild decrease in blood pressure may be desirable because myocardial work is reduced and wide variations in blood pressure, especially in response to manipulation or movement of the blocked area, may be prevented. Additionally, decreased intraoperative bleeding and perioperative blood replacement are reported benefits of neural sympathectomy, probably due to the combination of stable hemodynamics and dilation of venous capacitance vessels.[10] Perioperative thromboembolism is also reduced, not only for the above reasons but also because patients with effective analgesia tend to ambulate earlier.[11]

Modification of the neurohumoral response to surgery and trauma is the subject of much attention and effort.[12–14] The *stress response* is a protective reflex in which acute injury or stress triggers a tremendous sympathetic discharge, which then results in elevated plasma catecholamines, cortisol, glucose, antidiuretic hormone, and acute-phase proteins. These changes produce tachycardia, vasoconstriction, hypertension, increased oxygen consumption, negative nitrogen balance, and salt and water retention. In 1914, George W. Crile and William E. Lower coined the term "anoci-association" to describe the physiological changes associated with injury, and correctly predicted that the changes may be detrimental and retard the healing process.[15] Most efforts to attenuate the surgical stress response have been directed toward treating the consequences of the efferent sympathetic activity (eg, tachycardia, hypertension, increased myocardial oxygen consumption, and myocardial ischemia and infarction).[16–18] This practice may be expected to contribute to improved outcome and therefore has changed the way many anesthesiologists practice. Neural blockade, however, may go one step further by blocking somatic and sympathetic afferent activity, which serves to prevent the neurohumoral response to injury rather than to treat it after the fact. Outcome data are incomplete, but evidence[14] indicates that morbidity and mortality are reduced in high-risk surgical patients.

Neural blockade improves decreased respiratory function after trauma or operation.[19] Both lung volumes (ie, functional residual capacity [FRC] and forced expiratory volume in 1 second [FEV_1]) increase, in some cases to near baseline levels.[20] This improvement is greater than that achieved with intramuscular or epidural opioid analgesia, even if complete pain relief is obtained.[21] The mechanism of improvement is probably related not only to inhibition of segmental spinal reflexes that cause skeletal muscle spasm or splinting but also to superior pain relief. Improved respiratory mechanics support normal blood gases, pulmonary toilet, and decreased incidence of atelectasis and infection.

Nerve blocks using higher concentrations of local anesthetics (ie, lidocaine 1.5%–2.0% or bupivacaine 0.5%–0.75%) may produce motor neuron blockade and skeletal muscle relaxation. Dilute solutions of local anesthetics may block only sympathetic and sensory nerve fibers, and may spare motor nerves because of their larger size and greater myelinization. Skeletal muscle relaxation inhibits patient movement and ambulation, which may be distressing to the uninformed patient, but is desirable in certain conditions such as muscle spasm. The relaxation of muscle spasm by neural blockade also improves blood flow through the muscle tissue, which may permit metabolic products associated with muscle ischemia to wash out. This may break the pain–spasm–ischemic pain–continued spasm cycle and prevent sensitization of sensory receptors. Immobility of limbs for a short while after surgery may also prevent disruption of repair caused by excessive patient movement.

Properly administered neural blockade promotes a stable hemodynamic profile. Blockade of somatic and sympathetic afferent fibers attenuate increases in heart rate, blood pressure, and myocardial work in response to pain.[22–24] Nerve blocks may also prevent elevation of plasma epinephrine, norepinephrine, antidiuretic hormone, cortisol, and other chemical mediators, which minimizes secondary changes in hemodynamic parameters.[12] Circulatory changes in response to stimulation such as patient movement or procedures (eg, changing surgical dressings) may also be minimized. Indirectly, nerve blocks promote hemodynamic stability by enabling patients to be extubated soon after surgery and thus avoid the circulatory changes associated with prolonged intubation and mechanical ventilation. Although sympathetic blockade may cause systemic arterial hypotension, this does not usually occur unless a major conduction block (eg, spinal or epidural anesthesia) is used and extends to the midthoracic or higher level of the spine. Systemic arterial hypotension may be minimized by adequate intravascular volume loading prior to the block.

Neural blockade may also obviate the need for other analgesics, sedatives, and anesthetics. Alternative methods of analgesia may provide not only suboptimal analgesia but also incur the risks of the alternative therapy. Systemic opioids, for example, exhibit tremendous variation in interpatient analgesic response, especially when given intramuscularly on an intermittent or as-needed dosage schedule.[25] Systemic side effects of opioids include sedation, depression of ventilatory response to carbon dioxide, nausea, pruritus, and constipation.[26] Continuous or on-demand administration of opioids by mechanical patient-controlled analgesia pumps may minimize side effects.[26,27] The interpatient variability of opioids administered by the epidural or intrathecal route is also unpredictable.[28] Because a patient's response to a prescribed dose of opioid cannot be predicted, opioids should be administered with caution, regardless of route, and side effects treated promptly. The use of continued intubation and mechanical ventilation for analgesia after surgery risks complications caused by prolonged airway instrumentation and positive pressure ventilation.

LOCAL ANESTHETICS

Chemical Structures and Physicochemical Properties

Local anesthetics are chemical compounds that cause reversible blockade of nerve impulses. Commonly used local anesthetics are tertiary or secondary amines bound to an aromatic ring by either an amide or an ester chemical linkage. This distinction divides these drugs into two groups: aminoamides and aminoesters (Figure 12-1). These compounds exhibit both lipophilic and hydrophilic properties. The aromatic ring structure is the lipophilic portion

Agent	Aromatic Lipophilic	Intermediate Chain	Amine Hydrophilic	Molecular Weight (base)	pKa (25°C)	Partition Coefficient	% Protein Binding
Esters							
Procaine	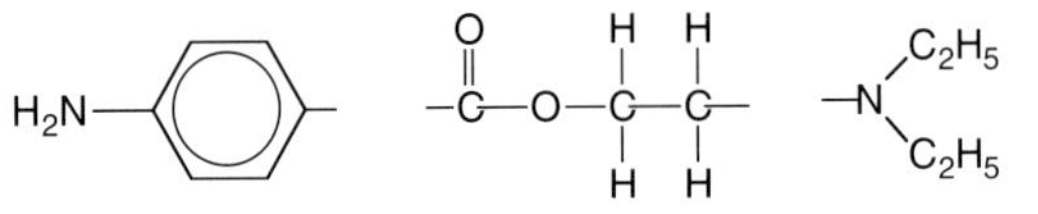			236	8.9	0.02	5.8
Tetracaine	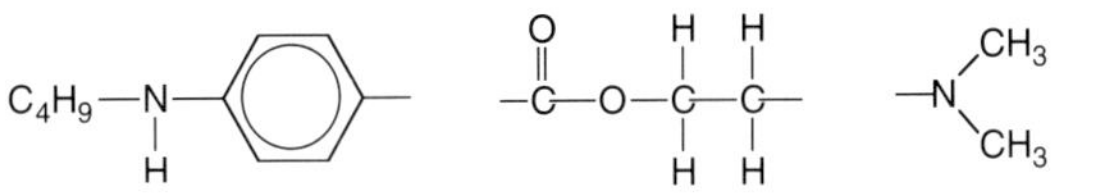			264	8.6	4.1	75.6
Chloroprocaine	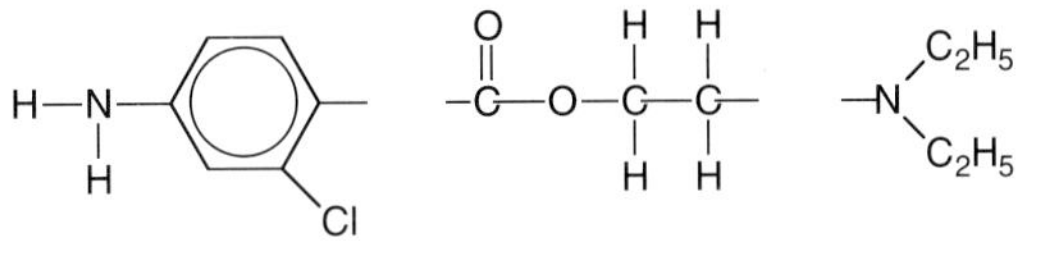			271	8.7	0.14	—
Amides							
Prilocaine	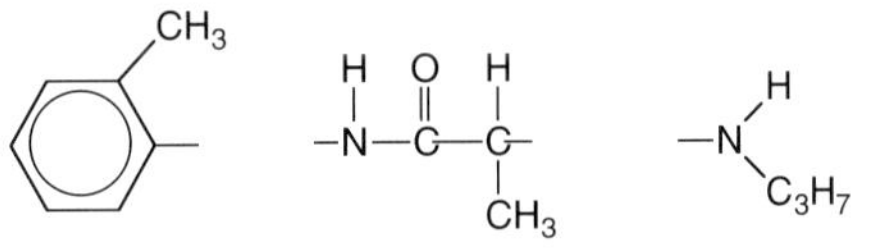			220	7.7	0.9	~55
Lidocaine	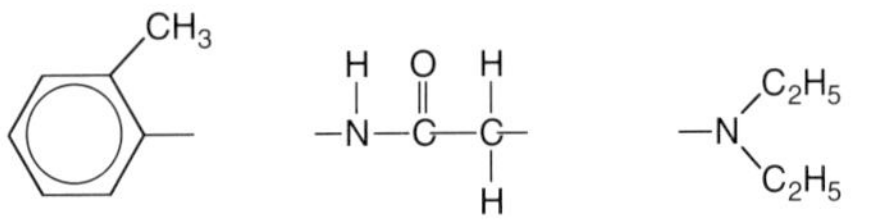			234	7.7	2.9	64.3
Mepivacaine	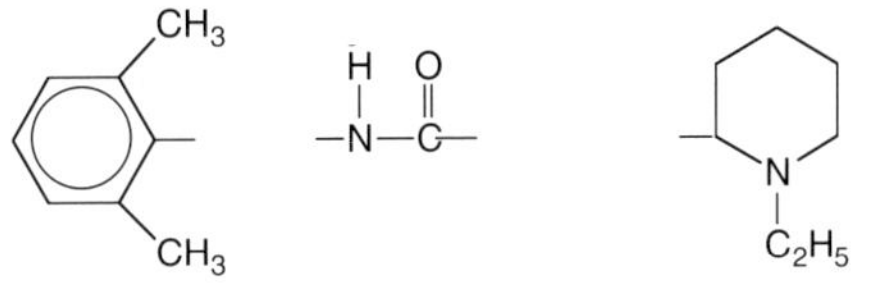			246	7.6	0.8	77.5
Bupivacaine	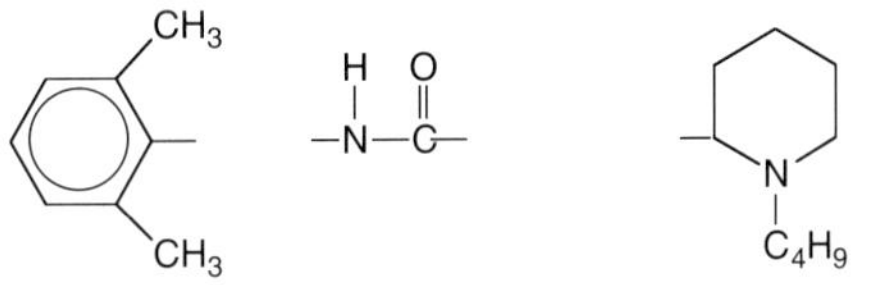			288	8.1	27.5	95.6
Etidocaine	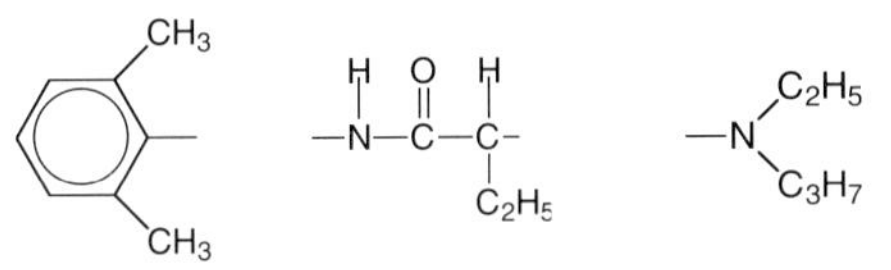			276	7.7	141	94

Fig. 12-1. Physicochemical properties of local anesthetics. Adapted with permission from Scott DB. *Techniques of Regional Anaesthesia.* Norwalk, Conn: Appleton & Lange; 1989: 16. © Mediglobe S.A., Fribourg, Switzerland.

of the molecule. The amine structure is the hydrophilic portion. Ionization of the amine portion to a positively charged species enhances the hydrophilic properties of the molecule.[29]

Local anesthetics are weak bases with pKa values between 7.5 and 9.0. Their physicochemical properties largely determine their clinical anesthetic characteristics. Inherent potency of all anesthetic compounds, including local anesthetics, correlates well with each compound's lipid solubility. Chloroprocaine, for example, is poorly soluble in lipid and has a relatively low anesthetic potency (concentrations of 2%–3% are required for clinical use). Bupivacaine, on the other hand, is lipid soluble and has greater anesthetic potency (more dilute solutions, 0.25%–0.5%, are clinically effective). Onset of action correlates roughly with a local anesthetic's pKa. The pKa of any compound is the pH at which equal amounts of nonionized and ionized species exist in equilibrium. The amount of each form at any given time depends on the local pH. This is illustrated by the formula

$$pKa = pH + \log (Bh^+/B)$$

Generally, the higher the pKa of these compounds, the greater the ionization at a physiological pH of 7.4, and the slower the onset of neural blockade.[30] Duration of anesthetic action is dependent on the local anesthetic's affinity for protein. Anesthetics that are highly protein bound (eg, bupivacaine) in general have a longer duration of action than those that are not (eg, procaine).

Physiology of Neural Blockade

Impulses are propagated along nerve cell axons by progressive depolarization of the cell membrane. Depolarization occurs when sodium rapidly enters the cell through sodium channels. Local anesthetics are thought to physically block, or to induce conformational changes within, these sodium channels by reversibly binding to receptors on the intracellular side of the membrane. While the sodium channel is inactive, nerve impulse conduction cannot occur.[31]

The nonionized lipophilic form of local anesthetic most easily crosses the myelin sheath and nerve cell membrane, but it is the ionized hydrophilic form that attaches to the receptor in the cell's sodium channel to block nerve impulse conduction.[32] This is why a local anesthetic with a high pKa (the ionized form is predominant at pH 7.4 and crosses the nerve membranes poorly) generally has a long onset time.

Local anesthetic duration of action correlates with the degree of protein binding because the local anesthetic receptor is thought to be a protein in or near the sodium channel. Anesthetics with high affinity for protein will dissociate from the receptor slowly and therefore the effect will be prolonged. Once dissociated from the receptor, the drug is taken up by the bloodstream and metabolized in the plasma (ester hydrolysis) or the liver (ester hydrolysis and amide microsomal degradation).[33]

Clinical Use

Onset of local anesthetic activity in vivo is dependent on several factors in addition to the pKa of the drug and the tissue pH. The number of molecules available for participation in neural blockade is important; therefore, higher concentrations and larger doses tend to speed onset. The addition of vasoconstrictors to the local anesthetic solution decreases the rate of anesthetic uptake by the bloodstream and, in effect, increases the local concentration, which shortens onset time.[33] Systemic absorption of epinephrine or phenylephrine used for this purpose may produce undesirable hemodynamic changes in the compromised patient. The addition of bicarbonate to the drug solution increases local tissue pH, which increases the amount of easily diffusible nonionized drug present and speeds onset. Carbonation of local anesthetic solutions also speeds the onset of action because carbon dioxide rapidly crosses the cell membrane and lowers intracellular pH. This acidosis favors ionization of intracellular local anesthetic molecules, which increases the activity of the drug by enhancing receptor binding.

Local anesthetic activity and duration of action are also enhanced by adding vasoconstrictors to the solution.[29] The anatomical location of the anesthetic injection affects the onset and duration of the local anesthetic action because the vascularity of the tissue and the regional blood flow determine the rate of local anesthetic uptake by the blood.[31] The local anesthetic concentrations in plasma after injection of a standard dose in different anatomic locations is shown in Figure 12-2. The highest plasma concentration occurs after injection into the intercostal space.

Tachyphylaxis (ie, the development of a decreased effect from a given dose of drug after repeated administration) may be caused by a gradual exhaustion of local tissue-buffering capacity, which is, in turn, caused by repeated injections of the relatively acidic local anesthetic salt solutions. Continuous infusion of anesthetic solution (rather than intermittent injection) or using a different local anesthetic may decrease tachyphylaxis.

Properties of Individual Drugs

The clinical uses and appropriate doses of commonly used local anesthetics are listed in Table 12-2. Although local anesthetics share a common mechanism of action, individual drugs have different indications, side effects, and other properties, such as addiction potential. Important properties of individual drugs are noted below.

Bupivacaine has a high affinity for protein (95% of the drug is bound to protein in plasma) and may be relatively more cardiotoxic than other local anesthetics, because dissociation from cardiac sodium channels may be very slow.[29] Bupivacaine may

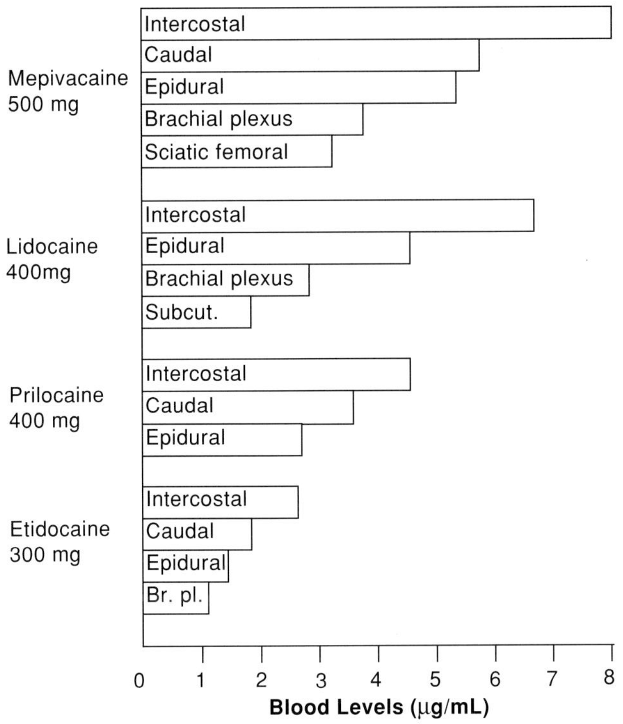

Fig. 12-2. Comparative peak blood levels of several local anesthetic agents. Reprinted with permission from Covino BG, Vassallo HG. *Local Anesthetics: Mechanism of Action and Clinical Use.* New York, NY: Grune and Stratton; 1976: 97. In: Carpenter RL, Mackey DC. Local anesthetics. In: Barash PG, Cullen BF, Stoelting RK. *Clinical Anesthesia.* Philadelphia, Pa: JP Lippincott; 1989: 384.

produce sensory blockade without motor blockade (ie, selective sensory block) at low concentrations.

Chloroprocaine is rapidly metabolized in plasma by pseudocholinesterases and therefore has a short duration of action and low toxicity potential. Patients with abnormal or decreased plasma cholinesterase may have a prolonged duration of action. Use of chloroprocaine may prolong the effect of other drugs metabolized by cholinesterases (eg, succinylcholine).

Cocaine is used exclusively for topical anesthesia of the nose and throat. It causes vasoconstriction, CNS stimulation, and is highly addictive.[30] Addition of a vasoconstrictor is both unnecessary and undesirable.

Etidocaine and lidocaine are structurally similar and have similar onsets of action. Etidocaine's duration of action is longer than lidocaine's and the degree of motor blockade is greater. Lidocaine has the largest number of clinical uses and may be used for topical, infiltration, plexus, epidural, and spinal anesthesia; and intravenous treatment of cardiac dysrhythmias.

Mepivacaine is not effective when used topically. It is also not desirable for use in obstetric anesthesia because neonatal metabolism of mepivacaine is five times slower than in the adult. Because U.S. military forces are used increasingly in operations other than war (OOTW, eg, peacekeeping missions), anesthetic procedures used with obstetric, neonatal, and pediatric patients are assuming greater relevance to military medicine.

Prilocaine may produce methemoglobinemia due to the accumulation of a metabolite, *o*-toluidine, which oxidizes hemoglobin to methemoglobin. This may occur after high doses of prilocaine, usually greater than 600 mg, have been administered. If methemoglobinemia occurs, it can be treated by administering reducing agents (eg, methylene blue 1 mg/kg).[29]

Adverse Reactions to Local Anesthetic

True allergy to local anesthetic drugs is extremely rare. When it occurs, it is usually due to hypersensitivity to a preservative (eg, *p*-aminobenzoic acid) or a metabolite of local anesthetics. Most reactions assumed to be allergic are actually due to

- systemic effects of toxic plasma concentrations of local anesthetic as a result of relative overdosage, or to intravascular injection of an otherwise appropriate dose;
- systemic epinephrine effects;
- a vasovagal reaction; or
- total spinal blockade (ie, high spinal causing cardiopulmonary collapse, which may mimic anaphylactic shock).

The cause of the adverse reaction must be determined quickly before appropriate treatment can be instituted.

Toxic plasma concentrations are manifest by CNS signs: first tinnitus, circumoral numbness, metallic taste, and then with increasing plasma concentration, tremulousness that may progress to seizure activity. A very small dose of local anesthetic may cause CNS signs if injected into an artery that perfuses the brain (eg, the vertebral artery). These CNS signs may be followed by cardiovascular effects, which require higher plasma concentrations. Direct depression of myocardial inotropy and chronotropy occur, in addition to systemic arterial vasodilation. Cardiac dysrhythmias and cardiovascular collapse may occur secondary to acidosis and hypoxia caused by seizure activity when local anesthetic plasma concentration is below cardiotoxic

TABLE 12-2

COMMONLY USED LOCAL ANESTHETICS: CLINICAL USES AND APPROPRIATE DOSES

Agent	Concentration (%)	Clinical Use	Onset	Usual Duration (h)	Recommended Maximum Single Dose (mg)	Comments	pH of Plain Solutions*
Amides							
Lidocaine	0.5–1.0	Infiltration	Fast	1.0–2.0	300	Most versatile agent.	6.5
	0.25–0.5	IV Regional			500 + Epi		
	1.0–1.5	Periph nerve blocks	Fast	1.0–3.0	500 + Epi		
	1.5–2.0	Epidural	Fast	1.0–2.0	500 + Epi		
	4	Topical	Mod	0.5–1.0	500 + Epi		
	5	Spinal	Fast	0.5–1.5	100		
Prilocaine	0.5–1.0	Infiltration	Fast	1.0–2.0	600	Least toxic amide agent.	4.5
	0.25–0.5	IV Regional			600	Methemoglobinemia usually occurs above 600 mg.	
	1.5–2.0	Periph nerve blocks	Fast	1.5–3.0	600		
	2.0–3.0	Epidural	Fast	1.0–3.0			
Mepivacaine	0.5–1.0	Infiltration	Fast	1.5–3.0	400 500 + Epi	Plain mepivacaine solution has longer duration than plain lidocaine solution. Useful when epinephrine is contra-indicated.	4.5
	1.0–1.5	Periph nerve blocks	Fast	2.0–3.0			
	1.5–2.0	Epidural	Fast	1.5–3.0			
	4.0	Spinal	Fast	1.0–1.5	100		
Bupivacaine	0.25	Infiltration	Fast	2.0–4.0	175 225 + Epi	Lower concentrations provide differential sensory/motor block. Ventricular arrhythmias and sudden cardiovascular collapse reported following rapid IV injection.	4.5
	0.25–0.5	Periph nerve blocks	Slow	4.0–12.0	225 + Epi		
	0.25–0.5	Obstetric epidural	Mod	2.0–4.0	225 + Epi		
	0.5–0.75	Surgical epidural	Mod	2.0–5.0	225 + Epi		
	0.5–0.75	Spinal	Fast	2.0–4.0	20		
Etidocaine	0.5	Infiltration	Fast	2.0–4.0	300 400 + Epi	Profound motor block useful for surgical but not for obstetric analgesia.	4.5
	0.5–1.0	Peripheral	Fast	3.0–12.0	400 + Epi		
	1.0–1.5	Surgical epidural	Fast	2.0–4.0	400 + Epi		
Dibucaine	0.25–0.5	Spinal (hyperbaric)	Fast	2.0–4.0	10	Recommended only for spinal and topical use.	—
	0.00067	Spinal (hypobaric)	Fast	2.0–4.0	10		
	1.0	Topical	Slow	0.5–1.0	50		
Esters							
Procaine	1.0	Infiltration	Fast	0.5–1.0	1,000	Used mainly for infiltration and differential spinal blocks. Allergic potential after repeated use.	5–6.5
	1.0–2.0	Periph nerve blocks	Slow	0.5–1.0	1,000		
	2.0	Epidural	Slow	0.5–1.0	1,000		
	10.0	Spinal	Mod	0.5–1.0	200		
Chloroprocaine	1.0	Infiltration	Fast	0.5–1.0	800 1,000 + Epi	Lowest systemic toxicity of all local anesthetics.	2.7–4
	2.0	Periph nerve block	Fast	0.5–1.0	1,000 + Epi	Intrathecal injection may be associated with sensory/motor deficits.	—
	2.0–3.0	Epidural	Fast	0.5–1.0	1,000 + Epi		
Tetracaine	0.5	Spinal	Fast	2.0–4.0	20	Use is limited primarily to spinal and topical anesthesia.	4.5–6.5
	2.0	Topical	Slow	0.5–1.0	20		
Cocaine	4.0–10.0	Topical	Slow	0.5–1.0	150	Topical use only. Addictive, causes vasoconstriction. CNS toxicity initially features marked excitation (fight or flight response). May cause cardiac arrhythmias owing to sympathetic stimulation.	—
Benzocaine	≤ 20	Topical	Slow	0.5–1.0	200	Useful only for topical anesthesia.	—

*Epinephrine-containing solutions have a pH 1 to 1.5 units lower than plain solutions.
Epi: epinephrine; IV: intravenous; Mod: moderate; Periph: peripheral; CNS: central nervous system
Adapted with permission from Covino BG. Clinical pharmacology of local anesthetic agents. In: Cousins MJ, Bridenbaugh PO, eds. *Neural Blockade*. 2nd ed. Philadelphia, Pa: JB Lippincott; 1988: 112–113.

levels. In general, treatment for toxic local anesthetic reactions is supportive until the drug is redistributed or metabolized, and the tissue levels decrease. The injection of local anesthetic should cease immediately, the airway be supported, and supplemental oxygen be administered. Tracheal intubation and pharmacological treatment of seizures is rarely required.

Intravascular absorption of epinephrine may cause tachycardia, hypertension, hypotension (a β-adrenergic effect), anxiety, restlessness, and a feeling of impending doom. These effects are often mistaken for local anesthetic toxicity. Treatment is supportive.

A vasovagal reaction may occur during needle placement or with injection of local anesthetic. Bradycardia, hypotension, sweating, and pallor precede fainting. Administration of atropine intravenously or intramuscularly and supportive measures are indicated.

True allergies to local anesthetics have been reported in a very small percentage of patients. These reactions are almost always due to hypersensitivity to the *p*-aminobenzoic acid metabolic derivatives of ester-type anesthetic drugs. Allergic reactions to amide-type drugs are extremely rare. Hypersensitivity to preservatives (eg, methylparaben) may also occur. Allergic reaction symptoms include urticaria and cutaneous flushing, wheezing, tachycardia, arterial hypotension, and cardiovascular collapse. Treatment consists of maintenance of a patent airway, ventilation with 100% oxygen, and administration of epinephrine that is titrated to maintain a normal blood pressure. Steroids and histamine blocking drugs may also be given.

REGIONAL ANESTHESIA FOR THORACIC AND ABDOMINAL SURGERY

Regional anesthesia for thoracic and abdominal surgery—except for superficial or lower-abdominal procedures—is usually used in combination with general anesthesia. Why should patients receive regional anesthesia if they are going to have a general anesthetic anyway? There are numerous advantages and disadvantages, and numerous and varied outcome studies have been performed. The advantages of combined general–regional anesthesia versus general anesthesia alone include the following:

- The general anesthetic requirement may be reduced, which may result in a reduction in dose-related general anesthetic effects, a faster emergence, earlier extubation, and shorter hospital stay.[14,34]
- The combined technique produces a smoother intraoperative course with more stable hemodynamic parameters and fewer changes of anesthetic depth required.[35,36]
- Noxious afferent input to the spinal cord may be minimized, which may reduce spinal cord sensitization, thereby decreasing or causing the development of permanent spinal cord sensitization, which may give rise to a chronic pain pathway. Thus the neurohumoral response to tissue injury is attenuated.[12]
- Postoperative analgesia may be provided by extending the nerve block technique after discontinuing general anesthesia.[34,35]
- The blockade of sympathetic nerve impulses to and from the spinal cord may be used to produce deliberate and controlled hypotension (to reduce bleeding) and may also provide analgesia for sympathetically mediated pain.[37]

The disadvantages of combined general–regional anesthesia versus general anesthesia alone include the following:

- The additional invasive procedure adds to the risk of anesthetic complications.[38]
- The nerve block procedure requires additional anesthetic preparation time. This is especially disadvantageous if the procedures are done in the operating room.
- The combination of major conduction nerve blocks and general anesthetic–induced myocardial depression may result in severe hypotension.[14,34]
- Some evidence[34] indicates that the combination of general and regional anesthesia is associated with a greater degree of intraoperative hypothermia than either technique used alone.
- There is a theoretical increased risk of intraoperative awareness if low concentrations of inhaled anesthetic agents are used.

Many outcome studies identify positive physiological effects of regional versus general anesthesia, including reduced intraoperative blood loss, improved postoperative respiratory function, maintenance of bowel motility, and more normal metabolic, immune, and hemostatic functions.[14,34,39,40] However, very few studies investigate whether these physiological changes (*a*) are clinically important or (*b*) affect patient outcome. Moreover, studies comparing the outcome of patients who undergo combination general–regional anesthesia versus general anesthesia only are fewer still.[14,36] Comparative studies have been hindered by a relative underutilization of local anesthetics in favor of opioids, inappropriate epidural catheter placement (eg, lumbar placement for thoracic or upper-abdominal surgery), and administration of lipophilic opioids at a spinal level (lumbar) distant from the site of action (thoracic).

Applied Anatomy for Regional Anesthesia of the Chest and Abdomen

Somatic Nerves

The chest and abdominal wall are innervated by branches of thoracic spinal nerves. Surgical procedures of the chest and abdomen involve almost exclusively areas innervated by nine pairs of spinal nerves, T-4 through T-12. T-1 is part of the brachial plexus, T-2 and T-3 innervate the chest wall above the level of the nipples, where thoracic surgery is rarely performed, and the lumbar spinal nerves involve only the peripheral (inguinal) lower abdomen. Each spinal nerve has a small dorsal ramus that innervates paraspinal muscles and skin, and a large ventral ramus that becomes the intercostal nerve and innervates skin, muscle, and bone in the distribution of the corresponding rib.[41]

Sympathetic and Parasympathetic Nerves

Sympathetic nerves to and from the chest and abdomen synapse in or pass through the paired sympathetic chain ganglia located anterior and lateral to the vertebral bodies from T-1 to L-5. Sympathetic outflow from the spinal cord reaches the sympathetic chain via the white rami communicantes; sympathetic afferents from the chain travel via the gray rami communicantes to the spinal cord. The greater, lesser, and least splanchnic nerves are formed by fibers from the sympathetic chain and synapse in the mesenteric ganglia.[41]

Afferent and efferent parasympathetic innervation of the chest and abdomen is largely via the paired vagal nerves.[41]

Applied Physiology for Regional Anesthesia of the Chest and Abdomen

Respiratory Effects

Control of ventilation is not inhibited by regional anesthesia.[42] Some evidence[43] suggests that systemic local anesthetics actually increase the ventilatory response to carbon dioxide.

The mechanics of ventilation are often disturbed after thoracic and abdominal surgery owing to decreased chest-wall compliance and diaphragm dysfunction.[34] Regional anesthesia does not affect motor nerves to the diaphragm (eg, the phrenic nerve, the most important contribution to which is from C-4), may rarely weaken some intercostal muscles, and has been shown to reduce diaphragm dysfunction after upper abdominal surgery.[39]

Increased airway resistance secondary to reduced sympathetic efferent activity to the lungs is a theoretical concern, although it has not been reported as a problem in patients with pulmonary disease who are undergoing thoracotomy. In fact, thoracic epidural anesthesia has been used to treat status asthmaticus, presumably by blocking sympathetic afferent fibers from the airways.[21]

Circulatory Effects

Cardiac Effects. Bradycardia, junctional rhythm, or heart block may be caused by blocking of sympathetic nerves to the heart, although complete blockade may be necessary for these effects.[15] Coronary artery blood flow, in normal and stenotic vessels, and cardiac function may increase dramatically owing to the sympathetic nerve block associated with thoracic epidural anesthesia.[44,45]

Systemic and Pulmonary Artery Blood Pressure. A decrease in systemic blood pressure is often associated with thoracolumbar sympathetic nerve block, largely due to dilation of venous capacitance vessels and decreased venous return to the heart.[44] Systemic vascular resistance is also reduced and cardiac output may increase if preload is maintained.[44] The degree of hypotension is dependent on the number of spinal segments blocked. Local anesthetics administered through a thoracic epidural catheter may cause less hypotension than a lumbar epidural catheter because some sympathetic outflow may be spared, innervation of the adrenal glands may be intact, and the pumping action of the lower extremity muscles to augment venous return may be functional.

A decrease in pulmonary artery pressure may be associated with blockade of sympathetic nerves to the chest unless pulmonary hypertension is caused by a mechanical resistance (ie, vascular changes or mitral valvular stenosis).[44] In this situation, the increased impedance offered is not affected by sympathetic blockade.

Endocrine, Gastrointestinal, and Urinary Effects

There is currently no better way to inhibit the neurohumoral response to tissue injury than via afferent neural blockade. This benefit may not be completely realized in thoracoabdominal surgery, however, because complete afferent blockade is not commonly attained owing to vagal afferents and humeral mediators such as cytokines.[12]

The sympathetic nerve block that may accompany regional anesthesia promotes gastrointestinal function by creating a predominant parasympathetic nerve influence on the gut, which increases peristalsis and gut motility.[40] This beneficial effect of regional anesthesia is often augmented by a reduced opioid requirement for adequate analgesia, and therefore, fewer opioid-induced side effects. These effects may combine to reduce the incidence of postoperative ileus.[34,35]

Urinary retention after surgery may be caused by residual general anesthetic effect, opioids, neural blockade, and other drugs. Like gut function, the ability to void may be maintained by segmental (thoracic) nerve blockade and the avoidance of opioid analgesics.[34,35]

Locomotion

Patients who have received regional anesthesia for thoracic and abdominal surgery should be able to ambulate earlier than patients who did not receive regional anesthesia. Motor nerves to the lower extremity originate in lumbar and sacral spinal nerves, which may be spared by segmental thoracic spinal nerve block. The superior analgesia provided by regional anesthesia, without the sedation caused by systemic analgesics, also promotes early ambulation.[34,35]

Specific Regional Anesthetic Techniques

The intelligent use of regional anesthesia for thoracic and abdominal surgery requires that the anesthesiologist have a thorough knowledge of (*a*) the anatomy and physiology related to neural blockade, (*b*) the patient's medical and surgical history, and (*c*) the planned surgical procedure. Techniques that may be useful for thoracic and abdominal surgery include thoracic epidural anesthesia, spinal anesthesia, intercostal nerve block, interpleural nerve block, and incisional local anesthetic infiltration. At least one of these techniques is usually indicated, regardless of the patient's condition or the surgical procedure planned. Characteristics of each technique are summarized in Table 12-3. Complications of regional anesthesia are discussed later in this chapter.

TABLE 12-3

REGIONAL ANESTHETIC TECHNIQUES FOR THORACIC AND ABDOMINAL SURGERY

Technique	Somatic Sensory Nerve Block	Sympathetic Nerve Block	Lower Extremity Motor Block
Epidural Anesthesia			
Thoracic	+	+	–
Lumbar	+	+	+
Spinal Anesthesia	+	+	+
Intercostal Nerve Block*			
Single	+	–	–
Continuous	+	–/+	–
Interpleural Nerve Block*	+	–/+	–
Paravertebral Nerve Block*	+	–/+	–
Peripheral Nerve Block	+	–	–

*Unilateral anesthesia: (+) = effect; (–) = no effect

Epidural Anesthesia

Epidural anesthesia is the most versatile regional anesthetic technique available in terms of surgical application, control of extent and duration of nerve block, and use for postoperative analgesia. Epidural anesthesia can produce segmental sympathetic, sensory, and motor block for many intrathoracic or intraabdominal procedures, lower extremity or abdominal surgery, analgesia during labor and delivery, and treatment of medical conditions such as Raynaud's phenomenon or postherpetic neuralgia.

Despite the advantages, thoracic epidural anesthesia should not be attempted by anesthesiologists who are unfamiliar with the technique. As an alternative, lumbar epidural anesthesia may be used for thoracic and abdominal surgery if local anesthetics are used intraoperatively to provide an adequate level of anesthesia but are discontinued postoperatively. Because high volumes of local anesthetic are required, the sympathectomy may be extensive, and motor block of the lower extremities will result. Epidural opioids may be used subsequently to provide postoperative analgesia without motor block, but this adds the potential for opioid side effects.

Owing to the close proximity of the underlying spinal cord, thoracic epidural anesthesia should not be routinely performed in anesthetized patients. As with any regional anesthetic technique, if needle insertion is difficult, multiple attempts should not be pursued because the incidence of complications increases inordinately. Know when to abandon the procedure and use an alternative technique.

Epidural anesthesia is contraindicated in the presence of informed patient refusal, local or severe systemic infection, abnormal coagulation, unstable neurological deficits, uncorrected hypovolemia, and possibly immunosuppression.

Technique. Epidural anesthesia may be performed at any level of the spine. The epidural space is identified by a characteristic loss of resistance to depression of the syringe plunger on entering the space (ie, *loss of resistance* technique) or by the disappearance of a drop of sterile saline from the needle hub on entering the space owing to the subatmospheric pressure of the space (ie, *hanging drop* technique). A *single-shot* technique may be used, in which one dose of anesthetic is injected into the space, or a *continuous* (usually intermittent injection) technique may be used, in which a catheter is threaded into the space through the needle; then the needle is removed. In the lumbar spine, a local anesthetic volume of approximately 1.5 to 2.0 mL per spinal segment is required for anesthesia. Epidural catheters may be kept in place for 48 to 72 hours or longer if the benefits of analgesia outweigh the risk of infection.

If local anesthetics will be used postoperatively, the tip of the epidural catheter should be placed as closely as possible to the midpoint of the range of spinal (thoracic) segments to be blocked. This location allows the use of lower volumes of local anesthetics, minimizes the extent of sympathetic nerve block, and is unlikely to cause lower-extremity motor block. Suggested levels of epidural catheter placement for given surgical procedures are listed in Table 12-4.

Local Anesthetic Drug Dosages. Local anesthetics must come into contact with the target nerves to exert their effect. Epidural dosing of local anesthetics is, therefore, largely based on volume. In the epidural space, local anesthetics spread in all directions from the catheter tip, but preferentially along lines of least resistance. The epidural space is smaller in the thoracic than in the lumbar spine, and the volume of anesthetic must be adjusted accordingly. General rules of thumb for adults are given in Table 12-5. The concentration of local anesthetic affects the speed of onset of block, degree of motor block, and duration of block. Motor-blocking strengths may be used intraoperatively, but the lowest con-

TABLE 12-4

LOCATION OF EPIDURAL CATHETER INSERTION

Site of Surgery	Epidural Catheter	Dose of Local Anesthetic (mL)
Thoracic	Upper thoracic spine (T-4 –T-7)	4–6
Upper abdominal	Mid thoracic spine (T-8–T-9)	6–8
Lower abdominal	Lower thoracic spine (T-10–T-11)	8–10

TABLE 12-5

EPIDURAL LOCAL ANESTHETIC DOSAGE GUIDELINES

Position of Catheter Tip	Volume Required per Spinal Segment (mL)	Volume Required for T-4 Level (mL)
Upper thoracic (T-4–T-7)	1.0	1–6
Mid thoracic (T-8–T-9)	1.5	8–10
Lower thoracic (T-10–T-12)	1.75	12–18
Lumbar (L-1–L-5)	2.0	20–28

centration that provides pain relief should be used postoperatively.

Opioid analgesics are usually administered on a milligram-per-kilogram basis. Lipophilic drugs, such as fentanyl, act via a spinal mechanism if placed in the thoracic epidural space, and via systemic absorption if placed in the lumbar epidural space.[46,47] Hydrophilic drugs, such as morphine or hydromorphone, spread more readily through the epidural space before absorption, act via a spinal mechanism, and are effective in the lumbar or thoracic epidural space.[48,49] Increased respiratory surveillance may be considered if a hydrophilic opioid is used in the upper-thoracic epidural space. Opioid dosage guidelines are given in Table 12-6.

Complications. The complications of epidural anesthesia are similar to those associated with spinal anesthesia (Table 12-7). Possible trauma caused by needle insertion may be greater owing to the larger needle size, and the risk of local anesthetic toxicity is greater owing to the larger doses used. Inadvertent dural puncture carries a high likelihood of post–dural-puncture headache. A "total" spinal (ie, the entire spinal cord has been blocked, at least to some extent) may result from intrathecal injection of a local anesthetic dose appropriate for epidural administration. As with spinal anesthesia, sympathetic nerve block may cause systemic hypotension, especially if the patient is hypovolemic. Bradycardia may occur if high thoracic spinal levels are blocked (ie, if cardioaccelerator fibers are anesthetized). Subarachnoid and epidural abscesses have been reported[41] after epidural needle or catheter insertion.

Spinal Anesthesia

Spinal anesthesia has many advantages compared to epidural anesthesia: much smaller local anesthetic doses are required, systemic vascular absorption and risk of systemic toxicity are negligible, onset of block is much faster, and the resultant nerve block is more complete, including motor blockade. Disadvantages include the inability to produce a segmental band of anesthesia, a more extensive virtual sympathectomy with more pronounced blood pressure changes, and fewer postoperative analgesic options.[50]

TABLE 12-6

EPIDURAL OPIOID DOSAGE GUIDELINES FOR A HEALTHY, 70-KG, ADULT PATIENT

Drug	Initial Dose (mg)	Injectate Volume* (mL)	Infusion Rate
Morphine	3–5	10	0.2–0.3 mg/h
Hydromorphone	0.5–1.0	10	60–150 µg/h
Fentanyl	75–150	10	30–100 µg/h
Sufentanil	25–50	10	5–15 µg/h

*Prepare opioid dose in preservative-free saline

TABLE 12-7

SPINAL VERSUS EPIDURAL ANESTHESIA

Characteristic	Spinal	Epidural
Onset	Fast	Slow
Local anesthetic dose	Small	Large
Local anesthetic plasma concentration	Nil	Nil
Density of block	Very dense	Less dense (spotty)
Need for supplementation	Less likely	More likely
Indication of needle placement	Reliable*	Less reliable†
Post–dural-puncture headache	Low risk	Possible
Hypotension	More likely	Less likely
Continuous technique	Less common	Very common
Postoperative analgesia	Possible (Duramorph‡)	Common

*By cerebrospinal fluid
†By loss of resistance
‡Morphine; manufactured by Elkins-Sinn, Cherry Hill, NJ

Spinal anesthesia may be used alone for many lower-abdominal procedures or lower-extremity surgery and may be combined with general anesthesia for upper-abdominal surgery. Spinal anesthesia is rarely used for thoracic surgery.

Spinal anesthesia is contraindicated for patients with coagulation abnormalities, infection at the site of needle placement, severe systemic infection, uncorrected hypovolemia, unstable neurological deficits, and possibly immunosuppression.

Technique. The basic technique for lumbar puncture may be found in any standard anesthesiology textbook. The injection of a single dose of local anesthetic through the spinal needle, a single-shot technique, is sufficient for many surgical techniques. The sensory and motor blockade produced by such a technique depends largely on the local anesthetic dosage, baricity, and location and speed of injection. Isobaric solutions (bupivacaine 0.5%, lidocaine 2%, and tetracaine 1%) are gaining popularity because neural blockade is independent of patient position, fewer spinal segments are blocked, and there are smaller reductions in systemic blood pressure. A continuous catheter technique may be used (*a*) to produce a slow onset of neural blockade by fractionating the total anesthetic dose and (*b*) to prolong neural blockade for long surgical procedures. Isobaric local anesthetic solutions are also useful in continuous catheter techniques because there is no tendency for the local anesthetic to accumulate in dependent portions of the subarachnoid space and thus potential neural toxicity (cauda equina syndrome) may be avoided.

The use of spinal catheters has diminished after reports of associated cauda equina syndrome.[51,52] The mechanism is thought to be related to uneven distribution of hyperbaric local anesthetic solutions in the spinal fluid and high (toxic) concentrations near the sacral nerve roots. To minimize the risk of neurological injury, spinal catheters should be inserted no more than 2 cm into the subarachnoid space, recommended maximum local anesthetic dosages should not be exceeded, and use of isobaric solutions should be considered.

Complications. The most common complication associated with spinal anesthesia is hypotension, which may be controlled by adequate fluid prehydration and the use of vasopressors. Nausea and vomiting may be minimized by good blood pressure control and small doses of antiemetics. Post–dural-puncture headache (also called spinal headache) may occur after any dural puncture (eg, for spinal tap, myelogram, spinal anesthesia) and may be minimized by using small-gauge, noncutting needles. Transient and persistent neurological deficits may rarely occur. Spinal hematoma or abscess are extremely rare but possible complications of spinal anesthesia.

Practical Points. Injection of hyperbaric local anesthetic solutions into the L-2–L-3 or L-3–L-4 interspace usually results in a T-4 level block, owing to the slope of the spinal curvature from the lumbar lordosis to thoracic kyphosis. Injection into the L-4–L-5 or L-5–S-1 interspace may result in a somewhat lower spinal level, owing to collection of some of the local anesthetic in the sacral spinal space.[53]

Isobaric local anesthetic solutions (eg, lidocaine 2%, tetracaine 1%, bupivacaine 0.5%) may result in a lower "highest" level, a smaller range of highest levels, and smaller blood pressure changes, compared to hyperbaric solutions.[53] The resultant spinal level of anesthesia is independent of patient position at the time of injection. Relatively large doses may be required to attain a high thoracic level.

Postoperative analgesia may be provided by longer acting opioids (eg, morphine 6–20 h) without causing motor block, but additional respiratory monitoring may be required postoperatively.[54,55] Spinal anesthesia or analgesia should not be used if local anesthetic block or prolonged analgesia (> 24 h) is required postoperatively. A continuous epidural or intercostal catheter technique may be more appropriate in this setting.

Intercostal Nerve Block

Intercostal nerve blocks may provide better postoperative analgesia than conventional opioid therapy. When the chest is open, the intercostal nerves can be injected under direct vision. Intercostal block has no effect on visceral structures, so by itself it is inadequate for surgery.

Intercostal nerve block should not be used in the presence of local or severe systemic infection, coagulation abnormality, severe pulmonary disease, or obesity or other physical condition that may make rib palpation difficult.

Anatomy. There are 12 pairs of thoracic anterior primary rami: the upper 11 comprise the intercostal nerves and the 12th is termed the subcostal nerve.[56] The 3rd through 11th pairs are responsible for the innervation of the muscles of the intercostal spaces and of the anterior abdominal wall, and for the cutaneous supply of the skin of the medial aspect of the upper arm and of the anterior and lateral aspects of the trunk from the level of the angle of Louis to just above the groin. The 1st, 2nd, and 12th pairs differ from the others and must be considered separately when intercostal nerve block is desired:

- The 1st intercostal nerve sends a large contribution, which passes across the front of the neck of the first rub, lateral to the superior intercostal artery, to enter the composition of the brachial plexus.
- The 2nd intercostal nerve differs from the typical intercostal nerves in that its lateral cutaneous branch crosses the axilla to supply the skin over the medial aspect of the upper arm. This branch is called the intercostobrachial nerve.
- The 12th thoracic nerve runs along the lower border of the 12th rib below the subcostal vessels, passes behind the lateral arcuate ligament to run in front of quadratus lumborum behind the kidney and colon.[56]

A typical intercostal nerve has four significant branches. The first branch is the gray ramus communicans, which passes anteriorly to the sympathetic ganglion. The second branch arises as the posterior cutaneous branch. This nerve supplies skin and muscles in the paravertebral region. The third branch is the lateral cutaneous division, which arises just anterior to the midaxillary line. This branch sends subcutaneous fibers posteriorly and anteriorly to supply skin of much of the chest and abdominal wall. The fourth and terminal branch of an intercostal nerve is the anterior cutaneous branch,[41] which innervates the ventral side of the chest and the abdominal wall.

Each nerve is joined to its corresponding thoracic sympathetic ganglion by a white and grey ramus communicans.[56] Distal to the rami communicantes, the nerve trunk divides into the dorsal and the ventral branches. The dorsal branch supplies the skin of the back, the muscles of the back, and the periosteum of the vertebrae through its lateral and medial branches.[57]

The ventral branch follows the rib into the costal sulcus, into the dorsal thoracic region and between the two laminae of the intercostal muscles in the intercostal space, and into the lateral and ventral portions of the thorax. The ventral branches each give off a lateral cutaneous branch, first to fifth in the posterior axillary line and sixth to twelfth in the anterior axillary line.[57]

The lateral cutaneous branches of intercostal nerves 7 through 12 participate in sensory and motor innervation of the anterior abdominal wall (skin, muscles, parietal peritoneum).[57]

At the angle of the rib (6–8 cm from the spinous processes), the nerve comes to lie between the internal intercostal muscle and the intercostalis intimus muscle. The costal groove is broadest and deepest at this point. The nerve is accompanied by an intercostal vein and artery, which lie superior to the nerve in the inferior groove of each rib. The costal groove forms a sharp angle with the rib. At this point, the intercostal groove ceases to exist, the lateral cutaneous branch is given off, and the intercostal nerve lies more inferiorly and moves toward the center of the intercostal space.[41]

Technique. The intercostal nerve block may be performed at several possible sites along the course of the nerve, using the following equipment:

- short, beveled, 23- or 25-gauge needle, and
- 10-mL syringe.

The most common site is in the region of the angle of the ribs just lateral to the sacrospinalis group of muscles (Figure 12-3).[41]

Skin markings can be made at the lateral edge of the sacrospinalis muscle (6–8 cm from the midline). The line may be curved medially and superiorly to avoid the scapulae. Skin at the lower edge of the rib

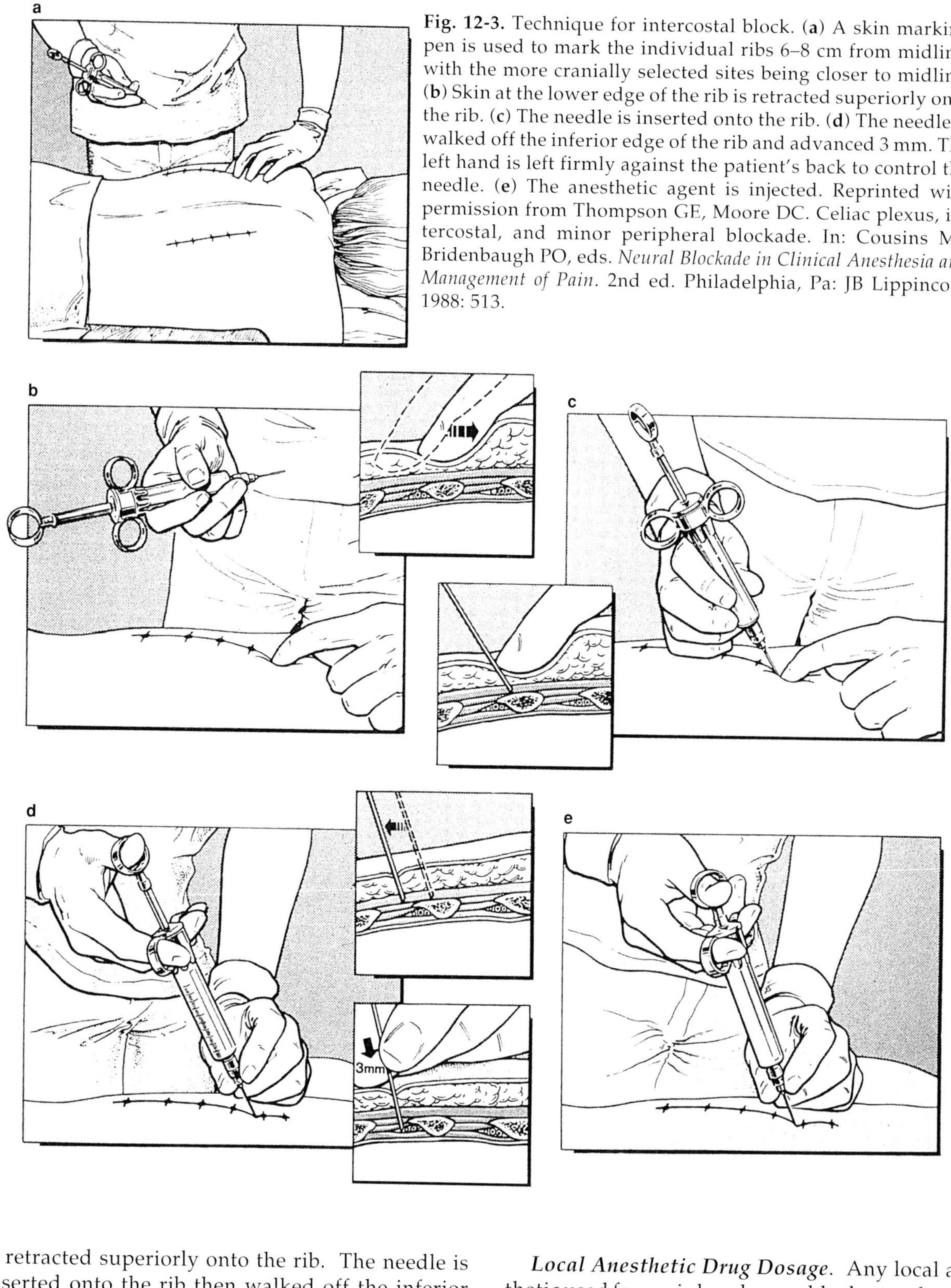

Fig. 12-3. Technique for intercostal block. (**a**) A skin marking pen is used to mark the individual ribs 6–8 cm from midline, with the more cranially selected sites being closer to midline. (**b**) Skin at the lower edge of the rib is retracted superiorly onto the rib. (**c**) The needle is inserted onto the rib. (**d**) The needle is walked off the inferior edge of the rib and advanced 3 mm. The left hand is left firmly against the patient's back to control the needle. (**e**) The anesthetic agent is injected. Reprinted with permission from Thompson GE, Moore DC. Celiac plexus, intercostal, and minor peripheral blockade. In: Cousins MJ, Bridenbaugh PO, eds. *Neural Blockade in Clinical Anesthesia and Management of Pain*. 2nd ed. Philadelphia, Pa: JB Lippincott; 1988: 513.

is retracted superiorly onto the rib. The needle is inserted onto the rib then walked off the inferior edge and advanced 3 mm toward the sulcus of the rib.[41] Aspirate before injecting 3 to 5 mL per segment.[41,57] The patient should hold his breath during the injection.

Local Anesthetic Drug Dosage. Any local anesthetic used for peripheral nerve blocks may be used, such as 0.5% bupivacaine or 1% etidocaine, in the amount of 3 to 5 mL.[57]

Complications. Pneumothorax is the most feared complication.[41] Blood levels of anesthetic agent are higher after this block because of the proximity to vessels, which can lead to toxic concentrations of local anesthetics if the patient receives an overdose of drug. Hemothorax could occur if the intercostal vessels are damaged.

Practical Points. A catheter technique has many advantages compared to multiple single injections: a one-time-only risk of pneumothorax, the ability to provide prolonged continuous analgesia, and blockade of sympathetic nerve fibers.[58,59]

Since large volumes (20–30 mL/h) of local anesthetic solutions may be required, use of a drug with low toxicity potential should be considered. We have used 1% chloroprocaine with success, although tachyphylaxis may develop.

Interpleural Nerve Block

Injection of local anesthetics between the visceral and parietal pleurae provides somatic nerve block by diffusion to the intercostal nerves, and sympathetic nerve block by spread to the paravertebral area.[60,61] Interpleural nerve block may be used for unilateral anesthesia of the upper abdomen. This approach to surgical anesthesia is less useful for thoracic procedures, especially if the pleurae have been disrupted or if thoracostomy drainage tubes are used.[62,63]

The effects of interpleural nerve block are similar to those of continuous intercostal nerve block.[64] Compared with continuous intercostal nerve block, interpleural block is patient-position dependent, has a higher incidence of pneumothorax, requires a higher local anesthetic dose, and results in higher plasma concentration of local anesthetics.[65–67] These characteristics favor use of continuous intercostal nerve block for unilateral procedures of the upper abdomen and flank.

Interpleural nerve block should not be used in the presence of local or severe systemic infection, coagulation abnormality, severe pulmonary disease, or pleural abnormality.

Peripheral Nerve Blocks

Peripheral nerve blocks and incisional infiltration with local anesthetics provide local somatic anesthesia. These anesthetic techniques may be used as the sole anesthesia for extremely limited procedures, to supplement general anesthesia, or to provide several hours of postoperative analgesia.

Infiltration of the surgical wound with a local anesthetic drug is an extremely under-utilized technique. It does not require technical expertise, is safe, and can provide a "bridge" of analgesia between general anesthesia and postoperative analgesia.[68] Some evidence suggests that infiltration of the surgical site prior to incision provides preemptive analgesia (ie, it prevents spinal cord activation and hyperalgesia by blocking afferent nerves from the site of injury).[69]

Peripheral or infiltration blocks are contra-indicated in the presence of local infection or allergy to the local anesthetic.

SPECIFIC NERVE BLOCK TECHNIQUES

Regional anesthesia provides operative anesthesia and postoperative analgesia for selected casualties receiving surgery during wartime. Use of regional anesthesia in this casualty population may prevent some sequelae of general anesthesia (eg, nausea and vomiting) and should decrease labor requirements for patient care in the post operative recovery area. It is conceivable that inducing sympathetic blockade in selected cases (eg, after extremity injury on the battlefield) may decrease the incidence of phantom limb pain or reflex sympathetic dystrophy. This would be especially likely if the ultralong duration, microencapsulated local anesthetics prove useful in clinical practice, so that a one-time blockade procedure could induce a sympathectomy with several days' duration. Specific nerve block techniques are outlined below, separated by anatomical region.

Regional Anesthesia of the Head and Neck

Regional anesthesia of the head and neck has application during trigeminal or occipital nerve blocks for diagnostic or therapeutic applications for pain syndromes. Cervical plexus blockade is useful for surgical procedures on the neck and shoulder. Maxillary, mandibular, and ocular nerve blocks are used for procedures on the face.

Cervical Plexus Block

The cervical plexus is formed by loops between the ventral rami of the upper four cervical nerves. These emerge as four distinct nerves from the posterior border of the sternomastoid at approximately its midpoint. The first branch radiates upward and backward as the lesser occipital nerve to supply part of the posterior surface of the upper part of the ear and the skin behind the ear; the second branch runs upward and forward as the great auricular nerve, which supplies skin over the posterior surface of the ear and the anterior lower third of the ear, and the angle of the mandible; the third branch, the anterior cutaneous nerve of the neck, supplies the skin from the chin to the suprasternal notch; and the fourth branch, the supraclavicular nerve, supplies the skin over the inferior aspect of the neck and clavicle down as far as the area over the second rib. Laterally, these supraclavicular nerves supply the skin over the deltoid muscle and posteriorly as far as the spine of the scapula.[41]

The branches of the plexus are divided into superficial and deep. The superficial branches pierce the cervical fascia just posterior to the sternomastoid and supply the skin of the side of the face and neck. The deep branches contribute primarily efferent (ie, motor) fibers to the muscles of the neck and the phrenic nerve.

Indications. Cervical plexus blockade is useful for operations on the lateral or anterior neck such as carotid endarterectomy or thyroidectomy.[70] It is useful for treatment of pain syndromes such as reflex sympathetic dystrophy.

Anatomy. The dorsal rami supply the muscles of the back of the head and neck and innervate the skin from the vertex to the shoulders.[71] The ventral rami of the upper four cervical nerves form the cervical plexus. This plexus innervates the skin of the front of the neck, the shoulders, and the upper chest, together with the neck muscles. The plexus lies over the upper four cervical vertebrae, deep to the internal jugular vein and the sternomastoid muscle, and anterior to the scalenus medius and levator scapulae. The branches of the plexus divide into superficial and deep. The superficial branches supply the skin of the side of the face and neck. The deep branches contribute motor nerve fibers to the muscles of the neck and phrenic nerve.[72]

Technique. Both superficial and deep cervical plexus blockades can be accomplished using the following equipment:

- 5-cm, 22-gauge needles; and
- 3 or 4 mL of 1% lidocaine or its equivalent.[41]

All four branches of the superficial cervical plexus can be blocked by infiltration at the midpoint of the posterior border of the sternomastoid. Lidocaine, 1% or its equivalent, can be infiltrated at this area; 5 to 10 mL will be required. This will produce cutaneous analgesia of the anterior and lateral neck from the mandible to the clavicle.[41]

The deep cervical plexus blockade is a para-vertebral block of spinal nerves C-2 through C-4 as they emerge from the foramina in the cervical vertebrae (Figure 12-4). Each nerve lies in the sulcus in the transverse processes of these vertebrae.[41] A line is drawn from the mastoid process to Chassaignac's tubercle (C-6). This line crosses a line drawn laterally from the cricoid cartilage, which is at the level of C-4.

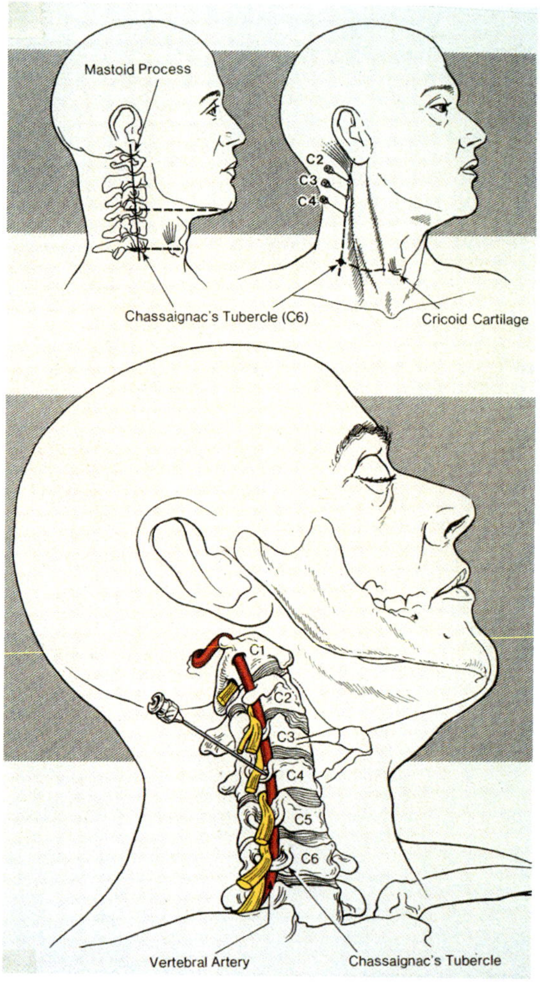

Fig. 12-4. When performing a deep cervical plexus block, note that caudad direction of the needle is essential to avoid penetration of an intervertebral foramen. Frequent aspiration is necessary to prevent injection into the vertebral artery. Reprinted with permission from Murphy TM. Somatic blockade of head and neck. In: Cousins MJ, Bridenbaugh PO, eds. *Neural Blockade in Clinical Anesthesia and Management of Pain.* 2nd ed. Philadelphia, Pa: JB Lippincott; 1988: 553.

The C-3 and C-2 nerve roots can be located by dividing the distance between the mastoid and horizontal line into thirds.[41] The C-5 nerve root lies midway between the C-6 line at Chassaignac's tubercle and C-4.

The needles are directed medially and caudally. Caudad direction is to avoid unintentionally entering the intervertebral foramen and producing a spinal block. The needle is advanced until the transverse process is contacted or paresthesias are obtained. Adequate anesthesia is provided by 3 to 4 mL of 1% lidocaine or the equivalent on each nerve. Deep cervical plexus block can often be obtained with injections at just one level with a larger volume, such as 6 to 8 mL.[41]

Complications. Complications of cervical plexus block include phrenic nerve block (a reason to avoid bilateral cervical plexus block), vertebral artery injection, epidural injection, subarachnoid injection, and recurrent laryngeal nerve block.[44]

Occipital Nerve Block

The skin over the posterior extensor muscles of the neck and occiput is supplied by the posterior rami of the cervical nerves.[41] The greater occipital nerve is the most prominent nerve supplying this area. It is sometimes blocked in the treatment of occipital tension headaches.

Anatomy. The greater occipital nerve can be blocked as it crosses the superior nuchal line. This line is identified by locating the greater occipital protuberance and the mastoid process. The greater occipital nerve crosses the superior nuchal line one third of the way between the external occipital protuberance and the mastoid process.[41]

Technique. Occipital nerve block is accomplished using a short needle (2–3 cm, 22- to 25-gauge) after a sterile skin preparation (Figure 12-5). The greater occipital nerve is located one third of the way between the greater occipital protuberance and the mastoid process.[41] It lies adjacent (medial) to the occipital artery, which can be palpated. Infiltration of 2 to 10 mL of 0.25% bupivacaine or its equivalent around the artery will provide a block of the greater occipital nerve.[57]

The lesser occipital nerve lies approximately 2.5 cm lateral to the greater occipital nerve. It can be blocked directly above and behind the mastoid process. This block is done by entering the skin vertically, directly at the exit point of the nerve behind the mastoid process. After definite bony contact has been established, 2 to 10 mL of local anesthetic is infiltrated (0.25% bupivacaine or its equivalent).

Complications. The occipital nerve block is associated with few complications, but inadvertent intravenous injection is possible.

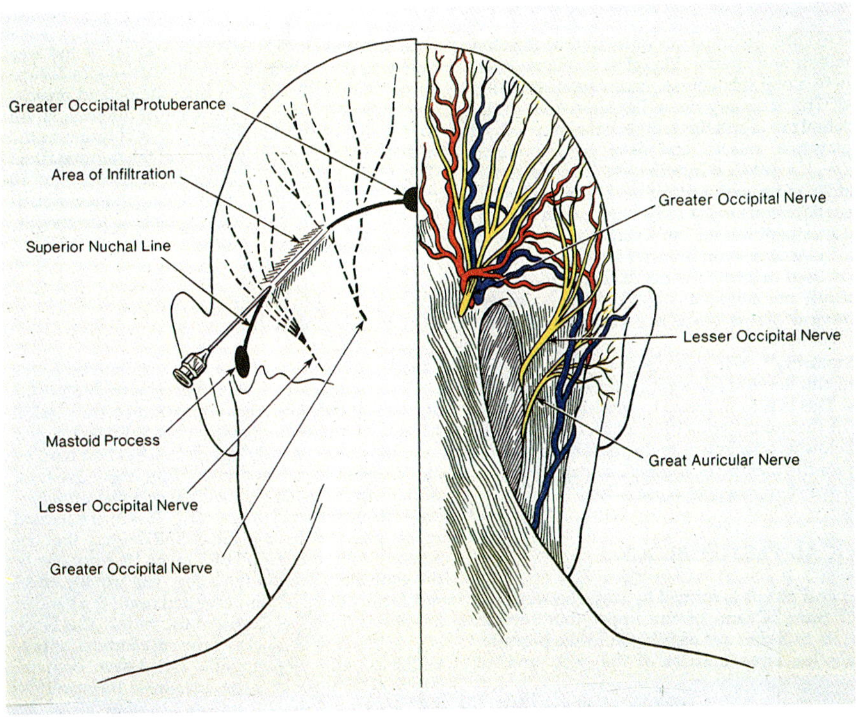

Fig. 12-5. In an occipital nerve block, the anesthetic agent is injected along an imaginary curved line extending between the mastoid process and the greater occipital protuberance. Reprinted with permission from Murphy TM. Somatic blockade of head and neck. In: Cousins MJ, Bridenbaugh PO, eds. *Neural Blockade in Clinical Anesthesia and Management of Pain*. 2nd ed. Philadelphia, Pa: JB Lippincott; 1988: 552.

Maxillary Nerve Block

Block of the maxillary nerve will anesthetize the skin and deep structures of the middle face including the nasal cavity, the maxillary bone and sinus, the upper teeth, and the upper part of the mouth and oral cavity. Indications for maxillary nerve block include trigeminal neuralgia of the second branch, pain of maxillary neoplasm, postoperative pain, atypical facial neuralgia, acute herpes zoster, and cluster headache.[57]

Anatomy. The maxillary nerve leaves the cranium through the foramen rotundum, crosses the pterygopalatine fossa, and enters the orbit through the inferior orbital fissure, where it becomes the infraorbital nerve.[50,71] Branches of the maxillary nerve include the posterior, middle, and anterior superior alveolar nerves.[57,72]

Technique and Local Anesthetic Drug Dosage. A 7-cm needle is inserted medially at the junction of the zygoma and the anterior edge of the ramus. The needle is inclined cephalad and posteriorly. The needle is advanced to the depth of the sphenoid bone.[57,72] A dose of 4 mL of 1% lidocaine or 0.25% bupivacaine is used to achieve anesthesia.[57]

Complications. The only reported complications are hemorrhage due to injury of the maxillary artery and subarachnoid injection.[57,72]

Mandibular Nerve Block

Block of the mandibular nerve will anesthetize the lower jaw and the skin and tissues of the lower face. The mandibular nerve, which is the largest branch of the trigeminal nerve, is sensory to the skin over the lower jaw, posterior face, lower lip, lower teeth and gums.[72] It supplies the motor fibers to the muscles of mastication.

Anatomy. The nerve divides into an anterior and a posterior trunk after leaving the foramen ovale. The sensory fibers of the anterior trunk run in the buccal nerve, which is distributed with branches of the facial nerve supplying the skin and mucous membrane on either side of the buccinator muscle. The posterior trunk divides into three branches: the auriculotemporal, the lingual, and the inferior alveolar nerves.[72] The auriculotemporal supplies the skin over the temporal region and external auditory meatus. The lingual supplies the mucous membrane of the floor of the mouth and anterior two thirds of the tongue, in addition to the lingual surface of the lower gums.[72] The inferior alveolar enters the mandibular foramen and runs in the mandibular canal supplying the lower teeth. At the mental foramen it gives off a lateral branch, the mental nerve, which supplies the skin over the anterior jaw and lower lip.[72]

Technique and Local Anesthetic Drug Dosage. To perform this block, a wheal is raised 0.5 cm below the zygomatic arch between the coronoid process and the condyle of the mandible. The needle is inserted at right angles to the skin until it contracts the pterygoid plate at a depth of 3 to 4 cm. It is then withdrawn a few millimeters and redirected 20° posteriorly until a paresthesia is elicited. Anesthetic drugs such as 5 mL of 2% lidocaine or 0.5% bupivacaine or their equivalent are used.[72]

Trigeminal Nerve Block

The trigeminal nerve, the largest of the cranial nerves, can be blocked for treatment of trigeminal neuralgia or postherpetic pain. The sensory supply to the face and anterior two thirds of the scalp is from the trigeminal nerve. It is formed by the union of a sensory and a motor root. This union is called the trigeminal, or Gasserian, ganglion. The trigeminal nerve supplies the skin of the face and scalp and the muscles of mastication via its three main branches: (1) the ophthalmic nerve, which leaves the cranium through the superior orbital fissure; (2) the maxillary nerve, which leaves through the foramen rotundum; and (3) the mandibular nerve, which leaves through the foramen ovale. All three nerves can be blocked with a single injection through the foramen ovale.[72]

Because the trigeminal nerve block is complex and possible complications include subarachnoid injection of local anesthetic at the base of the brain, we recommend that this block should *not* be performed in far-forward battlefield conditions. Radiographic capabilities to perform the block under radiographic control are required.

Ocular Nerves

Surgery of the eye can be done by numerous local techniques, including the following[72]:

- The cornea can be anesthetized by topical local anesthesia.
- The conjunctiva can be anesthetized by local infiltration.
- The globe can be anesthetized by retrobulbar injection.

- The nasociliary nerve supplies the skin and mucous membrane of the nose, cornea and conjunctiva; it can be blocked at the medial wall of the orbit.
- The supraorbital nerve supplies the upper eyelid and conjunctiva; it can be blocked at the supraorbital foramen.
- The infraorbital nerve supplies the skin of the ala of the nose, the lower eyelid, the cheek, and the upper lip; it can be blocked as it enters the face through the infraorbital foramen.

These procedures are not commonly done by most anesthetists, and it is recommended that they be performed only by personnel who are facile with local ophthalmic anesthesia.

Regional Anesthesia of the Airway

The nasal mucosa is innervated by fibers of the sphenopalatine ganglion via a branch of the middle division of the fifth cranial nerve. Branches of the fifth cranial nerve continue caudad to provide sensory innervation to the superior pharynx, uvula, and tonsils. Transmucosal topical application of local anesthetic can be used to anesthetize this region.[70]

Sensory innervation of the oral pharynx and supraglottic regions below the sphenopalatine fiber distribution is from branches of the glossopharyngeal nerve. These nerves lie laterally on each side of the pharynx in the region of the posterior tonsillar pillars. Topical anesthesia of these branches in the mouth and throat is an effective method of providing anesthesia to the submucosal branches of the glossopharyngeal nerve.[70]

The larynx is innervated by the superior laryngeal branch of the vagus nerve above the vocal cords. Below the vocal cords, the recurrent laryngeal nerve provides sensory innervation and supplies motor innervation for all but one intrinsic laryngeal muscle.[70]

Superior Laryngeal Nerve Block

The superior laryngeal branch of the vagus nerve is blocked as it sweeps around the inferior border of the greater cornu of the hyoid bone.[41] This can be palpated by pressing on the opposite greater cornu of the hyoid bone, which will displace the opposite cornu toward the side to be blocked.[41] A 2.5-cm, 25-gauge needle is walked from the inferior border of the greater cornu of the hyoid near its tip, and 3 mL of local anesthetic is infiltrated both superficially and deep to the thyrohyoid membrane (Figure 12-6). This procedure is repeated bilaterally. This block will produce anesthesia over the inferior aspect of the epiglottis and laryngeal inlet as far down as the vocal cords.[41]

Transtracheal Block

To produce anesthesia below the cords, a transtracheal puncture can be performed. A 20-gauge catheter is introduced through the cricothyroid membrane in the midline. After entry into the trachea is confirmed by aspiration of air, the catheter is advanced from the needle. Correct placement is confirmed again by aspiration of air, followed by rapid injection of 3 to 5 mL of local anesthetic, which produces a cough reflex. For this block, 2% to 4% lidocaine is commonly employed. Complications of the transtracheal block include the possibility of aspiration in certain patients due to the loss of the protective airway reflexes.

Nerve Blocks for Upper Extremity Surgery

Injuries to the upper extremities are common during wartime and may be amenable to regional anesthetic techniques during surgical repair. Regional anesthesia has the advantage of providing postoperative pain control and blockade of the sympathetic nervous system with selected blocks. Knowledge of the anatomy of the upper extremity is crucial for performance of regional anesthetic blockade.

The brachial plexus can be blocked at three locations[41]:

1. the interscalene approach, in which a needle is inserted in the interscalene groove at the level of the cricoid cartilage and advanced until the tubercle of C-6 is contacted or until a paresthesia is elicited;
2. the supraclavicular approach, in which the needle is inserted into the interscalene groove 1 cm or until a paresthesia is elicited; and
3. the axillary approach, which carries the least risk of pneumothorax.

The interscalene and supraclavicular approaches are more difficult to perform and therefore are less frequently used than the axillary approach.

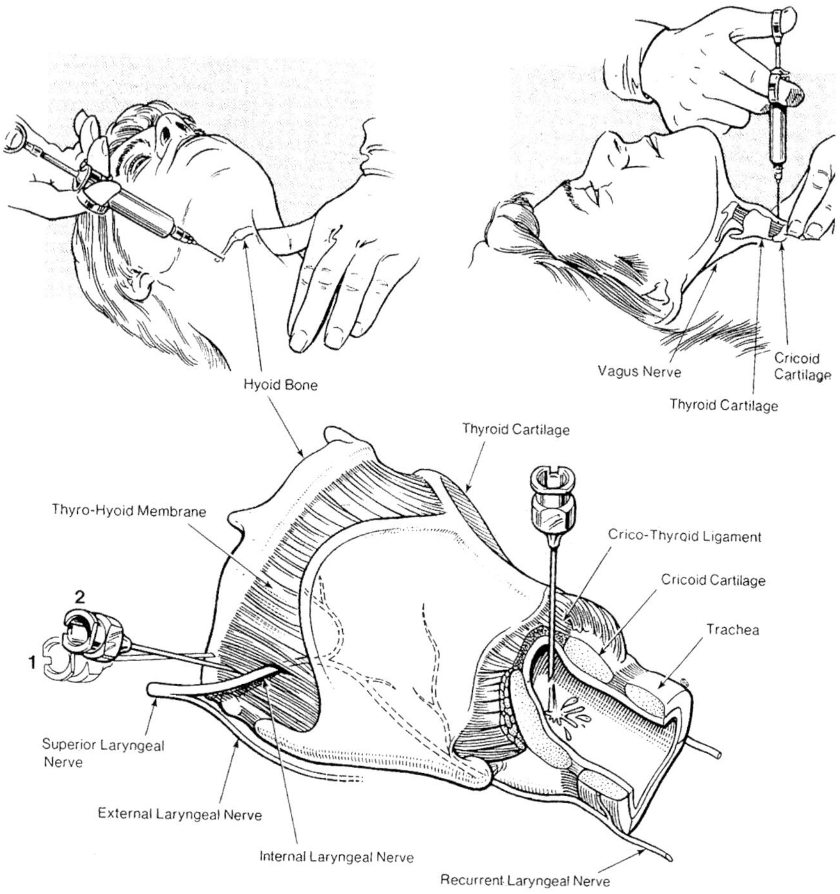

Fig. 12-6. Technique for anesthetizing the larynx and trachea such as might be used in performing bronchoscopy. The superior laryngeal nerve is blocked as it passes anterior and inferior to the posterior cornu of the hyoid bone. Anesthesia of the tracheal mucosa is obtained by injecting the agent directly through the space between the thyroid and cricoid cartilages. Reprinted with permission from Murphy TM. Somatic blockade of head and neck. In: Cousins MJ, Bridenbaugh PO. *Neural Blockade in Clinical Anesthesia and Management of Pain.* 2nd ed. Philadelphia, Pa: JB Lippincott; 1988: 549

Brachial Plexus Block: The Axillary Approach

Innervation of the upper extremity is from nerve roots of C-5 through T-1, which form the brachial plexus. The median and musculocutaneous nerves lie above the axillary artery; the ulnar and radial nerves lie below and behind the artery.

Technique. The axillary approach to a brachial plexus block is performed using the following equipment:

- 23-gauge, 1½-in., short, beveled needle;
- extension tubing; and
- 20-mL syringes.

The patient is in the supine position with the arm abducted and elbow flexed (Figure 12-7). The arm is externally rotated, so that the hand lies alongside the patient's head. The axilla is prepared and draped for surgery. The axillary artery is located as high as is practical in the axilla as it courses in the groove between the coracobrachialis and triceps muscles. The needle is advanced through the artery, which is deliberately entered. The needle is advanced until aspiration confirms it has passed just posterior to (ie, through) the artery, at which time one half of the local anesthetic solution is injected. The needle is then withdrawn until aspiration confirms it is just anterior to the artery; then the other half of the solution is injected.

The musculocutaneous nerve is blocked by infiltration of 5 mL of anesthetic into the coracobrachial muscle. Median cutaneous and intercostobrachial nerves can be blocked by subcutaneous infiltration of 10 mL of anesthetic solution in a half-ring around the medial aspect of the arm.

Local Anesthetic Drug Dosages. To achieve nerve blockade, the anesthesiologist should inject 30 to 40 mL of local anesthetic solution (1% lidocaine, 0.25% bupivacaine, 1.5% mepivacaine); in children, 10 to 20 mL should be injected.

Complications. When the axillary approach is used, complications are rare but include neuropathy, hematoma, and intravascular injection.

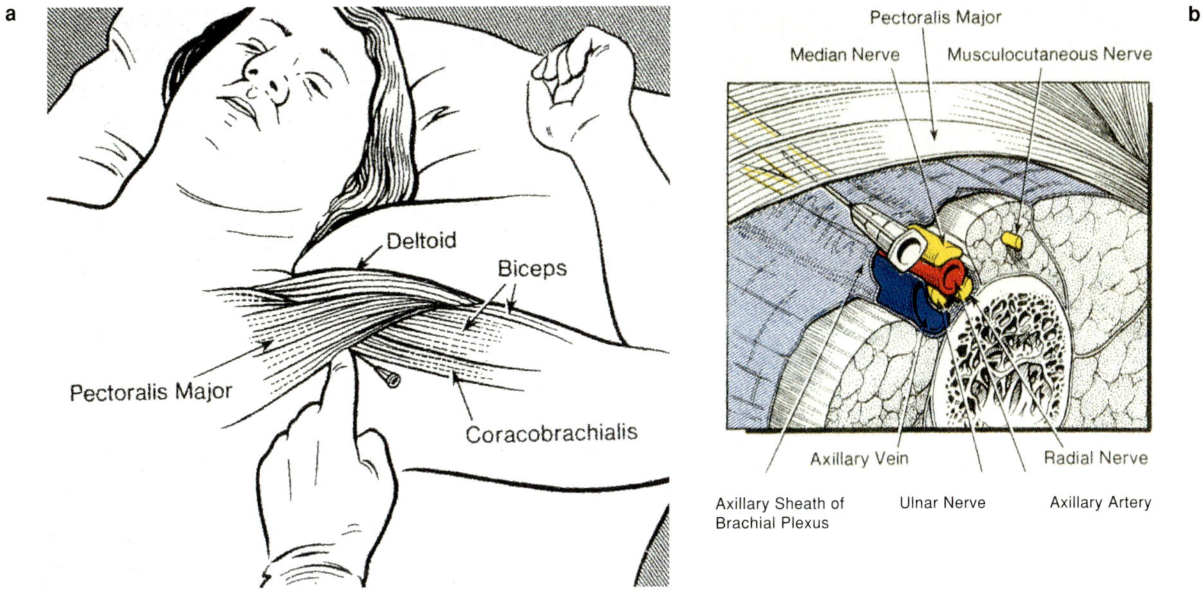

Fig. 12-7. The axillary approach to producing brachial plexus blockade. (**a**) The edge of the pectoralis major muscle and the axillary artery are the anatomical landmarks. (**b**) The anesthetic agent is injected deep to the axillary sheath of the brachial plexus. Reprinted with permission from Bridenbaugh LD. The upper extremity: somatic blockage. In: Cousins MJ, Bridenbaugh PO, eds. *Neural Blockade in Clinical Anesthesia and Management of Pain*. 2nd ed. Philadelphia, Pa: JB Lippincott; 1988: 401.

Brachial Plexus Block: The Interscalene Approach

The brachial plexus runs between the anterior and middle scalene muscles in the neck, where their fascia forms a perivascular sheath. The perivascular sheath is reached during this approach to a brachial plexus block by inserting a needle into the sheath at the sixth cervical vertebra, which corresponds to the level of the cricoid cartilage.

Technique. The patient is in the supine position, with the head rotated away from the side to be blocked (Figure 12-8). The groove between the anterior and middle scalene muscles is palpated behind the sternocleidomastoid muscle. The anterior scalene is immediately behind the sternomastoid, and a groove is palpable between the anterior and the middle scalene muscles.

A 3- to 4-cm needle is inserted perpendicular to the skin at the level of the cricoid cartilage (C-6) in the interscalene groove. The needle is slowly advanced until a paresthesia felt below the shoulder is elicited or a transverse spinous process is felt. If bone is contacted, the needle can be walked laterally along the transverse process until a paresthesia is elicited. A nerve stimulator with insulated needle may be used, instead of the anesthesiologist's relying on the casualty's perception of paresthesia. When it is in close proximity to the plexus, the nerve stimulator should elicit muscle twitching in the arm or hand.[72]

With an assistant using frequent aspiration, 30 to 40 mL of 1.5% mepivacaine (or its equivalent) is injected in fractionated doses. The patient's perception of pain while the anesthetic is being injected may indicate a direct intraneural injection, in which case the needle should be withdrawn about 1 mm and the injection should be repeated.

Complications. Complications of interscalene brachial plexus block include spinal or epidural blockade by inadvertent penetration of the epidural or dural spaces or entry via an intervertebral foramen, intraneural injection, and intraarterial or venous injection.

Brachial Plexus Block: The Supraclavicular Approach

The supraclavicular approach to brachial plexus block involves injecting local anesthetic into the perivascular sheath that surrounds the plexus at the level of the clavicle. When the brachial plexus passes between the clavicle and the first rib, it is joined by the subclavian artery, which runs deep to the anterior scalene muscle. The three trunks (superior, middle, and inferior) of the brachial plexus lie

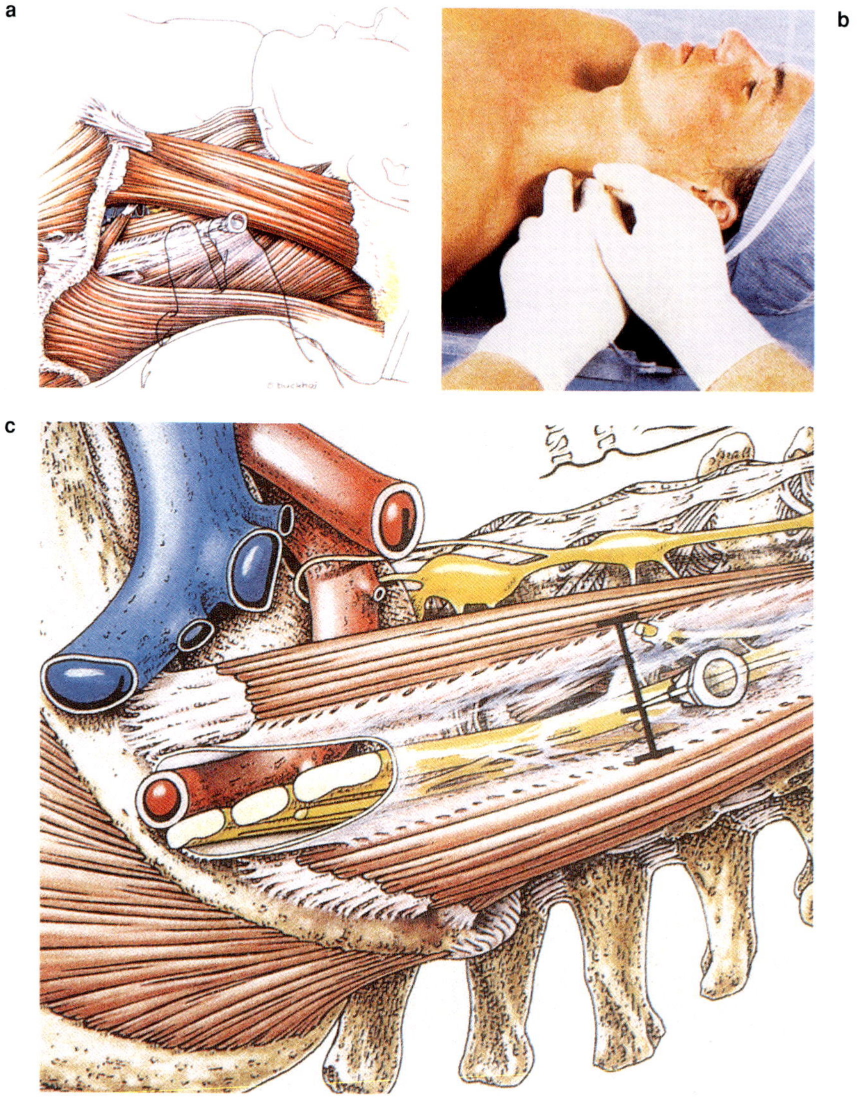

Fig. 12-8. (**a**) A needle is being placed in the perivascular sheath surrounding the brachial plexus. The anesthesiologist is palpating the interscalene groove to facilitate needle placement. (**b**) A flexible cannula is used during injection to ensure that the needle remains immobile after correct placement has been achieved. (**c**) The anatomy of the brachial plexus and its perivascular sheath at the C-6 level is seen in detail. Reprinted with permission from Scott DB. *Techniques of Regional Anaesthesia*. East Norwalk, Conn: Appleton & Lange; 1989: 93. Drawings by Paol Buckhöj.

in a vertical plane lateral to the subclavian artery.[72]

Technique. The patient is in the supine position, with the arm on the side to be injected pulled downward to depress the clavicle and shoulder (Figure 12-9). The subclavian artery can be palpated above the midportion of the clavicle. The interscalene groove is palpated posterior to the sternocleidomastoid muscle.

A 4-cm-long needle is inserted lateral to the subclavian artery and directed vertically and caudally. It is advanced slowly until the patient feels a paresthesia below the shoulder. If the needle contacts the first rib, the needle is withdrawn and the process is repeated as close as possible to the artery. A nerve stimulator can be used, and muscle movement in the arm or hand would indicate correct placement.[72]

When proper needle placement is obtained, fractionated doses of 1.5% mepivacaine (or its equivalent) are injected, using a flexible catheter, to a total dose of 44 mL.

Complications. Complications of this technique include arterial puncture, intraneural injection, pneumothorax, and spinal or epidural blockade.

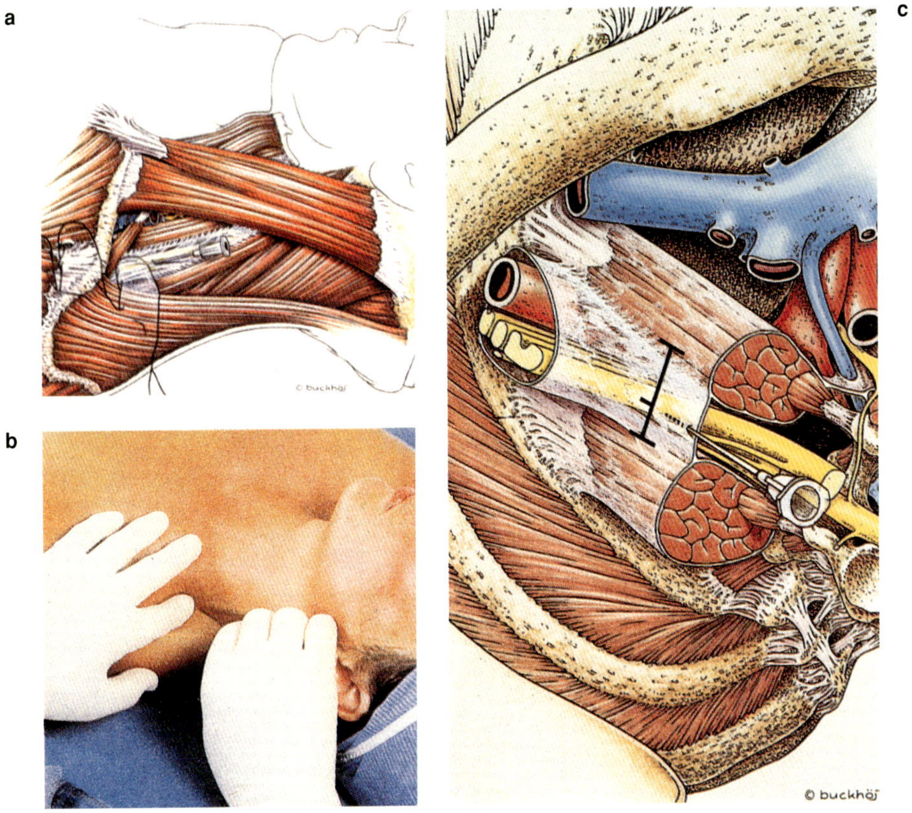

Fig. 12-9. (**a**) Needle placement into the perivascular sheath surrounding the brachial plexus and the subclavian artery at the level of the clavicle. (**b**) Palpation of the interscalene groove at the midportion of the clavicle and identification of the subclavian artery. (**c**) The three trunks of the brachial plexus and their relationship to the clavicle and interscalene muscles. Reprinted with permission from Scott DB. *Techniques of Regional Anaesthesia*. East Norwalk, Conn: Appleton & Lange; 1989: 99. Drawings by Paol Buckhöj.

Intravenous Regional Anesthesia: Bier's Method

Bier's method of achieving intravenous regional anesthesia (ie, the Bier block) allows analgesia and muscle relaxation in an extremity. It is performed by intravenously administering a local anesthetic distal to a tourniquet that provides complete vascular occlusion. We do *not* recommend the use of intravenous regional anesthesia for surgical procedures of the lower extremity. The high volumes of local anesthetic required to produce an adequate nerve block risk local anesthetic systemic toxicity and therefore make this technique a less desirable choice than specific nerve blocks.[73] Because the procedure is not infrequently used on the lower extremity, however, it is discussed here for the sake of completeness.

Technique. An intravenous catheter is placed in the distal extremity. A plastic extension tubing from the catheter is attached to a 50-mL syringe. A pneumatic double tourniquet is placed proximal to the operative site. The extremity is exsanguinated by the application of an Esmarch bandage or by elevation. The bandage is applied distal to proximal. The tourniquet is inflated after exsanguination and before removal of the bandage. The proximal pneumatic tourniquet is inflated above systolic pressure. Pulses are checked after inflation to confirm occlusion of circulation (usually 250–300 mm Hg in the arm and 350–400 mm Hg in the leg).

The local anesthetic solution is then injected. For short procedures, the intravenous catheter is removed at this point; for longer procedures, the cannula is left in place and the local anesthetic solution is reinjected after 90 minutes. The area anesthetized includes the distal extremity up to the area of the proximal tourniquet. If tourniquet discomfort begins, the distal tourniquet can be inflated, as this area is already anesthetized and the proximal tourniquet is deflated. Tourniquet pain is usually the limiting factor for success of this technique.

If surgery lasts longer than 40 minutes, the tourniquet can be deflated as a single maneuver. Between 20 and 40 minutes, the cuff can be deflated, reinflated immediately, and finally deflated after a minute to reduce the sudden absorption of anesthetic into the systemic circulation. The tourniquet is left inflated for at least 20 minutes.[70]

A separate intravenous site for injection of resuscitation drugs is needed for this block, as well as ready availability of all needed equipment.

Anesthetic Drug Dosages and Complications. The duration of action of the local anesthetic agent is limited by tourniquet time rather than the agent. The amount of drug given depends on the size of the extremity. Average doses are 40 to 50 mL of 0.5% lidocaine for an arm, and 100 mL of 0.25% lidocaine for a leg. Agents should not be mixed with vasoconstrictors. Local anesthetic drug toxicity can be seen if the tourniquet fails or is relieved too quickly. Nerve damage secondary to tourniquet application can be seen. Tourniquet time should not exceed 2 hours.

Relative Contraindications. Relative contraindications to the Bier block include distal infection of the extremity, ischemia of the involved extremity, heart block, and seizure disorder.

Sole-Anesthetic Nerve Blocks for Lower Extremity Surgery

Neural blockade of the lower extremity may be useful to provide preoperative analgesia, intraoperative anesthesia as the sole anesthetic or as a supplement to general anesthesia, and postoperative analgesia.[73] Some nerve blocks are suited for all three of these uses, while others provide good analgesia but may not be acceptable for intraoperative anesthesia.

As has been described earlier in this chapter, lower extremity anesthesia can be obtained by spinal or epidural techniques. Additional nerve blocks that may be useful for preoperative analgesia, intraoperative general anesthesia supplementation, postoperative analgesia, or as the sole anesthetic are described in this section. Combined peripheral nerve block techniques are indicated if spinal or epidural anesthesia are undesirable.[73] Advantages of a combined peripheral nerve block technique include the blockade of only one leg, smaller hemodynamic changes owing to the limited sympathectomy, and avoidance of major conduction anesthesia. The major disadvantage of the technique is the need for at least two needle insertions to block separately the peripheral nerves formed by the lumbar plexus and those formed by the sacral plexus. Individual techniques are discussed in the following section.

Lumbar Plexus Block

Blockade of the lumbar plexus provides unilateral analgesia in the distribution of the femoral, lateral femoral cutaneous, and obturator nerves. Patients with trauma to or surgical procedures of the hip or thigh may therefore benefit from this block. Lumbar plexus block is contraindicated in

a

b

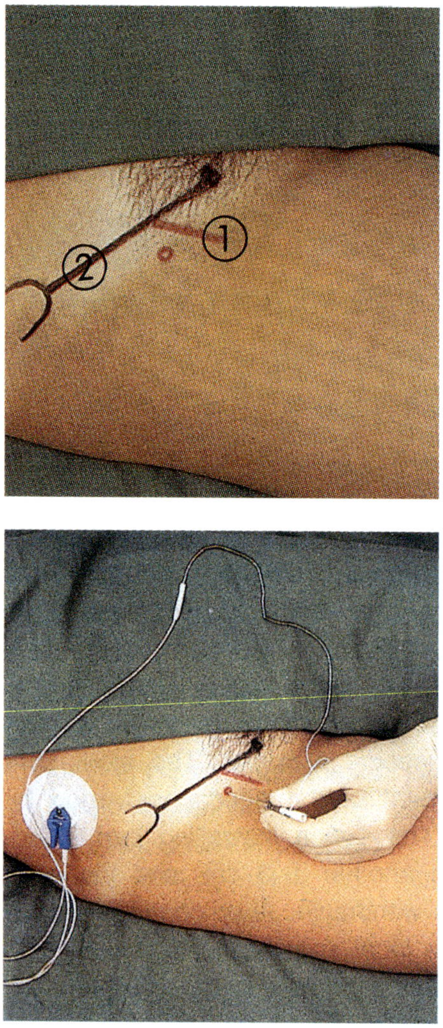

Fig. 12-10. The 3-in-1 lumbar plexus blockade. (**a**) The anatomical landmarks are the inguinal ligament (2) as it extends between the anterior superior iliac spine and pubic tubercle and the femoral artery (1). (**b**) The needle is inserted 1 to 1.5 cm laterally to the femoral artery and advanced in a cranial direction. Continuous infusion of anesthetic agent through a catheter is desirable. Reprinted with permission from Astra Chemicals GmbH, Zenz M, Hoerster W, Niesel HC, Kreuscher H, eds; DeKornfeld TJ, trans. *Regional Anesthesia*. 2nd ed. St. Louis, Mo: Mosby-Year Book; 1990: 109, 111.

the presence of local infection, coagulation abnormality, immunosuppression, and perhaps neurological deficits involving the ipsilateral limb. Two techniques have been described: the Winnie "3-in-1" paravascular approach from the femoral canal,[74] and the lumbar paravertebral approach to the lumbar plexus blockade.[73]

Winnie 3-in-1 Paravascular Approach. The Winnie 3-in-1 blockade can be performed with the patient in the supine position (Figure 12-10). This technique utilizes the fascial plane that the femoral nerve travels in as it crosses the pelvis. A large quantity of local anesthetic is injected in this plane so that it will spread upward into the pelvis and anesthetize the obturator and lateral femoral cutaneous nerves where they travel in conjunction with the femoral nerve. Paresthesias are usually necessary for this approach, as it is essential to have the needle exactly in the plane of the nerve. This block is performed by inserting the needle in a cephalad manner alongside the femoral artery angled at about 45° so that it passes under the inguinal ligament. After obtaining a paresthesia, 40 mL of anesthetic solution is injected incrementally.[70] During the injection, the anesthesiologist's index finger is moved to a point just distal to the needle, where firm pressure is applied to prevent retrograde flow of the injected local anesthetic.

Lumbar Paravertebral Approach. The lumbar paravertebral approach to the lumbar blockade may be used if the patient can be turned, because this approach is more often successful in blocking the obturator nerve (Figure 12-11). For continuous blockade, a Tuohy needle is inserted 3 cm lateral to the midline at the level of the L-3–L-4 interspace and is advanced until the transverse process of

b

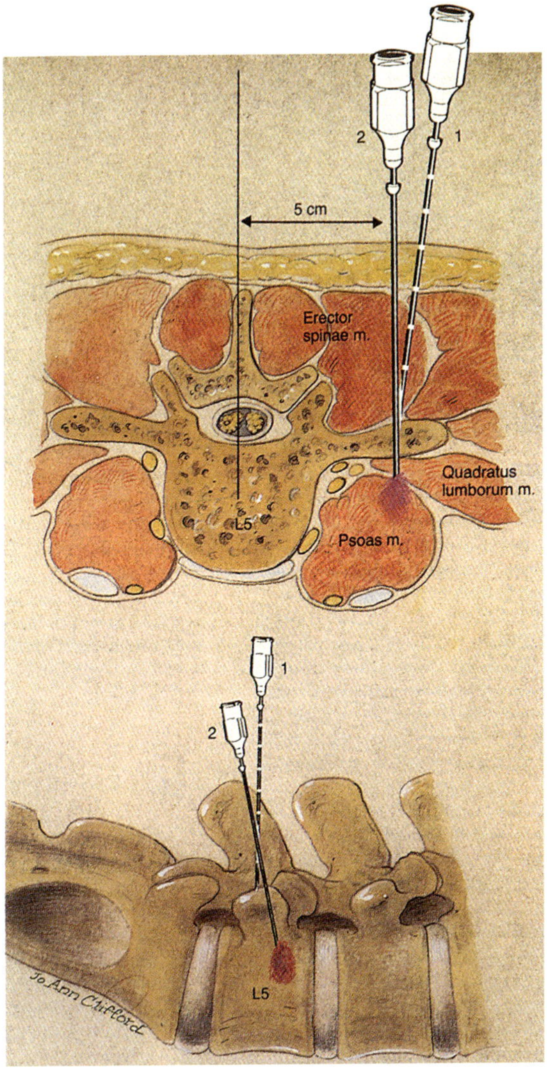

Fig. 12-11. Lumbar plexus block at the psoas compartment. (**a**) The iliac crests are used to determine the spinous process of the 4th lumbar vertebra. (**b**) A 15-cm long needle is inserted at a point 5 cm lateral to midline and 3 cm caudad to the 4th lumbar spinous process. The needle is advanced until the lateral process of the 5th lumbar vertebra is reached (needle point 1). The needle is then advanced in a cranial direction superior to the vertebral process and an injection made (needle point 2). Reprinted with permission from Brown DL. *Atlas of Regional Anesthesia*. Philadelphia, Pa: WB Saunders; 1992: 77, 78.

a

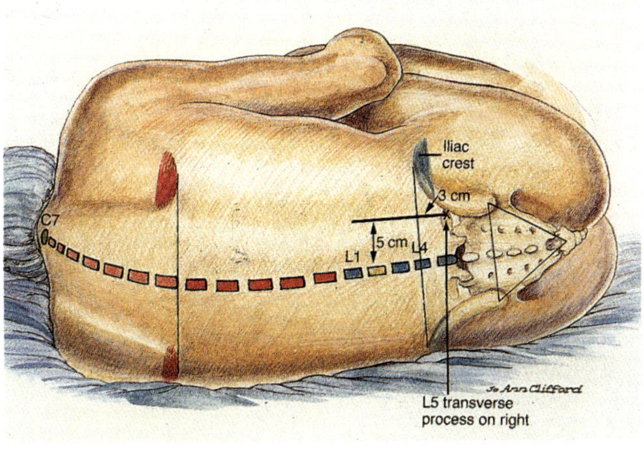

L-4 is contacted. The needle is then walked superiorly and laterally into the substance of the quadratus lumborum muscle, and is then advanced, using the loss-of-resistance technique, into the fascial plane between the quadratus lumborum and psoas muscles. The lumbar plexus lies within this psoas compartment. An epidural catheter may be passed into the compartment. Injection of 0.5 mL/kg of local anesthetic solution should provide a reliable block. The concentration of local anesthetic used depends on the degree of motor block desired. Continuous infusions of local anesthetic at 0.25 mL/kg/h may be used to continue the block.[73]

Femoral Nerve Block

Surgical use of femoral nerve block includes operations of the anterior portion of the thigh, both superficial and deep (Figure 12-12).[41] As with sciatic nerve block, the femoral nerve block is usually part of the combined block approach, incorporating not only sciatic but also lateral femoral cutaneous and obturator nerves.

The femoral nerve (which is composed of fibers arising from the spinal segments L-2–L-4) proceeds from the lumbar plexus in the groove between the psoas major and iliac muscles, where it enters the thigh by passing deep to the inguinal ligament. The femoral nerve lies anterior to the iliopsoas muscle and slightly lateral to the femoral artery.

Technique. The femoral nerve block may be accomplished using the following equipment:

- 1½-in., 22-gauge needle; and
- 20-mL syringe.

Palpate the femoral artery just below the inguinal ligament, and advance the needle toward the lateral border of the artery.[41] If a paresthesia is not obtained, redirect the needle to fan medial to lateral until a paresthesia is obtained. Then stabilize the needle and, after negative aspiration, inject 10 to 15 mL of local anesthetic solution. If a paresthesia is not obtained, the nerve can be blocked by injecting in a fanwise manner, medial to lateral, from the lateral border of the femoral artery.

Local Anesthetic Drug Dosages and Complications. Any anesthetic agent suitable for peripheral nerve blockade, 10 to 20 mL, is suitable. Hematoma at the site is possible because of the proximity to a major artery and vein. Residual nerve involvement is possible but rare, causing a dysesthesia or paresis.

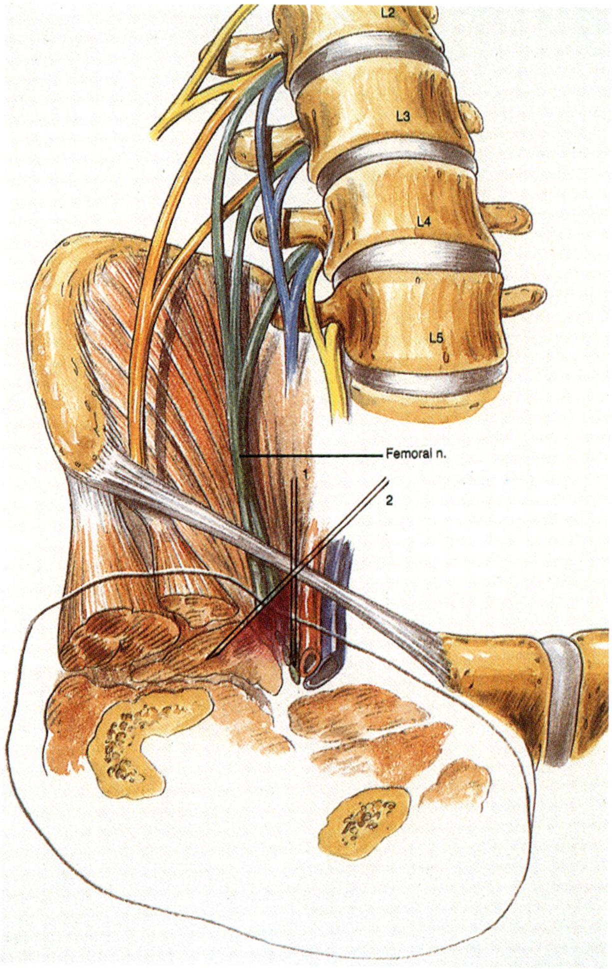

Fig. 12-12. Anatomy of the femoral nerve block. The inguinal ligament and the femoral artery are the landmarks. Injection is made lateral to the artery (2) after a femoral nerve paresthesia is produced (1). Reprinted with permission from Brown DL. *Atlas of Regional Anesthesia*. Philadelphia, Pa: WB Saunders; 1992: 95.

Sciatic Nerve Block

Sciatic nerve block is usually combined with femoral, obturator, or lateral femoral cutaneous nerve block to provide complete anesthesia of the lower extremity.[73] The sciatic nerve supplies sensory innervation to the posterior thigh and the entire leg and foot from just below the knee. The nerve (from spinal segments L-4–S-3) arises from the sacral plexus and passes from the pelvis through the sacrosciatic foramen beneath the lower margin of the piriformis muscle and between the tuberosity of the ischium and the greater trochanter of the femur (Figure 12-13).[41] The sciatic nerve becomes superficial at the lower border of the gluteus maximus muscle. From there, it courses down the posterior aspect of the thigh to the popliteal fossa, where it divides into the tibial and common peroneal nerves.[73]

Technique. The sciatic nerve block is performed with the following equipment:

- 21- or 22-gauge needle, 10 to 20 cm long; or
- 22-gauge, Teflon-coated (polytetrafluoroethylene, manufactured by Du Pont Polymers, Wilmington, Del.) stimulator needle with nerve stimulator; and
- 10-mL syringe.

The patient is relaxed and lying on the side that is not to be blocked. The upper leg is flexed at the hip and at the knee so that the heel rests on the knee of the lower, extended leg. The landmarks are connected with a line (greater trochanter, superior–posterior iliac spine). From the middle of this line, a line is drawn inferiorly at right angles and intersects a line drawn between the tip of the coccyx and the greater trochanter at about 3 cm. This point is marked for needle insertion. A 22-gauge, 15-cm long needle is introduced through a skin wheal at right angles to the skin and is advanced in the direction of the sacrosciatic foramen, through the gluteus maximus. Paresthesias, which may extend to the sole of the foot, prove the correct position of the needle. Electrical stimulation with a needle stimulator facilitates placement. After aspiration, 20 to 30 mL of the local anesthetic is injected.

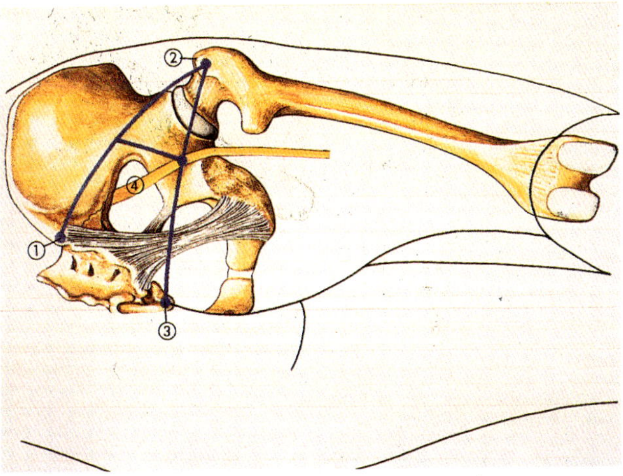

Fig. 12-13. The sciatic nerve block. A line is drawn between the posterior superior iliac spine and the greater trochanter. Then a line is dropped from its midpoint at right angles, which intersects a line drawn between the tip of the coccyx and the greater trochanter at about 3 cm. 1: posterior-superior iliac spine; 2: greater trochanter muscle; 3: tip of coccyx; 4: sciatic nerve. Reprinted with permission from Astra Chemicals GmbH, Zenz M, Hoerster W, Hiesel HC, Kreuscher H, eds; DeKornfeld TJ, trans. *Regional Anesthesia.* 2nd ed. St. Louis, Mo: Mosby–Year Book; 1990: 116, 117.

Local Anesthetic Drug Dosages and Complications. The sciatic nerve block can be achieved with 20 to 30 mL of 1.5% lidocaine or 0.5% bupivacaine. No significant complications secondary to this block have been documented. Residual dysesthesias have been reported but are usually self-remitting.[41]

Sciatic Nerve Block at the Popliteal Fossa

Sciatic nerve block from the popliteal fossa approach will provide unilateral anesthesia for procedures below the level of the knee, with the exception of the saphenous nerve distribution, which is a continuation of the femoral nerve, originating from the lumbar plexus (Figure 12-14).[41,73] The popliteal approach is especially amenable to a catheter technique.

Technique. Sciatic nerve block from the popliteal fossa approach can be accomplished using the following equipment:

- 18-gauge, 2½-in. catheter; and
- 20-gauge epidural catheter.

Insert the catheter over a blunt stylet 10 cm above the popliteal crease in the midline at an angle of approximately 30° to the skin. The needle is advanced in an anterior and cephalad direction until a fascial "pop" is felt. The stylet is then withdrawn and 20 mL of local anesthetic solution is injected through the catheter in incremental doses. A 20-gauge epidural catheter is then threaded through the short catheter; the short catheter is removed; and the epidural catheter is fixed in place using a sterile, transparent dressing. The sciatic nerve is anesthetized at its bifurcation to the common peroneal and tibial nerves.

Contraindications. Sciatic nerve block from the popliteal fossa approach is contraindicated in the presence of local or systemic infection, coagulation abnormality, immunosuppression, and unstable neurological deficits.[41]

Complications. The sciatic nerve block may be complicated by needle trauma, infection, and inadequate nerve block.

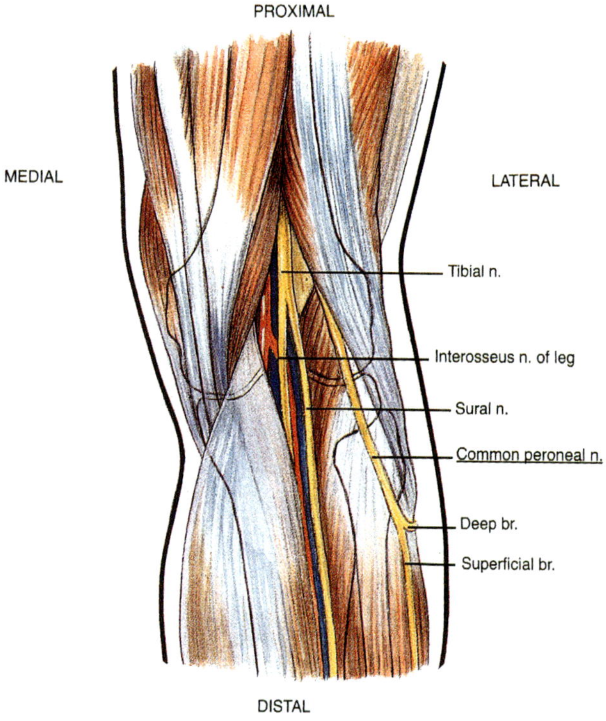

Fig. 12-14. Sciatic nerve block at the popliteal fossa. The injection is made in the posterior midline about 10 cm cranial to the transverse crease in the skin of the popliteal fossa. Reprinted with permission from Brown DL. *Atlas of Regional Anesthesia*. Philadelphia, Pa: WB Saunders; 1992: 112.

Lateral Femoral Cutaneous Nerve Block

The lateral femoral cutaneous nerve supplies the skin over the anterolateral aspect of the thigh as low as the knee. A posterior branch pierces the fascia lata and passes backward to supply the skin on the lateral side of the thigh. One of the terminal anterior branches forms part of the patellar plexus and must also be blocked for operations on the knee.

The lateral femoral cutaneous nerve (L-2–L-3) emerges at the lateral border of the psoas muscle at a level lower than the ilioinguinal nerve.[41] It passes obliquely under the iliac fascia and across the iliac muscle to enter the thigh deep to the inguinal ligament at a point 1 to 2 cm medial to the anterior superior iliac spine.

Technique. Lateral femoral cutaneous nerve block can be accomplished using the following equipment:

- 22-gauge, 1½ in. needle; and
- 10-mL syringe.

The patient is placed in the supine position. After palpation of the anterior superior iliac spine, a skin wheal is placed 2 to 3 cm inferior and 2 to 3 cm medial to it.[41] A 3- to 4-cm needle with syringe attached is inserted perpendicular to the skin (Figure 12-15). After the needle passes through the skin, the anesthesiologist feels firm fascia lata, followed by a sudden release as the needle passes through.

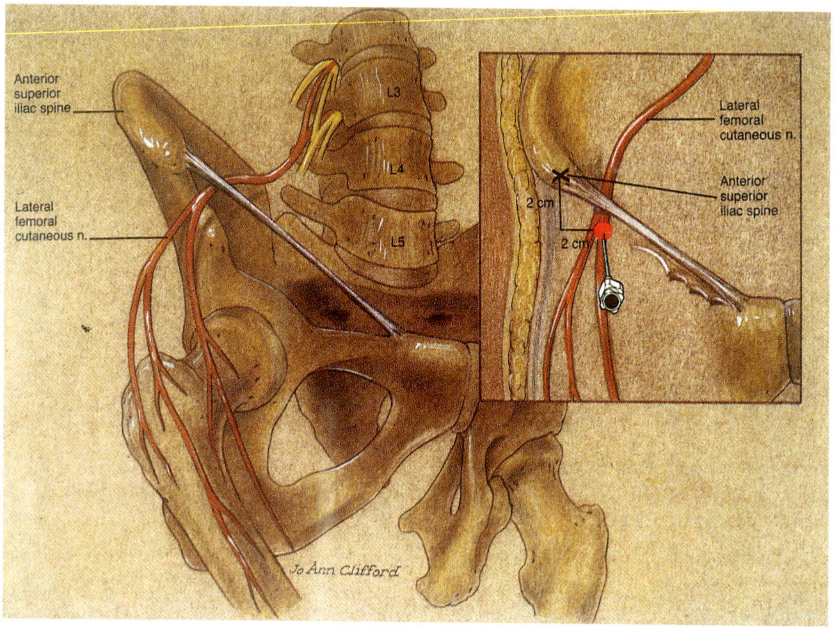

Fig. 12-15. The lateral femoral cutaneous nerve block as it passes under the inguinal ligament at a point about 2 to 3 cm inferior and 2 to 3 cm medial to the anterior superior iliac crest. Reprinted with permission from Brown DL. *Atlas of Regional Anesthesia*. Philadelphia, Pa: WB Saunders; 1992: 100.

Ten milliliters of a local anesthetic solution can be deposited fanwise as the needle is moved upward and downward, depositing solution both above and below the fascia.

An alternative technique is to direct the needle through the skin wheal in a slightly lateral and cephalad direction to strike the iliac bone just medial and inferior to the anterior superior iliac spine where the nerve emerges. Ten milliliters of local anesthetic is deposited in a medial fanwise fashion at this point.

Local Anesthetic Dosage and Complications. Any anesthetic agent suitable for peripheral nerve block can be used, in the amount of 10 mL. With the exception of remotely possible dysesthesia or hypoesthesia, there are no known risks with this nerve block.[41]

Ankle Block

The ankle block provides anesthesia for the foot by blocking five nerves at the level of the malleoli: the posterior tibial, sural, superficial peroneal, deep peroneal, and saphenous nerves.[41] The latter three innervate the dorsum of the foot (Figure 12-16).

The tibial nerve (composed of fibers from L-4–S-3), the larger of the two branches of the sciatic nerve, reaches the distal part of the leg from the medial side of the Achilles tendon, where it lies behind the posterior tibial artery.[41] The medial branch supplies the medial two thirds of the sole and plantar portion of the medial three and one half toes, up to the nail. The lateral branch supplies the lateral one third of the sole and plantar portion of the lateral one and one half toes.

The sural nerve is a cutaneous nerve that arises through the union of a branch from the tibial nerve and one from the common peroneal nerve. It proceeds subcutaneously along the short saphenous vein behind and below the lateral malleolus to supply the lower posterolateral surface of the leg, the lateral side of the foot, and the lateral part of the fifth toe.

The superficial peroneal nerve (composed of fibers from L-4–S-2) perforates the deep fascia on the anterior aspect of the distal two thirds of the leg and runs subcutaneously to supply the dorsum of the foot and toes, except for the contiguous surfaces of the great and second toes.

The deep peroneal nerve (composed of fibers from L-4–S-2) courses down the anterior aspect of the interosseous membrane of the leg and continues midway between the malleoli onto the dorsum of the foot. It innervates the short extensors of the toes as well as the skin on the adjacent areas of the first and second toes. The anterior tibial artery lies medial to the nerve, as does the tendon of the extensor hallucis longus muscle.

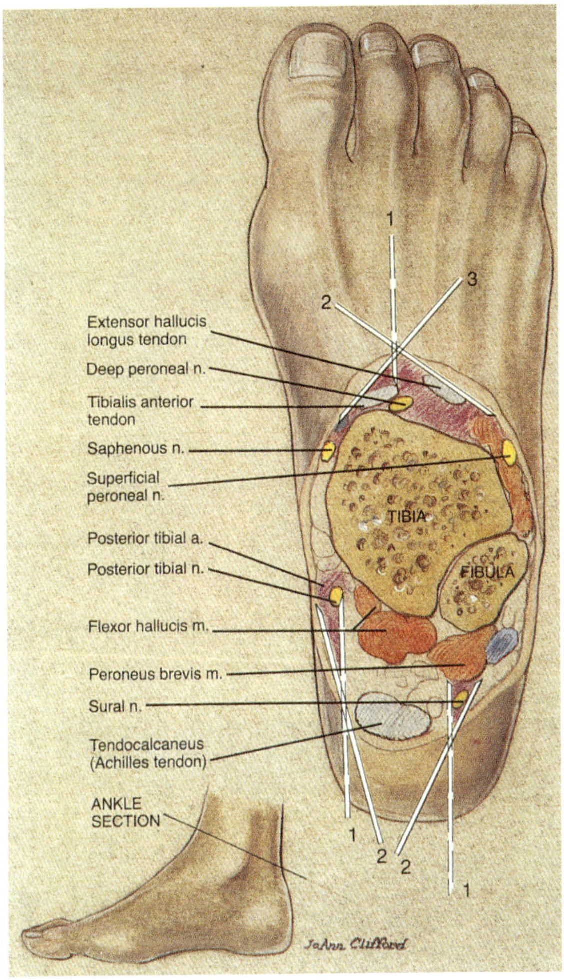

Fig. 12-16. Complete anesthesia of the foot can be obtained by blocking five nerves as they pass caudad to the ankle. The posterior tibial nerve is blocked near the posterior tibial artery as it passes the medial malleolus. The deep peroneal nerve is blocked near the dorsalis pedis artery. The same anterior needle site on the dorsum of the foot is used to infiltrate the tissues around the saphenous and superficial peroneal nerves. The sural nerve is blocked near the lateral malleolus. Needles labeled 1, 2, and 3 show sequence of infiltration. Reprinted with permission from Brown DL. *Atlas of Regional Anesthesia*. Philadelphia, Pa: WB Saunders; 1992: 119.

The saphenous nerve is the sensory terminal branch of the femoral nerve. It becomes subcutaneous at the lateral side of the knee joint. It follows the great saphenous vein to the medial malleolus and supplies the cutaneous area over the medial side of the lower leg anterior to the medial malleolus and the medial part of the foot.[41]

Technique. The ankle block can be accomplished using the following equipment:

- 22- to 25-gauge, 1½ in. needle; and
- 10-mL syringe.

The technique is modified according to the nerve to be blocked.

Posterior Tibial Nerve. The needle is introduced just posterior to the posterior tibial artery and is advanced until a paresthesia to the sole of the foot is elicited, at which point 5 mL of local anesthetic solution is injected.[41]

Sural Nerve. The needle is advanced into the groove between the lateral malleolus and the calcaneus, where 5 mL of local anesthetic solution is injected.

Saphenous Nerve. Infiltration of 5 mL of local anesthetic solution in the area where the saphenous vein passes anterior to the medial malleolus blocks this nerve.

Deep Peroneal Nerve. This is the major nerve to the dorsum of the foot, and it is blocked by placement of 5 mL of local anesthetic solution just lateral to the anterior tibial artery.

Superficial Peroneal Branches. A subcutaneous ridge of anesthetic solution (5–10 mL) is placed between the anterior tibial artery and the lateral malleolus.

Local Anesthetic Drug Dosages and Complications. Any anesthetic agents suitable for peripheral nerve block can be used, in the amounts specified above. Epinephrine-containing solutions are not used because of possible end-artery vasoconstriction and subsequent tissue ischemia. No major complications have been reported.[41]

SUMMARY

The techniques for regional anesthesia find potential application in several phases of combat casualty care: analgesia in the preoperative phase, intraoperative use as the sole anesthetic or as a supplement to general anesthesia, and analgesia in the postoperative phase. The most important benefit of regional anesthesia is that the deleterious effects of general anesthesia, such as loss of airway reflexes and respiratory depression requiring prolonged observation, are avoided. Furthermore, the quality of analgesia provided by regional blockade is superior to other forms of pain relief because local anesthetics completely block afferent and efferent nerve impulses.

Blockade of afferent impulses may have benefits that go beyond simple analgesia; the neurohormonal response to injury is itself blunted. The chemical agents used in regional anesthetics consist of a hydrophilic secondary or tertiary amine group bound to a lipophilic aromatic ring joined by either an amide or an ester linkage. The propensity for the hydrophilic group to ionize, as measured by the pKa, is an important determinate of potency; the higher the pKa, the greater the ionization and the longer the duration of action. This relationship arises from the fact that although passage of the anesthetic agent through the lipid myelin sheath of a nerve fiber depends upon lipid solubility, analgesia is caused by alterations in the structure of the proteins that constitute the sodium channels of the nerve axon. This latter effect depends on the binding of the ionized form of the hydrophilic group with receptor proteins.

Regional anesthetic techniques are determined by knowledge of anatomy and the nature of the planned surgery. Since the extremities are the most common site of war wounds, regional techniques would appear to be especially applicable. The epidural and spinal techniques are the most versatile regional procedures. They can be used for extensive abdominal and lower extremity operations, although they are contraindicated in the presence of severe systemic infection or uncorrected hypovolemia. Nerve blocks for specific anatomical regions, which with an experienced provider might find application in combat casualty care, are the brachial plexus block for injuries of the upper extremity and the sciatic and femoral nerve blocks for injuries of the legs. Intravenous regional anesthesia using the Bier method is especially useful in treating isolated injuries of the hand or forearm. Perhaps the most common technique using local anesthetics is also the simplest: local infiltration of the wounds, which is especially useful when a few, small, soft-tissue wounds require treatment.

REFERENCES

1. Wound Data and Munitions Effectiveness Team: The WDMET study. Original data are in the possession of the Uniformed Services University of the Health Sciences, Bethesda, MD 20814-4799. Three summary volumes contain extensive abstracts of the statistical data and can be obtained from: Defense Documentation Center, Cameron Station, Alexandria, VA 22304-6145. Volume 3, Table 4-7-9.

2. Wildsmith JAW. Developments in local anaesthetic drugs and techniques for pain relief. *Br J Anaesth.* 1989; 63:159–164.

3. Raja SN, Meyer RA, Campbell JN. Peripheral mechanisms of somatic pain. *Anesthesiology.* 1988;68:571–590.

4. Cousins MJ. Acute pain and the injury response. Immediate and prolonged effects. *Reg Anaesth.* 1989;14:162–179.

5. Yaksh TL. Pharmacology of spinal adrenergic systems which modulate spinal nociceptive processing. *Pharmacol Biochem Behav.* 1985;22:845–858.

6. Bridenbaugh PO, DuPen SL, Moore DC, Bridenbaugh LD, Thompson GE. Postoperative intercostal nerve block analgesia versus narcotic analgesia. *Anesth Analg.* 1973;52:81–85.

7. Cuschieri RJ, Morran CG, Howie JC, McArdle CS. Postoperative pain and pulmonary complications: comparison of three analgesic regimens. *Br J Surg.* 1985;72:495–498.

8. Sanchez V, Segedin ER, Moser M, Pallares VS. Role of lumbar sympathectomy in the pediatric intensive care unit. *Anesth Analg.* 1988;67:794–797.

9. Walsh JA, Glynn CJ, Cousins MJ, Basedow RW. Blood flow, sympathetic activity and pain relief following lumbar sympathetic blockade or surgical sympathectomy. *Anaesth Intensive Care.* 1984;13:18–24.

10. Blunnie WP, McIlroy PD, Marrett JD, Dundee JW. Cardiovascular and biochemical evidence of stress during major surgery associated with different techniques of anaesthesia. *Br J Anaesth.* 1983;55:611–618.

11. Modig J, Borg T, Karlstrom G, Maripuu E, Sahlstedt B. Thromboembolism after total hip replacement: role of epidural and general anaesthesia. *Anesth Analg.* 1983;62:174–180.

12. Kehlet H. Neurohumoral response to surgery and pain in man. In: Bond MR, Charlton JE, Woolf CJ, eds. *Proceedings of the 6th World Congress on Pain.* Philadelphia, Pa: Elsevier Science Publishers; 1991:35–40.

13. Roizen MF. Should we all have a sympathectomy at birth? Or at least preoperatively? *Anesthesiology.* 1988;68:482–484.

14. Yeager MP, Glass DD, Neff RK, Brinck-Johnson T. Epidural anesthesia and analgesia in high-risk surgical patients. *Anesthesiology.* 1987;66:729–736.

15. Crile GW, Lower WE. *Anoci-association.* Philadelphia, Pa: WB Saunders; 1914: 223–225.

16. Ghignone M, Calvillo O, Quintin L. Anesthesia and hypertension: The effect of clonidine on perioperative hemodynamics and isoflurane requirements. *Anesthesiology.* 1987;67:901–908.

17. Norris RM, Clarke ED, Sammel NL, Smith WM, Williams B. Protective effect of propranolol in threatened myocardial infarction. *Lancet.* 1978;2:907–909.

18. Stone JG, Foex P, Sear JW, Johnson LL, Khambatta HJ, Triner L. Myocardial ischemia in untreated hypertensive patients: Effect of a single small oral dose of a beta-adrenergic blocking agent. *Anesthesiology.* 1988;68:495–500.

19. Spence AA, Logan DA. Respiratory effects of extradural nerve block in the postoperative period. *Br J Anaesth.* 1975;47:281–284.

20. Pflug AE, Murphy TM, Butler SH, Tucker GT. The effects of postoperative peridural analgesia on pulmonary therapy and pulmonary complications. *Anesthesiology.* 1974;41:8–17.

21. Bromage PR, Camporesi E, Chestnut D. Epidural narcotics for postoperative analgesia. *Anesth Analg.* 1980; 59:473–477.

22. Hillman DR, Rung GW, Thompson WR, Davis NJ. The effect of bupivacaine scalp infiltration on the hemodynamic response to craniotomy under general anesthesia. *Anesthesiology.* 1987;67:1001–1003.

23. Hoar PF, Hickey RF, Ullyot DJ. Systemic hypertension following myocardial revascularization. A method of treatment using epidural anesthesia. *J Thorac Cardiovasc Surg.* 1976;71:859–864.

24. Klassen GA, Bramwell RS, Bromage PR, Zborowska-Sluis DT. Effect of acute sympathectomy by epidural anesthesia on the canine coronary circulation. *Anesthesiology.* 1980;52:8–15.

25. Austin KL, Stapleton JV, Mather LE. Multiple intramuscular injections: A major source of variability in analgesic response to meperidine. *Pain.* 1980;8:47–62.

26. Bennett RL, Batenhorst RL, Bivins BA, Bell RM, Groves DA, Foster TS. Patient–controlled analgesia—a new concept of postoperative pain relief. *Ann Surg.* 1982;195:700–705.

27. White PF. Use of patient-controlled analgesia for management of acute pain. *JAMA.* 1988;259:243–247.

28. Cousins MJ, Mather LE. Intrathecal and epidural administration of opioids. *Anesthesiology.* 1984;61:276–310.

29. Hondeghem LM, Miller RD. Local anesthetics. In: Katzung BG, ed. *Basic and Clinical Pharmacology.* East Norwalk, Conn: Appleton & Lange; 1989: 315–322.

30. Savarese JJ, Covino BG. Basic and clinical pharmacology of local anesthetic drugs. In: Miller RD, ed. *Anesthesia.* 2nd ed. New York: Churchill Livingstone; 1986: 1237–1242.

31. Covino BG, Vassalo HG. *Local Anesthetics Mechanisms of Action and Clinical Use.* Boston, Mass: Grune and Stratton; 1976.

32. Hondeghem LM, Mason JW. Agents used in cardiac arrhythmias. In: Katzung BG, ed. *Basic and Clinical Pharmacology.* East Norwalk, Conn: Appleton & Lange; 1989: 209–227.

33. Ritchie JM, Greene NM. Local anesthetics. In: Goodman LS, Gilman AG, eds. *The Pharmacological Basis of Therapeutics*, 6th ed. New York, NY: MacMillan; 1980: 300–321.

34. O'Connor CJ. Thoracic epidural analgesia: Physiologic effects and clinical applications. *J Cardiothorac Vasc Anesth.* 1993;7:595–609.

35. Lema MJ, Sinha I. Thoracic epidural anesthesia and analgesia. *Pain Digest.* 1994;4:3–11.

36. Tuman KJ, McCarthy RJ, March RJ, et al. Effects of epidural anesthesia and analgesia on coagulation and outcome after major vascular surgery. *Anesth Analg.* 1991;73:696–704.

37. Sharrock NE, Mineo R, Urquhart B, Salvati EA. The effect of two levels of hypotension on intraoperative blood loss during total hip arthroplasty performed under lumbar epidural anesthesia. *Anesth Analg.* 1993;76:580–584.

38. Scherer R, Schmutzler M, Giebler R, Erhard J, Stocker L, Kox WJ. Complications related to thoracic epidural analgesia: a prospective study in 1071 surgical patients. *Acta Anaesthesiol Scand.* 1993;37:370–374.

39. Pansard JL, Mankikian B, Bertrand M, et al: Effects of thoracic extradural block on diaphragmatic electrical activity and contractility after upper abdominal surgery. *Anesthesiology.* 1993;78:63–71.

40. Schnitzler M, Kilbride MJ, Senagore A. Effect of epidural analgesia on colorectal anastomotic healing and colonic motility. *Reg Anaesth.* 1992;17:143–147.

41. Cousins MJ, Bridenbaugh PO, eds. *Neural Blockade in Clinical Anesthesia and Management of Pain.* 2nd ed. Philadelphia, Pa: JB Lippincott; 1988.

42. Bromage PR. *Epidural analgesia.* Philadelphia, Pa: WB Saunders; 1978: 443–650.

43. Johnson A, Lofstrom JB. Influence of local anesthetics on ventilation. *Reg Anaesth.* 1991;16:7–12.

44. Blomberg S, Emanuelsson H, Kvist H, et al. Effects of thoracic epidural anesthesia on coronary arteries and arterioles in patients with coronary artery disease. *Anesthesiology.* 1990;73:840–847.

45. Reiz S. Circulatory effects of epidural anesthesia in patients with cardiac disease. *Acta Anaesthiol Belg.* 1988;39:21–27.

46. Guinard J, Mavrocordatos P, Chiolero R, Carpenter R. A randomized comparison of intravenous versus lumbar and thoracic epidural fentanyl for analgesia after thoracotomy. *Anesthesiology.* 1992;77:1108–1115.

47. Sandler AN, Stringer D, Panos L, et al. A randomized double-blind comparison of lumbar epidural and intravenous fentanyl infusions for postthoracotomy pain relief. *Anesthesiology.* 1992;77:626–634.

48. Fromme G, Steidl L, Danielson D. Comparison of lumbar and thoracic epidural morphine for relief of postthoracotomy pain. *Anesth Analg.* 1985;64:454–455.

49. Hakanson E, Bengtsson M, Rutberg H, Ulrick A. Epidural morphine by the thoracic or lumbar routes in cholecystectomy. Effect on postoperative pain and respiratory variables. *Anaesth Intensive Care.* 1989;17:166–169.

50. Boswell MV, Iacono RP, Guthkelch AN. Sites of action of subarachnoid lidocaine and tetracaine: Observations with evoked potential monitoring during spinal cord stimulator implantation. *Reg Anaesth.* 1992;17:37–42.

51. Lambert DH, Hurley RJ. Cauda equina syndrome and continuous spinal anesthesia. *Anesth Analg.* 1991;72:817–819.

52. Rigler ML, Drasner K, Krejcie TC, et al. Cauda equina syndrome after continuous spinal anesthesia. *Anesth Analg.* 1991;72:275–281.

53. VanGessel EF, Forster A, Schweizer A, et al. Comparison of hypobaric, hyperbaric, and isobaric solutions of bupivacaine during continuous spinal anesthesia. *Anesth Analg.* 1991;72:779–784.

54 Etches R, Sandler A, Daley M. Respiratory depression and spinal opioids. *Can J Anaesth.*1989;36:165–185.

55. Stoelting R. Intrathecal morphine—an underused combination for postoperative pain management. *Anesth Analg.* 1989;68:707–709.

56. Ellis H, ed. *Anatomy for Anaesthetists.* 6th ed. Oxford, England: Blackwell Scientific Publications; 1993.

57. Hoerster W, ed. *Regional Anesthesia.* 2nd ed. St Louis, Mo: Mosby–Year Book; 1990.

58. Murphy DF. Intercostal nerve blockade for fractured ribs and postoperative analgesia: Description of a new technique. *Reg Anaesth.* 1983;8:151–153.

59. Nunn JF, Slavin G. Posterior intercostal nerve block for pain relief after thoracotomy. *Br J Anaesth.* 1980;52:253–260.

60. Kambam J, Hammon J, Parris W, Lupinetti F. Intrapleural analgesia for postthoracotomy pain and blood levels of bupivacaine following intrapleural injection. *Can J Anaesth*. 1989;36:106–109.

61. Reiestad F, Stromskag K. Interpleural catheter in the management of postoperative pain. *Reg Anaesth*. 1986;11:89–91.

62. Rosenburg P, Scheinin B, Lepantalo M, Lindfors O. Continuous intrapleural infusion of bupivacaine for analgesia after thoracotomy. *Anesthesiology*. 1987;67:811–813.

63. Stromskag K, Reiestad F, Holmquist E, Ogenstad S. Intrapleural administration of 0.25%, 0.375%, and 0.5% bupivacaine with epinephrine after cholecystectomy. *Anesth Analg*. 1988;67:430–434.

64. Murphy DF. Interpleural analgesia. *Br J Anaesth*. 1933;71:426–434.

65. Lee V, Abram S. Intrapleural administration of bupivacaine for postthoracotomy analgesia. *Anesthesiology*. 1987;66:586

66. Moore D, Bridenbaugh L. Pneumothorax: Its incidence following intercostal nerve block. *JAMA*. 1962; 1005–1008.

67. Stromskag K, Steen P. Side effects and complications related to interpleural analgesia: An update. *Acta Anaesthesiol Scand*. 1990;34:1250–1254.

68. Partridge B, Stabile B. The effects of incisional bupivacaine on postoperative narcotic requirements, oxygen saturation and length of stay in the postanesthesia care unit. *Acta Anaesthesiol Scand*. 1990;34:486–491.

69. Ejlersen E, Andersen H, Eliasen K, Mogensen T. A comparison between preincisional and postincisional lidocaine infiltration and postoperative pain. *Anesth Analg*. 1992;74:495–498.

70. Barash P, ed. *Clinical Anesthesia*. Philadelphia, Pa: JB Lippincott; 1989.

71. Bridenbaugh LD. The upper extremity somatic blockade. In: Cousins MJ, Bridenbaugh PO, eds. *Neural Blockade in Clinical Anesthesia and Management of Pain*. 2nd ed. New York, NY: JB Lippincott; 1988: 387–416.

72 Scott B. *Techniques of Regional Anaesthesia*. Sydney, Australia: Prentice-Hall; 1989.

73. Rung G. Nerve blocks for lower extremity surgery. Presented at the Astra Regional Anesthesia Workshop; 1993; Chicago, Ill.

74. Winnie AP, Ramamurthy S, Durrani Z. The inguinal paravascular technique of lumbar plexus anesthesia: The "3-in-1 block." *Anesth Analg*. 1973;52:989–996.

Chapter 13

PERIOPERATIVE PAIN MANAGEMENT

JOHN M. STAMATOS, M.D.*; BEN H. BOEDEKER, D.V.M., M.D., PH.D.†; AND FRANK D. CROWL, M.D.‡

*Formerly, Captain, Medical Corps, U.S. Army; Chief, Pain Management Services, Department of Anesthesiology, Walter Reed Army Medical Center, Washington, D. C. 20307-5001; currently, Associate Director, The New York Center for Pain Management and Rehabilitation, St. Vincent's Hospital and Medical Center of New York, 130 West 12th Street, New York, New York 10011

†Major, Medical Corps, U.S. Army; Assistant Professor, Department of Anesthesiology, Uniformed Services University of the Health Sciences, Bethesda, Maryland 20814-4799; and Assistant Clinical Professor, Pennsylvania State University, College of Medicine, Department of Anesthesia, Hershey Medical Center, Hershey, Pennsylvania 17033

‡Formerly, Major, Medical Corps, U.S. Army; Department of Anesthesiology, Walter Reed Army Medical Center, Washington, D. C. 20307-5001; currently, Anesthesia Department, Holy Cross Hospital, 1500 Forest Glen Road, Silver Spring, Maryland 20910

INTRODUCTION

Pain control has become an integral part of the anesthesiologist's professional responsibilities. The physiological and humanitarian ramifications of inadequate pain relief can be catastrophic. Postinjury pain control in past wars has not always been optimal; in many instances, there has been none. Every war has its own descriptions of the suffering of untreated casualties, and it was the sound of casualties dying on the battlefield of Solferino in 1859 that motivated Henri Dunant to take the first steps that led to the formation of the International Red Cross:

> The stillness of the night was broken by groans, by stifled sighs of anguish and suffering. Heart-rending voices kept calling for help. Who could ever describe the agonies of that fearful night![1(p41)]

More than humanitarian concerns are relevant to managing pain, however; postinjury or postoperative pain relief also blunts the trauma-induced neuroendocrine response that leads to detrimental metabolic, respiratory, and cardiovascular derangements. Thus, effective analgesia can both make the casualty more comfortable and decrease morbidity.

Although this chapter is oriented toward the management of pain in postoperative, hospitalized, combat casualties, military anesthesia providers need to know not only the full dimensions of providing analgesia to combat casualties but also what specifically can and should be done in the echelons below the corps level. The landmark battlefield study on pain in combat casualties was carried out by members of the U.S. Army Medical Corps in Italy in late 1943 and 1944.[2] The impetus for this study came from the observation that, at corps-level hospitals, increasing numbers of casualties were being seen who had obvious clinical signs and symptoms of morphine overdose and even lethal poisoning. This problem was soon shown to be due to the practice by field medical personnel of injecting morphine—in 30-mg increments, subcutaneously or intramuscularly—soon after the casualty had been wounded. Absorption of the morphine from the site of injection was sluggish because the weather was cold and many of the casualties were hypovolemic or even in shock. Thus, repeated doses were given to relieve pain. On arriving at the hospital level and with the initiation of resuscitation, the morphine that was deposited in peripheral tissue was rapidly absorbed into the circulation—sometimes with fatal results.

By studying the prevalence of pain in combat casualties, the investigators set about determining how much morphine was really needed to obtain an acceptable degree of pain relief. On arriving at the corps hospital, casualties were asked to describe their pain, if any, using the following scale: none, slight, moderate, or severe. Casualties who admitted to pain of any degree were then asked if they wanted something to relieve it. Two hundred twenty-five casualties, representative of the more severely injured, were studied. Of these, 10 were subsequently excluded because their state of consciousness was altered. The remaining casualties were stratified into five groups according to the nature of their wounds: (1) fractures of extremity bone, (2) extensive soft-tissue injuries, (3) penetrating wounds of thorax, (4) penetrating wounds of abdomen, and (5) wounds of the head or brain or both (Figure 13-1 and Table 13-1). Ethical considerations precluded a study design in which one population would serve as an unmedicated control group; thus, most casualties had received morphine before reaching the hospital level.

Two striking findings emerged from this study. When seen at the hospital and evaluated for pain (7–14 h after their injuries, which was not a remarkably long time by World War II standards, and at least 5 h after last receiving morphine),

- approximately 75% of the casualties had no desire for medication for pain relief, and
- approximately 75% of the casualties had no pain or pain that was slight to moderate in intensity.

Because the amount of morphine administered was not different for those with or without pain and those who did or did not desire an analgesic, the investigators believed that the intensity of pain could not be explained on the basis of the amount of morphine administered. They concluded that

- most combat casualties do not need an analgesic prior to arrival at the hospital level, with the probable exception of casualties with abdominal wounds, in whom pain relief would appear to be usually indicated; and

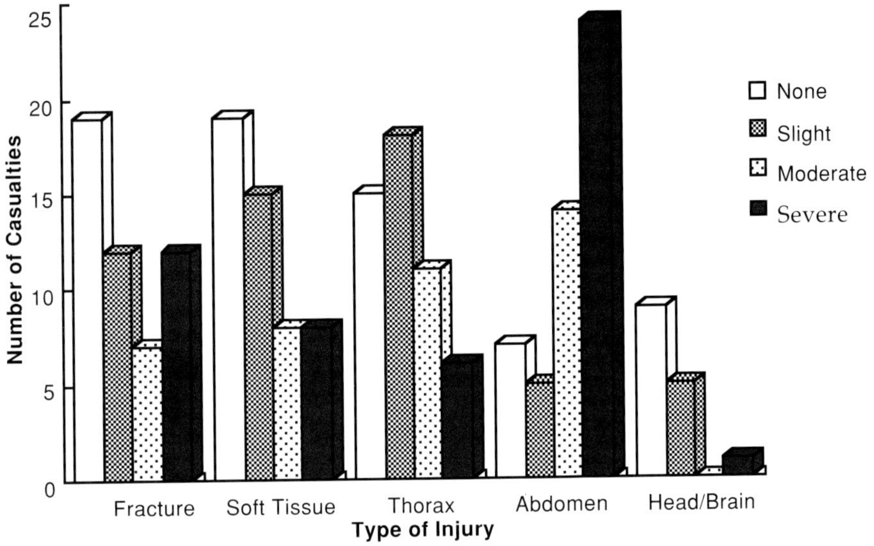

Fig. 13-1. When the nature of pain—assessed on admission to third-echelon hospitals—was studied in combat casualties who were wounded in Italy during World War II, the distribution of pain intensity could be plotted as a function of wound type. Most casualties with fractures, soft-tissue, and thoracic injuries reported little pain; most casualties with head wounds reported little or no pain. Only casualties with abdominal wounds demonstrated a great need for analgesia. Data source: Beecher HK. The control of pain in men wounded in battle. In: DeBakey ME, ed. *General Surgery*. Vol 2. In: Coates JB Jr, ed. *Surgery in World War II*. Washington, DC: US Department of the Army, Medical Department, Office of The Surgeon General; 1955: 4–49.

- if morphine is required, it should be administered intravenously (which, of course, may not be practicable on the battlefield).

At the hospital level and especially following surgical intervention, a patient's degree of pain is often difficult to assess. The recovery room personnel's assessment of the casualty's pain is usually subjective. A patient's communication skills and cultural background will influence the ability to express his or her level of discomfort. Several pain scores have been developed to help eliminate

TABLE 13-1

EPIDEMIOLOGICAL ASPECTS OF A WORLD WAR II COMBAT CASUALTY PAIN STUDY

Type of Injury	Time Since Injury (h) (m ± sd)	Total Dose of Morphine (mg) (m ± sd)	Time Since Last Dose (h) (m ± sd)	Request Further Pain Relief (%)
Fractured extremity bone (n = 50)	12.5 ± 1.3	27 ± 1.5	7.0 ± 0.8	22
Extensive soft-tissue extremity injury (n = 50)	11.4 ± 1.4	27 ± 2.7	7.2 ± 0.6	18
Penetrating, of thorax (n = 50)	9.8 ± 1.0	25.0 ± 1.8	6.5 ± 0.6	20
Penetrating, of abdomen (n = 50)	7.2 ± 0.7	29.0 ± 2.2	4.8 ± 0.7	54
Head and/or brain (n = 15)	7.9 ± 1.4	19.8 ± 4.2	6.2 ± 1.5	7

Adapted from Beecher HK. The control of pain in men wounded in battle. In: DeBakey ME, ed. *General Surgery*. Vol 2. In: Coates JB Jr, ed. *Surgery in World War II*. Washington, DC: US Department of the Army, Medical Department, Office of The Surgeon General; 1955: 45.

the subjectivity in the assessment of acute pain, but these are much more useful in a research setting or a civilian hospital than on the battlefield.[3]

Fortunately for casualties of modern warfare, many techniques and drugs are now available that provide considerable analgesia. Some, such as patient-controlled analgesia (PCA), will allow the casualty more autonomy with respect to narcotics administration, which will simultaneously reduce the demand for nursing care.[4,5] Administration of narcotics by the epidural or intrathecal routes will provide sustained pain relief far beyond that obtained with the more traditional intramuscular or intravenous routes.[6] By employing dilute concentrations of local anesthetics, regional blocks can be used to provide pain relief with a minimal decrement of motor function.[7] New nonsteroidal antiinflammatory drugs (NSAIDs), which are nearly as effective as the narcotics used in prior wars but are not addictive, can be given intramuscularly or intravenously and act as an adjunct in the therapy of the injured soldier.[8] By taking advantage of the newer techniques, military anesthesiologists can help soldiers who are injured on the battlefield to recover from surgery with minimal—or at least greatly reduced—discomfort.

Military trauma anesthesiologists must be able to meet the soldiers' postoperative pain requirements, have a sound working knowledge of the drugs at our disposal, and be adept in the use of the different modes of delivery and administration. The battlefield is not the ideal setting in which to treat patients. Therefore, we must be able to adapt to the situation and adequately treat the casualties as they present, using innovative ideas and combinations of treatment modalities to care for these soldiers.

PATHOPHYSIOLOGY OF PAIN

Visceral pain originates from organs of the abdominal cavity and thorax. The receptors cover large areas and the impulses travel through unmyelinated sympathetic fibers. These nerves respond to stretch, crush, ischemia, and displacement. The pain generated from these areas is dull, aching, and difficult to localize. The normal causes of visceral pain are distention of the viscera or renal pelvis secondary to obstruction. Somatic pain, in contrast, is transmitted in unmyelinated C fibers and small, myelinated, A-delta fibers, the impulse arising in receptors in skin, fasciae, bones, and joint spaces. These receptors innervate small discrete areas and are able to pinpoint noxious stimuli. Myelinated somatic nerve fibers, which are called A fibers, are the largest in diameter and conduct impulses the most rapidly. A fibers are further divided, by their progressively decreasing sizes, into alpha, beta, gamma, and delta fibers. The alpha and beta fibers convey motor and proprioception information. The gamma fibers control muscle spindle tone. The delta fibers, which are the A fibers with the smallest diameter, transmit messages concerning pain, temperature, and touch (Table 13-2).[9]

The thinly myelinated B fibers are smaller than the alpha fibers and have a preganglionic autonomic function for both sympathetic and parasympathetic systems.[9] The unmyelinated C fibers are the smallest diameter nerve fibers. They have the lowest rate of impulse conduction velocity and contain postganglionic autonomic axons as well as axons conveying pain, temperature and touch information.[10]

Three major types of receptors are stimulated by nociceptive input: low-threshold mechanoreceptors, high-threshold mechanoreceptors, and polymodal nociceptors. Low-threshold mechanoreceptors respond to mechanical stimulation like pressure. These receptors are carried on A-delta fibers and transmit the stimuli at about 20 m/s.[11] As the input increases, the firing rate increases. High-threshold mechanoreceptors respond to noxious mechanical stimulation. As they are on low-threshold mechanoreceptors, impulses to high-threshold mechanoreceptors are carried on A-delta fibers. Polymodal nociceptors transmit impulses through unmyelinated C fibers. These receptors respond to many different kinds of nociceptive input including chemical, thermal, and mechanical. The receptive fields are larger than those of the A-delta fibers, and stimulation of these fibers lasts longer than with the other receptors.[12] The generally accepted paradigm for pain perception, modulators, and transmitters is shown in Figure 13-2.

Local Transmitters of Pain

The many different biochemical transmitters of pain include potassium and hydrogen ions, serotonin, histamine, bradykinin, substance P, and leukotrienes.[13] When injected locally, all these substances either (*a*) are responsible for the transmission of noxious stimulation or (*b*) decrease the threshold of the pain transmission.[14]

Both potassium and hydrogen ions sensitize nerve endings and are usually released from cells when

TABLE 13-2

CLASSIFICATION OF NERVE FIBERS

Fiber Type	Diameter (μm)	Conduction Rate (m/s)	Anatomical Location	Function
A				
Alpha	12–20	100	Afferent to and efferent from muscles and joints	Large motor and proprioception
Beta	5–12	30–85	Afferent to and efferent from muscles and joints	Small motor, muscle tone, touch, pressure
Gamma	3–6	15–35	Efferent to muscle spindles	Muscle tone
Delta	2–5	3–25	Sensory roots and afferent peripheral nerves	Sharp pain, temperature, touch
B				
	3	3–15	Preganglionic autonomic	Vasomotor Visceromotor Suromotor Pilomotor
C				
sC	0.3–1.3	0.7–1.3	Postganglionic sympathetic	Vasomotor Visceromotor Suromotor Pilomotor
drC	0.4–1.2	0.1–2.0	Sensory roots and afferent peripheral nerves	Dull pain Temperature Touch

Data sources: (1) Raj P. *Practical Management of Pain*. 2nd ed. St. Louis, Mo: Mosby–Year Book; 1992: 139. (2) Barash PG, Cullen BF, Stoelting RK, eds. *Clinical Anesthesia*. Philadelphia, Pa: JB Lippincott; 1989: 374.

they are damaged during injury. Activity of peripheral pain receptors are regulated by, among other substances, serotonin and histamine. Serotonin is also a neurotransmitter for the descending inhibitory pathways. Bradykinin, a 9–amino acid peptide, is produced by enzymatic activity at the site of cell breakdown. Binding sites for bradykinins have also been found in the dorsal columns. Substance P, an 11–amino acid peptide, is synthesized in the dorsal root ganglia, from where it is transferred both centrally and peripherally along the nerve. In the peripheral locale—a nerve ending—substance P activates an enzyme that catalyzes the formation of arachidonic acid, which, in turn, serves as the substrate of the enzyme cyclooxygenase. This results in the production of prostaglandin E_2, an eicosanoid, that not only increases the sensitivity of nerve endings to chemical agents and mechanical injuries but also, by itself, causes hyperalgesia.[15] Substance P is also indirectly responsible for the vasodilation associated with local injury.[16] The leukotrienes are also derivatives of arachidonic acid, but that reaction is catalyzed by lipoxygenase. There are many different leukotrienes, and most are associated with lowering the threshold of the nerves associated with the transmission of pain.

Transmission of Pain

The events leading to the transmission of pain were first reported in 1927 and described as a triple response: intense vasodilation, local edema or wheal, and secondary vasodilation spreading to the local area.[17] This response is mediated by the transmitters of pain and stimulates the nociceptor fibers to fire. These fibers then synapse in the dorsal column of the spinal cord. There, the impulses are modulated and transmitted to the contralateral spinothalamic tract up into the cerebral cortex. The spinothalamic tract is subdivided into subtracts, one of which, the *lateral* subtract (found

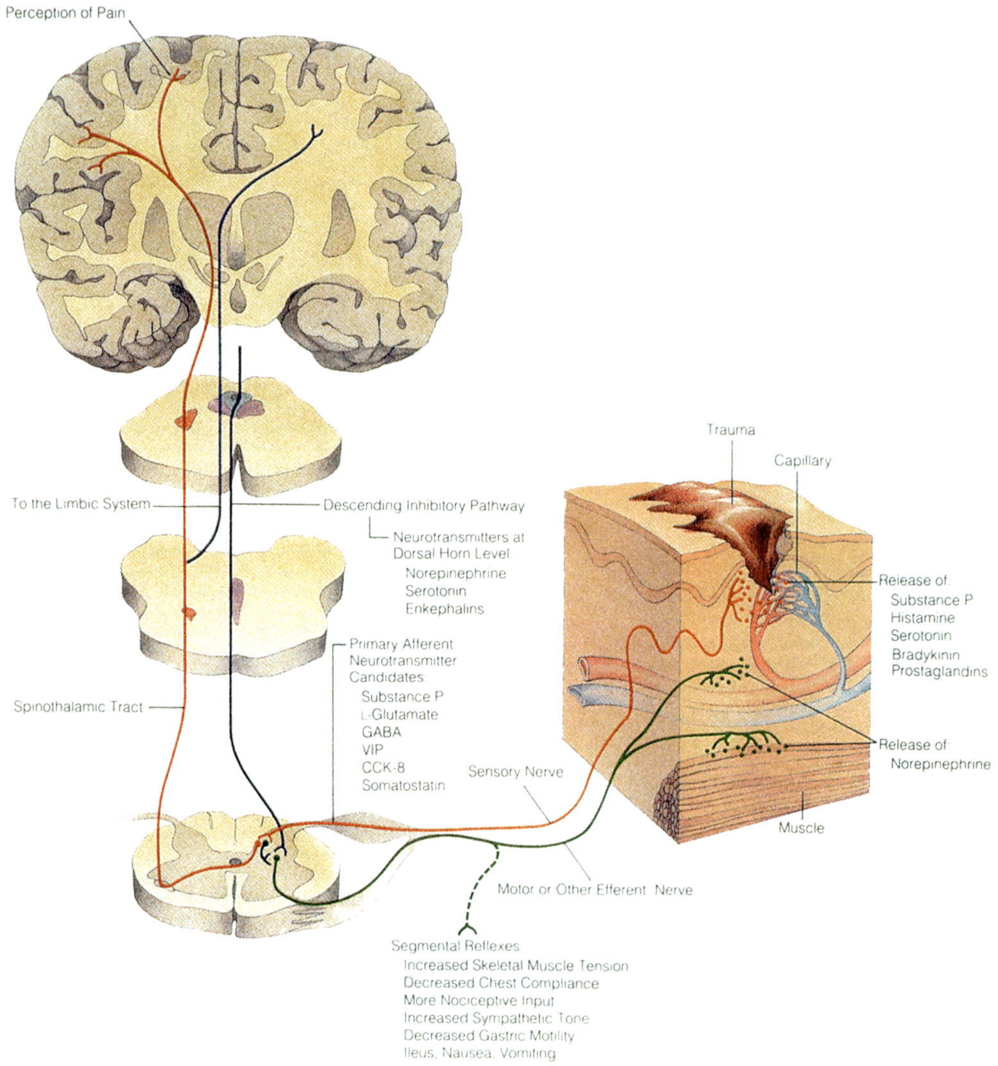

Fig. 13-2. Pain perception depends on the integrated function of three neurological pathways. First, peripheral nerves connect pain receptors in the injured tissue with neurons in the dorsal horn of the spinal cord. Second, nerve fibers pass from the dorsal horn neurons to the contralateral side of the cord, where they ascend to the cerebral cortex. The third component consists of tracts that arise in the upper brain stem and descend to the dorsal horn neurons, the function of which is thereby modulated. The ascending tract also has a component that passes to the limbic system and no doubt is important in modifying the emotional response to pain. A large number of transmitters are believed to be important in transmitting information about pain; several of these are discussed in text. GABA: γ-aminobutyric acid; VIP: vasoactive intestinal polypeptide; CCK-8: cholecystokinin-8. Reprinted with permission from Kehlet H. Postoperative pain. In: Wilmore DW, Brennan MF, Harken AH, Holcroft JW, Meakins JL, eds. *Critical Care*. Vol 1. In: *American College of Surgeons: Care of the Surgical Patient*. New York, NY: Scientific American, Inc; 1988–1993: II-12-10.

only in advanced primates), is probably responsible for the pinpoint perception of traumatic injury. As the impulses travel to the sensory tract of the cerebral cortex, they pass through the thalamus where they are again modulated. Once in the sensory cortex, the painful impulse is perceived and the body's response is determined. Thus, the major areas of the body in which pain is modulated are the dorsal columns, the spinothalamic tract, the thalamus, and the sensory cortex. The treatment of pain needs to focus on these areas.

Descending inhibitory pathways originate in the sensory cortex and terminate in the dorsal horn. These pathways are responsible for down-regulation of painful stimuli by releasing serotonin, norepinephrine, and enkephalins, which inhibit the activity of neurons that give rise to the fibers found in the spinothalamic tract. The release of substance P also causes the release of vasoactive substances (serotonin, bradykinin, histamine) at the site of injury. These substances stimulate both a hyperemic response and a hyperalgesic state at the injured site. Prostaglandins that are present in the cell membranes are also released in response to noxious stimuli. These substances do not themselves cause pain, but they do potentiate the noxious effects of the other substances that are present.[18]

The pharmacological treatment of pain is targeted to work on these sites of action. *Opioids* (ie, any natural or synthetic drug that has morphinelike pharmacological properties,[19] including the naturally occurring endorphins and enkephalins) activate both of the descending inhibitory pathways and bind presynaptically to the opioid receptors of the neurons in the dorsal horn. Opioids act to reduce the amount of substance P present.[20] Local anesthetics work by blocking the axonal transmission of pain.[21] Antipsychotics work to increase the level of serotonin in the dorsal horn and thus downregulate the pain transmissions.[22] NSAIDs stop the production of prostaglandin E_2 from prostacyclin.[23] Alpha-2 adrenergic agonists inhibit substance P by stimulating presynaptic and postsynaptic spinal cord receptors, which, in turn, inhibit pain transmission with a mechanism of action that is different from that of narcotics.[24]

SECONDARY MANIFESTATIONS OF ACUTE PAIN

The rationale for relieving pain transcends the anesthesiologist's professional mandate to alleviate suffering. Pain by itself has many deleterious effects, of which the inability to rest and sleep are the most obvious. Less obvious but of greater medical importance are such effects as pain-induced spasm of injured muscle, especially splinting of respiratory muscles; reflex stimulation of the autonomic nervous system, which causes hypertension and the release of catabolic hormones; and inhibition of the normal functions of the gut and urinary tract.

Respiratory System

The respiratory system is most often affected in injuries to the thoracic region or the upper abdomen. Casualties who remain in pain postoperatively splint when trying to breathe. This can cause decreased lung volumes and atelectasis, and can progress to lung collapse and pneumonia. The recognition of the importance of relieving pain in casualties with thoracic trauma was one of the most important advances in thoracic surgery during World War II:

> [P]ain was an almost constant accompaniment of any wound of the chest. The relief of pain had a vital bearing on hastening recovery.... [U]ntil it had been accomplished, the patient was unwilling to breathe deeply or cough, because of the discomfort which followed both acts, and fluid substances therefore accumulated in the tracheobronchial tree, which led to wet lung.[25(p244)]

Similar observations regarding pain in thoracic surgery have been made in civilian practice; pulmonary function greatly improves when adequate analgesia is provided.[26]

Cardiovascular System

Pain causes the amount of circulating catecholamines to increase. The effects of catecholamines on the cardiovascular system include increased (*a*) heart rate, (*b*) blood pressure, (*c*) cardiac output, and (*d*) systemic vascular resistance. Taken by itself, the increased heart rate, by limiting the time available for diastolic flow to occur, will cause a decrease in coronary blood flow. The usual concomitant increase in arterial pressure and coronary vasodilation caused by a catechol-mediated increase in cardiac metabolism negate the isolated effect of heart rate. Thus, coronary flow increases during tachycardia. Cardiac output may or may not change, depending on peripheral impedance. Increased systemic resistance will cause an increase in the workload for the heart. Together, these factors lead to increased myocardial oxygen consumption and, therefore, to an increased risk of myocardial ischemia in patients with limited cardiac reserve.[27] However, due to their age and physical condition, most injured soldiers should be able to tolerate this hemodynamic stress.

Gastrointestinal and Genitourinary Systems

Untreated pain will lead to decreased gastrointestinal motility with associated anorexia, nausea, and vomiting.[28] This places the patient at increased risk of pulmonary aspiration, and anastomotic and incisional dehiscence, and complicates the manage-

TABLE 13-3

NEUROENDOCRINE AND METABOLIC RESPONSES TO TRAUMA

Response	Effect	Cause
Endocrine	Catabolic	*Increased* ACTH, cortisol, ADH, GH, catecholamines, renin, angiotensin II, aldosterone, glucagon, interleukin-1
	Anabolic	*Decreased* insulin, testosterone
Metabolic		
Carbohydrate	Hyperglycemia, glucose intolerance, insulin resistance	*Increased* hepatic glycogenolysis (epinephrine, glucagon)
		Increased hepatic gluconeogenesis (cortisol, glucagon, growth hormone, epinephrine, free fatty acids)
		Decreased insulin secretion/action
Protein	Muscle protein catabolism, increased synthesis of acute-phase proteins	*Increased* cortisol, epinephrine, glucagon, interleukin-1
Fat	Increased lipolysis and oxidation	*Increased* catecholamines, cortisol, glucagon, growth hormone
Water and Electrolyte Flux	Retention of H_2O and Na^+, increased excretion of K^+, decreased functional extracellular fluid with shifts to intracellular compartments	*Increased* catecholamines, aldosterone, ADH, cortisol, angiotensin II, prostaglandins, and other factors

ACTH: adrenocorticotropic hormone; ADH: antidiuretic hormone; GH: growth hormone. Adapted with permission from Cousins M. Acute and postoperative pain. In: Wall PD, Melzac R. *Textbook of Pain*. New York, NY: Churchill Livingstone; 1989: Chap 18: 294.

ment of the casualty who needs to be returned to the operating room for additional surgery. Furthermore, sluggish gastrointestinal function delays the resumption of enteral nutrition. Unrelieved pain has a similar effect on the function of the urinary tract: persistent bladder retention necessitating prolonged urinary catheterization.

Endocrine and Metabolic Systems

Increased pain causes a stress response that manifests as an increase in the release of endogenous catecholamines, cortisol, and other mediators of the sympathetic response that promote harmful protein catabolism, glucose intolerance, and insulin resistance.[29]

An all-inclusive review of the endocrine response to postoperative pain is not within the scope of this chapter. Suffice it to say that the endocrine response to trauma—whether surgical or otherwise—is profound. Every system in the body is affected by these changes, most of which are secondary to circulating catecholamines released from the sympathetic nervous system (Table 13-3). Anabolism, catabolism, and substrate requirements all increase. The dual goals of postoperative pain control are the alleviation of pain and the subsequent decrease in the levels of circulating catecholamines.

CLINICAL PHARMACOLOGY OF OPIOID ANALGESICS

The opioids, of which morphine is the prototype, are the best known and most useful narcotic analgesics available. Morphine was first isolated from opium—the gum obtained by drying the milky juice made from the seedpod of the poppy plant *Papaver somniferum*—in 1803.[19]

Opioids act at two distinct anatomical sites: the supraspinal area and the spinal cord. In the supraspinal area, the drugs bind at receptor sites in the periventricular and periaqueductal gray area to modulate pain perception. In the spinal cord, the action is in the substantia gelatinosa of the dorsal horn. Here, the drugs block the release of the mediators of pain by binding to presynaptic receptors of afferent nerve terminals.[20]

Whether synthetic or derived from opium, these drugs are described by their effects at specific opioid receptors in the central nervous system (CNS). Four distinct opioid receptors have been identified in humans: mu, delta, kappa, and sigma.

The mu receptors are further subdivided into mu 1 and mu 2. Mu 1 receptors are located in the spinal cord and in the supraspinal area. Stimulation of these receptors produces analgesia. Morphine and beta-endorphin are agonists for this receptor. Mu 2 receptors cause ventilatory depression, decreased heart rate, euphoria, miosis, and physical dependence. Agonists of this group include fentanyl and meperidine.

The delta receptors, which have no intrinsic function, function as modulators of the mu receptors. Leuenkephalin is an agonist in this group.

The kappa receptors are located in the cerebral cortex and their activation causes analgesia, sedation, miosis, and some depression of ventilation. Agonists of this group include nalbuphine and butorphanol.

The sigma receptors are the latest of the opioid receptors to be described. Activation of this receptor stimulates dysphoria, tachycardia, and tachypnea. This may be the site of ketamine's action. Naloxone is an antagonist for all the opioid receptors.[30]

Opioid Agonists

Morphine

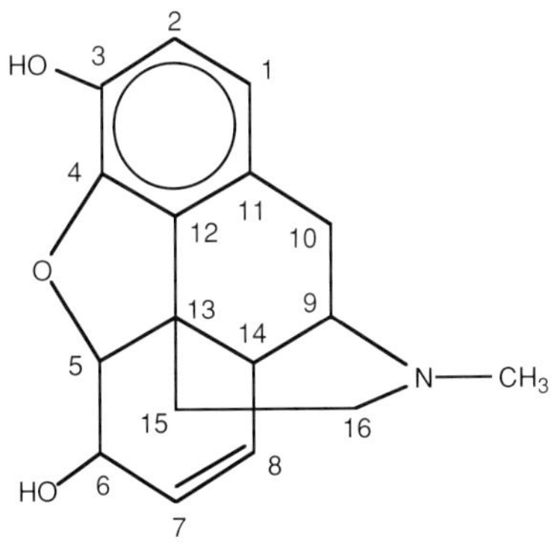

Morphine, the major phenanthrene alkaloid of opium, and codeine are the medically useful opioids derived from opium. Although codeine can be administered orally, it is not as potent as morphine and therefore will not be further discussed in this chapter.

An opioid agonist, morphine has demonstrated mu 1 activity in the periaqueductal gray matter. These receptors modulate noxious stimuli and send transmissions to the medullary nuclei. Spinal mu receptors also reduce the amount of substance P in the dorsal horn.

Morphine can be administered via the intravenous, intramuscular, epidural, and intrathecal routes. When delivered intravenously, morphine has a peak effect about 20 minutes after injection. Intramuscularly, an initial effect is seen in 15 to 30 minutes and the peak effect in 45 to 90 minutes. Orally administered morphine is not reliably absorbed. When given epidurally, the onset of pain relief tends to occur approximately 60 minutes later, and pain relief can last 16 to 24 hours. With intrathecal injections, the onset of pain relief tends to occur in approximately 10 to 15 minutes, which coincides with the peak level of drug in the cerebrospinal fluid.[30] Regardless of the mode of administration, the pain relief is relative to the concentration of the drug in the cerebrospinal fluid; pain relief is not always proportional to the blood levels.[31] The drug is eliminated from the body primarily by conjugation with glucuronic acid at hepatic and extrahepatic sites. A small amount of the dose is excreted unchanged in urine. Only 7% to 10% of morphine is eliminated by biliary excretion; the rest is excreted by the kidneys.[30]

Respiratory Side Effects. Mu 2 receptors in the pontine and medullary centers are responsible for respiratory depression.[32] The agonists produce a dose-related depression of respiration, the evidence of which is increased $Pa{CO_2}$. When morphine is administered in small doses, the respiratory rate usually decreases, which is compensated for by an increase in the tidal volume. With increasing doses of morphine, however, the tidal volume will decrease. Maximal respiratory depression occurs approximately 7 minutes after intravenous administration, 30 minutes after intramuscular injection, 90 minutes after subcutaneous administration, and up to 16 hours after epidural or intrathecal administration.[30]

Cardiovascular Side Effects. Morphine administration will decrease sympathetic outflow. No adverse effect will probably be seen in a supine, normovolemic patient, but a casualty who is standing or a supine casualty who is hypovolemic might suffer from hypotension. Morphine can also stimulate histamine release, causing peripheral vasodilation and hypotension. The histamine release can be attenuated by limiting the rate of infusion to less than 5 mg/min or by administering H_1 or H_2 blocking agents.[33] Morphine can also cause bradycardia, probably by stimulating the vagal nuclei in the medulla, and by exerting a depressing effect on the sinoatrial node. Although there are no known direct myocardial depressant effects of morphine, it causes a decrease in myocardial oxygen consumption. The mechanism is probably related to peripheral vasodilation and bradycardia. There is no direct effect on the cerebral circulation, but the secondary effect of the increased $Paco_2$ due to associated hypoventilation will cause cerebral vasodilation that could thereby increase intracranial pressure in the patient with neurotrauma.

Gastrointestinal Side Effects. Pain may cause decreased gastric emptying and motility. Morphine may enhance this dysmotility and lead to ileus. In addition, the tone of the ileocecal and anal sphincters is also increased. All these factors lead to decreased motility of and increased water absorption from the gut. Opioids will also cause spasm in the biliary smooth muscle (eg, the sphincter of Oddi). This spasm may mimic the pain of angina pectoris.

Nausea and vomiting are caused by direct stimulation of the chemoreceptor trigger zone of the medulla oblongata. This side effect can be treated with an antiemetic without reversing the analgesic effect of the morphine.

Genitourinary Side Effects. Morphine will cause increased peristalsis of the ureters, but the tone of the vesicle sphincter is also increased. The combination of these effects makes it more difficult for patients who are not catheterized to urinate. In some patients, morphine may also inhibit the urge to urinate.

Cutaneous Side Effects. Morphine will cause venodilation in the peripheral vessels of the extremities. The histamine release can also cause an erythema.

Pruritus, which is more pronounced in epidural and intrathecal use, can be pronounced and is secondary to a CNS effect of the drug. Pruritus can be reversed by titrating small amounts of an antagonist (eg, naloxone).[30]

Physical Dependence. All opioids can cause physical dependence. This complication occurs more often with agonists than with drugs that have combined agonist–antagonist effects. Although it usually takes longer, dependence can occur after as few as 72 hours of use. However, the possibility of dependence should not be a factor in limiting the use of a narcotic in the acutely injured soldier.

Dosage and Administration. For postoperative pain control, morphine should be titrated for effect. For intravenous or intramuscular injections, 0.05 to 0.1 mg/kg should provide adequate analgesia. Following this dose, the patient should be monitored for adequacy of pain control, changes in blood pressure and pulse, and respiratory rate. If the patient's pain is not controlled, then more narcotic can be administered; again, the patient's vital signs should be observed. When used intravenously or intramuscularly, morphine should be given every 3 to 6 hours.[34] Strict adherence to dosing intervals is needed to maintain therapeutic drug levels.

Epidurally or intrathecally administered morphine can provide pain relief for 16 to 24 hours with a single dose. It is important to remember that morphine's respiratory depression might not manifest itself for up to 20 hours after an injection. For acute pain, the doses of epidural morphine are 0.05 to 0.07 mg/kg, and can be administered every 12 hours as needed.[35] The anesthesiologist must bear in mind that morphine delivered via the epidural route requires up to 1 hour before the onset of pain relief. Morphine can be continuously infused at a rate of 0.005 to 0.01 mg/kg/h. Intrathecal narcotics also have the benefit of extended pain relief from a single injection. The usual dose of intrathecal morphine is 0.3 to 1 mg. The onset of action is almost immediate and the duration of a single injection is 12 to 24 hours.[6,35–37]

Fentanyl

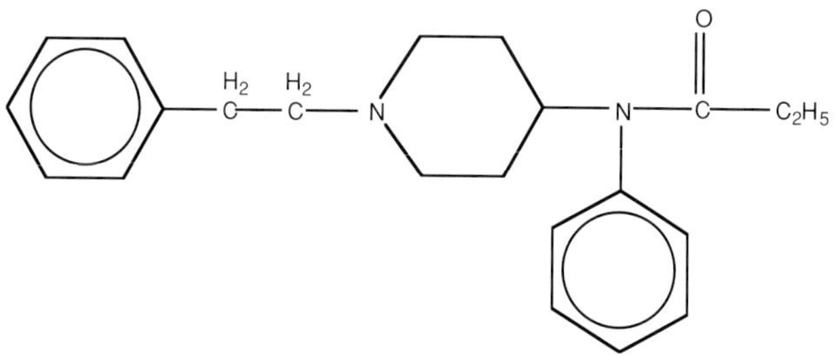

The opioid fentanyl is chemically similar to morphine. However, this synthetic narcotic is 75- to 125-fold more potent than morphine and, due to its high lipid solubility, it crosses the blood–brain barrier faster than morphine. The onset of action is approximately 30 seconds. The duration of action of the drug is also shorter than that of morphine, owing to fentanyl's rapid uptake by inactive tissue. Because of this uptake and subsequent release, when fentanyl has been given in repeated doses, its action can continue and be prolonged after the medication has been discontinued.[38] Fentanyl is metabolized by dealkylation, hydroxylation, and amide hydrolysis into inactive metabolites. The drug is excreted in the urine and feces.

Side Effects. The side effects of fentanyl are similar to those of morphine. Of note, less histamine is released than with morphine, but there is greater potential for physical dependence. Muscular rigidity, specifically of the chest wall, has also been associated with rapidly administered doses of fentanyl.[30]

Dosage and Administration. For the postoperative patient with acute pain, 1 to 2 μg/kg of fentanyl will give fast relief. Fentanyl's advantage over morphine is its speed of onset. However, the pain relief will not last as long as that from a dose of morphine, and fentanyl probably is not the best medication if prolonged use of intermittent boluses is anticipated. However, fentanyl can be given as an intravenous infusion to maintain pain relief. A starting dose of 1 to 2 μg/kg/h is adequate, but can be titrated as necessary.[30] Epidural administration of fentanyl is another useful option. A single injection of 1 to 2 μg/kg in the lumbar epidural space will give excellent relief from pain that originates in the abdomen or lower extremities. Long-term relief can be achieved with 10 μg/mL of fentanyl infusing at a rate of 1 to 2 μg/kg/h.[39,40] As with epidural administration of morphine, the patient's respiratory rate must be monitored throughout the duration of infusion, although the delayed respiratory depression seen with morphine has not been demonstrated with fentanyl. Intrathecal fentanyl can also be used for pain from the abdomen and lower extremities. A dose of 0.1 to 0.2 μg/kg is adequate. The risk for respiratory depression lasts approximately 4 hours—approximately as long as the pain relief from a single dose.[39,40]

Meperidine

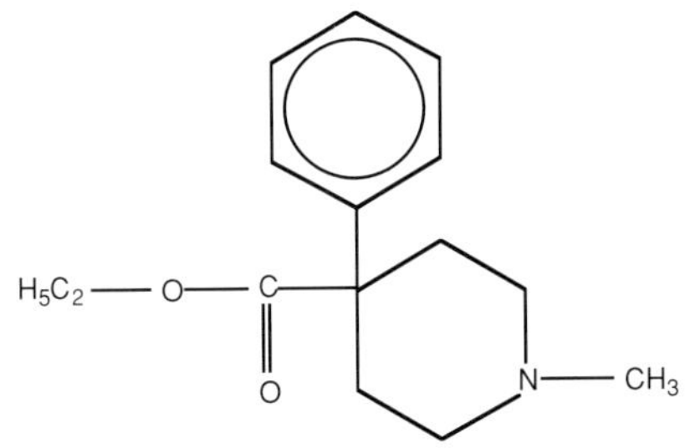

Although it is structurally different from morphine, meperidine has many of the same properties. Meperidine is approximately one tenth the strength of morphine when given as an intravenous or intramuscular injection, but is much better absorbed by the gastrointestinal system. Analgesic effects are noted approximately 15 minutes after an oral dose and 10 minutes after an intramuscular injection. The peak effect is usually seen within 2 hours after oral administration and 1 hour after an intramuscular injection. The effective length of analgesia is 2 to 4 hours. Meperidine is metabolized in the liver to normeperidine. The accumulation of the normeperidine is associated with increased CNS excitation. In large or frequently repeated doses, meperidine has caused seizures in humans. Normeperidine is excreted renally and will accumulate in patients with renal failure.[30]

Side Effects. Meperidine's side effects, like fentanyl's, are similar to morphine's, but with some differences. Large doses exert a myocardial depressant effect that will decrease myocardial contractility and stroke volume. This will lead to increased left ventricular filling pressures.[41] The incidence of nausea and vomiting associated with meperidine is equivalent to that of morphine, but patients who experience nausea and vomiting with morphine might not with meperidine.

Dosage and Administration. As mentioned above, meperidine is approximately one tenth as potent as morphine when given by intravenous or intramuscular injection. Thus, for acute post-operative pain relief, a starting dose of 0.25 to 0.5 mg/kg should be adequate. Also, owing to meperidine's better absorption, it is a good choice as an oral adjunct. The possibility for seizures exists with prolonged or high-dosage oral use of meperidine.[30]

Opioid Agonist–Antagonists

Butorphanol

Butorphanol exerts its analgesic effect by being an agonist of both the kappa and sigma receptors. It is an antagonist of the mu receptors. A dose of 2 to 3 mg is equipotent to 10 mg of morphine. The onset, peak effect, and duration of action of butorphanol are similar to those of morphine. Therapeutic dosages produce increased pulmonary artery pressure, cardiac output, and systemic blood pressure.[34]

Side Effects. In the low-dose, therapeutic range, the respiratory side effects of butorphanol are similar to those of morphine. The cardiovascular effects are the same as those described for meperidine. The drug will cause sedation, nausea, and diaphoresis in most people, and dysphoria in a small number of patients. Butorphanol will also antagonize mu agonists, thus making the choice of the proper dose of agonists difficult in the patient who is receiving butorphanol and will be returning to the operating room.

Dosage and Administration. Butorphanol is not available for enteral use. The suggested intravenous dose is 7 to 15 µg/kg, and the suggested intramuscular dose is 15 to 30 µg/kg. Butorphanol should be readministered every 3 to 4 hours.[34]

Nalbuphine

Nalbuphine is an agonist at the kappa and sigma receptors and an antagonist at the mu receptors. A dose of 10 mg of nalbuphine is equipotent to 10 mg of morphine. Unlike butorphanol, nalbuphine does not increase cardiac output or blood pressure. One advantage of this drug is its *ceiling effect* on respiratory depression[42]: the dose-related decrease in respiratory drive will not worsen with doses greater than 30 mg. Also, because nalbuphine is a mu antagonist, the drug can be used to reverse the respiratory depression of morphine or fentanyl without decreasing analgesia. The onset, peak effect, and duration of action are similar to those of morphine.

For postoperative pain relief, nalbuphine should be titrated for effect. For intravenous or intramuscular injections, 0.05 to 0.1 mg/kg should provide adequate analgesia. Whether administered via the intravenous or intramuscular route, nalbuphine should be given every 3 to 6 hours for pain control.[30]

Mixed Agonists

Dezocine

Dezocine is a new, mixed agonist with activity at the mu, kappa, and delta receptors. Its affinity for the mu receptors is 10-fold greater than for the delta receptors, and 40-fold greater than for the kappa receptors. This drug's advantage over other opioids is its ceiling effect on respiratory depression. Additionally, it is not a *scheduled* drug (ie, a federal narcotics license is not required). Its physical dependence has not been described. The hemodynamic effects are equivalent to those of morphine. The onset, peak effect, and duration of action are also similar to those of morphine.[43] Minimal side effects have been found in the clinical studies so far reported, but the number of patients reported is small.

The recommended dose for dezocine is 70 to 150 µg/kg intravenously and 70 to 200 µg/kg intramuscularly. It is suggested that dezocine be readministered every 3 to 4 hours.[43]

Naloxone

Naloxone is a competitive inhibitor of the mu, delta, kappa, and sigma receptors. After an intravenous injection, the onset of action is 1 to 2 minutes. The duration of action is 1 to 4 hours but is dose dependent. Naloxone can reverse the effects of *all* opioid agonists. It can also cause increased heart rate and systolic blood pressure. Acute pulmonary edema has been associated with narcotic reversal with naloxone, although this is a relatively rare complication. The case reports of pulmonary edema following naloxone administration have been in young healthy patients, and the reported doses have been as low as 80 µg.[44,45]

The recommended dose is 0.5 to 1 µg/kg, with doses being repeated until the desired effect is achieved. If the opioid being reversed has a longer half-life than naloxone, then it is important to start a naloxone infusion. The recommended rate of infusion is 5 to 10 µg/kg/h, but this rate can be titrated for effect.[46,47]

Adjunct Medications

Promethazine is an H_1 receptor antagonist that has been used in conjunction with narcotics to reduce the narcotic-associated nausea. The recommended dose to control nausea in patients is 12.5 to 25 mg every 4 to 6 hours. The dose is given as an intramuscular injection.

Droperidol is a powerful antiemetic owing to its inhibition of the dopaminergic receptors in the chemoreceptor trigger zone of the medulla. A dose of 0.625 to 1.25 mg given to a 70-kg adult is considered adequate to prevent nausea. Side effects of the drug include drowsiness and, in a small number of patients, extrapyramidal reactions. Droperidol may also cause increased sedation in the patient emerging from anesthesia.

CLINICAL PHARMACOLOGY OF NONSTEROIDAL ANTIINFLAMMATORY DRUGS

Nonsteroidal antiinflammatory drugs (NSAIDs) act by interrupting the inflammatory response.[48] This interruption is thought to be due to their inhibition of prostaglandin biosynthesis. Aspirin (acetylsalicylic acid) is the prototype of the nonopioid analgesic, antipyretic, and antiinflammatory drugs.[49]

NSAIDs are most often used

TABLE 13-4

SPECIFIC NONSTEROIDAL ANTIINFLAMMATORY AGENTS BY CLASS

Generic Name	Trade Name	Common Adult Dose for Pain
Salicylates		
Aspirin		325–650 mg/4 h PO
Choline/magnesium trisalicylate	Trilisate	1,000 mg, PO bid
Diflunisal	Dolobid	500 mg PO q 12 h
Salsalate	Disalcid	3,000 mg/d total dose divided as tid or bid
Propionic Acid Derivatives		
Fenoprofen	Nalfon)	200 mg qid or tid
Flurbiprofen	Ansaid	200–300 mg total daily dose divided bid, tid, or qid
Ibuprofen	Advil, Medipren, Midol, Nuprin, Motrin	300–800 mg tid to qid PO
Ketoprofen	Orudis	25–50 mg tid to qid PO
Naproxen	Naprosyn	250 mg tid to qid PO
Naproxen sodium	Anaprox	275 mg tid to qid
Indoles/Pyrroles		
Indomethacin	Indocin	25–50 mg bid to tid
Sulindac	Clinoril	150 mg bid
Tolmetin	Tolectin	400 mg tid
Ketorolac	Toradol	30–60 mg IM loading dose, then 15–30 mg IM qid
Oxicams		
Piroxicam	Feldene	20 mg qid
Anthranilic Acid Derivatives		
Meclofenamate sodium	Meclomen	50 mg tid to qid
Mefenamic acid	Ponstel	250 mg qid
Phenylacetic Acid Derivatives		
Diclofenac sodium	Voltaren	50 mg tid or qid or 75 mg bid
Pyrazolone Derivatives		
Phenylbutazone	Butazolidin	100 mg qid

IM: intramuscularly; PO: by mouth; bid: twice daily; tid: three times daily; qid: four times daily
Data sources: (1) *Physicians' Desk Reference*. 48th ed. Montvale, NJ: Medical Economics Data; 1994. (2) DiGregorio G. *Handbook of Pain Management*. 3rd ed. West Chester, Pa: Medical Surveillance Inc; 1991.

- as analgesics, to provide symptomatic relief of low-intensity pain associated with headache and musculoskeletal disorders (eg, osteoarthritis and rheumatoid arthritis),
- as antipyretics,
- to inhibit platelet aggregation in patients vulnerable to vascular obstruction from emboli,
- to inhibit synthesis of prostaglandins in neonates to evoke closure of the ductus arteriosus, and
- to treat excessive production of prostaglandins (eg, in Bartter's syndrome).[49]

Important information regarding generic names, trade names, and adult dosages of selected NSAIDs is summarized in Table 13-4; pharmacokinetic data are presented in Table 13-5.

TABLE 13-5

PHARMACOKINETIC DATA OF SELECTED NONSTEROIDAL ANTIINFLAMMATORY DRUGS

Name	Time to Peak Plasma Concentration (h)	Elimination Half-life (h)	Duration of Action (h)	Effective Plasma Concentration (μg/mL)
Aspirin	0.5–1	0.25–0.35	4–6	20
Choline/magnesium	1–2	9–17	12	150–300
Ibuprofen	1–2	2	4–6	—*
Indomethacin	2	2–3	4–6	0.3–1.0
Ketorolac	0.5	4–6	4–6	—
Sulindac	2	7–18	8–12	—
Piroxicam	3–5	30–80	48–72	1.5–2
Meclofenamate sodium	0.5–1	2	2	—
Diclofenac sodium	1–4	2	2	1–2
Phenylbutazone	1–3	60–100	80	50–150
Naproxen	1–2	10–17	8–12	25–75

*[—] Indicates data not available

Adapted with permission from Digregorio GJ, Barbieri EJ, Sterling GH, Camp JF, Prout MF. *Handbook of Pain Management.* 3rd ed. West Chester, Pa: Medical Surveillance Inc; 1991: 129.

Mechanisms of Action

The primary actions of NSAIDs—producing analgesia, acting as an antipyretic, and exerting an antiinflammatory effect—result from different mechanisms. These actions and mechanisms are discussed below.

Analgesia

NSAIDs produce analgesia by inhibiting the activity of cyclooxygenase (prostaglandin synthetase), an enzyme that leads to a decrease in the synthesis and release of prostaglandins from cells. Individual classes of NSAIDs have different methods of inhibiting the cyclooxygenase enzyme.[49] Prostaglandins enhance the potency of algesic substances such as bradykinin or substance P, which may stimulate nerve endings of unmyelinated C fibers and small-diameter A-delta fibers to elicit noxious afferent input. Bradykinin stimulates formation and release of more prostaglandins.[50] NSAIDs appear to reduce this potentiation of algesic activity of prostaglandins by blocking their synthesis.

In contrast to that produced by opioids, which act centrally, the analgesia produced by aspirinlike drugs is a peripheral phenomenon. Pain is produced when prostaglandins are produced locally around sensitive nerve endings, as seen with inflammation. NSAIDs are effective in relieving this pain by blocking prostaglandin synthesis. NSAIDs are not effective as analgesics when inflammation is not present (ie, there is no increase in prostaglandin synthesis in the area) or for the sharp, stabbing pain that is caused by direct stimulation of sensory nerves (ie, visceral pain).[49]

Antipyresis

NSAIDs exert an antipyretic action via a CNS mechanism. Fever is thought to occur because endogenous pyrogens cause a shift in the temperature-regulating system in the preoptic hypothalamus. NSAIDs are postulated to reduce the effect of endogenous pyrogens on the hypothalamus. In therapeutic doses, NSAIDs do not affect either normal body temperature or an increase in temperature associated with exercise, drugs, or hypothalamic lesions to which pyrogen does not contribute. Salicylates, acetaminophen, and ibuprofen are the only drugs approved in the United States as antipyretics, although indomethacin and naproxen have been recommended as drugs to lower fever of neoplastic disease that is uncontrolled by other antipyretics.[50]

Antiinflammatory Effect

Since prostaglandins induce symptoms of inflammation and enhance the effects of bradykinin and histamine, a reduction of prostaglandins at sites of inflammation is thought to decrease the inflammatory response. In arthritic diseases, NSAIDs reduce inflammation and swelling, thereby providing relief.[50]

Side Effects

Gastrointestinal System

All NSAIDs can cause gastrointestinal pathology, including gastritis, nausea, vomiting, diarrhea, constipation, and occult blood in the stool.[48,49] Gastrointestinal problems are more common with aspirin, indomethacin, and mefenamic acid[49] although nonacetylated salicylates may be less irritating.[50] Alcohol ingestion increases the likelihood that gastrointestinal side effects will occur.[49] The United States Pharmacopeia recommends that all NSAIDs be taken with a full glass of water.[49] NSAID-associated gastropathy has been proposed as the most frequent, serious, adverse drug effect in the United States; the risk of gastrointestinal problems is greater in elderly and debilitated patients.[50]

Aspirin should be avoided by patients with a history of ulcers and should not be used with agents that promote ulcer formation (eg, alcohol). The mechanisms of gastrointestinal bleeding and NSAID-induced ulceration are due in part to irritation from direct contact with mucosal cells and cyclooxygenase inhibition after absorption, which weakens the gastric-acid barrier. Chronic inhibition of prostaglandin synthesis appears to decrease mucosal cytoprotection. It is likely that aspirin-induced bleeding is aggravated by its effect on platelet aggregation.[50]

Renal System

Renal prostaglandins are important to ensure adequate renal perfusion and function in certain disease states, including congestive heart failure, cirrhosis with ascites, nephrotic syndrome, and dehydration. In these patient groups, NSAIDs may precipitate acute renal failure. Long-term use of high-dose NSAIDs may cause renal medullary ischemia and papillary necrosis. This was more common when phenacetin was used, especially in combination with aspirin, caffeine, and acetaminophen. Phenacetin has been replaced with acetaminophen, which may also be a risk factor for papillary necrosis. Renal prostaglandins inhibit tubular reabsorption of Na^+ and water, and inhibit renin secretion. In patients with poor renal perfusion states, NSAIDs may cause fluid retention, impaired responsiveness to diuretic therapy, and hyperkalemia.[50]

Respiratory System

Inhibition of bronchodilator prostaglandins by NSAIDs may leave the leukotriene pathway uncontested and lead to bronchospasm.[49] This may be a consideration in susceptible patients such as asthmatics. Full therapeutic doses of salicylates increase oxygen consumption and carbon dioxide production in skeletal muscle. Higher doses result in medullary stimulation, causing hyperventilation with a respiratory alkalosis. This is compensated for by excretion of bicarbonate by the kidneys, which leads to a compensated respiratory alkalosis. Toxic doses of salicylate depress the medulla, leading to an uncompensated respiratory acidosis in a patient with high renal bicarbonate excretion, which, in turn, leads to a coexisting metabolic acidosis.[48]

Hematological Effects

NSAIDs inhibit both thromboxane A_2 synthesis within platelets and prostacyclin synthesis within endothelial cells. Thromboxane A_2, a potent vasoconstrictor, stimulates platelet aggregation, which promotes clotting. Prostacyclin, a potent vasodilator, inhibits platelet aggregation, which promotes bleeding. NSAIDs inhibit the synthesis of both thromboxane A_2 and prostaglandin I_2. The net balance determines the tendency towards bleeding or clotting.[51]

Aspirin irreversibly inhibits platelet cyclooxygenase which prevents the formation of thromboxane A_2, thereby inhibiting platelet aggregation. The bleeding time is prolonged for the lifetime of the platelet. All other NSAIDs reversibly inhibit platelet cyclooxygenase, so that five half-lives are required to clear all the drug from the body and restore normal platelet function.[51]

Reye's Syndrome

Reye's syndrome, a childhood illness that develops after recovery from influenza or chickenpox, is characterized by vomiting, liver abnormalities, and encephalopathy. Nearly all victims of Reye's syndrome had received salicylates for management of the viral illness. If an analgesic antipyretic is required for use in children with acute viral illness, acetaminophen should be used, as there is no evidence of an association between acetaminophen and Reye's syndrome.[50]

CLINICAL PHARMACOLOGY OF LOCAL ANESTHETICS

Since prehistoric times, the natives of Peru have chewed the leaves of the indigenous plant *Erythroxylon coca*, the source of cocaine, to obtain a feeling of well-being and to reduce fatigue.[9,52] Chewing of the coca leaves caused a reversible perioral numbness, and subsequent investigation of the coca leaf allowed the identification of cocaine, the active ingredient. Cocaine was used as a topical ocular anesthesia and for nerve blocks during the latter 18th century.[49] Addictive properties and toxicity limited the use of cocaine for local anesthesia, but this finding stimulated research for more ideal local anesthetic agents. Einhorn introduced the esters procaine in 1905 and tetracaine in 1932, and Lofgren introduced lidocaine, an amide, in 1932.[9]

Local anesthetics are important adjuncts to the management of postoperative pain; they significantly reduce the amount of narcotics necessary to maintain a pain-free state in the postoperative patient.[7] A simple system governs the naming of local anesthetic drugs: those spelled with one *i* in the name are esters (eg, procaine, 2-chloroprocaine, tetracaine); those with two are amides (eg, lidocaine, mepivacaine, bupivacaine). Among the amides, stereoisomers of etidocaine, mepivacaine, bupivacaine, prilocaine, and ropivacaine have been recognized. Although the S forms of these molecules are generally less toxic and have a longer duration of action,[53] the chiral forms of local anesthetics are not discussed in this chapter.

Very dilute solutions of a local anesthetic combined with an opiate produce anesthesia comparable to that produced by more-concentrated solutions of plain local anesthetics. Use of dilute solution of local anesthetic causes less motor blockade, which facilitates postoperative ambulation. The interaction of opiates and local anesthetics is postulated to be due to a synergistic action of the drugs (administered epidurally) acting in two or more different sites to decrease sensory input. The local anesthetics act at the dorsal root ganglion while the opiates act on the dorsal horn of the spinal cord.[53]

Chemical and Physical Properties

The potency, onset of action, and duration of local anesthetic action are directly related to the physical properties of lipid solubility, pKa (ie, ionization), and protein binding (Figure 13-3).[53] Local anesthetics consist of a lipophilic, unsaturated, benzene-ring aromatic group; and a hydrophilic, tertiary amine separated by a hydrocarbon connecting chain (Figure 13-4). Clinically useful local anesthetic agents fall into two chemically distinct groups, based on the linkage between the aromatic portion and the intermediate chain.[52] This linkage can be via an ester (–CO–) or an amide (–HNC–) bond. The ester and amide compounds differ in their chemical stability, metabolic cycles, and allergic potentials.

In general, the greater the length of the connecting group and the more complicated the aromatic and amine structures, the greater the potency and the toxicity of the local anesthetic.[48] The addition of more complicated side chains to local anesthetics causes an increase in their tissue-protein binding ability and also makes the drug more fat soluble, thereby increasing the duration of action.[49]

Lipid Solubility

The aromatic group (ie, the benzene ring) that is present at one end of the molecule is the major determinant of the lipid solubility of local anesthetic drugs. The more-lipid-soluble drugs are the more-potent local anesthetics, probably because the lipid-soluble uncharged base form can pass through the lipid-containing nerve membrane to reach its site of action.[53]

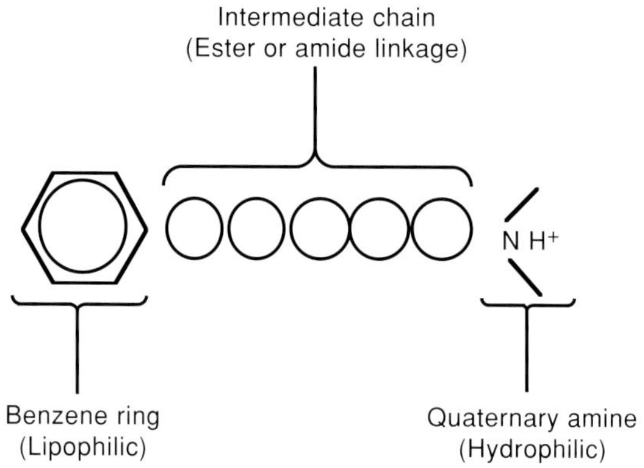

Fig. 13-3. The general structure of a local anesthetic molecule.

Amino Esters

Cocaine

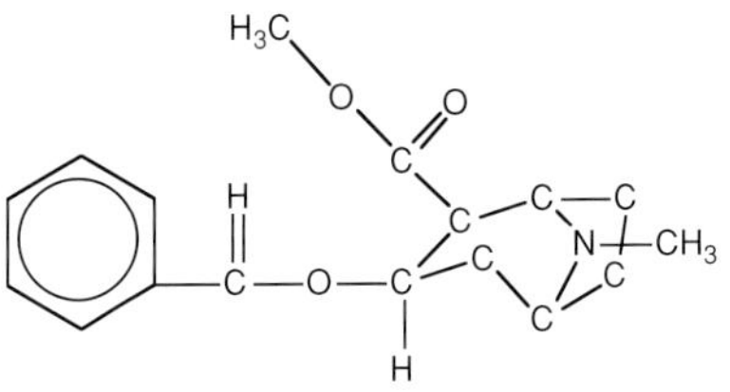

Procaine

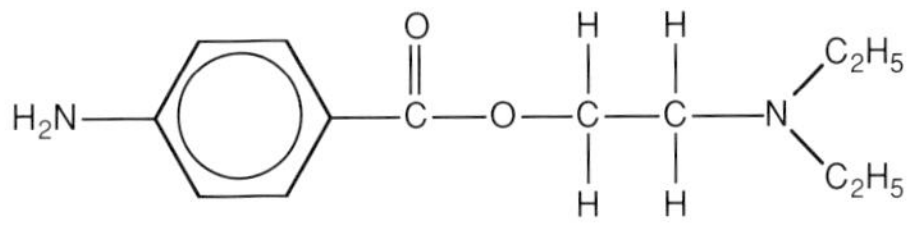

2-Chloroprocaine

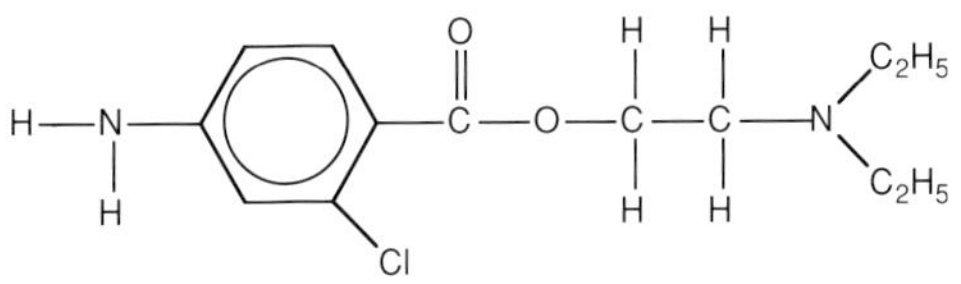

Tetracaine

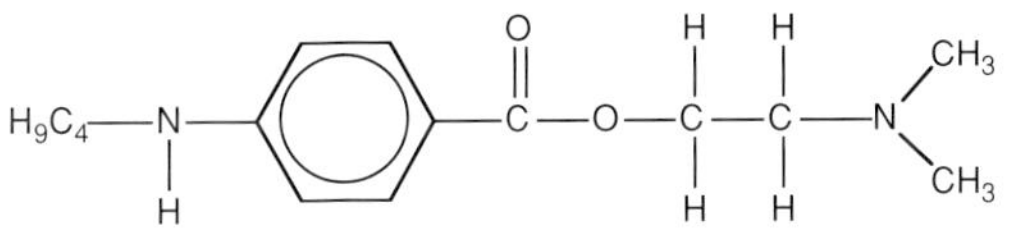

Amino Amides

Lidocaine

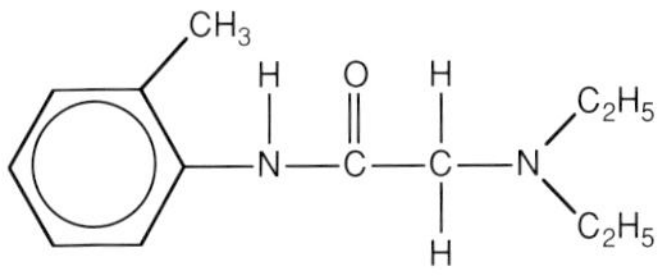

Prilocaine

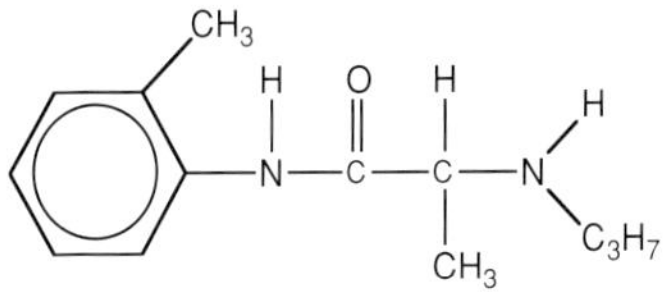

Etidocaine

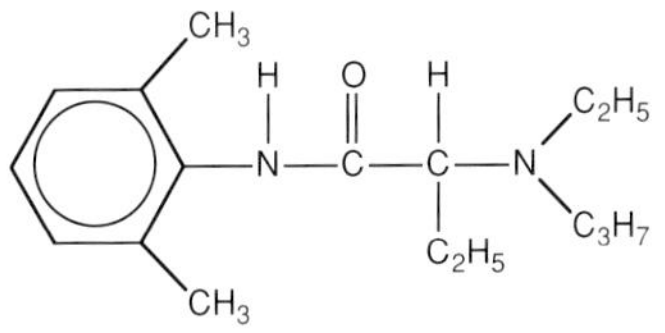

Mepivacaine

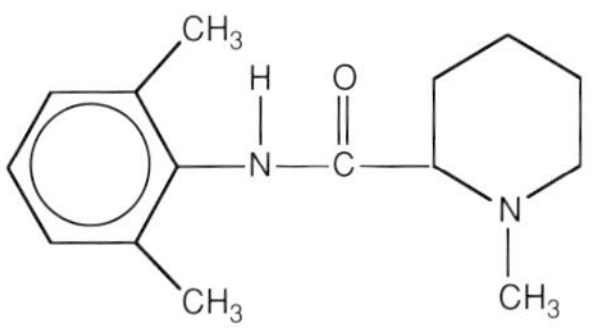

Bupivacaine

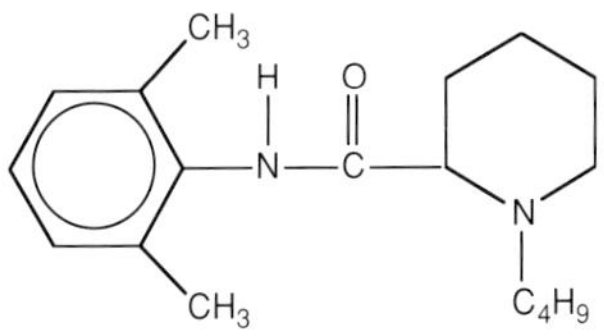

Ropivacaine

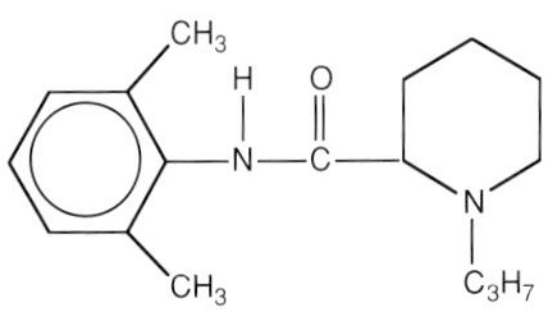

Fig. 13-4. Chemical structures of commonly used local anesthetics.

Ionization

Local anesthetic molecules contain an amino group, which determines the hydrophilic activity and ionization of the molecule. The amino group is capable of accepting a hydrogen ion, which converts the nonionized base form of the drug into the cationic (ie, charged) form. The proportion of each form (nonionized base and cation) present is determined by the pKa of the drug and the pH of the solution (pKa is defined as the pH at which 50% of the drug is ionized and 50% is present as the free base). The nonionized (free base) form penetrates the nerve membrane and the ionized (cationic) form produces blockade of the sodium channel. With many local anesthetics, the speed of onset can be related to the degree of difference between the pKa of the drug and the pH of the normal human body.[53]

As a general rule, the lower the pKa of the local anesthetic, the shorter the onset time for induction of anesthesia. The closer the pH of the injected solution of local anesthetic is to body pH, the shorter the onset time. Commercial preparations of local anesthetics are made more acidic to enhance stability, which favors the formation of the cationic form (Figure 13-5).[53]

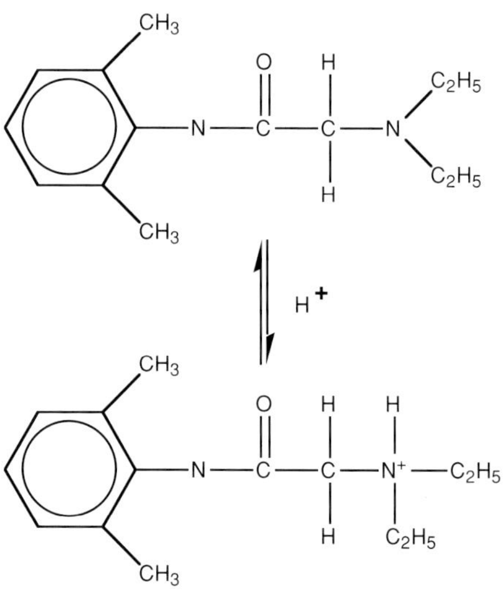

Fig. 13-5. Equilibrium between the base and the cationic forms of a local anesthetic.

Protein Binding

Anesthetics are not pharmacologically active while in their protein-bound form. In the plasma, local anesthetics bind to albumin (a low-affinity, high-capacity binding) and to α_1-acid glycoprotein (a high-affinity, low-capacity binding). The binding of local anesthetics to proteins is concentration-dependent and decreases in a curvilinear manner as the local anesthetic concentration in plasma increases. So the potential for toxicity increases disproportionally with increases in plasma concentration.[53]

Protein binding of local anesthetics is influenced by the pH of the plasma. The percentage of bound drug decreases as the pH decreases. Therefore, acidosis potentiates the toxicity of local anesthetics by increasing the fraction of the active form of the drug—both in the circulation and at the active site.[53] Protein binding of local anesthetics, which is decreased in newborns and pregnant women, causes an increase in the free fraction of local anesthetic.[53] α_1-Acid glycoprotein is decreased in elderly individuals, pregnant women, and newborns. Premature infants have approximately one half the α_1-acid glycoprotein that is present in newborns.[53] The fraction of drug that is bound to protein in plasma correlates with the duration of activity of the local anesthetic. Bupivacaine and etidocaine are 95% protein bound. These drugs last longer than lidocaine, which is 65% protein bound. Recently, researchers have speculated that there may be a similarity between the binding of the local anesthetic molecule to plasma protein and the binding to the receptor protein in the sodium channel.[54]

Mode of Action

The local anesthetics in clinical use today are sodium channel–blocking agents. They exert their effect by inhibiting the influx of Na^+ across the neuronal cell membrane. This produces a conduction blockade of nerve impulses by preventing increases in permeability of nerve membranes to Na^+ If the permeability to Na^+ fails to increase, the rate of depolarization will slow such that the threshold potential is not reached and an action potential is not propagated. The ionic gradients and the resting-membrane potential of the nerve are unchanged, but the increase in Na^+ permeability that is associated with the nerve impulse is inhibited. Local anesthetics do not alter the resting transmembrane potential or the threshold potential.[52]

The theories of the mechanism of action include (*a*) the displacement of Ca^{++} from a membrane site that controls Na^+ permeability, (*b*) the Meyer-Overton rule of anesthesia, (*c*) a change in surface charge, and (*d*) the specific-receptor theory.

Displacement of Calcium

A low calcium concentration outside the neuron enhances local anesthetic activity, while an increasing external calcium concentration antagonizes local anesthetic activity. However, the direct actions of calcium and local anesthetic appear to be independent of each other.[9]

Meyer-Overton Rule

The Meyer-Overton rule of anesthesia postulates that diffusion of the relatively lipophilic anesthetic molecules into the lipid component of the neuronal membrane expands the membrane to a critical volume and interferes with sodium conductance. Local anesthetics have been shown to increase the volume of lipid membranes and increase their degree of disorder. High-pressure antagonism of the anesthetic activity of certain uncharged local-anesthetic molecules such as benzyl alcohol and benzocaine has been seen. Pressure reversal has not been shown to occur in the case of charged local anesthetics. These findings indicate charged and uncharged local anesthetics may have separate sites of action.[9,55]

Change in Surface Charge

A third proposal for the mechanism of action of local anesthetics involves the induction of alterations in the membrane surface charge. The cationic molecule neutralizes, to a variable degree, the fixed negative charges on the inside membrane surface, altering the transmembrane potential. If the molecule of local anesthetic is absorbed into the extracellular side of the axonal membrane, the extra positive charges add to the already relatively positive extracellular charge and hyperpolarize the membrane. This hyperpolarization makes it harder for a nerve impulse to raise the transmembrane potential to the depolarization threshold. If the local anesthetic is absorbed into the intracellular side of the axonal membrane, the increase in positive charge could prevent sufficient repolarization of the membrane interior to allow reactivation of the sodium channels that were inactivated by a previous action potential. The surface-charge theory could account for the antagonism between divalent cations such as calcium and local anesthetics.[9]

Specific-Receptor Theory

The specific-receptor theory postulates that local anesthetics interact directly with specific receptors in the neuronal membrane. This interaction affects specific ion channels of the neuronal membrane in such a fashion that the ionic flux needed for initiation and propagation of the action potential is inhibited. The structure of the sodium channel is that of a lipoglycoprotein that spans the neuronal membrane and contains an aqueous pore that is able to discriminate between sodium and other ions, being selectively more permeable to sodium.[9] Intrinsic electrical properties of the macromolecules that compose the channel allow it to change configuration in response to changes in the membrane potential, thus determining the conductance of sodium ions across the axolemma.

The sodium channel can exist in three states: closed (ie, resting), open, and inactivated.[10] When a nerve impulse occurs and the sodium channel goes through the open to the inactivated state, it carries another impulse until it repolarizes and returns to the resting state. Immediately following an action potential, many of the sodium channels are in the inactivated state and cannot be reopened by a subsequent voltage change. So once an excitable membrane has been depolarized by an action potential, it cannot conduct a second impulse until it has first repolarized and allowed inactivated sodium channels to return to their resting state. If an adequate number of sodium channels are not present in the resting state, sodium current sufficient for a second action potential cannot be generated.[9,10]

Frequency-Dependent Blockade

The property of frequency-dependent blockade (ie, use-dependent blockade), in which neuronal blockade by charged local anesthetic molecules increases with repetitive, brief, membrane depolarizations, is one phenomenon that suggests direct interaction between sodium channel receptors and the charged local anesthetic molecules. It is postulated that frequency-dependent blockade develops because charged, hydrophobic, anesthetic molecules inhibit Na^+ conductance through the sodium channel by gaining access to a channel receptor located within the channel itself, while the pore of the sodium channel is open. For this reason, selective conduction blockade of nerve fibers by local anesthetics may be related to the nerve's characteristic frequencies of activity (ie, selective conduction blockade occurs more readily in a rapidly firing nerve).[9,10] Reversal of the inhibitory effect of the local anesthetic also requires an open channel pore to facilitate the dissociation of the molecule of local anesthetic. Consequently, a closed channel containing a local anesthetic molecule would be slow to return to its uninhibited state.[9,10]

In contrast to charged anesthetics, neutral anesthetics exhibit much less frequency-dependent blockade; this may be because they are not restricted to the aqueous phase and can gain access through the lipid milieu of the membrane interior. Local anesthetics may also shift the sodium channel population to a nonconducting state by binding channels that have already been inactivated, preventing their return to the resting depolarization-susceptible configuration. A weak tonic (ie, resting) block may be induced by binding with channels in the resting (closed) state to prevent their voltage-induced activation.

The discovery that the blocking potency of local anesthetic molecules is much greater when the interaction is with receptors of open and inactivated channels, as compared to those of closed channels, has led to the modulated-receptor hypothesis of local anesthetic receptor binding. According to the modulated-receptor hypothesis, local anesthetics have a higher affinity for open and inactivated sodium channels than for closed channels. During stimulation, channels that are open and inactivated bind local anesthetics more tightly. This binding stabilizes the channels in a nonconducting state, and increasingly so with each stimulating pulse.[9] The variable state of the local anesthetic receptor determines the strength of its interaction with the local anesthetic molecule. An excitable membrane with a higher depolarization frequency will be more sensitive to the blocking effects of local anesthetics. This theory offers an explanation for frequency-dependent blockade.

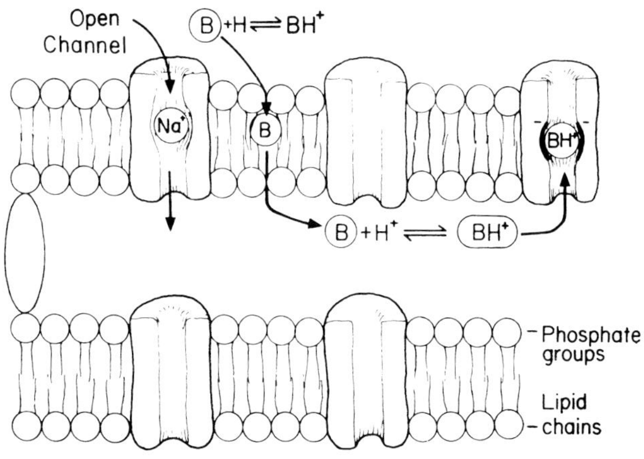

Fig. 13-6. A molecule of local anesthetic moves through a lipid bilayer and enters the sodium channel. On the drawing, B represents the base form of a local anesthetic and BH^+ represents the cationic form. Reprinted with permission from DiFazio CA, Woods AM. Drugs commonly used for nerve blocking. Pharmacology of local anesthetics. In: Raj PP, ed. *Practical Management of Pain.* St. Louis, Mo: Mosby–Year Book; 1992: 690.

Receptor Sites in the Sodium Channel

It is uncertain as to exactly where in the sodium channel the local-anesthetic receptors are located. Three sites of binding are postulated[9,10]:

1. near the interior opening; this area has an affinity for charged local anesthetic molecules;
2. at the interface between the channel and membrane lipid; this area has an affinity for uncharged molecules; and
3. at the outer aspect of the sodium channel; this area is the site of actions of toxins such as tetrodotoxin.

Figure 13-6 shows the nonionized base form of the local anesthetic molecule diffusing through the neural lipid bilayer. Inside the nerve, the equilibrium is established between the free base and cationic forms of the local anesthetic. The ionized cationic form enters the sodium channel from the intracellular side of the nerve membrane, binding to an anionic site, which blocks the sodium channel.[53]

Actions of Local Anesthetics on Nerve Fibers

Actions of local anesthetics on nerve fibers generally depend on the diameter of the fiber and the length of the fiber exposed to the agent. These two related characteristics are discussed below.

Minimum Length of Exposed Nerve

A minimum length of myelinated nerve fiber must be exposed to an adequate concentration of local anesthetic for nerve block to occur. Conduction blockade is predictably present if at least three successive nodes of Ranvier are exposed to adequate concentration of local anesthetic.[49] Both types of pain-conducting fibers (ie, myelinated type A-delta and nonmyelinated type C fibers) are blocked by similar concentrations of local anesthetics despite their differences in diameter. Preganglionic type B fibers are more readily blocked by local anesthetics than any other fiber, even though these fibers are larger in diameter than type C fibers (type B fibers are myelinated; type C are not).

Differential Blockade

It has long been a clinical observation that all neuronal functions are not affected equally by local anesthetics. Blockade of the components of a peripheral nerve may proceed at different rates, with loss of sympathetic function first, followed by pinprick sensation, touch and temperature, and, lastly, motor function. Or there may be relative sparing of one neuronal function over another (eg, low-dose bupivacaine labor epidural, with its relatively intact motor tone). There are several potential explanations for differential blockade:

1. The fiber's diameter is inversely proportional to the fiber's susceptibility to local anesthetic blockade.
2. Internodal distance is proportional to the axon diameter, so the equivalent spread of local anesthetic may produce conduction blockade of a thin axon but not of the adjacent thick axon (Figure 13-7).
3. C fibers may be blocked faster, owing to the relatively unimpeded local anesthetic access to the axon.
4. The slower local anesthetic block of A fibers depends on the pKa and the lipid partition coefficient of the local anesthetic molecule.

The lower the pKa (the greater the percentage of lipophilic uncharged molecules at physiological pH) and the greater the lipid partition coefficient of the local anesthetic molecule, the more rapid the onset of block in A fibers. In high concentrations, even a relatively hydrophilic local anesthetic can produce a rapid block of A fibers because of the greater diffusion gradient, causing a rapid transit across the myelin sheath. Thus, the use of a less–lipid-soluble local anesthetic would most likely result in differential block of A-delta and C fibers at the onset of the nerve block. The differential block seen with bupivacaine is believed to be due to the relatively high pKa of this agent, such that fewer uncharged molecules are available to penetrate the diffusion barriers surrounding large A fibers. Differential blockade may be the manifestation of a frequency-dependent process with more–rapid-firing axons being sensory and slower-firing axons being somatic motor efferents.

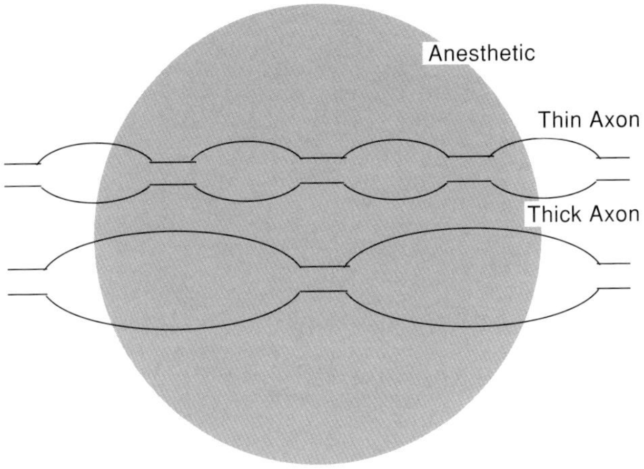

Fig. 13-7. Differential blockade of myelinated nerve fibers of different diameters. Internodal distance is proportional to axon diameter. Conduction blockade occurs when at least three adjacent nodes of Ranvier are blocked. This drawing shows the blockade of a thin myelinated axon occurring before a block will be established in a thicker myelinated fiber. Adapted with permission from Franz DN, Perry RS. Mechanisms for differential block among single myelinated and non-myelinated axons by procaine. *J Physiol.* 1974;236:207.

Differential block may also be a reflection of the geographical arrangement of the nerve fibers within the peripheral nerve, with the outermost fibers being blocked preferentially if the local anesthetic solution is dilute. The local anesthetic diffuses from the outer surface (ie, the mantle) toward the center (the core) along a concentration gradient. The mantle is blocked first. These are the more proximal structures. The core is the more distal structure. Skeletal muscle paralysis may precede the onset of sensory blockade if motor nerve fibers are distributed peripheral to sensory fibers in the mixed peripheral nerve (Figure 13-8).

Pharmacokinetics

Pharmacokinetics denotes the movement of a drug through the body: movement into the bloodstream, movement from blood into tissues, and movement out of the body by metabolism and excretion. When regional anesthesia is sought, the local anesthetic is injected in close proximity to the site of desired effect so that local, physical factors become more important than systemic pharmacokinetic factors for predicting the desired pharmacodynamic effects. The concentration of local anesthetic that develops in neural tissue is affected by the proximity of the injected anesthetic to the nerve, the flow of anesthetic around the nerve tissue, diffusion across

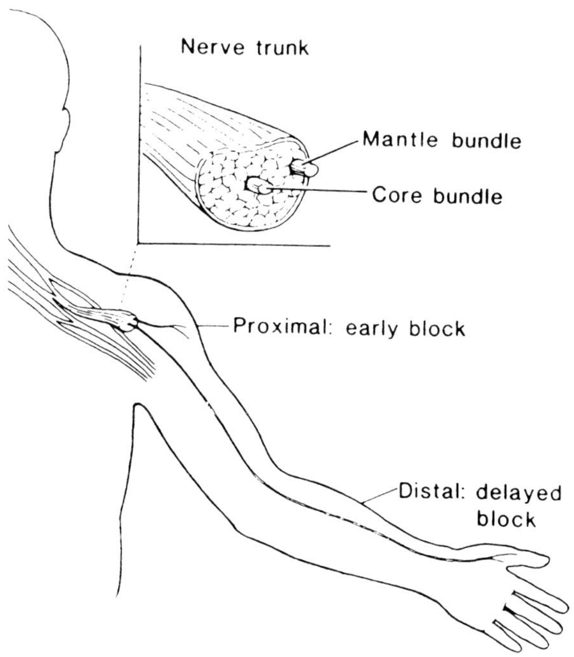

Fig. 13-8. Somatotropic arrangement of fibers in a neuron. Local anesthetics diffuse along a concentration gradient to block the mantle fibers before the core bundle. This is the explanation for anesthesia occurring in more proximal areas of the extremity first. Reprinted with permission from Stoelting R, Miller R. *Basics of Anesthesia*. 2nd ed. Philadelphia, Pa; JB Lippincott; 1989: 84.

the tissue barriers and into the nerve, binding to nonneural tissues, and absorption into the vascular and lymph system.

Both local carbon dioxide partial pressure and temperature are determinants of the pharmacokinetics of local anesthetics. Making local anesthetics from the carbonate salt rather than the hydrochloride salt and adding carbon dioxide to the solution yields a better-quality neural blockade. This approach both shortens the time of onset and improves the neural blockade. This effect may be due to (1) elevated carbon dioxide, which causes a direct neural blockade, and (2) increased carbon dioxide in the axoplasm, which causes an increase in ion trapping of the local anesthetic in the axoplasm by favoring the shift of nonionized free base form to the impermeable ionized form of local anesthetic.[53] Warming the local anesthetic solution increases the pKa of the local anesthetic so that at a constant pH, warming results in an increase in the fraction of free base available. Warming the local anesthetic solution causes a consistently faster onset of action.[53]

Bulk Flow

A large volume of local anesthetic solution will spread by bulk flow to a greater extent and produce a greater spread of nerve block. Concentration (or total mass of drug) also affects the spread, probably by influencing diffusion gradients. Separating the effects of volume, concentration, and mass is difficult. A minimum volume is probably necessary to provide adequate spread around the nerve. A minimum concentration is necessary to provide an adequate diffusion gradient to penetrate the nerve. Once these minimum values have been attained, the total mass of drug becomes important.

Diffusion and Binding

The rapidity and extent of diffusion depends to largest extent on the pKa of the local anesthetic, the concentration injected, and the lipid solubility. The ionized form of the drug diffuses poorly, whereas, the nonionized free base is freely diffusible. Alkalinization of the injected solution will increase the proportion of nonionized drug and should facilitate diffusion. Acidosis from local infection will retard diffusion of local anesthetic because of increased ionization. Local anesthetics with high lipid solubility can penetrate neural membranes more readily but they also have more nonspecific binding, which can impede diffusion to the specific site of action.

Systemic Absorption

The most important factors affecting peak blood level (C_{max}) are (*a*) the total dose of local anesthetic, which is almost a linear relationship, and (*b*) the site of injection (see Chapter 12, Regional Anesthesia, Figure 12-2), in the following relationship:

intercostal > caudal > epidural >
brachial plexus > sciatic or femoral

When a 1 mg/kg dose of local anesthetic is given as an epidural or caudal injection, a peak blood level of approximately 1 µg/mL results. When a 1 mg/kg dose of local anesthetic is given in a less-vascular area (eg, the brachial plexus) or as a subcutaneous infiltration, a peak blood level of approximately 0.5 µg/mL is seen. During an intercostal block, a peak blood level of 1.5 µg/mL occurs. Peak blood levels may be seen 10 to 30 minutes after injection.[53]

The peak blood levels that are seen after injection are affected by the rate of local anesthetic biotransformation and elimination. For amides, this effect is small. For example, 70% of the lidocaine presented to the liver undergoes hepatic extraction. This is limited by hepatic blood flow and the low concentration of local anesthetic in the plasma after a nerve block is performed.[53] Biotransformation is the primary determinant of the very low plasma levels that occur after a nerve block by an ester local anesthetic. Due to their metabolism by plasma cholinesterase, esters such as 2-chloroprocaine have a plasma half-life of approximately 45 seconds.[53]

Distribution, Metabolism, and Elimination

Once a local anesthetic is absorbed into the blood, it is distributed first to the lung, where local anesthetics have a high solubility. On reaching the systemic circulation, distribution is determined by tissue blood flow. The local anesthetics go first to vessel-rich groups and then are redistributed into tissues with lower relative perfusions.

The amide local anesthetics are extremely stable agents; esters are relatively unstable in solution. Amino esters are hydrolyzed in plasma by plasma cholinesterase. Patients with atypical plasma cholinesterase may be at increased risk for developing excessive plasma concentrations of ester local anesthetics. Amide compounds undergo hepatic microsomal metabolism. Hepatic disease or reductions in hepatic blood blow—such as those that occur with congestive heart failure or during general anesthesia—can reduce the rate of local clearance of amide local anesthetics.

If a patient develops seizures and becomes acidotic, the local anesthetic that has accumulated in the brain will be more ionized and unable to cross the lipid blood–brain barrier for redistribution. Acidosis also modifies the pharmacokinetics of local anesthetics in the fetus. When a fetus is depressed and more acidotic, the uncharged, absorbed local anesthetic that crosses the placenta will become ionized and be trapped in the fetus.[49]

Expedited Onset and Prolongation of Action

Expedited Onset. Onset of local anesthesia can be expedited by increasing the nonionized lipid-soluble form of local anesthetic. As discussed previously, this is the form of local anesthetic that can penetrate the nerve membrane. The fraction of the free base (nonionized) form and the cationic (ionized) form is determined by the pKa of the drug and the pH of the drug solution, and the pH of the tissue in which the drug is injected.[53] Adjustment of the pH by alkalinizing the injectate shifts the equilibrium towards the nonionized free-base form of the local anesthetic, so that more molecules are available to penetrate the nerve membrane. Increases in the amount of free base in solution are limited by the solubility of the free base in solution. After a saturated solution of free base is achieved, further alkalinization will result in precipitation of the drug.[53] Local anesthetics often fail to work in areas of local acidosis (eg, an abscess). In these areas, the equilibrium between charged and uncharged forms of the anesthetic is shifted in favor of the charged form as a result of the abundance of hydrogen ions. This decreases the amount of uncharged local anesthetic available to diffuse through the neural membrane to initiate anesthesia.[49]

Prolongation of Action with Epinephrine. The addition of epinephrine (1:200,000, 5 µg/mL) or phenylephrine (2 mg) to local anesthetic solutions that are to be injected produces local tissue vasoconstriction, which limits systemic absorption, and prolongs the duration of action by keeping the local anesthetic in contact with nerve fibers.[52]

In the presence of volatile anesthetics, systemic absorption of epinephrine may contribute to cardiac dysrhythmias, or accentuate hypertension in selected patients (eg, those with preeclampsia or thyrotoxicosis). Addition of epinephrine is not recommended[52] in patients with

- unstable angina pectoris,
- cardiac dysrhythmias,
- uncontrolled hypertension,
- uteroplacental insufficiency,
- peripheral nerve block in areas lacking collateral blood flow (eg, the digits, penis, nose), or
- those receiving intravenous regional anesthesia.

Commercially prepared local anesthetic solutions with epinephrine are pH-adjusted to a more acidic environment, which creates stability for the epinephrine (see Table 12-2 for appropriate doses of commonly used local anesthetics).[53] Alkalinization of these solutions improves onset time for anesthesia. If epinephrine is added to plain local anesthetic solution, the onset time is improved because the pH of the plain solution is higher (pH 6.5) than the pH of the commercially prepared, pH-adjusted, epinephrine-containing local anesthetic solution (pH 4.5).[53]

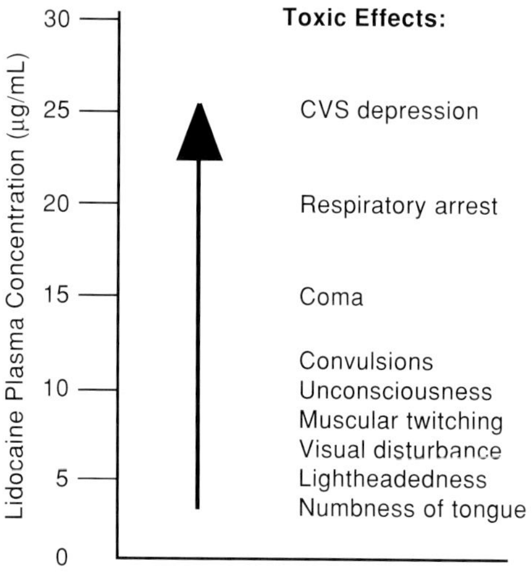

Fig. 13-9. Toxic effects of local anesthetics produced by increasing lidocaine plasma levels. CVS: cardiovascular system. Reprinted with permission from Carpenter RL, Mackey DC. Local anesthetics. In: Barash PG, Cullen BF, Stoelting RK, eds. *Clinical Anesthesia*. Philadelphia, Pa: JB Lippincott; 1989: 389.

Toxicity

Central nervous system (CNS) toxicity in the form of seizures occurs at a lower blood level than cardiac toxicity (Figure 13-9). Excessively high blood levels of local anesthetic can result from various mishaps, including the following:

- accidental intravascular injection of a large amount of local anesthetic,
- premature release of a tourniquet during a Bier block,
- administration of an improper dose for the site of administration (absorption into the bloodstream depends on the site of administration), and
- administration of a local anesthetic to a patient with an allergy to the drug.

Toxicity should be prevented by the means described in Exhibit 13-1. Table 13-6 compares safe doses (in mg/kg) of local anesthetics between various agents and areas of injection. Peripheral blocks are slowly absorbed, which allows administration of a higher dose, compared with an intercostal block, which is rapidly absorbed.

Blood levels of lidocaine of 1 to 5 µg/mL are therapeutic for treating cardiac arrhythmias and as a supplement to general anesthesia. With levels of 3 to 5 µg/mL, systemic symptoms such as circumoral numbness and buzzing or ringing in the ears may be seen. With levels of 10 to 12 µg/kg, seizures are seen, which are due to selective blockade of inhibitory pathways in the brain, leaving facilitatory neurons unopposed. Before the onset of seizures, patients have slow speech, jerky movements, tremors, and hallucinations. Cardiac toxicity is seen with levels of 20 to 25 µg/kg.[53]

Bupivacaine blood levels of 4 µg/mL causes seizures, while with higher doses (6 µg/mL), cardiac toxicity is seen.[53]

Central Nervous System Toxicity

CNS toxicity manifests as seizure activity. If seizure activity is not rapidly stopped, acidosis progresses due to anoxia, which decreases protein binding of the local anesthetic, creating more free (unbound) active drug. This is treated primarily by preventing the detrimental effects of hypoxia and is accomplished by the following protocol[53]:

- Ventilate with 100% oxygen.
- Suppress the seizures by raising the seizure threshold of the CNS with intravenous thiopental (50–100 mg if myocardial function is not depressed), midazolam (1–2 mg), or diazepam (5–10 mg).
- Patients with severe toxicity should be intubated. Succinylcholine may be used to facilitate intubation.
- Termination of the tonic clonic muscle activity with muscle paralysis will prevent further acidosis due to increased muscle activity.

Cardiotoxicity

All local anesthetics cause a dose-dependent depression of contractility of cardiac muscle. This cardiodepressant effect on contractility parallels the anesthetic potency of local anesthetics in blocking peripheral nerves (bupivacaine has 4-fold more cardiac toxicity than lidocaine).[53]

Progressive prolongation of ventricular conduction predisposes to reentrant phenomena. Widened QRS is followed by a sudden onset of ventricular fibrillation. All local anesthetics produce a dose-dependent depression of conduction velocity in cardiac tissue, including intraatrial, AV nodal, His-Purkinje, and intraventricular pathways.[53]

Bupivacaine is 4-fold more cardiotoxic than lidocaine, perhaps because with depolarization of the cardiac sodium and calcium channels, lidocaine

EXHIBIT 13-1

PREVENTION OF LOCAL ANESTHETIC–INDUCED TOXICITY

1. Be familiar with the local anesthetic agent being used.
2. Select a dose that should be associated with clinically safe blood levels at the site of injection.
3. Administer the drug in a manner that identifies an unintended intravascular injection:
   - Fractionate the dose by injecting 3- to 5-mL increments of local anesthetic so that an intravenous or intrathecal injection can be identified before a large amount of drug has been administered.
   - Aspirate frequently during injection to identify intravenous or intrathecal injections.
   - Maintain verbal contact with the patient to identify early subjective sensations such as circumoral tingling and ringing in the ears.
   - Inject a small test dose of epinephrine in a 1:200,000 concentration to elicit an increase in heart rate with inadvertent intravascular injection.
   - Injecting a small amount of air before injecting local anesthetic, combined with precordial Doppler monitoring, may detect intravenous injections.
   - Have resuscitation equipment available when local or regional anesthesia is performed.
4. Have a knowledge of the patient's medical history (hepatic/renal disease or allergy to *p*-aminobenzoic acid).

Data source: Warfield D. *Manual of Pain Management*. Philadelphia, Pa: JB Lippincott; 1991.

rapidly enters and leaves the open channels (ie, the fast-in, fast-out effect). Bupivacaine, on the other hand, rapidly enters the channels but binds the proteins in the channel causing a fast-in, slow-out effect, which strongly blocks inactivated open cardiac channels. This prevents the channels from recovering during diastole, leading to increased susceptibility to reentrant dysrhythmias.[53]

TABLE 13-6

COMPARABLE SAFE DOSES OF LOCAL ANESTHETICS (MG/KG)*

	Areas Injected			
		Central Blocks†		Intercostal Blocks§
Drugs	Peripheral Blocks‡	Plain	With Epi 1:200,000	with Epi 1:200,000
2-Chloroprocaine	—	20	25	—
Procaine	—	14	18	—
Lidocaine	20	7	9	6
Mepivacaine	20	7	9	6
Bupivacaine	5	2	2	2
Tetracaine	—	2	2	—

*Estimated to produce peak plasma levels that are less than half the plasma levels at which seizures could occur
†Areas of moderate vascularity (ie, caudal epidural blocks)
‡Areas of low vascularity (ie, axillary blocks using local anesthetic solutions containing 1:200,000 epi)
§Areas of high vascularity (ie, intercostal blocks using local anesthetic solutions containing 1:200,000 epi)
Epi: epinephrine
Reprinted with permission from DiFazio CA, Woods AM. Drugs commonly used for nerve blocking. Pharmacology of local anesthetics. In: Raj PP, ed. *Practical Management of Pain*. St. Louis, Mo: Mosby–Year Book; 1992: 695.

Acidosis increases cardiotoxicity of local anesthetics by decreasing protein binding, which increases the free (active) fraction of the drug. Acidosis also increases the ionized form of the local anesthetic, which is the active form in blocking cardiac channels.[53]

Therapy for local anesthetic–induced cardiotoxicity employs the following protocol:

- Institute adequate ventilation.
- Terminate the seizures.
- Support blood pressure with fluids, vasopressors, or cardiopulmonary resuscitation.
- Institute antiarrhythmia therapy with bretylium or magnesium sulfate.
- In some cases, remove the offending agent by means of iontophoresis.

Cardiotoxicity of the long-acting local anesthetics may be increased in the patient who is pregnant. Lower doses of bupivacaine are required to produce cardiotoxicity in pregnant ewes compared to nonpregnant controls.[53] This may be due, in part, to the fact that protein binding is decreased during pregnancy, causing an increased fraction of free drug.

Allergy to Local Anesthetics

p-Aminobenzoic acid is one of the metabolites of esters and related compounds that can induce allergic reactions in some patients. Amino amides, on the other hand, are not metabolized to *p*-aminobenzoic acid, and reports of allergic reactions to these agents are extremely rare.

SELECTION OF LOCAL ANESTHETICS

Local anesthetics are selected based on (*a*) the duration of anesthesia needed, (*b*) the need for motor blockade, and (*c*) the speed of their onset of action.[53]

Esters

Procaine

Procaine, the first synthetic local anesthetic, is characterized by slow onset and short duration of action. It penetrates tissue barriers poorly. Procaine is metabolized to *p*-aminobenzoic acid, which has allergenic potential.

2-Chloroprocaine

The 2-chloro- derivative of procaine, 2-chloroprocaine has a rapid onset of action and a short (30–60 min) duration of activity. Its half-life is 45 seconds in the plasma. 2-chloroprocaine has a low potential for systemic toxicity owing to its rapid breakdown. Sensory deficits have occurred with inadvertent intrathecal administration due to bisulfite, the preservative that was added. Bisulfite is an acidic solution that releases sulfur dioxide, forming neurotoxic sulfurous acid. Bisulfite has been removed from the preparation and ethyl-enediaminetetraacetic acid (EDTA) substituted. EDTA may cause spasm of back muscles after epidural administration owing to EDTA's binding of calcium in the paraspinal muscles.[53]

Tetracaine

Tetracaine, the butyl aminobenzoic acid derivative of procaine, is potent and long acting. This drug is usually used for spinal analgesia in a dose of 6 to 15 mg. The high degree of motor block tetracaine produces may outlast the sensory blockade.

Cocaine

Cocaine is an ester of benzoic acid. It produces topical anesthesia and vasoconstriction. In addition to its local anesthetic activity, cocaine causes CNS stimulation that manifests initially as euphoria and sometimes dysphoria. This is followed by poststimulatory depression. Cocaine's cardiovascular effects are caused by the drug's blocking the uptake of catecholamines at adrenergic nerve terminals. This block can cause sympathetically mediated tachycardia, vasoconstriction leading to hypertension, myocardial ischemia, and dysrhythmias. Administration of epinephrine or volatile anesthetics may sensitize the myocardium to the effects of cocaine. Cocaine is metabolized by plasma cholinesterase.

Preparations of this drug consist of 4% to 10% concentrations for topical anesthesia of the nose, pharynx, and tracheobronchial tree.[48] The usual topical dose is 1 to 3 mg/kg.[10]

The fatal dose of cocaine has been approximated at 1.2 g, although severe toxic effects have been reported from doses as low as 20 mg.[56] In well-premedicated, extensively monitored, anesthetized patients presenting for cardiac surgery, no sympathomimetic effect was seen due to nasal topical cocaine (1.5 mg/kg).[57] Treatment of toxicity from cocaine consists of the following protocol:

- Cardiotoxicity may be treated with esmolol to control the heart rate.
- Labetalol offers hypertension control with alpha and beta blockade.[57]
- Seizures from cocaine may respond to benzodiazepines.[52]

Amides

Lidocaine

Lidocaine was the first amide-derived local anesthetic. It has excellent tissue penetration, a rapid onset, and intermediate duration (1–2 h). The addition of epinephrine improves the quality of the block and decreases absorption from the site of injection while also prolonging the duration of anesthesia.

Mepivacaine

Mepivacaine is similar to lidocaine in activity and toxicity, and has an intermediate duration of action. This drug is poorly metabolized by the fetal liver, so therefore is infrequently used for obstetric anesthesia. It is not effective topically.

Prilocaine

Prilocaine in doses higher than 600 mg may result in accumulation of the metabolite *o*-toluidine, an oxidizing compound that converts hemoglobin to methemoglobin. This methemoglobin production is reversed with methylene blue 1 to 2 mg/kg administered intravenously.

Bupivacaine

Bupivacaine was developed from mepivacaine. It has good separation of motor and sensory anesthesia. Bupivacaine has a slow onset, with a long (3 h) duration of action. It is often used for postoperative analgesia because of the motor–sensory separation. Hepatic enzymes for bupivacaine metabolism are present in the fetus, so it may be used in obstetrical anesthesia. Bupivacaine is commonly used for subarachnoid anesthesia in hyperbaric (0.75% bupivacaine with glucose) or isobaric (0.5% bupivacaine) forms.

Etidocaine

Etidocaine is structurally similar to lidocaine. It has a rapid onset of action and a prolonged duration. Its motor block may outlast its sensory block.

Ropivacaine

Ropivacaine is currently undergoing clinical trials. It has properties similar to bupivacaine but may have less cardiotoxicity. Ropivacaine has a similar pKa and protein-binding characteristics as bupivacaine. It is less lipid soluble than bupivacaine, with similar onset and duration. It comes as 0.75% to 1% concentrations. Ropivacaine has good separation of sensory and motor block.

MODE OF ADMINISTRATION OF ANALGESIC DRUGS

Under battlefield conditions, the postoperative care of casualties should be as simple as possible. Whenever possible, casualties should take an active role in their own care, thus limiting the amount of support services needed. Monitored recovery areas are small in wartime, compared with the number of patients who will need operations. The task of the recovery-area staff is to provide safe, adequate pain relief that allows the casualty to be returned to an unmonitored setting as quickly as possible.

Intramuscular and Intravenous Routes

The mainstay of postoperative pain relief will probably be narcotics administered via the intravenous and intramuscular routes. Their mechanisms of actions are well defined, they are easily administered, they are effective for acute pain, and their effects can easily be reversed with an antagonist like naloxone. Morphine and meperidine in particular are well-known drugs and most medical personnel are familiar with the dosing regimens (Tables 13-7 and 13-8).

Intravenous narcotics can also be delivered via a PCA pump. The pump can be loaded with a supply of narcotics that will last many hours, and, within preset time limits (during which time the patient is effectively locked out of the system), the patient can

TABLE 13-7

INTRAMUSCULAR MEDICATIONS

Drug	Dose (mg/kg)	Peak Onset (min)	Duration (h)
Narcotics			
Morphine	0.05–0.10	45–90	3–6
Meperidine	0.25–0.50	60	2–4
Agonist–Antagonists			
Butorphanol	0.015–0.030	45–90	3–4
Nalbuphine	0.05–0.10	45–90	3–6
Mixed Agonists			
Dezocine	0.070–0.20	45–90	3–6
Nonsteroidal Antiinflammatory Drugs			
Ketorolac	30–60 mg	90	6–12

control the administration. Many authorities[4,5,58,59] consider the pain relief from the pump to be superior to other forms of narcotics administration. The added advantage of the PCA pump is that the patient feels a sense of control over his or her own care.[4] This administration technique would be very useful in a field hospital. The drugs commonly used in PCA pump are meperidine and morphine, both in standard concentrations. Once the patient's PCA pump is programmed, it needs only to be checked every 8 hours. The patient needs to be observed every hour to check respiratory rate only. This means that the personnel monitoring these patients will have more time to function in other capacities. For an adult, the starting dose can be 1 mg per dose for morphine and 5 mg per dose for meperidine. The lockout interval should be 8 to 12 minutes. The dose can be increased as needed according to the patient's needs. If the clinical picture mandates, a continuous infusion of narcotics can also be considered.

The usefulness of agonist–antagonists in the field is limited. The major disadvantage of these medications is that the dose–response curves are usually

TABLE 13-8

INTRAVENOUS MEDICATIONS

Drug	Dose (mg/kg)	Peak Onset (min)	Duration (h)
Narcotics			
Morphine	0.05–0.10	20	3–6
Fentanyl	0.001–0.002	10	1–3
Meperidine	0.25–0.50	20–30	2–4
Agonist–Antagonists			
Butorphanol	0.007–0.015	20–30	3–4
Nalbuphine	0.05–0.10	20–30	3–6
Mixed Agonists			
Dezocine	0.070–0.15	20–30	3–6

shaped like an inverted U: the pain relief reaches a plateau, then decreases with higher doses. With lower doses, the agonist effects of the drugs predominate and the patient will obtain pain relief. However, if the pain is intense and the patient needs large doses of narcotic, the antagonist effect of the drug tends to predominate and the patient will not obtain relief.[30] The next dilemma that the medical officer encounters is that the agonist–antagonist opioid will also inhibit the activity of other narcotics that would be used to alleviate the patient's pain. Thus, it would be very difficult to give the correct amount of narcotics. Because of these problems, agonist–antagonist drugs would have limited usefulness in the field for intravenous or intramuscular administration.

Another drug that could have a useful postoperative role in field hospitals is ketorolac, administered intramuscularly. This drug has been used successfully for acute postoperative pain.[60] Its advantages are that it is not a controlled substance and it can be administered in conjunction with narcotics for additive pain relief without additive side effects. Ketorolac would be a good adjunct to the therapy of patients whose pain cannot be controlled with large doses of narcotics. Once the patients are tolerating oral intake, they can be switched to an oral NSAID.

Epidural and Intrathecal Routes

Intrathecal or epidural delivery of narcotics should be considered whenever possible. The advantage of these modes of administration is the small amount of observation necessary for the maintenance of good postoperative pain relief. The prolonged and profound pain relief obtained from medication delivered via these modes makes them ideal for use in field hospitals. After epidural or intrathecal administration, patient care includes observation for respiratory depression and side effects common to narcotics. Depending on the type of injury, catheters can be placed in the epidural space for long-term narcotic administration. Not only will the patient be able to obtain narcotics for pain relief, but if the patient needs to be returned to the operating suite, the catheter can be used to provide anesthesia for subsequent operations.

After the narcotics have been administered, the patient can return to a minimally monitored setting for continued postoperative care. The patient can receive either intermittent boluses of a long-acting narcotic, or a continuous infusion of a shorter-acting substance (Table 13-9). The side effects of narcotics have been described above. The most dangerous side effect is respiratory depression but its true incidence is difficult to determine. Current studies indicate that it ranges from 1:32 to 1:260, depending on the dose.[6] The predisposing factors to respiratory depression are advanced age, CNS depression or concomitant systemic narcotic use, increased intrathoracic pressure, and thoracic extradural administration.[6,36,37] The healthy, young adults who comprise most of the military patient population are at less potential risk for respiratory depression. A well-tolerated treatment of narcotic side effects is a naloxone infusion: the effects of respiratory depression and the other side effects can be reversed without also reversing the analgesic effects of the narcotics.

If the need for an epidural catheter is anticipated for postoperative pain relief, and if the patient is to remain at relative bed rest, then epidurally administered local anesthetics can be considered. Administering 0.125% to 0.25% solutions of bupivacaine will not only increase the pain relief to the prescribed area, but will also increase the blood flow. However, for this route to be of use, injury has to be located in a nerve distribution that can be blocked safely by an infusion of local anesthetic through an epidural catheter.[7]

TABLE 13-9

POSTOPERATIVE OPIOID DOSES

Drug	Intravenous Dose (mg)	Epidural Dose (mg)	Subarachnoid Dose (mg)
Morphine	5–10	2–5	0.20–0.50
Meperidine	50–100	30–50	10–20
Fentanyl	0.10–0.15	0.10–0.20	0.075–0.15

SUMMARY

Eliminating perioperative pain is justified not only by medical ethics—the imperative to relieve pain and alleviate suffering—but also because severe and unremitting pain can accentuate the potentially dangerous alterations in metabolism and the function of various organs that are caused by severe trauma. Foremost among the metabolic effects is hypermetabolism, leading to catabolism of muscle protein and decreased lean body mass. Similarly, unrelieved pain from thoracic or upper-abdominal trauma may, by causing splinting of respiratory muscles, prevent normal pulmonary gas exchange and clearance of tracheobronchial secretions. Thus, morbidity may be reduced by eliminating pain.

The neurological pathway by which we are made aware of painful stimuli arising in peripheral tissue begins in peripheral pain receptors, which connect via peripheral nerves with ascending pathways that arise in the dorsal horn cells of the spinal cord. From here, information travels in the anterolateral portion of the spinal cord through the brain stem and hypothalamus to the cerebral cortex. The activity of the ascending tracts is modified by impulses that descend from higher centers via descending tracts that synapse with neurons in the dorsal horn. Neurotransmitters are found along the neurological pathway—from substance P and histamine at the peripheral pain receptors to serotonin and enkephalins in the CNS.

Therapeutic interventions that are likely to be useful in treating combat casualties with painful trauma are of two classes: those such as local anesthetics, which prevent transmission of impulses along nerves either in the periphery or in proximity to the spinal cord; and those that either interfere with the synthesis and function of neurotransmitters or directly inhibit neurons in the CNS, which transmit painful stimuli from the periphery. The NSAIDs are examples of substances that alter neurotransmitter activity, while morphine and other opiates, by acting on cells in the spinal cord, decrease traffic passing up the ascending tracts. Opiates also activate the descending inhibitor tracts and act at sites along the neurological pathways for pain in the brain stem and cerebrum.

The spectrum of pain-relieving interventions that are available to military anesthesia providers ranges from orally administered NSAIDs, through intravenous morphine, through regional or epidural blocks with local anesthetics, to epidural analgesia with opioids. Opioids have the advantage of being both potent and, by not blocking sympathetic and motor pathways, selective. There is, however, a risk of respiratory depression. Epidural block with a local anesthetic stops all afferent nerve traffic, one consequence of which is peripheral vasodilation in the affected body parts, which may give rise to potentially dangerous hypotension.

REFERENCES

1. Dunant H. *A Memory of Solferino*. Geneva, Switzerland: International Committee of the Red Cross; 1986.

2. Beecher HK. The control of pain in men wounded in battle. In: DeBakey ME, ed. *General Surgery*. Vol 2. In: Coates JB Jr, ed. *Surgery in World War II*. Washington, DC: US Department of the Army, Medical Department, Office of The Surgeon General; 1955: 4–49.

3. Mitchell RWD, Smith G. The control of acute postoperative pain. *Br J Anaesth*. 1989;63:147–158.

4 Bullingham RES. Optimum management of postoperative pain. *Drugs*. 1985;29:376–386.

5. Rose PG, Piver MS, Batista E, Lau T. Patient-controlled analgesia in gynecologic oncology. *J Reprod Med*. 1989;34:651–654.

6. Morgan M. The rational use of intrathecal and extradural opioids. *Br J Anaesth*. 1989;63:165–188.

7. Wildsmith JAW. Developments in local anaesthetic drugs and techniques for pain relief. *Br J Anaesth*. 1989;63:159–164.

8. Smith G. Management of postoperative pain. *Can J Anaesth*. 1989;36:S1–S4.

9. Cousins M, Bridenbaugh P, eds. *Neural Blockade in Clinical Anesthesia and Management of Pain*. 2nd ed. Philadelphia, Pa: JB Lippincott; 1988.

10. Barash, P, Cullen BF, Stoelting RR. *Clinical Anesthesia*. Philadelphia, Pa: JB Lippincott; 1989.

11. Adriaesen H, Gybels J, Handwerker H, Van Hees J. Response properties of thin myelinated (A-delta) fibers in human skin nerves. *J Neurophysiol*. 1969;32:1025–1031.

12. Van Hees J, Gybels JM. Pain related to single afferent C fibers from human skin. *Acta Physiol Scand*. 1974;92:374–380.

13. Juan H, Lembeck F. Action of peptides and other algesic agents on perivascular pain receptors of the isolated perfused rabbit ear. *Naunyn-Schmiedeberg's Arch Pharmacol*. 1974;283:151–164.

14. LaMotte RH, Campbell JN. Comparison of responses of warm and nociceptive C-fiber afferents in monkey with human judgement of thermal pain. *J Neurophysiol*. 1979;41:509–515.

15. Mariott DR, Wilkin GP, Wood JN. Substance P–induced release of prostaglandins from astrocytes: Regional specialization and correlation with phosphoinositol metabolism. *J Neurochem*. 1991;56:259–265.

16. Gamse R, Petsche U, Lemback F, Jancso G. Capsaicin applied to peripheral nerve inhibits axoplasmic transport of substance P and somatostatin. *Brain Res*. 1982;239:447–456.

17. Lewis T. *Pain*. New York, NY: Macmillan; 1942: 17.

18. Terenius L. Biochemical mediators of pain. *Triangle*. 1981;20:19–25.

19. Jaffe JH, Martin WR. Narcotic analgesics and antagonists. In: Goodman LS, Gilman A. *The Pharmacological Basis of Therapeutics*. 5th ed. New York, NY: Macmillan; 1975: 245.

20. Yaksh TL, Rudy TY. Studies on the direct spinal action of narcotics in the production of analgesia in rats. *J Pharmacol Exp Ther*. 1977;202:411–428.

21. Richie JM, Greene NM. Local anesthetics. In: Gilman AG, Goodman LS, eds. *The Pharmacological Basis of Therapeutics*. New York, NY: Macmillan; 1985: 302–321.

22. Rosenblatt RM, Reich J, Dehring D. Tricyclic antidepressants in the treatment of depression and chronic pain. *Anesth Analg*. 1984;63:1025–1032.

23. Flower RJ, Moncada S, Vane JR. Analgesic–antipyretics and anti-inflammatory agents: Drugs employed in the treatment of gout. In: Gilman AG, Goodman LS, eds. *The Pharmacological Basis of Therapeutics*. New York, NY: Macmillan; 1985: 674–715.

24. Eisenach JC, Dewan DM, Rose JC, Angela JM. Epidural clonidine produces antinociception, but not hypotension, in sheep. *Anesthesiology*. 1987;66:496–501.

25. Brewer LA III. Resuscitation and preoperative preparation. In: Berry FB, ed. *Thoracic Surgery*. Vol 1. In: Coates JB Jr, ed. *Surgery in World War II*. Washington, DC: US Department of the Army, Medical Department, Office of The Surgeon General; 1963.

26. Bromage PR. *Epidural Analgesia*. Philadelphia, Pa: WB Saunders; 1978.

27. Yeager MP, Glass DD, Neff RK, Brinck-Johnsen T. Epidural anesthesia and analgesia in high-risk surgical patients. *Anesthesiology*. 1987;66:729–736.

28. Nimmo WS. Effects of anesthesia on gastric motility and emptying. *Br J Anaesth*. 1984;56:29–37.

29. Kehlet M. Modification of responses to surgery by neural blockade: Clinical implications. In: Cousins MJ, Bridenbaugh PO, eds. *Neural Blockade in Clinical Anesthesia and Management of Pain*. 2nd ed. Philadelphia, Pa: JB Lippincott; 1988: 145–188.

30. Stoelting RK. Opioids, agonists, and antagonists. In: Stoelting RK, ed. *Pharmacology and Physiology in Anesthetic Practice*. New York, NY: JB Lippincott; 1987: 69–95.

31. Hug CC, Murphy MR, Rigel EP, Olson WA. Pharmacokinetics of morphine injected intravenously into the anesthetized dog. *Anesthesiology*. 1981;54:38–47.

32. Mueller RA, Lundberg DB, Breese GR, Medner J, Medner T, Jonason J. The neuropharmacology of respiratory control. *Pharmacol Rev*. 1982;34:255–285.

33. Rosow CE, Moss J, Philbin DM, Savarese JJ. Histamine release during morphine and fentanyl anesthesia. *Anesthesiology*. 1982;56:93–96.

34. Jaffe JH, Martin WR. Opioid analgesics and antagonists. In: Gilman AG, Goodman LS, eds. *The Pharmacological Basis of Therapeutics*. New York, NY: Macmillan; 1985: 473–490.

35. Cousins MJ, Mather LE. Intrathecal and epidural administration of opioids. *Anesthesiology*. 1984;61:276–310.

36. Gwirtz KH. Intraspinal narcotics in the management of postoperative pain. *Anesthesiology Rev*. 1990;17:16–28.

37. Martin R, Lamarche Y, Tetrault JP. Epidural and intrathecal narcotics. *Can J Anaes*. 1983;30:662–673.

38. Hug CC, Murphy MR. Tissue redistribution of fentanyl and termination of its effects in rats. *Anesthesiology*. 1981;55:369–375.

39. Rutter DV, Skewers G, Morgan M. Extradural opioids for postoperative analgesia: A double-blinded comparison of pethidine, fentanyl, and morphine. *Br J Anaesth*. 1981;53:915–929.

40. Torda TA, Pybus DA. Comparison of four narcotics for extradural analgesia. *Br J Anaesth*. 1982;54:291–295.

41. Freye E. Cardiovascular effects of high dosage of fentanyl, meperidine and naloxone in dogs. *Anesth Analg*. 1974;53:40–47.

42. Gal TJ, DiFazio CA, Moscicki J. Analgesic and respiratory depressant activity of nalbuphine: A comparison with morphine. *Anesthesiology*. 1982;57:367–374.

43. DiFazio CA. Pharmacology and narcotic analgesics. *The Clinical Journal of Pain*. 1989;5(suppl 1):S5–S7.

44. Prough DS, Roy R, Bumgarner J, Shannon G. Acute pulmonary edema in healthy teenagers following conservative doses of intravenous naloxone. *Anesthesiology*. 1984;60:485–486.

45. Partridge BL, Ward CF. Pulmonary edema following low-dose naloxone administration. *Anesthesiology*. 1986;65:709–710.

46. Ravel N, Schott U, Dahlstrom B, et al. Influence of naloxone infusion on analgesia and respiratory depression following epidural morphine. *Anesthesiology*. 1986;64:194–201.

47. Thind GS, Wells CD, Wilkes RG. The effects of continuous intravenous naloxone on epidural morphine analgesia. *Anesthesia*. 1986;41:582–585.

48. Jacob L. *Pharmacology*. 2nd ed. New York, NY: John Wiley; 1987.

49. Warfield C. *Manual of Pain Management*. Philadelphia, Pa: JB Lippincott; 1991.

50. Clark W. *Goth's Medical Pharmacology*. St. Louis, Mo: Mosby–Year Book. 1992; 356–373.

51. Ferrante FM. NSAIDs. In: *Comprehensive Review of Pain Management*. Richmond, Va: American Society of Regional Anesthesia; 1994: 199–226.

52. Stoelting R, Miller R. *Basics of Anesthesia*. 3rd ed. New York, NY: Churchill Livingstone; 1994.

53. Raj P. *Practical Management of Pain*. 2nd ed. St. Louis, Mo: Mosby–Year Book; 1992.

54. DiFazio CA, Woods AM. Drugs commonly used for nerve blocking. Pharmacology of local anesthetics. In: Raj PP, ed. *Practical Management of Pain*. St. Louis, Mo: Mosby–Year Book; 1992: 685–700.

55. McLaughlen S. Local anesthetics and the electrical properties of phospholipid bilayer membranes. In: Fink BR, ed. *Molecular Mechanisms of Anesthesia*. New York, NY: Raven Press; 1975: 193–220.

56. *Physicians' Desk Reference*. 48th ed. Montville, NJ: Medical Economics Data; 1994.

57. Barash P. *Cocaine: Therapeutic Uses and Problems Anesthetizing the Abuser*. Richmond, Va: ASA Annual Refresher Course Lectures. October 19, 1991.

58. Hecker BR, Albert L. Patient-controlled analgesia: A randomized, prospective comparison between two commercially available PCA pumps and conventional analgesia therapy for postoperative pain. *Pain*. 1988;35:115–120.

59. Zacharias M, Pfeifer MV, Herbison P. Comparison of two methods of intravenous administration of morphine for postoperative pain relief. *Anaesth Intensive Care*. 1990;18:205–209.

60. Brown CR, Moodie JE, Yee JP. Efficacy of intramuscular ketorolac and meperidine in pain following major oral surgery. *Clin Pharmacol Ther*. 1988;43:161–165.

Chapter 14

TRANSFUSION THERAPY

NORIG ELLISON, M.D.*

*Professor of Anesthesia and Vice Chairman, Department of Anesthesia, University of Pennsylvania School of Medicine, 3400 Spruce Street, Philadelphia, Pennsylvania 19104-4283

INTRODUCTION

In the foreword to the U.S. Army Medical Department's official history, *Blood Program in World War II*, Lieutenant General Leonard D. Heaton states:

> If any single medical program can be credited with the saving of countless lives in World War II and in the Korean War, it was the prompt and liberal use of whole blood.[1(p ix)]

Many physicians who served in the Korean and Vietnam wars would certainly confirm that observation. We need only to observe the effect of a rapid, multiple-unit transfusion via both femoral veins in restoring a modicum of hemodynamic stability to an exsanguinated, seemingly pulseless, but previously healthy young combat casualty to appreciate the validity of the American Red Cross slogan that the gift of a unit of blood is, indeed, the gift of life.

Earlier, Edward D. Churchill, in his World War II memoir *Surgeon to Soldiers*, observed: "The goal of resuscitation...is not solely to save life but to prepare for necessary surgery. This will in turn be accompanied by further loss of blood."[2(p37)] This statement was written during the early days of the North African campaign, when the policy called for liberal use of *plasma*, not blood, because

> (1) An interval of time is necessary [for cross-matching]. (2) Preservation can be for a relatively short period [initially 8 days, later extended to 21 days] and transportaion is difficult because of the need of bulky and heavy apparatus for proper refrigeration. (3) The addition of red cells to the blood stream is often undesirable, especially when large quantities of blood are necessary (1,000 cc. or more)....[2(p43)]

This third point is most astonishing in view of recent combat and civilian experience and reflects the body of knowledge against which Churchill made his observation.

To study any clinical problem where many variables are involved, a large number of patients are needed. Fortunately, the need for resuscitation involving a massive transfusion (defined as > 1.0 estimated blood volume [EBV]) is rare in civilian practice; thus, three classic papers—one published in 1954 and based on the Korean War experience,[3] the other two published in 1973 and 1974 and based on the Vietnam War experience[4,5]—are frequently cited. The paper from the Korean War described almost exclusive use of low-titer, group O, Rh-positive "universal-donor" blood and warned that the use of type-specific whole blood following the administration of universal-donor whole blood carried with it the risk of hemolytic transfusion reaction.[3] It may be a reflection of the increasing sophistication of the U.S. Army Medical Department that during the Vietnam War, type-specific blood was usually used without undue risk of hemolytic transfusion reaction at field and evacuation hospitals. Clearing companies and forward surgical hospitals continued to use group O, low-titer, Rh(d) whole blood, and patients who received more than four such units continued to receive this type on evacuation until laboratory results demonstrated that the administration of type-specific red blood cells (RBCs) would not produce a hemolytic transfusion reaction.[6,7]

Table 14-1 lists the 14 issues addressed in either or both papers that describe transfusion practice during the Vietnam War.[4,5] The marked similarity in the problems perceived and the solutions to them is not surprising. In fact, except for the issue of coagulopathy in relation to volume of blood transfused, the conclusions in the two papers are essentially identical.

LOGISTICS

One of the major problems facing the severely traumatized patient in need of massive transfusion is logistical, which includes obtaining and transporting whole blood and blood components to the treatment center, as well as securing sufficient large-bore intravenous lines to permit rapid infusion.

Collection, Distribution, and Administration of Blood

The problems unique to a combat situation such as existed in Vietnam include highly variable demand rates. From fewer than 100 units per month in

TABLE 14-1

PROBLEMS ASSOCIATED WITH MASSIVE TRANSFUSION

	Discussed in this Chapter?	Discussed in Collins?[1]	Discussed in Miller?[2]
Acid-base balance	Yes	Yes	Yes
Altered 2,3 diphosphoglycerate	No	Yes	No
Citrate toxicity	Yes	Yes	Yes
Coagulation	Yes	Yes	Yes
Denatured protein	No	Yes	No
Mathematics of blood replacement	Yes	Yes	No
New additives	No	Yes	No
Other sources of blood	Yes	No	Yes
Plasticizers	No	Yes	No
Posttransfusion hepatitis	Yes	No	Yes
Potassium, ammonia, phosphate	Yes	Yes	Yes
Pulmonary effects, microemboli	Yes	Yes	Yes
Temperature regulation	Yes	Yes	Yes
Vasoactive substances	No	Yes	No

Data sources: (1) Collins JA. Problems associated with the massive transfusion of stored blood. *Surgery*. 1974;75:274–295. (2) Miller RD. Complications of massive blood transfusions. *Anesthesiology*. 1973;39:82–93.

1965, the demand peaked in February 1969 at 38,000 units per month (Figure 14-1), with very long supply lines.[6] To ensure that blood will arrive in country as soon as possible after collection, some of this blood was actually processed while being flown to Vietnam from the 42 donor centers set up in the

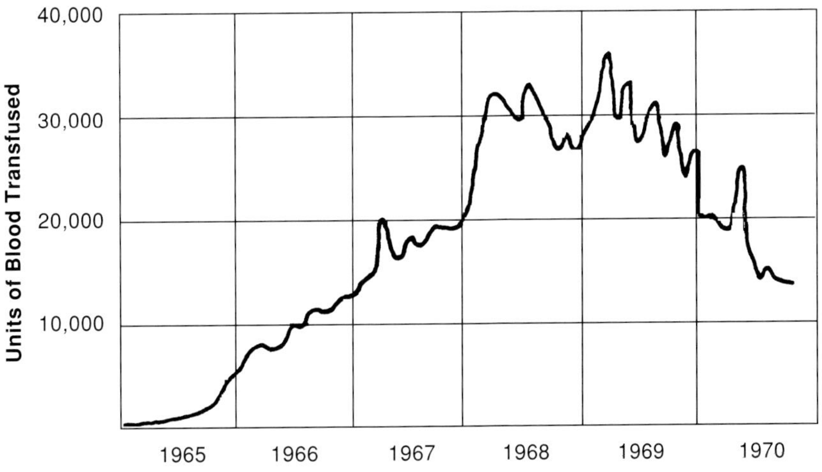

Fig. 14-1. Units of blood used in South Vietnam, January 1965 through December 1970. Reprinted from Neel S. *Medical Support of the US Army in Vietnam, 1965–1970*. Washington, DC: Department of the Army; 1973: 115.

United States and Japan. Nevertheless, blood was approximately 7 days old when received in Vietnam, and further time-consuming shipment forward was required.

Such combat-unique situations do not exist in a civilian setting. However, the supply-to-demand ratio for blood remains perilously thin. An editorial published in 1975 stated that only 5% of the population provided more than 95% of the blood administered in the United States and wishfully surmised that if the number of donors could be doubled, then the problem of blood shortages would become history.[8] In the interim, improved technical capabilities have (*a*) almost doubled the number of units collected, (*b*) increased utilization by extending shelf life from 21 to 42 days, and (*c*) increased fractionation nationwide, thus permitting the blood supply to be extended even further. Nevertheless, the supply of blood barely meets the demand. Why? There are three reasons: (1) the development of more invasive procedures such as liver transplants and radical cancer surgery, and (2) the use of highly aggressive treatment protocols (especially those used in oncology patients), both of which require more platelets to prevent iatrogenic hemorrhage; and (3) more recently, the irrational fear in a significant portion of the potential donor population that the act of donating blood carries with it a risk of contracting blood-borne infectious diseases such as acquired immunodeficiency syndrome (AIDS).

To avoid a hemolytic transfusion reaction, a system of patient-to-specimen identification and marriage is essential, especially so in mass casualty situations. The most common cause of death due to hemolytic transfusion reaction in peacetime is clerical error that occurs outside the blood bank and results in a patient's receiving an ABO-incompatible unit of blood.[9] In trauma centers, the assignment of a specific "trauma number" to each patient immediately on arrival has proven an effective way to begin a patient-identification system.

Although the Seldinger technique for inserting large catheters into blood vessels was originally described in 1951, the technique was not commonly used outside angiographic suites and cardiac catheterization laboratories until the mid-1970s,[10] and surgical cutdowns on the saphenous, femoral, or antecubital veins were used during the Vietnam War to provide adequate venous access to facilitate rapid, large-volume transfusion. In civilian trauma centers today, the subclavian and internal or external jugular veins are the vessels most commonly used, and the Seldinger technique is employed to insert large-bore catheters. Also, the inflatable pressure bags that were formerly employed have largely been replaced by rapid-infusion systems, a by-product of the heart-lung machine. Because the American College of Surgeons' Advanced Trauma Life Support (ATLS) practice guidelines are used by the military's deployable medical facilities, fluid resuscitation of combat casualties will most commonly involve percutaneous access through an antecubital vein or an extremity cutdown rather than a central venous catheterization.

Component Therapy Versus Whole Blood

The three classic wartime studies[3–5] dealt with the use of whole blood. Currently in the United States, however, more than 80% of blood is fractionated at the time of collection. This may not leave sufficient whole blood for use in trauma and other instances of massive blood loss where many clinicians believe whole blood is desirable, if not essential. The issue is one that has plagued the relationship between anesthesiologists and blood-bank specialists for some time, as the following comments illustrate:

> There will be little variation in response from the blood bank: You will ask for whole blood, and they will send you packed cells, even though people bleed only whole blood,... you will be stuck with the time-consuming reconstitution of each cold sludgy unit.[11(p94)]
>
> . . . .
>
> I believe that in an active general-hospital practice, half the transfusions should be given as whole blood. A greater use of cells perpetuates the make work cycle and at least doubles the cost to the patient.[12(p1411)]

The principal arguments for the use of component therapy are (1) it permits specific, goal-directed therapy, and (2) at the same time, each unit of blood can be used to treat several patients. In particular, if Factor VIII is removed to treat patients with hemophilia, and if platelets are removed to permit more aggressive chemotherapy in oncology patients, a by-product will be packed RBCs; many surgical patients are suitable candidates to receive this by-product, not just those in whom volume overload is a consideration. One investigator[13] has suggested that if fewer than four units are needed, RBCs diluted with crystalloid or colloid solutions will suffice; if more than four are required, whole blood would be preferred. Others[14] have approached this problem differently: after they remove the platelets and cryoprecipitate from a unit of whole blood, they return the remaining plasma to the RBCs, producing *modified* whole blood. The effectiveness of this product in treating trauma patients without increasing hemostatic problems has been demonstrated, and more widespread use of modified whole blood would seem indicated.

PURPOSES OF TRANSFUSION

There are two major purposes for transfusion therapy: (1) to improve the oxygen-carrying capacity of the cardiovascular system and (2) to restore hemostasis by increasing coagulation factor and platelet concentrations to hemostatic levels.

Increase Oxygen-Carrying Capacity

Oxygen transport is a prime function of the cardiopulmonary system. There are a number of factors that are determinants of oxygen transport (eg, the RBC mass and the circulating blood volume). The body's defense mechanism to maintain a normal intravascular volume in the presence of blood loss will mobilize interstitial fluid and then shift it into the intravascular space, but this process takes hours. In contrast, the body's attempt to maintain cardiac output (ie, constriction of systemic venules and small veins and, when blood loss continues, constriction of the vascular sphincters in circulatory beds of skin, skeletal muscle, kidney, and splanchnic viscera) occurs within 60 to 120 seconds of an acute hemorrhage. The maintenance of cardiac output is mediated by the adrenergic system and circulating catecholamines, and by the renin-angiotensin system and the secretion of vasopressin. As a result, hemoglobin levels will remain falsely high if volume-for-volume replacement is not carried out on an ongoing basis. Preservation of blood flow to the heart and brain, two organs capable of regulating their own flow over a wide range of arterial pressure, will be preserved until the loss exceeds the ability to compensate.[15]

Allowable Blood Loss and Normovolemia

Although circulating blood volume is lost during hemorrhage, increased venous tone and augmented contractility may bring about an increase in cardiac output, which will make possible maintenance of normal oxygen transport. Therefore, volume replacement is not a reason for blood or blood-component transfusion if a compensatory increase in cardiac output has resulted in maintenance of normal oxygen delivery. Indeed, it is a common practice in elective surgery to permit patients to lose blood down to a predetermined hemoglobin level before blood transfusion begins, based on the formula

$$\text{Allowable blood loss} = \frac{Hb_{initial} - Hb_{target}}{Hb_{initial}} \bullet EBV$$

where $Hb_{initial}$ represents the hemoglobin at the start of surgery, Hb_{target} represents the target hemoglobin level at which point blood transfusion will be started, and *EBV* represents the estimated blood volume.[16]

A rough estimation of EBV may be calculated by multiplying body weight by the figures given in Table 14-2, which also incorporate corrections that need to be made for gender and body habitus. This allowable blood loss formula has a built-in safety factor, in that each successive milliliter of blood lost will be more dilute than the one lost before.

In using this formula, the maintenance of normovolemia by replacing the ongoing blood loss on a 1:1 basis with colloid solution, or a 1:3 basis with crystalloid solution, is assumed and is crucial. Failure to replace ongoing loss will result in hypovolemia, which is followed quickly by hypotension and tachycardia. In an acute trauma patient in whom bleeding has been ongoing in the absence of significant asanguineous fluid replacement (as is common with combat casualties), neither the measured hemoglobin level nor the blood volume estimated from Table 14-2 will reflect the actual circu-

TABLE 14-2

ESTIMATED BLOOD VOLUME, BASED ON BODY WEIGHT AND HABITUS

Body Habitus	Blood Volume as % of Body Weight: Female	Male
Obese	5.5	6.0
Asthenic	6.0	6.5
Lean	6.5	7.0
Muscular	7.0	7.5

lating RBC mass. Thus, in contrast to the practice in elective operations, intentional hemodilution in a trauma patient is probably ill advised.

Hemoglobin Level and the "Transfusion Trigger"

Far more controversial than the need to maintain normovolemia is the issue of what constitutes a safe lower level of hemoglobin. It was formerly a common practice to use 10.0 g of hemoglobin per deciliter of blood as the minimum acceptable hemoglobin level. Below this level, patients would be transfused before anesthesia was induced. At this level, if the patient was already anesthetized and had lost sufficient blood, blood transfusion would begin with simultaneous replacement of crystalloid or colloid solution to reach a hemoglobin level of 10.0 g/dL. This practice frequently created conflict between anesthesiologists and surgeons, as the following statement implies:

> Anesthesia needs a careful reevaluation of the minimum hemoglobin level below which the administration of anesthesia is not safe. It is not the same for all patients nor for all procedures. We request intelligent individualization.[17(p302]

Today, especially in the acutely traumatized patient, there is no minimum acceptable level, no "magic" number. The 1988 National Institutes of Health Consensus Development Conference on Perioperative Red Blood Cells Transfusion[18] specifically recommended a decrease in the "transfusion trigger" (ie, the point that must be reached before a transfusion is necessary) from 10.0 g/dL, but did not set a lower limit. A 70-kg man will consume approximately 250 mL of oxygen per minute, and oxygen delivery is approximately 1,000 mL/min, resulting in an oxygen-extraction ratio of 25%. This ratio reflects only part of the reserves the body can call on when oxygen consumption increases or the hemoglobin level decreases. A combination of increased oxygen extraction and cardiac output, as well as preservation of blood flow to vital organs, will provide adequate oxygen delivery in the presence of profound anemia. A hematocrit of 0.10 (equivalent to a hemoglobin level of 3.3 g/dL) and an oxygen extraction ratio of 50% have been suggested[19] as the crucial points below which survival is questionable. An earlier researcher[20] had kept anesthetized young pigs alive for 45 minutes with hematocrits of 0.004 by administering 100% oxygen at 3 atm in a hyperbaric chamber.

While it is doubtful that clinicians will ever have to deal with either of these values, hemoglobin levels of 7 to 9 g/dL are commonly used today as the point that must be reached—in the stable posttrauma patient—before allogenic blood will be administered. Two groups of patients have forced clinicians to alter their transfusion practices: those with renal failure, and members of the religious group Jehovah's Witnesses. Considerable clinical experience with both groups has repeatedly demonstrated that patients can tolerate much lower hemoglobin levels without either impaired wound healing or delayed convalescence.

Restore Hemostasis

Effective hemostasis depends on the triad of vascular integrity, an adequate number of functional platelets, and a minimal level of each coagulation factor. A defect in vascular integrity is the common precipitating event resulting in the need for blood transfusion in any trauma or other surgical patient,

TABLE 14-3

COAGULATION FACTOR LEVELS AT 21 DAYS OF STORAGE AS FRESH FROZEN PLASMA AND THE MINIMAL HEMOSTATIC LEVELS

Coagulation Factor	Remaining After 21-Day Storage (%)	Minimal Level for Hemostasis (%)
I	99	50–100
II	93	20–40
V	51*	10–15
VII	82*	5–10
VIII	29†	10–40
IX	95	10–40
X	89*	10–15
XI	88*	10–40
XII	100	—
XIII	100	1–5

*Decrease is statistically but not clinically significant
†Decrease is significant both statistically and clinically
Data sources: (1) Hondow JA, Russell WJ, Duncan BM, et al. The stability of coagulation factors in stored blood. *Aust N Z J Surg.* 1982;52:265–269. (2) Pisciott PT, ed. *Blood Transfusion Therapy: A Physician Handbook.* 3rd ed. Arlington, Va: American Association of Blood Banks; 1989.

and restoration of vascular integrity is primarily a surgical responsibility. However, no matter how meticulous a surgeon is in meeting that responsibility, patients will continue to bleed if an adequate number of normally functioning platelets and a minimal level of the 11 coagulation factors are not present. *Microvascular bleeding* (MVB) is the term used to describe the diffuse hemorrhagic syndrome, which is not surgically correctable.

The minimal levels of platelets and coagulation factors necessary for effective hemostasis, and the levels present after 21 days of storage in a blood bank, are shown in Table 14-3. Clearly, with the possible exception of factor VIII, a deficiency of which produces the clinical syndrome of hemophilia A, none of the coagulation factors will decay to clinically significant levels, although a statistically significant decay occurs in the levels of factors V, VII, X, and XI.[21]

The concentrations of platelets and coagulation factors are peculiarly sensitive to dilutional effects arising from volume replacement—with either packed RBCs or asanguineous fluid. The effect of dilution is best understood when viewed in terms of the mathematics of blood replacement, which are illustrated in Figure 14-2. In the controlled and idealized situation, where replacement volume matches ongoing blood loss, replacement of 1.0 EBV will allow 36.8% of the original blood, including platelets and coagulation factors, to remain.[5] This calculation is based on four assumptions that constitute the ideal:

1. mixing is instantaneous and complete,
2. initial blood volume equals final blood volume,
3. the recipient is essentially a closed system (ie, the patient is no longer continuing to lose blood), and
4. the transfused blood is uniform.

Obviously, the idealized situation never exists; in the more common trauma situation (ie, patients B or C in Figure 14-2), patients are received in a hypovolemic state and must be transfused back to their original blood volume.

Platelets and Dilutional Thrombocytopenia

In contrast to the hemostatic efficiency of the coagulation factors, which is maintained even at low temperatures, the hemostatic efficiency of platelets declines rapidly below a critically low platelet count. For this reason, a dilutional thrombocytopenia is the most common cause of bleeding in patients who receive a massive transfusion. This is true whether the patient receives whole blood, modified whole blood, or RBCs.[14] In 21 combat casualties who received more than 15 units of blood (described in one of the two studies done during the Vietnam War era),[4] the researchers correlated how closely the decrease in platelets approximates a washout equation—as if the units administered were platelet-free. In four casualties whose MVB did not

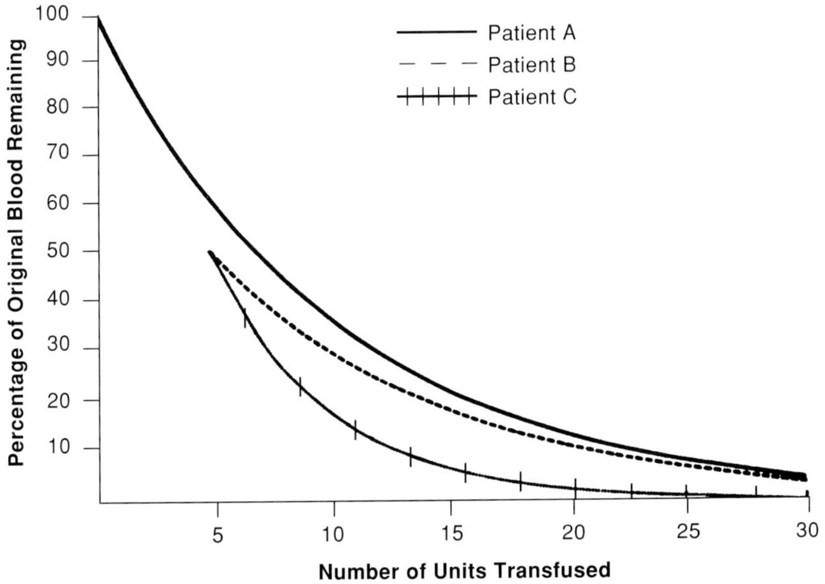

Fig. 14-2. Percentage of original blood remaining in each of three hypothetical recipients, all beginning and ending with a blood volume of 5 L, assuming that each unit of blood contains 500 mL, and using formulas and assumptions for continuous exchange described in text. Patient A remains normovolemic throughout. Patients B and C sustain a loss of one half their normal blood volume before transfusion begins. In Patient B, this loss is replaced immediately; subsequent hemorrhage and transfusion occur with a normal blood volume. In Patient C, the initial loss is replaced only after hemorrhage has stopped. Reprinted with permission from Collins JA. Problems associated with the massive transfusion of stored blood. *Surgery*. 1974;75:277.

decrease after the administration of fresh frozen plasma (FFP), the administration of 3 to 4 units of fresh whole blood resulted in a marked increase in platelet count and a decrease in bleeding.[4] The other study from the Vietnam War[5] did not find so strict a relation between volume of blood transfused and MVB; these researchers concluded that, in general, the most seriously injured casualties exhibited the most abnormal coagulation patterns, and earlier, complete resuscitation prevented the bleeding complications.

Fresh Frozen Plasma

When only RBCs are administered, reconstitution of the RBCs with crystalloid or colloid solutions other than FFP may accelerate the decrease in the levels of coagulation factors and contribute to MVB.[22] However, no formula for units of FFP per units of RBC transfused has been demonstrated to be effective in preventing MVB, nor are routine coagulation tests useful as predictors of MVB and the need for FFP.[23] Indeed, in massive transfusion, an abnormality of these tests may be considered the norm, and test results must be correlated with the clinical picture to determine whether the administration of platelets or coagulation factors is required.[24] Researchers using modified whole blood found that platelet counts lower than 50 • 10^9/L or fibrinogen levels lower than 80 mg/dL were associated with increased bleeding. They also echoed the call for whole blood to treat patients who require massive transfusion.[25]

The 1984 National Institutes of Health Consensus Development Conference on Fresh Frozen Plasma listed six indications and four nonindications for the use of FFP (Exhibit 14-1). In particular, the Consensus Development Conference strongly condemned the use of prophylactic FFP in patients who require massive transfusion, while at the same time acknowledging that

> [t]he use of fresh frozen plasma in massive blood transfusion, for which there is less credible evidence of efficacy, appears to have increased in frequency, possibly due in part to the relative unavailability of whole blood.[26(p552)]

If FFP is to be used in these patients, no absolute rule can be proposed to govern its administration. A review article discussing the use of FFP in patients with hepatic disease and who have massive blood transfusion suggested only broad general guidelines (Exhibit 14-2).[27]

EXHIBIT 14-1

NATIONAL INSTITUTES OF HEALTH CONSENSUS DEVELOPMENT CONFERENCE RECOMMENDATIONS ON FRESH FROZEN PLASMA

Indications for Fresh Frozen Plasma

1. Replacement of factors II, V, VII, X, and XI (concentrates are available for factors VIII and IX)
2. Neutralization of coumarin intercoagulation
3. Massive blood transfusion
4. Source of antithrombin III
5. Treatment of immune deficiencies in infants due to severe protein-losing enteropathy when total parenteral nutrition is ineffective
6. Treatment of thrombotic thrombocytopenic purpura

Nonindications for Fresh Frozen Plasma

1. Volume expansion
2. Nutritional supplement
3. Postcardiopulmonary bypass prophylaxis
4. Massive blood transfusion prophylaxis

Source: Consensus Development Conference. Fresh-frozen plasma: Indications and risks. *JAMA*. 1985;253:551–553.

Disseminated Intravascular Coagulation

Disseminated intravascular coagulation (DIC) is a relatively recently recognized entity, first appearing in *Index Medicus* in 1973, but one for which numerous etiologies have long produced recognizable clinical syndromes—ranging from the bleeding seen in women with abruptio placenta to that which can follow a hemolytic transfusion reaction. Treatment of DIC requires treatment of the primary cause as well as restoration of an effective hemostatic process. The triad of decreased platelet count, increased prothrombin time, and decreased fibrinogen in the absence of transfusion can be considered diagnostic for DIC. If only two of the three are present, an increase in fibrin split products is necessary. Indeed, in the appropriate clinical setting, a decrease in platelet count and fibrinogen is sufficient to make the diagnosis.[24] Shock and acidosis are commonly seen in the trauma patient and are also potential contributors to initiating DIC.

EXHIBIT 14-2

GUIDELINES FOR USING FRESH FROZEN PLASMA IN MASSIVE TRANSFUSION

1. The initial volume required for significant effect on the coagulation status needs to be large and administered rapidly (ie, 600–2,000 mL over 1–2 h).
2. There is probably no indication for administering fresh frozen plasma (FFP) to patients with severe liver disease and abnormal levels of coagulation factors who are not actively bleeding or facing a hemostatic challenge (any surgical procedure is considered to be a hemostatic challenge).
3. FFP is not likely to help trauma and postoperative patients who are not actively bleeding or patients undergoing elective operations with moderate blood replacement unassociated with shock.
4. FFP may help control abnormal bleeding in trauma patients receiving massive transfusion. Large volumes, rapidly administered, are necessary. Particular attention to platelet levels is more important because dilutional thrombocytopenia is a more common cause of bleeding in this setting.
5. Although there is no shortage of set schedules for administration of FFP, most are unreferenced and anecdotal, and not one regimen has proven effective.
6. Rigid use of the activated partial thromboplastin time or prothrombin time to anticipate the probability of beneficial effect of FFP is not justified. Although these tests may help in individual cases, their poor predictive value for the development of abnormal bleeding diminishes their usefulness.

Source: Braunstein AH, Oberman HA. Transfusion of plasma components. *Transfusion.* 1984;24:281–285.

Surgical Hemostasis

The third element in effective hemostasis, vascular integrity, is usually ignored or relegated to the domain of the surgeon. However, several physiological defense mechanisms will limit blood loss in the body's attempt to maintain homeostasis. Initially, vasoconstriction to decrease the size of the defect and anastomotic dilation to shunt blood away from the defect will limit loss. Furthermore, as blood loss continues without replacement, blood pressure will progressively decrease, thereby minimizing or even halting blood loss. Anesthesiologists can best contribute to the maintenance of vascular integrity by providing adequate anesthesia to avoid hypertension and, where appropriate, using vasoactive agents such as sodium nitroprusside to decrease blood loss by inducing hypotension.

POTENTIAL ADVERSE EFFECTS OF TRANSFUSION

Acid–Base Abnormalities

Patients who require massive blood transfusion become acidotic for two reasons[23]:

1. The need for a large-volume transfusion indicates a massive blood loss, which is consistently associated with decreased blood pressure and perfusion, which in turn may lead to anaerobic metabolism and increasing acidosis.
2. The preservative solutions in which blood is collected are all acidotic, and blood pH at the time of collection will be 7.16. Continued carbon dioxide and lactic acid production without means of escape for the former will decrease the pH to 6.87 at 21 days and 6.73 at 35 days.

Previously, some authorities recommended giving bicarbonate empirically (eg, 44.6 mEq for every five units of whole blood). However, the need for bicarbonate cannot be based on any empirical formula.[28,29] If transfusion in any volume restores hemodynamic stability, then there will be no need for bicarbonate. In the patient who remains in shock, anaerobic metabolism will persist and acidosis will worsen. In such patients, the administration of bicarbonate is better determined by an arterial blood gas analysis than by an empirical formula.

Hypothermia

Blood is stored at 4°C, and approximately 15 kcal are required to raise each unit of whole blood to 37°C, approximately one half that needed for one unit of RBCs.[5] This is not a problem when 1 to 3 units are administered over several hours.[23] However, in massive transfusion, marked hypothermia can occur if the blood is not warmed. Except for possibly decreasing oxygen demand, little good can result from hypothermia (Exhibit 14-3). Even the beneficial effects of decreased oxygen demand are offset by the increased oxygen demand that results from shivering, which can occur with a decrease of 0.5°C to 1.0°C in esophageal temperature.

Warming of blood is best accomplished by means of a high-capacity fluid warmer. There is no shortage of blood warmers available, and their use can avoid or markedly ameliorate the problem of hypothermia in the patient receiving a massive transfusion.[30] This problem is best treated prophylactically.

Hyperkalemia and Hypocalcemia

While blood is stored, potassium concentration progressively increases in plasma as potassium leaches out of the cells, increasing in concentration from 12 mEq/L at 7 days to more than 32 mEq/L at 21 days. This rarely produced a clinical problem in the past, because the blood would have to have been administered at a rate greater than 120 mL/min—a rate that was rarely achieved before rapid-transfusion devices were developed. However, cardiac arrest was recently reported in a patient who received such a transfusion; the rate peaked at 420 mL/min just prior to the arrest. Potassium was 10.7 mEq/L just prior to the arrest and 12.6 mEq/L immediately after.[31]

While the development of hyperkalemia is not a problem in most transfusions, electrocardiographic signs of hyperkalemia, particularly high-peaked T waves and a shortened QT interval, occur initially (serum potassium level 6.0 mEq/L). At serum potassium levels higher than 6.5 mEq/L, the QRS complex widens, simulating left bundle branch block, and the PR interval increases at levels higher than 7.0 mEq/L. Potassium levels higher than 10 to 12 mEq/L produce ventricular fibrillation or asystole. Prophylactic treatment with calcium is not recommended. However, in response to electrocardiographic changes, calcium administration is certainly indicated. Preventive measures include using fresh blood (ie, < 5 d old), rarely a practical solution, or washing the RBCs with saline in a cell saver just before transfusion.[31] The latter has the potential of decreasing potassium once potassium equilibrates sufficiently to produce hypokalemia, which has its own dysrhythmic problems.

As blood is collected in donor bags, chelation of calcium prevents the formation of clots. This has

EXHIBIT 14-3

ADVERSE EFFECTS OF HYPOTHERMIA

1. Metabolism is impaired:
   - citrate and lactate: may lead to hypocalcemia and acidosis.
   - narcotics and anesthetic agents: result in prolonged half-life and delayed awakening, especially undesirable in anesthesia.
2. Release of potassium from intracellular space is promoted. This potassium could be additive with that released in an acidotic state; increased potassium will impair cardiac function.
3. The affinity of hemoglobin for oxygen is increased, thereby decreasing the availability of oxygen stores at the tissue level.
4. Increased risk of dysrhythmias, especially at temperatures < 30°C. Theoretically, rapid transfusion through large central catheters may preferentially cool the myocarcium, resulting in dysrhythmias at body temperatures well above < 30°C.
5. Shivering will increase oxygen demands, producing an increase of oxygen demand and cardiac output.

Source: Collins JA. Problems associated with the massive transfusion of stored blood. *Surgery*. 1974;75:274–295.

been the fundamental principle on which anticoagulation in transfusion medicine is based, whether the anticoagulant is acid citrate dextrose, citrate phosphate dextrose (shelf life 3 wk), or an adenine-containing anticoagulant such as citrate phosphate dextrose–adenine 1 (CPDA-1, shelf life 5 wk), or adenine solution number 1 (ADSOL, manufactured by Baxter Healthcare Corp, Roundlake, Ill; shelf life 6 wk). ADSOL is the chemical preservative most frequently used by the American Red Cross. The U.S. military continues to use CPDA-1. Blood prepared with the latter has a slight logistical advantage because it has a hematocrit of 0.80; the hematocrit of ADSOL-preserved blood is 0.60. Because citrate is always present in excess of the ionized calcium in the unit collected to ensure adequate anticoagulation, the administration of a unit of whole blood or plasma may decrease the ionized calcium in the plasma. This possibility prompted a recommendation to administer ionized calcium on an empirical basis. However, the increased citrate toxicity level is extremely transient because of rapid hepatic metabolism. Indeed, J. P. Bunker's[32] original conclusion that citrate toxicity was a potential problem in patients with impaired hepatic function (made in 1955, a decade before the advent of the ionized calcium electrode) is explained by that patient population's inability to metabolize citrate rapidly. The conclusion remains valid today. The inverse relationship between citrate and ionized calcium levels, as well as the transient nature of any depression on ionized calcium levels after calcium is discontinued, have been shown clearly.[33]

Therefore, the anesthesiologist should remember that *routine* calcium administration is not indicated. If electrocardiographic signs of hypocalcemia develop, manifested by widening of the QRS complex, then calcium administration is indicated. The clinical manifestation of hypocalcemia is, in fact, decreased myocardial contractility, not a hemorrhagic diathesis. Both hemodynamics and the electrical activity of the heart will usually improve promptly as citrate levels decrease. Calcium administration is rarely required.

Transmission of Infection

In 1943, B. B. Beeson[34] reported seven cases of jaundice occurring 1 to 7 months after blood transfusion, the first recognition that infection could be transmitted via blood products. In 1975, the U.S. Food and Drug Administration began requiring that all deaths associated with blood transfusions be reported; during the next decade, 355 deaths were so implicated. Of these deaths, 97 (27.3%) were due to disease transmission, including 3 related to AIDS.[35] Because AIDS was only beginning to surface as a transfusion-associated disease by 1985, with the first death reported in the literature during 1983, the percentage of transfusion-associated AIDS deaths will undoubtedly increase.

Although viral, bacterial, and parasitic diseases can all be transmitted by blood transfusion, the transmission of viral diseases is the major problem. Blood from donors with undetected infections can unintentionally be collected for transfusion in the following circumstances:

1. The donor is either an asymptomatic carrier, or has a clinically inapparent disease, or is in the prodromal stage of infection. Otherwise, the potential donor would have been rejected from donating blood on the basis of the history or physical examination.
2. The disease is in the early stage, where serologic markers of infection have not developed (the "window"), or the disease is one for which routine screening is not yet available.

Viral Diseases

Hepatitis. The demonstration that blood obtained commercially was associated with higher incidences of posttransfusion hepatitis (PTH) than that collected from voluntary donors provided the impetus for an all-volunteer blood-donor system. This was the first positive step to decrease the incidence of PTH. Two studies,[36,37] published 7 years apart, on patients who had cardiac surgery at the National Institutes of Health, Bethesda, Maryland, are revealing. The first, published in 1965, in which the patients had received large volumes of allogenic blood during the early 1960s, demonstrated that patients who receive primarily commercial blood developed either icteric or nonicteric hepatitis in 50% of the cases.[36] In the second, published in 1972, in which the patients received exclusively volunteer blood that was negative for hepatitis A–antigen, the incidence of PTH dropped to 7.1%.[37]

Even in the 1990s, PTH, which produces long- as well as short-term morbidity and mortality, remains the most common infection associated with allogenic blood transfusion. The identified viruses are hepatitis A, B, C (the most recently identified), and delta. During the mid-1960s, two groups of researchers contributed significantly to our knowledge of hepatitis. Saul Krugman and associates[38] clearly distinguished two types of hepatitis, infectious and serum, on the basis of incubation period, history, and duration. At the same time, B. S. Blumberg and associates[39] identified the antigen responsible for serum hepatitis, the so-called "Australian antigen," which originally was found in an Australian aborigine. This antigen is now known to be the unassembled viral coat or surface antigen, HBsAg.

Hepatitis A (infectious hepatitis), caused by the hepatitis A virus (HAV), is a rare cause of PTH for three reasons: (1) there is only a brief (7- to 10-d) viremia during the prodromal phase when patients would be acceptable donors, (2) passively transfused anti-HAV antibodies from other transfused units would prevent HAV from infecting a recipient, and (3) there is no carrier state for HAV.

Hepatitis B, caused by the hepatitis B virus (HBV), remains a source of PTH with an estimated frequency of 1:200 to 1:300, despite the existence since 1971 of a serologic test.[18] Administering blood in emergencies without testing, or collecting blood during the window before serologic markers develop, or both, explain the continued production of PTH by HBV. Of all patients who develop HBV, 90% will have a self-limited course, with the majority being asymptomatic (70% nonicteric); 5% to 10% will go on to a chronic state; and 1% will have a fulminant form of hepatitis with a mortality higher than 50%. Of the 10% who develop a chronic state, one half will evidence one of the chronic forms of hepatitis and the remainder will become asymptomatic carriers.[40] This last cohort is the group without symptoms or history of hepatitis whose blood would transmit HBV were it not for the hepatitis B surgace antigen (HBsAg) test. Two other HBV antigens have been identified: the inner protein core (HBc) and the e antigen (HBeAg), which is a free protein in serum. The development of antibody to HBsAg indicates that immunity to HBV has developed and resolution of the acute infection is occurring, while failure to develop anti-HBs and the persistence of detectable anti-HBc and HBsAg indicate chronic infection.

Hepatitis C, caused by the hepatitis C virus (HCV), has now been identified, having previously been known by the unwieldy term non-A, non-B (NANB) hepatitis, and it is quite likely that some as-yet-undetermined portion of NANB hepatitis is not due to HCV.[41] This virus has a shorter incubation period than HBV (35–70 d) and a milder initial course, with 75% of patients being nonicteric; but 50% of patients will develop a chronic state and 10% will progress to cirrhosis.[42]

Evidence for the role of blood transfusion in the induction of chronic liver disease and the inability to develop a specific NANB hepatitis assay prompted the adoption of surrogate tests for the detection of NANB hepatitis carriers. These were serum alanine aminotransferase and anti-HBc. It was estimated that these surrogate markers would reduce the incidence of NANB hepatitis by 50%, based on retrospective studies conducted at the National Institutes of Health.[40] The effect of the development of a specific assay of HCV is unresolved, as is whether it will negate the use of surrogate tests.

Human Immunodeficiency Virus. Human immunodeficiency virus (HIV) is a ribonucleic acid (RNA) retrovirus first reported to be transmitted by transfusion when a 20-month-old child, who had received blood products from 19 donors in the first month of life during exchange transfusions to treat hemolytic disease of the newborn, developed AIDS.[43] The 1984 Centers for Disease Control (CDC) report received widespread publicity and created, for want of a better term, hysteria in many patients, whose fear of blood transfusion was totally irrational.[44] At the same time, this hysteria has had two positive effects: conservative blood transfusion practices have been promoted, and donor screening has been intensified. The screening, which was initiated to exclude groups at high risk for HIV infection from the donor population, has also served to exclude one primary source of donors transmitting viral hepatitis. Today, approximately 2% of AIDS cases are attributed to the transfusion of single-donor products, and 1% to clotting concentrates in patients with hemophilia.[18,45] Most of these cases were the result of blood transfusions prior to the advent of serologic testing in March 1985, and it is believed that this incidence will decrease in the future. Five steps have been taken to decrease the risk of transfusion-associated AIDS:

1. High-risk groups such as intravenous drug users, sexually active homosexual or bisexual males, individuals with symptoms suggestive of AIDS, and sexual partners of persons with or at risk for HIV infection are excluded.
2. Donors' confidential designation of their blood "for laboratory use only" has been

added to the voluntary self-deferment to avoid potential donor embarrassment or peer pressure to donate.
3. All donor units are screened for HIV antibodies.
4. Blood products manufactured from pooled donor plasma are heated or chemically treated to inactivate HIV and other viruses that might be present.
5. All cases of transfusion-associated AIDS are completely investigated to identify asymptomatic donors. When donors develop AIDS, recipients of all their prior donations should be investigated as part of the American Red Cross' Look-Back Program.[46]

The fact that transfusion recipients of AIDS are infected involuntarily and unknowingly, in contrast to persons who have become infected through risky behavior, has made transfusion-associated AIDS an explosive public issue. Many recipients first became aware of infection through the Look-Back Program and, based in part on that program, it is estimated that 12,000 blood transfusion recipients became infected prior to antibody testing in 1985.[47] The current estimate of transfusion-associated AIDS is between 1:40,000 and 1:1,000,000.[18] These cases are primarily attributed to blood donation during the 6- to 14-week window between infection and the development of HIV antibodies.

Cytomegalovirus. Cytomegalovirus (CMV) is a member of the herpes family, which are all DNA viruses found intracellularly in leukocytes. Thus, there is little risk of transfusion from acellular blood components such as plasma or cryoprecipitate, and minimal risk with leukocyte-poor RBCs. CMV infection is common, with 50% of donors having demonstrated prior exposure as manifested by antibodies, but only 5% to 12% of seropositive donors may be infectious.[48] Normally, only a mild febrile illness is associated with viremia and viruria, followed by seroconversion 13 to 16 weeks later. In contrast to the mild infection described above, immunocompromised patients may develop serious, often fatal, multisystem disease. Infants whose birth weight is low (< 1,250 g), whose mothers are seronegative (ie, no transplacental passive immunization), and who receive seropositive blood are similarly at great risk.

Epstein-Barr Virus. Epstein-Barr virus may be a potential cause of fever in patients without detectable CMV antibodies. More than 90% of donors have antibodies to Epstein-Barr virus,[49] and blood is not screened for them because most individuals are immune to this virus and not susceptible to infection.

Bacterial Diseases

Bacterial contaminants do not present a problem in transfusion practice because both the preservative and the storage temperature (4°C) are bacteriostatic for almost all species. Meticulous cleansing of the puncture site and use of a closed-bag system for collection will continue to make bacterial contaminants a rarity. The final step in preventing the infusion of blood contaminated with bacteria is an inspection of the unit prior to the administration. Hemolyzed or cloudy units should be returned to the blood bank for examination and culture.

Following RBC administration between April 1987 and May 1989, *Yersinia enterocolitica* produced seven cases of sepsis, with five fatalities. These deaths occurred in patients who had received units of RBCs that had been stored for 26 to 40 days prior to transfusion.[50] The bacterium *Y enterocolitica* is unique in that 4°C is not bacteriostatic. Whether these cases are just the tip of the iceberg is uncertain at this time, and the steps to be taken to prevent additional occurrences are not clear. Obviously, a return to 21-day shelf life would solve the problem. However, the impact of that action on the available blood supply would be likely to create more problems than it solves.

Syphilis is no longer common and *Treponema pallidum* is unlikely to survive more than 72 hours in citrated blood stored at 4°C. For that reason, the American Association of Blood Banking standards dropped the requirement for serologic testing for syphilis in 1981. However, federal law, which takes precedence over the American Association of Blood Banking standards, still requires such testing. Because individuals with syphilis may engage in sexual practices that make them at higher risk for HIV infection, serologic testing may further protect the blood supply from transfusion-transmitted hepatitis and AIDS.

For 20 years, it has been the practice to store platelets at room temperature. Bacteremia following platelet transfusion was not recognized until 1981, when new plastic storage containers were introduced; these improved gas exchange and permitted shelf life to be extended from 5 to 7 days. Unfortunately, the longer shelf life also made possible the growth of any contaminating bacteria. As a result of the potential for transfusion-related sepsis, shelf life was returned to 5 days.[51]

Immunosuppression

In 1982, L. Burrows and P. Tartter[52] suggested that blood transfusion adversely affected survival in colorectal cancer. A logical conclusion—that the need for blood suggests a more advanced cancer—has been refuted by other detailed studies.[53,54] These studies suggested that not only colorectal cancer but also cancer of the lung, prostate, kidney, and other organs were adversely affected by blood transfusion. This effect is seen more markedly following transfusion of whole blood transfusion than of RBCs, and has been attributed to an as-yet-unidentified component of stored plasma (or associated cellular-damage debris).[53] Currently, perioperative transfusions have now been correlated with early recurrence and poor prognosis in several forms of malignancy, as well as with increased risk of bacterial infection.[54] Patients receiving exchange transfusions as newborns, during cardiac surgery, or with ulcerative colitis have all demonstrated alterations in their immune parameters; most startlingly, these alterations may persist for 20 years.

There is a beneficial effect of blood transfusion on immunosuppression: recipients of renal transplants who have received previous transfusions are less likely to reject their donor kidneys.

Hemolytic Transfusion Reactions

Traditionally, hemolysis has been thought of as occurring intravascularly or extravascularly. When hemolysis is intravascular (ie, acute), it is associated with complement activation and release of free hemoglobin into the plasma. Extravascular (ie, chronic) hemolysis occurs when macrophages of the reticuloendothelial system destroy RBCs outside the intravascular space; this is the normal mechanism whereby senescent or otherwise nonviable erythrocytes are removed from circulation. Hemolytic transfusion reaction occurs in both types of hemolysis and in both awake and anesthetized patients (Exhibit 14-4).[42] Fever is the most common symptom in both categories of patients; thus, a hemolytic transfusion should be considered any time a febrile reaction follows a transfusion. Similarly, hives and skin rash do not occur in patients who are undergoing hemolytic reactions, which distinguishes this serious reaction from the more common, mild, allergic reactions. Many of these early symptoms are not readily apparent in the anesthetized patient. Indeed, blood oozing from surgical or cannulation sites, hemoglobinuria, and inappropriate hypotension are often the first signs of a hemolytic transfusion reaction under anesthesia. Frequently, such patients are given additional units of incompatible blood before medical personnel realize that a hemolytic transfusion reaction has occurred.

Therapy for the hemolytic transfusion reaction is aimed at preventing renal failure and DIC. Although mannitol has been the traditional drug of choice, volume loading with crystalloid solution and the intravenous administration of furosemide to increase renal blood flow and urinary output are now recommended. Of course, the transfusion must be stopped as soon as the reaction is suspected. Both that unit of blood and all others should be

EXHIBIT 14-4

HEMOLYTIC TRANSFUSION REACTION SYMPTOMATOLOGY

Acute Intravascular Hemolysis

Awake Patients

- Fever
- Tachycardia
- Hemoglobinuria
- Diffuse bleeding
- Back pain
- Nausea
- Flushing
- Dyspnea
- Apprehension
- Chest pain
- Chills

Anesthetized Patients

- Fever
- Tachycardia
- Hemoglobinuria
- Diffuse bleeding
- Hypotension

Chronic Extravascular Hemolysis and Delayed Hemolytic Transfusion Reaction

- Anemia
- Mild jaundice

Reprinted with permission from Ellison N, Faust RJ. Complications of blood transfusion. In: Saidman L, Benumof J, eds. *Anesthesia and Perioperative Complications*. St. Louis, Mo: Mosby–Year Book; 1992: 511.

rechecked in the blood bank, because a systematic clerical error may have cleared all units that were cross-matched at the same time. The coagulation system must be monitored for the development of DIC; platelet concentrates and FFP may be indicated if DIC develops.

Allergic Reactions

Signs and symptoms of an allergic reaction occur in 1% to 2% of recipients and vary from localized urticaria to (rarely) severe anaphylactic reaction. The latter has an estimated incidence of 1 per 20,000 to 1 per 50,000 transfusions. Most allergic reactions are thought to be caused by antibodies against plasma proteins; most are mild and respond to antihistamines.

Severe reactions, manifested by bronchospasm, dyspnea, and pulmonary edema, require treatment with epinephrine and steroids. These reactions may be caused by immunoglobulin (Ig) G or antibodies to IgA in an IgA-deficient patient. If IgA antibodies are found in recipients' serum, only extensively washed RBCs and IgA-deficient plasma should subsequently be administered to that patient.

Febrile Reactions

Approximately 1% of all transfusions are accompanied by a temperature elevation with or without chills. These reactions are usually caused by antibodies to leukocytes or platelets and occur in patients who have been sensitized previously. Leukocyte-poor components will prevent these reactions.

There is no definitive test with which to make the diagnosis of a benign febrile reaction, which may also be the first sign of a hemolytic reaction or the infusion of a grossly contaminated unit of blood. For this reason, temperature elevation requires that more ominous causes be ruled out. When necessary, the fever can usually be treated with antipyretic medication.

ALTERNATIVE SOLUTIONS FOR VOLUME REPLACEMENT

The establishment of an intravenous line is an essential part of the management of almost every patient to be anesthetized. Through that line, a crystalloid solution is commonly administered. There is no controversy over those two steps. The controversy centers around whether to administer crystalloid or colloid solutions to patients, especially those who are experiencing large fluid losses. Table 14-4 compares extracellular fluid with the various replacement fluids. Crystalloid solutions freely cross capillary membranes, and within minutes, 60% to 80% of the solution is found in the interstitial space, with only 20% to 40% remaining intravascular. The failure of crystalloid solutions to provide long-term intravascular expansion has led some clinicians to advocate the use of colloid solutions.

Albumin, 5% or 25% in saline, has an intravascular half-life of 24 hours, as does plasma protein fraction, which contains approximately 80% albu-

TABLE 14-4

COMPARISON OF EXTRACELLULAR FLUID AND VARIOUS REPLACEMENT SOLUTIONS

Solution	Na^+ (mEq/L)	K^+ (mEq/L)	Cl^- (mEq/L)	Total Base (mEq/L)	pH	Ca^{++} (mEq/L)	Mg^+ (mEq/L)	Calories per Liter
Extracellular Fluid	138	5	108	27	7.4	5	3	12
5% Dextrose in Water	0	0	0	0	4.5	0	0	200
Normal Saline	154	0	154	0	6.0	0	0	0
Lactated Ringer's	130	4	109	28	6.5	3	0	9
Normosol	140	5	98	50	7.4	0	3	24
5% Albumin	145	0	90	—	7.4	—	—	—
Heta starch	154	0	154	0	5.5	—	—	—

Reprinted with permission from Ellison N. Fluid and electrolytes and managing blood loss. In: Longnecker DE, Murphy FL, eds. *Introduction to Anesthesia: The Principles of Safe Practice*. 8th ed. Philadelphia, Pa: WB Saunders; 1992: Chap 15: 171.

min and 20% globulin. The latter is less widely used because of hypotension associated with rapid administration of large volumes.[55] Two commercial colloid preparations are available. Dextran is a polymerized glucose molecule with a molecular weight of 40,000 to 70,000 and an intravascular half-life of approximately 6 hours. Doses in excess of 1.5 g/kg/d may be associated with hemostatic disorders and will also interfere with blood typing and cross-matching, owing to coating of the RBCs with dextran. Hydroxyethyl starch is a synthetic polymer composed mainly of amylopectin and has a intravascular half-life longer than 24 hours. The maximum recommended dose is 20/mL/kg/d.

As previously mentioned, tolerance of blood loss down to a predetermined target hemoglobin level is a well-accepted and routine part of the fluid management of any patient undergoing elective surgery. In the patient who is bleeding massively, ideal formulas frequently fail to work and blood replacement is necessary. In these cases, autologous blood—other than that obtained by intraoperative scavenging—is rarely available. In terms of volume administration, the need to provide adequate oxygen transport is really the only requirement for RBCs. As previously discussed, platelets and procoagulate proteins may be necessary to secure hemostasis.

PRINCIPLES OF GOOD CIVILIAN TRANSFUSION PRACTICE

The maintenance of normovolemia is essential for the preservation of homeostasis in the anesthetized patient. While the administration of blood or blood products is often required to maintain normovolemia, their administration may have lethal consequences, as the many complications cited attest. Nevertheless, more than 12 million units of blood or blood components are administered annually to more than 4 million patients in the United States. Their administration is lifesaving in many cases.

The three National Institutes of Health Consensus Development Conferences on Blood Product Administration developed four common themes that are especially applicable to civilian practice[56]:

1. Conservation is the most important way to avoid the risks associated with transfusion of blood products, and every effort should be made to avoid or decrease the need to administer allogenic blood products. Meticulous attention to hemostasis by surgeons and tolerance of lower hemoglobin levels by anesthesiologists are examples of appropriate conservative management.
2. There is a surprising, even appalling, lack of adequate studies on the value of and indications for the blood products in question. This lack is in contrast to the usual well-controlled studies that have accompanied the introduction of other therapeutic maneuvers.
3. Educational efforts, directed at both patients and physicians, are essential. These include, at the local level, strong proponents of modern transfusion practices to disseminate available data and current recommendations.
4. Future research is required to answer basic questions such as the role of platelets in hemostasis, and clinical questions such as the indications for administering RBCs, platelets, and the coagulation factors in plasma.

SUMMARY

In cases of massive blood loss, there is no substitute for the transfusion of allogenic blood. However, there are really only two indications for transfusion: (1) to increase oxygen-carrying capacity, for which RBCs (ideally) and whole blood (alternatively) are indicted; and (2) to secure hemostasis, for which platelets and plasma are indicated.

The administration of allogenic blood is not without risk. Among the several risks associated with blood transfusion, hemolytic transfusion reaction and disease transmission are the most feared. The former can be obviated by careful identification and marriage of the patient's blood sample and the donor unit at the time a blood sample is collected, during the cross-match, and again at the time the donor unit is administered to the patient. Disease transmission cannot always be avoided, for there is always the possibility that the donor has recently been infected and has not yet developed serologic markers of infection. For this reason, it is essential that patients receive only the minimum number of units required to provide adequate oxygen-carrying capacity and to secure hemostasis.

REFERENCES

1. Heaton LD. Foreword. In: Coates JB Jr, ed. *Blood Program in World War II.* Washington, DC: US Army Medical Department, Office of The Surgeon General; 1964: ix.

2. Churchill ED. *Surgeon to Soldiers.* Philadelphia, Pa: JB Lippincott; 1972: 36–58.

3. Crosby WH, Akeroyd JH. Some immunohematologic results of large transfusions of group O blood and recipients of other blood groups. *Blood.* 1954;9:103–116.

4. Miller RD. Complications of massive blood transfusions. *Anesthesiology.* 1973;39:82–93.

5. Collins JA. Problems associated with the massive transfusion of stored blood. *Surgery.* 1974;75:274–295.

6. Neel S. *Medical Support of the US Army in Vietnam, 1965–1970.* Washington, DC: Department of the Army; 1973: 114–126.

7. Barnes A, Allen TE. Transfusion subsequent to administration of universal-donor blood in Vietnam. *JAMA.* 1968;204:147–149.

8. Ellison N, Wurzel HA. The blood shortage: Is other transfusion an answer? *Anesthesiology.* 1975;43:288–290.

9. Myhre BA, Bove JR, Schmidt PJ. Wrong blood—a needless cause of surgical deaths. *Anesth Analg.* 1981;60: 777–778.

10. Ellison N. Central venous access, a mixed blessing. *Semin Anesth.* 1990;9:288–297.

11. Courington FW. Anesthesia guidelines for the trauma patient. *Semin Anesth.* 1985;4:92–101.

12. Schmidt PJ. Red cells for transfusion. *N Engl J Med.* 1978;299:1411–1412.

13. Schmidt PJ. Component therapy. *Int Anesthesiol Clin.* 1982;20:23–43.

14. Counts RB, Haisch C, Simon TL. Hemostasis in massively transfused patients. *Ann Surg.* 1979;190:91–99.

15. Stehling LC, Zauder HL. How low can we go? Is there a way to know? *Transfusion.* 1990;30:1–3.

16. Stehling LC, Zauder HL. Acute normovolemic hemodilution. *Transfusion.* 1991;31:857–868.

17. Ballinger CA, Collins JA. Experts opine. *Surg Anesth.* 1975;19:301–302.

18. Consensus Development Conference. Perioperative red blood cell transfusion. *JAMA.* 1988;260:2700–2703.

19. Levine E, Rosen A, Schgal L, et al. Physiologic effects of acute anemia implications for reduced transfusion trigger. *Transfusion.* 1990;30:11–14.

20. Boerema I, Meyre NG, Brummelkamp WK, et al. Life without blood. *J Cardiovasc Surg.* 1960;1:133–146.

21. Hondow JA, Russell WJ, Duncan BM, et al. The stability of coagulation factors in stored blood. *Aust N Z J Surg.* 1982;52:265–269.

22. Murray DJ, Olson J, Strauss R, Tinker JH. Coagulation changes during packed red cell replacement of major blood loss. *Anesthesiology.* 1988;69:839–845.

23. Pisciott PT, ed. *Blood Transfusion Therapy: A Physician Handbook.* 3rd ed. Arlington, Va: American Association of Blood Banks; 1989.

24. Ellison N. Hemostasis in the trauma patient. *Semin Anesth.* 1985;4:163–176.

25. Ciavarella D, Reed RL, Counts RB, et al. Clotting factor levels and the risk of diffuse microvascular bleeding in the massively transfused patient. *Br J Haematol.* 1987;67:365–368.

26. Consensus Development Conference. Fresh-frozen plasma: Indications and risks. *JAMA.* 1985;253:551–553.

27. Braunstein AH, Oberman HA. Transfusion of plasma components. *Transfusion.* 1984;24:281–285.

28. Collins JA, Simmons RL, James PM, et al. Acid–base status of seriously wounded casualties, II: Resuscitation with stored blood. *Ann Surg.* 1971;173:6–10.

29. Miller RD, Tong MJ, Robbins TO. Effects of massive transfusion of blood on acid–base balance. *JAMA.* 1971;216:1762–1765.

30. Zauder HL. Massive transfusion. *Int Anesthesiol Clin.* 1982;20:157–170.

31. Jameson LC, Popic PM, Harris BA. Hyperkalemic death during use of high-capacity fluid warmer for massive transfusion. *Anesthesiology.* 1990;73:1050–1052.

32. Bunker JP, Stetson JB, Coe RC, et al. Citric acid intoxication. *JAMA.* 1955;157:1361–1363.

33. Denlinger JK, Nahrwold ML, Gibbs DS, Lecky JH. Hypocalcemia during rapid blood transfusion in anesthetized man. *Br J Anaesth.* 1976;78:995–1000.

34. Beeson BB. Jaundice occurring one to four months after transfusion of blood or plasma: Report of seven cases. *JAMA.* 1943;121:1332–1333.

35. Sazama K: Report of three hundred fifty-five transfusion-associated deaths: 1976–1985. *Transfusion.* 1990;30:583–590.

36. Walsh JH, Purcell RH, Morrow AG. Post-transfusion hepatitis after open heart operations. *JAMA.* 1965;211:261–265.

37. Alter HJ, Holland PV, Purcell RH, et al. Post-transfusion hepatitis after exclusion of commercial and hepatitis-B antigen donors. *Ann Intern Med.* 1972;77:691–699.

38. Krugman S, Giles JP, Hammond J. Infectious hepatitis: Evidence for two distinctive clinical, epidemiological, and immunological types of infections. *JAMA.* 1967;200:365–367.

39. Blumberg BS, Gerstley BJS, Hungerford DA, London T, Sutnick AI. A serum antigen (Australia antigen) in Down's syndrome, leukemia, and hepatitis. *Ann Intern Med.* 1967;66:924–931.

40. Rutherford CJ. Transfusion-associated disease. In: Churchill WH, Kurtz SR, eds. *Transfusion Medicine.* Cambridge, Mass: Blackwell Scientific Publications; 1988: 107–127.

41. Kuo G, Choo O-L, Alter HJ, et al. An assay for circulating antibodies to a major etiologic virus of non-A, non-B hepatitis. *Science.* 1989;244:362–364.

42. Ellison N, Faust RJ. Complications of blood transfusion. In: Saidman L, Benumof J, eds. *Anesthesia and Perioperative Complications.* St. Louis, Mo: Mosby–Year Book; 1992: Chap 21.

43. Ammann AJ, Cowan MJ, Wara DW, et al. Acquired immune deficiency in an infant: Possible transmission by means of blood products. *Lancet.* 1983;1:956–958.

44. Curran JW, Lawrence DN, Jaffe H, et al. Acquired immune deficiency syndrome (AIDS) associated with transfusions. *N Engl J Med.* 1984;310:69–75.

45. Busch MP, Young MJ, Samson SM, et al. Risk of human immunodeficiency virus (HIV) transmission by blood transfusions before the implementation of HIV-1 antibody screening. *Transfusion*. 1991;31:4–11.

46. Busch MP. Let's look at human immunodeficiency virus look-back before leaping into hepatitis C virus look-back. *Transfusion*. 1991;31:655–661.

47. Peterman TA, Lui K-J, Lawrence DN, Allan JR. Estimating the risks of transfusion-associated acquired immune deficiency syndrome in humans. *Transfusion*. 1987;27:371–374.

48. Prince AM, Szmuness W, Millian SJ, David D. A serologic study of cytomegalic virus infections associated with blood transfusion. *N Engl J Med*. 1971;284:1125–1131.

49. Henle W, Henle G. Epstein-Barr virus and blood transfusions. *Prog Clin Biol Res*. 1985;182:201–209.

50. Tipple MA, Bland LA, Murphy JJ, et al. Sepsis associated with transfusion of red cells contaminated with *Yersinia enterocolitica*. *Transfusion*. 1990;26:209–213.

51. Food and Drug Administration. Reduction of the maximum platelet storage period to five days in an approved container. *FDA Bulletin*. Washington, DC: Food and Drug Administration; June 2, 1986.

52. Burrows L, Tartter P. Effect of blood transfusions on colonic malignancy recurrence rate. *Lancet*. 1982;2:662.

53. Blumberg N, Heal JM. Transfusion and recipient immune function. *Arch Pathol Lab Med*. 1989;113:246–253.

54. Schriemer PA, Longnecker DE, Mintz PD. The possible immunosuppressive effects of perioperative blood transfusion in cancer patients. *Anesthesiology*. 1988;68:422–428.

55. Ellison N, Behar M, MacVaugh H III, Marshall BE. Bradycardia, plasma protein fraction, and hypotension. *Ann Thorac Surg*. 1980;29:15–19.

56. Ellison N. A commentary on three NIH Consensus Development Conferences on transfusion medicine. *Anesth Clin NA*. 1990;8:609–624.

Chapter 15

MILITARY TRANSFUSION PRACTICE

CHARLES D. BOLAN, Jr., M.D.*; and NOEL R. WEBSTER, M.S.†

*Major, Medical Corps, U.S. Army; Assistant Chief of Medicine, Walter Reed Army Medical Center, Washington, D. C. 20307-5001
†Lieutenant Colonel, Medical Service, U.S. Army; Deputy Director, Armed Services Blood Program Office, Falls Church, Virginia 22041

INTRODUCTION

Transfusion support of resuscitation and surgery in the combat zone is a cornerstone of military medicine.[1–8] Military doctrine includes planning for blood products and the provision of blood components in the combat zone, but it does not include implementation of patient care. This chapter describes a safe and effective transfusion service for the combat zone. It covers clinical, technical, and military aspects of planning and training, including blood component therapy, the variety of transfusion practices in the four echelons of care, the special requirements for women, and the possible impact of research on military blood programs.

Military doctrine for health service support and blood management in a theater of operations is outlined in manuals such as U.S. Army Field Manual 8-55, *Planning for Health Service Support* (FM 8-55).[9] The principles for transfusion practice by echelon are shown in Table 15-1. Doctrine for availability of blood components in theater and for planning factors for blood products is shown in Tables 15-2 and 15-3, respectively. The material in this chapter outlines the implementation of doctrine.

The definition of echelons of care varies according to military service and mission; it is best viewed as a continuum of care rather than as care delivered within rigid, fixed boundaries.[10] In general, second-echelon units (constituted by the medical company/battalion and its organic units) support battalion aid stations, casualty collection points, and other first-echelon of care units. In the army and marines, "second-echelon" corresponds to "division-level" units (eg, clearing stations) that support the medical platoons of maneuver battalions, and the terms are sometimes used interchangeably. Second-echelon units, which are authorized to transfuse only universal-donor (ie, blood group O packed

TABLE 15-1

BLOOD TRANSFUSION PRACTICES BY ECHELON

Echelon/ MMS	Blood Product	ABO and Rh Group	Transfusion Service Procedures	Storage Capacity	Blood Resupply
First	none	—	—	—	—
Second	PRBCs	O, Rh +/–	ABO group donor RBCs†	50 units RBC per field medical refrigerator	Third-echelon BSU
Third					
D304*	PRBCs	O, A, B, Rh +/–	ABO and Rh-group patient and donor RBCs† Major side, immediate spin cross-match	480 units liquid RBCs	Third-echelon BSU
D404*	PRBCs	O, A, B, Rh +/–	Same as D404	Same as D304, plus 475 units frozen	Third-echelon BSU
	FFP	A, B, AB, Rh +/–	None	20 units	Third-echelon BSU
	PLT	O, A, Rh +/–	None	5 units‡	Third-echelon BSU or MTF
Fourth	Same as D404	Same as D404	Same as D404	Same as D404	Fourth-echelon BSU

*Capability to collect and perform the ABO and Rh group determination on 180 units of whole blood for extreme emergencies. D304 is liquid-only DEPMEDS module. D404 is hybrid liquid-frozen DEPMEDS module. D405 is a frozen-blood augmentation set that converts the D304 to D404 capability.
†Not necessary if Armed Services Whole Blood Processing Laboratory has verified the ABO group.
‡One unit = one 6-pack
BSU: blood supply unit; DEPMEDS: Deployable Medical Systems; FFP: fresh frozen plasma; MMS: medical material set; MTF: medical treatment facility; PLT: platelet concentrate; PRBCs: packed red blood cells
Adapted from US Department of the Army. *Planning for Health Service Support*. Washington, DC: Headquarters, DA; approved final draft January 1994. Field Manual 8–55: 8-6–8-7.

TABLE 15-2

BLOOD PRODUCTS AVAILABLE TO THE THEATER

Product	Unit of Issue	Storage	Shelf Life for Transfusion	Echelon Availability	Blood Group Availability O +/–	A +/–	B +/–	AB +/–
Liquid PRBCs	~ 250 mL	35 d	35 d	Second & third (MASH)	100%	—	—	—
				Third (CSH) & fourth	50%	40%	10%	—
Frozen/deglycerolized RBCs	~ 250 mL	10 y	3 d (postwash)	Third & fourth	100%	—	—	—
FFP	~ 250 mL	1 y	24 h (postthaw)	Third & fourth	—	50%	25%	25%
Platelet concentrate	~ 60 mL	5 d	5 d	Third & fourth	50%	50%	—*	—*

*Will be provided by blood bank platoon and medical treatment facilities by in-theater blood collections
CSH: combat support hospital; FFP: fresh frozen plasma; MASH: mobile army surgical hospital; PRBCs: packed red blood cells; RBCs: red blood cells
Adapted from US Department of the Army. *Planning for Health Service Support*. Washington, DC: Headquarters, DA; approved final draft January 1994. Field Manual 8-55: 8-6.

red blood cells ([PRBCs]), have limited patient-holding, laboratory, and radiological capabilities. Located forward of hospitals and lacking surgical capability unless augmented by a forward surgical team, second-echelon units are strategically situated for triage, resuscitation, and stabilization of casualties before they are medically evacuated to higher echelons of care.

Third-echelon facilities (mobile army surgical hospitals [MASHs] and combat support hospitals [CSHs]) provide resuscitative and definitive surgery and have much more extensive laboratory, radiological, patient holding, and nursing support than second-echelon units. As presently configured, the MASH provides liquid group O red blood cells, but not platelets or fresh frozen plasma (FFP). Platelets and FFP are available at CSHs as well as at the fourth echelon. MASHs, CSHs, and fourth-echelon facilities are all authorized for *emergency* collection of limited units of whole blood. Fourth-echelon facilities, such as field hospitals (FH) and general hospitals (GH), have blood banking support similar to that found in a civilian medical center.

Military transfusion therapy is directed to best meet the clinical needs of the casualty within the operational constraints of the tactical situation. The current concept of medical support within a theater of operations is being revised, and units such as MASH, CSH, GH and FH are being reconfigured.

TABLE 15-3

BLOOD PLANNING FACTORS

Blood Component	Planning Factor
Red blood cells	4 units for each WIA and each NBI casualty initially admitted to a hospital*
Fresh frozen plasma	0.08 units for each hospitalized WIA or NBI casualty
Platelet concentrate	0.04 units for each hospitalized WIA or NBI casualty

*For blood-planning purposes, only count the WIA or NBI once in the system, not each time the patient is seen or admitted
NBI: nonbattle injury; WIA: wounded in action
Reprinted from US Department of the Army. *Planning for Health Service Support*. Washington, DC: Headquarters, DA; approved final draft January 1994. Field Manual 8-55: 8-11.

For purposes of this chapter, *second-echelon transfusion capability* refers to the use of group O PRBCs to support resuscitation, and *third-echelon transfusion capability* refers to support of resuscitative surgery without benefit of a full, tertiary care, blood banking capability. In practice, these arbitrary guidelines blur. Resuscitation with blood remains an integral component of surgery at any echelon, and forward surgical treatment squads may be assigned to augment a division clearing station. Conversely, a medical clearing company may augment a CSH, a MASH, or a GH to provide resuscitation and second-echelon medical support in the corps support zone or the communication zone.

BLOOD TRANSFUSION AT THE SECOND ECHELON

Second-echelon medical units are authorized liquid group O PRBCs for initial resuscitation and stabilization. These units thus bring blood the farthest forward on the battlefield and the closest to the casualties. This approach is not new. During World War II, the need for whole blood was recognized and was at least occasionally available at clearing stations (Figure 15-1). The ideal, of course, is to provide blood as close as possible to the location where the casualty was injured, but logistical considerations make this difficult.

Second-echelon blood transfusion conforms with two principles taught in the American College of Surgeons' Advanced Trauma Life Support (ATLS) course[11]:

1. Resuscitation begins as soon as possible (ie, the civilian "Golden Hour", but in military medicine this critical time is much shorter; see Chapter 1, Combat Trauma Overview).
2. Resuscitation with blood is given for hemorrhage of more than 25% to 30% of a casualty's blood volume (Figure 15-2). Casualties with this degree of hemorrhage need the restoration of oxygen-carrying capability that only red blood cells provide; volume expansion with plasma, crystalloid solutions, or albumin will not be sufficient to treat hypovolemic shock.

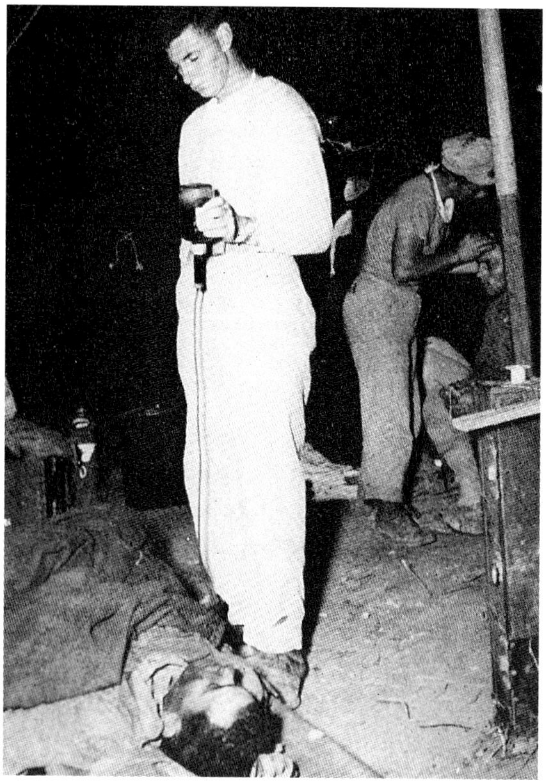

Fig. 15-1. Whole blood is being administered on 21 April 1945 to a casualty at a clearing station of the 102nd Medical Battalion during the savage Okinawa Campaign. Historically, the emphasis has been on giving blood at the surgical level; this photograph reminds us that blood can be given far forward, near the point where casualties are injured. In fact, during the D-day invasion in June 1944, U.S. Navy assault surgeons who landed with U.S. Army troops on Normandy beachheads each carried units of whole blood packed in ice, intending to administer it at the first echelon. Sources: (1) Ben Eiseman, MD, Rear Admiral, Medical Corps, US Navy Reserve (ret), Denver, Colo. Personal communication, June 1995. (2) Photograph: Reprinted from Flick JB, Raine F, Robertson RC. Pacific Ocean areas. In: Carter NB, ed. *Activities of Surgical Consultants*. Vol 2. In: Coates JB Jr, ed. *Surgery in World War II*. Washington, DC: US Army Medical Department, Office of The Surgeon General; 1964: 680.

Transfusion Experience From Previous Wars

The transfusion of red blood cells, either for stabilization prior to medical evacuation or perioperatively, is an essential element of military medical therapy in forward locations. The experiences that follow, of U.S. Army medical officers during World War II, the Korean War, the Vietnam War, and the Persian Gulf War, all (*a*) describe the use of blood at the second echelon and (*b*) further the rationale for the use of blood in forward areas.

World War II

[T]ransfusions...were not ordinarily given in battalion aid stations or in collecting and clearing stations, though occasionally as during the rapid advance at Anzio, these installations were so far ahead of field hospitals that blood was sent to them.[12(p406)]

. . . .

[I]f hemorrhage had occurred, only whole blood could meet the situation. Blood had been used extensively as far forward as battalion aid stations. Given over a 24-hour period, 5,000 cc. could completely change the appearance and outlook of a critically wounded casualty.[12(p635)]

. . . .

When whole blood was immediately available as far forward as clearing companies and portable surgical hospitals, it became the practice to use plasma only when blood was not at hand.

By March of 1945, it was routine for invasion forces to carry blood ashore with them, and it was not uncommon, on reading a casualty's Emergency Medical Tag in a rear hospital, to find that he had received 1 or more pints of bank blood at a clearing company. Some casualties received as much as 6 pints in an hour.[12(p634)]

. . . .

Colonel Churchill had himself supervised the development of the program from his arrival in North Africa in March 1943. His first recommendations were the result of his personal verification of the need for whole blood by his own examination of wounded casualties in clearing stations and forward hospitals.[12(p443)]

Korea

Our military surgeons have become increasingly bold in the use of blood for resuscitation of casualties.[3(p439)]

. . . .

[T]he use of universal blood in the combat zone is a valuable military expedient.... Small but effective banks of blood can be established at the forward aid stations.[3(p455)]

. . . .

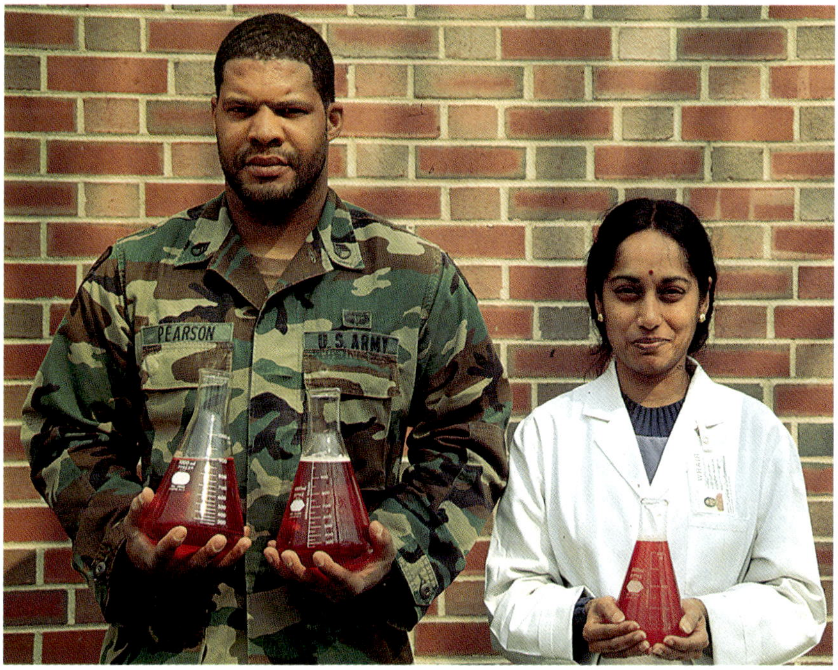

Fig. 15-2. The flasks that this man and woman hold contain fluid representing approximately 25% of their blood volume, based on their gender and weight. Casualties who lose more than this amount of blood require transfusion support with red blood cells to prevent shock.

> In Korea—a stable situation—we sent group O blood forward to the aid stations, where it was stored in wet ice boxes.[13]

Vietnam

> As the troop strength built up, so did the number of medical units receiving blood, ranging from front-line clearing companies to 400-bed evacuation hospitals. By February of 1966 there were 26 separate medical units receiving blood, including 15 medical clearing companies, 3 surgical hospitals etc....[5(p1478)]
>
> ....
>
> During the Plei Me battle, one clearing company of the 1st Air Cavalry Division handled most of the patients, giving 154 units to 94 patients, including 15 units to one soldier with wounds of the arm and throat.[5(p1479)]

Persian Gulf War

> [T]he entire concept and technical details of [administering] blood at the division clearing station have largely been ignored.... [S]ince most patients in the Vietnam war overflew clearing stations and went directly to corps-level hospitals, the institutional memory and clinical art of division blood management suffered a nearly 40-year lapse.[14]

Case Presentation

During Operation Desert Shield of the Persian Gulf War, a 7-year-old boy stepped on a land mine near Al Nasiryah, Iraq, and suffered a near total amputation of his left leg. He was taken by his father to the aid station of 1st Battalion, 504th Parachute Infantry Regiment, 82nd Airborne Division, where bleeding was controlled and intravenous crystalloid solution administered. Despite this initial resuscitation, the child remained in shock. Air evacuation was not available, and he was transported as an emergency via ground ambulance to the medical clearing station in direct support of the brigade.

On arrival at the medical clearing station, the patient remained pale and lethargic. The pulse was more than 150 beats per minute and barely palpable at the femoral artery. The skin was cool and clammy. There was no bleeding from the wound, which was properly bandaged and splinted; two intravenous lines were open, and normal saline was being administered.

One unit of group O PRBCs was administered. The patient's mental status improved and his pink color returned. The pulse became stronger and slowed toward the normal range. A second unit of group O blood was administered and the patient transferred to a holding tent to await routine evacuation.

The management of this casualty illustrates the important role played by maintaining a blood transfusion capability in a second-echelon facility. Clinically, the child was in severe hemorrhagic shock and responded only to replacement of lost blood volume with circulating red blood cells. Large-volume resuscitation with normal saline failed to reverse shock. Plasma, albumin, or other colloid may raise blood pressure and provide temporary improvement, but fail to control shock without red blood cell replacement.[6,11] Logistically, after resuscitation with blood and stabilization, the patient required only routine evacuation, thus reducing the burden on aeromedical evacuation when it resumed.

Field Administration of Group O Packed Red Blood Cells

Basic technical details such as supply and storage requirements; inspection, record-keeping, and inventory procedures; and clinical principles such as technique and patient evaluation must be considered when group O PRBCs are to be administered in the field (Exhibit 15-1 and Figure 15-3). The critical importance of training is discussed later in this chapter.

Technical Factors

Technical factors involve maintaining appropriate transfusion supplies as well as the storage and record keeping required to maintain 30 to 60 units of blood available for transfusion. Infusion sets, normal saline, and group O blood stored in a small thermostabilizer constitute all the supplies necessary to maintain a second-echelon transfusion capability (Figure 15-4). Units of PRBCs can also be safely stored in rigid polystyrene plastic chests containing wet ice. Since all supplies can be stored in the equivalent space of two small chests, a second-echelon transfusion program is entirely consistent with the mobility of a light infantry or airborne unit. The transfusion log is essential; in it, records are kept of unit numbers, blood types, inspections, temperatures, expiration dates, and information about the recipient (Figure 15-5). However, log books are not available for field use—especially at the second echelon—and must be adapted by hand from standard-issue notebooks.

The temperature of the blood must be maintained between 1°C and 6°C—this must be ensured with daily inspections of blood stored in refriger-

EXHIBIT 15-1

FIELD ADMINISTRATION OF GROUP O PACKED RED BLOOD CELLS

Technical Factors

- *Required Supplies.* Infusion sets (eg, from the Blood Chest Packing List of the 307th Medical Battalion [Airborne] Sets, Kits, and Outfits Components Listing, the Chest Med Inst & Supply No. 5, National Stock Number [NSN] 6545-00-914-3500, and Blood Recipient Set Y-Type, NSN 6515-01-128-1407), normal saline, blood log books, blood refrigerator, and group O packed red blood cells (PRBCs) are required.
- *Storage.* Maintain temperature between 1°C and 6°C. Shelf life is 35 days after collection for citrate phosphate dextrose adenine (CPDA-1) PRBCs. Blood will be safe if it remains with wet ice. Consider putting blood in plastic bags to protect label legibility.
- *Inspection.* Inspect daily for temperature and for evidence of hemolysis, package breakdown, or infection.
- *Records.* For all units, record dates, unit numbers, ABO group and Rh type, expiration date, and results of daily inspection. When a unit is infused, record unit information as above, along with the date of transfusion and the casualty's name, service number, and military unit.
- *Inventory.* Maintain 30 to 60 units for a clearing station, 500 or more units at higher echelons. *Coordinate closely with the blood supplier.* Determine how quickly inventory can be reconstituted.
- *Reports.* Report information on inventory, numbers of blood groups, and expiration dates of units on hand. Figure 15-3 is sample blood report.

Clinical Factors

- *Technique.* Infuse intravenously using an infusion set and normal saline.
  - When group O PRBCs are used, it is not necessary to check the casualty's ABO blood group.
  - If the casualty is a woman, make sure Rh factor is correctly matched. Transfuse with Rh-negative blood if Rh factor is unknown.
- *Annotation.* Record the transfusion in the transfusion log and on the casualty's field aid card. Consider pinning the empty unit package to the casualty's clothing for transfer with the casualty to the next echelon of care.
- *Transfusion Volume. Follow clinical, not laboratory, criteria for response.* Look for return of pink color and blood pressure higher than 80 mm Hg systolic. Do not use field laboratory tests to guide transfusion. Consider whether the casualty is likely to be bleeding internally. Avoid excessive transfusion both to conserve blood and to possibly reduce blood loss.

ated or thermostabilized containers, or by keeping blood stored with wet ice. If placed with wet ice, the units may be first placed in a plastic bag to protect against water damage. The expiration date for PRBCs collected in citrate-phosphate-dextrose-adenine (CPDA-1) solution shall not exceed 35 days after phlebotomy. Units must be inspected daily for evidence of hemolysis and package integrity. It is crucial that the number, type, and expiration dates of all units be recorded in the daily log. The recipient's patient identification number, name, military unit, and the date should also be recorded when a unit is transfused. It is imperative that each unit received have a final record of disposition (eg, the unit was transfused, destroyed, shipped to another facility, etc) and that the record be maintained indefinitely. In prior conflicts, some physicians have stored blood for up to 10 days past expiration when daily inspections remained normal for use as a last resort in a mass casualty situation. Personnel must quickly determine the frequency and format of desired reports and procedures for resupply with the blood-supply program (these are discussed later in this chapter under Planning and Training).

Clinical Factors

Since the major cause of transfusion reactions is the inadvertent administration of correctly typed and cross-matched blood to *the wrong patient*, it is

______________________________ This is ______________________ Blood Report Over
(Addressee) (Originator)

Addressee answers, then originator responds: This is ______________________

FLASH **IMMEDIATE** **PRIORITY** **ROUTINE** **(Underline and transmit the precedence of this message.)**

TOP SECRET **SECRET** **CONFIDENTIAL** **UNCLASSIFIED** **(Underline and transmit the security classification of this message.)**

BLOOD REPORT

Line 1 (or as of) ______________________ (Day-time-zone of this report. Use Zulu time!)

Line 2 (or unit) ______________________ (Reporting unit's name or designator code.)

Line 3 (or activity) ______________________ (Reporting unit's activity brevity code letter.)

Line 4 (or location) ______________________ (Unit location in LAT/LONG, UTM, or place name.)

Line 5 (or rendezvous) ______________________ (NAVAL VESSELS ONLY: Projected location in LAT/LONG or place name for delivery of blood products.)

Line 6 (or arrival) ______________________ (NAVAL VESSELS ONLY: Estimated time of arrival [day, time, time zone, month, year] at the projected location.)

Lines 7–12 may be repeated as a group when more than one activity must be reported in a message.

Line 7 (or status of) ______________________ (Name or designator code of the unit of activity reporting status of blood supplies if other than message originator.)

Line 8 (or activity) ______________________ (Reporting unit's activity brevity code letter if other than message originator.)

Line 9 (or on hand) ______________________ (Number and code of each blood product on hand.)

Line 10 (or needed) ______________________ (Number and code of each blood product requested.)

Line 11 (or expiration) ______________________ (Estimate of total number of blood products by group and of those that will expire in the next 7 days.)

Line 12 (or resupply) ______________________ (Estimate of total number of blood products by group and type required for resupply in the next 7 days.)

Line 13 (or narrative) ____

____

Line 14 (or time) ______________________ (Message hour-minute-zone when required. Use Zulu Time!)

Line 15 (or authentication is) ______________________ (Message authentication IAW JTF procedures.)

MESSAGE MODIFIERS

Management Offices:
A Joint Blood Program Office
B Area Joint Blood Program Office

Facilities:
C Armed Services Whole Blood Processing Laboratory
D Blood Donor Center
E Blood Products Depot
F Blood Transshipment Center
G Blood Supply Unit
H Medical Treatment Facility
I Naval Vessel

Blood Products:
J Red Blood Cells (Packed)
K Whole Blood
L Frozen Red Blood Cells
M Fresh Frozen Plasma
N Frozen Platelets

Blood Groups:
O To Be Determined
P To Be Determined
Q Random Group and Types O, A, B
R Random Group and Types O, A
S Group O
T Group A
U Group B
V Group AB

Time Frame:
W Required Within 12 Hours
X Required Within 24 Hours
Y Required Within 48 Hours

Miscellaneous:
Z Not Applicable, or See Remarks

Fig. 15-3. Sample Blood Report used by the 655th Medical Company (–), USAREUR Blood Bank, Operation Desert Shield, Fall, 1990.

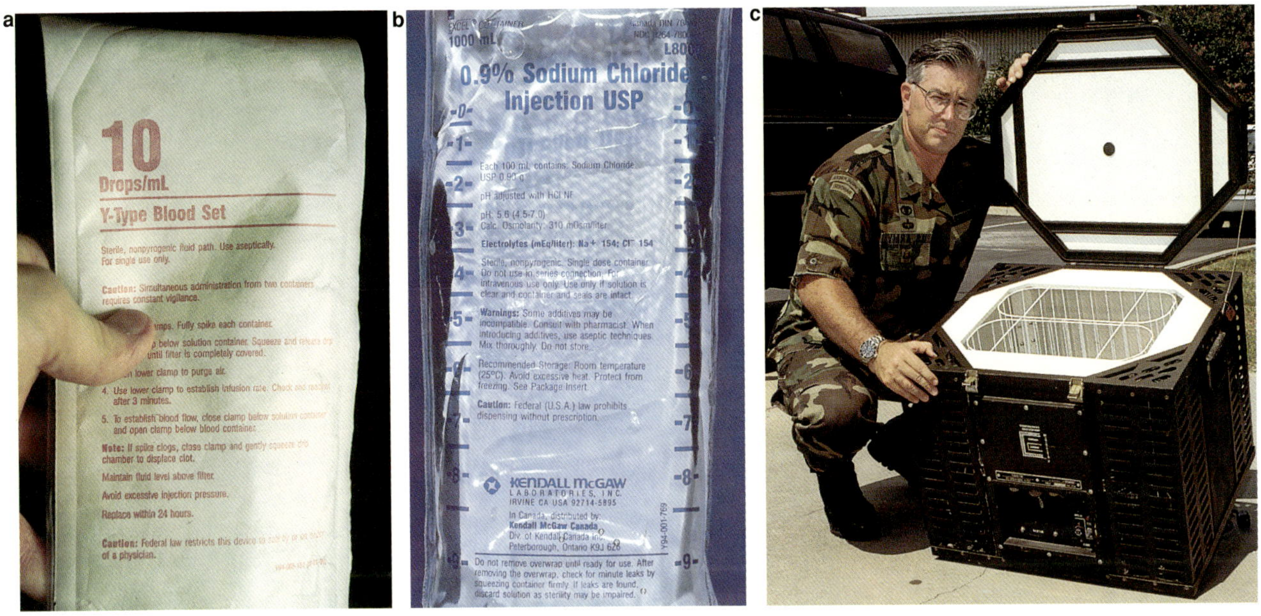

Fig. 15-4. Blood supplies and refrigerator (thermostabilizer, also called the blood box) for field transfusion of packed red blood cells (PRBCs). (**a**) Infusion set needed to administer blood, which should be infused with normal saline through a simple intravenous catheter. (**b**) Normal saline; blood should not be transfused through the same catheter with hypotonic fluid or lactated Ringer's solution. (**c**) The thermostabilizer is manufactured by Thermopol, Inc, Chicago, Ill; weight: 83 lb; dimensions: 25 in. (w) x 21 in. (l) x 22.5 in. (h). This chest can be connected to either generator power or the direct current of a vehicle battery. These items, the transfusion log book and reports seen in Figure 15-5, and group O PRBCs constitute all the supplies required to run an effective second-echelon transfusion program.

imperative to use only group O PRBCs obtained through established blood program channels at second-echelon facilities. The appropriate connections between patient, infusion set, and donor unit should be mastered and practiced in advance in mock situations with simulated patients before being used on casualties.

Normal saline is the only crystalloid fluid to be infused with blood during a transfusion. Hypotonic solutions such as dextrose in water or half-normal saline can cause hemolysis. Calcium in lactated Ringer's solution will complex citrate and may cause coagulation.[15] The American Association of Blood Banks' *Technical Manual* recommends that lactated Ringer's solution not be infused with blood.[16]

The volume of blood required for transfusion is determined *clinically* and should be an amount that restores mentation, circulatory stability, pink color, and a systolic blood pressure of about 80 mm Hg to the patient. Continued infusion after these criteria have been met can promote further bleeding in patients with internal injuries, and waste limited supplies of blood.[2] Recent studies suggest that immediate, full-volume resuscitation may not be optimal for patients with penetrating chest injuries,[17] and the proper timing and amount of fluid resuscitation is not yet known with certainty.[18] Laboratory tests such as measuring the hematocrit are not appropriate measures of response to transfusion in trauma patients in a field setting.

After transfusion, the unit's number and blood type should be noted on the casualty's field aid card (ie, the emergency medical tag); the empty unit should be pinned to the patient's clothing while the patient is being transported. Knowledge of the number and type of previously transfused units may be useful in guiding therapy for possible subsequent transfusions at higher echelons.

Field Management of Transfusion Reactions

The signs and symptoms of a transfusion reaction can be subtle.[19] The diagnosis may be especially difficult in a field setting and in casualties with internal injuries and dirty wounds. However, abrupt fever, chills, hypotension, hemoglobinuria, hemoglobinemia (in plasma), or shortness of breath in the appropriate setting may provide sufficient evidence of hemolysis to initiate therapy (Exhibit 15-2). Infusion of the unit of blood should be stopped while the intravenous catheter remains in place infusing normal saline. Every attempt should be made to maintain blood pressure and urinary out-

Blood Inventory Tracking Operation

Name of Medical Care Facility

1. Unit Number	2. Expiration Date	3. Product Type	4. Cryovial Location	5. BSU	6. Medical Unit	7. Date Issued	8. Disposition Date	9. Reason	10. Method	11. Location	12. Report to JBPO

1. Input number of unit of blood
2. Input the expiration date of unit of blood
3. Input ABO/Rh of unit
4. If frozen units are deglycerolized, indicate the location of the cryovial if known
5. Indicate the name of the BSU that supplied the unit of blood
6. Medical care facility dispositioning the blood
7. Date blood was issued by the BSU, or received by the medical facility
8. Date blood was disposed or shipped
9. Indicate the reason that the blood was dispositioned (ie, expired, shipped)
10. Means of disposal (ie, incinerated, autoclaved)
11. Where the blood was dispositioned (ie, afloat)
12. JBPO will indicate date when report is received

Frequency of transmission of reports will be determined by the JBPO.

At the least, the disposition of units must be submitted on redeployment of the MTF.

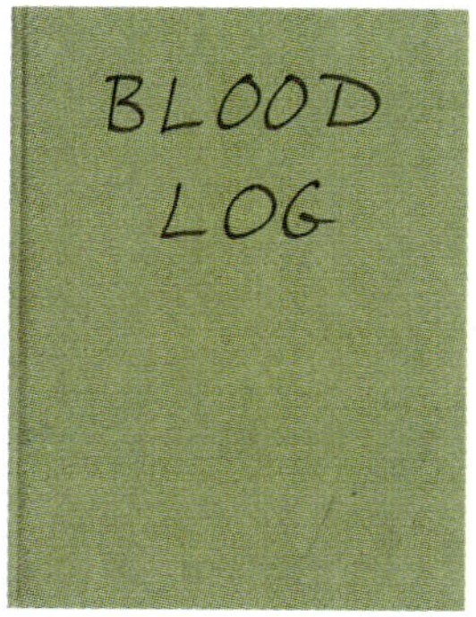

Blood Inventory Tracking Operation

Transfused Units

1. Unit Number	2. Expiration Date	3. Product Type	4. Cryovial Location	5. BSU	6. Medical Unit	7. Date Transfused	8. Patient's Name	9. Patient's SSN	10. Note	11. Report to JBPO

1. Input number of blood unit transfused
2. Input the expiration date of the blood unit transfused
3. Input ABO/Rh of unit transfused
4. If deglycerolized red cells are transfused, indicate thelocation of the cryovial if known
5. Input name of BSU supplying blood; if unknown, leave blank
6. Medical care facility transfusing the blood
7. Date of blood transfusion
8. If unknown, indicate nationality or branch or service (ie, Haitian 1)
9. If unknown, indicate patient's nationality (ie, Haitian)
10. Indicate the reason for the transfusion (ie, gunshot wound)
11. JBPO will indicate date when report is received

Frequency of submission of reports will be determined by the JBPO.

At the least, the disposition of transfused units must be submitted on redeployment of the MTF.

Fig. 15-5. Blood Inventory tracking operation reports. Blood log is a standard-issue notebook adapted for use with hand-drawn labels and report sheets. Blood Inventory Tracking Operation reports adapted from US Department of the Army. *Planning for Health Service Support*. Washington, DC: Headquarters, DA; approved final draft January 1994. Field Manual 8-55: Chap 8, Section V.

EXHIBIT 15-2

FIELD MANAGEMENT OF A TRANSFUSION REACTION

- Stop the infusion of blood. Continue to infuse normal saline through the intravenous line.
- Examine the urine for hemoglobinuria. Examine plasma for hemoglobinemia.
- Maintain blood pressure and urinary output with saline. Consider administering mannitol or furosemide after volume repletion if the patient is oliguric.
- Reexamine the donor unit for seal integrity, evidence of hemolysis or infection, and recheck the transfusion log for clerical error.
- Annotate the field medical card with a description of the suspected reaction and the therapy provided. Transfer the unit suspected of causing the reaction to the next echelon of care with the casualty.

put with continued saline infusion; if urinary output decreases, then furosemide or mannitol may improve renal function. Benadryl (diphenhydramine hydrochloride, manufactured by Parke-Davis, Morris Plains, N.J.) may be useful for treating hives and itching.

The donor unit should be reexamined for compatibility with the blood type of the recipient as well as for evidence of infection, loss of package integrity, hemolysis, and, in winter, freezing, which can cause hemolysis. The suspected reaction and its management should be annotated both on the casualty's field aid card and in the transfusion log; if possible, the unit of blood should be transferred with the casualty during evacuation to the next echelon of care.

TRANSFUSION SUPPORT AT THE THIRD AND FOURTH ECHELONS

Because blood transfusion is an integral part of surgery, third- and fourth-echelon facilities perform all aspects of transfusion therapy with PRBCs described for second-echelon facilities. Third- and fourth-echelon facilities have improved laboratory and blood banking capability, and are responsible for more complex transfusion practices (Table 15-4). Some third-echelon, and all fourth-echelon facilities may be required to support surgery with random-mix instead of universal-donor group O PRBCs (see Tables 15-1 and 15-2). Compared with the use of group O universal-donor PRBCs, the use of random-mix blood greatly increases the risk of transfusion reactions and requires testing of the recipient's blood group—with attendant delays in therapy as well as increasing the requirement for laboratory testing. Random-mix blood must only be used with trained and tested personnel in authorized laboratories. Some experienced military clinicians[13] argue strongly that only group O universal-donor PRBCs should be available within the entire combat zone; this, however, is not present doctrine. Support with frozen blood and other blood products such as platelets and FFP may also be authorized. Finally, third- and fourth-echelon units are authorized by doctrine to perform emergency collection and transfusion of blood that is collected in the field when blood products are unavailable through regular channels.

Logistical Aspects

The requirements for liquid PRBCs have already been described. Additional blood banking capa-

TABLE 15-4

MEDICAL LABORATORY PROCEDURES, BLOOD BANK

Description	MASH	CSH	FH	GH
Perform blood group and type (ABO, Rh)	x	x	x	x
Perform blood cross-matches		x	x	x
Thaw fresh frozen plasma		x	x	x
Issue platelet concentrate		x	x	x

Reprinted from US Department of the Army. *Planning for Health Service Support*. Washington, DC: Headquarters, DA; approved final draft January 1994. Field Manual 8–55: 7-5.

bility for military medical facilities in the Department of Defense's Deployable Medical Systems (DEPMEDS) configurations is determined by the blood bank section. The Liquid Blood Bank Medical Material Set (MMS) D304 can store 500 units of PRBCs, and can perform ABO grouping, Rh typing, and a single-tube (major-side saline, immediate spin) cross-match on each patient. The Liquid/Frozen Blood Bank MMS D404 has the same capacity for liquid PRBCs as the MMS D304, but can also store 485 units of frozen PRBCs, 10 units of FFP, and 5 units of platelets (each unit of platelets contains six platelet packs). The MMS D404, when fully staffed and supplied, should be capable of reconstituting 180 units of frozen PRBCs in 24 hours. Both blood bank sections should be able to issue up to 250 units of banked PRBCs in 24 hours, and are authorized to collect and type 180 units of fresh whole blood for extreme emergencies.[10] (See Chapter 6, Deployable Hospitals, for a more complete discussion of MMSs and their use in DEPMEDS-equipped hospitals.)

The use of frozen red blood cells allows large amounts of universal-donor blood to be prepositioned at military medical facilities outside the continental United States (OCONUS), which has the theoretical potential to minimize long supply lines from CONUS. However, frozen red blood cells require storage in –80°C freezers, as well as large volumes of sterile crystalloid, special processing equipment, trained personnel, and, after being thawed, at least 1 hour per unit to process for deglycerolization. After they are thawed, frozen red blood cells have a shelf life of only 24 hours; however, this time may be extended under emergency military conditions to 72 hours.[20] Although future research may improve the utility of frozen blood, at present these factors may limit its use in forward locations.[20,21] Frozen blood remains an integral part of doctrine. Medical officers assigned to areas that utilize frozen blood resources should be especially careful to start early, hands-on planning and realistic training to determine the system's clinical utility.

Platelets require storage at 20°C to 24°C with continuous gentle agitation, and have a 5-day viable shelf life after collection. One unit of FFP contains one unit of all clotting factors per milliliter, and must be stored at –18°C or colder. FFP has a shelf life of 12 months when stored at this temperature and must be administered within 24 hours after being thawed. Given these constraints, the availability of FFP and, especially, platelets may be limited in the combat zone.[9]

Effect of Massive Transfusion

Resuscitation and surgery of the severely wounded casualty may require large amounts of blood. Massive, large-volume transfusions can rapidly reduce a medical treatment facility's blood supplies. This may also lead to subsequent difficulties in patient management, including dilutional coagulopathy and selection of appropriate blood group for further transfusion. The management of a dilutional coagulopathy is described in Chapter 14, Transfusion Therapy.

The *subsequent* transfusion management of the patient who survives surgery with massive transfusion requires that attention be paid to both the patient's ABO blood group and the blood group of the units previously transfused.[22] Patients with A, B, or AB blood groups who have received more than 4 units of group O whole blood, or 8 units of group O PRBCs, should be transfused with group O blood if further transfusions are needed for at least 2 weeks or until their serum is compatible with the donor blood type as determined by a full compatibility test.[22,23]

Emergency Collection and Transfusion of Whole Blood Donated in the Field

Collection and transfusion of fresh, whole blood in the field (authorized by doctrine at third- and fourth-echelon facilities *under emergency conditions only*) is a source of platelets, plasma, and red blood cells. Because whole blood contains plasma with antibodies to the antigens not present on the donor's red blood cells, it is necessary to do full ABO group determination on both the donor's and the recipient's blood. The principles involved in performing an emergency collection of whole blood in the field are outlined in Exhibit 15-3.

When performing an emergency collection, a key factor is the potential risk of infection. Infections may be caused by viruses (such as the human immunodeficiency virus, parvovirus, or hepatitis) or other organisms (such as those that cause malaria or syphilis) transmitted via the donor's blood, or bacterial skin flora contracted by the use of improper sterile technique. Sterility is best ensured by using (*a*) Betadine Solution (povidone-iodine, 10%, manufactured by Purdue Frederick, Norwalk, Conn.) to scrub the donor's arm and (*b*) the appropriate collection technique. Blood must be collected into a sterile, closed, blood-collecting and -dispensing bag. Because blood is a fertile culture medium, small amounts of contaminating bacteria may grow rap-

EXHIBIT 15-3

EMERGENCY COLLECTION AND TRANSFUSION OF BLOOD DONATED IN THE FIELD

This collection and transfusion technique should be used in extreme emergencies after all efforts to obtain adequate supplies of blood collected by blood banks have failed. Emergency collection should *never* be performed in lieu of securing blood through normal channels. Although the following information is provided so that the technique can be performed as safely as possible in this contingency, the emphasis should be on careful planning to obtain an adequate supply of blood-bank-procured blood.

Donor Factors

Lab tests for transmissible infection may not be available in the field. Careful screening of a donor's *risk* for infection is thus essential. Strongly consider recruiting volunteers who were active blood bank donors prior to deployment—their blood and their risk for infection will have been checked repeatedly during that period. Recognize that military units may place pressure on their members to donate; give a donor a chance to decline in private in case he or she is unwilling to admit to potentially risky behavior. Donations may be obtained every 6 to 8 weeks from healthy male donors. After donating, the donor should be given oral fluid replenishment and, if possible, light duty for 12 to 24 hours. Donors screened in the field should be questioned regarding the following topics:

- history of intravenous drug use,
- history of hepatitis,
- history of high-risk sexual behavior,
- exposure to malaria, dengue fever, or recent febrile illness,
- prior blood transfusion, and
- prior or current pregnancy.

Collection Factors

Scrupulously scrub the donor's vein with Betadine Solution (povidone-iodine, 10%, manufactured by Purdue Frederick, Norwalk, Conn.). The collecting unit is a closed system, with a measured amount of sterile anticoagulant and preservative already in place. A volume of 450 to 500 mL should be collected. The unit of whole blood should be cooled immediately and used as soon as possible. Assign the collected unit an identification number, and enter the number in the blood log. A tube of serum from the donor should be saved indefinitely for future testing and tracking. The appropriate supplies, listed below, must be available in advance:

- blood collection sets;
- Betadine swabs to sterilize the collection site;
- appropriate markers to label and identify the collected unit;
- typing sera for groups A and B blood, which must be kept cool with blood in the refrigerator;
- glass slides, mixing swabs, wax pencils, and lab slips;
- purple-top blood tube (containing ethylehediaminetetraacetic acid [EDTA] anticoagulant); and
- red-top tube for serum sample.

Transfusion Factors

Transfusion of whole blood must be fully ABO specific because the plasma in the donor's blood may have high levels of antibodies to the recipient's antigens. (Universal-donor group O whole blood, as used in the Korean and Vietnam wars, was checked to ensure that the antibody titer was not elevated prior to shipment to a combat zone.) Full blood typing, with determination of Rh, and cross-matching should be performed on both the donor unit and the recipient.

idly, especially if the unit is warm and not used immediately. Thus, scrupulous sterile technique is essential, and the collected unit should be labeled, cooled, and used as soon as possible. The collected unit should (*a*) be given a unique unit-identification number (eg, the social security number of the donor) and (*b*) be added to the blood inventory and disposition records.

Currently, laboratory tests to screen the donor unit for infectious diseases are not available in the field setting, although some may be developed in the near future. *Questions to determine the donor's potential risk for transmissible infections* (eg, a history of drug use, high-risk sexual behavior, hepatitis, or recent febrile illness) are thus *critical to selection of the safest donor in a field environment*. Current policy mandates that a sample tube of serum from the donor be retained and stored for future testing and tracking if necessary. The physician should also consider a potential donor's time in country and possible exposure to endemic disease such as malaria. The individuals who can most safely donate are those who give a negative response to these questions and who have been successfully screened and used as regular blood donors prior to deployment. Although there will be heavy peer pressure on potential donors to provide blood for their wounded comrades, they should be given a chance to decline in private, according to procedures established in civilian blood banks. Again, the technique of emergency collection and transfusion of whole blood should only be used under dire circumstances when there is absolutely no other source of blood and when the casualty would die without transfusion.

MILITARILY UNIQUE CONSIDERATIONS

The administration of group-specific blood, proper use of identity tags, and clinical relevance of the Rh blood group for female casualties pose challenges for military physicians in the combat zone. Research is active and the development of new products and technology can be anticipated. Integration of these factors into appropriate planning and training exercises is critical to successful military transfusion practice.

Group-Specific Transfusion and Random-Mix Blood

Universal-donor group O PRBCs are the optimal resuscitation fluid for a combat casualty; however, the supply may be limited in a combat zone. Liquid group O PRBCs comprise only 50% of blood collected and shipped to a combat zone. Because second-echelon units are authorized by doctrine to receive only group O PRBCs, the supply of universal-donor group O PRBCs may be more limited at third- and fourth-echelon units, and may become limited at second-echelon facilities during peak demand for blood.

Group-specific transfusion refers to blood that is matched on the basis of the donor's and the recipient's ABO groups alone. Random-mix blood refers to a supply of PRBCs that has been collected from donors of all blood groups. Administration of group-specific, random-mix blood requires correct determination of the recipient's ABO blood group *and* the correct administration of the appropriate unit to the recipient. In contrast, group O PRBCs may be transfused in an emergency without regard for either testing the recipient[24,25] or matching the appropriate unit with the recipient.

The determination of the recipient's blood group and the safe transfusion of random-mix blood under combat or mass casualty conditions, even with the laboratory capability of a fourth-echelon tertiary facility, require extensive, careful planning and training. The potential risks and logistical problems may be understood by considering the nature of the ABO blood groups.

The ABO blood groups are named for the antigen or antigens that are present on the surface of red blood cells (Figure 15-6).[26] Shortly after birth, we develop immunoglobulin (Ig) M antibodies directed against the antigen or antigens that are not present on our own red blood cells. Thus, individuals with group O blood have neither the A or the B antigen present on their red blood cells, but have antibodies against both A and B antigens in their plasma. Individuals with group A blood have only the A antigen present on the red cells, and have antibodies to the B antigen in the plasma. These IgM antibodies are present shortly after birth and efficiently activate complement when combined with antigen. An ABO-mismatched transfusion is immediately life-threatening and may cause hemolysis, hemoglobinuria, hypotension, renal failure, and death.[19]

Group O PRBCs, which comprise approximately 40% to 50% of the blood supply, can safely be infused into casualties of any ABO blood group regardless of the recipient's blood group. Group O *whole* blood, which was used as universal-donor blood during World War II and the Korean and Vietnam wars, can also be safely infused if special laboratory techniques demonstrate that the donor plasma (which is infused with the unit of whole blood) does not have high-titer anti-A or anti-B antibodies.[5,12] However, transfusion of whole blood or PRBCs of the A, B, and AB blood groups can only be given to casualties who have these same blood antigens present on their red cells. Thus, transfusion of PRBCs of any blood group other than O

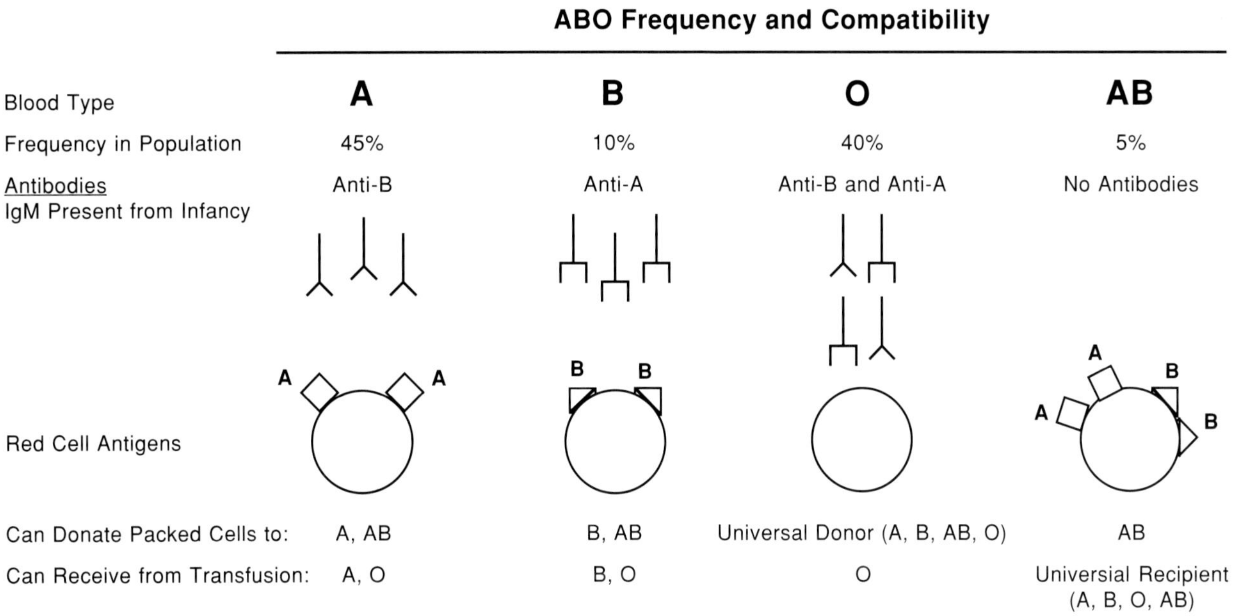

Fig. 15-6. The nature of blood and the ABO blood groups.

requires knowledge and confirmation of both the recipient's and the donor's blood groups.

Identification Tags

Determination of blood groups for identification tags (ie, dog tags) is not done in medical laboratories, and there may be a 3% to 6% error rate in either the ABO or the Rh blood groups,[27] although a recent study[28] indicates that the risk may be lower. During World War II, however,

> when blood had to be given in emergencies in forward hospitals and tests for compatibility were impractical, the blood group of the recipient had to be accepted on the basis of his identification tag, in which the known error was from 5 to 25 percent.[12(p429)]

Previously, these percentages of error had been acknowledged in the context that dog tags were designed only to identify *potential* donors and were not designed to be used for transfusions on individual patients.[12,27] However, even contemporary medical officers who are unfamiliar with this philosophy may assume that identity tags are provided to guide transfusions without confirmatory testing, as World War II–era medical officers did:

> Circular Letter No. 170, Office of The Surgeon General, War Department, Services of Supply. In this letter [dated 2 December 1942], it was pointed out that the policy of blood grouping of military personnel and its purpose seems to have been misunderstood by some medical officers.... [T]he assumption that the first [dog tag or identification tag] typing test would be the only one performed was based on a false premise. To correct the misconception it was pointed out again that the purpose of the program was to simplify assembling donors whose blood would probably crossmatch with that of intended recipients.[12(p235)]
>
> . . . .
>
> Our physicians were amazed to learn, well into development of our blood program, that the error rate in dog tags was as high as 5–10%, and that dog tags were not designed to be a field expedient means to transfuse random mix blood. We also found that we did not know the blood type for civilian casualties.[29]

In addition, civilian casualties will not have identity tags, which further illustrates the inappropriateness of using identity tags for type-specific blood transfusion.

Finally, identity tags may be used in the future in second-echelon facilities, which use universal-donor group O PRBCs, to match the Rh group of the casualty with that of the donor unit (this subject is discussed in greater detail later in this chapter). Priority for Rh-negative blood will be given to female casualties.[30] This strategy would (*a*) decrease exposure and sensitization of Rh-negative female casualties to Rh-positive blood, (*b*) represent a significant change in the doctrinal use of identity tags, and (*c*) require improved testing capability and further education and training.

Female Casualties and Rh Blood Groups

Military medical officers must carefully consider the relevance of the Rh blood group system and the different clinical implications of Rh-mismatched blood transfusions when administered to male or to female combat casualties. The Rh blood groups and antibodies differ clinically from those in the ABO system; they were not identified until more than 30 years after discovery of the ABO blood groups, when they were determined to be the major cause of hemolytic disease of the newborn. Approximately 85% of the population is Rh positive; 15% is Rh negative.[31] Acute intravascular hemo-lytic reactions in Rh-mismatched transfusions are rare, because antibodies formed against Rh antigens are IgG, and unlike IgM–ABO antibodies, do not activate complement efficiently. Additionally, these IgG antibodies appear in Rh-negative patients only after exposure (ie, sensitization) to Rh-positive blood and are not present from birth like the antibodies to ABO antigens. Sensitization occurs most frequently in Rh-negative women after exposure to the blood of an Rh-positive fetus at childbirth. Rh-mismatched transfusion reactions are thus usually not immediately life threatening, and are manifest by chronic, extravascular hemolysis that appears several weeks after exposure to Rh-positive blood. However, unlike ABO antibodies, these IgG antibodies do cross the placenta, and, in the Rh-positive fetus of an Rh-negative, previously sensitized mother, will cause chronic extravascular hemolysis or hemolytic disease of the newborn (Figure 15-7).

Thousands of Rh-negative male combat casualties have been transfused with Rh-positive blood without clinically significant consequences.[5,12] There is a much smaller experience with transfusion of Rh-mismatched blood to female civilian trauma casualties,[32,33] including cases that have resulted in legal action.[34] In the future, medical officers will likely care for more female casualties in combat. Some major clinical factors that should be considered are discussed in Exhibit 15-4.

Active Research Efforts

A major goal of military research is to develop blood products for field use, thus providing essential support for resuscitation of the wounded soldier immediately or within the first few hours after the injury is sustained. The research and development for such products is being conducted in universities, by the American Red Cross, and in

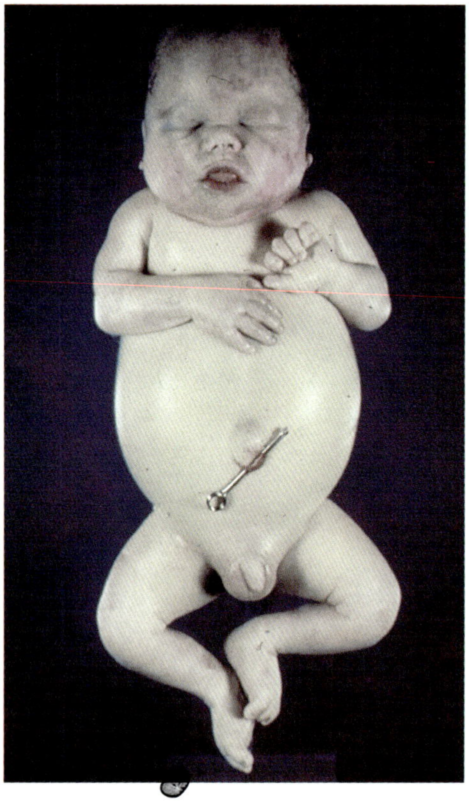

Fig. 15-7. The consequences of administering Rh-positive blood to Rh-negative women are not immediately apparent but neither are they benign. This third-trimester fetus died of chronic hemolytic disease of the newborn, which occurs in Rh incompatibility when an Rh-positive fetus is conceived in an Rh-negative, but sensitized, mother. The immunoglobulin G antibodies in the mother's blood cross the placenta and cause chronic hemolysis with hyperbilirubinemia and enlargement of the fetus' blood-forming organs. Antibodies to Rh groups form only after an Rh-negative individual is exposed to Rh-positive blood. This occurs most commonly in women after they give birth to an Rh-positive child. *Sensitization and antibody formation will also occur in Rh-negative battlefield casualties who receive transfusions of Rh-positive blood.* Owing to the relative frequency of Rh-negative individuals in the general population, Rh-mismatched blood transfusions have been given widely in prior wars; however, the casualties were male. In both men and sensitized women, the immediate consequences of an Rh-mismatched transfusion are clinically mild and at the time of future surgery can be managed routinely with modern blood banking techniques. However, women who are sensitized will be at risk for severe complications of pregnancy in an Rh-positive fetus. Photograph: Courtesy of Colonel John Pierce, MD, Medical Corps, US Army; Chief of Pediatrics, Walter Reed Army Medical Center, Washington, DC.

EXHIBIT 15-4

TRANSFUSION SUPPORT OF FEMALE COMBAT CASUALTIES: CLINICAL IMPORTANCE OF THE RH BLOOD GROUP

Universal-donor blood is used for resuscitation in the field.

Blood typing and cross-matching are not feasible in forward combat mass casualty situations. Universal-donor transfusions, defined as group O without Rh specificity, have been safe and effective when administered to male casualties in prior conflicts. During World War II, experience with multiple Rh-incompatible transfusions demonstrated that serious reactions to Rh-incompatible blood were rare in men, although the survival of incompatible red cells was poor.[1] In Vietnam, over 100,000 universal-donor transfusions were given without a single fatal reaction.[2]

Rh-positive blood is used in universal donor transfusions.

All group O units shipped to Korea were Rh positive.[1] Group O, Rh-negative blood was distributed to fixed hospitals in Japan. This policy was developed to maintain Rh-negative blood at facilities with the capability to identify Rh-negative individuals and to prevent further transfusions with Rh-incompatible units. Current doctrine does not discriminate between Rh-positive and Rh-negative group O units distributed for universal transfusion at forward units. Thus, 85% of all units transfused in these areas will be Rh positive.

Women deployed to forward combat units who require transfusion may therefore receive Rh-incompatible blood.

Using manpower data from the Persian Gulf War[3] and current military doctrine,[4,5] up to 10% of universal donor transfusions given to female casualties are predicted to be Rh incompatible (ie, Rh-positive blood is transfused into an Rh-negative recipient).

Rh-incompatible transfusions in women can be less efficacious and cause anti-Rh antibodies that compromise future pregnancies.

Approximately 35% of deployed women have been pregnant.[3] If sensitized, Rh-incompatible cells will survive poorly in these women and cause a delayed transfusion reaction. Virtually any Rh-negative patient transfused with Rh-positive blood develops anti-Rh antibodies. IgG anti-Rh antibodies can cross the placenta during future pregnancies and cause severe, fatal consequences to the fetus.

The risk of transfusing Rh-incompatible blood to women can be minimized.

Based on the supply of O-negative blood and the number of expected female casualties, adequate stocks of O-negative blood should be available to transfuse most female casualties who receive universal-donor transfusions. In the future, development of hemoglobin-based oxygen carriers, enzymatic removal of Rh antigen from stored liquid red cells, or improved logistical aspects of frozen group O, Rh-negative blood may decrease the incidence of Rh-incompatible blood transfusion. At present, in situations where a casualty's Rh blood group cannot be determined, reserving Rh-negative units whenever possible for transfusion to women will not expose men to any more danger than in prior wars but will limit the dangers involved to women. Department of Defense policy is now being revised to call for using identity tags to match the blood type and Rh factor of the donor unit and the recipient in forward mass casualty situations where universal-donor group O blood is used.[6] NOTE: identity tags should *never* be used to match the ABO blood group of donor and recipient.

(1) Kendrick DD. *Blood Program in World War II*. Washington, DC: Department of the Army, Medical Department, Office of The Surgeon General; 1964: 748. (2) Camp FR, Conte NF, Brewer JR. Military blood banking 1941–1973: Lessons Learned Applicable to Civil Disasters and Other Considerations. Fort Knox, Ky: US Army Medical Research Laboratory; 1973. (3) Scheflen KC. Defense Manpower Data Center, Monterey, Calif. Personal communication, 21 April 1990. (4) Scotti MJ, chairman. Defense Medical Standardization Board. *DEPMEDS Policies/Guidelines: Treatment Briefs*. Fort Detrick, Frederick, Md: Defense Medical Standardization Board; 1990. (5) Rosenblatt MS, Hirsch EF, Valeri RC. Frozen red blood cells in combat casualty care: Clinical and logistical considerations. *Milit Med*. 1994;159:392–397. (6) Joseph SC, Assistant Secretary of Defense (Health Affairs). *Policy for the Use of ID Tags and ID Cards for Emergency Transfusion at the Second Echelon of Medical Care and the Validation of Those Parameters*. Washington, DC: Department of Defense. Memorandum for Secretaries of the Military Departments, Chairman of the Joint Chiefs of Staff, 21 April 1995.

Exhibit prepared for this textbook by Janiine Babcock, MD, Major, Medical Corps, US Army; Blood Research Detachment, Walter Reed Army Institute of Research, Washington, DC 20307-5100.

the commercial sector, as well as through research programs in the U.S. Army and the U.S. Navy. An essential ingredient for the rapid success of these efforts is close communication among these organizations so that appropriate information can be shared and duplication of effort does not occur.

Current efforts are mainly directed toward improving the shelf life and storage properties of PRBCs or developing a blood substitute to simplify the use of blood on the battlefield. Other efforts are directed toward improving early hemostasis and improving access to platelets and other blood products at third- and fourth-echelon areas (Exhibit 15-5). Some of these goals may be met without developing new technology by adapting existing technology to the field environment. One method could be the use of portable blood pheresis units to produce platelets and FFP without removal of the donor's red blood cells (Figure 15-8 and Exhibit 15-6).

EXHIBIT 15-5

DEVELOPMENT OF BLOOD PRODUCTS FOR FUTURE FIELD USE

The following blood products and specific component therapies are being developed for field use:

Hemoglobin-Based Oxygen Carriers

A temporary replacement for red cells in the field may be hemoglobin-based oxygen carriers. These might be prepared in solutions of 10% virally inactivated hemoglobin that has been cross-linked to avoid the dissociation of the 64-kd tetrameric form into 32-kd dimers, which can induce renal failure. The hemoglobin can be purified from human red blood cells or produced in a recombinant form; hemoglobin that has undergone polymerization in addition to cross-linking (or that has been encapsulated in liposomes) appears to have a prolonged survival time in the circulation and to have reduced vasoactivity. Thus, multiple products or forms of hemoglobin may eventually be licensed. Such products, which are being produced by at least four companies, are in phase I or phase II clinical trials in the United States and abroad. Hemoglobin-based oxygen carriers could presumably be used in liquid form in the second echelon; perhaps, for ease of storage, they could also be prepared in lyophilized form as well.

Platelets

The short, 5-day dating period for platelets, as well as the requirement that they be maintained at 22°C with continuous gentle agitation, precludes their use in far-forward positions. The ideal platelet preparation would be one that could be virally inactivated and then (*a*) lyophilized under controlled conditions and (*b*) reconstituted and infused. Alternatively, platelet concentrates could be stored indefinitely in a frozen form utilizing nontoxic cryoprotectants; they could then be thawed and directly infused into recipients.

Fibrin Sealant

Fibrin sealant comprised of purified, virally inactivated human fibrinogen and human thrombin is now commercially available in Europe and Canada, although the product has not been approved for use in the United States by the U.S. Food and Drug Administration. Fibrin sealant could be used on the field, delivered on bandages to control massive bleeding from organs such as the liver or spleen or from open wounds. Such preparations in cruder form were actually used successfully during World War II. Once such preparations are licensed, their use will undoubtedly be extended to many types of surgical situations.

Plasma

Plasma that has undergone viral inactivation by pasteurization or by solvent detergent treatment is now available in other countries. Such plasma could be prepared in freeze-dried form and then reconstituted in the field for treatment of casualties.

Modifications in Red Blood Cell Storage

Efforts are being made to extend the survival of PRBCs up to 6 to 8 weeks after collection, thus allowing longer storage time after reaching their destination in the theater of operations. Additional research efforts include (*a*) prolonging the storage time of frozen cells that have undergone deglycerolization and (*b*) converting the Rh(D) antigen to produce Rh-negative cells.

Exhibit prepared for this textbook by Barbara Alving, MD, Colonel, Medical Corps, US Army; Chief, Department of Hematology and Vascular Biology, Walter Reed Army Institute of Research, Washington, DC 20307-5100.

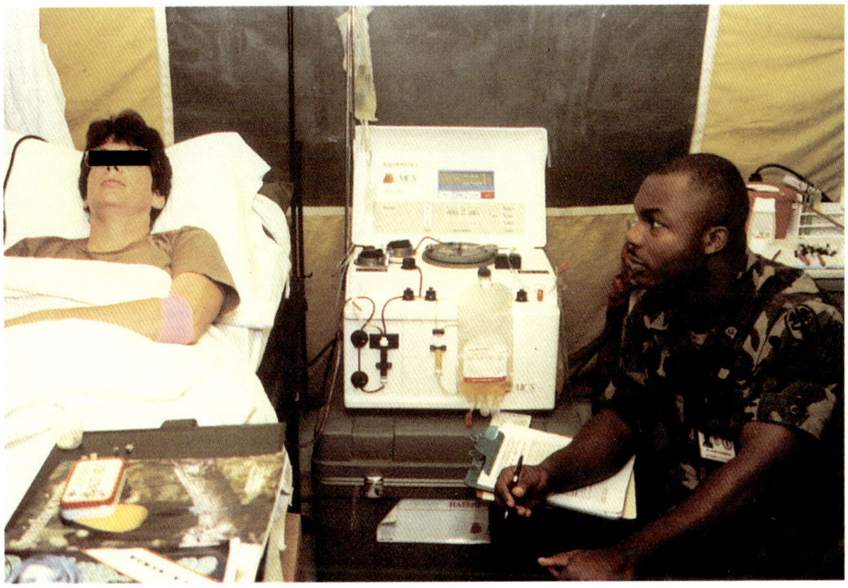

Fig. 15-8. Collection of platelets with a portable pheresis unit from a volunteer donor in a Department of Defense Deployable Medical Systems (DEPMEDS) environment. Approximately 2 hours are required for the donation. The pheresis unit uses generator power and is the size of a medium-sized television set. A volume of platelets equivalent to a six-pack was collected from this single donor, but the red blood cells were returned. Platelets can be collected in this fashion every 2 weeks.

EXHIBIT 15-6

HEMOPHERESIS: A FUTURE SOURCE OF PLATELETS IN THE FIELD?

The need for platelets during contingencies is small; however, there are times when platelets are required to save lives. Because platelets have only a 5-day storage life, it is very difficult to transport them from the continental United States to other parts of the world within the time allowed. Current research is investigating ways to extend the shelf life of platelets to longer than 5 days (see Exhibit 15-5), although final development and licensure by the U.S. Food and Drug Administration may take years.

In the meantime, the only way to provide platelets in the field has been emergency donor collections of whole blood at field hospitals. This form of collection has increased risks due to the inability to pretest the donors for transfusion-transmitted diseases, and many donors must be available to provide enough platelets for even one casualty.

To minimize the need for this form of collection and to alleviate risks and reduce stress, the U.S. military is studying the possible use of portable plateletpheresis capabilities for use in the field. Today's technology has plateletpheresis machines that are very light (55 lb), durable, and easy to transport. One plateletpheresis donor unit has the equivalent of platelets obtained from six to eight regular whole-blood donors. This scheme has several advantages:

- Pretested donors can be ready to donate, allowing for a safer product.
- Fewer donors are required, as plateletpheresis donors can donate every 3 to 7 days, compared with 8 weeks for regular blood donors.
- A superior product is provided, virtually free from red blood cells and more concentrated, reducing possible inadvertent hypervolemia.

The disadvantages include the following:

- Laboratory technicians must be trained to do plateletpheresis, which is a time-consuming and expensive process.
- Approximately 1.5 to 2 hours per patient is required for each plateletpheresis donation.

A concept that may possibly be used in the future is having plateletpheresis capability on hospital ships and at army blood supply units. These units would then supply other third- and fourth-echelon hospitals with platelets when emergency situations require.

PLANNING AND TRAINING

A successful military transfusion program must blend operational, clinical, and blood-distribution system factors (Figure 15-9), each of which requires consideration of these three critical elements:

1. education of personnel, with hands-on, realistic training,
2. review of doctrine in FM 8-55 and other manuals, and
3. real-time interaction with the blood-distribution system before and during the deployment.

Detailed guidelines for interacting with the military blood-distribution program have been prepared for this textbook; these are included at the end of this chapter.

Adjustments From Civilian Medicine

The needs and practices of military medicine require that medical officers make both a philosophical and a clinical adjustment (Figure 15-10). After they have been educated, leaders should review doctrine and incorporate blood product management into their training exercises.

Leaders from prior wars with experience in planning and training for a military blood transfusion

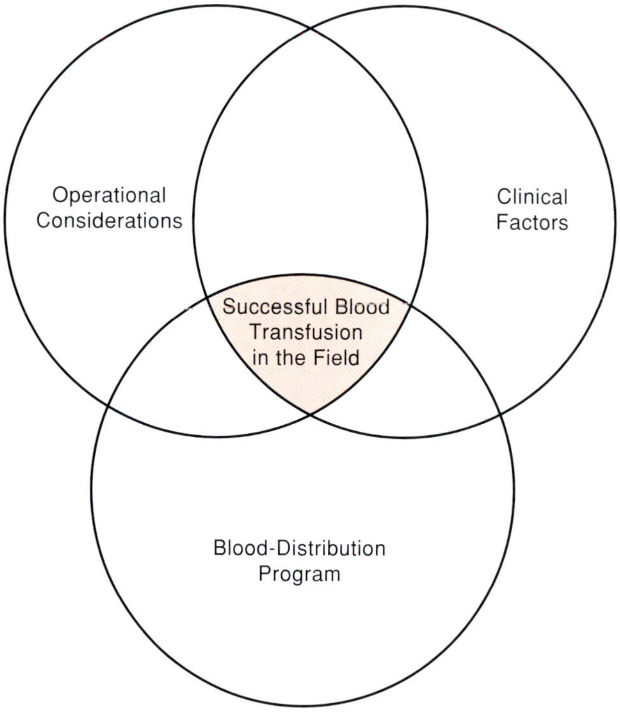

Fig. 15-9. Planning and training for a successful military transfusion program. Operational, clinical, and blood-distribution program factors must blend together smoothly and should be incorporated into all training exercises.

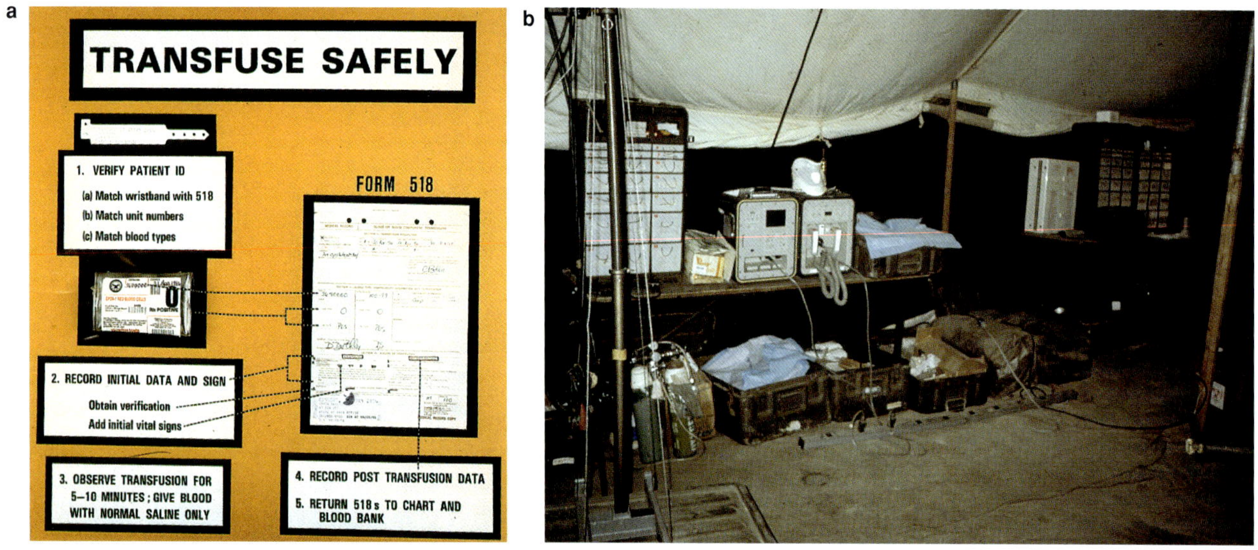

Fig. 15-10. Military hospital and field transfusion environments. (**a**) The poster describes safe transfusion practice in the hospital; after the medical officer orders the blood, the entire process is handled by other medical personnel such as nurses and laboratory workers. (**b**) In the resuscitation tent of a clearing station, the medical officer will not have access to the hospital personnel who routinely handle the blood (as indicated in the poster). When medical officers move from the hospital to the field, they must adjust not only to the changes in physical environment but also to the absence of these personnel.

program have described the philosophical and clinical readjustments they found necessary as they made the transition from civilian to military medicine:

> Division clearing stations are not emergency rooms. Ambience is different, triage is different, problems are different. The rules must be different and the reasons for this must be part of the indoctrination of the medical officers in the combat zone and the pathologists who operate the blood supply.[13]
>
> . . . .
>
> [From World War II:] Intravenous therapy (transfusion therapy) is a medical specialty, training in which is not provided in a routine medical education.... [T]he civilian physician, if all goes smoothly, is completely unaware of the organization and painstaking control that make the use of parenteral fluids safe. When, however, he enters the Medical Corps, he is called upon to practice more intravenous therapy than he employed in civilian life.... Military medicine presents special problems in intravenous therapy as compared with civilian practice: the incidence of shock, hemorrhage, and burns is many times greater, as is their severity. In their treatment, the methods of civilian medicine must be modified by considerations of transport, equipment, and environment.... If a medical officer were to attempt to accumulate a store of whole blood, he would find that none of the methods in use in civilian practice could be applied directly to his military problem without modifications.[12(p77)]
>
> . . . .
>
> [From the Persian Gulf War:] Modern physicians don't handle blood.... It has become so specialized that physicians (clinicians) have lost experience dealing with blood. The contemporary technical information available on blood management was focused largely on theater and corps hospital blood receipt and storage.[14]

Hands-On Practice: Lessons Learned, Lost, and Learned Again

Hands-on training at the patient level is critical to the successful implementation of military transfusion practice (Figure 15-11). Medical personnel should walk through demonstrations that simulate transfusing blood to mock casualties in realistic training situations, including mass casualty exercises. Blood and the appropriate supplies should be taken to the field during training, and all daily inspections, inventories, and reports performed. The senior medical officer at the Second-Brigade Clearing Station during the Persian Gulf War (1990–1991) recalls:

> We maintained a blood capability in our clearing station for a 3-month period before the ground war started. Our resupply of blood was frequently random-mix, with expiration dates only a few days from the date of our receipt. Our biggest advantage was having practiced a random-mix scheme at division level, and knowing that it was highly unsatisfactory; we therefore insisted on group O blood, often returning to the blood-supply unit several times to obtain it.
>
> When I returned to the 82nd as Division Surgeon less than 3 years after the Persian Gulf War, medics

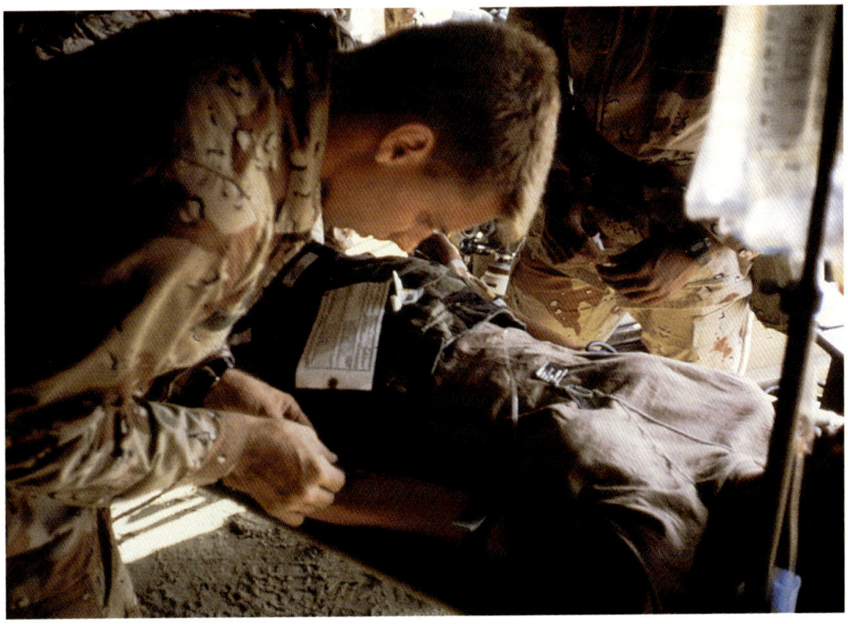

Fig. 15-11. Hands-on practice with second-echelon blood transfusion. Soldiers of B Company, 307th medical battalion, 82nd Airborne division, practice their division-level blood transfusion program. The "combat casualty" is simulated.

> had already stopped practicing with blood because it was not "safe." During one exercise, I noted that the blood was in our forward (alpha) echelon; however, the infusion sets were in our second (bravo) echelon. The soldiers who had done the packing had never administered a unit of blood.
>
> For our airfield seizure role at present, our planning is much simpler: we jump in with group O blood in ice and melted water in Styrofoam boxes. There is occasionally some difficulty obtaining blood prior to jumping, but not so much as during the Persian Gulf War because now we are the only game in town.[35]

And during Operation Restore Hope in Somalia (1993), an emergency blood drive was performed to obtain plasma and platelets for a patient who was hurt in a vehicle accident. The 86th Evacuation Hospital laboratory personnel did an excellent job and saved a life. In their afteraction review, they stated that they were not as well trained as they should have been but understood that it is difficult to train for specific emergency conditions. They also stated that trying to collect blood at a time of extreme emergency, with little time, is very difficult and stressful, especially when there also are increased demands placed elsewhere in the laboratory.[36]

A Second-Echelon Transfusion Strategy

Figure 15-12 depicts a strategy that was developed for transfusion of blood for male and female casualties in the 82nd Airborne division during the Persian Gulf War.[37] At this time, division clearing stations were supported by the 307th medical battalion and could be augmented with a forward surgical support team. At the onset of deployment, group O PRBCs were in short supply, and division units frequently received random-mix blood. Initially, an A/O system, as had previously been used in Vietnam, was chosen, owing to a shortage of

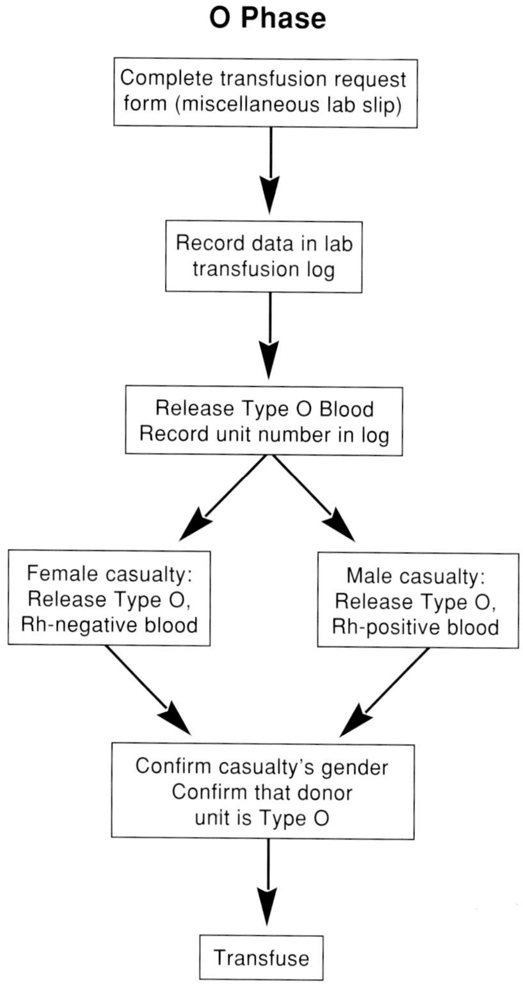

Fig. 15-12. This second-echelon blood transfusion program was developed for men and women in the 82nd Airborne division during the Persian Gulf War. Group O packed red blood cells (PRBCs) were used. In this setting, no determination of the recipient blood group was necessary. Data were recorded and the unit transfused. Women were to receive Rh-negative blood and men Rh-positive blood. When universal-donor blood was not available in the early stages of the deployment, and only random-mix blood was available, an A/O phase was planned. After practicing the A/O system, division medical companies carried only group O blood and used the system illustrated here. The A/O system, which was intended to be reserved for use only in emergencies, was never actually used.

EXHIBIT 15-7

NEW POLICY FOR USING IDENTIFICATION TAGS AND CARDS FOR EMERGENCY BLOOD TRANSFUSION AT THE SECOND ECHELON

On 21 April 1995, the Assistant Secretary of Defense for Health Affairs issued a memorandum for the secretaries of the military departments and the chairman of the joint chiefs of staff to establish new Department of Defense policy for transfusing Rh-negative blood and for using identification tags and cards for second-echelon blood transfusions:

> Effective immediately, during contingencies, the Services will provide Rh negative packed red cells to Rh negative male and female patients based on the Rh blood type on their ID tag or card at the second echelon of medical care. Third echelon and higher level of care medical treatment facilities have the capability and are expected to group, type and crossmatch blood with group specific Rh negative packed red cells selected for both Rh negative female and male patients prior to transfusion. Priority of Rh negative blood for transfusion should be given to Rh negative females if shortages of Rh negative blood arise. This new policy will also reduce the same sensitization to Rh negative males, although the impact of sensitization on males and the health care system is not as great.
>
> With implementation of the above policy and as a result of acceptable high error rates of the ABO group and Rh type placed on ID cards and tags, it is imperative that the Services review their procedures for verifying and validating that the ABO group and Rh type on each service member's ID tags and cards matches laboratory testing results as documented in each service member's medical records. These procedures should also require that this verification be performed during the processing just prior to deployment.
>
> The Services are to implement this policy immediately and provide their plans for verifying and validating service members' ID tags and cards concerning blood groups and types within 60 days of the date of this memorandum.

Reprinted from Joseph SC. Assistant Secretary of Defense (Health Affairs). *Policy for the Use of ID Tags and ID Cards for Emergency Transfusion at the Second Echelon of Medical Care and the Validation of Those Parameters.* Washington, DC: Department of Defense. Memorandum for Secretaries of the Military Departments, Chairman of the Joint Chiefs of Staff, 21 April 1995.

universal-donor PRBCs for use at the division level. We decided to transfuse female casualties with Rh-negative blood and to use Rh-positive blood in males, as had been practiced previously.

Since this deployment, new policy is being established to transfuse group O PRBCs to casualties at the second-echelon, according to the Rh group on their identity tags (Exhibit 15-7).[30]

The chief value of this system was that it *gave a structure for practice*. Although the A/O system appeared simple in theory, the added complexity of (*a*) performing a single slide test for the A antigen on the recipient's cells and (*b*) correctly assigning the result of the test to a casualty in a resuscitation tent greatly increased the risk of a transfusion reaction and slowed the pace of patient care—even when practiced under controlled training conditions. All units in the division, therefore, vigorously pursued a supply of group O PRBCs. The A/O system was reserved as an emergency back-up system but was never used.

Planning at the Third and Fourth Echelons

Although third- and fourth-echelon facilities have improved blood banking capabilities, planning and training are just as critical to a successful transfusion policy in these facilities as they are at the second echelon. The clinical environment may vary considerably according to the location and operational situation where the hospital is deployed. Two personal experiences relate different blood banking procedures (Exhibits 15-8 and 15-9). The transfusion practice in each setting was successful because the clinical policies were tailored for the operational setting, and the personnel were familiar with policies because their preparation, planning, and training had been extensive.

SUMMARY

Treatment of battlefield injuries with blood transfusion in an operational environment is a cornerstone of military medicine. The practice has saved thousands of lives and gave rise to the civilian blood banking industry shortly after World War II. Since then, transfusion medicine has become increasingly sophisticated and specialized, and physicians in peacetime medicine are no longer trained

EXHIBIT 15-8

PREPARING BLOOD BANKS FOR MASS CASUALTY INCIDENTS

Fourth-echelon and other military general hospitals should be capable of providing blood bank services that are comparable to those of a civilian medical center. In a mass casualty incident, these services should include protocols for the selection of blood products for massive transfusions, positive blood-sample identification systems, a complete blood-component service, and procedures for the releasing of un–cross-matched universal-donor blood.

The following guidelines, based on previous military and civilian experiences,[1–5] are intended to provide a framework for addressing these issues.

Protocols for Managing Severe Blood Loss

Past experiences indicate that in mass casualty situations, physicians are likely to request the same quantities and types of blood products that they have become accustomed to using in the management of similar cases.[1,2] For this reason, protocols that are intended to be used during a mass casualty incident should be implemented in advance as part of routine operations. The concept of stockpiling special blood products, blood substitutes, or plasma expanders to be used only in a mass casualty incident introduces the risk of delays while clinicians accommodate themselves to unfamiliar clinical responses and reactions.

Separate Donor-Related and Casualty-Related Services

In a mass casualty incident, the blood bank staff should be unencumbered by blood-donor and -supply problems and should focus their efforts on providing safe, serologically compatible blood products in a timely manner. The current standard of practice in civilian and military hospitals requires all blood products intended for transfusion to be tested for multiple infectious disease markers, including anti–human immunodeficiency virus and hepatitis B surface antigen.[6] The former practice of collecting units of blood at the hospital and transfusing them as ABO-matched, but otherwise untested, warm blood is outdated and is not recommended.

Ideally, all blood donor–related functions should be conducted in a separate facility that is sufficiently distant from the hospital to allow a surge of blood donors to respond to the incident without congesting access to the hospital. The distinct functions of a hospital transfusion service (eg, cross-matching, blood typing) compared with a blood-donor service (eg, phlebotomy, infectious-disease testing, component preparation) should be recognized in the planning process. The optimal result would be a physical separation that would allow each service to conduct its specialized functions without competing for resources.

Positive Identification Systems

A system that positively identifies each casualty, blood sample, and blood product intended for transfusion is essential for safe management of a mass casualty incident. Wristband systems with uniquely numbered sticky labels are marketed commercially and have been used successfully by civilian transfusion services in a wide range of emergency situations.

Universal-Donor Blood and Abbreviated Cross-Matching

The blood bank should have a standing operating procedure that defines the requirements for releasing group O-positive (or O-negative) universal-donor blood without a cross-match. Criteria should also be specified for switching from the standard 60-minute cross-match to an abbreviated 5- to 15-minute cross-match. If group O whole blood or fresh frozen plasma is transfused to a group A or B recipient, then guidelines should be specified for safe reversion to ABO group-specific red blood cell transfusions.

(1) Sandler SG, Sharon R, Hermoni D, Superstein E. Blood transfusion therapy in the rear hospital during the Yom Kippur War (October 1973). *Milit Med.* 1977;141:49, 52–53. (2) Sandler SG. Strategies for blood services in mass casualty incidents. In: Cowley RA, Edelstein S, Silverstein M, eds. *Mass Casualties: A Lesson Learned Approach. Accidents, Civil Disorders, Natural Disasters.* Washington, DC: US Department of Transportation. 1982: 229–233. DOT HS 806 302; October 1982. Proceedings, First International Assembly on Emergency Medical Services; June 1982. (3) Sandler SG. Blood utilization during the October 1973 (Yom Kippur) war. Presented at Combat Casualty Care Research Program; US Army Medical Research Development, Acquisition and Logistics Command (Provisional); 8–9 November 1993; Fort Detrick, Frederick, Md. (4) Camp FR, Conte NF, Brewer JR. *Military Blood Banking 1941–1973: Lessons Learned Applicable to Civil Disasters and Other Considerations.* Fort Knox, Ky: US Army Medical Research Laboratory; 1973. (5) Kendrick DD. *Blood Program in World War II.* Washington, DC: Department of the Army, Medical Department, Office of The Surgeon General; 1964. (6) Standard E5.000/Tests intended to prevent disease transmission. In: *Standards for Blood Banks and Transfusion Services.* 16th ed. Bethesda, Md: American Association of Blood Banks; 1994: 14.

Exhibit prepared for this textbook by S. Gerald Sandler, MD, Professor of Medicine and Pathology, and Director, Blood Bank and Blood Donor Service, Georgetown University Medical Center, Washington, DC 20007.

EXHIBIT 15-9

BLOOD BANKING IN AN ISOLATED THEATER OF OPERATIONS: EXPERIENCE OF THE 46TH COMBAT SUPPORT HOSPITAL, MOGADISHU, SOMALIA, 1993

Background

- Blood supply system: from Armed Services Whole Blood Processing Laboratory (ASWBPL), Maguire Air Force Base, New Jersey. Daily reports submitted. Routine shipments arrived weekly. About 72 hours from request to delivery of blood products.
- Available blood products:
  - random-mix packed red blood cells (liquid)
  - fresh frozen plasma; about one fourth to one half of bags cracked and unsuitable for use after rewarming
  - platelets not available
- Inventory: started with 50 units of packed red blood cells, increased to 200 units
- Blood banking personnel:
  - one M-4 blood bank–qualified technician
  - one laboratory officer
  - no pathologists or blood bank fellowship–trained officers
- Nearest civilian hospitals: Cairo, Egypt, and Nairobi, Kenya
- Emergency collection of whole blood: blood was drawn only when the demand was expected to increase. The donation and collection systems were kept separate from the dispensing function of the blood bank.

Training and Preparation

Civilian mass casualties were treated at least weekly. All aspects of trauma medicine were exercised, including the blood bank and the use of whole blood. After treatment, all aspects of trauma care, including the blood bank, were reviewed and improved if needed. The following amounts of blood were administered from 30 September through 4 October 1993:

Date	Incident or Injury	Blood Products Administered
30 September	Shark bite, one casualty	> 50 units of fresh frozen plasma and packed red blood cells; > 20 units of fresh whole blood, type O
2 October	Land mine exploded under a jeep; four casualties, including one woman	> 20 units of fresh whole blood, type O; Rh-negative blood used for the woman
3–4 October	Rangers pinned down after a failed raid in Mogadishu; > 20 casualties	> 70 units of fresh whole blood, type O

Impressions

The use of whole blood maintained a reserve inventory of ASWBPL blood products. Surgeons preferred whole blood to component therapy, especially as platelets were not available. Hemostasis was subjectively improved. All blood donors had been tested for antigens to the human immunodeficiency virus prior to deployment, but (*a*) identifying potential donors in advance of deployment and (*b*) having access to field test kits for blood-borne pathogens would have been useful.

Exhibit prepared for this textbook by (1) Denver Perkins, MD, Colonel, Medical Corps, US Army; Director for Clinical Services 46th Combat Support Hospital; Assistant Chief of Anesthesia, Walter Reed Army Medical Center. (2) David Elliot, MD, Lieutenant Colonel, Medical Corps, US Army; Chief of Surgery 46th Combat Support Hospital; Chief of Critical Care, Walter Reed Army Medical Center. (3) Hector Velasquez, Captain, Medical Service, US Army; Chief Laboratory Officer 46th Combat Support Hospital, Chief of Clinical Microscopy, Walter Reed Army Medical Center, Washington, DC 20307-5001.

in nor practice routine blood banking skills. The complex principles of transfusion support of civilian trauma patients in a fixed facility with a modern blood bank are detailed in Chapter 14, Transfusion Therapy. However, military casualties, wounded in a dangerous, austere environment, continue to suffer from injuries that require blood product therapy. There is increasing emphasis on moving resuscitation and surgery even farther forward on the battlefield with mobile surgical teams. In addition, military personnel continue to be deployed to isolated areas lacking access to fixed facilities with modern blood banking resources. Thus, the ability to bring these resources as safely as possible to forward and remote areas in an operational emergency military situation remains imperative.

This chapter describes the theory and practice of the unique aspects of military transfusion medicine. Emphasis is on planning and training, becoming familiar with military terms and doctrine, integrating operational and clinical factors with the blood-supply system, and making the adjustment from the civilian clinician's relative isolation from the laboratory and the blood bank. Medical officers must understand the availability of blood products according to doctrine and the echelons of care so they can anticipate the clinical needs of casualties—from resuscitation to definitive surgery and postoperative care. Technical factors related to the safe operation of a small emergency blood bank in the field must be mastered by clinical personnel who may be unfamiliar with their peacetime use.

The frequency of the ABO and Rh blood groups in the general donor population acquire unique military significance, and the immediate and delayed effects of massive transfusion occur frequently. The treatment of female casualties in the field poses additional unique military considerations and is mandating further changes in doctrine, which include the proper use and interpretation of identity tags.

Blood products have a finite shelf life and require special storage, handling, and monitoring, which may limit their use in a rapidly evolving operational scenario. Thus, research is active in the areas of developing a blood substitute, controlling hemorrhage early on the battlefield with products such as fibrin glue, and providing platelet support.

Most importantly, successful military transfusion medicine requires practice and planning. The learning curve is steep and cannot be mastered for the first time on actual casualties. Leaders should use blood products as realistically as possible during training exercises. Early interaction with the blood-supply system is critical. Only when clinical, technical, and operational factors are recognized early and then practiced can medical officers safely provide blood products and meet what should be the standard of care for emergency treatment of men and women injured in battle.

Acknowledgments

The authors thank Colonel William H. Crosby, Medical Corps, U.S. Army (ret); Colonel Robert J. T. Joy, Medical Corps, U.S. Army (ret); Colonel Louis Diehl, Medical Corps, U.S. Army, Walter Reed Army Institute of Research and Walter Reed Army Medical Center; the personnel of the 307th Medical Battalion and the 82nd Airborne Division, who developed the division's blood policy during the Persian Gulf War; Colonel Craig Llewellyn, Medical Corps, U.S. Army (ret); Captain Evan Renz, Medical Service, U.S. Army; Commander Kevin Yeskey, U.S. Public Health Service; Captain Gerald McGlothlen, Medical Service Corps, U.S. Navy Reserves; Commander David Reichman, Medical Service Corps, U.S. Navy; and Colonel Anthony Polk, Medical Service, U.S. Army (ret), Director, Armed Services Blood Program Office, during the Persian Gulf War.

REFERENCES

1. Robertson LB. A contribution on blood transfusion in war surgery. *Lancet*. 1918;1:759–762.

2. Beecher HK. Preparation of battle casualties for surgery. *Ann Surg*. 1945;121:769–792.

3. Crosby WH, Howard JM. The hematologic response to wounding and to resuscitation accomplished by large transfusions of stored blood: A study of battle casualties in Korea. *Blood*. 1954;9:439–460.

4. Heaton LD. Foreword. In: Kendrick DD. *Blood Program in World War II*. Washington, DC: Department of the Army, Medical Department, Office of The Surgeon General; 1964.

5. Kiel F. Development of a blood program in Viet Nam. *Milit Med*. 1966;131:1469–1482.

6. Churchill ED. *Surgeon to Soldiers*. Philadelphia, Pa: JP Lippincott; Philadelphia, Pa: 1972: 36–58.

7. Frishberg DP. Historical review: Highlights in the development of combat transfusion programs. *Journal of Military Medical Laboratory Science*. 1989;18:41–44, 66–71.

8. Crosby WH. World War II's war within a war: What delayed the delivery of whole blood to overseas combat troops. *MD*. 1991;Dec:35–39.

9. US Department of the Army. *Planning for Health Service Support*. Washington, DC: Headquarters, DA; approved final draft January 1994. Field Manual 8–55.

10. Scotti MJ, chairman. Defense Medical Standardization Board. *DEPMEDS Policies/Guidelines: Treatment Briefs*. Fort Detrick, Frederick, Md: Defense Medical Standardization Board; 1990.

11. Committee on Trauma, American College of Surgeons. *Advanced Trauma Life Support Program for Physicians: Instructor Manual*. 5th ed. Chicago, Ill: American College of Surgeons; 1993.

12. Kendrick DD. *Blood Program in World War II*. Washington, DC: Department of the Army, Medical Department, Office of The Surgeon General; 1964: 406, 443, 634, 635.

13. Crosby WH. Colonel, Medical Corps, US Army (ret). Personal communication, September 1994.

14. Gerber FE. *Employment of the 307th Medical Battalion (Airborne) in Operations Desert Shield and Desert Storm: A Personal Experience*. Carlisle, Pa: US Army War College, Military Studies Program; May 1992. Monograph.

15. Ryden SE, Oberman HA. Compatibility of common intravenous solutions with CPD blood. *Transfusion*. 1975;15:250–255.

16. Walker RH, ed. Blood transfusion practice. In: *Technical Manual*. 11th ed. Bethesda, Md: American Association of Blood Banks; 1993: 421.

17. Bickell WH, Matthew MJ, Pepe PE, et al. Immediate versus delayed fluid resuscitation for hypotensive patients with penetrating torso injuries. *N Engl J Med*. 1994;331:1105–1109.

18. Jacobs LM. Timing of fluid resuscitation in trauma. *N Engl J Med*. 1994;331:1153–1154. Editorial.

19. Walker RH, ed. Adverse effects of blood transfusion. In: *Technical Manual*. 11th ed. Bethesda, Md: American Association of Blood Banks; 1993: 471.

20. Rosenblatt MS, Hirsch EF, Valeri RC. Frozen red blood cells in combat casualty care: Clinical and logistical considerations. *Milit Med*. 1994;159:392–397.

21. Crosby WH. Frozen blood for military transfusion service. *Milit Med*. 1967;132:119–121.

22. Crosby WH, Akeroyd JH. Some immunohematologic results of large transfusions of group O blood in recipients of other blood groups: A study of battle casualties in Korea. *Blood*. 1954;9(2):103–116.

23. Barnes A, Allen TE. Transfusions subsequent to administration of universal donor blood in Vietnam. *JAMA*. 1968;204:695–697.

24. Walker RH, ed. Pretransfusion testing. In: *Technical Manual*. 11th ed. Bethesda, Md: American Association of Blood Banks; 1993: 312.

25. Walker RH, ed. Blood grouping and typing. In: *Technical Manual*. 11th ed. Bethesda, Md: American Association of Blood Banks; 1993: 621.

26. Walker RH, ed. ABO, H, and P blood groups. In: *Technical Manual*. 11th ed. Bethesda, Md: American Association of Blood Banks; 1993: 203–228.

27. Gaydos JC, Cowan DS, Polk AJ, et al. Blood typing errors on US Army identification cards and tags. *Milit Med*. 1988;153:618–620.

28. Ensign BG, Dougherty TH, Bowlus IN, Konecki EA. ABO and Rh blood type errors on Air Force identification cards. *Milit Med*. 1995;160(6):288–290.

29. Jaques D. Lieutenant Colonel, Medical Corps, US Army; Senior Medical Officer, 307th Medical Battalion, 82nd Airborne, Persian Gulf War; Chief of Surgery, Department of Surgery, Walter Reed Army Medical Center, Washington, DC. Personal communication, June 1994.

30. Joseph SC, Assistant Secretary of Defense (Health Affairs). *Policy for the Use of ID Tags and ID Cards for Emergency Transfusion at the Second Echelon of Medical Care and the Validation of Those Parameters*. Washington, DC: Department of Defense. Memorandum for Secretaries of the Military Departments, Chairman of the Joint Chiefs of Staff, 21 April 1995.

31. Mollison PL, Engelfriet CP, Contreras M, eds. The Rh blood group system. In: *Blood Transfusion in Clinical Medicine*. 9th ed. Boston, Mass: Blackwell Scientific Publications; 1992: 543–591.

32. Lefebre J, McLellan BA, Coovadia AS. Seven years experience with group O unmatched packed red blood cells in a regional trauma unit. *Ann Emerg Med*. 1987;16:1344–1349.

33. Schmidt PJ, Leparc GF, Samia CT. Use of Rh positive blood in emergency situations. *Surg Gynecol Obstet*. 1988;167:229–233.

34. Engle HL. Medicolegal considerations in transfusion medicine. In: Petz LD, Swisher SN, eds. *Clinical Practice of Transfusion Medicine*. 2nd ed. New York, NY: Churchill Livingstone; 1989: 355–362.

35. Clark J. Major, Medical Corps, US Army. Senior Medical Officer, 2nd Brigade Clearing Station, 82nd Airborne Persian Gulf War. Division Surgeon 82nd Airborne. Personal communication, December 1994.

36. Kozar M. First Lieutenant, Medical Service, US Army. Laboratory officer, 86th Evacuation Hospital, Mogadishu, Somalia. Personal communication, May 1995.

37. Bolan CD, Strawder G. 82nd Airborne Division blood policy. In: Gerber FE. *Employment of the 307th Medical Battalion (Airborne) in Operations Desert Shield and Desert Storm: A Personal Experience*. Carlisle Pa: US Army War College, Military Studies Program; May 1992. Monograph.

GUIDELINES FOR INTERACTING WITH THE BLOOD-DISTRIBUTION SYSTEM

Crossing the bridge between the medical officers who treat the casualties and the blood-distribution system that supports them takes planning, coordination, and teamwork. The successful blood product distributions that we have had recently in operations other than war and during combat operations are due largely to the foresight, hard work, and sacrifice of many people. They have read and understood the history of the use of blood products, have actually played a part in making the system work, have used blood products in battlefield conditions, and have seen the miracles that blood provides. Above all, we must teach from these lessons of history in order to train as a team, train as realistically as possible, and then train again so that we are always prepared.

All medical officers who work in a field environment where they will be transfusing blood products must understand the Armed Services Blood Program (ASBP) blood-distribution system (Guidelines Exhibit 1). Interestingly, the adoption of a permanent ASBP evolved from lessons learned from the Korean War, where

> [n]o single medical item was more important than blood, and its supply was a specialized program stretching from the zone of the interior to the battlefield.[1(p243)]
>
> . . . .
>
> At the end of World War II, well-founded, detailed recommendations for a transfusion service had been prepared and submitted through channels to the proper authorities. Time, manpower, effort, money, and lives could all have been spared in Korea if these recommendations had been utilized as a basis for postwar planning. As it was, the newly developed plans were not ready for implementation when the Korean combat began.[2(p xiii)]

The existence of an ASBP and its blood-distribution doctrine has since provided excellent support—from the Vietnam War, to the Persian Gulf War, to Operation Uphold Democracy (1994) in Haiti. Blood products were used in each of these operations. What has changed are the amounts and types of blood products as well as the transfusion procedures. This trend will also continue as new blood products and possible blood substitutes become licensed.

As important as support to the blood program, however, is the fact that the *who, what, where, when,* and *how* change for every operation and situation. Thus, prior planning and coordination as well as training are required to make things work as they should. The medical officer at the field medical treatment facility (MTF) or the forward medical company must be aware that blood products will not suddenly appear at their facility. For the system to work, the medical team must plan for and request blood products through the right communications and coordination channels.

Who Should Medical Officers Talk to When Blood Products Are Required?

The chain of command is always the main communication channel for making things happen. Commanders are responsible for what happens in their units. Good commanders also realize that they are not expert in everything. They defer to lawyers on legal issues, to logisticians on logistical issues, and should also should defer blood-distribution and technical blood issues to the blood expert.

Once he has coordinated the medical officer's requirements with the blood expert, the commander will usually allow the two to communicate directly, requiring status updates to keep himself informed.

At certain levels of command, the commander will have a Surgeon's staff. The commander will appoint or designate a person to be the blood program officer. For example, a Joint Blood Program Officer (JBPO) can be found at each Unified Command Surgeon's Office. JBPOs are usually laboratory officers who are specialists in blood banking and are well trained in the blood-distribution system. These blood program officers are directly involved with planning the blood-distribution system for operations within their unified command.

Depending on its size or based on the operation, the unified command may designate Area Joint Blood Program Officers (AJBP0s). These officers are used quite often with Joint Task Forces (JTFs) and work for the JTF Surgeon. They plan, coordinate, and communicate in much the same way as the JBPO but within a much more defined geographical area. They, too, are laboratory officers specialized in blood banking procedures. They are good assets for answering any blood-distribution questions that arise. Their main purposes are to

- monitor blood requirements from treatment facilities within their designated area,
- coordinate deliveries of blood products to those facilities, and
- report to the JBPO as well as their respective command element.

The AJBPO is responsible for making sure the blood-distribution system is working. The AJBPO is also responsible for monitoring blood-supply units (BSUs) and blood transshipment centers that provide storage of blood products for further shipment to MTFs.

BSUs are designated in the operations plans or orders. They can be an army blood platoon, a marine fluids platoon, a fixed MTF, a medical ship offshore, or a field MTF. They are designated specific missions depending on their capabilities. They will usually have a laboratory officer who may or may not be specialized in blood banking.

GUIDELINES EXHIBIT 1

ARMED SERVICES BLOOD-DISTRIBUTION SYSTEM: OPERATIONAL DESCRIPTION

Blood product requirements are preplanned and established in each unified command operations plan. The daily blood report (BLDREP), which includes a request for blood products and the status of the inventory, activates the execution of those plans. Information copies of the BLDREP and the blood shipment report (BLDSHIPREP) are provided in accordance with local command operational plans. The blood-distribution system is the standard doctrine. However, it is very flexible and, based on the situation, changes can be made with coordination with the Armed Services Blood Program Office (ASBPO). The numbers inside the boxes correspond to the numbered guidelines below.

1. Each medical treatment facility (MTF) or element, including a naval vessel, that requires blood products submits a daily blood report (BLDREP) to a designated unified command component blood-supply unit (BSU). The MTF may be located in the second, third, or fourth echelon of medical support.
2. Each designated unified command component BSU issues blood products to the requesting MTFs. If directed, a BSU may serve MTFs of more than one service. The BSU may be located in the third or fourth echelon of medical support.
3. Each component BSU submits a daily BLDREP to a designated Area Joint Blood Program Office (AJBPO).
4. Each blood transshipment center (BTC) or transportable blood transshipment center (TBTC) issues blood products to each designated component BSU based on daily allocation guidelines established by the AJBPO or, if no AJBPO exists, the Joint Blood Program Office (JBPO).
5. Each BTC or TBTC submits a daily BLDREP to the designated AJBPO.
6. Each AJBPO manages blood products between component BSUs and submits a daily BLDREP to the JBPO.
7. The JBPO manages blood products between blood program areas in the unified command and submits a daily BLDREP to the Armed Services Blood Program Office (ASBPO).
8. The ASBPO directs the designated Armed Services Whole Blood Processing Laboratory (ASWBPL) to ship blood products, based on the ASWBPL situation report (ASWBPLSITREP).
9. Each ASWBPL ships blood products to designated unified command BTC or TBTC.
10. Military blood donor centers (BDCs) in the continental United States (CONUS) ship blood products to resupply designated ASWBPLs as directed by the respective Service Blood Program Office (SBPO). Defense Logistics Agency contracts with civilian blood agencies are activated when Armed Services Blood Program shortfalls are experienced.
11. Prepositioned frozen blood products stored in unified command armed services blood product depots (BPDs) are issued to BSUs as directed by the JBPO.
12. The JBPO provides, on a continuous basis, information on the status of the theater blood program to the unified command surgeon, who, in turn, coordinates with the Joint Staff.
13. The ASBPO is chartered to ensure implementation of the Armed Services Blood Program polices established by the Assistant Secretary of Defense for Health Affairs, and to coordinate the provision of blood products to the unified commands in concert with the Joint Staff. The U.S. Army is the Executive Agent for the ASBPO. An ASBPO situation report (ASBPOSITREP) is provided in accordance with mobilization plans.

Guidelines Exhibit 1 *continues*

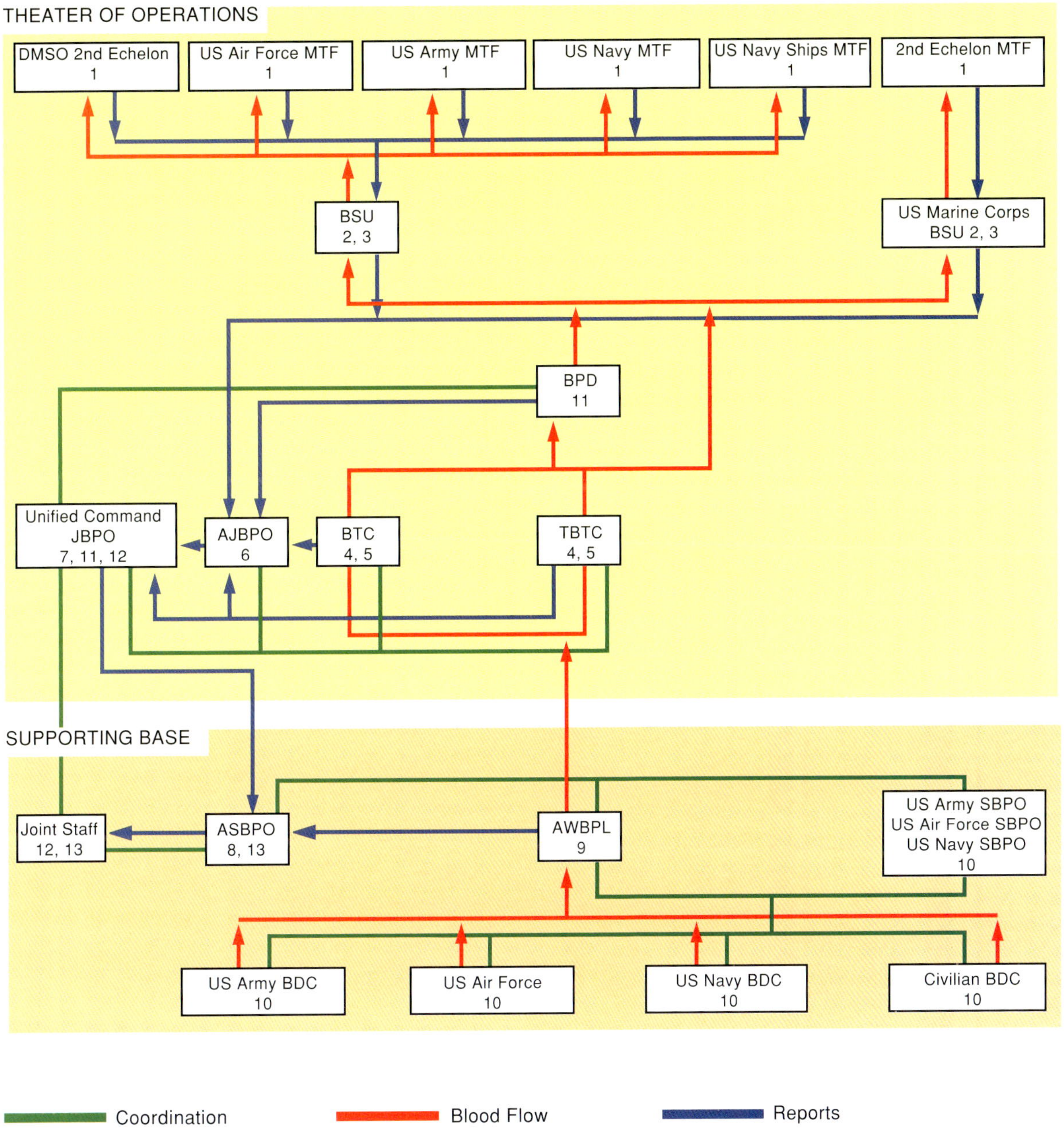

AJBPO:	Area Joint Blood Program Office
ASBP:	Armed Services Blood Program
ASBPO:	Armed Services Blood Program Office
ASBPOSITREP:	ASBPO situation report
ASWBPL:	Armed Services Whole Blood Processing Laboratory
ASWBPLSITREP:	ASWBPL situation report
BDCs:	blood donor centers
BLDREP:	blood report
BLDSHIPREP:	blood shipment report
BPD:	blood product depot
BSU:	blood supply unit
BTC:	blood transshipment center
CONUS:	continental United States
JBPO:	Joint Blood Program Office
JTF:	Joint Task Forces
MTF:	medical treatment facility
POC:	point of contact
SBPO:	Service Blood Program Office
TBTC:	transportable blood transshipment center

However, they are trained to store and distribute blood products to MTFs. They are usually the MTF's and the medical officer's prime point of contact to the blood-distribution system.

So medical officers need to know that they will be supported by a BSU, who is monitored by an AJBPO, who reports to a JBPO within the unified command. These players in the blood-distribution system need to be able to communicate directly.

How Do Medical Officers Communicate With Their Points of Contact?

Once medical officers know who their direct points of contact are, how do they communicate their blood requirements? The Department of Defense has standardized message formats so that each service can communicate with the other services. Two of these standardized messages are the blood report (BLDREP) and the blood shipment report (BLDSHIPREP).

Each MTF is required to submit a daily BLDREP to its supplier of blood products. This report can be sent by the fastest means of communication available. In some situations, this can be by courier. In other situations, telephones, radios, or satellite communications may be used. This report can also be sent by the message center nearest the MTF. The means by which the report is sent is dictated by the communications capabilities that exist within the MTF and within the supporting communications network.

A standard BLDREP will provide the facility's current blood inventory, the amount of blood products required within the next 12 to 48 hours, the amount of blood that will expire in the next 7 days, and the estimate of blood products required in the next 7 days. It may give the location of the MTF, and it has a narrative section to address any problems and to provide any other information required by higher commands. For example, transfusions may be addressed by stating the blood-unit donor number, matched to the patient transfused by the casualty's social security number.

A standard BLDSHIPREP will alert the receiver of blood products as to when a blood shipment will be arriving. It will also provide the number of blood products being shipped, by their ABO group and Rh type. If the shipment is arriving by air, it will usually have a mission number and a transportation control number to specify which plane the blood products will be arriving on. It will give the shipper's address and the point of contact.

Examples of BLDREPs and BLDSHIPREPs, with codes for using these reports, are explained in *Planning for Health Service Support*[3] and *Health Service Support Logistics in Joint Operations*.[4] It is imperative that medical officers who require blood products for their facilities make sure that their staffs are trained on the exact procedure to follow when submitting these reports.

How Do Medical Officers Receive Their Blood Products?

The best part of the blood-distribution system is that it has at its service all the transportation capabilities that the Department of Defense has available. The problem is that these resources can become limited. Therefore, communication of requirements and coordination of transportation assets becomes very important.

Fortunately, this blood-distribution system is used daily for peacetime transportation of blood products around the world. Thus, personnel involved especially with the strategic lift capabilities are always ready to implement contingency blood-distribution procedures. Medical officers must realize that because strategic lift is limited, good coordination of blood requirements with sufficient advanced notice is also required.

Tactical transportation capabilities are also sufficiently flexible to meet requirements. Blood products can be shipped directly to the MTF (ie, unit distribution) or MTF personnel may have to go to a specific location to receive their blood products (ie, point distribution). In these routine instances, wheeled vehicles (assets organic to the unit) are used. Problems arise when distance, terrain, security, and time become factors.

When wheeled-vehicle transport is not useful, helicopters fill the void. Medical-evacuation helicopters have a secondary mission to ship blood products forward to MTFs. Helicopter support to ships that receive casualties needs to be coordinated. Helicopters can carry blood products via sling-load when more blood is required than can be held within the helicopter.

When helicopter capability is limited due to security, distance, and increased demands, tactical airlift via aircraft such as C-130s must be coordinated well. The JBPOs and AJBPOs should know these capabilities and be able to coordinate shipments as required. It is *their* responsibility to coordinate these capabilities for the MTFs.

When Can Medical Officers Get Blood From the Armed Services Blood Program?

Each of the military's different types of operations is unique as to when the MTFs will require blood products. Medical officers may find themselves involved in a forward surgical element that is being deployed as part of the first wave of assault troops. In this case, the medical officer will need to deploy with blood products. In other cases, the medical officer may deploy with an MTF that will be deployed in a second iteration of troop movements and will not have to take on casualties until days after entering the area of operations. In this case, it would not be reasonable to deploy with blood products; rather, they should be requested just before casualties are expected. In all cases, the medical officer needs to ask these questions: When is the blood required? and When can I get it?

The blood-distribution system can accommodate the treatment facilities as long as there has been coordination and advanced notice. For example, the Joint Task Force Surgeon for Operation Uphold Democracy was able to bring players together prior to the operation to plan all aspects of the medical support. Major Noel Webster, from the Armed Services Blood Program Office, was able to meet with the 82nd Airborne Division Surgeon, Lieutenant Colonel Jeffrey Clark, to coordinate some of the Division's unique requirements for blood support. Major Webster gave him some recommendations, and points of contact (POCs) were established to set up the distribution system. The POCs worked agreements among themselves, and Lieutenant Colonel Clark had the POCs train and exercise the distribution prior to deploying to make sure any problems were identified and resolved. When the 82nd Airborne Division was ready to deploy, all systems were go and the blood was ready and prepared without a hitch.

In other circumstances, the JBPO would be the POC coordinating the planning prior to and during an operation. For example, the U.S. Central Command (CENTCOM) Surgeon's JBPO, Commander Barbara Fieldman, was heavily involved in identifying BSUs for supporting medical treatment during the Persian Gulf War. In this operation, MTFs did not have to deploy with blood; instead, a blood-distribution infrastructure of BTCs and BSUs was in place to provide blood products for them. Commander Fieldman coordinated with the MTF commanders personally to make sure they were being supported.

REFERENCES

1. Crowley AE. *The Medics' War: United States Army in the Korean War*. Washington, DC: Center of Military History, US Army; 1987: 243.

2. Kendrick DD. Preface. In: *Blood Program in World War II*. Washington, DC: Department of the Army, Medical Department, Office of The Surgeon General; 1964: xiii.

3. US Department of the Army. *Planning for Health Service Support*. Washington, DC: Headquarters, DA; approved final draft, January 1994. Field Manual 8-55.

4. Joint Chiefs of Staff. *Joint Tactics, Techniques, and Procedures for Health Service Support Logistics in Joint Operations*. Washington, DC: US Departments of the Army, Navy, Navy US Marine Corps, and Air Force; initial draft 15 August 1993. Joint Pub 4-20.1.

Chapter 16

NEUROLOGICAL INJURIES

JEFFREY M. BERMAN, M.D.*; JOHN F. BUTTERWORTH IV, M.D.†; AND DONALD S. PROUGH, M.D.‡

*Captain, Medical Corps, U.S. Navy Ready Reserve; Instructor of Anesthesia, Department of Anesthesia, Bowman Gray School of Medicine, Medical Center Boulevard, Winston-Salem, North Carolina 27157-1009

†Associate Professor of Anesthesia and Vice Chairman for Research, Department of Anesthesia, Bowman Gray School of Medicine, Medical Center Boulevard, Winston-Salem, North Carolina 27157-1009

‡Captain, Medical Corps, U.S. Navy Ready Reserve; Professor and Chairman, Department of Anesthesiology, The University of Texas Medical Branch, 301 University Boulevard, Galveston, Texas 77555-0591

INTRODUCTION

Traumatic brain injury is classified as *open* or *closed*. Closed head trauma is further subdivided into *severe* (characterized by prolonged coma; ie, inability to obey simple verbal commands), *moderate* (either requiring craniotomy or producing coma of short duration), and *minor* (neither requiring surgery nor resulting in coma). Because of the enormous economic and social toll exacted by vehicular trauma, closed head injury, which is a common cause of death after civilian blunt trauma, has been extensively studied in patients and in experimental models. Open head injury, which is more relevant to military trauma, has been studied much less well. Therefore, many of the principles of nonoperative management of penetrating brain injury are based on the assumption that knowledge gained from clinical or experimental closed brain injury can be extrapolated to injuries caused by penetrating missiles. One central assumption is that secondary brain injury—an often-preventable consequence of hypotension, hypercarbia, hypoxemia, or intracranial hypertension—contributes heavily to death or disability caused by the original injury.[1,2]

Penetrating injuries to the spinal cord do not play a large role in military medicine: most casualties whose spinal cords are transected are killed when the missile (bullet or fragment) continues on its path and injures nearby organs (eg, the heart and great vessels, liver, spleen). In addition, data gathered during the Vietnam War by the Wound Data and Munitions Effectiveness Team (WDMET) indicate that 98% of soldiers with gunshot wounds of the cervical spine that included the cord were fatally injured.[3] Closed injuries to a soldier's spinal cord are not different from those that occur to civilians, and occur for the same reasons (eg, blunt trauma due to vehicular accidents and falls). There are far more casualties with brain than spinal cord injuries; furthermore, the chances that therapeutic intervention will effect improved results are greater with brain than with spinal cord injuries. For these reasons, most of this chapter pertains to traumatic brain injury; spinal cord injury is treated much less extensively.

This chapter discusses the perioperative care of the neurologically injured patient as it is practiced today in medical centers. Because the equipment and facilities found in the Department of Defense's Deployable Medical Systems (DEPMEDS) hospitals replicate to some extent the sophistication of civilian trauma centers, we have included descriptions of state-of-the-art systems and management techniques. However, we also provide practical suggestions for use when advanced support systems are not available.

THE NATURE OF HEAD INJURIES SUSTAINED IN COMBAT

Combat casualties with head trauma will present with either open or closed injuries. In open injuries, the scalp is lacerated and the bone is fractured, usually with significant depression, thereby exposing the dura; this in turn is usually lacerated, exposing the cortex, which is almost invariably damaged as well. Closed head injuries may or may not involve laceration of the scalp, but if a laceration is present, the calvarium either will be uninjured or will have no more than a simple, nondepressed, linear fracture. In most cases of closed head injury, there is no scalp laceration or skull fracture at all.

Combat casualties with head trauma can also be classified as having either *blunt* or *penetrating* injuries, depending on the mechanism of injury. Blunt trauma usually results in closed injuries, while penetrating wounds are almost always open. In the combat zone, the overwhelming majority of battle casualties with head trauma have penetrating missile wounds made either by fragments from explosive munitions or bullets fired by small arms. Most of the latter wounds are open in the sense that the dura has been lacerated and the cranial contents are exposed. When closed injuries due to blunt trauma occur in the combat zone, they are usually due to accidents not related to hostile action. Such casualties are classified as having *nonbattle* injuries.

Penetrating missile wounds of the head are extremely lethal. WDMET data from the Vietnam War indicate that the probability of being fatally wounded by a missile—either fragment or bullet—that hit the skull was close to 4 out of 5 (Chapter 1, Combat Trauma Overview, discusses the WDMET data more fully). Bullet wounds to the head made by assault rifles were fatal in about 95% of cases.[3] Combat casualties with penetrating head trauma who survive to reach a deployable hospital fall into two categories: (1) most commonly, a small fragment wound, with injuries to one cerebral lobe; or (2) less commonly, a tangential gunshot wound, in which the bullet causes a depressed skull fracture, which, in turn, actually lacerates the dura and the brain. Depending on how deeply the bullet has penetrated into the intracranial compartment, it may or may not, in and of itself, directly injure the brain parenchyma. Neurosurgical practice in the combat zone consists of managing both these categories of casualties and those with multiple lobe injuries, such as those caused by bullets. These casualties are in addition to those who demonstrate the spectrum of closed injury, which can range from transient loss of consciousness to deep coma.

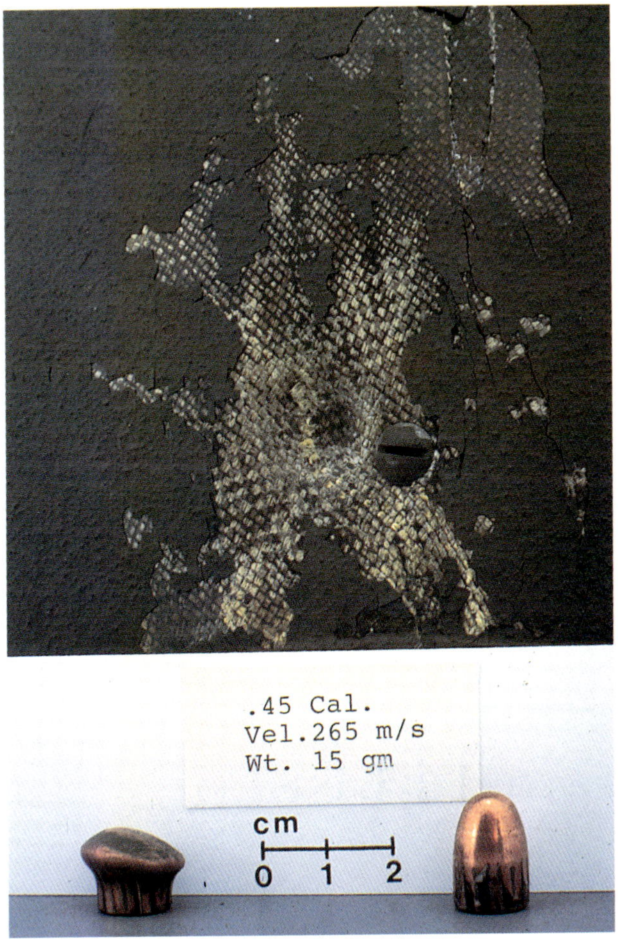

Fig. 16-1. The protection provided by Kevlar helmets is impressive: this helmet, seen close up, was struck by an 0.45 ACP (automatic Colt pistol) at a range of 3 m. The defeated bullet is shown on the left; an unfired bullet is shown on the right. By way of contrast, the 9 x 19-mm Parabellum round will usually perforate a Kevlar helmet. Photograph: Wound Ballistics Laboratory, Letterman Army Institute of Research, Presidio of San Francisco, Calif.

Given the dismal outcome of penetrating missile wounds to the head, preventive measures such as protective helmets have long been recognized to be of great importance. The presently fielded military helmet will stop most fragments produced by improved fragmentation munitions as well as certain types of bullets fired from pistols (Figure 16-1). Fielded helmets will rarely stop a bullet fired from a rifle or machine gun unless the bullet's performance has been severely degraded by passing through a solid object (such as another casualty), has ricocheted off an object and is traveling sideways, or is at the end of its trajectory (1,000 m or so) (Figure 16-2).

During the Persian Gulf War, the Kevlar helmet was found to be extremely beneficial and was associated with a significant diminution of open head injuries, compared to what would have been expected and considering the number of injuries seen to other parts of the body, particularly when compared to the number of injuries to the face and eyes.[4] For this reason, we might well expect that in future conflicts (in which explosive munitions are the predominant source of penetrating missiles, as they were during the

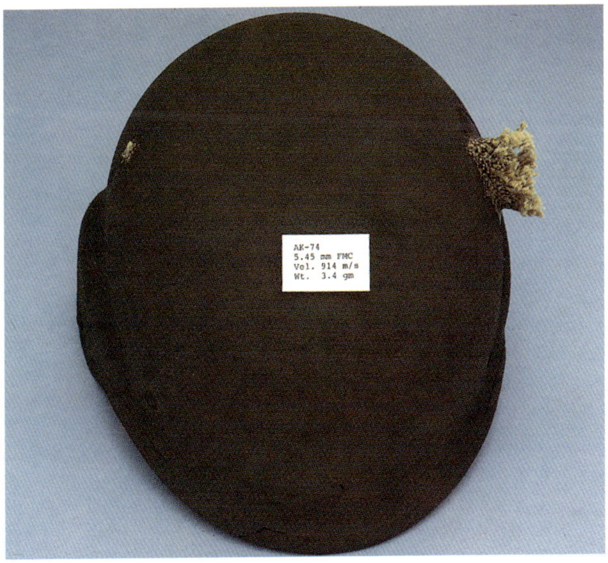

Fig. 16-2. Both sides of this Kevlar helmet have been perforated by a 5.45-mm bullet (fired by an AK74 at range of 3 m), which entered from the viewer's left. Notice the mushroomlike mass of disrupted Kevlar at the site of the bullet's exit. Kevlar fibers have been found lining tissue wound tracts in experimental ballistic studies. Photograph: Wound Ballistics Laboratory, Letterman Army Institute of Research, Presidio of San Francisco, Calif.

Persian Gulf War), a greater percentage of hospitalized casualties will have closed rather than open head injuries.

Casualties who have sustained closed head injuries and survive to reach the hospital level often suffer more significant brain injury than do those who have sustained open injuries. This is due, in part, to the fact that open injuries generally allow some decompression of the immediately surrounding cerebral substance through the break in the skull. In closed injuries, in contrast, the additional volume of blood clot and cerebral swelling must be accommodated within the space of the bony intracranial compartment, which does not change in volume. Therefore, the brain tissue itself is subjected to the total obligatory compression (aside from the small amount that is accommodated by the vessels and the ventricles).

In addition, the physical factors that determine whether an injury will actually break the calvarium are generally associated with a more focal and less diffuse distribution of kinetic energy. The injury is, therefore, usually greater at a small, focal area. The casualty with a significant closed head injury will usually present in coma, with or without lateralizing signs such as extraocular motility and pupillary pareses or asymmetrical posturing. Closed or open facial injuries may well be present also, and airway obstruction must always be the first consideration. Injuries to other parts of the body must be suspected and searched for. Although most casualties with a significant, life-threatening head injury will be comatose when they are evaluated initially, a significant number will be awake but will subsequently deteriorate; a patient with mental status changes, focal neurological findings (particularly those suggestive of a seizure), or even a good history for significant head injury must be observed very carefully.

Casualties with open head injuries may appear more frightening, particularly if brain is exposed, but as noted above, they may have less diffuse brain injury than casualties with closed head injuries. Casualties with open head injuries (and even exposed and injured brain) may be wide awake and alert, often with only a minor, focal, neurological deficit—or no deficit at all. On the other hand, a wound to the brain made by a small fragment or a bullet that has not glanced may well have only a small wound of entrance with extremely little surface tissue damage. These wounds are often much more serious than those involving much more significant surface tissue damage, mostly because in the latter case, the kinetic energy imparted to the head at the wound of entrance is often superficial and tangential. A computed tomography (CT) scan of the former type of wound will often disclose significant intracranial injury that was belied by the relatively benign appearances of the scalp and bone injuries. Such a scan will usually demonstrate significantly greater tissue injury at the wound of exit, especially when the penetrating missile is a bullet. The reason for the greater damage at a bullet's wound of exit is that yaw and tumbling are much more prominent here than at the wound of entrance. For this reason, if the bullet or an irregular fragment has actually exited through the side opposite the wound of entrance, or is lying near the inner surface of the calvarium on the opposite side, that side should generally be addressed first at the time of surgery—as soon as any life-threatening superficial bleeding has been stopped at the wound of entrance. The technique will be discussed in greater detail later in this chapter.

A casualty with a glancing or a relatively shallow injury will often present with much more extensive superficial tissue damage. Here the cerebral damage will be relatively superficial and usually not involve the deeper structures. An example of this would be two different types of self-inflicted gunshot wounds. In the first instance, the individual would point the barrel of the gun directly at his temporal region, then pull the trigger. On leaving the barrel of the gun, the bullet would enter immediately, pass through both hemispheres, and exit the calvarium at the other side. In all likelihood, the greater cerebral damage would be just inside the wound of exit. The superficial damage at the wound of entrance would be relatively slight. In the second instance, consider that the individual flinched at the last instant, turning the barrel so that it was nearly parallel to the plane that was tangential to the skull at the site of the wound. Here, extensive scalp damage would occur and the depressed skull fracture would traverse the the calvarium up to the point where the tangent plane was no longer in contact with the skull. The cerebral damage would be limited to the surface and perhaps a centimeter or so in depth. Keeping these two examples in mind will allow the medical officer to interpret the clinical significance of the appearance of different types of penetrating injury.

GOALS OF NEUROSURGICAL INTERVENTION

Aside from debridement, treatment modalities for casualties with head injuries are, for the most part, nonsurgical. Injury to central nervous system substance cannot be repaired by any primary physical intervention (analogous to suturing for the repair or reanastomosis of a lacerated abdominal organ). If central neural fibers are cut or definitively crushed, there is no treatment, surgical or otherwise, that will restore function. If, on the other hand, the substance of central neural fibers is intact but their function is reversibly impaired (ie, a situation analogous to that of neuropraxia in the peripheral nervous system), certain interventions seem to be capable of altering the physiological environment to make it more conducive to the reversal of the dysfunction. Consequently, nonsurgical treatment of casualties with head injuries is emphasized in this chapter, although several surgical considerations require discussion.

The goal of surgery in closed head injury is generally limited to decompressing the brain parenchyma by removing a mass lesion, which will almost invariably be a hematoma. The only exceptions to this procedure would be the relatively rare circumstances in which (*a*) a lobectomy would be performed to remove edematous brain or (*b*) a cerebrospinal fluid leak would be repaired. The former would usually be a delayed procedure, necessitated at the time of peak swelling (48–72 h after the injury); the latter would almost invariably be delayed well beyond that time.

In open or penetrating head injury, the goals are generally very clearly defined; unlike the usual situation with closed head injury, at least some degree of surgical treatment is almost invariably indicated. Perhaps the first truly comprehensive description of modern neurosurgical techniques in open head injury can be found in Harvey Cushing's 106-page article published in 1918 in the *British Journal of Surgery*,[5] in which he chronicles his extensive experience obtained on the World War I battlefields of France. This, along with his companion article published the same year in the *British Medical Journal*,[6] set the procedural standards, which remained essentially unchanged (aside from the development of certain new hemostatic techniques) until the work of Arnold M. Meirowsky,[7] published half a century later in an official history of the U.S. Army Medical Department, and based on his Korean War experience. Meirowsky's article remained the clear standard until a reasonable update was suggested by Benny Brandvold and colleagues[8] in 1990, writing of their experiences with casualties evacuated to Rambam Maimonides Medical Center, Haifa, Israel.

The first priority in any trauma surgery is invariably the control of hemorrhage; the second is the removal of contaminated material and nonviable tissue. In this regard, open head injury is no exception and initial hemorrhage control is straightforward. Purely on the basis of cerebral compression, it is virtually impossible to exsanguinate into the substance of the brain (unlike into the abdomen or most other regions of the body). The only exception is in the newborn, with its large intracranial volume relative to the rest of its body, and its widely expansive cranial sutures. It is also impossible for hemorrhage deep in the cerebral substance to continually drain a penetrating wound, as the brain will swell and shut off such egress very rapidly. All exsanguinating hemorrhage in open head injury must then emanate from skin, bone, the dural sinuses, or extremely superficial cortical vessels. The scalp is well vascularized, and exsanguination from a scalp laceration alone is possible. Bleeding from the diploic spaces of fractured calvarium is generally limited to a moderately brisk ooze, at most, but over time this can be significant. Unless instantly tamponaded by a depressed bone fragment, bleeding from a lacerated dural sinus would generally result in exsanguination after a few minutes. The surgeon will therefore see this kind of hemorrhage only after an appropriately situated, depressed fracture is elevated. Brisk bleeding from a cortical (pial) vessel is often seen on elevation of depressed bone.

The first steps of surgical treatment will therefore be the control of hemorrhage from the sources described above. Tricks that help the surgeon depend on a familiarity with the anatomy and character of the vessels in each of these areas. Cessation of scalp bleeding, for example, requires coagulation of individual vessels that are found immediately deep to the galea. Grabbing the galea with forceps will disclose these structures quite easily. Bone hemostasis can readily be obtained by rubbing a small amount of bone wax over the cut edge. Dural sinus bleeding will be extremely profuse as soon as the tamponading bone has been removed, but it can be slowed down considerably by simply elevating the head of the table (ie, putting the patient into a reverse Trendelenburg's position). Too much elevation, on the other hand, can allow air to be entrained into the sinus, which is rigidly supported by the dura. This can easily lead to an air embolus. The trick, therefore, is to elevate the head of the bed just enough to allow a slow egress of blood, which will permit the surgeon to repair the sinus with direct suture or a patch of cadaver dura or fascia. The bony diploë also contain blood-filled spaces that will entrain air if the head of the bed is high enough. Rapid and accurate use of wax is extremely important here. Bleeding from the superficial cortex is generally from vessels immediately deep to the pia mater, and most of these can be identified and cauterized.

Once life-threatening hemorrhage has been controlled, the surgeon's attention is turned to debridement of the projectile tract. Contaminated cerebral substance that is oozing out of the wound site is totally nonviable and will never regain function. It can therefore be removed without condemning the patient to further deficit. If left in place, it will undoubtedly lead to further necrosis, cerebritis, and abscess formation. All devitalized brain tissue must therefore be removed by suction, which is continued until the tract remains open and does not immediately swell shut.

Meirowsky believed that the entire wound tract absolutely required radical debridement, and that *all* foreign material, aside from the metal itself, required complete removal. For many years, all bone was searched for, even if it meant increasing the deficit, as surgeons believed that any retained bone would unquestionably lead to abscess formation. However, the Vietnam Head Injury Study[9] has suggested that, although careful debridement is indicated, small amounts of bone left in place may not lead to quite as dangerous a situation as Meirowsky had previously suggested. More recently, experience in the the Israeli–Lebanese War has suggested that with mandatory monitoring a slightly more conservative approach may be acceptable, as long as the threshold for emergent intervention remains low.[8] Presumably, newer antibiotics and better imaging techniques have been instrumental in this change in philosophy (Figure 16-3).

As Cushing pointed out in 1918, failure to close (or patch) the dura will lead to the development of fungus cerebri (ie, an ulcerated cerebral hernia with granulation protruding from the scalp wound). Inattention to dural tears at the base of the skull will lead to cerebrospinal fluid leaks through the nose or ear, which may lead to a need for subsequent surgical repair. Closed head injuries may also require delayed surgical treatment for cerebrospinal fluid rhinorrhea or otorrhea.

Once these surgical considerations have been addressed, the nonsurgical interventions, which can improve the physiological environment so as to promote neural survival and recovery (as well as the survival and recovery of the casualty) may be entertained. Future surgical considerations will be limited to unfortunate circumstances such as delayed brain swelling (rarely requiring lobectomy), further cerebrospinal fluid leaks, or abscess formation.

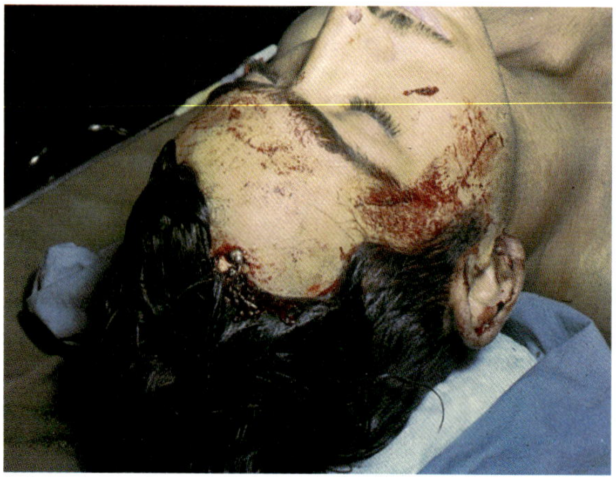

a

Fig. 16-3. This combat casualty has a typical penetrating head wound (made by a preformed fragment from an improved fragmentation grenade). At the time of operation, the casualty was alert and able to move his extremities normally. (**a**) The casualty before induction of anesthesia. The wound of entrance is seen in the right frontal region. The radiographs demonstrate that the fragment (**b**) has crossed the midline and (**c**) has come to rest in the superficial portion of the casualty's left parietal cortex. (**d**) A craniectomy has been performed and (**e**) the missile tract at the wound of entrance has been debrided. (**f**) The craniectomy site has been closed with a fascial graft. (**g**) An anteroposterior radiograph of the skull shows the large defect left by the craniectomy. The fragment is still present. The tissue damage and resulting heightened neurological defect caused by its removal would probably not have been justified by the resultant decrease in the risk of complications such as sepsis arising from a retained foreign body. In contrast to bullets, fragments usually cause more tissue damage where they enter the brain substance than they cause in the more distant parts of their pathway. Photographs: Swan Vietnam Surgical Slide Collection.

b

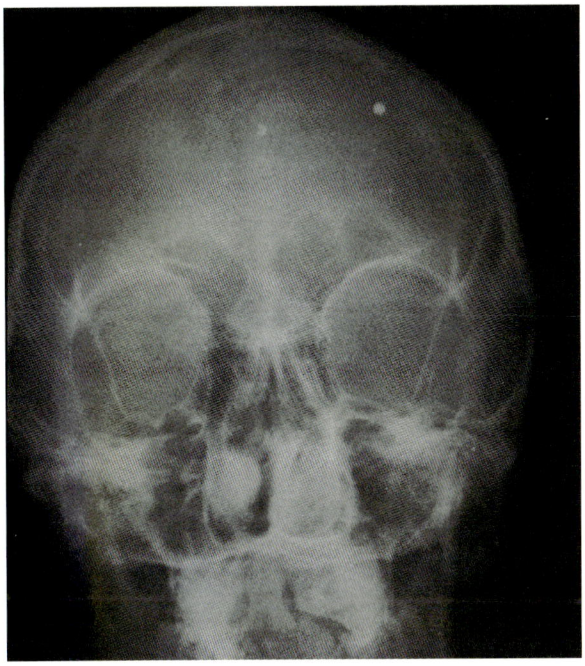

c

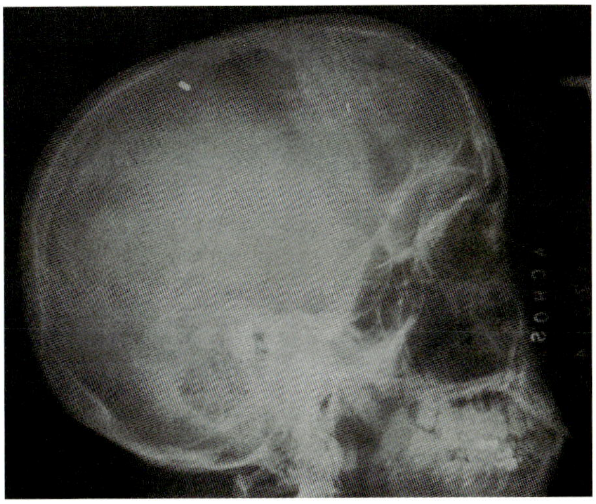

e

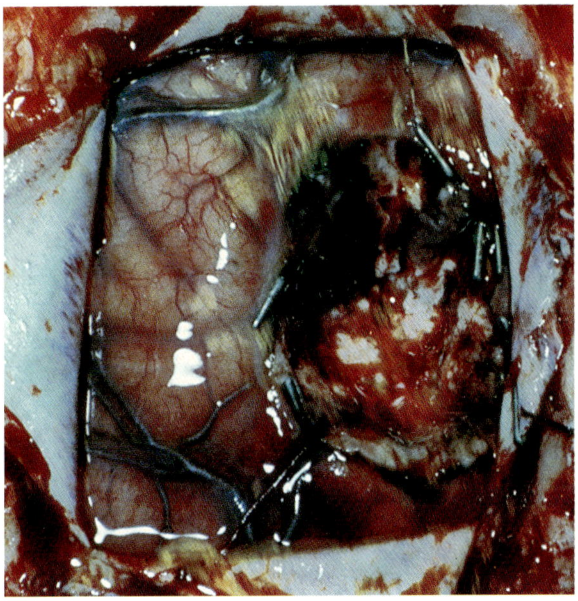

d

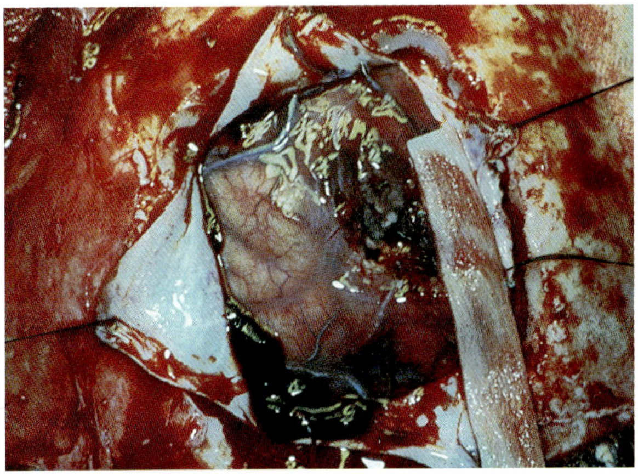

g

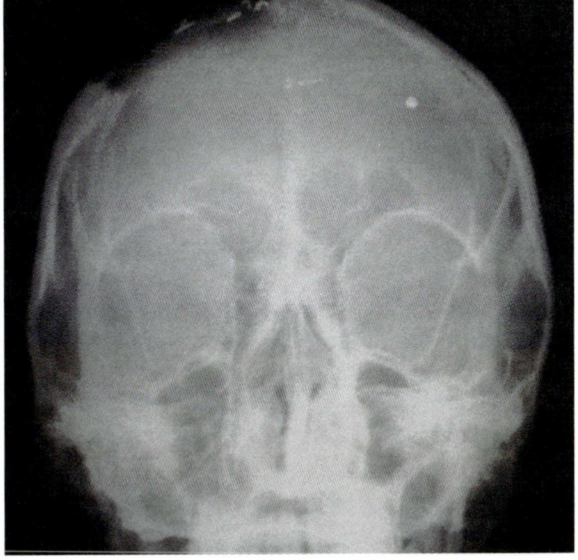

f

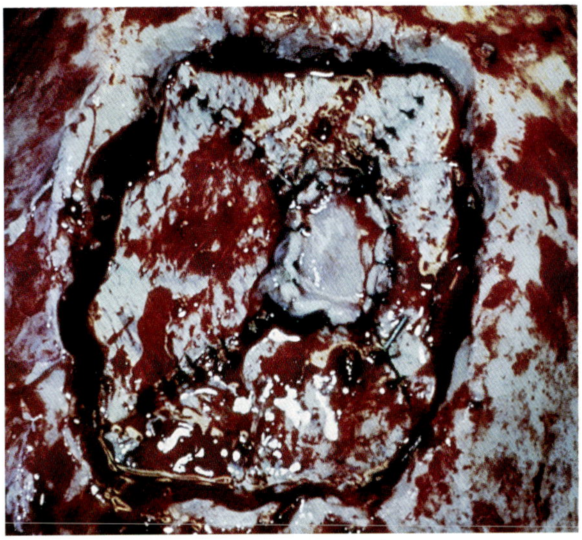

PATHOLOGICAL ANATOMY AND PHYSIOLOGY OF TRAUMATIC BRAIN INJURY

Traumatic brain injuries are diffuse or focal. Comatose trauma patients who demonstrate no focal lesions by CT or magnetic resonance imaging (MRI) during initial diagnostic assessment are said to have diffuse brain injury. Diffuse injury includes diffuse axonal injury, hypoxic brain injury, diffuse brain swelling, and diffuse punctuate brain hemorrhages; focal brain injury includes contusions, avulsions, hematomas, hemorrhages, infarctions, and infections. Diffuse injuries produce coma through damage to the brainstem or cerebral cortex. Focal injuries produce coma by brain compression, brain shift, or herniation. Patients with diffuse brain injury are much less likely than those with focal injuries to have sustained a skull fracture or cerebral contusion, to develop signs of sustained intracranial hypertension, or to have a lucid interval after injury before becoming comatose.[2]

Hypoxic cerebral damage, a common postmortem finding after blunt head trauma,[10,11] is associated with arterial hypoxemia or cerebral hypoperfusion, occurring as a consequence of shock, sustained intracranial hypertension, or cerebral vasospasm.

Both cerebral edema and cerebral swelling occur after brain trauma. Vasogenic cerebral edema results when damage to the blood–brain barrier leads to increased accumulation of interstitial water. Cytotoxic edema, characterized by cellular water accumulation, may follow cerebral hypoxia. In contrast, diffuse cerebral swelling represents vascular congestion, evident on CT scan as symmetrical effacement of the lateral ventricles and the basal cisterns, and normal or increased white matter density.

Ten percent of patients with closed head injuries and Glasgow coma scale (GCS) scores of 13 will require surgery for intracranial lesions. This decision, will, of course, be made on a combination of clinical and radiographic (ie, CT) criteria. The most common focal injuries are cerebral contusions, intraaxial (within the substance of the neuraxis) hematomas, and extraaxial (subdural and epidural) hematomas. Extraaxial hematomas are rarely detected in patients who have both a GCS score of 15 and no focal neurological deficits.[12] On CT, subdural hematomas tend to be crescent shaped, spreading out across the brain surface. In contrast, the typical epidural hematoma has a biconvex (ie, lens-shaped) appearance. Delayed intracerebral hematomas may follow a combined traumatic and anoxic insult.

Closed Brain Injury

Most forms of acute brain injury in humans result from sudden cranial impact or angular cranial acceleration. Impact injuries deform and sometimes fracture the skull, initiating shock waves that are transmitted throughout the brain. When brain tissue strikes bony intracranial prominences, disruption of vascular integrity may produce focal injuries. The clinical spectrum of anatomical findings in minor, moderate, and severe diffuse brain injuries has been reproduced experimentally.[13] Neurological outcome after experimental head trauma correlates with the degree of parenchymal brain injury, especially the extent of primary axonal injury. Traumatic brain injury also alters the cerebral vasculature and disrupts the blood–brain barrier. This disruption may represent the most fundamental response of the brain vasculature to injury and may be a primary mechanism of concussion.[14]

The systemic physiological responses to experimental brain injury include an immediate period of apnea, the duration of which increases with increasing severity of injury.[15] Hypertension and bradycardia immediately follow moderate-to-severe injury, even if mechanical ventilation prevents apnea. Intracranial hypertension consistently accompanies the arterial hypertension; however, intracranial pressure (ICP) returns to normal before the arterial blood pressure. Intracranial hypertension is usually not sustained after experimental head injury.

Penetrating Brain Injury

The pathophysiology of experimental penetrating brain injury has been less extensively investigated than closed head injury. The duration of injury-induced apnea increases in proportion to the muzzle energy of the projectile. Blood pressure and cerebral perfusion pressure (CPP) tend to increase steadily after wounding.[16] In monkeys, missile wounds produce dramatic, immediate increases in ICP (to 40–60 mm Hg) that persist for at least 10 minutes after impact. As CPP falls to approximately 50% of preinjury levels, cerebral blood flow (CBF) declines to approximately 60% of baseline.[17]

Enhanced Vulnerability to Secondary Ischemic Brain Injury

Current clinical and experimental data leave little doubt that the traumatized brain is uniquely vulnerable to posttraumatic ischemic insults. Disability and death arising from insults such as hypotension and hypoxemia are important because they occur after patients have entered the medical care system. Consequently, prevention and effective treatment of secondary ischemic insults should limit morbidity and mortality.

Secondary ischemic brain injury appears to contribute to poor outcome after traumatic brain injury. In one study,[11] nearly 90% of patients who died after traumatic brain injury showed ischemic lesions in a variety of patterns. Diffuse ischemic injury was evident in 23.5%, arterial boundary-zone ischemic injury in 7.5%, ischemia in a specific arterial territory in 10.5%, and hippocampal ischemic injury in 45%.

Hypotension and hypoxemia—systemic insults that can induce cerebral hypoperfusion—worsen outcome, both in terms of higher mortality and worse neurological recovery, after head injury. In 1981, researchers[2] examined the effects of a variety of potential secondary insults on the incidence of unfavorable outcome (ie, severe disability, persistent vegetative state, or death) after severe traumatic brain injury and found that a systolic blood pressure of 90 mm Hg or lower on admission to the hospital was associated with an increase in the incidence of unfavorable outcomes, from 35% to 65%; and hypoxemia (≤ 60 mm Hg on admission) was associated with an increase in unfavorable outcomes, from 35% to 59%. A retrospective review published in 1993[1] of the experience of the Trauma Coma Data Bank even more strongly suggests that hypotension is a powerful predictor of poor outcome after head injury.

Experimental brain injury is followed by a decrease in brain pH and, under certain circumstances, both a decline in high-energy phosphate compounds and an increase in tissue lactate levels. Posttraumatic deterioration in cerebral aerobic metabolism is aggravated by concurrent hypoxia or hypotension. After experimental injury, severe hypoxemia ($Pa{O_2}$ < 40 mm Hg) worsens neurological deficits and brain ischemia, increases tissue inorganic phosphate, and reduces phosphocreatine and adenosine triphosphate.[18] Similarly, hypotension that alone would not alter the cerebral energy state (assessed by magnetic resonance spectroscopy) reduces brain intracellular pH, adenosine triphosphate, and phosphocreatine, and increases the concentration of inorganic phosphate after brain trauma.[19] On the other hand, a study with animals published in 1993[20] demonstrates the existence of an impact level beyond which the head-injured subject never fully recovers from the initial postinjury drop in blood pressure. The deterioration of brain metabolism that follows the combination of hypoxemia or hypotension with experimental brain injury underscores the necessity for prompt restoration of oxygenation, perfusion pressure, and ventilation in patients with head injuries.

Traumatic brain injury initiates a variety of additional biochemical changes, each of which could contribute to enhanced vulnerability to subsequent vascular or tissue injury. Free oxygen radicals may interfere with the normal ability of the cerebral vasculature to dilate in response to declining blood pressure.[21] In cats subjected to head injury, hemorrhagic hypotension reduces CBF more than in control animals.[22,23] Compensatory cerebral vasodilation also fails to occur in response to hemodilutional resuscitation after hemorrhage and head trauma.[24]

Increases in excitatory amino acids such as glutamate and aspartate, which activate *N*-methyl-D-aspartate (NMDA) receptors (among others), correlate with the severity of brain injury in rats and with reduced availability of high-energy phosphate compounds.[25] Evidence also suggests that cholinergic mechanisms mediate enhanced vulnerability to global cerebral ischemia after experimental head injury.[26] The metabolism of cell membrane lipids generates prostaglandins, leukotrienes, and oxygen free radicals. The presence of extravascular blood also generates free radicals. Experimental brain injury increases thromboxane A_2, a powerful vasoconstrictor and platelet aggregator, and also increases brain levels of prostaglandin E_2, a compound that has been associated with reduced motor activity.[27] Finally, some classes of endogenous and exogenous opioid agonists and antagonists may aggravate, while others may limit, brain injury. For example, naloxone, a nonspecific opiate antagonist, significantly worsens outcome after fluid-percussion head injury in rats, whereas morphine reduces deficits.[28]

Although preadmission hypotension and hypoxemia are associated with worse outcome, such insults continue to occur after admission to the hospital, raising the possibility of limiting secondary ischemic injury, either through effective prevention or through preischemic pharmacological intervention. Among a series of 100 patients in an intensive care unit after mild, moderate, or severe traumatic brain injury, hypotension (mean arterial pressure [MAP] ≤ 70 mm Hg) occurred in 76%; reduced CPP (≤ 60 mm Hg), defined as MAP minus ICP, occurred in 78%; and hypoxemia (≤ 90% hemoglobin saturation) occurred in 43%.[29] In eight patients who underwent ICP monitoring after severe traumatic brain injury without evidence on cranial CT of intracranial hypertension, ICP exceeded 20 mm Hg for more than 5 minutes in seven patients, and CPP was less than 60 mm Hg for more than 5 minutes in five patients.[30] Therefore, systemic insults that could worsen outcome by inducing cerebral ischemia occur commonly in patients with head injuries, both at the time of admission to the hospital and during intensive care.

To further support the likelihood that postadmission cerebral ischemia contributes to poor outcome after traumatic brain injury, patients who survived head injury demonstrated evidence of ischemic injury on CT. In 1987, researchers[31] monitored the cerebral metabolic rate for oxygen ($CMRO_2$) and the cerebral metabolic rate for lactate in 44 patients with severe head injuries, and correlated those results with changes in cranial CT scans. Although 27 patients developed low-density areas surrounding intracranial hematomas, 6 others developed evidence of cerebral infarction not associated with hematomas. Low $CMRO_2$ and net cerebral lactate production were found to be weak predictors of later infarction.

Recognition (via continuous monitoring) of cerebral ischemia during intensive care offers the possibility of prompt intervention. Several investigators have examined the ability of jugular venous bulb monitoring to detect ischemia. The jugular venous bulb provides "mixed" cerebral venous blood, relatively uncontaminated by extracranial venous effluent. Like mixed systemic venous sampling, cerebral venous oxygenation provides information that suggests but does not prove cerebral ischemia. In 45 patients cared for in intensive care units after traumatic brain injury, 33 episodes of jugular desaturation below 50% were documented.[32] One researcher[33] reported 121 episodes of combined arterial and jugular venous desaturation during intensive monitoring of 69 patients with severe head injuries; of the 121 episodes, 32 (26.5%) responded poorly to treatment. Prolonged desaturation was associated with deterioration of the GCS score.[33] More importantly, among 102 patients with GCS scores below 9 on admission or on the first day thereafter, one episode of jugular venous desaturation (< 50% for > 10 min) was associated with good recovery or moderate disability in 23%, more than one episode with good recovery or moderate disability in 12%, and the absence of jugular venous desaturation with good recovery or moderate disability in 46%.[34]

Systemic and Organ-System Responses

Clinical head injury is associated with sympathetically mediated hypertension, tachycardia, and increased cardiac output. The more severe the level of isolated clinical head injury (ie, the lower the GCS score), the greater the increase in plasma norepinephrine levels and heart rate.[35] However, experimental data[20] suggest that beyond a threshold impact level, the increase in catecholamines no longer linearly correlates with the intensity of the impact. In sympathetically stimulated patients with head injuries, β adrenergic blockade reduces heart rate, cardiac index, and circulating catecholamines.[36]

In addition to the characteristic hyperdynamic response associated with head injury, hypertension also accompanies severe increases in ICP, a response first recognized by Cushing in 1903[37] and now known as the Cushing phenomenon. If permitted to progress and depending on the direction in which the brain expands, increasing intracranial hypertension may produce medullary compression and precipitous systemic hypotension. Management of the Cushing phenomenon consists of therapy to reduce ICP, thereby interrupting the reflex response. If systemic hypertension is secondary to the Cushing phenomenon, attempts to control blood pressure using vasodilators may both reduce MAP and increase ICP, thereby further compromising cerebral perfusion.

Patients with head injuries also undergo stress-induced hyperglycemia and accelerated protein wasting. The frequent occurrence of fever and hypoalbuminemia has been attributed to endothelial cell injury.[38]

Pulmonary Effects

Acute head injury is associated with a variety of respiratory problems, some potentially fatal (eg, apnea, central neurogenic pulmonary edema, and altered breathing patterns), as a result of associated injuries, fat embolism syndrome, pulmonary contusion, and hemopneumothorax. Hypoxemia may occur even in patients who lack auscultatory or radiographic evidence of pulmonary compromise, apparently because of failure of mechanisms that regulate ventilation–perfusion matching.[39] Central neurogenic pulmonary edema, a rare, acutely life-threatening complication usually seen accompanying severe injury, may result from acute left atrial hypertension or increased pulmonary capillary permeability.[40] Management of central neurogenic pulmonary edema necessitates prompt correction of intracranial hypertension, if present, in addition to therapy to improve oxygenation.

Coagulopathy

Laboratory evidence of disseminated intravascular coagulation is reported in nearly one fourth of patients with head injuries.[41] Patients with higher concentrations of fibrin degradation products have poorer functional outcomes and are more likely to develop the adult respiratory distress syndrome.[42]

Cerebral Circulatory Responses

Acute head injury of sufficient severity to produce coma is associated with moderately decreased CBF, markedly depressed $CMRo_2$, and highly variable autoregulation and carbon dioxide reactivity. The uninjured cerebral circulation is responsive to changes in metabolic demand; CPP; the partial pressure of carbon dioxide, arterial ($Paco_2$); and the partial pressure of oxygen, arterial (Pao_2). Cerebral blood flow normally is coupled to $CMRo_2$, which varies directly with body temperature and the level of brain activation; that is, $CMRo_2$ is increased by fever, seizures, or pain. Cerebral blood flow remains constant (approximately 50 mL/100 g/min in adults) in the normal brain as CPP changes over a range of approximately 50 to approximately 130 mm Hg. In normal individuals, over a range of $Paco_2$ from 20 to 80 mm Hg, CBF will be acutely halved if $Paco_2$ is halved and will double if $Paco_2$ is doubled. That relationship is apparently intact in most patients with head injuries. Pao_2 exerts little effect on CBF unless Pao_2 declines below 60 mm Hg (hemoglobin saturation < 90%). Below that level, CBF increases abruptly.

In 1991, one group of researchers[43] reported that CBF was less than a critical value of 18 mL/100 g/min in one third of measurements made within 6 hours of injury in 106 patients with head injuries. Moreover, the average difference in cerebral arteriovenous oxygen content ($AVDo_2$) was greater than normal during this critical early interval (Figure 16-4), suggesting that CBF was indeed inadequate.[43] Later, in the days after injury, some patients with head injury demonstrate depressed levels of both $CMRo_2$ and CBF, while others demonstrate uncoupling, with CBF substantially in excess of $CMRo_2$ (Figure 16-5).[44] Nearly 90% of patients younger than 18 years of age demonstrate relative cerebral hyperemia, defined as CBF that exceeds metabolic demand, or even exceeds normal values, at some point during intensive monitoring.[45]

Experimental and clinical data[46] demonstrate that CBF after head trauma frequently is MAP dependent rather than MAP independent (Figure 16-6). Most patients with mass lesions demonstrate defective autoregulation; conversely, autoregulation remains intact in many patients without intracranial mass lesions.[46] In patients with head injuries in whom autoregulation is intact, mannitol reduces ICP and does not change CBF; if autoregulation is defective, ICP changes little and CBF increases.[47]

In many patients, reduced CBF appears to represent appropriate coupling between low $CMRo_2$ and low CBF rather than cerebral ischemia.[44] However, patients with low but coupled CBF may be vulnerable to excessive vasoconstriction during acute hyperventilation. Nearly 20% of patients develop a wide cerebral $AVDo_2$ during hyperventilation, sug-

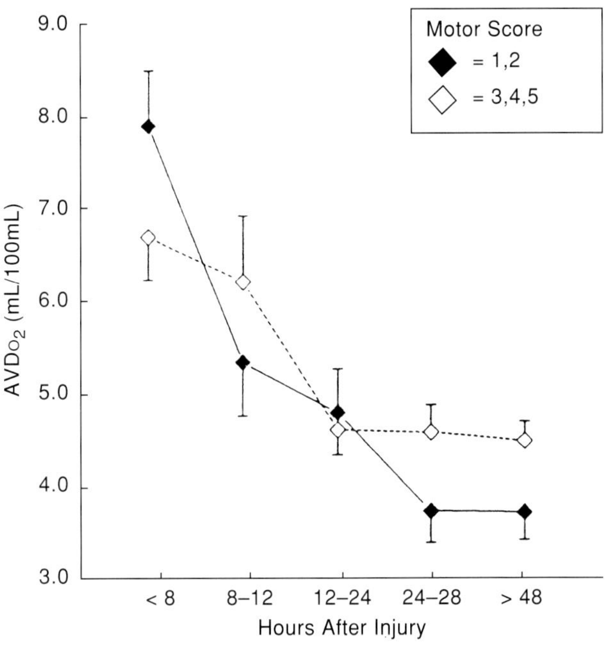

Fig. 16-4. Time course of mean arteriovenous oxygen difference ($AVDo_2$) in patients with head injuries and with motor scores of 1 or 2, and those with motor scores of 3 to 5 (motor score is measured as the best response to a painful stimulus: 1 = no response; 2 = extension; 3 = abnormal flexion; 4 = flexion withdrawal; 5 = localizing response). Error bars represent the standard error of the mean. Reprinted with permission from Bouma GJ, Muizelaar JP, Choi SC, Newlon PG, Young HF. Cerebral circulation and metabolism after severe traumatic brain injury: The elusive role of ischemia. *J Neurosurg*. 1991;75:688.

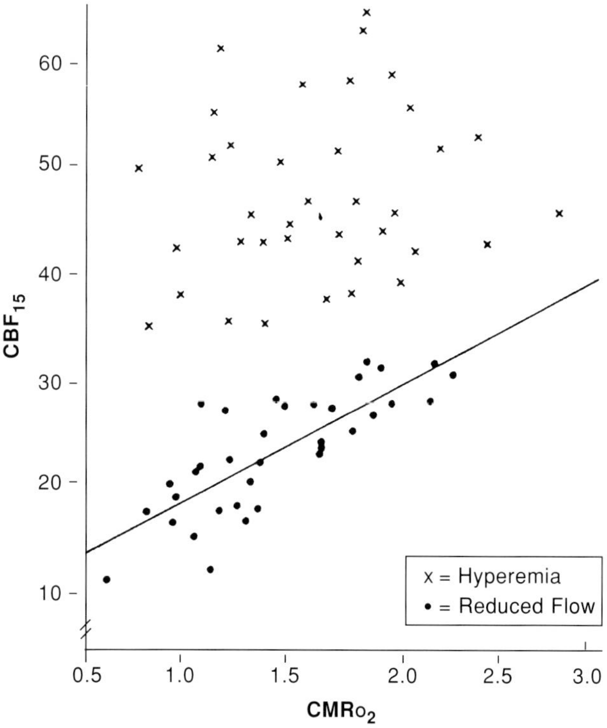

Fig. 16-5. In patients who have sustained closed head injury, both the cerebral metabolic rate of oxygen consumption ($CMRO_2$, the abscissa) and cerebral blood flow (CBF, based on ^{133}Xe clearance integrated over 15 min, the ordinate) are reduced. (Normal values are 3.4 mL/100 g/min and 50 mL/100 g/min, respectively). In some patients (closed circles), $CMRO_2$ and CBF appear to be reduced to a similar extent (ie, coupled). In others (represented by the x's), global CBF is higher than apparently is necessary to meet metabolic demand (uncoupled). Reprinted with permission from Obrist WD, Langfitt TW, Jaggi JL, Cruz J, Gennarelli TA. Cerebral blood flow and metabolism in comatose patients with acute head injury: Relationship to intracranial hypertension. *J Neurosurg.* 1984;61;247.

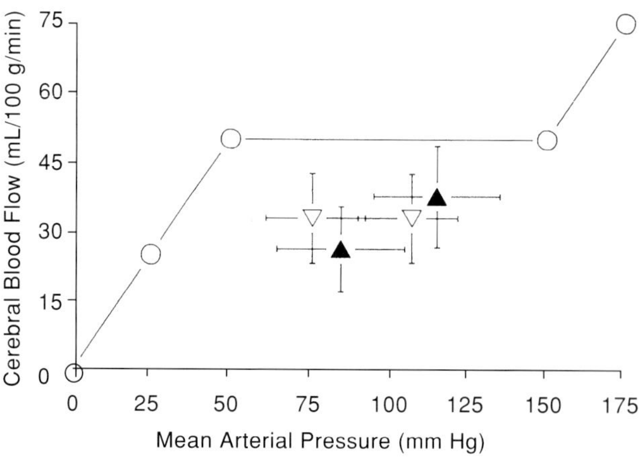

Fig. 16-6. In comparison to the normal autoregulatory curve (open circles), adult patients who have sustained closed head injury have reduced flow, and in some cases (closed triangles), impaired autoregulation. Other patients have reduced flow and preserved autoregulation (open triangles). Data source: Muizelaar JP, Lutz HA III, Becker DP. Effect of mannitol on ICP and CBF and correlation with pressure autoregulation in severely head-injured patients. *J Neurosurg.* 1984;61:700–706.

gesting that hyperventilation therapy occasionally may adversely influence cerebral perfusion (Table 16-1).[44] If increased ICP develops in patients with a wide cerebral $AVDO_2$, other measures to reduce ICP, such as sedation or osmotic diuresis, produce better matching of cerebral oxygen supply and demand than further hyperventilation. If CBF measurements are unavailable, the calculation of the cerebral oxygen extraction or the lactate extraction may provide clinically useful information regarding the adequacy of cerebral oxygen delivery.[31–33,48–50]

TABLE 16-1

FINDINGS IN 10 PATIENTS WITH WIDE ARTERIOVENOUS OXYGEN DIFFERENCES AFTER HEAD INJURY*

Hemodynamic Variable	Hyperventilated Patients*	Normal Value ($Paco_2 \approx 40$ mm Hg)
$CMRO_2$	1.9 ± 0.5	3.3 ± 0.4
CBF_{15}	18.6 ± 4.4	53.3 ± 6.8
$AVDO_2$	10.5 ± 0.7	6.3 ± 1.2
VPO_2	22.3 ± 1.8	37.5 ± 5.6

*Values are means ± standard deviations obtained 10 to 85 h after the injury
$AVDO_2$: arteriovenous oxygen differences (in vol %); CBF_{15}: mean cerebral blood flow based on ^{133}Xe clearance integrated over 15 min; $CMRO_2$: cerebral metabolic rate for oxygen (in mL/100 g/min); VPO_2: jugular venous oxygen tension (in mm Hg)
Reprinted with permission from Obrist WD, Langfitt TW, Jaggi JL, Cruz J, Gennarelli TA. Cerebral blood flow and metabolism in comatose patients with acute head injury: Relationship to intracranial hypertension. *J Neurosurg.* 1984;61:251.

CARE OF THE PATIENT WITH TRAUMATIC BRAIN INJURY

Initial Care

Two assessment systems can be used to understand the reports that characterize the initial management of traumatic brain injury. The first, the GCS, was originally developed to permit comparisons among series of patients with traumatic brain injuries, based on their initial clinical presentation (Table 16-2).[51] Consisting of three major categories (eye opening [1–4 points], verbal responses [1–5 points], and motor function [1–6 points, assessed in the best responding limb]), the GCS score ranges from 3 to 15. Mild head injury is defined as scores ranging from 13 to 15, moderate as scores from 9 to 12, and severe as 8 or less. The GCS constitutes a reliable index of overall brain function with minimal interobserver variability. The second system, the Glasgow outcome scale (GOS) defines five categories: good recovery, moderate disability, severe disability, persistent vegetative state, and death (Table 16-3).[52] Defined in these terms, about 2,000 to 3,000 patients per million population per year come to medical attention; 85% to 90% are in the mild category, 5% to 10% in the moderate, and 5% in the severe.[29] The GCS is a powerful predictor of the final outcome (Table 16-4).[53]

Prompt application of basic life support may prevent secondary hypoxic brain damage.[54] Secondary insults such as anemia, hypotension, hypoxemia, and hypercarbia, alone or in combination, occur in nearly 50% of comatose patients with head injuries (Table 16-5).[2] Thus, tracheal intubation, positive-pressure ventilation with oxygen, and systemic hemodynamic resuscitation should be initiated promptly when indicated, and should not be

TABLE 16-2

GLASGOW COMA SCORE

Component	Response	Score
Eye Opening	Spontaneously	4
	To verbal command	3
	To pain	2
	None	1
	Subtotal	**(1–4)**
Motor Response (best extremity)	Obeys verbal command	6
	Localizes pain	5
	Flexion-withdrawal	4
	Flexion (decortication)	3
	Extension (decerebration)	2
	No response (flaccid)	1
	Subtotal	**(1–6)**
Best Verbal Response	Oriented and converses	5
	Disoriented and converses	4
	Inappropriate words	3
	Incomprehensible sounds	2
	No verbal response	1
	Subtotal	**(1–5)**
	Total	**(3–15)**

Reprinted with permission from Teasdale G, Jennett B. Assessment of coma and impaired consciousness. *Lancet*. 1974;2:81–84.

TABLE 16-3

GLASGOW OUTCOME SCALE

Patient Outcome	Description
Good Recovery	Normal or minimally impaired patients who have returned to school, university, or former occupation, or are capable of managing their households
Moderate Disability	Patients who can perform the tasks of daily living but are no longer able to work or attend school
Severe Disability	Patients who require assistance to perform the tasks of daily living but do not require institutional care
Persistent Vegetative State	Patients remain unresponsive and speechless for weeks or months; absent function in the cerebral cortex (as judged behaviorally) although cortex may appear structurally intact
Death	Patients do not regain consciousness; most deaths occur within 48 h

Reprinted with permission from Jennett B, Bond M. Assessment of outcome after severe brain damage: A practical scale. *Lancet*. 1975;1:480–484.

TABLE 16-4

RELATION OF ACUTE GLASGOW COMA SCALE SCORE TO GLASGOW OUTCOME SCALE SCORE*

GOS Score	GCS Score 3–4	GCS Score 5–6	GCS Score 7–9	Total Cases
	No. (%) of Cases			
Dead/PVS	15 (78.9%)	19 (45.2%)	9 (25.7%)	43
SD/MD/GR	4 (21.2%)	23 (54.8%)	26 (74.3%)	53
Total Cases	19	42	35	96

*Significance: $P < .0001$ (chi-square)
GCS: Glascow Coma Scale; GOS: Glasgow Outcome Scale; PVS: persistent vegetative state; SD: severe disability; MD: moderate disability; GR: good recovery
Reprinted with permission from Jaggi JL, Obrist WD, Gennarelli TA, Langfitt TW. Relationship of early cerebral blood flow and metabolism to outcome in acute head injury. *J Neurosurg*. 1990;72:178.

deferred until the patient arrives at a trauma center.

Intubation of patients with head injuries, who also may have unrecognized cervical spine injuries, presents a challenge in which several therapeutic conflicts must be balanced. Inadequate ventilation and oxygenation must be promptly reversed. Ideally, profound sedation and muscle relaxation limit increases in ICP associated with endotracheal intubation; however, hypovolemia resulting from associated injuries may contraindicate effective sedation. Intubation may be technically difficult owing to trauma to facial structures or to trismus. In such cases (and if time permits), it may be practical to secure an airway using a fiberoptic endoscope. Occasionally, cricothyroidotomy, transcricothyroid oxygen insufflation, or formal tracheostomy may be required. Facial fractures constitute a relative contraindication to nasotracheal intubation.[55]

Despite legitimate concern that the depolarizing muscle relaxant succinylcholine may increase ICP,[56] its more rapid onset of action, compared with that of nondepolarizing muscle relaxants, may make it necessary to use succinylcholine for immediate intubation of an unstable patient. After intubation, the patient should be ventilated with an oxygen-

TABLE 16-5

INFLUENCE OF REMEDIABLE CAUSES OF SECONDARY INJURY ON OUTCOME AFTER HEAD INJURY

Secondary Insult	Definition	Poor Outcome* (%)
Hypoxemia	$Pa{O_2} < 60$ mm Hg	59
Hypotension	SBP < 90 mm Hg	65
Anemia	Hct < 30%	62
Hypercarbia	$Pa{CO_2} > 45$ mm Hg	78
Intracranial hypertension	ICP > 20, reducible	45
	ICP > 20, not reducible	95

*Poor outcome: severe disability, persistent vegetative state, or death
Hct: hematocrit; ICP: intracranial pressure; SBP: systolic blood pressure
Adapted with permission from Miller JD, Butterworth JF, Gudeman SK, et al. Further experience in the management of severe head injury. *J Neurosurg*. 1981;54:292.

enriched gas mixture. Minute ventilation should be adjusted to maintain Pa_{CO_2} at or below 40 mm Hg unless clinical evaluation or monitoring indicates severe, acute, intracranial hypertension. Routine hyperventilation may not improve outcome and may even be deleterious.[57]

No resuscitation fluid has proven ideal in patients with multiple trauma and head injury. Several studies with animals have demonstrated lower ICP or higher CBF when hypertonic saline solutions are substituted for isotonic fluids (Figure 16-7).[58,59] Clearly, hypotonic solutions, which increase brain tissue volume, should be avoided. The role of colloid-containing solutions is controversial. Although for years clinicians have considered colloids less likely to increase ICP after head injury, data suggest that changes in colloid osmotic pressure exert minimal effects on brain water or ICP in animals both with and without intracranial pathology.[60,61] Although rapid resuscitation with 6.0% hydroxyethyl starch increases ICP less than hemodynamically comparable resuscitation using lactated Ringer's solution,[62] the difference is probably due to the fact that lactated Ringer's solution is slightly hypotonic.

The neurological examination, preferably conducted before induction of neuromuscular paralysis, should assign a GCS score and, in all comatose patients, assess brainstem function, (ie, pupillary light responses and oculocephalic or vestibuloocular reflexes). Patients should undergo a more complete neurological examination as time permits, but as expeditiously as possible. Changes in the examination may be localizing and may dictate intervention, even if they do not change the GCS score.

Clearly, the highest priority for comatose patients with head injuries is to determine the need for craniotomy. Patients with open or penetrating inju-

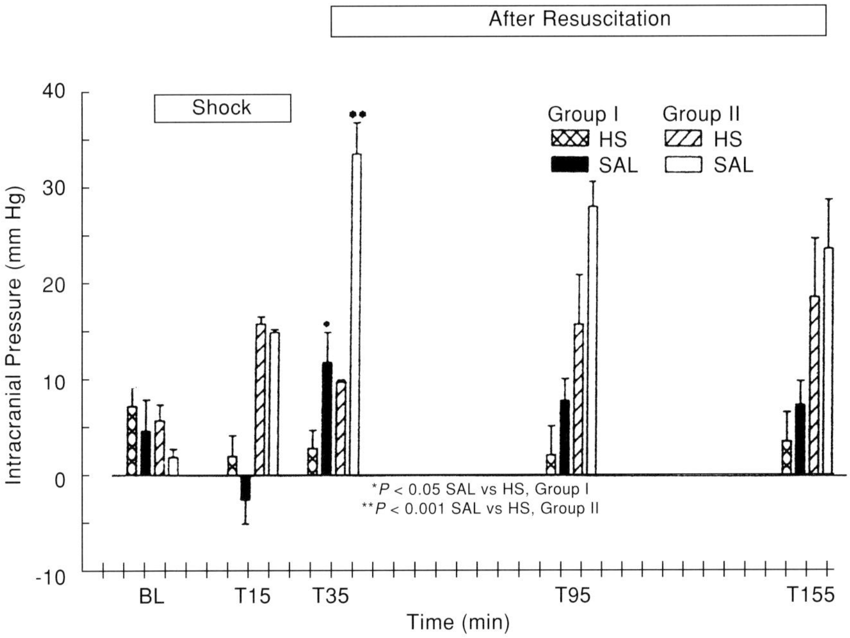

Fig. 16-7. Response of intracranial pressure (ICP) to resuscitation from shock with 7.2% hypertonic saline (HS) or 0.8% saline (SAL) in animals without (Group 1) and with (Group 2) a right hemispheric intracranial mass. Intracranial hypertension (15 mm Hg) in Group 2 was induced by inflation of a right-hemispheric subdural balloon to which additional saline was added as necessary to maintain ICP at 15 mm Hg during shock. Shock extended from 0 time to T30 (30 min after initiation of shock). BL denotes baseline; T15 refers to 15 min after the beginning of a 30-min shock interval; T35, T95, and T155 refer to 5, 60, and 120 min after a single-bolus resuscitation. After a 30-min interval of hemorrhagic shock at a mean cerebral perfusion pressure of 35 mm Hg, rapid resuscitation consisted of 0.8% SAL (54 mL/kg) or 7.2% HS (6.0 mL/kg). In animals both with and without intracranial mass lesions, ICP was significantly greater immediately after resuscitation in animals resuscitated with 0.8% SAL than in those resuscitated with 7.2% HS; differences quickly became statistically insignificant. Reprinted with permission from Prough DS, Whitley JW, Taylor CL, Deal DD, DeWitt DS. Regional cerebral blood flow following resuscitation from hemorrhagic shock with hypertonic saline: Influence of a subdural mass. *Anesthesiology*. 1991;75:323.

ries require prompt surgical debridement or, if local facilities are limited and the patient is sufficiently stable to transport, transfer to a secondary- or tertiary-care facility. All patients who do not obey simple commands (in the absence of drug or alcohol intoxication) require prompt CT scanning to exclude intracranial mass lesions. Patients who require evacuation of subdural hematomas but whose craniotomy is delayed have a far worse outcome than those patients whose hematomas are promptly evacuated.[63] Before the widespread availability of CT and MRI, neuroradiological evaluation could rapidly be accomplished through either cerebral angiography or air ventriculography. These latter two techniques, now rarely used, should be considered if immediate scanning is unavailable, as may well be true under battlefield conditions. In such circumstances, a single-shot arteriogram, performed on initial evaluation of a patient with a high likelihood of an intracranial mass lesion, could be lifesaving. The use of near-infrared spectroscopy to diagnose acute intracranial hematomas is yet to be completely evaluated, although preliminary data[64] are encouraging.

Adult patients who have *briefly* lost consciousness, but who subsequently have a completely normal neurological examination, probably do not need a CT scan in the absence of other clinical indications. The management of patients who have intermediate levels of injury requires repeated evaluation and careful observation.

Diagnostic priorities for other organ systems should proceed as indicated by the description of the traumatic event and by the general physical examination. In all comatose patients with head injuries, unless they are known to have suffered *only* an isolated head injury, abdominal CT scan or diagnostic peritoneal lavage[65] should be performed to detect occult intraabdominal injury. Patients should be considered to have cervical spine fractures until this possibility has been excluded by a cross-table lateral neck radiograph (or a cervical CT scan) that adequately shows all cervical vertebrae. Some degree of immobilization (eg, using a hard collar) should be maintained until the patient is sufficiently cooperative to perform his own neck manipulation for flexion and extension films.

Although shock sometimes occurs in association with an isolated head injury, other causes of hypotension that must be excluded[65] include intraabdominal hemorrhage (evaluated by CT scan or diagnostic peritoneal lavage), intrathoracic hemorrhage (evaluated by chest radiography, CT scan, or aortography), long-bone fractures (assessed using a skeletal survey), myocardial ischemia or cardiac decompensation (evaluated using electrocardiography or pulmonary arterial catheterization), and pericardial tamponade (suggested by a paradoxical pulse, central venous or pulmonary artery pressure monitoring, chest radiography, echocardiography, or pericardiocentesis). Untreated shock portends a worse prognosis.[1]

Anesthetic Management

Military trauma anesthesia personnel may be confronted with a spectrum of casualties with head injuries, from those who arrive from the battlefield only moments after injury to those who have been thoroughly evaluated and stabilized. The patient may be intubated, sedated, and paralyzed, or may be awake but combative. Surgery may be required for emergent evacuation of an intracranial hematoma or may be directed at treatment of injuries to other organ systems. Therefore, it is obvious that anesthesia personnel participate in a continuum of care that includes the considerations discussed elsewhere in this chapter. However, for purposes of brevity, this section will address questions of anesthetic management as they apply to unintubated patients presenting for surgery with moderate-to-severe head injuries.

Preoperatively, little time may be available for evaluation. Therefore, the following assumptions are appropriate. Airway obstruction, hypoventilation, and hypoxia are likely, and oxygen requirements are increased. Both depression of consciousness and injury increase the risk of aspiration of stomach contents. Hypotension, uncommon in a patient with an isolated head injury, implies hemorrhage from associated injuries or spinal cord injury and markedly increases the risk of secondary cerebral ischemia in patients with head injuries. Many patients with head injuries are hypertensive because of catecholamine release. Some patients are hypertensive because of physiological reflexes that attempt to maintain CPP as ICP increases. Only severe hypertension necessitates treatment; reflex hypertension caused by intracranial hypertension requires treatment of increased ICP. Direct vasodilators (ie, nitroglycerine, nitroprusside, and hydralazine) increase CBF and ICP. β-Adrenergic blocking agents such as esmolol or propranolol or mixed α- and β-adrenergic blocking agents such as labetalol minimally affect ICP.

Monitoring should be determined by the severity of the injuries and the availability of technologically sophisticated equipment. Resuscitation and stabilization should not be delayed in an effort to establish better monitoring. If time and circumstances permit, direct arterial pressure monitoring and central venous pressure monitoring are valuable. Pulse oximetry and capnography provide early warning of deterioration in gas exchange. Automated, noninvasive blood pressure monitoring may free anesthesia personnel for other activities. If practical, ICP monitoring may be useful if a patient with severe head injuries requires extensive surgery for other injuries.

Volume resuscitation should not be constrained by fears of increasing cerebral edema. At the present time, the most appropriate fluid for the initial treatment of hemorrhagic shock in a patient with head injuries is 0.9% saline, a slightly hypertonic solution that should result in no increase in brain water or ICP in areas of brain in which the blood–brain barrier is intact. Blood products should be given as indicated and available. More highly hypertonic solutions, which decrease brain water and ICP in experimental animals and decrease ICP in humans, may become the treatment of choice in the future.

Anesthetic induction must preserve CPP. Avoidance of hypotension is more important than reduction of small increases in ICP. Potential induction agents include thiopental, etomidate, benzodiazepines, and ketamine. Barbiturates decrease $CMRO_2$, reduce CBF, and reduce ICP. However, large dosages of barbiturates may reduce blood pressure, especially in hypovolemic patients, and may slow emergence from general anesthesia. Etomidate provides prompt induction and is usually well tolerated even in moderately hypovolemic patients. Benzodiazepines decrease $CMRO_2$ and CBF, and usually preserve blood pressure. Large dosages may slow emergence. Ketamine, which increases CBF and ICP, would rarely be appropriate in a patient with head injuries. Cricoid pressure should be applied during induction and intubation.

In a patient who is hemodynamically resuscitated, a reasonable sequence is to administer succinylcholine (or a large dose of a nondepolarizing agent), thiopental, and fentanyl while maintaining cricoid pressure. In a severely hypovolemic patient, succinylcholine and a small dose of a narcotic or intravenous lidocaine to blunt the hemodynamic response to intubation would be preferable. Although succinylcholine may increase ICP, expeditious control of the airway is more important.

Volatile anesthetics decrease $CMRO_2$, but they also increase CBF and should only be administered to patients at risk of intracranial hypertension after hyperventilation has been established. Isoflurane appears to be most satisfactory. Although nitrous oxide causes small increases in CBF and $CMRO_2$, the reduced fraction of inspired oxygen (FIO_2) necessitated by nitrous oxide administration limits its use in patients with lung injury.

Management in the Intensive Care Unit

The primary goals of management in the intensive care unit are to prevent secondary neurological injury and to limit complications that develop in other organ systems.

Cerebral Circulatory Considerations

Much of the management of casualties with acute head injuries is intended to maintain adequate cerebral perfusion. Because CBF is not routinely measured, most cerebral circulatory information is inferred from measurements of $PaCO_2$, blood pressure, and ICP. Measurement of ICP, combined with measurement of MAP, permits calculation of CPP according to the equation:

$$CPP = MAP - ICP$$

Cerebral ischemia, defined as inadequate cerebral oxygen delivery (CDO_2), can result from a critical reduction of any of the components, including CBF, hemoglobin concentration, and arterial hemoglobin saturation (SaO_2). Uniquely susceptible to oxygen deprivation, the brain constitutes only approximately 2% of total body weight, but it receives 15% of the cardiac output and accounts for 15% to 20% of total oxygen consumption.

Brain Monitoring

Most global cerebral insults, occurring secondary to hypotension, hypoxemia, or cardiac arrest, are readily detected by systemic monitors. Therefore, brain-specific monitors can provide additional information primarily in situations such as cerebral trauma, in which regional cerebral oxygenation may be impaired despite adequate systemic oxygenation and perfusion.

Monitoring devices facilitate early recognition of physiological derangements that would produce complications unless effective treatment were provided. The application of brain-monitoring devices in patients with head injuries therefore presupposes certain assumptions:

1. Reduced C_{DO_2} (CBF • arterial O_2 content) is associated with avoidable neurological morbidity.
2. The proportion of patients who will develop avoidable injury is sufficiently large to justify extensive application of brain-monitoring devices.
3. Thresholds for intervention can be defined based on experimental and clinical evidence.

Brain monitors assess, directly or indirectly, cerebral function, cerebral perfusion, or brain metabolism (Exhibit 16-1). The role of brain monitoring has been incompletely defined in acute head injury. Many brain monitors, such as those that record CBF, evoked potentials, and computer-processed electroencephalograms, are technically challenging and difficult to apply in combat situations unless specifically trained personnel are available. More importantly, no generally accepted protocols have been developed that establish clinically important thresholds for monitored variables other than ICP, define appropriate interventions to improve the monitored variables, and have been proven to improve outcome.

EXHIBIT 16-1

TYPES OF CEREBRAL MONITORING

Function

- Evoked potentials
- Electroencephalogram
  - Raw
  - Processed

Perfusion

- Cerebral blood flow
  - Velocity
  - Intracranial pressure

Metabolism

- Oxygen extraction
- Jugular bulb saturation
- Near-infrared spectroscopy

Operational Characteristics of Monitors

Thresholds of CBF that correlate with various clinical outcomes, physiological changes, and changes in monitored variables have been defined (Table 16-6). It is impossible to predict with certainty if even severe changes in function will be followed by further cerebral damage. Moreover, because various brain regions are selectively vulnerable to injury, regional ischemia and infarction may develop without producing changes in monitored variables. The complexity and heterogeneity of brain tissue virtually preclude development of a single, perfectly predictive brain monitor.

Evoked Potentials. Sensory evoked potentials (EPs), which include somatosensory evoked potentials (SSEPs), brainstem auditory evoked potentials (BAEPs), and visual evoked potentials (VEPs), and, more recently, motor evoked potentials (MEPs), provide a visual representation of the response of

TABLE 16-6

CLINICAL, PATHOPHYSIOLOGICAL, AND MONITORING THRESHOLDS IN CEREBRAL ISCHEMIA

Cerebral Blood Flow (mL/100 g/min)	Clinical Findings	Pathophysiological Changes	Electrophysiological Changes
50	Normal		
23	Reversible paralysis		EEG slowing, EP change
20		Na^+/K^+ pump dysfunction	
18	Permanent paralysis		EEG flat
15			EP absent
10		K^+ efflux, Ca^{++} influx	

EEG: electroencephalogram; EP: evoked potentials

neural structures to stimulation. EPs are generated by integrated neural networks, including the initial sensory structure, the transmitting pathways, and cortical and subcortical stimulus-processing centers. As the response to a stimulus is transmitted centrally, characteristic waveforms are generated that correspond to structures through which the stimulus passes. EPs, especially BAEPs and MEPs, are relatively refractory to insult, although they are modified by sedatives, narcotics, and anesthetics, as well as by trauma, hypoxia, or ischemia. Because obliteration of EPs occurs only under conditions of profound cerebral ischemia or mechanical trauma, EP monitoring is one of the most specific ways to assess neurological integrity. However, EPs are less sensitive to smaller changes in cerebral (or spinal cord) oxygen availability.

In patients with head trauma[66,67] or spinal cord injury,[68,69] EP monitoring has been employed primarily as a diagnostic and prognostic aid. Multimodality EPs improve the prognostic accuracy of the clinical examination and measurement of ICP in patients with head injuries.[67] With impending brain death, cortical SSEPs disappear first; BAEPs disappear only when brain death is imminent.[70] Because BAEPs are resistant to the effects of barbiturates, EPs assist in assessing neurological status even in patients in barbiturate coma.

Electroencephalographic Monitoring. Computerized compression of electroencephalographic (EEG) data permits frequent, repetitive assessment with a minimum of specific training. In the most commonly employed software programs, the data are displayed as a compressed spectral array (CSA) or density spectral array (DSA). Because the EEG is sensitive to drug effects, either unprocessed or processed EEG monitoring can be used to assess sedation in critically ill patients as well as to provide early evidence of seizure activity or cerebral ischemia.

This equipment remains relatively expensive, depends on the availability of dedicated technicians, and requires a modest level of sophistication for interpretation of changes. Like EP monitoring, EEG monitoring appears to have little value for either surveillance or goal-directed therapy in patients with head injuries, in contrast to its possible value for intraoperative monitoring.

Cerebral Blood Flow Monitoring. Although measuring the cerebral blood flow via xenon 133 clearance is a powerful research tool, these measurements do not yet constitute a clinically useful monitor. Despite the prognostic value of CBF measurements in patients who have suffered closed head injury, no role has developed for primary diagnosis, surveillance, or goal-directed management. Among the obstacles to wider use are the necessity for administering a radionuclide; the technically demanding nature of the measurements; and the relatively long interval (5–15 min) of stable conditions required to perform a single measurement, after which an additional several minutes must pass before subsequent measurements can be performed.

Intracranial Pressure Monitoring. Because ICP functions as the outflow pressure for the cerebral circulation (assuming jugular venous pressure is lower), ICP bears an important relationship to CBF, although CBF cannot be directly inferred from knowledge of ICP and MAP. In more than one third of patients with head injuries, ICP exceeds 20 mm Hg, a level thought to be a critical threshold for clinical intervention.[71] If untreated, intracranial hypertension will increase brain injury by causing herniation or cerebral hypoperfusion. Although ICP monitoring has been credited by some investigators[72] with an improving prognosis from acute closed head injury, others[73] question whether concurrent improvements in management, rather than ICP monitoring, explain the improvement. Although the subarachnoid screw[74] occasionally generates erroneous information,[75] measurement of ICP is usually considered to be a fundamental part of the care of patients with severe closed head injury (ie, GCS score ≤ 8).[76] A practical, reliable fiberoptic ICP monitor has been developed (manufactured by Camino Laboratories, San Diego, Calif.) that works well as an intraventricular, subdural, or brain tissue monitor[77] and has relatively little drift of calibration over periods of 5 days or less.[78]

Unlike the other modalities previously discussed, ICP monitoring has been used for surveillance and for goal-directed therapy. The information is especially valuable in patients in whom neuromuscular blocking agents are administered as part of treatment to reduce ICP, because such agents preclude a comprehensive neurological examination. Clinicians have applied systematic, although institutionally specific, protocols for avoidance of intracranial hypertension and for reduction of increased ICP when a threshold of 15 or 20 mm Hg is exceeded. Decisions about diuretics, hyperventilation, changes in the patient's position, and additional diagnostic procedures may be influenced by ICP information. If intracranial hypertension is refractory to conventional therapy, ICP monitoring is one of the alternative techniques used to titrate barbiturate coma,[79] although prophylactic barbiturate coma has failed to improve neurological outcome after head injury.[80] Whenever ICP monitoring is employed, the potential complications, the most important of which is infection, must be considered. The risk of intracranial infection appears to be less with subarachnoid bolts than with ventriculostomies, although subcutaneous tunneling may diminish the risk of infection in the latter procedure.

Brain Metabolic Monitoring. Two forms of brain metabolic monitoring are available: jugular venous saturation and near-infrared spectroscopy. Blood obtained from the jugular venous bulb provides the cerebral equivalent of "mixed venous" blood. Clinical venipuncture of the jugular venous bulb was first performed more than 60 years ago.[81] Today, retrograde cannulation of the jugular bulb is a safe, technically simple procedure.[82] CBF, $CMRo_2$, arterial oxygen content (Cao_2), and jugular venous oxygen content ($Cjvo_2$) are related according to the following equation:

$$(Cao_2 - Cjvo_2) \bullet CBF = CMRo_2$$

Rearranged, the equation becomes

$$Cjvo_2 = Cao_2 - CMRo_2 \div CBF$$

Therefore, $Cjvo_2$ is a function of CBF, $CMRo_2$, and arterial oxygenation. $Sjvo_2$, which, together with hemoglobin, determines $Cjvo_2$, is a potential monitor of the cerebral circulation. Mixed cerebral venous blood, like mixed systemic blood, is a global average of effluent from a variety of brain regions and may not reflect even severe *regional* hypoperfusion. Therefore, low $Sjvo_2$ is abnormal and suggests the possibility of cerebral ischemia; but while normal or elevated $Sjvo_2$ is reassuring, it is not adequate evidence of satisfactory cerebral perfusion. Recent experience with jugular venous bulb monitoring suggests that the technique may be appropriate to guide management.[31–33,48–50]

Near-infrared spectroscopy, a noninvasive technique that quantifies brain hemoglobin saturation, may eventually offer the opportunity to provide effective monitoring for surveillance or goal-directed therapy. Near-infrared light penetrates the skull and, during transmission through or reflection from brain tissue, undergoes changes in optical density proportional to the relative concentrations of oxygenated and deoxygenated hemoglobin in the tissue beneath the field.[83] Although considerable animal and clinical data demonstrate the sensitivity of the technique for the detection of qualitative changes in brain oxygenation,[84] clinical application has been delayed because of uncertainties regarding quantification of the signal. Recent data[85] suggest that quantification of the signal may be practical and that a noninvasive, continuous monitor of cerebral circulatory adequacy will be possible. The availability of an inexpensive, simple-to-operate surveillance monitor as well as a monitor that could be used for goal-directed therapy provides an opportunity to manage the cerebral circulation as comprehensively as the systemic circulation can now be managed.

General Supportive Care

The essential elements of general supportive care include airway support, administration of maintenance fluids, provision of sedation and analgesia, careful head positioning, and frequent turning. If airway reflexes are impaired, intubation may prevent aspiration and reduce the likelihood of hypoxemia or hypocapnia. Pulse oximetry and capnography facilitate prompt detection of hypoxemia or hypercarbia. Fluid restriction to 50% to 75% of calculated maintenance has long been considered appropriate. Recently, this belief has been challenged,[61] and greater emphasis is now placed on osmolality rather than fluid restriction. Because agitation or pain increases $CMRo_2$ and CBF, and can precipitate intracranial hypertension, adequate analgesia is particularly important in patients with not only head injuries but also other painful injuries (eg, surgical wounds or fractured long bones or ribs). In noncomatose patients in whom repeated neurological evaluation or direct observation of mental status is essential, sedatives and analgesics must be used with great caution. Neuromuscular blockade necessitates generous, empirical administration of sedatives and narcotic analgesics.

The head should not be rotated excessively. Although compression of the jugular venous system by head rotation produces no change in ICP in normal individuals, it may impede cerebral venous drainage and increase ICP in those with reduced intracranial compliance. Despite the demonstration that head elevation actually reduces CPP in some patients,[86] most patients appear to tolerate a 15° to 30° elevated-head position well.[87]

An essential aspect of the nursing care of patients with head injuries is frequent, systematic turning:

from the right lateral decubitus position, to the supine, to the left lateral decubitus position. This turning reduces decubitus ulceration and pulmonary retention of secretions. If turning-induced increases in ICP prevent adequate positioning, the use of a laterally rotating kinetic bed may both facilitate pulmonary toilet and limit the incidence of decubitus ulcers. In patients who do not require the kinetic bed, appropriate skin care includes the use of a low-pressure mattress pad.

Management of Intracranial Hypertension

Because of the spatial constraints imposed by the rigid skull, the brain, cerebrospinal fluid, and cerebral blood volume have little room to expand without increasing ICP. Head injury may increase intracranial volume, and therefore ICP, by the mechanisms listed in Table 16-7. Through extensive monitoring of ventricular fluid pressure in patients who had chronic intracranial mass lesions such as gliomas, Nils Lundberg and associates[88] demonstrated in 1965 that ICP is not static but rather is subject to periodic wave phenomena, the most dangerous of which is the plateau wave. Plateau waves (sometimes called Lundberg waves), which often precipitate acute neurological deterioration, appear to result from cerebral vasodilation[89] (Figure 16-8) and increases in cerebral hemispheric blood volume accompanied by a decline in CBF.[90]

Intracranial hypertension can be managed using a variety of strategies, all of which are based on the central concept that reduction of ICP (or improvement of intracranial compliance) can be accomplished by reducing one of the three intracranial constituents: blood volume, tissue volume, or cerebrospinal fluid volume.

Cerebral blood volume can be reduced using several techniques. Endotracheal intubation limits the likelihood of increases in CBF induced by hypoxemia or hypercarbia. Neuromuscular blockade prevents increases in cerebral venous volume as a consequence of coughing, straining, or actively exhaling, but neuromuscular blockade has not been associated with improved outcome in clinical head injury.[91] Head elevation facilitates cerebral venous drainage but, by reducing venous return, cardiac output, and MAP, may actually reduce CPP.[86] Adequate sedation and analgesia attenuate increases in $CMRo_2$ and CBF that are produced by painful or noxious stimulation. Control of fever limits increases in $CMRo_2$ and the accompanying increases in CBF. Passive hyperventilation, probably overused in the past, acutely reduces CBF and cerebral blood volume, although CBF tends to return to original levels despite continued hyperventilation. Selective diminution of blood volume in the pial

TABLE 16-7

CAUSES OF INTRACRANIAL HYPERTENSION AFTER HEAD TRAUMA

Cause	Mechanism
Mass Lesions	Local expansion
Intracerebral hematoma	
Extraaxial hematoma	
Brain Swelling	Vascular congestion, hyperemia
Brain Edema	
Cytotoxic	Cellular swelling secondary to hypoxia or ischemia
Vasogenic	Breakdown of blood–brain barrier, interstitial accumulation of protein
Interstitial	Hydrocephalus
Secondary Vasodilation	
Hypercarbia	Increased extracellular hydrogen ion concentration
Hypoxia	Mechanism unclear; possibly increased local metabolite (adenosine?) concentration
Hypertension	Impaired autoregulation

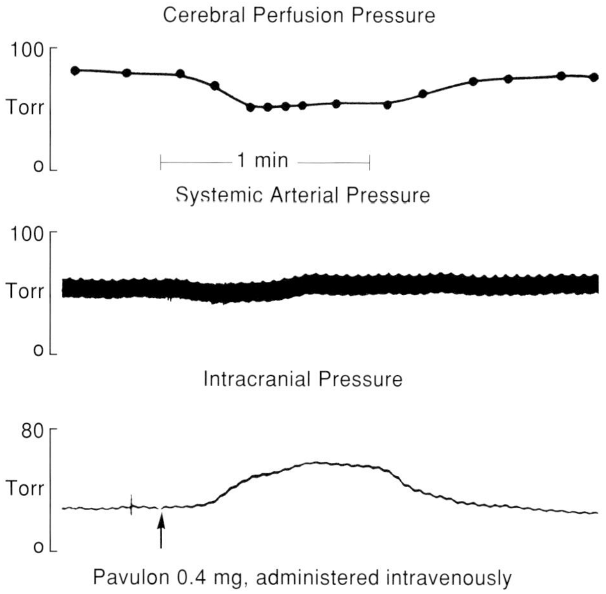

Fig. 16-8. Plateau wave during intracranial pressure recording. Shortly after receiving pancuronium (Pavulon, manufactured by Organon, Inc, West Orange, NJ) 0.4 mg administered intravenously, systemic arterial pressure declined slightly. Almost immediately, intracranial pressure increased dramatically, causing a marked decline in cerebral perfusion pressure. Reprinted with permission from Rosner MJ, Becker DP. Origin and evolution of plateau waves: Experimental observations and a theoretical model. *J Neurosurg*. 1984;60:317.

veins has been demonstrated in experimental animals with α_2-adrenergic receptor agonists.[92]

Reduction of brain tissue volume is conventionally achieved by diuresis. Osmotic diuresis, usually accomplished using mannitol, reduces brain water primarily in normal brain. A continuous intravenous infusion of mannitol significantly increases regional CBF without increasing blood pressure or reducing ICP.[93] Maximal reduction of ICP appears to be achieved by larger dosages of mannitol administered rapidly, particularly if followed by furosemide.[94] Fluid restriction, a conventional part of therapy, does not reduce brain tissue volume or ICP in experimental animals.[61] Another method that has been used to reduce brain tissue water and therefore to manage refractory intracranial hypertension is the administration of hypertonic saline. In anecdotal reports,[95] small volumes of a saline solution approximating 30% (5.0 mmol/mL) have produced a prolonged reduction in ICP and improved prerenal azotemia. In children with head injuries, a 3.0% saline solution reduced ICP significantly.[96] If intracranial hypertension is refractory to pharmacological therapy, subtemporal decompression may reduce mortality.[97] Glucocorticoids, expected to reduce cerebral edema and ICP, have been ineffective in clinical trials.[98,99]

Regardless of whether ICP can be reduced, an intervention that can reduce cerebral oxygen consumption should be therapeutically desirable. Barbiturates in sufficient dosages suppress both $CMRO_2$ and CBF.[93–100] Although barbiturates have been used to control ICP in patients with head injuries, routine administration of barbiturates did not reduce the incidence of intracranial hypertension or improve outcome in a well-designed randomized clinical trial[80]; in fact, the occurrence of barbiturate-induced hypotension prompted the investigators to suggest caution. Barbiturates still may have a role in selected patients who have refractory intracranial hypertension.[79]

Systemic Circulatory Management

Treatment of hypertension requires careful distinction of the life-threatening Cushing response from hypertension associated with the typical hyperdynamic response to head injury. Many commonly used antihypertensive agents, including sodium nitroprusside, nitroglycerin, and hydralazine, may increase ICP. Although those drugs may be used if ICP is monitored, alternative agents (such as the long-acting α-adrenergic and β-adrenergic antagonist, labetalol) may be preferable. Labetalol reduces blood pressure without increasing ICP. Acutely, esmolol may provide rapidly reversible control of blood pressure and heart rate. Adequate sedation and analgesia may also reduce hypertension and tachycardia.

Ventilatory Management

Although many patients with severe head injury will ventilate and oxygenate normally if they are provided with a secure airway, many clinicians prefer mechanical ventilation. Hyperventilation, though useful in reducing life-threatening intracranial hypertension, may lead to inadequate CBF as evidenced by excessive cerebral oxygen extraction[44] and, when used as routine therapy, actually worsen neurological outcome and mortality in comparison to normocarbia.[57] Positive end-expiratory pressure (PEEP) may be used to manage hypoxemia in patients with head injuries. PEEP-related increases in ICP are avoided both clinically and experimentally by head elevation.[101,102]

Many clinicians in North America routinely paralyze patients for at least the first several days of intensive care to prevent decerebrate and decorticate posturing and active expiration, each of which is associated with increases in MAP, central venous pressure, and ICP. The primary disadvantage of neuromuscular blockade is that it interferes with clinical neurological examination. However, recent reports[103] warn of prolonged neuromuscular dysfunction in patients who have been paralyzed for extended intervals. More importantly, evidence[92] suggests that neuromuscular blockade may extend the duration of intensive care of patients with head injuries without improving outcome.

Seizure Prophylaxis

Although the overall incidence of posttraumatic seizures is low, most clinicians provide seizure prophylaxis in the acute interval after head injury, particularly for patients with skull fractures or intracranial hematomas.[104] In adults, the prophylactic seizure medication most commonly employed is phenytoin, in a dose of 100 mg administered three times daily (therapeutic serum concentration 10–20 µg/mL). Phenobarbital is commonly added. For the management of acute seizures, diazepam, lorazepam, or phenytoin are usually chosen.

MEDICAL COMPLICATIONS OF HEAD TRAUMA

In addition to their head trauma per se, casualties with brain injuries are also at risk for gastrointestinal and pulmonary complications, infections, and electrolyte and fluid imbalances. Enteral or parenteral nutritional support is usually required.

The incidence of stress-induced gastrointestinal bleeding in patients with head injuries is directly proportional to the severity of the injury.[105] Although aggressive antacid therapy or frequent administration of histamine type 2 blocking agents may be necessary to increase gastric pH, recent data[106] demonstrate that gastric bacterial overgrowth accompanies loss of gastric acidity. Sucralfate, which provides effective prophylaxis without causing gastric alkalinization, may be preferable for ulcer prophylaxis.[107]

Patients with severe head injury are at risk for aspiration pneumonitis, noncardiac pulmonary edema, pulmonary embolism, and barotrauma. Prevention of aspiration requires gastric decompression and the use of an appropriately inflated, cuffed endotracheal tube. To limit secretion retention, atelectasis, and secondary infection, mandatory turning and positioning are essential.

An occasional patient with severe head injury develops the adult respiratory distress syndrome secondary to either infection or severe intracranial injury (in which case the syndrome is often called central neurogenic pulmonary edema). The management of adult respiratory distress syndrome consists of ventilatory support with PEEP and relief of intracranial hypertension, if present.

Patients with severe head injury also are at risk for nonpulmonary infections. Urinary tract infection may result from urinary catheterization. Maxillary sinusitis is surprisingly common among nasotracheally intubated patients with head trauma,[108] although a prospective trial showed that orally intubated patients also have a substantial incidence.[109] Ventriculitis and meningitis complicate trauma, surgical procedures that violate the dura, and indwelling intraventricular monitoring devices.

Abnormalities of sodium metabolism are common in patients with acute head injury. Hypernatremia may result from diabetes insipidus (DI) secondary to trauma or transection of the pituitary stalk. Typically, traumatic DI follows a three-phase course, with polyuria occurring initially, followed by reduced urinary output as stored antidiuretic hormone is released from the damaged pituitary, followed finally by prolonged DI.[110] Partial deficits of antidiuretic hormone also occur. The diagnosis of DI necessitates the demonstration that polyuria is a physiologically inappropriate response, which is usually confirmed by the development of hypovolemia or hypernatremia. If hypernatremia develops, the free-water deficit should be corrected slowly. Antidiuretic hormone replacement can be provided in the form of either aqueous vasopressin (5–10 units administered intramuscularly every 6–8 h), lysine vasopressin, or desmopressin (DDAVP, 0.1 mL administered intranasally every 12 to 24 h).

Patients with head injuries frequently develop hyponatremia, occasionally as the result of the syndrome of inappropriate antidiuretic hormone secretion (SIADH)[111] or excessive intravenous administration of free water, or occasionally, excessive production of atrial natriuretic peptide.[112] The treatment of hyponatremia depends on its cause. Hyponatremia associated with hypovolemia should be managed with intravenous fluid administration of isotonic fluids. Conversely, patients with SIADH usually respond to water restriction. Occasionally, demeclocycline may be necessary to correct SIADH.[113]

Despite extensive documentation of hypermetabolism after head injury, the appropriate route and composition of nutritional support have yet to be defined. Many questions remain unanswered. However, most clinicians tend to initiate either enteral or parenteral nutrition as soon as possible after acute head injury, generally preferring enteral nutrition if tolerated. Because patients with a GCS score of 4 to 5 require nearly 70% more than normal predicted resting metabolic requirements,[114] positive nitrogen balance may be difficult to achieve.[115] Fever further increases metabolic requirements. Glucocorticoids increase nitrogen wasting.[116] When feeding patients with head injuries, the possibility of hyperglycemia should be anticipated and glucose should be controlled. Although only descriptive data[117] implicate hyperglycemia in worse neurological outcome after head trauma, considerable experimental and clinical data[118] suggest that hyperglycemia worsens injury in some, but not all, models of focal and global neurological ischemia.

RECOVERY AND OUTCOME FOLLOWING TRAUMATIC BRAIN INJURY

Despite good neurological recovery, patients with head injuries often have persistent cognitive or emotional deficits or personality changes, particularly if posttraumatic coma results from diffuse brain injury rather than discrete focal lesions. Recovery of the verbal intelligence quotient usually begins within a few months and becomes stable more rapidly than the performance intelligence quotient, which may continue to improve for a year or more.[119] Memory deficits, which may impair social interactions and interfere with work performance, usually persist only briefly after minor injuries. In contrast, patients with severe injuries, particularly those involving both temporal lobes, may have persisting, profound difficulty with both long- and short-term memory.[120]

The most common major neurological findings in patients who survive head injury are unilateral cerebral hemispheric dysfunction and cranial nerve palsies. Factors associated with an increased risk of epilepsy after closed head injury include intracranial hematomas and depressed skull fractures. Of patients who develop seizures within 5 years of injury, nearly 75% will have their first seizure during the first year after injury.[104]

Good recovery to moderate disability can be anticipated for approximately 50% of adult patients who enter the hospital with GCS scores of 8 or lower.[2,72] Studies consistently demonstrate increasing mortality with declining GCS scores.[2,67,121] Overall, the level of consciousness (as assessed by the GCS) and brainstem reflexes (pupillary light responses and vestibuloocular or oculocephalic reflexes) correlate highly with patient outcome.[2,67] Bilaterally impaired pupillary light responses or impaired eye movements are associated with a mortality exceeding 75%.[2,67] In patients with intracranial hematomas, signs of brainstem failure, which would ordinarily predict a dismal outcome, may reverse rapidly after evacuation of a hematoma.[2,67,122] Factors unrelated to the neurological examination that adversely influence outcome include advanced age, which also correlates with an increasing risk of medical complications; hypoxemia, hypocarbia, hypotension, or anemia on admission to the hospital; and the presence of an intracranial mass lesion on CT scan.[1,2,67]

Patients who sustain focal lesions tend to have a worse outcome than those presenting with diffuse injury and a similar level of consciousness.[123] Patients in whom subdural hematomas are promptly evacuated (ie, within 4 h) have a 30% mortality; those operated on later have a 90% mortality.[63] More timely diagnosis of epidural hematoma using CT appears to have reduced mortality.[28] More prolonged and severe intracranial hypertension is associated with worse outcome after all head injuries. Patients in whom ICP consistently exceeds 20 mm Hg have a mortality exceeding 50%, whereas patients in whom ICP remains continuously lower than 20 mm Hg have a mortality of only 16%.[2,72] Mortality approaches 100% if intracranial hypertension cannot be controlled medically.

To increase cost-effectiveness, future research should seek to identify those patients who are so severely impaired that intensive therapy offers no benefit. A recently tested prognostic scale successfully predicted a fatal outcome (without a single falsely pessimistic prediction) in 23 of 52 severely patients with head injuries.[124] If confirmed in larger studies, such data would permit physicians to make informed, ethical decisions to withhold therapy from certain well-defined categories of patients, thereby more effectively allocating increasingly scarce resources.

SPINAL CORD INJURY

Each year in the United States, 10,000 victims of acute spinal cord injury become paraplegic or quadriplegic. The economic cost of caring for 180,000 acutely and chronically disabled persons is $4 billion per year.[125] Most victims of spinal cord injury are young, usually between 15 and 35 years of age,[126] and male. Patients whose neurological level of injury is above C-7 are unlikely to return to an independent existence (Table 16-8).[127]

Three factors appear to have reduced the acute mortality of patients with spinal cord injury and have improved life expectancy[127]:

1. Patients are more quickly given emergency care.
2. They are then frequently transferred to specialized trauma centers, followed by transfer to specialized rehabilitation facilities.
3. The medical management of cardiovascular, pulmonary, gastrointestinal, and urinary systems has improved, as has skin care and the management of infections.

Spinal anatomy can be divided into three biomechanical categories.[126] The first portion, the vertebral unit, includes the bones, ligaments, and muscles. The second unit is composed of the spinal cord, nerve roots, and membranous elements, including the dura; and the third, the spinal cord vasculature. Although these arbitrary divisions are not strictly accurate, they are useful for conceptualizing spinal cord injury that results from anatomical damage to one or more elements.

The vertebral unit of the spinal column is composed of 7 cervical, 12 thoracic, 5 lumbar, and 5 fused sacral vertebrae, and 1 coccygeal element formed by the fusion of 4 separate bodies.[126] With the exception of the first two cervical and the sacral vertebrae, articulation is accomplished by the intervertebral discs, which stabilize the synarthroses between the vertebral bodies; and the posterolateral joints, which are stabilized by their capsules as well as the intrasupraspinous ligaments and the ligamentum flava. The structure promotes stability over a wide range of motion.

The segmental organization of the spinal cord, an extension of the brainstem, is apparent from the

TABLE 16-8

FUNCTIONAL ABILITY BASED ON LEVEL OF NEUROLOGICAL INJURY

Level of Injury	Functional Ability
C-2–C-4	No movement of upper extremities; some neck control C-2 requires ventilatory support
C-5	Use of biceps allows feeding and grooming with use of special equipment
C-6	Use of wrist allows independent grooming, driving, and simple meal preparation
C-7	Ability to extend arm can permit independent living
T-1–T-6	Normal hand ability; usually capable of independent living in wheelchair-adapted environment
T-12	Complete trunk control with good sitting balance Ambulation with long leg braces possible
L-4	Use of hip flexors and quadriceps Ambulation possible with short leg braces Spinal reflex activity regulating bladder and bowel usually present in T-12 or above but absent in L-1 or below

Reprinted with permission from Levinson W, Ward G. Care of spinal-cord injured patients after the acute period. *J Gen Int Med.* 1989;4:337.

paired spinal nerves, which are formed from the anterior (motor) roots and the posterior (sensory) roots, then exit through the intervertebral foramina. The spinal cord is suspended within the spinal fluid by nerve roots and ligaments. The pia mater, arachnoid, and dura mater constitute the spinal meninges. The dura, a fibrous membrane extending from the cranium, is firmly attached circumferentially at the foramen magnum, usually closely apposed to the posterior surfaces of the first and second cervical vertebrae, and loosely associated with the posterolongitudinal ligament in the lumbar and cervical regions. The 21 dentate ligaments, which extend from above the first cervical roots to the region of the last thoracic roots, attach to the inner surface of the dura and the lateral surface of the cord, securing and suspending the cord within the dura. Interposed between the spinal dura and the vertebral column is the epidural space, which contains veins, fatty tissue, and ligaments.

The vascular supply of the proximal spinal cord originates from the vertebral and posterior cerebellar arteries, supplemented regionally by branches from the thoracic and abdominal aorta and the deep cervical, intercostal, lumbar, and lateral sacral arteries. These arteries and branches give origin to lateral spinal arteries, which, in turn, give rise to anterior and posterior radicular arteries. The paired anterior radicular arteries enter the spinal cord with each anterior (motor) root and pass caudad to join the anterior spinal artery.

The severity of spinal cord injury is determined by two pathophysiological events: primary mechanical injury and secondary injury. Disruption of the bony and ligamentous elements of the spinal canal through flexion, extension, compression, rotation, shear, or traction injures vascular structures and axons in direct proportion to the magnitude of the disruptive force. Secondary injury worsens the primary mechanical injury as a result of the deleterious effects of hypoxia, hypotension, and progressive vascular and biochemical events that follow injury. Shortly after experimental cord compression, hyperemia and small hemorrhages appear in the central gray matter. These areas subsequently expand, further compromising cord perfusion. Within 8 hours, edema and infarction spread to the white matter. The end result of this sequence is swelling, edema, necrosis, extensive demyelinization, and severe neuronal loss in the central gray matter.[128]

Many of the factors implicated in head injury have also been implicated in spinal cord injury (Figure 16-9), primary among which is the failure of cellular adenosine 5′-triphosphate (ATP) stores, followed by intracellular influx of calcium. With the influx of calcium, phospholipase A_2 is activated, forming arachidonic acid from membrane phospholipids derived from injured cells. Arachidonic acid disrupts cellular integrity; decreases mitochondrial ATP synthesis; and is metabolized to form prostaglandins, thromboxanes, leukotrienes, and free radicals. The free radicals then act directly to destroy normal cellular components, mediate platelet aggregation, initiate vasospasm, inhibit neurotransmitter release, and cause the release of lysosomal enzymes.[129] The complex pathophysiological effects of secondary injury have suggested a multiplicity of possible therapeutic interventions.

Experimental evidence[130] suggests that hyperglycemia is associated with worsened neurological outcome after experimental spinal cord ischemia, as it is with cerebral ischemia. In contrast, insulin-induced hypoglycemia improves recovery of electrophysiological function after spinal cord ischemia.[131] Ethanol, commonly involved in spinal cord injury, interferes with spinal cord autoregulation, thereby worsening neurological outcome in ethanol-intoxicated animals.[132]

After trauma to the vertebral column, neurologically injured patients may be asymptomatic or they may have complete or incomplete spinal cord injury syndromes. The four most common incomplete syndromes are the Brown-Sequard, acute central cord, anterior cord, and posterior cord syndromes (Table 16-9).[133]

Physiological Responses

Cardiovascular

The immediate cardiovascular response to spinal cord injury is sympathetically mediated tachycardia and hypertension, followed by hypotension secondary to acute sympathectomy if the lesion is above T-5. Acute sympathectomy results in slightly decreased systemic vascular resistance and marked dilation of the venous capacitance vessels. If the cord lesion is cephalad to T-4, the input to cardiac accelerator fibers also is lost, reducing or eliminating compensatory increases in heart rate in response to hypotension. At times, bradycardia produced by unopposed vagal tone may result in cardiac arrest, particularly in association with hypoxemia.[134]

Pulmonary edema occurs in up to 50% of patients with cervical spinal cord injury. In experimental animals, pulmonary edema may result from severe vasoconstriction and acute pulmonary venous hy-

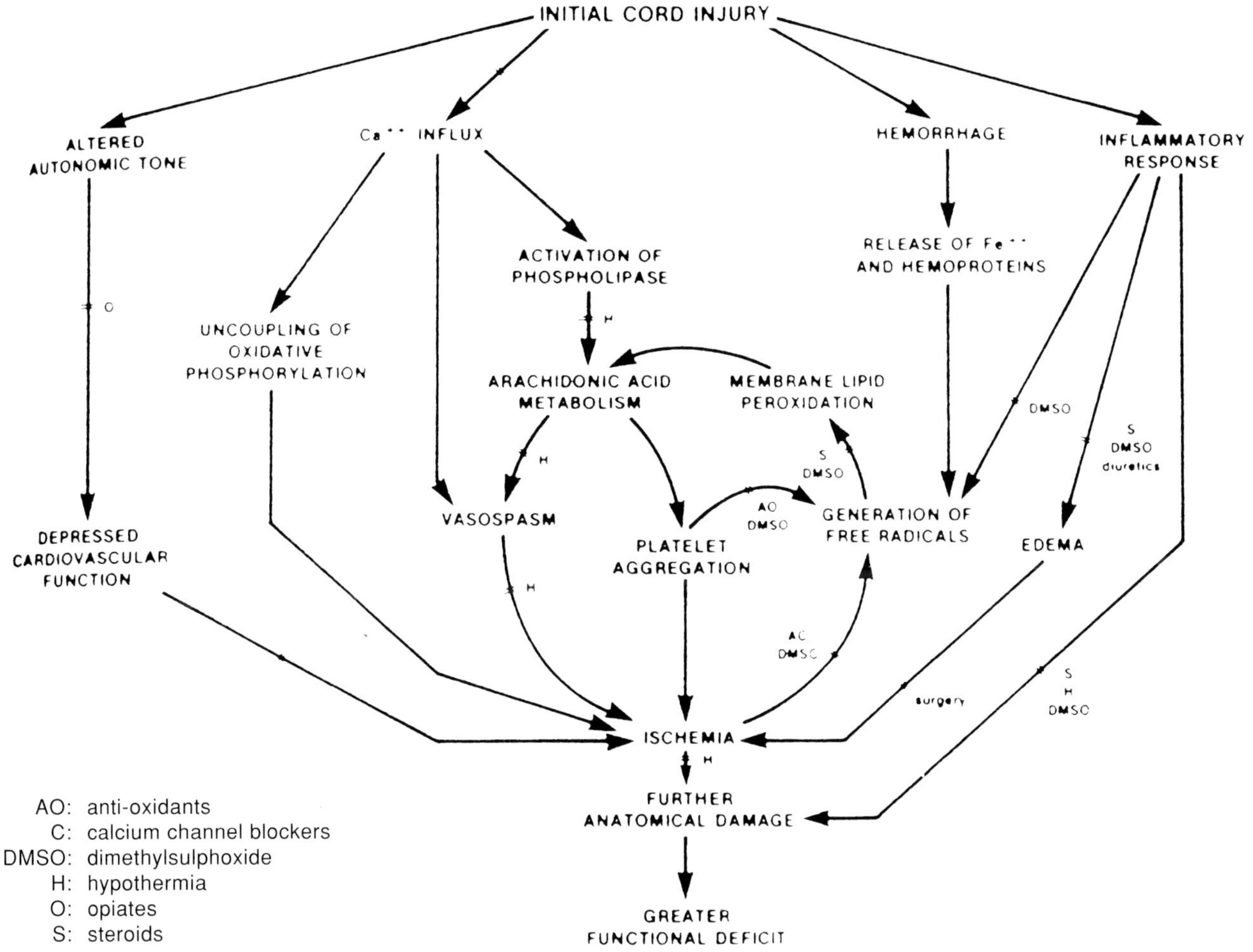

Fig. 16-9. Schematic illustration of proposed mechanisms of secondary spinal cord injury. The processes interact, ultimately producing a greater deficit than could be attributed to the primary injury alone. Potential sites at which these interactive pathways could be interrupted are illustrated. Reprinted with permission from Janssen L, Hansebout RR. Pathogenesis of spinal cord injury and newer treatments: A review. *Spine.* 1991;14:25.

pertension accompanying massive sympathetic discharge after high spinal cord injury.[135] Researchers[136] have demonstrated that experimental transection of the spinal cord at the level of C-4 initiates a transient, sympathetically mediated response characterized by a marked increase in MAP followed by hypotension and increases in pulmonary artery occlusion pressure and extravascular lung water. A variety of electrocardiographic changes have been reported, including subendocardial ischemia, shifting pacemaker, atrial fibrillation, ventricular tachycardia, ST-T wave changes, and multifocal premature ventricular contractions.

Although acute spinal cord injury exerts no direct effects on myocardial function, the loss of sympathetic innervation reduces the ability of the myocardium to tolerate sudden increases in preload and afterload. In patients in whom hemodynamic problems persist, particularly if pulmonary edema is present, pulmonary artery catheterization may clarify the need for additional intravascular volume replacement versus the need for inotropic support.[137]

Autonomic Hyperreflexia. As sympathetic nervous system function begins to recover and spinal shock resolves, usually within 2 to 3 weeks after injury, patients with spinal cord injury cephalad to the level of splanchnic sympathetic innervation (T-4–T-6) may manifest autonomic hyperreflexia (Exhibit 16-2).[138] The pathogenesis of this disorder is the loss of neurogenic control distal to the level of the lesion, which, in response to noxious stimuli (usually visceral) below the level of the lesion, leads to profound vasoconstriction. Subsequent reflex

TABLE 16-9

NEUROLOGICAL SYNDROMES POSSIBLE WITH CERVICAL SPINE INJURY

Syndromes	Findings
Brown-Sequard	Ipsilateral paralysis Ipsilateral position and vibration sense loss Contralateral temperature and pain sense loss
Acute Central Cord	Bilateral motor loss, weakness in upper extremities exceeds weakness weakness in lower extremities Bladder control loss Variable sensory loss
Anterior Cord	Bilateral motor, pain, and temperature loss Preserved position and vibration sense Hyperesthesia below the level of the lesion
Posterior Cord	All motor and sensory functions preserved except touch and temperature

Adapted with permission from Hastings RH, Marks JD. Airway management for trauma patients with potential cervical spine injuries. *Anesth Analg*. 1991;73:473.

EXHIBIT 16-2

SIGNS AND SYMPTOMS OF AUTONOMIC HYPERREFLEXIA

- Hypertension
  - Vasoconstriction (below lesion)
  - Vasodilation (above lesion)
- Bradycardia
- Dysrhythmia (ectopic beats occurring during period of heart block)
- Sweating (below lesion)
- Piloerection (below lesion)
- Headache
- Shortness of breath
- Flushed face and neck
- Nausea
- Blurred vision
- Muscle fasciculations
- Convulsions
- Loss of consciousness

Adapted with permission from Schreibman DL, Mackenzie CF. The trauma victim with an acute spinal cord injury. *Problems in Anesthesia*. 1990;4:472

TABLE 16-10

PULMONARY AND RESPIRATORY MUSCLE FUNCTION IN QUADRIPLEGIC PATIENTS WITH CERVICAL SPINAL CORD INJURY AT C-4 THROUGH C-7

Variable	Predicted Normal Value (%)
Vital capacity	52 ± 11
FEV_1/FVC (%)	85 ± 3
Inspiratory capacity	71 ± 16
Expiratory reserve volume	21 ± 12
Total lung capacity	70 ± 4
Functional residual capacity	86 ± 14
Residual volume	141 ± 20
Maximum voluntary ventilation	49 ± 10
PI_{max} (cm H_2O)	64 ± 12*
PE_{max} (cm H_2O)	41 ± 22*

*Values are expressed as absolute units, not as percentages of predicted normal values

FEV_1: forced expiratory volume in 1 s; FEV: forced vital capacity; PI_{max}: maximum inspiratory pressure; PE_{max}: maximum expiratory pressure

Adapted with permission from Findley LJ, Rochester DF. The lungs and neuromuscular and chest wall diseases. In: Murray JF, Nadel JA, eds. *Textbook of Respiratory Medicine*. Philadelphia, Pa: WB Saunders; 1988: 1949.

activity of the carotid and aortic baroreceptors produces vasodilation above the level of the lesion, ventricular dysrhythmias, bradycardia, and, occasionally, heart block. Of patients with lesions above T-7, 66% to 85% manifest hyperreflexia at some time.[138,139] Although the potential for autonomic hyperreflexia is maximal at approximately 4 weeks after injury, any patient with spinal cord injury above T-7 is at risk of exposure to a variety of visceral stimuli, most commonly distention of a hollow viscus.[140–143] Medical management is first directed toward eliminating the causative stimuli, using direct-acting vasodilators such as sodium nitroprusside, controlling cardiac arrhythmias, or, during surgery, deepening anesthesia.

Pulmonary System

A lesion at the level of T-1 eliminates the contributions of the intercostal muscles to both inspiration and expiration and of the abdominal oblique muscles to expiration. Inspiratory reserve volume and total lung capacity are thereby reduced, as are expiratory reserve volume and forced vital capacity (FVC). Table 16-10 illustrates typical pulmonary function tests from patients with acute injury to the mid-to-lower spinal cord.[144] Although functional residual capacity increases in both normal and quadriplegic patients as they are tilted upward, the increase in normal persons is accomplished by an increase in expiratory reserve volume, whereas in quadriplegic patients, who are unable to assist expiration by actively contracting the abdominal musculature, the increase is produced by an increase in residual volume.[145] Within the first few days after acute spinal cord injury, FVC typically decreases somewhat, then begins to recover. Five months later, both peak expiratory flow rates and FVC are substantially greater than during the first week after injury (Figure 16-10).[146]

Despite considerable compromise of the respiratory musculature, most patients who are able to generate a normal or nearly normal tidal volume remain normocarbic. However, hypoxemia occurs when FVC is lower than 15 mL/kg because coughing and sighing are inadequate. Acute onset of aspiration, atelectasis, or pneumonia may result in sudden respiratory compromise.

Spinal Cord Blood Flow

Despite extensive experimental work demonstrating the relationship between acute spinal cord injury and reduced spinal cord blood flow (SCBF), the relationship between spinal cord ischemia and the progression of neurological deficits is unclear. Because of the unique circulation of the spinal cord, "watershed" areas exist at midpoints of the spinal arterial circulation, equidistant from the radicular arteries. Arterial blood flow in the spinal cord comes from opposite directions, from the cervical cord vessels above and the paired anterior and posterior spinal arteries below.[147] The lower cervical area, most distant from collateral pathways, is most vulnerable to ischemia. Researchers[148] demonstrated that in monkeys, the area most vulnerable to ischemia was at the level of C-6, resulting from the compartmental division of blood flow up and down the anterior spinal artery. Because of limited collateral flow from the vertebral and intercostal arteries, the cervical cord between C-5 and C-8 would be the area most vulnerable to ischemia when MAP falls below the lower limit for autoregulation. Another area of special concern is the variable portion of the thoracic spinal cord supplied by the radicularis magna.

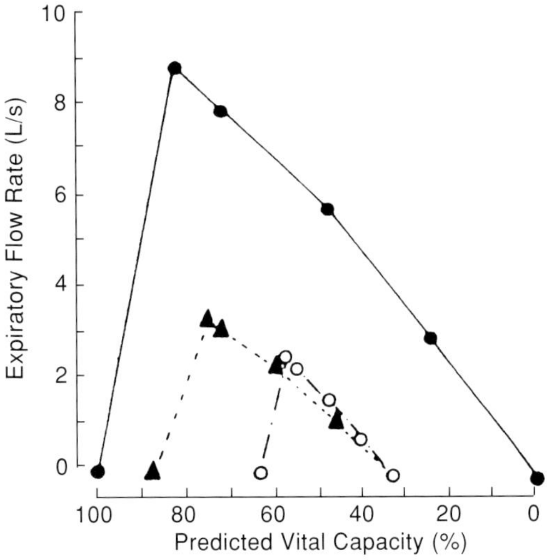

Fig. 16-10. A comparison of predicted expiratory flow rates as a function of predicted vital capacity (closed circles). Open circles represent data from 11 patients in the first week after injury; closed triangles represent data from the same 11 patients 5 months after injury. Reprinted with permission from Ledsome JR, Sharp JN. Pulmonary function in acute cervical cord injury. *Am Rev Respir Dis.* 1981;124:43.

SCBF autoregulation has been described as similar to that of cerebral autoregulation, with the range of 60 to 120 mm Hg representing the autoregulatory plateau (Figure 16-11).[149] Although it is unclear whether autoregulation of SCBF is impaired after cord injury, it is likely that the traumatized spinal

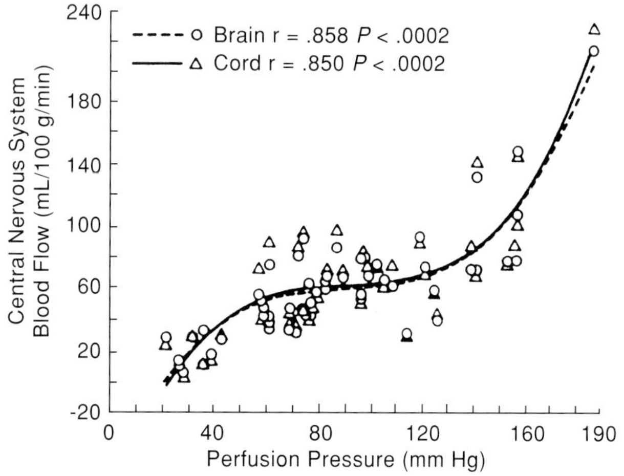

Fig. 16-11. Autoregulation of blood flow is similar in both spinal cord and brain in rats anesthetized with pentobarbital. In both tissues, the autoregulatory plateau extends from 60 to 120 mm Hg perfusion pressure. Reprinted with permission from Hickey R, Albin MS, Bunegin L, Gelineau J. Autoregulation of spinal cord blood flow: Is the cord a microcosm of the brain? *Stroke.* 1986;17:1184.

cord, like the traumatized brain, is extremely vulnerable to hypotension.

Initial Care

Initial care of the patient with potential or evident spinal cord injury consists of three parts: clinical evaluation and stabilization, radiological evaluation, and, when necessary, airway management. Of course, depending on the severity of respiratory compromise, securing the airway may be the first priority.

Clinical Evaluation and Stabilization

Meticulously detailed neurological examinations must be performed as soon as possible. Serial examinations will characterize the initial spinal cord insult, herald extension of injury, and provide prognostic in-formation. Based on knowledge of the neurological level of injury, physiological responses can be anticipated.

It is imperative that patients with spinal cord injury rapidly enter a system in which care is provided by adequately trained, technically proficient personnel who are attuned to the importance of the basic principles of trauma care and the importance of immobilization of the spine, especially if airway intervention is required. Respiratory support and the prompt reversal of shock by the intravenous administration of fluids are essential to reducing morbidity and mortality. During evaluation and management, appropriate use of cervical collars, backboards or vacuum mattresses, sand bags, and 3-in. tape will immobilize the spine and minimize exacerbation of the injury to the cord until adequate radiological studies have ruled out injury. Such studies may not be possible for days or weeks in patients with multiple trauma.

Once the level of the neurological deficit is established, problems can be anticipated and managed. Among these, the acute level-dependent systemic complications of acute spinal cord injury include, as discussed earlier, loss of sympathetic control of the vascular tree, left ventricular dysfunction, and respiratory compromise. Long-term problems include autonomic hyperreflexia, decreased gastrointestinal motility, nutritional depletion, genitourinary problems, and metabolic dysfunction.

After treating any life-threatening conditions recognized in the primary survey, the medical officer should then proceed to a secondary survey and meticulous head-to-toe physical examination. In comatose patients, concomitant spinal cord injury may be overlooked, especially if a meticulous neurological exam is not conducted. However, neck pain is a sensitive, specific indication of cervical spine injury in awake, cooperative patients (Table 16-11).[133] Because 25% to 60% of patients who have sustained vertebral column injuries have other injuries,[137] a high index of suspicion must be maintained, even when evaluating an alert, cooperative patient, because the patient may be insensate to an injury below the level of the injury to the spinal cord. Of patients who have spinal cord injuries, 49% also have a concomitant closed head injury.[150] Retrospective studies detect a much lower incidence (6%) of total head injuries associated with spinal cord injuries, and approximately a 2% incidence of severe closed head injury (GCS score ≤ 8).[151] Injuries of the thoracic spine are associated with multiple rib fractures, flail chest, or aortic disruption.

In summary, during initial evaluation, a rapid assessment of spinal cord, head, and other injuries should be made; the airway and adequate ventilation assured; supplemental oxygen applied; intravenous access secured; fluid resuscitation initiated; and expeditious transport arranged to a definitive care facility, ideally a trauma or spinal cord injury center.

Radiological Evaluation

In the recent past, a single, cross-table lateral, plain cervical spine X-ray examination, which in-

TABLE 16-11

CERVICAL SPINE INJURY AND NECK PAIN IN ALERT TRAUMA PATIENTS

Primary Study	Number of Patients With C-Spine Injury	Number of Patients With Neck Pain	Study	Number of Patients Primary C-Spine Injury	Number of Patients Without Neck Pain
Fisher (1984)*	5	5	Fisher	0	328
Roberge (1988)	6	6	Roberge	0	141
Bayless (1989)	2	2	Bayless	0	122
Bachulis (1987)	65	65	Neifeld (1988)	0	145
Ringenberg (1988)	253	247†	Kreipke (1989)	0	324
Lally (1989)‡	16	16			
Rachesky (1987)‡	21	21			

*Numbers in parentheses are the years in which the primary source was published
†Six patients with other painful injuries did not report neck pain
‡Pediatric trauma
Adapted with permission from Hastings RH, Marks JD. Airway management for trauma patients with potential cervical spine injuries. *Anesth Analg*. 1991;73:473.

cluded all seven cervical vertebrae and the C-7–T-1 interspace, was considered sufficient to assess cervical spine integrity. However, the sensitivity of this single view is only 74% to 92% (Table 16-12). A three-view evaluation, including anteroposterior and odontoid views, permits better assessment of vertical alignment of the spinous and articular process and of abnormalities in the joint and disk spaces.[133] If a patient is able to follow commands, lateral flexion-extension views should be obtained, as the patient controls head motion. Until then, rigid immobilization with a hard cervical collar (eg, the Philadelphia collar, manufactured by Philadelphia Collar, Westville, N.J.) is

TABLE 16-12

SENSIVITY OF CERVICAL SPINE X-RAY STUDIES

Primary Study	View	Number of Patients With Cervical Spine Injury	Sensitivity* (%)
Streitwieser (1983)†	CTL	44	82
	3 Views	38	92
Shaffer (1981)	CTL	35	74
Bachulis (1987)	CTL	90	77
Ross (1987)	CTL	13	85
	3 Views	13	92
MacDonald (1990)	CTL	92	92
Freemyer (1989)	3 Views	33	91

*Sensitivity = true positives ÷ (true positives + false negatives) • 100
†Numbers in parentheses are the years in which the primary sources were published
CTL: cross-table lateral view; 3 views: cross-table lateral, anteroposterior, and open-mouth
Adapted with permission from Hastings RH, Marks JD. Airway management for trauma patients with potential cervical spine injuries. *Anesth Analg*. 1991;73:476.

indicated, if there is any clinical suspicion of neck injury.

Computed or conventional tomography supplements plain radiographs that are equivocal or negative despite clinical evidence of cord injury.[152–154] The occurrence of spinal cord injury without radiographic evidence of vertebral injury or instability can be as high as 15% to 70%.[155,156] Although MRI is superior for evaluation of injury to soft tissues, including paravertebral tissue, intervertebral discs and ligaments, the complexity involved in obtaining MRI scans precludes its use in most acute circumstances.

Airway Management

Despite the simultaneous risks of inadequate pulmonary function and aggravation of spinal cord damage, there are no universally accepted approaches to airway management in patients with acute spinal cord injury. The method chosen in a specific situation is determined by a variety of factors, among them the severity of physiological compromise, the clinician's experience and ability, the availability of specialized equipment, the magnitude and type of associated injuries, the presence of hemodynamic stability, and the availability of definitive diagnostic information about the cervical spine.[133,157] Because the need to secure the airway emergently cannot be predicted in advance, a cart containing necessary equipment should be readily available (Exhibit 16-3).

The choice among various methods of airway management depends on the severity of physiological compromise. If a patient is unable to maintain normoxia and normocarbia, or is actively vomiting and unable to protect the airway, then direct visualization and orotracheal intubation should be attempted first. Adjunctive medications, such as sedatives, induction agents, or muscle relaxants, should be used as dictated by the patient's hemodynamic status. Cricoid pressure may be used if necessary, but its vigorous application could produce subluxation at the injury site. Immobilization of the cervical spine can be accomplished with manual in-line axial traction (MIAT),[157] a method associated with no evidence of new or worsened neurological injury resulting from intubation in more than 3,000 patients.[158] Gardner-Wells tongs can also be used for cervical spine immobilization. If the oral route is impractical because of injury, edema, or oropharyngeal bleeding, and an artificial airway is required, emergent surgical cricothyrotomy can be performed; alternatively, percutaneous needle cricothyrotomy can be used as a temporizing measure.

If the need for an artificial airway is less acute, nasotracheal intubation may be performed either blindly or using fiberoptic guidance. The nasal route should not be used in the presence of basilar skull fracture, midface instability, or nasoseptal injury because of the risk that the endotracheal tube will enter the brain[55] or cause serious hemorrhage. Vasoconstriction of the nasal mucosa can be achieved with the application of nasal decongestant spray (eg, Afrin, manufactured by Shearing-Plough Health Care Products, Inc., Memphis, Tenn.) or phenylephrine. Topical anesthesia may alleviate discomfort even in a semicomatose patient who might otherwise react vigorously to noxious airway stimulation, thereby precipitating extension of the spinal cord injury. Fiberoptic bronchoscopy can be used to facilitate nasotracheal intubation, assuming that the intubator is skilled and that there is little blood or foreign material in the oropharynx.

The nasal route does have some important disadvantages, however. Any mechanical airway manipulation may provoke hypertension, a particular hazard in a patient with closed head injury and decreased intracranial compliance. Epistaxis may be severe, especially in patients who have coagulopathies. When performed blindly, nasotracheal intubation may damage the larynx. Either blind or fiberoptically guided nasotracheal intubation may be time-consuming. Semicomatose,

EXHIBIT 16-3

NECESSARY EQUIPMENT FOR EMERGENCY AIRWAY MANAGEMENT

- Laryngoscope with blades of various sizes and shapes
- Endotracheal tubes of various sizes
- Endotracheal tube stylet
- Oral and nasal airways
- Face masks of various sizes
- Tonsil-tipped suction handle or suction source
- Ambu bag (attached to oxygen source)
- Pharmacological adjuncts (drugs drawn up in syringes)

Reprinted with permission from Grande CM. Airway management of the trauma patient in the resuscitation area of the trauma center. *Trauma Q*. 1988;5(1):38.

inebriated, or frightened patients may react combatively, risking further injury to the spinal cord. Prolonged nasotracheal intubation is associated with maxillary sinusitis and occasional sepsis.

Other methods of placing oral tracheal tubes such as retrograde wires may be challenging because of associated injuries. Thus, even in circumstances that are not emergent, the method of choice for tracheal intubation may be orotracheal intubation in conjunction with MIAT, after denitrogenation, supplemented by a carefully titrated dose of thiopental, midazolam, or etomidate, and a neuromuscular blocking agent. Succinylcholine is appropriate if the injury is less than 48 hours old; after 48 hours, the risk of succinylcholine-induced hyperkalemia, potentially a fatal event,[159] increases dramatically. A nondepolarizing agent such as vecuronium is preferable if more than 48 hours have elapsed.

Anesthetic Management

Anesthesia personnel may be confronted with patients with spinal cord injury at any stage of resuscitation, just as they may with patients with head injuries. This section addresses the anesthetic management of the patient with spinal cord injuries who does not have a secure airway.

Preoperatively, the most important considerations relate to respiratory compromise, hypotension, and the possibility of associated injuries. Respiratory compromise may not be evident on initial examination but may be apparent if the patient is asked to perform a vital-capacity maneuver. Hypotension is secondary to venodilation and impairment of the usual reflex increase in heart rate that occurs with hypotension in patients in whom sympathetic pathways are intact. Associated injuries below the level of the injury may not be recognized because of the absence of pain. Before induction of anesthesia, blood pressure should be restored with the use of volume expansion. Pressors may occasionally be necessary. Dopamine tends to constrict the venous system and increase heart rate. Ephedrine may be useful for short-term stabilization. Atropine is especially useful if bradycardia is a major factor in hypotension or if severe bradycardia follows airway stimulation.

Monitoring during anesthesia should be determined by the severity of associated injuries and the availability of equipment. If time and circumstances permit, direct arterial pressure monitoring will warn promptly of hypotension. Central venous pressure monitoring may provide information about the relationship between blood volume and expanded venous capacitance. Pulse oximetry and capnography provide early warning of deterioration in gas exchange. Automated, noninvasive blood pressure monitoring may free anesthesia personnel for other activities.

Anesthetic induction must preserve hemodynamic stability while securing the airway with minimal risk of aggravating the cervical spine injury. The initial decision is whether to intubate the patient awake (fiberoptically or blindly) or whether to proceed with a rapid-sequence induction. Either should be accompanied by MIAT. Awake intubation, in the absence of MIAT, risks cervical movement when the endotracheal tube enters the trachea and stimulates coughing. On the other hand, vigorous head movements during direct laryngoscopy also risk excessive cervical motion.

Potential anesthesia induction agents include thiopental, etomidate, benzodiazepines, and ketamine. The effects of anesthetics on perfusion of the injured spinal cord are not well known. Most clinicians assume that the effects are similar to the effects of agents on CBF and $CMRO_2$. Large dosages of barbiturates may reduce blood pressure, especially in hypovolemic patients. Etomidate provides prompt induction and is usually well tolerated even in some hypotensive patients. Benzodiazepines usually preserve blood pressure. Large dosages may slow emergence. Cricoid pressure should be applied during induction and intubation. In a hemodynamically resuscitated patient with acute spinal cord injuries, a reasonable sequence is to administer thiopental and fentanyl followed by succinylcholine, all while maintaining cricoid pressure. Hyperkalemia resulting from succinylcholine administration is unlikely after recent (< 24-h old) spinal cord injury. The incidence increases after 24 hours and plateaus by 12 days. For maintenance, the effects of volatile anesthetics on spinal perfusion also appear to parallel their effects on CBF and $CMRO_2$.

Postoperatively, the ability to extubate the patient with a spinal cord injury depends on preoperative respiratory compromise and on the magnitude and site of surgery. Before extubating the patient with a cervical cord injury, it is wise to determine FVC and peak negative pressure.

Management in the Intensive Care Unit

Management in the intensive care unit is intended to limit neurological disability and reduce the morbidity and mortality of the complica-

TABLE 16-13

CAUSE OF DEATH IN THE FIRST MONTH AFTER SPINAL CORD INJURY

Cause of Death	Actual Deaths	SMR	95% Confidence Limit of SMR
Septicemia	5	500.0	61.7–938.3
Cancer	0	0.0	0.0–0.0
Ischemic heart disease	4	7.7	0.2–15.2
Other heart disease	8	133.3	40.9–225.7
Cerebrovascular disease	4	33.3	0.6–66.0
Diseases of arteries	2	50.0	0.0–119.3
Venous thrombosis and embolism	10	500.0	190.1–809.9
Influenza and pneumonia	12	300.0	130.3–469.7
Other respiratory disease	4	66.7	1.4–132.0
Diseases of digestive system	4	66.7	1.4–132.0
Diseases of urinary system	4	200.0	4.0–396.0
Symptoms and ill-defined conditions	11	275.0	112.5–437.5
Unintentional injuries and suicides	0	0.0	0.0–0.0
Residual	7	24.1	6.2–42.0
Unknown	1		

SMR: standardized mortality ratio (actual deaths ÷ predicted deaths • 100)
Adapted with permission from DeVivo MJ, Kartus PL, Stover SL, Rutt RD, Fine PR. Cause of death for patients with spinal cord injuries. *Arch Intern Med.* 1989;149:1765.

tions that accompany acute spinal cord injury. It is necessary to prevent further damage to the patient's spinal cord, manage cardiovascular and pulmonary complications, and control pain. In the first month after spinal cord injury, which includes the time during which patients are most likely to be admitted to the intensive care unit, pneumonia, pulmonary embolism, and sepsis are the most common factors contributing to death (Table 16-13).[160]

In the intensive care unit, monitoring of patients with acute spinal cord injury consists of careful cardiovascular monitoring, monitoring of gas exchange, and the use of EPs for diagnosis and prognosis. Pulmonary monitoring is the same as that used for other critically ill patients, consisting of pulse oximetry, capnography, and, as necessary, arterial catheterization to obtain arterial blood gases. Pulse oximetry may be of particular value in those patients who become bradycardic in response to hypoxemia.

Somatosensory evoked potentials (SSEPs), noninvasive tests of the integrity of spinal cord transmission, have developed into important diagnostic and prognostic tools in patients with acute spinal cord injury.[161,162] Strictly speaking, SSEPs cannot be used to monitor acute injuries. Not surprisingly, preservation of SSEPs after injury is consistent with incomplete spinal cord transection and portends a more favorable outcome than loss of SSEPs.[163] When combined with clinical evaluation of motor function, sensation to pinprick, and joint position, SSEPs provide greater prognostic value.[69] Although techniques for the use of MEPs have been developed for humans, few data quantify the likely diagnostic and prognostic value of this modality.[164]

Spinal Cord Protection

Because of the progressive hemorrhagic infarction of the spinal cord that sometimes follows acute trauma, the pathophysiology of secondary, progressive injury has been extensively investigated (see Figure 16-9). Of the great variety of interventions that have been attempted after acute spinal cord injury, several have received particularly intense scrutiny, including localized spinal cord hypothermia, endogenous opioid antagonists, glucocorticoids, free radical scavengers, and G_{M1} ganglioside.

Topical Hypothermia. Topical hypothermia was first investigated more than 25 years ago,[165] based on the assumption that hypothermia would reduce spinal cord metabolism, thereby decreasing the risk of infarction, and presumably decreasing the rate of formation of toxic metabolites.[166] Despite experimental evidence in favor of topical hypothermia, the results in humans have been inconsistent and discouraging,[126] perhaps because of the heterogeneity of human spinal cord injury and the substantial delay before most patients reach treatment facilities.

Opiate Antagonists. Researchers[167,168] first reported in the 1980s that endorphins (endogenous opioids) are involved in the progression of spinal cord injury and that the administration of naloxone, an opiate antagonist, increased blood pressure and SCBF and improved neurological recovery in comparison to results in animals given a saline control. Thyrotropin-releasing hormone, an opiate antagonist that does not reverse opioid-mediated analgesia, also exerts a beneficial effect in experimental spinal cord injury.[168,169] However, other researchers[170] conclusively demonstrated that, in humans, naloxone (given as a bolus of 5.4 mg/kg, followed by an infusion at a rate of 4.0 mg/kg/h for 23 h) failed to improve neurological outcome in comparison with placebo and methylprednisolone (discussed below) (Table 16-14).

Glucocorticoids. In animals subjected to spinal cord trauma, glucocorticoids, including dexamethasone and methylprednisolone, have generally exerted therapeutic benefit. As a consequence of promising data from studies with animals, a multicenter, double-blind, randomized clinical trial[171] compared patients who received "standard"-dose glucocorticoids (100 mg as a bolus followed by daily administration of 100 mg for 10 d) and patients who received "high"-dose glucocorticoids (a 1,000-mg bolus followed by 1,000 mg daily for 10 d). There were

TABLE 16-14

NEUROLOGICAL OUTCOME AT 6 WEEKS AND 6 MONTHS IN PATIENTS TREATED WITHIN 8 HOURS OF INJURY

	6 Weeks			6 Months		
Category of Injury and Measure*	**MP**	**Naloxone**	**Placebo†**	**MP**	**Naloxone**	**Placebo†**
Plegic with total sensory loss						
Number of patients	*47*	*37*	*46*	*45*	*34*	*44*
Motor	6.2‡	3.2	1.3	10.5‡	7.5	4.2
Pinprick	5.9	3.0	2.2	9.4‡	4.2	4.0
Touch	6.8‡	3.7	2.6	9.7‡	7.1	4.7
Plegic with partial sensory loss						
Number of patients	*5*	*12*	*6*	*5*	*11*	*6*
Motor	14.4	14.1	18.0	23.0	28.9	26.5
Pinprick	11.8	13.9‡	4.0	11.6	18.4	9.8
Touch	4.4	7.1	0.3	0.0	13.5	5.2
Paretic with variable sensory loss						
Number of patients	*14*	*12*	*17*	*12*	*11*	*17*
Motor	18.3‡	12.7	10.8	24.3‡	14.5	12.9
Pinprick	10.7	8.2	7.5	14.3	9.6	7.5
Touch	3.8	6.1	1.2	7.6	6.2	1.0

*Scores for motor function range from 0 to 70; scores for sensations of pinprick and touch each range from 29 to 87
†Placebo value is used as the control (reference value) to which MP and naloxone were compared, using an analysis of variance
‡$P < .05$
MP: methylprednisolone
Adapted with permission from Bracken MB, Shephard MJ, Collins WF, et al. A randomized, controlled trial of methylprednisolone or naloxone in the treatment of acute spinal-cord injury. *N Engl J Med.* 1990;322:1409.

no differences in neurological recovery between the two groups, but wound infections were more prevalent in the patients receiving the higher dose.

A second, randomized, controlled clinical trial[170] compared placebo, naloxone, and methylprednisolone given as a bolus of 30 mg/kg, followed by a 23-hour infusion at a rate of 5.4 mg/kg/h. The protocol differed from the earlier trial[171] in two key respects. First, the initial daily dose was much greater. Second, the drug was given for only 1 day, based on the rationale that short-term administration would be associated with fewer wound complications and infections, but would still provide maximal glucocorticoid effect during the most critical interval. The subjects who received methylprednisolone within 8 hours of injury showed a significantly greater improvement in motor function and sensation to pinprick and touch than those who received the placebo, naloxone, or methylprednisolone more than 8 hours after injury (see Table 16-14).[170] Although the differences in the second clinical methylprednisolone trial were statistically significant, they were not dramatic; however, even small differences in motor function may result in major differences in the rehabilitation and quality of life of patients with spinal cord injury. In this study, the short-term administration of glucocorticoid was not associated with increased risk of infection or gastrointestinal bleeding.

Free Radical Scavengers. Considerable experimental evidence suggests that postischemic oxidative injury may contribute to neurological damage. A variety of methods have been used in an attempt to reduce oxidative stress, particularly to reduce the accumulation of oxygen free radicals in injured tissue. One of the more effective experimental interventions has been the use of 21-aminosteroids, compounds that are derived chemically from glucocorticoids, but lack glucocorticoid activity and are potent inhibitors of iron-dependent lipid perioxidation.[172]

G_{M1} Ganglioside. Most of the pharmacological interventions that have been directed at acute spinal cord injury have been designed to reduce the rapid hemorrhage and infarction of the spinal gray matter that occur in the first few hours after injury. However, an alternative strategy is to attempt to preserve the axons passing through white matter adjacent to the site of injury.[173] Experimental data suggest that preservation of as few as 6% of axons prevents distal muscle paralysis and preserves normal movement.[174] Enhanced recovery or repair of damage to long tracts in the spinal cord potentially can be initiated 72 hours or more after the primary injury.[175] In a prospective, randomized, placebo-controlled, double-blind trial, G_{M1} ganglioside (monosialotetrahexosylganglioside), a compound that enhances neurological recovery after experimental spinal cord injury,[176] substantially enhanced improvement, assessed using the Frankel scale and the American Spinal Injury Association (ASIA) motor scores, after 1 year of follow-up.[173] The improvement appeared to be attributable to restoration of useful motor function in initially paralyzed muscles rather than to improving strength in paretic muscles. The overall improvement in ASIA motor score (Figure 16-12) reflects a trend toward greater improvement in lower extremity function than in upper extremity function (Figure 16-13). The magnitude of the beneficial effect of G_{M1} ganglioside in this study was approximately twice as great as that reported earlier with high-dose methylprednisolone. Because the patients in the G_{M1} ganglioside trial received relatively small, probably ineffective, dosages of methylprednisolone, these data raise the exciting possibility that the combination of acutely administered high-dose glucocorticoids and the subsequent administration of G_{M1} ganglioside could produce greater improvement than either agent alone.

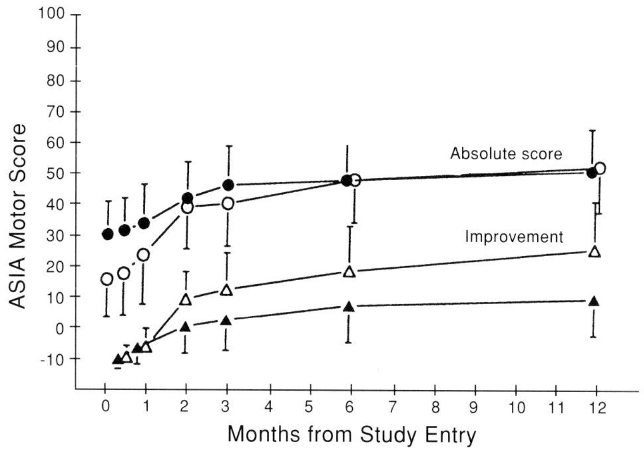

Fig. 16-12. Changes in the American Spinal Injury Association (ASIA) motor score in patients treated with G_{M1} ganglioside (open symbols) and a placebo (solid symbols) in the 12 months after their entry into the study. The upper curves (circles) show unadjusted improvement and demonstrate that the two groups were significantly different at admission into the study (ie, the patients receiving G_{M1} ganglioside were more severely injured). After adjustment for the imbalance in scores at entry, the improvement is apparent. The error bars represent 95% confidence intervals. Reprinted with permission from Geisler FH, Dorsey FC, Coleman WP. Recovery of motor function after spinal-cord injury—a randomized, placebo-controlled trial with GM-1 ganglioside. *N Engl J Med.* 1991;324:1835.

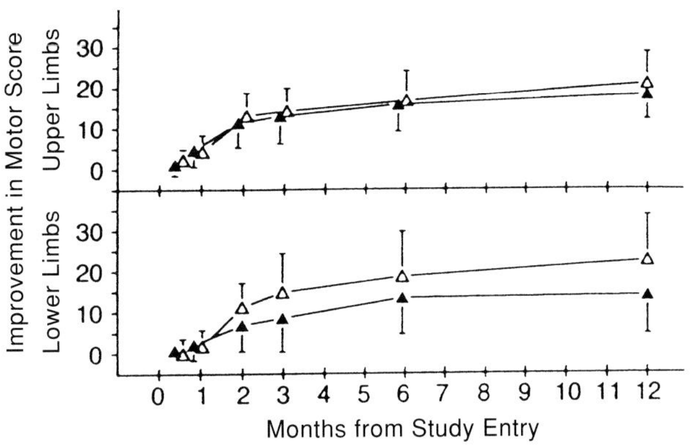

Fig. 16-13. Comparison in the improvement of motor score, assessed using the American Spinal Injuries Association (ASIA) score, in the upper and lower limbs in patients with cervical injuries who were randomized to receive G_{M1} ganglioside (open triangles) and a placebo (solid triangles). A trend toward a drug effect in the score for the lower extremities was not observed in the upper extremities. The error bars represent 95% confidence intervals. Reprinted with permission from Geisler FH, Dorsey FC, Coleman WP. Recovery of motor function after spinal-cord injury—a randomized, placebo-controlled trial with GM-1 ganglioside. *N Engl J Med.* 1991;324:1836.

Cardiovascular Management

Cardiovascular management in the intensive care unit is directed at maintaining intravascular volume, providing inotropic support as needed, avoiding excessive fluid administration, and carefully avoiding or promptly treating bradycardia—especially that associated with suctioning in hypoxic patients. The syndrome of spinal shock, which may continue to be a problem for as long as 6 weeks after injury, requires adequate intravascular volume expansion and, in some cases, vasoactive drugs such as dopamine (which, even in low dosages, acts as a venoconstrictor). Particular care should be taken with the positioning of patients in the spinal shock phase of acute spinal cord injury, because sudden changes in position, particularly to the upright position, may result in sudden hemodynamic instability.[177,178] Hemodynamic deterioration resulting from bradycardia may necessitate intermittent or prophylactic treatment with atropine, especially during vagotonic maneuvers such as tracheal suctioning, endotracheal intubation, or rectal examination.

In the acute phase of management, an arterial catheter may be useful for blood pressure monitoring and management of blood gases. Pulmonary artery catheterization may be useful for short-term assessment of intervascular volume and cardiac output during the acute phase of spinal shock. However, because of the significant contribution of infection to morbidity and mortality in patients with spinal cord injury, invasive monitoring should be used judiciously. Fluid challenges have been recommended to assess cardiac function in conjunction with pulmonary artery catheterization.[137] Using this approach, fluid is administered in 250-mL increments at 50 mL/min until cardiac filling pressures rise and remain at least 2.0 mm Hg greater than the preinfusion level. Fluid challenges help to define the need for inotropic support as well as for additional volume administration in hypotensive patients.

Pulmonary Management

In patients with spinal cord injury, the major cause of early death—respiratory failure secondary to muscle paralysis—depends on the level of injury, and may either progress or regress over time. Frequently, diaphragmatic function gradually and progressively deteriorates for up to 5 days after injury, often accelerated by other pulmonary complications such as pulmonary edema or aspiration of vomitus. Serial measurements of FVC and peak negative inspiratory pressure permit early recognition of deterioration and prompt intubation and mechanical ventilation before hypoxemia and hypercarbia occur. In general, patients with spinal cord injury require ventilatory assistance when FVC is lower than 15 mL/kg or when a peak negative inspiratory pressure of –25 cm H_2O cannot be attained. Likewise, measurements of FVC and peak negative inspiratory pressure used to guide weaning from mechanical ventilation (Table 16-15).[138]

Nosocomial pulmonary infections occur not only as a result of respiratory compromise but also because of the relative immunocompromise that accompanies severe trauma. Close attention to pulmonary toilet, including chest physiotherapy, positioning, and tracheal suctioning, is essential,[179] especially in those patients in whom postinjury FVC barely exceeds the threshold for intubation (15 mL/kg). The use of rotating beds, especially for patients in cervical traction, may promote better pulmonary toilet, although controlled studies[180] of this expensive intervention in patients with head injuries have been less encouraging than earlier, uncontrolled studies. Care must be taken during rotational therapy to maintain hemodynamic stability in patients who have high cervical lesions or spinal shock.

TABLE 16-15

WEANING CRITERIA FOR REMOVAL FROM MECHANICAL VENTILATION

Weaning Criterion	Acceptable Value
Maximum inspiratory force	> −20 cm H_2O
Maximum expiratory force	> +20 cm H_2O
Vital capacity	> 1,000 mL
Expiratory value	> 10 L/s (level dependent)
$Pa{O_2}/F{IO_2}$	> 250
Lung/thoracic cage compliance	> 30 mL/cm H_2O

Adapted with permission from Schreibman DL, Mackenzie CF. The trauma victim with an acute spinal cord injury. *Problems in Anesthesia.* 1990;4:471.

For patients who require intubation for pulmonary support, the choice of neuromuscular blocking agents is important. After the first 24 to 48 hours after injury, succinylcholine-induced hyperkalemia can be life threatening.[159,181] Although the exact onset of this response in humans has not been elucidated, studies[182] in a primate model suggest that the critical time may be as soon as 4 days after injury, with half of the peak increases (approximately 2.8 mEq/L above baseline) in serum potassium occurring at 8 days, and peak increases (approximately 5.5 mEq/L above baseline) occurring at 14 days after injury. The interval during which patients with spinal cord injury remain vulnerable to the hyperkalemic response to succinylcholine is unclear but certainly extends more than 6 months after injury.

Prevention of venous thrombosis and pulmonary embolism, major causes of morbidity and mortality after spinal cord injury,[177] is an important part of the management of patients with acute injury to the spinal cord. Low-molecular-weight heparin is safer and more effective than conventional heparin in the prevention of thromboembolism in patients who have complete motor paralysis.[183]

Pain Syndromes

Three types of pain syndromes commonly develop in the postacute phase of spinal cord injury[127,184]:

1. Pain at the site of trauma is usually well localized, tender and responds well to analgesics, heat, and transcutaneous electrical nerve stimulation (TENS).
2. Radicular or dermatomal pain presumably results from irritation of nerve roots by adhesive arachnoiditis. Variable symptoms include sharp, burning pain with hypersensitivity in a radicular distribution. TENS may be effective. Carbamazepine is also often effective. Other analgesics are sometimes helpful, but often not.
3. Posttraumatic spinal deafferentation pain is a diffuse burning or dysesthesia below the level of injury. Often difficult to control, deafferentation pain is resistant to analgesics but may respond to phenytoin, carbamazepine, or amitriptyline. Approaches such as dorsal root entry zone (DREZ) surgery are reserved for refractory cases.

The specific management of pain associated with spinal injury beyond the acute stages is beyond the scope of this chapter, which deals with trauma anesthesia for combat casualties, not their rehabilitation. However, *Rehabilitation of the Injured Soldier,*[185] a volume in the *Textbook of Military Medicine* series, discusses the problem in detail.

Medical Complications

The sequelae of spinal cord injury include numerous and varied medical complications, such as those of the gastrointestinal and genitourinary systems, electrolyte abnormalities, decubitus ulcers, and the need for nutritional and emotional support.

Gastrointestinal System

Gastric atony usually accompanies spinal shock; intestinal motility may be reduced for several weeks after injury. Because air swallowing leading to gastric distention is frequently a problem in the early course of hospitalization after spinal cord injury, placement of a nasogastric tube is mandatory. Replacement of nasogastric drainage is important to prevent hypokalemic, hypochloremic metabolic alkalosis. Prophylaxis against stress gastritis and ulceration can be accomplished using antacids, H_2 blocking agents, or sucralfate. In 1989, researchers[186] reported that early provision of total energy requirements through adequate oral or parenteral nutrition decreased the incidence of gastrointestinal bleeding in patients with spinal cord injury.

In cervical and high–thoracic spinal cord injury, the sympathetic control of the transverse colon and rectum is disrupted, as is parasympathetic control of the descending and rectosigmoid colon. Loss of voluntary control of the external anal sphincter, pelvic floor, and abdominal wall impairs normal bowel evacuation. Early after the injury, reflex emptying of the colon usually occurs. Later, fecal impaction secondary to ineffective distal colonic peristalsis can manifest as absent bowel movements or diarrheal flow around an obstructing fecal mass.[127] Rarely, colonic distention may result in autonomic hyperreflexia. A high-fiber diet, generous fluid intake, and stool softeners usually adequately prevent fecal impaction.

Genitourinary System

All patients with complete spinal cord injury and many patients with incomplete cord injury syndromes require urinary bladder drainage to relieve distention. Because of recurrent urinary tract infections associated with long-term, indwelling bladder catheters, intermittent bladder catheterization is initiated after initial stabilization. Recurrent, chronic urinary tract infections remain a cause of morbidity and mortality.[127,177,178] Renal function often deteriorates as a result of repeated urinary tract infections and stone formation, which may be secondary to either infection or hypercalciuria. Pyelonephritis and chronic renal insufficiency or failure may lead to proteinuria, electrolyte losses, and uremia.

Electrolyte Abnormalities

Immobility stimulates calcium release from bone and, therefore, hypercalcemia usually manifests within 2 weeks after spinal cord injury; hypercalcemia eventually leads to nephrolithiasis and frequently becomes a chronic problem. Because of osteoporosis, a consequence of bone demineralization, patients with spinal cord injuries are vulnerable to fractures that occur with minimal trauma. Care must be taken when these patients are transferred and positioned in association with their routine care, examinations, or surgery.

Hyponatremia, a mild, common complication after spinal cord injury, occasionally results in severe water intoxication.[187] In part, this reflects a tendency of patients with spinal cord injuries toward high fluid intake, in addition to impaired free-water excretion.

Decubitus Ulceration

Pressure sores are a common, potentially expensive, and morbid complication of spinal cord injury.[127] Typically occurring over bony prominences, decubitus ulcers can be prevented by proper skin care, compulsive skin inspection, and judicious application of weight-relieving equipment. Patients in the intensive care unit should be repositioned every 2 hours, both to prevent decubitus ulceration and to prevent stasis of secretions. Air-bladder beds such as Roto-rest R and Kin-air R beds (manufactured by Hill-ROM, Charlotte, N.C.) are usually the best solution.

Nutritional Support

Adequate provision of calories and nitrogen prevents muscle wasting and therefore facilitates management of pulmonary status and later rehabilitation. Although not specifically demonstrated in patients with spinal cord injury, improved nutritional status and limitation of catabolism should reduce morbidity and mortality. Early use of the gastrointestinal tract, which can be accomplished with small nasoenteric tubes, feeding jejunostomy tubes placed during surgery, or, in some instances, conventional nasogastric tubes, is preferable to intravenous hyperalimentation. Metoclopramide may facilitate feeding by improving gastric emptying. Intravenous hyperalimentation should be considered only a short-term alternative used to reduce catabolism in patients unable to tolerate enteral feedings.

Emotional Support

The psychological impact of spinal cord injury cannot be overstated. Most casualties with spinal cord injury are young, previously healthy, active individuals; they all require psychological and emotional support in dealing with sudden disability and prolonged rehabilitation. Early involvement of patients, friends, and family is imperative.[188] Without consistent support, rehabilitation may prove difficult or futile.

SUMMARY

Advances in strategic planning, logistical support, and the miniaturization of devices permit the modern fighting force to have relatively sophisticated medical services in close support of forward operations. Despite the fact that mobile army surgical hospitals or equivalent hospital units may be located close to the front lines of engagement, thereby reducing evacuation time and facilitating the initiation of definitive care, combat conditions do not always permit immediate evacuation. Initial triage and treatment may be required in technologically constrained circumstances. At this level, the art of medicine must be most critically practiced within the strict guidelines of military triage. Thus, when confronted with the neurologically injured patient, time or other injuries may already have rendered the casualty with head or spinal cord injuries unsalvageable owing to intervening hypoxia, hypercarbia, or hypotension. Regardless of the apparent prognosis, resuscitation should proceed aggressively, keeping in mind the vulnerability of the acutely injured central nervous system to systemic insults.

Airway obstruction, hypoventilation, and hypoxia should be presumed to be present in any comatose patient with a head injury. Concomitant spinal cord injury should be suspected. The airway should be secured quickly. Oral intubation is best accomplished with accompanying manual in-line cervical traction. Nasal intubation is relatively contraindicated in the patient with apparent facial fractures. During intubation, cricoid pressure may limit the likelihood of aspiration of stomach contents. Ventilation should account for increased oxygen consumption.

Hemodynamic resuscitation must be accomplished promptly. Cerebral ischemia or intracranial hypertension may result from inadequately treated hypotension. Volume administration, especially in the form of 0.9% saline or more hypertonic solutions, is unlikely to increase ICP. If hypotension and bradycardia are related to acute spinal cord injury, then volume expansion, ephedrine, and atropine will restore perfusion pressure. Hypertension, a common physiological response to acute head injury, usually requires no treatment and may represent a physiological reflex that maintains CPP in the face of increased ICP.

If intracranial hypertension is suspected, then hyperventilation should be used; however, routine hyperventilation is unnecessary and ineffective. Mannitol, with or without furosemide, helps to maintain high serum osmolality, which is the key to reducing the volume of normal brain tissue, thereby lowering ICP.

Although barbiturates (which decrease CMR_{O_2}, act as cerebral vasoconstrictors, and reduce ICP) may be useful in inducing anesthesia in normovolemic patients, they do not improve outcome if used routinely in all patients with head injuries. Benzodiazepines or etomidate represent appropriate alternatives for induction of anesthesia or sedation during intubation. Etomidate may be particularly useful in patients who are hypovolemic.

Working in an austere combat environment with limited material and equipment can be stressful to military medical personnel; however, the lives of many critically injured individuals can be saved and their neurological function preserved.

Contributing Author

Colonel William Bergman, M.D., Medical Corps, U.S. Army, Neurosurgical Consultant to The Surgeon General, Walter Reed Army Medical Center, Washington, D. C. 20307-5001

REFERENCES

1. Chesnut RM, Marshall LF, Klauber MR, et al. The role of secondary brain injury in determining outcome from severe head injury. *J Trauma*. 1993;34:216–222.

2. Miller JD, Butterworth JF, Gudeman SK, et al. Further experience in the management of severe head injury. *J Neurosurg*. 1981;54:289–299.

3. Bellamy RF. Colonel, Medical Corps, US Army. Personal communication, July 1994. The single most useful database describing combat wounds and the circumstances of wounding is the Wound Data and Munitions Effectiveness Team (WDMET) study prepared by the U.S. Army Materiel Command during the Vietnam War. These data are stored at the National Naval Medical Center, Bethesda, Maryland. Access is controlled by the Uniformed Services University of the Health Sciences, Bethesda, Maryland 20814-4799; telephone (301) 295-6262. Three summary volumes contain extensive abstracts of the statistical data and can be obtained from Defense Documentation Center, Cameron Station, Alexandria, Virginia 22304-6145; telephone (703) 545-6700 and (703) 274-7633.

4. Carey ME. Analysis of wounds incurred by US Army Seventh Corps personnel who were treated in Corps hospitals during Operation desert Storm, 20 February to 10 March 1991. *J Trauma*. 1995;in press. Presented at the Seventh International Symposium of Weapons Traumatology and Wound Ballistics; September 1994; St. Petersburg, Russia.

5. Cushing H. A study of a series of wounds involving the brain and its enveloping structures. *Br J Surg*. 1918;5:558–684.

6. Cushing H. Notes on penetrating wounds of the brain. *Br Med J*. 1918;221–226.

7. Meirowsky AM, ed. *Neurological Surgery of Trauma*. Washington, DC: Department of the Army, Office of The Surgeon General; 1965.

8. Brandvold B, Levi L, Feinsod M, George ED. Penetrating craniocerebral injuries in the Israeli involvement in the Lebanese conflict, 1982–1985. *J Neurosurg*. 1990;72:15–21.

9. Myers PW, Brophy A, Salazar AM, Jones B. Retained bone fragments after penetrating brain wounds: Long-term follow-up in Vietnam veterans. Presented at the Annual Meeting of the American Association of Neurological Surgeons, April, 1989. *J Neurosurg*. 1989;70:319A. Abstract.

10. Adams JH, Graham DI, Scott G, Parker LS, Doyle D. Brain damage in fatal nonmissile head injury. *J Clin Pathol*. 1980;33:1132–1145.

11. Graham DI, Ford I, Adams JH, et al. Ischaemic brain damage is still common in fatal non-missile head injury. *J Neurol Neurosurg Psychiatry*. 1989;52:346–350.

12. Stein SC, Ross SE. The value of computed tomographic scans in patients with low-risk head injuries. *Neurosurgery*. 1990;26:638–640.

13. Gennarelli TA, Thibault LE. Biological models of head injury. In: Becker DP, Povlishock JT, eds. *Central Nervous System Trauma Status Report*. Bethesda, Md: National Institutes of Health; 1985: 391–404.

14. Povlishock JT, Becker DP, Miller JD, Jenkins LW, Dietrich WD. The morphopathologic substrates of concussion. *Acta Neuropathol*. 1979;47:1–11.

15. Sullivan HG, Martinez J, Becker DP, Miller JD, Griffith R, Wist AO. Fluid-percussion model of mechanical brain injury in the cat. *J Neurosurg*. 1976;45:521–534.

16. Carey ME, Sarna GS, Farrell JB, Happel LT. Experimental missile wound to the brain. *J Neurosurg*. 1989;71:754–764.

17. Crockard A, Johns L, Levett J, Brown F, Mullan S. "Brainstem" effects of experimental cerebral missile injury. In: Popp AJ, Bourke RS, Nelson LR, Kimelberg KH, eds. *Neural Trauma*. New York, NY: Raven Press; 1979: 19–25.

18. Ishige N, Pitts LH, Pogliani L, et al. Effect of hypoxia on traumatic brain injury in rats, II: Changes in high energy phosphate metabolism. *Neurosurgery*. 1987;20:854–858.

19. Ishige N, Pitts LH, Berry I, Nishimura MC, James TL. The effects of hypovolemic hypotension on high-energy phosphate metabolism of traumatized brain in rats. *J Neurosurg*. 1988;68:129–136.

20. Yuan X-Q, Bergman WC, Bruttig SP, Henson G, Ferris C, Bowerson JC. Identification of a turning point in the impact level which alters the early physiological responses to fluid percussion brain injury in the swine. *FASEB J*. 1993;7:353A.

21. Wei EP, Kontos HA, Christman CW, DeWitt DS, Povlishock JT. Superoxide generation and reversal of acetylcholine-induced cerebral arteriolar dilation after acute hypertension. *Circ Res*. 1985;57:781–787.

22. Lewelt W, Jenkins LW, Miller JD. Autoregulation of cerebral blood flow after experimental fluid percussion injury of the brain. *J Neurosurg*. 1980;53:500–511.

23. DeWitt DS, Prough DS, Taylor CL, Whitley JM, Deal DD, Vines SM. Regional cerebrovascular responses to progressive hypotension after traumatic brain injury in cats. *Am J Physiol*. (*Heart Circ Physiol*). 1992;32: H1276–H1284.

24. DeWitt DS, Prough DS, Taylor CL, Whitley JM. Reduced cerebral blood flow, oxygen delivery, and electroencephalographic activity after traumatic brain injury and mild hemorrhage in cats. *J Neurosurg*. 1992;76:812–821.

25. McIntosh TK, Vink R, Soares H, Simon R. Possible role of excitatory amino acid neurotransmitters in pathophysiology of experimental brain injury. *J Cereb Blood Flow Metab*. 1989;9:S77.

26. Jenkins LW, Lyeth BG, Lewelt W, et al. Combined pretrauma scopolamine and phencyclidine attenuate posttraumatic increased sensitivity to delayed secondary ischemia. *J Neurotrauma*. 1988;5:275–287.

27. DeWitt DS, Kong DL, Lyeth BG, et al. Experimental traumatic brain injury elevates brain prostaglandin E_2 and thromboxane B_2 levels in rats. *J Neurotrauma*. 1988;5:303–313.

28. Hayes RL, Lyeth BG, Jenkins LW, et al. Possible protective effect of endogenous opioids in traumatic brain injury. *J Neurosurg*. 1990;72:252–261.

29. Miller JD. Head injury. *J Neurol Neurosurg Psychiatry*. 1993;56:440–447.

30. O'Sullivan MG, Statham PF, Jones PA, et al. Role of intracranial pressure monitoring in severely head-injured patients without signs of intracranial hypertension on initial computerized tomography. *J Neurosurg*. 1994;80:46–50.

31. Robertson CS, Grossman RG, Goodman JC, Narayan RK. The predictive value of cerebral anaerobic metabolism with cerebral infarction after head injury. *J Neurosurg*. 1987;67:361–368.

32. Sheinberg M, Kanter MJ, Robertson CS, Contant CF, Narayan RK, Grossman RG. Continuous monitoring of jugular venous oxygen saturation in head-injured patients. *J Neurosurg*. 1992;76:212–217.

33. Cruz J. On-line monitoring of global cerebral hypoxia in acute brain injury: Relationship to intracranial hypertension. *J Neurosurg*. 1993;79:228–233.

34. Robertson CS. *Br J Intens Care*. 1992;1(suppl):12.

35. Clifton GL, Ziegler MG, Grossman RG. Circulating catecholamines and sympathetic activity after head injury. *Neurosurgery*. 1981;8:10–14.

36. Robertson CS, Clifton GL, Taylor AA, Grossman RG. Treatment of hypertension associated with head injury. *J Neurosurg*. 1983;59:455–460.

37. Cushing H. The blood-pressure reaction of acute cerebral compression, illustrated by cases of intracranial hemorrhage. *Am J Med Sci*. 1903;125:1017–1044.

38. McClain CJ, Hennig B, Ott LG, Goldblum S, Young B. Mechanisms and implications of hypoalbuminemia in head-injured patients. *J Neurosurg*. 1988;69:386–392.

39. Schumacker PT, Rhodes GR, Newell JC, et al. Ventilation–perfusion imbalance after head trauma. *Am Rev Respir Dis.* 1979;119:33–43.

40. Malik AB. Mechanisms of neurogenic pulmonary edema. *Circ Res.* 1985;57:1–18.

41. Kumura E, Sato M, Fukuda A, Takemoto Y, Tanaka S, Kohama A. Coagulation disorders following acute head injury. *Acta Neurochir.* 1987;85:23–28.

42. Crone KR, Lee KS, Kelly DL Jr. Correlation of admission fibrin degradation products with outcome and respiratory failure in patients with severe head injury. *Neurosurgery.* 1987;21:532–536.

43. Bouma GJ, Muizelaar JP, Choi SC, Newlon PG, Young HF. Cerebral circulation and metabolism after severe traumatic brain injury: The elusive role of ischemia. *J Neurosurg.* 1991;75:685–693.

44. Obrist WD, Langfitt TW, Jaggi JL, Cruz J, Gennarelli TA. Cerebral blood flow and metabolism in comatose patients with acute head injury. Relationship to intracranial hypertension. *J Neurosurg.* 1984;61:241–253.

45. Muizelaar JP, Marmarou A, DeSalles AF, et al. Cerebral blood flow and metabolism in severely head-injured children, I: Relationship with GCS score, outcome, and PVI. *J Neurosurg.* 1989;71:63–71.

46. Bruce DA, Langfitt TW, Miller JD, et al. Regional cerebral blood flow, intracranial pressure, and brain metabolism in comatose patients. *J Neurosurg.* 1973;38:131–144.

47. Muizelaar JP, Lutz HA III, Becker DP. Effect of mannitol on ICP and CBF and correlation with pressure autoregulation in severely head-injured patients. *J Neurosurg.* 1984;61:700–706.

48. Robertson CS, Narayan RK, Gokaslan ZL, et al. Cerebral arteriovenous oxygen difference as an estimate of cerebral blood flow in comatose patients. *J Neurosurg.* 1989;70:222–230.

49. Cruz J, Miner ME, Allen SJ, Alves WM, Gennarelli TA. Continuous monitoring of cerebral oxygenation in acute brain injury: Injection of mannitol during hyperventilation. *J Neurosurg.* 1990;73:725–730.

50. Diehl JT, Lester JL III, Cosgrove DM. Clinical comparison of hetastarch and albumin in postoperative cardiac patients. *Surg Forum.* 1981;32:260–262.

51. Teasdale G, Jennett B. Assessment of coma and impaired consciousness: A practical scale. *Lancet.* 1974;2:81–84.

52. Jennett B, Bond M. Assessment of outcome after severe brain damage: A practical scale. *Lancet.* 1975;1:480–484.

53. Jaggi JL, Obrist WD, Gennarelli TA, Langfitt TW. Relationship of early cerebral blood flow and metabolism to outcome in acute head injury. *J Neurosurg.* 1990;72:176–182.

54. Levine JE, Becker D, Chun T. Reversal of incipient brain death from head-injury apnea at the scene of accidents. *N Engl J Med.* 1979;301:109.

55. Muzzi DA, Losasso TJ, Cucchiara RF. Complication from a nasopharyngeal airway in a patient with a basilar skull fracture. *Anesthesiology.* 1991;74:366–368.

56. Lanier WL, Iaizzo PA, Milde JH. Cerebral function and muscle afferent activity following intravenous succinylcholine in dogs anesthetized with halothane: The effects of pretreatment with a defasciculating dose of pancuronium. *Anesthesiology.* 1989;71:87–95.

57. Muizelaar JP, Marmarou A, Ward JD, et al. Adverse effects of prolonged hyperventilation in patients with severe head injury: A randomized clinical trial. *J Neurosurg.* 1991;75:731–739.

58. Prough DS, Johnson JC, Stump DA, Stullken EH, Poole GV Jr, Howard G. Effects of hypertonic saline versus lactated Ringer's solution on cerebral oxygen transport during resuscitation from hemorrhagic shock. *J Neurosurg*. 1986;64:627–632.

59. Prough DS, Whitley JM, Taylor CL, Deal DD, DeWitt DS. Regional cerebral blood flow following resuscitation from hemorrhagic shock with hypertonic saline. *Anesthesiology*. 1991;75:319–327.

60. Zornow MH, Todd MM, Moore SS. The acute cerebral effects of changes in plasma osmolality and oncotic pressure. *Anesthesiology*. 1987;67:936–941.

61. Shapira Y, Artru AA, Cotev S, Muggia-Sulam M, Freund HR. Brain edema and neurologic status following head trauma in the rat: No effect from large volumes of isotonic or hypertonic intravenous fluids, with or without glucose. *Anesthesiology*. 1992;77:79–85.

62. Poole GV, Prough DS, Johnson JC, Stullken EH, Stump DA, Howard G. Effects of resuscitation from hemorrhagic shock on cerebral hemodynamics in the presence of an intracranial mass. *J Trauma*. 1987;27:18–23.

63. Seelig JM, Becker DP, Miller JD, Greenberg RP, Ward JD, Choi SC. Traumatic acute subdural hematoma: Major mortality reduction in comatose patients treated within four hours. *N Engl J Med*. 1981;304:1511–1518.

64. Gopinath SP, Robertson CS, Grossman RG, Chance B. Near-infrared spectroscopic localization of intracranial hematomas. *J Neurosurg*. 1993;79:43–47.

65. Butterworth JF IV, Maull KI, Miller JD, Becker DP. Detection of occult abdominal trauma in patients with severe head injuries. *Lancet*. 1980;2:759–762.

66. Greenberg RP, Newlon PG, Hyatt MS, Narayan RK, Becker DP. Prognostic implications of early multimodality evoked potentials in severely head-injured patients. *J Neurosurg*. 1981;55:227–236.

67. Narayan RK, Greenberg RP, Miller JD, et al. Improved confidence of outcome prediction in severe head injury: A comparative analysis of the clinical examination, multimodality evoked potentials, CT scanning, and intracranial pressure. *J Neurosurg*. 1981;54:751–762.

68. Powers SK, Bolger CA, Edwards MSB. Spinal cord pathways mediating somatosensory evoked potentials. *J Neurosurg*. 1982;57:472–482.

69. Li C, Houlden DA, Rowed DW. Somatosensory evoked potentials and neurological grades as predictors of outcome in acute spinal cord injury. *J Neurosurg*. 1990;72:600–609.

70. Garcia-Larrea L, Bertrand O, Artru F, Pernier J, Mauguiere F. Brain-stem monitoring, II: Preterminal BAEP changes observed until brain death in deeply comatose patients. *Electroencephalogr Clin Neurophysiol*. 1987;68:446–457.

71. Miller JD, Becker DP, Ward JD, Sullivan HG, Adams WE, Rosner MJ. Significance of intracranial hypertension in severe head injury. *J Neurosurg*. 1977;47:503–516.

72. Saul TG, Ducker TB. Effect of intracranial pressure monitoring and aggressive treatment on mortality in severe head injury. *J Neurosurg*. 1982;56:498–503.

73. Stuart GG, Merry GS, Smith JA, Yelland JDN. Severe head injury managed without intracranial pressure monitoring. *J Neurosurg*. 1983;59:601–605.

74. Vries JK, Becker DP, Young HF. A subarachnoid screw for monitoring intracranial pressure. *J Neurosurg*. 1973;39:416–419.

75. Miller JD, Bobo H, Kapp JP. Inaccurate pressure readings for subarachnoid bolts. *Neurosurgery*. 1986;19:253–255.

76. Ward JD. Intracranial pressure monitoring. In: Fuhrman BP, Shoemaker WC, eds. *Critical Care: State of the Art*. Fullerton, Calif: The Society of Critical Care Medicine; 1989: 173–185.

77. Chambers IR, Mendelow AD, Sinar EJ, et al. A clinical evaluation of the Camino subdural screw and ventricular monitoring kits. *Neurosurgery*. 1990;26:421.

78. Crutchfield JS, Narayan RK, Robertson CS, Michael LH. Evaluation of a fiberoptic intracranial pressure monitor. *J Neurosurg*. 1990;72:482–487.

79. Eisenberg HM, Frankowski RF, Contant CF, Marshall LF, Walker MD. High-dose barbiturate control of elevated intracranial pressure in patients with severe head injury. *J Neurosurg*. 1988;69:15–23.

80. Ward JD, Becker DP, Miller JD, et al. Failure of prophylactic barbiturate coma in the treatment of severe head injury. *J Neurosurg*. 1985;62:383–388.

81. Myerson A, Halloran RD, Hirsch HL. Technic for obtaining blood from the internal jugular vein and internal carotid artery. *Arch Neurol Psychiatry*. 1927;17:807–808.

82. Goetting MG, Preston G. Jugular bulb catheterization: Experience with 123 patients. *Crit Care Med*. 1990;18:1220–1223.

83. Kurth CD, Steven JM, Benaron D, Chance B. Near-infrared monitoring of the cerebral circulation. *J Clin Monit*. 1993;9:163–170.

84. Smith DS, Levy W, Maris M, Chance B. Reperfusion hyperoxia in brain after circulatory arrest in humans. *Anesthesiology*. 1990;73:12–19.

85. Pollard V, DeMelo E, Deyo DJ, Stoddard H, Hoffmann DJ, Prough DS. Generation and validation of an algorithm for brain oxygen monitoring. *Anesth Analg*. 1994;78:S343.

86. Rosner MJ, Coley IB. Cerebral perfusion pressure, intracranial pressure, and head elevation. *J Neurosurg*. 1986;65:636–641.

87. Feldman Z, Kanter MJ, Robertson CS, et al. Effect of head elevation on intracranial pressure, cerebral perfusion pressure, and cerebral blood flow in head-injured patients. *J Neurosurg*. 1992;76:207–211.

88. Lundberg N, Troupp H, Lorin H. Continuous recording of the ventricular fluid pressure in patients with severe acute traumatic brain injury. *J Neurosurg*. 1965;22:581–590.

89. Rosner MJ, Becker DP. Experimental brain injury: Successful therapy with the weak base, tromethamine, with an overview of CNS acidosis. *J Neurosurg*. 1984;60:961–971.

90. Hayashi M, Kobayashi H, Handa Y, Kawano H, Kabuto M. Brain blood volume and blood flow in patients with plateau waves. *J Neurosurg*. 1985;63:556–561.

91. Hsiang JK, Chesnut RM, Crisp CB, Klauber MR, Blunt BA, Marshall LF. Early, routine paralysis for intracranial pressure control in severe head injury: Is it necessary? *Crit Care Med*. 1994;22:1471–1476.

92. McCormick JM, McCormick PW, Zabramski JM, Spetzler RF. Intracranial pressure reduction by a central alpha-2 adrenoreceptor agonist after subarachnoid hemorrhage. *Neurosurgery*. 1993;32:974–979.

93. Jafar JJ, Johns LM, Mullan SF. The effect of mannitol on cerebral blood flow. *J Neurosurg*. 1986;64:754–759.

94. Roberts PA, Pollay M, Engles C, Pendleton B, Reynolds E, Stevens FA. Effect on intracranial pressure of furosemide combined with varying doses and administration rates of mannitol. *J Neurosurg*. 1987;66:440–446.

95. Worthley LIG, Cooper DJ, Jones N. Treatment of resistant intracranial hypertension with hypertonic saline: Report of two cases. *J Neurosurg*. 1988;68:478–481.

96. Fisher B, Thomas D, Peterson B. Hypertonic saline lowers raised intracranial pressure in children after head trauma. *J Neurosurg Anesth*. 1992;4:4–10.

97. Gower DJ, Lee KS, McWhorter JM. Role of subtemporal decompression in severe closed head injury. *Neurosurgery.* 1988;23:417–422.

98. Clifton GL, Robertson CS, Contant CF. Enteral hyperalimentation in head injury. *J Neurosurg.* 1985;62:186–193.

99. Dearden NM, Gibson JS, McDowall DG, Gibson RM, Cameron MM. Effect of high-dose dexamethasone on outcome from severe head injury. *J Neurosurg.* 1986;64:81–88.

100. Michenfelder JD. The interdependency of cerebral functional and metabolic effects following massive doses of thiopental in the dog. *Anesthesiology.* 1974;41:231–236.

101. Frost EAM. Effects of positive end-expiratory pressure on intracranial pressure and compliance in brain-injured patients. *J Neurosurg.* 1977;47:195–200.

102. Toung TJ, Miyabe M, McShane AJ, Rogers MC, Traystman RJ. Effect of PEEP and jugular venous compression on canine cerebral blood flow and oxygen consumption in the head elevated position. *Anesthesiology.* 1988;68:53–58.

103. Segredo V, Caldwell JE, Matthay MA, Sharma ML, Gruenke LD, Miller RD. Persistent paralysis in critically ill patients after long-term administration of vecuronium. *N Engl J Med.* 1992;327:524–528.

104. Jennett B, Miller JD, Braakman R. Epilepsy after nonmissile depressed skull fracture. *J Neurosurg.* 1974;41:208–216.

105. Kamada T, Fusamoto H, Kawano S, Noguchi M, Hiramatsu K. Gastrointestinal bleeding following head injury: A clinical study of 433 cases. *J Trauma.* 1977;17:44–47.

106. Driks MR, Craven DE, Celli BR, et al. Nosocomial pneumonia in intubated patients given sucralfate as compared with antacids or histamine type 2 blockers: The role of gastric colonization. *N Engl J Med.* 1987;317:1376–1382.

107. Tryba M. Risk of acute stress bleeding and nosocomial pneumonia in ventilated intensive care unit patients: Sucralfate versus antacids. *Am J Med.* 1987;83:117–124.

108. Humphrey MA, Simpson GT, Grindlinger GA. Clinical characteristics of nosocomial sinusitis. *Ann Otol Rhinol Laryngol.* 1987;96:687–690.

109. Holzapfel L, Chevret S, Madinier G, et al. Influence of long-term oro- or nasotracheal intubation on nosocomial maxillary sinusitis and pneumonia: Results of a prospective, randomized, clinical trial. *Crit Care Med.* 1993;21: 1132–1138.

110. Geheb MA. Clinical approach to the hyperosmolar patient. *Crit Care Clin.* 1987;3:797–815.

111. Doczi T, Tarjanyi J, Huszka E, Kiss J. Syndrome of inappropriate secretion of antidiuretic hormone (SIADH) after head injury. *Neurosurgery.* 1982;10:685–688.

112. Kiwit JC, Schroders C, Wambach G. Plasma ANP levels and its relation to electrolyte and water regulation in neurosurgical intensive care patients. *Z-Kardiol.* 1988;77:119–123.

113. Singer I, Rotenberg D. Demeclocycline induced nephrogenic diabetes insipidus: In-vivo and in-vitro studies. *Ann Intern Med.* 1973;79:679–683.

114. Robertson CS, Clifton GL, Grossman RG. Oxygen utilization and cardiovascular function in head-injured patients. *Neurosurgery.* 1984.15:307–314.

115. Clifton GL, Robertson CS, Grossman RG, Hodge S. The metabolic response to severe head injury. *J Neurosurg.* 1984;60:687–696.

116. Robertson CS, Clifton GL, Goodman JC. Steroid administration and nitrogen excretion in the head-injured patient. *J Neurosurg.* 1985;63:714–718.

117. Lam AM, Winn HR, Cullen BF, Sundling N. Hyperglycemia and neurological outcome in patients with head injury. *J Neurosurg*. 1991;75:545–551.

118. Lanier WL, Stangland KJ, Scheithauer BW, Milde JH, Michenfelder JD. The effects of dextrose infusion and head position on neurologic outcome after complete cerebral ischemia in primates: Examination of a model. *Anesthesiology*. 1987;66:39–48.

119. Brooks DN, Aughton ME, Bond MR, Jones P, Rizvi S. Cognitive sequelae in relationship to early indices of severity of brain damage after severe blunt head injury. *J Neurol Neurosurg Psychiatry*. 1980;43:529–534.

120. Levin HS, Goldstein FC, High WM Jr, Eisenberg HM. Disproportionately severe memory deficit in relation to normal intellectual functioning after closed head injury. *J Neurol Neurosurg Psychiatry*. 1988;51:1294–1301.

121. Butterworth JF IV, Selhorst JB, Greenberg RP, Miller JD, Gudeman SK. Flaccidity after head injury: Diagnosis, management, and outcome. *Neurosurgery*. 1981;9:242–248.

122. Seelig JM, Greenberg RP, Becker DP, Miller JD, Choi SC. Reversible brain-stem dysfunction following acute traumatic subdural hematoma: A clinical and electrophysiological study. *J Neurosurg*. 1981;55:516–523.

123. Gennarelli TA, Spielman GM, Langfitt TW, et al. Influence of the type of intracranial lesion on outcome from severe head injury. *J Neurosurg*. 1982;56:26–32.

124. Gibson RM, Stephenson GC. Aggressive management of severe closed head trauma: Time for reappraisal. *Lancet*. 1989;2:369–371.

125. Walker MD. Acute spinal-cord injury. *N Engl J Med*. 1991;324:1885–1887.

126. Albin MS, White RJ. Epidemiology, physiopathology, and experimental therapeutics of acute spinal cord injury. *Crit Care Clin*. 1987;3:441–452.

127. Levinson W, Ward G, Valleroy M. Care of spinal-cord-injured patients after the acute period. *J Gen Int Med*. 1989;4:336–348.

128. Albin MS, Bunegin L, Gilbert J, Babinski MF. Anesthesia for spinal cord injury. In: Porter SS, Kirby RR, Brown DL, eds. *Problems in Anesthesia: Neuroanesthesia*. Philadelphia, Pa: Lippincott; 1991: 138–154.

129. Janssen L, Hansebout RR. Pathogenesis of spinal cord injury and newer treatments: A review. *Spine*. 1989;14:23–32.

130. Drummond JC, Moore SS. The influence of dextrose administration on neurologic outcome after temporary spinal cord ischemia in the rabbit. *Anesthesiology*. 1989;70:64–70.

131. Robertson CS, Grossman RG. Protection against spinal cord ischemia with insulin-induced hypoglycemia. *J Neurosurg*. 1987;67:739–744.

132. Flamm ES, Demopoulos HB, Seligman ML, Tomasula JJ, DeCrescito V, Ransohoff J. Ethanol potentiation of central nervous system trauma. *J Neurosurg*. 1977;46:328–335.

133. Hastings RH, Marks JD. Airway management for trauma patients with potential cervical spine injuries. *Anesth Analg*. 1991;73:471–482.

134. Frankel HL, Mathias CJ, Spalding JM. Mechanisms of reflex cardiac arrest in tetraplegic patients. *Lancet*. 1975;2:1183–1185.

135. Theodore J, Robin ED. Speculations on neurogenic pulmonary edema (NPE). *Am Rev Respir Dis*. 1976;113:405–411.

136. Albin MS, Bunegin L, Wolf S. Brain and lungs at risk after cervical spinal cord transection: Intracranial pressure, brain water, blood–brain barrier permeability, cerebral blood flow, and extravascular lung water changes. *Surg Neurol*. 1985;24:191–205.

137. Mackenzie CF, Shin B, Krishnaprasad D, McCormack F, Illingworth W. Assessment of cardiac and respiratory function during surgery on patients with acute quadriplegia. *J Neurosurg*. 1985;62:843–849.

138. Schreibman DL, Mackenzie CF. The trauma victim with an acute spinal cord injury. *Problems in Anesthesia*. 1990;4:459–476.

139. Ciliberti BJ, Goldfein J, Rovenstine EA. Hypertension during anesthesia in patients with spinal cord injuries. *Anesthesiology*. 1954;15:273–279.

140. Wanner MB, Rageth CJ, Zäch GA. Pregnancy and autonomic hyperreflexia in patients with spinal cord lesions. *Paraplegia*. 1987;25:482–490.

141. Babinski MF. Anesthetic considerations in the patient with acute spinal cord injury. *Crit Care Clin*. 1987;3:619–636.

142. Stowe DF, Bernstein JS, Madsen KE, McDonald DJ, Ebert TJ. Autonomic hyperreflexia in spinal cord injured patients during extracorporeal shock wave lithotripsy. *Anesth Analg*. 1989;68:788–791.

143. Schonwald G, Fish KJ, Perkash I. Cardiovascular complications during anesthesia in chronic spinal cord injured patients. *Anesthesiology*. 1981;55:550–558.

144. Findley LJ, Rochester DF. The lungs and neuromuscular and chest wall diseases. In: Murray JF, Nadel JA, eds. *Textbook of Respiratory Medicine*. Philadelphia, Pa: WB Saunders; 1988: 1942–1971.

145. Fugl-Meyer AR. Effects of respiratory muscle paralysis in tetraplegic and paraplegic patients. *Scand J Rehabil Med*. 1971;3:141–150.

146. Ledsome JR, Sharp JM. Pulmonary function in acute cervical cord injury. *Am Rev Respir Dis*. 1981;124:41–44.

147. Di Chiro G, Fried LC. Blood flow currents in spinal cord arteries. *Neurology*. 1971;21:1088–1096.

148. Fried LC, Doppman JL, Di Chiro G. Direction of blood flow in the primate cervical spinal cord. *J Neurosurg*. 1970;33:325–330.

149. Hickey R, Albin MS, Bunegin L, Gelineau J. Autoregulation of spinal cord blood flow: Is the cord a microcosm of the brain? *Stroke*. 1986;17:1183–1189.

150. Davidoff G, Thomas P, Johnson M, Berent S, Dijkers M, Doljanac R. Closed head injury in acute traumatic spinal cord injury: Incidence and risk factors. *Arch Phys Med Rehabil*. 1988;69:869–872.

151. Michael DB, Guyot DR, Darmody WR. Coincidence of head and cervical spine injury. *J Neurotrauma*. 1989;6:177–189.

152. Mace S. Emergency evaluation of cervical spine injuries: CT versus plain radiographs. *Ann Emerg Med*. 1985;14:973–975.

153. Trafton PG, Boyd CA Jr. Computed tomography of thoracic and lumbar spine injuries. *J Trauma*. 1984;24:506–515.

154. Schaefer DM, Flanders A, Northrup BE, Doan HT, Osterholm JL. Magnetic resonance imaging of acute cervical spine trauma: Correlation with severity of neurologic injury. *Spine*. 1989;14:1090–1095.

155. Pang D, Wilberger JE. Spinal cord injury without radiographic abnormalties in children. *J Neurosurg*. 1982; 57:114–129.

156. Hardy AG. Cervical spinal cord injury without bony injury. *Paraplegia*. 1977;14:296–305.

157. Grande CM, Stene JK, Bernhard WN. Airway management: Considerations in the trauma patient. *Crit Care Clin*. 1990;6:37–59.

158. Grande CM, Barton CR, Stene JK. Appropriate techniques for airway management of emergency patients with suspected spinal cord injury. *Anesth Analg*. 1988;67:710–711.

159. Tobey RE. Paraplegia, succinylcholine and cardiac arrest. *Anesthesiology*. 1970;32:359–364.

160. DeVivo MJ, Kartus PL, Stover SL, Rutt RD, Fine PR. Cause of death for patients with spinal cord injuries. *Arch Intern Med*. 1989;149:1761–1766.

161. Albin MS. Resuscitation of the spinal cord. *Crit Care Med*. 1978;6:270–276.

162. Grundy BL, Friedman W. Electrophysiological evaluation of the patient with acute spinal cord injury. *Crit Care Clin*. 1987;3:519–548.

163. Rowed DW, McLean JAG, Tator CH. Somatosensory evoked potentials in acute spinal cord injury: Prognostic value. *Surg Neurol*. 1978;9:203–210.

164. Levy WJ, York DH, McCaffrey M, Tanzer F. Motor evoked potentials from transcranial stimulation of the motor cortex in humans. *Neurosurgery*. 1984;15:287–302.

165. Albin MS, White RJ, Locke GE, Kretchmer HE. Spinal cord hypothermia by localized perfusion cooling. *Nature*. 1966;210:1059–1060.

166. Albin MS, White RJ, Yashon D, Harris LS. Effects of localized cooling on spinal cord trauma. *J Trauma*. 1969;9:1000–1008.

167. Faden AI, Jacobs TP, Mougey E, Holaday JW. Endorphins in experimental spinal injury: Therapeutic effect of naloxone. *Ann Neurol*. 1981;10:326–332.

168. Faden AI. Pharmacotherapy in spinal cord injury: A critical review of recent developments. *Clin Neuropharmacol*. 1987;10:193–204.

169. Faden AI. Opiate antagonists and thyrotropin-releasing hormone, II: Potential role in the treatment of central nervous system injury. *JAMA*. 1984;252:1452–1454.

170. Bracken MB, Shephard MJ, Collins WF, et al. A randomized, controlled trial of methylprednisolone or naloxone in the treatment of acute spinal-cord injury. *N Engl J Med*. 1990;322:1405–1411.

171. Bracken MB, Collins WF, Freeman DF, et al. Efficacy of methylprednisolone in acute spinal cord injury. *JAMA*. 1984;251:45–52.

172. Anderson DK, Braughler JM, Hall ED, Waters TR, McCall JM, Means ED. Effects of treatment with U-74006F on neurological outcome following experimental spinal cord injury. *J Neurosurg*. 1988;69:562–567.

173. Geisler FH, Dorsey FC, Coleman WP. Recovery of motor function after spinal-cord injury—A randomized, placebo-controlled trial with GM-1 ganglioside. *N Engl J Med*. 1991;324:1829–1838.

174. Young W. Recovery mechanisms in spinal cord injury: Implications for regenerative therapy. In: Seil FJ, ed. *Neural Regeneration and Transplantation*. Vol 6. In: *Frontiers of Clinical Neuroscience*. New York, NY: Alan R. Liss; 1989: 157–169.

175. Blight AR, Young W. Central axons in injured cat spinal cord recover electrophysiological function following remyelination by Schwann cells. *J Neurol Sci*. 1989;91:15–34.

176. Gorio A, Di Guillo AM, Young W, et al. GM-1 effects on chemical traumatic and peripheral nerve induce lesions to the spinal cord. In: Goldberger ME, Gorio A, Murray M, eds. *Development and Plasticity of the Mammalian Spinal Cord*. Vol 3. Padua, Italy: Liviana Press; 1986: 227–242.

177. Luce JM. Medical management of spinal cord injury. *Crit Care Med*. 1985;13:126–131.

178. McVicar JP, Luce JM. Management of spinal cord injury in the critical care setting. *Crit Care Clin*. 1986;2:747–758.

179. McMichan JC, Michel L, Westbrook PR. Pulmonary dysfunction following traumatic quadriplegia. *JAMA*. 1980;243:528–531.

180. Clemmer TP, Green S, Ziegler B, et al. Effectiveness of the kinetic treatment table for preventing and treating pulmonary complications in severely head-injured patients. *Crit Care Med*. 1990;18:614–617.

181. Gronert GA, Theye RA. Pathophysiology of hyperkalemia induced by succinylcholine. *Anesthesiology*. 1975;43:89–99.

182. John DA, Tobey RE, Homer LD, Rice CL. Onset of succinylcholine-induced hyperkalemia following denervation. *Anesthesiology*. 1976;45:294–299.

183. Green D, Lee MY, Lim AC, et al. Prevention of thromboembolism after spinal cord injury using low-molecular-weight heparin. *Ann Intern Med*. 1990;113:571–574.

184. Davis R. Pain and suffering following spinal cord injury. *Clin Orthop*. 1975;112:76–80.

185. Dillingham TR, ed. *Rehabilitation of the Injured Soldier*. Part 4. In: Zajtchuk R, Bellamy RF, eds. *Textbook of Military Medicine*. Washington, DC: US Department of the Army, Office of The Surgeon General, and Borden Institute; in press.

186. Kuric J, Lucas CE, Ledgerwood AM, Kiraly A, Salciccioli GG, Sugawa C. Nutritional support: A prophylaxis against stress bleeding after spinal cord injury. *Paraplegia*. 1989;27:140–145.

187. Sica DA, Culpepper RM. Case report: Severe hyponatremia in spinal cord injury. *Am J Med Sci*. 198;289:331–333.

188. Brackett TO, Condon N, Kindelan KM, Bassett L. The emotional care of a person with a spinal cord injury. *JAMA*. 1984;252:793–795.

Chapter 17

EYE INJURIES

JOHN D. CURRENT, M.D.*

*Colonel, Medical Corps, U.S. Army Reserve; formerly, Chief, Anesthesia and Operative Service, Brooke Army Medical Center, Fort Sam Houston, Texas 78234; currently, Associate Professor, Department of Anesthesiology, University of Mississippi Medical Center, 2500 North State Street, Jackson, Mississippi 39216

INTRODUCTION

There are two basic types of eye injuries: penetrating (ie, open) and nonpenetrating. As a rule, nonpenetrating injuries are less severe than penetrating injuries, but either type can lead to blindness. Nonpenetrating eye injuries, in which the globe remains intact, are usually lesser anesthetic-management dilemmas than penetrating eye injuries, in which the globe is disrupted. Nonpenetrating eye injuries include injuries to the eye and orbit and can be as minor as a corneal abrasion or eyelid ecchymosis, or as severe as retinal detachment, vitreous hemorrhage, or optic nerve injury. Penetrating injuries—the major source of serious combat eye injuries—are more common than might be thought, given the small portion of the body surface area that the eyes occupy. In wars of this century, from 3% to 9% of surviving casualties have been treated for eye injuries.[1] The higher-than-expected frequency of eye injuries reflects not only the exposed position of the head in combat but also the vulnerability of the eyes. They are a "soft" target: an injury of the same magnitude in another part of the body might very well be ignored. Finally, the increased use on the modern battlefield of explosive munitions that are designed to produce large numbers of small fragments is an additional factor that predisposes to the unexpectedly high frequency of eye injuries.

Of combat eye casualties in the Vietnam War in whom the mechanism of their eye injury was known, 79% were injured by fragments, with rockets, mortars, mines, and grenades being the most common explosive munitions responsible; bullets were the source of only 6% of eye wounds.[1] This is interesting because in living casualties, bullets caused a much smaller proportion of eye injuries compared with their overall casualty-generating importance during the Vietnam War (ie, bullets were the wounding agents in 30%–50% of living casualties).[2] These percentages would seem to be contradictory, but the reason for the seeming contradiction is simple: compared with a small fragment, a bullet that injures the eye is much more likely to continue on into contiguous organs such as the brain, where it frequently causes a fatal injury.[2] The fragments that cause eye injuries in *living* casualties are, in fact, quite small: 70% of the fragments had a mass of 1 to 100 mg.[1]

Many combat casualties present with corneal foreign bodies, the removal of which rarely requires the participation of an anesthesiologist. In the Vietnam surgical experience, the most common indication (50%) for a major eye operation was the presence of a disrupted globe requiring an enucleation (Figure 17-1). Other common indications for operation were corneal or scleral lacerations (19%), the presence of an intraocular foreign body (15%), and the laceration of the ocular adnexa (11%). Outside the combat zone, the most common indications for a major eye operation in a combat casualty with an eye injury were the presence of an intraocular foreign body (37%) and the need for enucleation (35%). The indication for the latter was severe infection that had destroyed the globe or the threat of sympathetic ophthalmia.[1] To care properly for such patients, the military anesthesiologist must know of the anatomy and physiology of the eye.

ANATOMY AND PHYSIOLOGY OF THE EYE

The eye is divided into the posterior and anterior chambers by the iris and the pupil (Figure 17-2). Aqueous humor fills the anterior and posterior chambers. The aqueous humor is formed primarily by the ciliary processes, with some contribution from the iris. It flows forward through the pupil to the angle formed by the iris and cornea. There, a trabecular meshwork containing the spaces of Fontana (ie, the spatia anguli iridocornealis) is the site of absorption of the aqueous humor. The aqueous humor then flows through the canal of Schlemm (ie, the sinus venosus sclerae), eventually reaching the venous system. Hypercarbia results in the dilation of choroidal arteries.[3] The sclera forms a fairly rigid structure, restricting volume changes in the eye (ie, restricting compliance). The net effect is analogous to changes in intracranial pressure: hypercarbia causes increased intraocular pressure (IOP).[4] Similarly, hyperventilation causes choroidal arterial vasoconstriction with a concomitant decrease in IOP.[5] The surgeon may request hyperventilation by the anesthesiologist in hopes of reducing IOP. However, the effect is quantitatively small. There is only about a 0.1 torr change in IOP for every torr change in the partial pressure of carbon dioxide in the arteries ($Paco_2$), which limits the value of the practice.[6]

Hypoxia also causes choroidal arterial vasodilation and a rise in IOP. Interestingly enough, hypothermia does not increase IOP; on the contrary,

a b c d

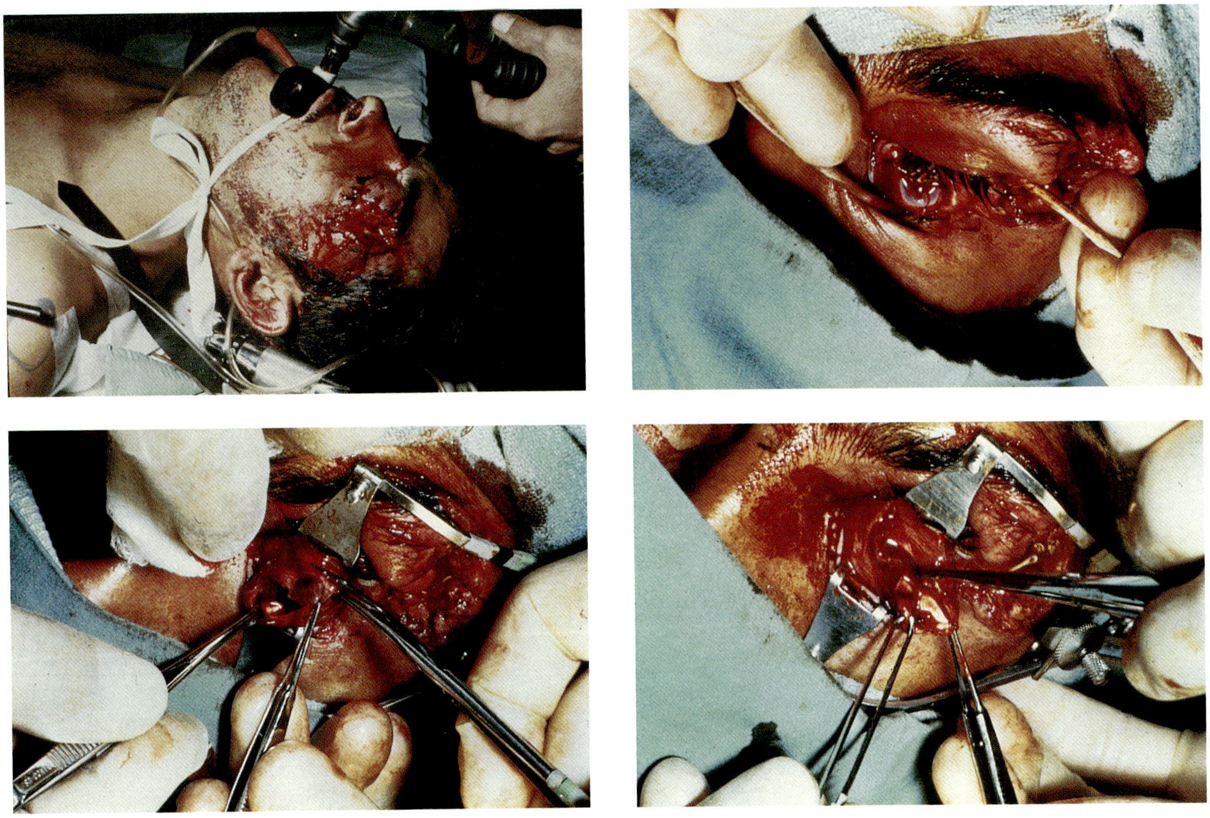

e

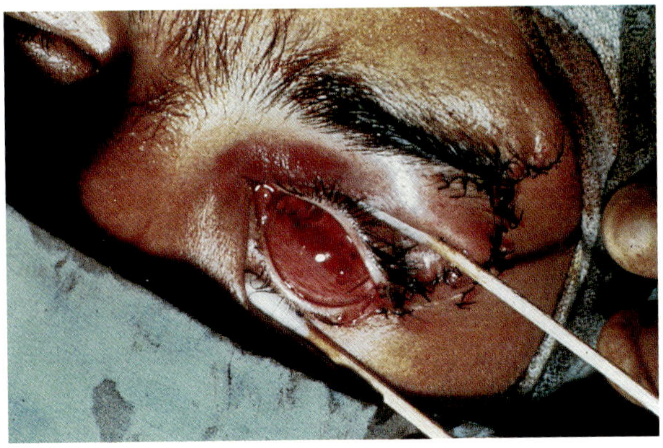

Fig. 17-1. This series of photographs, taken during the Vietnam War, shows the typical operative management of a disrupted globe. (**a**) The casualty, who suffered a destructive injury caused by multiple fragment wounds to the left side of his face, is intubated and ready for surgery. (**b**) The ophthalmologist is inspecting the casualty's eye; the globe is totally disrupted. (**c**) Enucleation is in progress. (**d**) The orbital contents are being extracted. (**e**) A prosthesis has been placed in the socket. Photographs: Swan Vietnam Surgical Slide Collection.

hypothermia reduces the production of aqueous humor and also causes vasoconstriction, which result in a lowered IOP.[7] Increasing venous pressure may profoundly increase IOP. This occurs by impeding outflow of aqueous humor through the canal of Schlemm, compression of the eye by episcleral veins, and dilation of choroidal vessels. Any straining, coughing, vomiting, and so forth during laryngoscopy or emergence from anesthesia may result in dramatic increases in IOP via this mechanism.[8] Increases of 30 to 40 torr have been recorded. External compression of the eye (eg, pressure from a mask or the increased tone of extraocular muscles) may increase IOP. This is particularly hazardous in the case of an open eye injury because the potential exists for loss of eye contents. However, when the globe is intact, the ophthalmologist may use several minutes of eye compression to reduce IOP and make the globe less rigid. This likely occurs owing to expression of aqueous humor from the anterior chamber.

The discussion of IOP has so far emphasized mechanical and vascular determinants. However, the normal mechanism for control of IOP involves the balance between production and drainage of the aqueous humor. Most pharmacological means to control IOP affect this balance. Normal IOP is 10 to 22 torr; IOP is considered abnormal if it exceeds 25

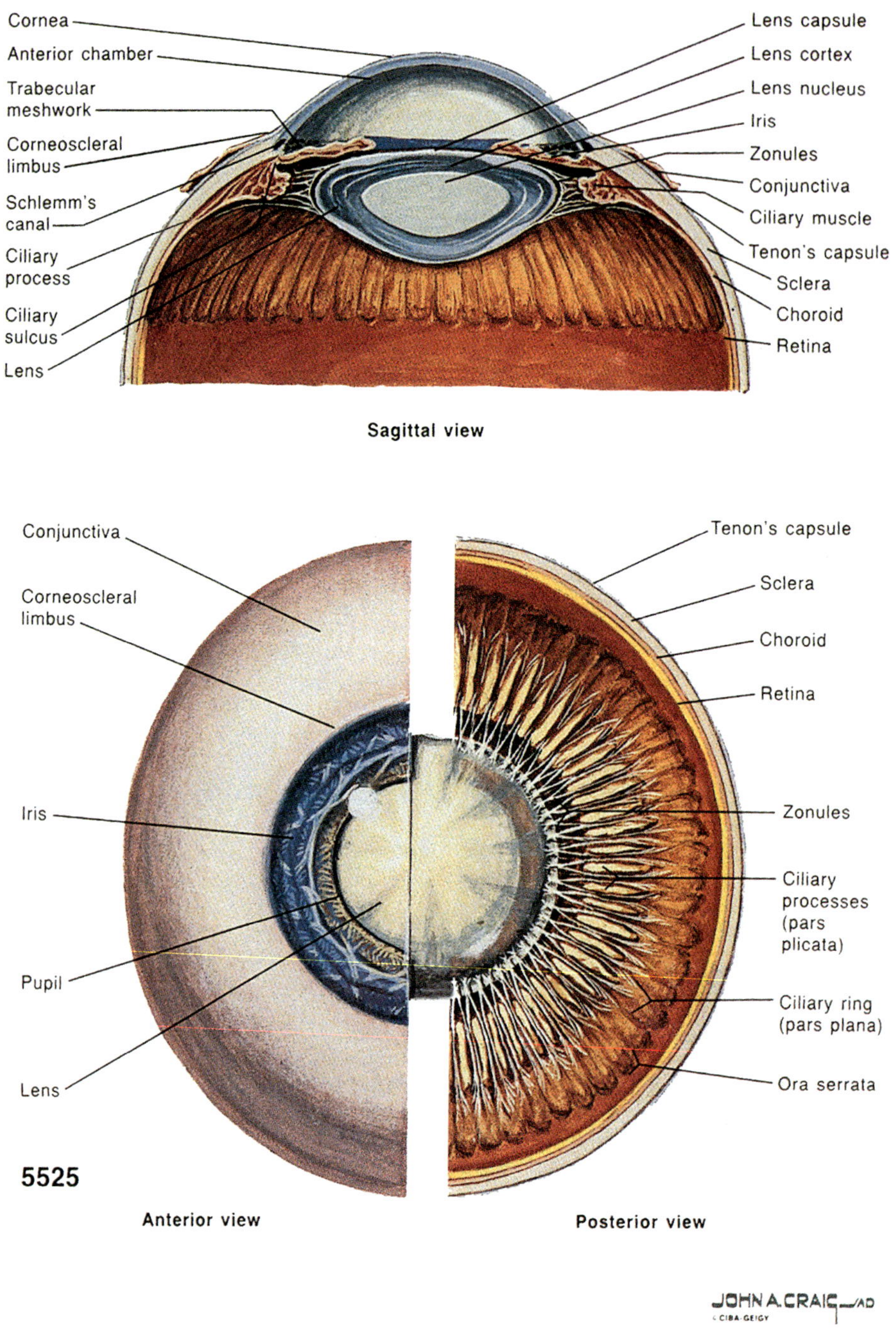

Fig. 17-2. Anterior segment of the eye. Reprinted with permission from Paton D, Craig JA. Management of cataracts. *Clinical Symposia*. 1990;42(4):6.

torr. The method of measurement may influence the IOP determined. Indentation (ie, Schiötz) tonometry may cause expression of aqueous humor and a reduction of IOP with repeated determinations. Older studies using indentation tonometry for measuring the effects of drugs and anesthetic agents on IOP have been called into question because of this. The more accepted and accurate method for determination of IOP is applanation tonometry, particularly if repeated measurements are necessary.[7]

EFFECT OF DRUGS ON INTRAOCULAR PRESSURE

Miotic agents such as echothiophate (Phospholine Iodide, manufactured by Wyeth-Ayerst Laboratories, Philadelphia, Pa.) and acetylcholine are used to lower IOP. The constriction of the pupil tightens the iris, stretching the trabecular meshwork of the spaces of Fontana. The net result is a facilitation of drainage of the aqueous humor and lowering of IOP. Aqueous humor production may be decreased with ophthalmic preparations of epinephrine, timolol, and acetazolamide. The production of aqueous humor is an active process using the carbonic anhydrase enzyme system. Therefore, acetazolamide can reduce IOP by reducing the production of aqueous humor by 50%. Acute lowering of IOP may be achieved through the use of osmotic agents. These drugs act to increase plasma oncotic pressure, which diminishes aqueous production, albeit transiently. Mannitol is the drug most commonly used, although urea and glycerol have also been used.[3] They all require catheter drainage of the urinary bladder intraoperatively. Furthermore, glycerol, given orally, increases the volume of stomach contents and adds a potential risk for regurgitation and aspiration under general anesthesia.

General anesthetic agents, particularly barbiturates and potent inhalational agents have consistently been shown[9–11] to reduce IOP. In humans, intravenous administration of etomidate has been shown[12] to consistently and significantly lower the IOP. Intravenous lidocaine has been shown[13] to reduce the IOP response to laryngoscopy and intubation. Ketamine, on the other hand, may increase the IOP or leave it unchanged. An intravenous bolus dose of ketamine has been found[14] to result in a 37% increase in IOP, with the maximum increase occurring 15 minutes after the injection. Other researchers[15,16] have presented data that suggest that heavily premedicated patients do not experience increases in IOP with ketamine. However, blepharospasm, nystagmus, or laryngospasm may make ketamine undesirable for ophthalmic surgery.

Succinylcholine has been found[17] to increase IOP. This increase is not temporally related to muscle fasciculations[18]; indeed, pretreatment with acetazolamide or propranolol have been reported[19] to prevent a rise in IOP after succinylcholine without preventing fasciculations. Increases in IOP with succinylcholine have been reported[20–24] after adequate pretreatment doses of nondepolarizing muscle relaxants. Attempts to use small, "self-taming" doses of succinylcholine have themselves resulted in elevation of IOP.[25] Furthermore, pretreatment with lidocaine does not prevent increases of IOP following succinylcholine administration.[26]

In contrast, nondepolarizing muscle relaxants consistently reduce—or at worst, do not change—IOP.[27–31] Intubating doses of atracurium and vecuronium do not raise IOP, but the intubation itself may.[32] The increase-in-IOP response to laryngoscopy and intubation in children was prevented by the addition of intravenous lidocaine (1.5 mg/kg) to the standard induction sequence of thiopental and pancuronium.[33]

ANESTHETIC MANAGEMENT OF THE CASUALTY WITH AN OPEN EYE INJURY

Anesthetic management may play an important role in the outcome of ophthalmic surgery. The surgeon requires a motionless eye and a bloodless field. Any coughing, bucking, straining, or vomiting by a patient with an open eye injury may result in hemorrhage and loss of vitreous or vision.[8] Eye injuries in which the globe is fully perforated require especially careful anesthetic management to avoid extrusion of intraocular contents and resultant permanent disability. The anesthesiologist must certainly avoid applying external pressure to the eye, such as during application of the face mask. It is also helpful to the surgeon to have the endotracheal tube out of the way, using a downward-directed tube such as a RAE (named for its developers: Ring, Adair, and Elwyn; manufactured by Mallinckrodt Critical Care, Great Falls, N.Y.) or an armored tube. Of simultaneous concern to the military anesthesiologist is the likelihood that the casualty will have a full stomach. If time and the patient's medical condition permits, aspiration prophylaxis should be considered. Oral or intramuscular histamine 2 blocking agents may be administered to the patient, preferably 1.5 to 2 hours prior to the procedure. Ranitidine 150 mg, administered orally, or 50 mg, administered intramuscularly (or alternatively, cimetidine 300 mg, administered orally, or 150 mg, administered intramuscularly), should increase the pH of the stomach contents. Famotidine 20 mg, administered orally or intravenously, will also reduce gastric volume and increase pH. Reglan 10 mg, administrated orally or intravenously, may reduce the volume of stomach contents by promotion of gastric emptying. Administration of a nonparticulate antacid (ie, Bicitra, manufactured by Baker Norton Pharmaceuticals, Inc, Miami, Fla., 30 mL, administered orally) will effectively increase the pH of stomach contents although at the expense of a small increase in gastric volume.

Intubation and Induction

Retrobulbar block is contraindicated due to the risk of external pressure causing extrusion of eye contents. Indeed, retrobulbar block itself may be complicated by global perforation.[34] Similarly, awake intubation is contraindicated due to the real risk of coughing during topical anesthesia or airway insertion. There is a general agreement that the best approach is to perform endotracheal intubation with a rapid-sequence induction of anesthesia and cricoid pressure.[35] Care must be taken in the application of cricoid pressure to avoid both occluding venous return from the head and, possibly, increasing the IOP. The controversy surrounds the choice of muscle relaxant selected to facilitate intubation. The thiopental-pancuronium induction sequence is the standard against which other techniques must be compared.[36] If hemodynamic stability permits, a relatively large dose of thiopental may lessen the likelihood of any patient reaction to laryngoscopy or intubation. Administration of pancuronium 0.15 mg/kg should allow intubation within 90 seconds. The patient should be counseled regarding the possibilities that the relaxation could outlast the procedure and therefore that postoperative intubation and ventilation might be required. The likelihood of tachycardia may make this technique undesirable in patients with coronary artery disease.[37]

Variations on this nondepolarizing sequence include (*a*) large-dose atracurium or vecuronium,[38] (*b*) Metubine-pancuronium combination (Metubine Iodide, manufactured by Dista Products Co., Indianapolis, Ind.), and (*c*) the priming principle. Researchers[39] who studied onset time and intubating conditions using atracurium 1.5 mg/kg and vecuronium 0.25 mg/kg found onset time of 95% twitch depression to average 56 and 64 seconds, respectively. Intubating conditions at 60 seconds were somewhat better with vecuronium, but were satisfactory with either regimen. They noted that 40% of the patients receiving that dose of atracurium suffered hypotension and tachycardia.

The Metubine-pancuronium combination takes advantage of the synergistic effect of these two drugs to reduce the amount of each necessary to achieve rapid relaxation. Pretreatment with Metubine 0.05 mg/kg followed by pancuronium 0.06 mg/kg gives adequate intubation conditions nearly as rapidly as the larger-dose pancuronium technique but does not produce so prolonged a period of paralysis. Other researchers[40] pretreated patients with metocurine 0.03 mg/kg and 3 minutes later administered pancuronium 0.08 mg/kg. They found that 95% depression of twitch height occurred in 70 seconds and all patients had good-to-excellent intubating conditions. However, these patients' recovery to 25% twitch height required 100 minutes.

The use of the priming principle has been advocated for patients with open eye injuries.[41] A defasciculating dose of an intermediate-duration nondepolarizer is followed 3 to 5 minutes later with a larger dose, 1.5- to 2-fold larger than the usual intubating dose.[36] This gives a fairly rapid onset of muscle relaxation but not as rapid as that produced by succinylcholine.

One group of researchers[42] found that additional thiopental improved intubating conditions when using the priming principle with atracurium. Furthermore, other researchers[43] found that priming with atracurium did not significantly improve intubating conditions, and recommended that it not be done. This may reflect the importance of deep anesthesia in securing favorable intubating conditions without increasing IOP.[42] The duration of the blockade is much shorter than that obtained with pancuronium, although postoperative ventilation could be necessary following short procedures. At recommended doses, atracurium may occasionally result in adverse hemodynamic changes. Therefore, I suggest the use of vecuronium 0.01 mg/kg as a priming dose, followed in 3 to 5 minutes with 0.2 mg/kg. There should be virtually no hemodynamic consequences from the vecuronium.

Whether succinylcholine should be used in the patient with open eye injuries remains an issue of debate. Although some researchers[44] have reported considerable experience with the use of a pretreatment dose of curare followed by succinylcholine in the patient with open eye injuries with neither loss of vitreous nor aspiration, others[45] consider this approach to be controversial. Nevertheless, investigators[46] reporting in 1990 suggest that the rapid-sequence induction technique modifies the effect of succinylcholine on IOP resulting in no loss of vitreous. They believe that both (*a*) scrupulous attention to adequate depth of anesthesia with thiopental and (*b*) waiting until complete paralysis is instituted with succinylcholine before laryngoscopy and intubation permit safe intubation, as had been demonstrated[44] in 1985. Adequate depth of anesthesia avoids the likelihood of coughing, straining, and grimace, which are likely to be more problematic than the effects of succinylcholine in the anesthetized patient.[46]

A large dose of thiopental should be used in the hemodynamically stable patient, assuring adequate depth of anesthesia and minimizing any response to laryngoscopy and intubation. The addition of alfentanil 20 µg/kg has been found useful in reducing the response to tracheal intubation.[47] Awake intubation is inadvisable in patients with open eye injuries because any cough or straining could result in loss of ocular contents. Similarly, retrobulbar block is contraindicated because the block itself may increase the IOP due to extrinsic pressure on the globe. Furthermore, blepharospasm, grimace, or perforation of the globe may occur,[48] and the operator may not be able to minimize hemorrhage by applying manual pressure.

Patients with severe hypovolemia from acute blood loss may not tolerate standard anesthetic-induction techniques. Severe hypotension or cardiac arrest may occur if the patient is given a hypnotic induction such as ketamine, which causes cardiac depression, or thiopental, which causes sympathetic and cardiac depression. The safest induction technique for these patients will generally be scopolamine and a muscle relaxant alone.

No single induction technique is suitable for all trauma situations. Often, the medical officer will be confronted with a combination of injuries and conditions that make choosing the best anesthetic-induction technique difficult. Examples would be a patient with a head injury and a full stomach, a patient with an open eye injury and a displaced mandibular fracture, and an uncooperative patient with bleeding and possible cervical spine injury. In situations such as these, the medical officer must decide which conditions are of overriding importance and select the most appropriate airway-management technique and anesthetic plan for those particular conditions.

Emergence

Although modern ophthalmic wound closure can withstand bucking and straining by the patient, it seems best to avoid these on awakening to minimize the risk of vitreous loss.[3] Deep extubation may be considered in the patient known to have an empty stomach but this is not the usual circumstance, as all battlefield casualties are assumed to have a full stomach. Intravenous lidocaine may be helpful in minimizing the patient's reaction to the endotracheal tube. A dose of 1.5 mg/kg should be used; this seldom causes prolonged emergence. Other measures that may be considered include emptying the stomach by gastric tube while the patient is still paralyzed and anesthetized, and using an antiemetic such as droperidol.

INTERACTIONS WITH OTHER DRUGS

Many of the ophthalmic agents introduced into the eye may be absorbed systemically, resulting in cardiovascular or metabolic effects. Timolol is a β-adrenergic blocking agent used in the treatment of glaucoma. The use of this agent may cause systemic beta-blockade, with bronchospasm or bradycardia possible. It is important that the military trauma anesthesiologist be aware of this fact, but, in most cases, timolol certainly does not need to be discontinued preoperatively. The ophthalmologist may apply phenylephrine eyedrops to dilate the pupil perioperatively. Concentrations as high as 10% are available; however, occasional systemic manifestations occur (hypertension or bradycardia or both). Caution in use is advised. Perhaps a diplomatic request to the surgeon to use the lowest effective concentration may be made. An ophthalmic drug very interesting to the anesthesiologist is the miotic agent Phospholine Iodide. This long-acting pseudocholinesterase inhibitor may still have systemic effects up to 6 weeks after discontinuation.[37] This drug prolongs the effects of succinylcholine, trimetaphan, and ester local anesthetics, all of which depend on pseudocholinesterase for termination of action.

PERIOPERATIVE OPHTHALMIC COMPLICATIONS

Corneal Abrasion

The most common perioperative ophthalmic complication is corneal abrasion, to which two factors contribute: basal tear production is greatly reduced, and the protective eyelid closure reflex is lost under general anesthesia. The corneal abrasion will often occur in the inferior one third of the globe, which is the area exposed when the eyelids are allowed to remain partially open. Preventive measures to avoid corneal abrasions include closure of the eyelids and instillation of some type of artificial tears. Many techniques have been suggested to keep the eyelids closed, including taping, suturing, or patching the eyelids. Aqueous artificial tear solutions have to be reapplied during long procedures, as they are not long retained in the eye. For this reason, bland ointments are more commonly used, although there may be a small likelihood of allergic reactions to preservatives used in these preparations.[6]

Acute Angle-Closure Glaucoma

In postoperative patients, it may be important to distinguish the painful eye associated with a corneal abrasion from that occurring with acute glaucoma. The corneal abrasion often is accompanied by pain aggravated by blinking and rapid eye movement, tearing, and the sensation of a foreign body. An area of dullness may be seen on examination. In acute glaucoma, the cornea may be dull and reddened, and the pupil may be dilated. The patient may complain of headache and pain around the eye. A loss of vision may be recorded.

There are two types of glaucoma: open angle and closed angle. Both have the common feature of abnormally elevated IOP. In closed-angle glaucoma, the iris is bulged or folded forward, blocking the aqueous flow into the trabecular meshwork. An acutely swollen lens or pupillary dilation may result from this aqueous humor obstruction. Anesthetic care of such patients includes instilling miotic agents,[8] which constrict the pupil and promote aqueous drainage; avoiding venous congestion (eg, keep the patient's head up, do not allow the patient to perform the Valsalva maneuver, and prevent the patient from bucking or coughing)[19]; and carefully managing intravenous fluid administration to prevent overhydration. Neither atropine nor glycopyrrolate in the usual premedication dosages have been found to worsen IOP with either type of glaucoma; nor have they been implicated when used in combination with anticholinesterases for reversal of neuromuscular blockade.[8] However, scopolamine has been found to have a greater mydriatic effect than atropine and should not be used in patients with glaucoma. This effect of scopolamine may be more problematic in white than in black patients.[49] Open-angle glaucoma is associated with scarring or endothelial thickening of the trabecular meshwork, resulting in obstruction to aqueous humor outflow. Anesthetic considerations are the same as with closed-angle glaucoma with the addition of avoiding hypotension, because these patients are prone to thrombosis of the retinal artery.

Supraorbital Nerve Compression

Another potential postoperative complication is supraorbital nerve compression. This may occur due to improper positioning of the patient or incorrect placement of the face mask or mask straps during anesthesia. The patient may complain of periorbital numbness and edema may be noted. Fortunately, this problem usually resolves without treatment, although it may require some weeks.

Retinal Artery Thrombosis

A much worse complication is retinal artery thrombosis. This complication is more likely to occur in the patient with elevated IOP (eg, in a patient with glaucoma). Retinal artery thrombosis has also been associated with the use of deliberate hypotension.[6] It is most important to ensure that no pressure is applied to the eye of the anesthetized patient, such as occurs in the prone position.

Oculocardiac Reflex

An oculocardiac reflex has been described and is occasionally seen in patients who are undergoing eye surgery. This reflex is elicited by traction on the extraocular muscles, pressure on the globe, pinching of the conjunctiva, or placement of a retrobulbar block. The afferent limb of this reflex involves the ciliary nerves and ganglion, the ophthalmic branch of the trigeminal nerve, the trigeminal ganglion, and, finally, the main sensory nucleus of the trigeminal nerve near the fourth ventricle.[6] The efferent impulses are conducted down the vagus nerve, resulting in bradycardia or arrhythmias such as junctional rhythm, atrioventricular block, ventricular bigeminy, or even cardiac standstill. This reflex is seen more frequently in children than in adults. Furthermore, hypercarbia or hypoxemia may increase the likelihood or severity of the response to the eliciting stimulus. Usual premedication doses of atropine given intramuscularly are of no value in preventing this reflex. However, intravenously administered atropine or glycopyrrolate, given prior to the application of a stimulus, modifies or prevents the response. Routine use is controversial in the adult and is seldom done. Rather, most anesthesiologists take advantage of the easy fatigability of this reflex in the management of bradycardia or arrhythmias resulting therefrom. Asking the surgeon to halt manipulations long enough for the reflex to diminish and then proceeding is feasible. Adequacy of oxygenation and ventilation should be checked. If the reflex recurs or is severe, then intravenous atropine may be given.[37]

SUMMARY

Penetrating missiles in the form of small fragments are the most common cause of eye injuries in combat casualties who require the services of military trauma anesthesiologists. Not only does the missile itself directly destroy ocular tissue, but the wound tract into the globe also serves as an opening through which intraocular contents may be extruded, causing irreversible injury. This secondary complication can occur when IOP is acutely elevated by coughing, bucking, or straining, and its occurrence has also been reported during intubation and emergence from anesthesia. IOP may also be altered pharmacologically. Miotic agents, barbiturates, inhalational anesthetic agents, and nondepolarizing muscle relaxants all decrease IOP, while an increase follows the use of succinylcholine.

The great majority of combat casualties with eye injuries will require general endotracheal anesthesia; for this, the thiopental-pancuronium induction sequence is the standard of choice, as it minimizes the risk of an acute increase in IOP. Bucking and straining during extubation should be avoided, but deep extubation is not usually possible because each battlefield casualty is assumed to have a full stomach.

Military trauma anesthesiologists need to be aware of the potential for such perioperative complications as corneal abrasions, acute angle-closure glaucoma, supraorbital nerve compression, retinal artery thrombosis, and the oculocardiac reflex. Careful planning and attention to detail by the military anesthesiologist will prevent or reduce loss of vision and promote the rapid return to duty of soldiers with eye injuries.

REFERENCES

1. LaPiana F. Colonel, Medical Corps, US Army, Walter Reed Army Medical Center, Washington, DC. Unpublished analysis prepared for the Center of Military History, US Department of the Army, Washington, DC, 1985.

2. Bellamy RF. Colonel, Medical Corps, US Army, Walter Reed Army Medical Center, Washington, DC. Unpublished analysis of Wound Data and Munitions Effectiveness Team database. Personal communication, June 1994.

3. Holloway KB. Control of the eye during general anaesthesia for intraocular surgery. *Br J Anaesth.* 1980;52:671–679.

4. Samuel JR, Beaugie A. Effect of carbon dioxide on the intraocular pressure in man during general anaesthesia. *Br J Ophthal.* 1974;58:62–67.

5. Adams AK, Barnett KC. Anaesthesia and intraocular pressure. *Anaesthesia.* 1966;21:202–210.

6. McCammon RL. Anesthetic considerations in the presence of ocular disease. In: *American Society of Anesthesiologists Refresher Courses in Anesthesiology.* Philadelphia, Pa: JB Lippincott; 1980: 127–137.

7. Cunningham AJ, Barry P. Intraocular pressure—physiology and implications for anaesthetic management. *Can Anaesth Soc J.* 1986;33:195–208.

8. Adams AK, Jones RM. Anaesthesia for eye surgery: General considerations. *Br J Anaesth.* 1980;52:663–669.

9. Schreuder M, Linssen GH. Intra-ocular pressure and anaesthesia. *Anaesthesia*. 1972;27:165–170.

10. Runciman JC, Bowen-Wright RM, Welsh NH, Downing JW. Intra-ocular pressure changes during halothane and enflurane anaesthesia. *Br J Anaesth*. 1978;50:371–374.

11. Magora F, Collins VJ. The influence of general anesthetic agents on intraocular pressure in man. *Arch Ophthalmol*. 1961;66:806–811.

12. Oji EO, Holdcroft A. The ocular effects of etomidate. *Anaesthesia*. 1979;34:245–249.

13. Lerman J, Kiskis AA. Lidocaine attenuates the intraocular pressure response to rapid intubation in children. *Can Anaesth Soc J*. 1985;32:339–345.

14. Yoshikawa K, Murai Y. The effect of ketamine on intraocular pressure in children. *Anesth Analg*. 1971;50:199–202.

15. Peuler M, Glass DD, Arens JF. Ketamine and intraocular pressure. *Anesthesiology*. 1975;43:575–578.

16. Ausinsch B, Rayburn RL, Munson ES, Levy NS. Ketamine and intraocular pressure in children. *Anesth Analg*. 1976;55:773–775.

17. Katz RL, Eakins KE. The actions of neuromuscular blocking agents on extraocular muscle and intraocular pressure. *Proc R Soc Med*. 1969;62:1217–1220.

18. Pandey K, Badola RP, Kumar S. Time course of intraocular hypertension produced by suxamethonium. *Br J Anaesth*. 1972;44:191–195.

19. Carballo AS. Succinylcholine and acetazolamide (Diamox) in anaesthesia for ocular surgery. *Can Anaesth Soc J*. 1965;12:486–498.

20. Donlon JV. Anesthesia factors affecting intraocular pressure. *Anesthesiol Rev*. 1981;8:13–18.

21. Cook JH. The effect of suxamethonium on intraocular pressure. *Anaesthesia*. 1981;36:359–365.

22. Meyers EF, Krupin T, Johnson M, Zink H. Failure of nondepolarizing neuromuscular blockers to inhibit succinylcholine-induced increased intraocular pressure. *Anesthesiology*. 1978;48:149–151.

23. Bowen DJ, McGrand JC, Hamilton AG. Intraocular pressures after suxamethonium and endotracheal intubation. *Anaesthesia*. 1978;33:518–522.

24. Bowen DJ, McGrand JC, Palmer RJ. Intraocular pressures after suxamethonium and endotracheal intubation in patients pretreated with pancuronium. *Br J Anaesth*. 1976;48:1201–1205.

25. Meyers EF, Singer P, Otto A. A controlled study of the effect of succinylcholine self-taming on intraocular pressure. *Anesthesiology*. 1980;53:72–74.

26. Smith B, Babinski M, Leano N. The effect of lidocaine on succinylcholine-induced rise in intraocular pressure. *Can Anaesth Soc J*. 1979;26:482–483.

27. Tattersall MP, Manus NJ, Jackson DM. The effect of atracurium or fazadinium on intra-ocular pressure. *Anaesthesia*. 1985;40:805–807.

28. Balamoutsos NG, Tsakona H, Kanakoudes PS, Iliadelis E, Georgiades CG. Alcuronium and intraocular pressure. *Anesth Analg*. 1983;62:521–523.

29. Couch JA, Eltringham RJ, Magauran DM. The effect of thiopentone and fazadinium on intraocular pressure. *Anaesthesia*. 1979;34:586–590.

30. George R, Nursingh A, Downing JW, Welsh NH. Non-depolarizing neuromuscular blockers and the eye: A study of intraocular pressure. *Br J Anaesth*. 1979;51:789–792.

31. Maharaj RJ, Humphrey D, Kaplan N, et al. Effects of atracurium on intraocular pressure. *Br J Anaesth*. 1984;56:459–462.

32. Schneider MJ, Stirt JA, Finholt DA. Atracurium, vecuronium and intraocular pressure in humans. *Anesth Analg*. 1986;65:877–882.

33. Lerman J, Kiskis AA. Lidocaine attenuates the intraocular pressure response to rapid intubation in children. *Can Anaesth Soc J*. 1985;32:339–345.

34. Ramsay RC, Knobloch WH. Ocular perforation following retrobulbar anesthesia for retinal detachment surgery. *Am J Ophthalmol*. 1978;86:61–64.

35. Barr AM, Thornley BA. Thiopentone and suxamethonium crash induction. *Anaesthesia*. 1976;31:23–29.

36. Barr AM, Thornley BA. Thiopentone and pancuronium crash induction. *Anaesthesia*. 1978;33:25–31.

37. McGoldrick KE. Current concepts in anesthesia for ophthalmic surgery. *Anesth Rev*. 1980;7:7–16.

38. Abbott MA, Samuel JR. The control of intra-ocular pressure during the induction of anaesthesia for emergency eye surgery. *Anaesthesia*. 1987;42:1008–1012.

39. Lennon RL, Olson RA, Gronert GA. Atracurium or vecuronium for rapid sequence endotracheal intubation. *Anesthesiology*. 1986;64:510–513.

40. Mehta MP, Choi WW, Gergis SD, Sokoll MD, Adolphson AJ. Facilitation of rapid endotracheal intubations with divided doses of nondepolarizing neuromuscular blocking drugs. *Anesthesiology*. 1985;62:392–395.

41. Schwarz S, Ilias W, Lackner F, Mayrhofer O, Foldes FF. Rapid tracheal intubation with vecuronium: The priming principle. *Anesthesiology*. 1985;62:388–391.

42. Naguib M, Abdulatif M, Gyasi HK, Absgood GH. Priming with atracurium: Improving intubating conditions with additional doses of thiopental. *Anesth Analg*. 1986;65:1295–1299.

43. Sosis M, Larijani G, Marr AT. Priming with atracurium. *Anesth Analg*. 1987;66:329–332.

44. Libonati MM, Leahy JJ, Ellison N. The use of succinylcholine in open eye surgery. *Anesthesiology*. 1985;62:637–640.

45. Weiner MJ, Olk RJ, Meyers EF. Anesthesia for open eye surgery. *Anesthesiology*. 1986;65:109–110.

46. Calobrisi BL, Lebowitz P. Muscle relaxants and the open globe. *Int Anesthesiol Clin*. 1990;28:83–87.

47. Morton NS, Hamilton WFD. Alfentanil in an anaesthetic technique for penetrating eye injuries. *Anaesthesia*. 1986;41:1148–1151.

48. Zaturansky B, Hyams S. Perforation of the globe during the injection of local anesthesia. *Ophthalmic Surg*. 1987;18:585–588.

49. Garde JF, Aston R, Endler GC, Sison OS. Racial mydriatic response to belladonna premedication. *Anesth Analg*. 1978;57:572–576.

Chapter 18

INJURIES TO THE FACE AND NECK

MICHAEL D. MATSON, M.D.*

*Lieutenant Colonel, Medical Corps, U.S. Army; Staff Anesthesiologist, Walter Reed Army Medical Center, Washington, D. C. 20307-5001

INTRODUCTION

Anesthesiologists in both the civilian and military communities sometimes encounter casualties with trauma to the face and neck. In the civilian sector, injuries to the face and neck are most commonly the result of blunt trauma from automobile and motorcycle accidents. In the military, injuries to the face and neck are primarily the result of penetrating missiles. During World War I, facial injuries often occurred when soldiers were (*a*) shot in the head as they peered out of their trenches[1] or (*b*) struck by large chunks of metal from the detonation of random-fragmentation shells. Such traumata were usually rapidly fatal because the missile, by virtue of its high kinetic energy, did not stop on entering the soldier's face or neck but continued on into the brain or cervical spine (Figure 18-1).[2]

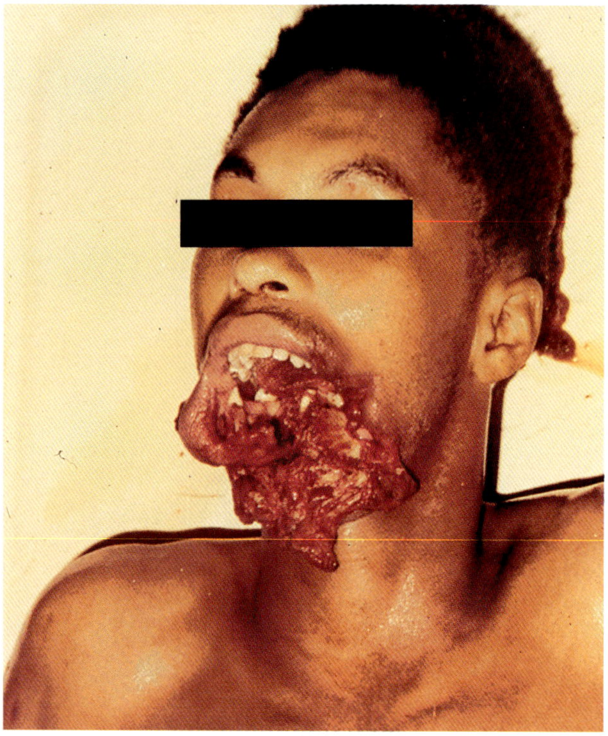

Fig. 18-1. Wounds of the face caused by high-velocity missiles have a propensity to involve the nearby anatomical structures. This soldier was killed during the Vietnam War when a bullet fired from an AK47 (7.62 mm) entered his lower jaw, passed through the fifth cervical vertebra, and transected his spinal cord. Photograph: Wound Data and Munitions Effectiveness Team slide collection.

Injuries to the face and neck in more recent military conflicts such as the Vietnam War have increasingly been the result of so-called improved fragmentation munitions such as grenades, mortars, and artillery shells.[1,3] Improved fragmentation munitions are designed to generate large numbers of small (< 1 cm), light (< 1 g) fragments. Thus, the typical *living* casualty in a modern war who has ballistic trauma to the face or neck—and who survives long enough to be evacuated from the battlefield—has one to a few benign-appearing wounds. The damage appears to be limited to a sinus, an orbit, a few teeth, or the soft tissue of the pharynx or neck. Nevertheless, these benign-appearing injuries may be life threatening (Figure 18-2).

Casualties with face and neck wounds can challenge the anesthesiologist. Establishment of an airway and adequate ventilation in these patients can be difficult (Figure 18-3), and supervenient factors such as the following can complicate management:

- hemorrhage,
- risk of aspiration,
- associated injuries,
- difficult intubation,
- tissue debris and foreign material obstructing the airway, and
- an unstable cervical spine.

Associated injuries—especially those of the head, but also those to other parts of the body—are common. Once the airway is secure, care of the associated injuries will frequently be more immediately important than care of the actual face and neck injuries themselves. Management of casualties with multiple injuries can be complicated by hemorrhage, hypovolemic shock, increased intracranial pressure, or disturbances of other body systems. The care of these patients, as with other trauma patients, should be in accordance with Advanced Trauma Life Support (ATLS) guidelines.[4] The perioperative management of casualties with injuries to the face and neck should follow this sequence of steps:

1. Assess the airway and establish patency, if necessary.
2. Assess breathing and provide or support ventilation, if necessary.

a

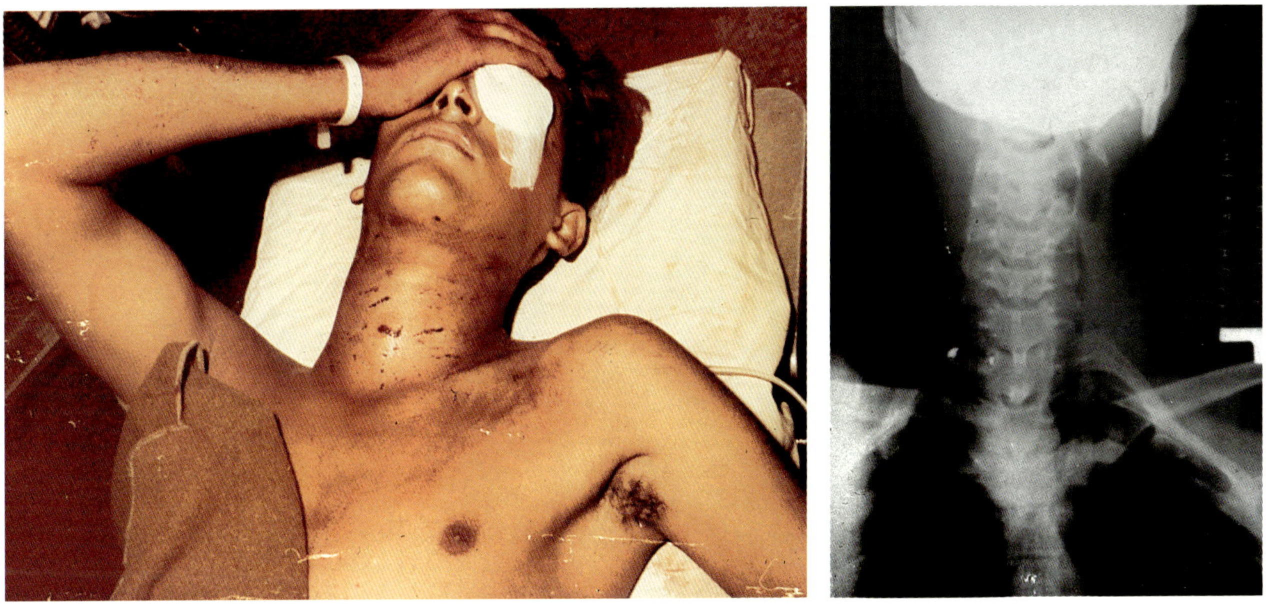

b

Fig. 18-2. (**a**) This casualty was wounded during the Vietnam War by three small fragments produced by an exploding, improved-fragmentation hand grenade. One fragment entered his left orbit and caused an injury that was treated by enucleation. Two additional fragments struck the right side of his neck, where one lacerated the right common carotid artery. (**b**) The radiograph (taken at the third-echelon surgical hospital) clearly shows how the expanding hematoma caused tracheal displacement. This casualty was treated before his airway was compromised. Photographs: Wound Data and Munitions Effectiveness Team slide collection.

a

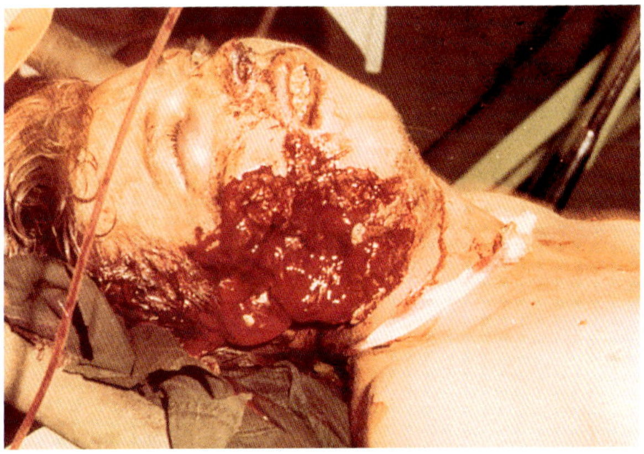

b

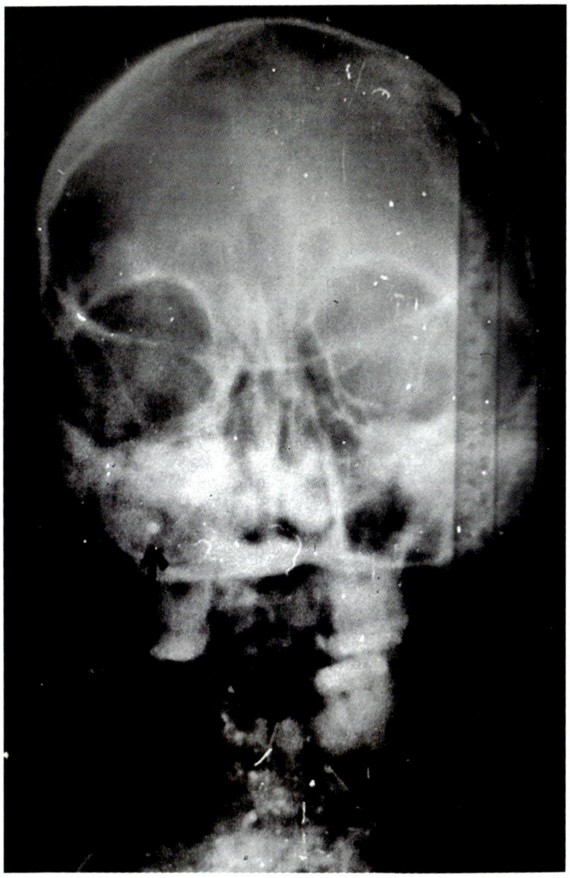

Fig. 18-3. (**a**) This casualty from the Vietnam War sustained a tangential gunshot wound of the right side of his face. Obstruction of his airway by blood and tissue fragments indicated the need for immediate airway control, but neither oral nor nasal intubation was possible in the field. The casualty was transported in the prone position (to prevent aspiration of blood) until an emergency tracheotomy could be performed at a third-echelon surgical hospital. (**b**) The great destruction caused by the gunshot wound is apparent in this anteroposterior radiograph. Note that a goodly portion of the right mandible is missing. Many artifacts are present in the radiograph; however, the arrow indicates a fragment in the casualty's maxillary sinus. Photographs: Wound Data and Munitions Effectiveness Team slide collection.

3. Assess circulation and control life-threatening bleeding.
4. Assess the level of consciousness and pupillary size and reaction.
5. Provide resuscitation as needed.
6. Evaluate in detail for
   - head and neurological injury,
   - maxillofacial injury,
   - neck injury,
   - chest injury,
   - abdominal injury,
   - genitorectal injury,
   - injury of the extremities, and
   - other injuries.
7. Prioritize injuries and plan coordinated, definitive care.

FACIAL FRACTURES

Fractures are common in facial trauma. Low-energy blunt impacts tend to cause isolated fractures (ie, fractures of the nose or mandible). High-energy blunt or penetrating impacts can cause panfacial or multiple fractures (ie, combinations of Le Fort fractures, naso-orbital-ethmoid fractures, and frontal bone fractures).

Mandibular Fractures

Mandibular fracture are common facial injuries. In the military, mandibular fractures can occur as a result of vehicular trauma, fragmentation blasts, and other causes. The force of the impact is redistributed as the mandible is fractured and displaced; thus, skull fractures are less common with mandibular fractures than with maxillary fractures.[1] Fractures of the mandible may be unilateral, bilateral, or comminuted. Unilateral fractures are relatively stable. Bilateral and comminuted fractures tend to be unstable. Patients with displaced fractures of the mandible present with malocclusion. They may also have pain, swelling, crepitation, and drooling. Loss of support for the base of the tongue can lead to airway obstruction, as can edema and hematomas. Trismus secondary to pain, edema, or hematomas can occur with mandibular fractures and can greatly complicate airway management. The swallowing mechanism can be impaired and that, combined with bleeding and hypersecretion of the salivary glands, can increase the risk of aspiration. Patients with mandibular fractures are also likely to require intermaxillary wiring, which further complicates perioperative airway management.

Nasal Fractures

Nasal fractures are also common facial injuries. Signs of nasal fracture include nasal deformity, epistaxis, hematoma of the nasal dorsum, and crepitance of the nasal bone. Significant hemorrhage can occur with nasal fractures and, in the obtunded patient, can lead to airway obstruction or aspiration. Obstruction of the nasal air passage can also occur as a result of bony deformities and edema. Blind nasal intubation should be avoided in patients with nasal fractures or intranasal injuries. If nasal intubation is required, then evaluation of the nasal passage via fiberscope or other means should precede tube placement.

Maxillary Fractures

Maxillary fractures are common in civilian practice (eg, automobile accidents). In the military, maxillary fractures might occur if a truck were to detonate a mine. These injuries are generally caused by high-energy trauma and are often associated with skull fractures or intracranial injuries. As the maxilla is a very vascular structure, fracture and disruption can cause significant bleeding both preoperatively and intraoperatively. Manifestations of maxillary fractures include malocclusion, marked facial swelling, mobility of the midface, palpable malalignment of the bone edges (ie, step-off deformities) at the fracture site, and ecchymosis. A variety of maxillary fracture patterns can occur in severe facial trauma, but classically three patterns, the Le Fort fractures, are described (Figure 18-4).[5]

The Le Fort I fracture involves the lower midface and may be unilateral or bilateral. The fracture line is located above the level of the teeth but below the nose. The teeth and hard palate are separated from the upper portions of the maxilla. The lower portion of the maxilla is mobile. Occasionally, the lower portion will be fractured at the midline into two segments.

The Le Fort II (ie, pyramidal) fracture is located at a higher level than Le Fort I fractures. The fracture line generally passes through the nasal bone, the lacrimal bone, the floor of the orbit, the infraorbital margin, and across the upper portion of the maxillary sinus and pterygoid plates to the pterygopalatine fossa. The maxilla is "free floating" in this fracture.

The Le Fort III fracture results in complete separation of the facial bones from their cranial attachments. The fracture line is high in position and extends across the nasofrontal suture and through the upper orbits. The main fracture segment is the entire midface. Le Fort II and III fractures are commonly associated with intracranial injuries, cribriform plate injuries, dural tears, and cerebrospinal fluid leaks.

Zygomatic Fractures

Fractures of the zygoma are less severe than maxillary fractures. However, displaced bony fragments may impinge on the coronoid process of the mandible and make opening the mouth difficult and painful. This can complicate airway management. Other signs of zygomatic fracture include ophthalmological abnormalities, flattening of the cheek, bony step-off deformity, and ecchymosis.

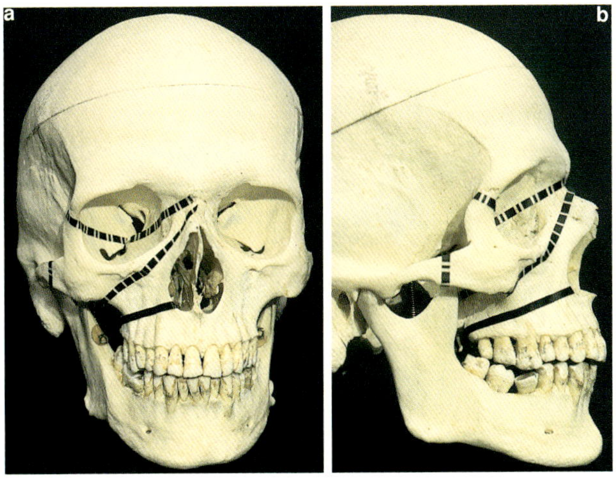

Fig. 18-4. (**a**) Anterior view of typical Le Fort I fracture lines (bottom line), Le Fort II fracture lines (center line), and Le Fort III fracture lines (top line). (**b**) Lateral view of the typical Le Fort fracture lines.

NECK INJURIES

The neck region contains a number of critical neurological, vascular, and airway structures in a relatively small space. Blunt and penetrating trauma to the neck can cause a wide variety of injuries, ranging from minor to severe to life threatening. Neck injuries in the military setting carry a 10% to 15% mortality.[6] Airway injury, vascular injury, and cervical spine injury can rapidly lead to death. If not properly managed, esophageal injuries can lead to serious infection, sepsis, and death. Quick and effective medical management can be lifesaving in some of these casualties.

The neck is commonly divided into three anatomical sections, one above the next.[7] Zone I, the lowest section, is the area behind the clavicles up to the cricoid cartilage. Zone I contains portions of the major vessels from the chest as well as portions of the lung apices, upper mediastinum, trachea, esophagus, and thoracic duct. This zone is partially protected by the clavicles. Zone II is bounded by horizontal planes at the level of the cricoid cartilage below and the angle of the mandible above. This section contains portions of the airway, esophagus, major blood vessels, cranial and peripheral nerves, cervical spine and spinal cord, and other structures. Zone II is relatively vulnerable to injury because the only bony protection is the cervical vertebral column to the rear. Zone III is the section between the angle of the mandible below and the base of the skull above. This zone contains many of the same structures as zone II, but surgical exposure is much more difficult in this region.

Neck injury can be caused by both blunt and penetrating trauma. Examples of blunt trauma are vehicular accidents and falls. Sources of penetrating trauma are gunshots, fragmentation blasts, knife wounds, and high-speed vehicular accidents.

Casualties with neck injuries require rapid evaluation to assess airway injury or compromise, ventilation, vascular injury, esophageal integrity, and neurological function. As with other injuries, the first priority is to ensure that the casualty has a secure airway and adequate ventilation. The possibility of cervical spine injury must be considered in every instance. In some cases, urgent intervention is required to stabilize the casualty. In others, the casualty can be monitored while injuries are evaluated in more detail and a surgical plan is developed. Expedient surgical exploration of penetrating neck injuries is indicated if the medical officer suspects vascular, airway, esophageal, or neurological injuries, or a missile path that crosses the midline.[8]

Airway Injuries

Potential injuries to the airway in neck trauma include crush injuries of the laryngeal structures and cricoid cartilage; tears, fistulae, lacerations, and transection of the trachea; bleeding and mucosal edema in the airway; and vocal cord obstruction due to nerve injury or arytenoid dislocation. The airway can also be compressed and obstructed by adjacent hematomas and subcutaneous emphysema in the neck.

Airway injuries can rapidly lead to death in the field before the casualty can be transported to a medical facility. Casualties with airway injuries may present for emergency treatment in severe respiratory distress. They can also present with what appears to be minor respiratory compromise and can, over a period of hours, insidiously develop airway obstruction from expanding hematomas or edema. The airway should be secured early if any signs of distress are present. This topic is discussed more fully in Chapter 3, Airway Management.

The integrity of the larynx can be disrupted by crush injuries from blunt trauma or from damage to the cartilage or supporting structures from penetrating trauma. Blunt trauma can also damage or collapse the cricoid cartilage and can cause tearing or total disruption of the cricotracheal junction. Penetrating trauma can tear, lacerate, or transect the trachea at any level. If the trachea or laryngeal structures are damaged, the airway must be secured below the lowest level of the injury. A tracheostomy can be done on an emergent basis, if necessary. Cricothyroidotomy is contraindicated if the cricothyroid area is damaged or if the trachea is damaged, as the canula could easily be placed into a false passage. With a tracheostomy, the surgeon may be able to get below the level of the tracheal injury and avoid placing the canula into a false passage. A transected trachea requires rapid surgical exploration and retrieval of the retracted distal segment. If time allows, casualties with airway injuries can potentially be intubated using a fiberoptic technique.

Vascular Injuries

Vascular injuries are common in penetrating neck trauma[9] and relatively uncommon in blunt neck trauma. Arterial injuries can lead to exsanguination, cerebral ischemia, and hematomas that can compress the airway. Venous injuries can lead to exsanguination or air embolism. Rapid exsanguination and loss of large volumes of blood into the chest can occur if the major vessels in zone I are disrupted. Fistulae from blood vessels to the airway can lead to massive pulmonary aspiration.

If time allows, preoperative angiography will help define the extent of the vascular injury. Early airway control will be needed if the patient has hemodynamic instability, neurological compromise, or bleeding into the airway. If the casualty is unstable, then rapid surgical control and resuscitation will be needed. The anesthesia team and surgical team must keep each other apprised of the patient's condition, ongoing blood loss, adequacy of control of bleeding, and the status of both blood-component and volume resuscitation.

Intraoperatively, continuous processed electroencephalography is valuable in monitoring for global cerebral ischemia during arterial clamping and repair. In addition, maintenance of a normal blood pressure will help maximize cerebral blood flow via collateral routes when one of the carotid or vertebral arteries is compromised.

There is a potential for air embolism if the internal jugular vein is disrupted. This can be a fatal complication if massive air aspiration occurs. The patient should be monitored for onset of air embolism with a precordial stethoscope, continuous respiratory-gas analysis, and precordial Doppler probe, if available. Transesophageal echocardiography is an extremely sensitive monitor of venous air embolism. Treatment of venous air embolism, should it occur, includes head-down positioning of the patient; flooding the surgical field; aspiration of air from the right atrium with a multiorifice central venous catheter; discontinuation of nitrous oxide, if it is being used; and hemodynamic support, if needed.

Nerve Injuries

Neurological structures that can be injured in neck trauma include the spinal cord, brachial plexus, phrenic nerves, cranial nerves, and sympathetic fibers. Spinal cord injuries are discussed below in the section on cervical spine injuries. Brachial plexus injuries can result in upper-extremity weakness and paresthesia. Causalgia is a common late complication of brachial plexus injury. Phrenic nerve injury leads to paralysis of the hemidiaphragm. Injury of the vagus nerve or the recurrent laryngeal nerve can result in vocal cord paralysis, which can contribute to airway obstruction. Injury of the vagus nerve or superior laryngeal nerve may abolish sensation above the vocal cords and can blunt protective airway reflexes.

Esophageal Injuries

Esophageal injuries occur more frequently with penetrating than with blunt neck trauma. Disruption of the esophagus can easily lead to infection that spreads to the mediastinum and becomes life threatening. Fistulae between the esophagus and the trachea, or between the esophagus and the blood vessels, occasionally occur. Esophageal tears and lacerations require early surgical diagnosis and repair.[10]

CERVICAL SPINE INJURIES

Injuries to the cervical vertebrae can occur when soldiers fall from a height, have direct penetrating trauma to the neck, or suffer head and face injuries or multiple trauma. The incidence of serious cervical spine injury in patients with major trauma varies from 1% to 3%.[11] Because of the potential for permanent injury to the cervical spinal cord, cervical spine trauma can be devastating. Medical personnel must carefully protect the cervical spine from the time of their first contact with the soldier until such time as injuries to the cervical vertebrae and spinal cord are either ruled out or definitively stabilized. Spinal cord injury can occur during field stabilization, transport to the hospital, airway management, or at any other time in the early phases of care. Initial care requires immobilization of the neck, control of the airway, assessment of cervical spine stability, and evaluation of neurological damage. Subsequent care involves restoration of anatomical integrity of the cervical vertebral column if required, continued protection of the cervical spinal cord, and rehabilitation. Injuries to the cervical spine and spinal cord are also discussed in Chapter 1, Combat Trauma Overview, and are the subject of Chapter 16, Neurological Injuries.

Cervical Vertebral Injuries

There are seven vertebrae (C-1 through C-7) in the neck. They provide support for the skull and protection for the cervical spinal cord. C-1 and C-2 are unique in structure and function. C-1, the atlas, consists of anterior and posterior arches and has no protruding articular processes. It articulates with the occipital condyles of the skull above and with C-2 below. C-2, the axis, has an anterior upward protrusion called the dens or odontoid process. C-2 has downward-protruding articular processes posteriorly. The dens and the articular surfaces articulate with C-1 above. C-2 articulates with C-3 via the articular surface of the body anteriorly and protruding articular processes posteriorly. C-3 through C-7 are similar in structure. Each vertebra consists of a body anteriorly, articular processes to the sides, and a spinous process posteriorly. Pedicles connect the body to the articular processes; laminae connect the articular processes to the spinous process. C-2 to C-7 articulate with each other via the posterior articular processes. The bodies of C-2 to C-7 are linked by intervertebral discs. The cervical vertebral column is strengthened by numerous ligaments.

The cervical spine is the most mobile and the least protected portion of the vertebral column, and is susceptible to injury from blunt and penetrating trauma. Instability of the cervical spine can result from fractures of portions of the vertebrae or disruption of the supporting ligaments. Compression fractures of the vertebral bodies and fracture-dislocations of the articular processes can cause cord compression and injury. Chin, mandibular, and zygomatic injuries are more commonly associated with injuries of the upper cervical spine, whereas upper-face and scalp injuries are more commonly associated with injuries of the lower cervical spine.

Cervical Spinal Cord Injuries

In the cervical region, the spinal cord occupies two thirds of the vertebral canal. Anterior and posterior nerve roots exit the spinal cord at intervals. The anterior roots have somatic fibers that control muscle movement, and the posterior roots have afferent fibers that carry sensory impulses.

Spinal cord trauma can occur directly, as a result of penetrating injury, or indirectly, from cord compression due to cervical fractures or dislocations. From 30% to 70% of patients with significant cervical spine injury may have associated spinal cord injury.[12] Compression of the spinal cord leads to vascular insufficiency, ischemia, edema, and neuronal cell death. Cord injuries can be complete, in which case no neurological impulses pass through the level of the injury, or they can be incomplete, in which case partial neurological deficits are present. Injuries to the brainstem or the upper cervical spinal cord are often fatal because of interruption of respiration and other vital functions. The innervation of the diaphragm is at the C-3 to C-5 level. Thus, injuries to the spinal cord at these levels or higher lead to respiratory failure. Injuries to the lower cervical spinal cord can interrupt intercostal muscle function, which seriously impairs pulmonary function.

Injury to the anterior portion of the spinal cord damages the spinothalamic and corticospinal tracts. Deficits include paralysis with loss of pain and temperature sensation. Injury to the posterior spinal cord is less common. Deficits include varying degrees of sensory loss and impairment of the positional and vibratory senses. In the Brown-Sequard syndrome, one side of the spinal cord is damaged. Deficits include motor weakness on the side with the lesion and pain and temperature sensory insensitivity on the side opposite the lesion. The Brown-Sequard syndrome can occur with penetrating trauma and with certain subluxation or dislocation injuries of the cervical vertebrae.

Spinal cord injury can cause a condition known as spinal shock. Disruption of the sympathetic fibers at the cervical cord level results in vasodilation, bradycardia, and hypotension. This condition occurs early in the injury and lasts several days to weeks. If spinal cord function does not recover, this syndrome gives way to autonomic hyperreflexia, a condition in which hyperresponsive autonomic reflex loops develop in the isolated lower level of the spinal cord. These conditions greatly complicate the perioperative management of casualties with spinal cord injuries.

Because spinal cord injuries are often permanent and devastating, every effort must be made to identify cervical spine instability and to protect the spinal cord during medical treatment.

Evaluation of Cervical Spine Injuries

Soldiers with any of the following conditions need radiological evaluation to rule out cervical spine injury[13]:

- multisystem trauma,
- blunt facial or head trauma,
- altered sensorium or neurological deficits,
- serious facial or scalp lacerations,
- fractures above the clavicles,
- traumatic neck pain or tenderness, or
- penetrating neck injuries.

An exception to this policy is patients who are fully alert, who do not have neck pain or tenderness, and who do not have other painful injuries that would mask neck pain. The standard radiological evaluation of the cervical spine consists of three views: cross-table lateral, anteroposterior, and open-mouth odontoid. All seven cervical vertebrae must be fully imaged on the cross-table lateral and anteroposterior views. Computed tomography views of the cervical vertebral column should be obtained if the plain views are inadequate or questionable, or if a neurological deficit is present.[13] Computed tomography is also indicated in patients with high-energy penetrating trauma to the cervical spine.[14]

Management of Blunt Cervical Spine Injuries

Initial care of soldiers with potential blunt cervical spine injuries should follow ATLS guidelines. At first contact with such a soldier, medical personnel should immobilize the neck, and, if necessary, the airway should be stabilized. Some casualties will require urgent airway intervention. Airway management must be approached with great caution because the risk of permanently injuring the cervical spinal cord is ever present. The most common methods of securing the airway in casualties with potential cervical spine injuries are oral intubation with cervical spine immobilization and blind nasal intubation. These techniques and other airway-management options are discussed later in this chapter.

Anesthesia providers must be concerned with more than just securing the airway in casualties with possible cervical spine injuries: they must carefully protect the cervical spine and the spinal cord during the perioperative period. The neck must be maintained in a neutral alignment during transport and positioning. Protection of the spinal cord also involves maintaining perfusion pressure and oxygenation. If spinal cord injury has occurred, high-dose methylprednisolone has been shown[15] to be of value in improving neurological outcome in some patients. Recovery from spinal cord injury depends on

- the extent of the initial injury,
- prevention of further injury, and
- avoidance of hypoxia and hypotension.

Spinal shock sometimes complicates the care of casualties with spinal cord injury. It is a syndrome that can be seen in the acute phase of spinal cord injury. The sympathetic system is disrupted by the injury and the casualty develops bradycardia, vasodilation, and hypotension. Profound hypotension is brought on by blood loss and positional changes. Fluid loading, atropine, and vasopressors may be required to treat spinal shock. Patients with spinal shock quickly develop pulmonary edema in response to fluid overload. Invasive monitoring can help guide fluid management in the perioperative period.

Over a period of days to weeks, the syndrome of spinal shock gives way to a chronic condition known as autonomic hyperreflexia. This is a syndrome of hyperreactive autonomic reflexes that sometimes develops in casualties with cord injuries above the T-6 level. Unchecked reflexes in the isolated spinal cord cause dramatic vasoconstriction and hypertension to occur in response to various stimuli. Autonomic hyperreflexia can be blocked by regional or general anesthesia and can be treated with potent vasodilators.

Patients with spinal cord injuries also have problems with temperature regulation. Careful temperature monitoring and meticulous patient warming are needed in the perioperative period.

Casualties with spinal cord injuries quickly develop the potential for a hyperkalemic response to succinylcholine administration. The rapid increase in serum potassium that occurs can cause fatal dysrhythmias. The dramatic potassium release results from a rapid increase in the neural receptors on the muscle membranes when normal neural tone is interrupted by spinal cord injury. Succinylcholine should be avoided in patients with spinal cord injuries more than a few hours old.

Casualties with cervical cord injuries can also develop respiratory dysfunction. Forced vital capacity is greatly reduced in patients with lower cervical cord injuries because of loss of intercostal and abdominal muscle function. Aspiration and pneumonia are common complications. Careful pulmonary care is required in these patients to minimize serious respiratory complications.

During surgical stabilization of cervical spine injuries, the anesthesia provider can contribute to the improved outcome of patients by providing evoked-potential monitoring. Extension of spinal cord injury can be prevented in some cases with this neurological monitor.[16]

ASSOCIATED INJURIES

Injuries to the face and neck are frequently dramatic in appearance. They can divert the medical team's attention away from other associated injuries. The associated injuries, although they are at times less obvious than face and neck injuries, can nonetheless be serious and potentially life threatening, and can greatly affect patient outcome and anesthetic management. Once the airway is secure and the cervical spine is stabilized, the most serious of the injuries must be dealt with.

The proximity of the face and neck to the major vessels and other important structures makes the possibility of serious associated injuries likely. The injuries most commonly seen in association with face and neck trauma are intracranial and ocular.

Neurological Injuries

Most patients with extensive facial injuries have associated neurological injuries.[1] Overt head trauma may be detected on initial observation and examination of the patient; however, serious intracranial injury can be present with only minimal external trauma. During the primary trauma survey, the patient's pupillary symmetry and response are assessed and the patient's level of consciousness is quickly evaluated.[4] The Glasgow coma scale is a convenient and accepted system for evaluating and documenting the patient's level of consciousness (also see Chapter 1, Combat Trauma Overview, Chapter 3, Airway Management, and Chapter 16, Neurological Injuries). If neurological abnormalities are detected on initial evaluation or if extensive face and neck injuries are present, then neurosurgical consultation should be obtained.[17] Examination by a neurosurgeon and skull radiographs, computed tomography, and nuclear magnetic imaging are indicated in most cases.[18] If sophisticated imaging systems are not readily available, which will be the case in most field environments, then management decisions will need to be based on clinical evaluation. The focus then will be on stabilization and transfer of the casualty to a medical treatment facility equipped for full neurosurgical evaluation and care.

Patients with head injury and an altered level of consciousness, especially those whose Glasgow coma scale score is lower than 9, are likely to have increased intracranial pressure. The presence of elevated intracranial pressure significantly influences the airway-management plan and the perioperative anesthetic management plan. Special monitoring is indicated in these patients. The use of intracranial pressure monitoring allows the military trauma anesthesiologist to monitor the effects of anesthetic interventions. The availability of continuous capnography permits precise control of blood carbon dioxide levels through adjustments in ventilatory support. Carbon dioxide levels directly affect intracranial blood flow, which, in turn, influences intracranial pressure. In the postoperative period, repeated neurological examinations as well as continued monitoring of intracranial pressure are of value. If postoperative mechanical ventilation is required, continued monitoring of exhaled carbon dioxide is important.

Ocular Injuries

Eye injuries are common in the military combat environment. There are many causes, but eye injuries in combat most commonly are the result of fragmentation blasts from artillery, mortars, or other munitions. Proper anesthetic management of the patient with eye injuries is critical: mismanagement can lead to permanent disability (also see Chapter 17, Eye Injuries).

There are two basic types of eye injuries: penetrating (ie, *open*) and nonpenetrating. As a rule, nonpenetrating injuries are less severe than penetrating injuries, but either type can lead to blindness. Nonpenetrating eye injuries, in which the globe remains intact, usually present a lesser anesthetic-management dilemma than penetrating eye injuries, in which the globe is disrupted. Nonpenetrating eye injuries include injuries to the eye and orbit and can be as minor as a corneal abrasion or eyelid ecchymosis, or as severe as retinal detachment, vitreous hemorrhage, or optic nerve injury. Penetrating injuries can cause a wide spectrum of damage to the eye and orbital structures. Eye injuries in which the globe is fully perforated require careful anesthetic management to avoid extrusion of intraocular contents and resultant permanent disability.

In managing casualties with eye injuries, the anesthesia care provider must (*a*) avoid increased intraocular pressure and (*b*) provide a motionless surgical field for the ophthalmologist. Increased intraocular pressure in the open eye can lead to displacement of intraocular contents and permanent eye injury. Intraocular pressure can be increased by the patient's coughing and straining during attempts to manage the airway. Succinylcholine also increases intraocular pressure, caused by the contraction of extraocular muscles as well as other less-well-defined mechanisms.[19]

General anesthesia is usually required in ophthalmic trauma surgery. Retrobulbar block, while perfectly adequate for most routine ophthalmic surgery, is contraindicated in the presence of an open eye injury because it can increase intraocular pressure. The ideal general-anesthesia induction technique for a patient with a penetrating eye injury is similar to that for a patient with increased intracranial pressure. A technique should be chosen that will ensure that the patient is deeply anesthetized and fully paralyzed before the airway is instrumented. This will minimize the likelihood that intraocular pressure will be increased. Unless strongly indicated for other reasons (eg, immediate airway control), succinylcholine should be avoided and a nondepolarizing relaxant should be used in its place. Nondepolarizing relaxants do not increase intraocular pressure.[20] During the maintenance phase of the anesthetic, the patient should continue to remain deeply anesthetized and well paralyzed to avoid any movement of the eye or any increase in intraocular pressure during surgery. A smooth emergence from anesthesia will minimize the stress on delicate ophthalmic surgical repairs.

Other Injuries

Injuries to structures other than the cervical spine, eyes, and head or central nervous system can certainly be present in casualties with injuries to the face and neck (eg, thoracic, intraabdominal, pelvic, and orthopedic injuries). The presence of multiple associated injuries complicates management. Casualties with these kinds of injuries require evaluation by appropriate surgical specialists. The care plan must be individualized for each casualty and requires careful coordination among all the specialists involved.

AIRWAY MANAGEMENT

As with other medical emergencies, airway management of combat casualties is of prime importance. The airway requires immediate attention; additional resuscitative efforts are wasted if airway management is ineffective or delayed. Casualties with injuries to the face and neck may present with acute airway obstruction, or they may develop airway obstruction at some point during their care. The airway can be obstructed by blood, vomitus, broken teeth or bone fragments, disrupted soft tissue, or other foreign bodies. In addition, the posterior portion of the tongue may fall back and obstruct the airway.[21] This can occur as a result of the decreased muscle tone that can be seen in neurological injury, or it might be secondary to loss of support of the base of the tongue due to an unstable fracture of the mandible. Edema and hematomas in the airway can cause partial or complete airway obstruction. Laryngeal and tracheal injuries can distort and block the airway. Laryngeal injuries may be occult or otherwise appear minimal at the time of injury, but can progress to cause airway obstruction over time.[22] If tracheal disruption is present, positive-pressure ventilation may lead to subcutaneous and mediastinal emphysema, which can further distort the airway. Neck injuries can cause edema and hematomas, which can compress the airway.

Airway management of these casualties is often complicated by associated injuries that may be present. Cervical spine injury, intracranial injury, blood loss, and the risk of aspiration all influence the way that the airway is managed.

Mask Ventilation

Mask ventilation may be required in emergent circumstances to stabilize casualties who have face or neck injuries. The following conditions interfere with effective mask ventilation by causing an obstruction or otherwise preventing an effective mask seal:

- facial lacerations,
- nasal fractures,
- maxillary fractures,
- mandibular fractures, and
- dental trauma.

If the casualty's airway is obstructed by the tongue, then forward displacement of the mandible may open the airway. Pulling the tongue forward with gauze, clamps, or sutures are other maneuvers that may relieve obstruction of the airway. These techniques tend to interfere with mask ventilation, but if the casualty is making spontaneous respiratory effort, the relief of obstruction may be all that is needed to restore adequate ventilation. (Placing the casualty in a lateral position may also correct the obstruction, but such movement could potentially injure the cervical spinal cord if the cervical spine is unstable.) In many cases, placing an oral airway device will relieve the obstruction, but blind placement in a casualty with potential intraoral or pharyngeal injury could be harmful and could potentially worsen the obstruction.

Mask ventilation should be considered a temporary technique to stabilize the casualty while provisions are made to obtain more definitive airway control. During mask ventilation, the patient's airway remains unprotected and aspiration is always a risk. Blood and food in the stomach, bleeding in the airway, and an altered level of consciousness are factors that are frequently present and that increase the likelihood of aspiration.

Cricoid pressure in the casualty whose protective airway reflexes are inadequate will normally prevent passive regurgitation. However, attempts to block active vomiting with cricoid pressure are likely to fail and may cause esophageal injury. Proper positioning of the casualty and rapid, effective suctioning are the best means of dealing with active vomiting. If the casualty can cooperate, or if he has a nasogastric or orogastric tube in place, then a clear antacid solution can be given to neutralize the stomach acid. Reducing the acidity of stomach contents will decrease the pulmonary inflammatory response if aspiration does occur.

Tracheal Intubation

Tracheal intubation of casualties with face or neck injuries can be difficult. The possibility of cervical spine instability in these patients further complicates airway management. Intubation alternatives for casualties with possible cervical spine injuries include the following:

- orotracheal intubation with cervical immobilization,
- blind nasotracheal intubation,
- fiberoptic tracheal intubation,
- lighted stylet orotracheal intubation, and
- retrograde wire tracheal intubation.

Orotracheal intubation under direct laryngoscopic visualization is a technique with which anesthesia providers are quite comfortable. Direct visualization of the airway is valuable in patients with facial injuries because airway injuries can be assessed. In addition, the risk of esophageal intubation is reduced. Intubation under direct laryngoscopic visualization can be dangerous in patients with cervical spine injuries if the neck is manipulated. Some authorities[23] believe that orotracheal intubation of patients with cervical spine injuries could damage the spinal cord. Others[24,25] are confident that, with meticulous cervical spine immobilization, orotracheal intubation is safe and reliable. Cervical collars do not provide adequate stabilization for oral intubation.[26] The recommended technique for immobilization of the cervical spine is to have a skilled practitioner apply moderate, manual, in-line traction and stabilization to the head and cervical spine.[27] Preferably, the surgeon in charge should provide the in-line traction.[4] If that is not feasible, another appropriately trained member of the trauma team may apply the traction. The neck should be maintained in a neutral position throughout the intubation. If orotracheal intubation in a casualty with a potential cervical spine injury requires that the neck be extended, then an alternative airway-management technique should be selected.

Some authorities[28] believe that blind nasotracheal intubation should be the primary initial intubation technique for patients with possible cervical spine injuries. Blind nasal intubation is a simple, rapid technique that is reasonably reliable. However, it is difficult to perform successfully in apneic patients, and it is contraindicated in patients with midface or basilar skull fractures.[29] Because this is a blind technique, it should not be used if the integrity of the airway has been disrupted. False placement into a tissue plane may cause airway obstruction. If nasal intubation is required in a patient with midfacial or nasal injuries, the nasal airway should be inspected with a fiberscope prior to intubation. A common complication of blind nasal intubation is epistaxis. Blood in the airway complicates subsequent attempts at airway management.

Fiberoptic tracheal intubation is an excellent technique for securing the airway in casualties with potential cervical spine injuries or with facial injuries.[30] The neck is maintained in a neutral position and the airway is visualized throughout the intubation. The nasal or the oral route can be used. The technique is quick and reliable in skilled hands. In casualties with face and neck trauma, the fiberoptic technique allows the anesthesia provider to evaluate the integrity of the airway. Drawbacks include equipment expense, impairment by blood and secretions, the length of setup time required, and the need for training and experience. For these reasons, fiberoptic intubation is used primarily in the controlled, as opposed to the emergent, setting.

Retrograde wire tracheal intubation is useful in some patients with facial or possible cervical spine injuries.[31] A catheter is placed percutaneously through the cricothyroid membrane, angling cephalad. A flexible guide wire is inserted through the catheter and advanced until it can be pulled out of the mouth. A tracheal tube exchanger, or a substitute such as a section of a nasogastric tube, is threaded over the wire and into the mouth. An endotracheal tube is then inserted over the tube exchanger. The wire is pulled out from the mouth end and the endotracheal tube is advanced off the tube exchanger and down the trachea. A variation of this technique is to use a long guide wire and thread it through the suction port of a fiberoptic bronchoscope.[32] The bronchoscope is advanced blindly over the guide wire and is directed by the guide wire into the trachea. The wire is then removed and the bronchoscope is advanced to the carina. The endotracheal tube that was placed over the fiberoptic bundle is then advanced into the airway. The retrograde wire technique is quick and reliable. Its primary advantage is that it can be performed even if the airway contains blood or secretions.

Lighted stylet tracheal intubation is quick and reliable in skilled hands,[33] although this is a blind technique and should not be used in casualties who may have airway injuries. The casualty's neck is maintained in a neutral position during the intubation. The technique involves placing the endotracheal tube over a malleable lighted stylet. The stylet is bent to approximately a right angle at the level of the endotracheal tube cuff. The casualty's tongue or mandible is displaced forward and the stylet is directed blindly toward the glottis. The anesthesia provider observes the neck and watches for a bright, midline transillumination at the level of the lower portion of the thyroid cartilage. The endotracheal tube is then advanced off the stylet and down the trachea. The success rate for lighted stylet intubation is related to the experience and training of the practitioner.

Tracheal intubation of the unconscious patient can generally be accomplished without any anesthetic agents. Intubation of the conscious patient will normally require some form of topical or general anesthesia. Topical anesthesia puts the patient at risk for aspiration of gastric contents. If topical anesthesia is incomplete, airway stimulation during intubation may induce vomiting or may cause the patient to move suddenly. Induction of general anesthesia also abolishes protective airway reflexes and can cause severe hemodynamic instability in casualties who are hypovolemic from blood loss. The anesthesia provider must select the technique that provides the best balance between the intubating conditions and the patient's stability. The subject is discussed in greater detail in Chapter 3, Airway Management.

Transtracheal Jet Ventilation

Transtracheal jet ventilation is a temporizing technique that stabilizes the patient and allows time for the practitioner to secure longer-term control of the airway. The technique involves placing a large intravenous catheter, such as a 14-gauge catheter, percutaneously through the neck into the upper trachea. This is connected to a high-pressure oxygen source (50 psi) with a tubing system that has an adjustable pressure regulator and a manual valve. The oxygen source can be a wall source, an oxygen tank, or the flush-valve output of the anesthesia machine. The breathing circuit of the anesthesia machine is not an acceptable gas source for transtracheal jet ventilation because the driving pressure is too low. Bag-valve systems are unacceptable for the same reason. The specific components that make up an effective transtracheal jet ventilation system are well described in the literature.[34] To be useful in emergencies, the system must available and already connected to an oxygen source.

The anesthesia provider provides manual ventilation for the patient, while also adjusting the driving pressure and watching the patient's chest rise and fall with each breath. The advantages of transtracheal jet ventilation are that it is fast, effective, and lifesaving. The disadvantages are the risk of bleeding from catheter placement, and the risk of pneumothorax if the driving pressure is too high or if the tracheal outlet is obstructed. Improper placement of the catheter may lead to subcutaneous emphysema. Inadequate alveolar ventilation will result in hypercarbia.

Cricothyroidotomy

In some casualties with face or neck injuries, adequate mask ventilation may be impossible, and tracheal intubation may be dangerous or unsuccessful. In the emergent situation, cricothyroidotomy is a rapid and effective means of airway control. Since cricothyroidotomy has a significant complication rate in the emergency setting,[35] it should be performed only when the airway cannot be secured by other methods.

If the anatomical landmarks are not distorted, a cricothyroidotomy incision can quickly be made between the thyroid cartilage and the cricoid cartilage. A small, cuffed endotracheal tube, or any makeshift stent, can be placed through the incision into the airway.

Most anesthesia providers prefer cricothyroidotomy to tracheostomy in emergent situations because

- the risk of bleeding is reduced,
- surgical access is quicker, and
- anatomical landmarks are more reliable.

Tracheostomy

Tracheostomy may be performed as the initial airway-management technique in selected casualties with face and neck injuries. If the casualty has (*a*) severe facial injuries that preclude safe or successful orotracheal or nasotracheal intubation and (*b*) injury to the cricothyroid region of the neck that distorts the anatomical landmarks, then emergent tracheostomy may be the best option. Tracheostomy may also be required if the cricothyroid region of the airway or the uppermost portion of the trachea is disrupted. In these cases, tracheostomy allows access to the airway below the area of injury. In some patients with specific combinations of facial fractures, tracheostomy may be required so that the surgery can be completed. If time allows and the patient is stable, awake tracheostomy at the beginning of the surgery may be safer than the anesthesia provider's attempting to perform orotracheal or nasotracheal intubation in the presence of multiple facial fractures and a potentially unstable cervical spine. In most cases where postoperative tracheostomy will be necessary, however, it is best to wait until near the conclusion of the surgery to perform the tracheostomy.

PERIOPERATIVE ANESTHETIC MANAGEMENT

In the management of patients with face and neck trauma, airway stabilization takes top priority. Other problems that require early attention (and are often a result of associated injuries) are hemorrhage and hypovolemic shock. Stabilization of these patients requires early and continued involvement of the anesthesia team, as well as the coordinated efforts of multiple surgical specialty teams when associated injuries are present.[18] Although the dramatic appearance of face and neck injuries may divert the attention of the medical personnel away from the casualty's other injuries, expedient care of the associated injuries may initially take precedence over repair of the face and neck injuries. The individual surgical teams may have distorted views of the priorities of medical care, and communication among the surgical teams—including the anesthesia team—is crucial to assure that proper priorities are maintained and that care proceeds appropriately. The anesthesia team must seek active involvement in the preparation and planning for surgery to ensure that the associated injuries are identified preoperatively, and that the patient is maximally resuscitated and stabilized preoperatively.

Numerous associated problems that can complicate perioperative anesthetic management may be present in patients with face and neck trauma:

- an inadequate airway,
- hemorrhage,
- intracranial injury,
- spinal injury,
- pulmonary contusion,
- pulmonary aspiration,
- pneumothorax,
- cardiac contusion,
- cardiac tamponade,
- intraabdominal injury, and
- renal injury.

Some problems, such as pneumothorax, cardiac tamponade, and external hemorrhage, should be corrected before the administration of general anesthesia, if at all possible. Other problems, such as intraabdominal injury, can be stabilized under general anesthesia, whereas problems like increased intracranial pressure, aspiration pneumonitis, and acute renal failure will have a significant impact on anesthetic management and will continue to require attention throughout the perioperative period. Safe anesthetic management depends on the ability to monitor affected organ systems during the resuscitative and operative phases of treatment.[18] Physiological monitoring of the patient with face and neck trauma may include such modalities as central venous lines, arterial lines, Foley catheters, repeated blood analysis, and possibly intracranial pressure monitoring, in addition to the usual anesthesia monitoring. Appropriate perioperative anesthesia monitoring may help identify ongoing renal, respiratory, and neurological injury.

Local and Regional Anesthesia

Not all face and neck trauma patients require general anesthesia. Patients with multiple injuries and patients with severe maxillofacial injuries will normally require general anesthesia, but patients with isolated and less-severe injuries may do well with regional and local anesthesia. Limited facial soft-tissue injuries can usually be repaired with local anesthesia alone. In fact, the use of epinephrine-containing local anesthetic will provide improved hemostasis compared with that provided by regional or general anesthesia. Local and regional anesthesia, however, can induce temporary paralysis of the facial nerve, which may interfere with the diagnosis of facial nerve injury. Regional anesthesia can be used for selected areas of the face and neck.

General Anesthesia

Patients who require extensive or lengthy procedures and patients who are uncooperative will need general anesthesia.[36] Anesthetic techniques and monitoring are influenced primarily by the associated injuries that are present. Anesthetic induction and intubation require careful evaluation of the airway and consideration of the side effects of the induction agents. Anesthetic induction is greatly simplified if the casualty's airway was intubated during the initial stabilization and resuscitation. Induction agents can then be selected and titrated to produce minimal adverse effects on the associated injured organ systems. If intubation is required in the operating room, then induction agents and techniques must be selected that provide maximally safe intubating conditions while at the same time minimize risk to injured organ systems. All factors must be considered, and each situation must be individualized.

The safest induction technique for patients at risk for aspiration, which includes most trauma victims, is usually a rapid-sequence induction using a hypnotic agent such as ketamine or sodium thiopental along with succinylcholine. However, in patients with possible cervical spine injury, which, again, includes many trauma patients, awake intubation with cervical spine immobilization is generally indicated, if time and conditions allow. Patients with increased intracranial pressure and patients with open eye injuries should have a slow, controlled, and complete induction of anesthesia with sodium thiopental or a similar hypnotic agent, a narcotic agent, and a nondepolarizing muscle relaxant prior to intubation of the airway. This technique minimizes the likelihood of a dangerous increase in intracranial pressure or intraocular pressure at the start of anesthesia.

Patients with severe hypovolemia from acute blood loss may not tolerate standard anesthetic-induction techniques. Severe hypotension or cardiac arrest may occur if the patient is given a hypnotic induction such as ketamine, which causes cardiac depression, or sodium thiopental, which causes sympathetic and cardiac depression. The safest induction technique for these patients will generally be scopolamine and a muscle relaxant alone.

No single induction technique is suitable for all trauma situations. Often, the medical officer will be confronted with a combination of injuries and conditions that make choosing the best anesthetic-induction technique difficult (eg, a patient with a head injury and a full stomach, a patient with an open eye injury and a displaced mandibular fracture, and an uncooperative patient with bleeding and possible cervical spine injury). In scenarios such as these, the anesthesia provider must first decide which conditions are of overriding importance and then select the most appropriate airway-management technique and anesthetic plan for those conditions. Careful clinical assessment is required for every case.

Intraoperative Airway Management

Completion of the initial intubation does not mean that the airway can then be ignored. Accidental extubation can easily occur when maxillofacial surgical procedures are in progress. It may be difficult to secure an orotracheal or nasotracheal tube in patients with facial injuries due to tissue disruption and surgical cleansing. Suturing the tracheal tube in place, monitoring the progress of surgery, communicating with the surgeons, assisting with head positioning, and continuously monitoring the patient's ventilation will all help to decrease the risk of accidental extubation.

Both the specific injuries and the specific surgical procedures planned have an impact on airway management. Orotracheal intubation is generally the preferred method for initial intubation, but some surgical procedures (ie, procedures requiring intermaxillary fixation) cannot be completed with an orotracheal tube in place. If intermaxillary fixation is required, then orotracheal intubation must be converted either to a nasotracheal placement or to a tracheostomy. Nasotracheal intubation is acceptable in patients who do not have nasal fractures, but if nasal fractures are present in conjunction with other fractures necessitating intermaxillary wiring, then a tracheostomy is likely to be needed. Tracheostomy in casualties with face and neck injuries is indicated[18] in patients

- who have significant intracranial injuries that require intermaxillary fixation;
- who have nasal fractures combined with maxillary or mandibular fractures that require intermaxillary fixation;
- who have significant pulmonary injuries or flail chest, and who also require intermaxillary fixation;
- whose massive soft-tissue swelling may interfere with reintubation;
- who were intubated emergently via a cricothyroidotomy; and
- who have injuries to the laryngeal or cricothyroid region.

The placement of a tracheostomy tube does not guarantee that the airway is secure. The tracheostomy tube can easily become dislodged and, if the tracheostomy was recently performed, emergent replacement of the tracheostomy tube may cause the tube tip to be placed into a blind tract between tissue planes. Placing "stay" sutures during the tracheostomy procedure will aid in (*a*) identifying the appropriate tissue planes and (*b*) replacing the tracheostomy tube if the tube becomes dislodged before the tracheostomy site has healed. An armored tube, sutured in place, may be more secure intraoperatively than a standard tracheostomy tube.

Postoperative Airway Management

Patients who are emerging from anesthesia and are recovering from surgical repair of their face and neck injuries require special attention. If the patient is to be extubated at the conclusion of the surgical procedure, airway protection must be assured. Caution is required in the patient with intermaxillary wiring. Intact airway reflexes must be present, although that alone does not guarantee that aspiration will not occur. Aspiration in the presence of intermaxillary wiring can easily be fatal.[37] Attention must focus on reducing the risk of emesis and rapidly dealing with it when it occurs. Evacuating gastric contents with a suction tube and giving an antiemetic agent prior to extubation will help. Wire cutters must be immediately available at the bedside and the specific locations of the wires to be cut should be made clear to personnel caring for the patient.

Even if the jaws are not wired, other problems can occur with extubation. If significant soft-tissue trauma has occurred, postoperative edema or hematomas may lead to progressive airway obstruction after extubation. If the patient remains intubated postoperatively, accidental extubation in an uncontrolled environment can lead to disaster. Vigilance must be maintained throughout the perioperative period well into the recovery period in patients with face and neck injuries.

SUMMARY

Casualties with face and neck injuries present challenging problems to the anesthesiologist. Airway management can be complicated. Serious associated injuries, especially head injuries, are often present and can have a significant impact on anesthetic care. Initial management should follow published ATLS guidelines. Securing the airway, protecting the cervical spine, and providing ventilation and controlling hemorrhage as needed are the top priorities. Subsequent management must be carefully planned and prioritized. This requires the coordinated effort of the anesthesia team and the various surgical subspecialty teams involved.

REFERENCES

1. Grande CM, Wyman CI, Bernhard WN. Perioperative anesthetic management of maxillofacial and ocular trauma: Injuries of the craniofacial complex. In: Stene JK, Grande CM, eds. *Trauma Anesthesia*. Baltimore, Md: Williams & Wilkins; 1991: 266–285.

2. Bellamy RF. Unpublished analysis of the Wound Data and Munitions Effectiveness Team database. Personal communication, September 1993.

3. Bellamy RF, Zajtchuk R. The weapons of conventional land warfare. In: Bellamy RF, Zajtchuk R, eds. *Conventional Warfare: Ballistic, Blast, and Burn Injuries*. Part 1, Vol 5. In: Zajtchuk R, Jenkins DP, Bellamy RF, eds. *Textbook of Military Medicine*. Washington, DC: US Department of Army, Office of The Surgeon General, and Borden Institute; 1991: Chap 1.

4. Committee on Trauma, American College of Surgeons. *Advanced Trauma Life Support Program for Physicians: Instructor Manual*. 5th ed. Chicago, Ill: American College of Surgeons; 1993.

5. Le Fort R. Etude experimentale sur les fractures de la machoire superieure. *Rev Chir*. 1901;23:208–227.

6. McSwain NE. Penetrating neck wounds: Major advances in the 1980's. In: Maull KI, Cleveland HC, Strauch GO, Wolferth CC, eds. *Advances in Trauma*. Chicago, Ill: Yearbook Medical Publishers; 1986: 135–140.

7. Ordog GJ, Albin D, Wasserberger J, et al. 110 bullet wounds to the neck. *J Trauma*. 1985;25:238–241.

8. Capan LM, Miller SM, Turndorf H. Management of neck injuries. In: Capan LM, Miller SM, Turndorf H, eds. *Trauma Anesthesia and Intensive Care*. Philadelphia, Pa: JB Lippincott; 1991: 409–446.

9. Ayuyao AM, Kaledzi YL, Parsa MH, Freeman HP. Penetrating neck wounds: Mandatory versus selective exploration. *Ann Surg*. 1985;202:563–566.

10. Richardson JD, Martin LF, Borzotta AP, Polk HC. Unifying concepts in treatment of esophageal leaks. *Am J Surg*. 1985;149:157–160.

11. Kreipke DL, Gillespie KR, McCarthy MC, Mail JT, Lappas JC, Broadie TA. Reliability of indications for cervical spine films in trauma patients. *J Trauma*. 1989;29:1438–1439.

12. Guthkelch AN, Fleischer A. Patterns of cervical spine injury and their associated lesions. *West J Med*. 1987;147:428–431.

13. Kellman R. The cervical spine in maxillofacial trauma. *Otolaryngol Clin North Am*. 1991;24:1–13.

14. Hastings RH, Marks JD. Airway management for trauma patients with potential cervical spine injuries. *Anesth Analg*. 1991;73:471–482.

15. Bracken MB, Shepard MJ, Collins WF, et al. Second National Acute Spinal Cord Injury Study. A randomized, controlled trial of methylprednisolone or naloxone in the treatment of acute spinal cord injury. *N Engl J Med*. 1990;322:1405–1411.

16. Rose DD, O'Hara CA, Fossum SR, Hanowell LH. Cervical spine injury: Perioperative patient care. *AORN J.* 1993;57:830–850.

17. Martin SH. Injury of the head and cervical spine. *Otolaryngol Clin North Am.* 1976;9:403–423.

18. Manson PN, Saunders JR. Anesthesia in head and neck surgery: Head and neck cancer surgery and maxillofacial trauma. *Clin Plast Surg.* 1985;12:115–122.

19. Wislicki L, Factors affecting intraocular pressure. *Proc R Soc Med.* 1977;70:372–374.

20. Calobrisi B, Lebowitz P. Muscle relaxants and the open globe. *Int Anesthesiol Clin.* 1990;28:83–85.

21. Strate RG, Boies LR. The emergency management of trauma. *Otolaryngol Clin North Am.* 1976;9:315–330.

22. Huff JS, Magielski JE. Surgical treatment of laryngeal injuries. *Otolaryngol Clin North Am.* 1976;9:393–401.

23. Bivins HG, Ford S, Bezmalinovic Z. The effect of axial traction during orotracheal intubation of the trauma victim with an unstable cervical spine. *Ann Emerg Med.* 1988;17:25–29.

24. Scannell G, Waxman K, Tominaga G, Barker S, Annas C. Orotracheal intubation in trauma patients with cervical fractures. *Arch Surg.* 1993;128:903–906.

25. Walls RN. Airway management. *Emerg Med Clin North Am.* 1993;11:53–60.

26. Aprahamian C, Thompson BM, Finger WA, et al. Experimental cervical spine injury model: Evaluation of airway management and splinting techniques. *Ann Emerg Med.* 1984;13:584–587.

27. Wood PR, Lawler PG. Managing the airway in cervical spine injury: A review of the advanced trauma life support protocol. *Anaesthesia.* 1992;47:792–797.

28. Jorden RC, Rosen P. Airway management in the acutely injured. In: Moore EE, Eisman B, VanWay EW, eds. *Critical Decision in Trauma.* St. Louis, Mo: CV Mosby; 1984: 30–35.

29. Rosenbaum P. Anesthesia for eye, head, and neck surgery. In: Firestone LL, Lebowitz PW, Cook CE, eds. *Clinical Anesthesia Procedures of the Massachusetts General Hospital.* Boston, Mass: Little, Brown; 1988: 346–365.

30. Ovassapian A, Dykes MH. The role of fiberoptic endoscopy for airway management. *Semin Anesth.* 1987;6:93–104.

31. Barriot P, Riou B. Retrograde technique for tracheal intubation in trauma patients. *Crit Care Med.* 1988;16:712–713.

32. Gupta B, McDonald JS, Brooks JH, Mendenhall J. Oral fiberoptic intubation over a retrograde wire. *Anesth Analg.* 1989;68:517–519.

33. Ellis DG, Stewart RD, Kaplan RM, et al. Success rates of blind orotracheal intubation using a transillumination technique with a lighted stylet. *Ann Emerg Med.* 1986;15:138–142.

34. Benumof JL, Scheller MS. The importance of transtracheal ventilation in the management of the difficult airway. *Anesthesiology.* 1989;71:769–778.

35. McGill J, Clinton JE, Ruiz E. Cricothyrotomy in the emergency department. *Ann Emerg Med.* 1982;11:361–364.

36. Dickinson JT, Jaquiss GW, Thompson JN. Soft tissue trauma. *Otolaryngol Clin North Am.* 1976;9:331–360.

37. Sims J, Giesecke AH. Airway management. In: Giesecke AH, ed. *Anesthesia for the Surgery of Trauma.* Philadelphia, Pa: FA Davis; 1976: 71–78.

Chapter 19

THORACIC INJURIES

LAWRENCE L. YEE, M.D.*; ALEXANDER S. RUBIN, M.D.†; AND RONALD F. BELLAMY, M.D.‡

*Formerly, Major, Medical Corps, U.S. Army; Staff Anesthesiologist, Walter Reed Army Medical Center, Washington, D. C. 20307-5001; currently, Staff Anesthesiologist, O'Connor Hospital, 2105 Forest Avenue, San Jose, California 95128

†Formerly, Major, Medical Corps, U.S. Army; Staff Anesthesiologist, Walter Reed Army Medical Center, Washington, D. C. 20307-5001; currently, Staff Anesthesiologist, Frederick Memorial Hospital, Frederick, Maryland 21702

‡Colonel, Medical Corps, U.S. Army; Managing Editor and Officer in Charge, Textbook of Military Medicine, Borden Institute, Walter Reed Army Medical Center, Washington, D. C. 20307-5001

INTRODUCTION

The casualty suffering thoracic trauma usually poses a lesser challenge to the military trauma anesthesiologist than might be supposed. As we discussed in Chapter 1, Combat Trauma Overview, the reasons for this are simple: (1) most casualties who are wounded in the chest die on the battlefield, and (2) only a minority of those who reach a medical treatment facility alive require a formal thoracotomy. Most survivors require only the insertion of a chest tube. Thus, thoracic trauma in combat casualties has some of the all-or-none characteristics of an airplane crash: the victim is either killed outright or has a injury that is treatable by simple interventions. Nevertheless, there are exceptions (eg, the casualty who suddenly exsanguinates when a mediastinal hematoma ruptures, the casualty whose tracheobronchial tree is filling with blood, the casualty who suddenly develops massive arterial air embolism when mechanical ventilation is started) that can push even the most competent anesthesiologists to their limits.

TYPES OF INJURY

Thoracic trauma can be the result of one or more of the four basic mechanisms of injury: penetrating (ballistic), blunt, blast, and thermal. Thermal injury resulting from the inhalation of hot, poisonous gases is an important cause of combat mortality and morbidity in the navy and among soldiers who crew armored fighting vehicles. Inhalation injury is discussed in Chapter 22, Burn Injuries; therefore, it will not be further discussed in this chapter.

Penetrating missiles have been far and away the major source of thoracic trauma in combat casualties, as seen in Table 19-1, which presents data from two countries and two wars. The data from the U.S. Army in the Vietnam War covers a 14-month period (September 1968–November 1969) at the 24th Evacuation Hospital.[1] During this interval, the hospital served as a specialty center for neurological, head and neck, and thoracic casualties. Data from the Rambam Medical Center covers the period 6 to 29 June 1982 (during the military operation in Lebanon that the Israelis call Peace in Galilee).[2]

Because penetrating trauma is the cause of the overwhelming majority of combat casualties with thoracic injuries, and because it is generally agreed that missile wounds are distributed randomly, the overall prevalence of thoracic trauma should approximate the fraction of the body surface area that overlies the thorax: about 16 in 100. Most casualties with thoracic trauma are killed; therefore, the actual percentage of the casualty population who will require treatment for thoracic trauma will be somewhat smaller and usually ranges between 5% and 10%.[3]

Penetrating Missiles

The nature of the medical problems caused by penetrating missiles, whether they are bullets from small arms or fragments from explosive munitions, is due to three factors:

1. the function of the organ or organs struck,
2. the physical characteristics of the missile, and
3. the biophysics of the interaction between the missile and the tissue that is struck.

It should be readily apparent that the first factor—the nature of the organ hit—is of paramount importance in determining the medical outcome of a ballistic injury. A missile wound of the brainstem is likely to be much more serious than a hit made by a similar missile to the little toe. Unfortunately, the thoracic cavity has more than its share of organs—the heart, great vessels, and lungs—the injury of which will be immediately catastrophic.

The second factor—the physical characteristics of the missile—is usually assessed in terms of kinetic energy (calculated as $\frac{1}{2}MV^2$, where *M* represents the projectile's mass and *V* its velocity). Tissue destruction caused by a ballistic injury is related in a general sense to the kinetic energy transferred to the target tissue such that

$$\frac{1}{2}M(V_{ent} - V_{ext})^2$$

where V_{ent} and V_{ext} represent the velocity of the missile when it enters and exits the body, respectively. When the missile does not exit but stops within the body, the kinetic energy transferred equals $\frac{1}{2}MV_{ent}^2$. Fragments usually do not exit from the body, while bullets, unless they deform or fragment, frequently cause perforating wounds. Bullets that fragment (ie, rounds fired from the M16 series of assault rifles) or deform (ie, many

TABLE 19-1

ETIOLOGY OF THORACIC TRAUMA

	24th Evacuation Hospital US Army, Vietnam[1]	Rambam Medical Center Haifa, Israel[2]
Total Casualties	7,500	938
Chest Trauma	900*	64
Intrathoracic Injury	547	63
Fragment	443	41
Bullet	76	7†
Blunt	28	6‡
Blast		6§

*Including superficial missile wounds as well as blunt trauma to the chest wall but without any intrathoracic component
†There were, in addition, two casualties with both bullet and fragment wounds
‡There was a seventh casualty with both fragment and blunt thoracic trauma
§All six casualties with pulmonary blast injury also had fragment wounds of the thorax
Data sources: (1) McNamara JJ, Messersmith JK, Dunn RA, Molot MD, Stremple JF. Thoracic injuries in combat casualties in Vietnam. *Ann Thor Surg*. 1970;10:389–401. (2) Rosenblatt M, Lemer M, Best LA, Peleg H. Thoracic wounds in Israeli battle casualties during the 1982 evacuation of wounded from Lebanon. *J Trauma*. 1985;25:350–354.

commonly available bullets used by civilian hunters and law-enforcement agencies) typically are associated with much greater energy transfer than occurs with intact bullets that cause perforating wounds.

A second important physical characteristic is the shape of the projectile. Streamlined bullets can pass through tissue with little reduction in velocity, while irregular fragments from explosive munitions slow rapidly and, therefore, can transfer a much greater fraction of their kinetic energy—with a corresponding increase in the potential for tissue damage.

The third factor determining the medical consequences of ballistic injury has to do with the interaction of the projectile and the tissue along its pathway. Obviously, the longer the wound tract, the more damage that is likely to occur. This is true because (*a*) the bullet passes through more tissue, and (*b*) it is more likely that the bullet will destabilize (either *yaw* [ie, the long axis of the bullet deviates from the direction of flight] or *tumble* [ie, the bullet flips end over end]), greatly increasing energy transfer. The density of the tissue is another determinant of the projectile–target interaction. The more dense the tissue, the more complete the energy transfer. Thus, projectile energy transfer is maximal in bone but minimal in the least-dense body tissue, the lung. (A more complete discussion of the biophysics of wound ballistics can be found in the Textbook of Military Medicine volume *Conventional Warfare: Ballistic, Blast, and Burn Injuries*.)[4]

Wound ballistics as it applies to the thorax is best summarized in the official history of thoracic surgery in World War II:

> [H]igh-velocity missiles that traverse the pulmonary tissue therefore often cause surprisingly little pulmonary damage. The high immediate lethality of high-velocity wounds of the chest is apparently directly related to the percentage chance of damage to vital structures, particularly the heart and great vessels. If the high-velocity missile does not inflict a mortal wound, then it often traverses the chest with considerably less damage to the thoracic contents than is caused by a low-velocity shell fragment.[5(p59)]

Blunt and Blast Injuries

In the field, nonpenetrating injuries to the chest are caused either by forceful contact with a blunt object or by blast overpressure. Blunt chest trauma such as may occur in motor vehicle accidents results from gross compression of the thorax, which may cause rib fractures and a variable degree of displacement of intrathoracic viscera such as the heart. In extreme circumstances, the heart may be so displaced that stretch-and-shear strain affecting the proximal descending aorta may cause it to rupture. With blunt trauma, but not with blast injury, the more serious the injury, the greater the likelihood of rib fractures. Fractures of the upper five ribs are usually associated with the most serious, and often occult, injuries.

The exact mechanisms that produce visceral injury within the thoracic cavity following blunt and blast injury are poorly understood, but it is no longer thought that acceleration–deceleration of the body is an important mechanism *per se*. Extensive experimental studies using living animals and human cadavers indicate that the probability of injury can best be understood in terms of (*a*) the magnitude of compression of the thorax and (*b*) the velocity at which the compression occurs (Figure 19-1).[6,7]

When compression is applied slowly (< 1 m/s; eg, in vigorous closed-chest cardiopulmonary resuscita-

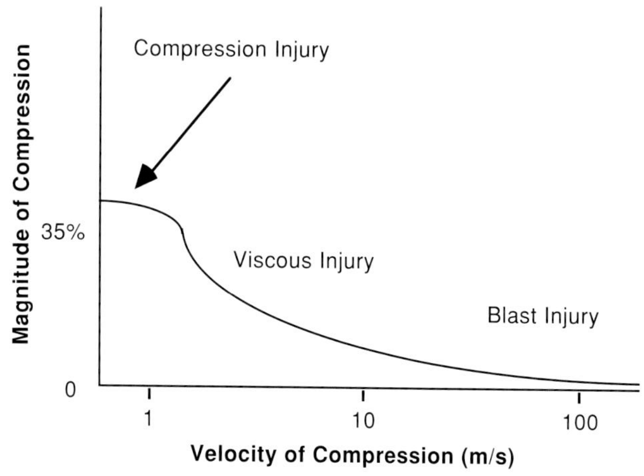

Fig. 19-1. In this depiction of the relation between the amount and the speed of compression, the curved line indicates a constant probability of the occurrence of a thoracic injury of a specified lethality. The magnitude of compression is given as the percentage of the anteroposterior diameter of the thorax. Data sources: (1) Viano DC, Lau IA. A viscous tolerance criterion for soft tissue injury assessment. *J Biomechanics.* 1988;21(5):387–399. (2) Viano DC. Live fire testing: Assessing blunt impact and acceleration injury vulnerabilities. *Milit Med.* 1991;156:589–595.

tion), a decrease in the thoracic anteroposterior diameter of at least one third must occur before there is a high risk of damage to internal viscera. However, when compression occurs at a faster velocity (> 3 m/s), the same injury can occur with much less compression. When compression is applied very slowly, the viscera have time to adjust to the distortion produced by their displacement. With more rapid compression, however, this compensation is impaired because it involves a time-dependent variable: namely, the internal displacement of layer upon layer of tissue as they slide over one another. The sliding is resisted by the inherent viscosity of the tissue much as a the viscosity of a flowing liquid causes hydraulic resistance. When the sliding cannot keep up with the velocity of compression, shearing forces arise that cause tissue laceration, rupture, or fractures. Such trauma, which results from a mechanical process that is determined by both the velocity of the compression and the viscoelasticity of the tissue, is known as a *viscous* injury.

Blast injury may be thought of as occupying the opposite end of the compression–velocity continuum depicted in Figure 19-1. With blast injury, the compression causes a tiny displacement (measured in a fraction of a millimeter) that occurs at a speed approaching that of sound. Blast overpressure is especially likely to injure very light, feebly supported structures such as the alveolar capillaries and tympanic membranes.

OVERVIEW OF COMBAT THORACIC TRAUMA

As seen in reports from three recent wars (the experience of the U.S. Army's 24th Evacuation Hospital in Vietnam[1]; Rambam Medical Center in Haifa, Israel[2]; and the Basrah, Iraq, Teaching Hospital in a 6-month period in 1981 during the Iran–Iraq War[3]), the most common thoracic clinical problems were combined hemothorax and pneumothorax, hemothorax, pneumothorax, pulmonary contusion, cardiac tamponade, pulmonary hematoma, rib or sternal fractures or both, perforation of the diaphragm, and laceration of the heart or great vessels (Table 19-2). These data clearly show that the most common medical treatment problems—collections of blood and air within the pleural space—are the result of pulmonary lacerations. It is important to recognize that the thoracic injury is unlikely to be the only injury present: 85% of the casualties in the 24th Evacuation Hospital report[1] and 80% of the casualties reported from Rambam[2] had one or more additional injuries involving another part of the body.

The specific nature of the medical interventions required to treat combat casualties with thoracic injuries is shown in Table 19-3. It is apparent that only a minority of thoracic casualties required a formal thoracotomy.

When treating a casualty with a thoracic injury, the military trauma anesthesiologist is much more likely to provide anesthesia for a major operation in some other body part than for an operation on the thorax. Published series, with the exception of the work of one surgeon in Lebanon (which is discussed below), indicate that a formal thoracotomy is needed in only about 10% to 20% of casualties with thoracic injuries who reach a military hospital alive.[8] In most thoracic casualties, the interventions required for the treatment of the thoracic injury consist of inserting a chest tube and providing local care to the wounds of entrance and exit. However, military trauma anesthesiologists should be aware that some thoracic surgeons perform what is really

TABLE 19-2

DIAGNOSIS OF THORACIC CASUALTIES

Diagnosis	24th Evac. Hospital US Army, Vietnam[1]	Rambam Medical Center Haifa, Israel[2]	Basrah Teaching Hospital, Iraq[3]
Combined hemo- and pneumothorax	230	15	
Hemothorax	199	9	81
Pneumothorax	100	13	37
Pulmonary contusion	99	5	20
Cardiac tamponade	7	1	4
Pulmonary hematoma		15	
Rib/sternal fractures		14	12*
Diaphragmatic perforation			17
Heart or great-vessel laceration			4

*Listed as flail chest

Data sources: (1) McNamara JJ, Messersmith JK, Dunn RA, Molot MD, Stremple JF. Thoracic injuries in combat casualties in Vietnam. Ann Thor Surg. 1970;10:389–401. (2) Rosenblatt M, Lemer M, Best LA, Peleg H. Thoracic wounds in Israeli battle casualties during the 1982 evacuation of wounded from Lebanon. J Trauma. 1985;25:350–354. (3) Suleman ND, Rasoul HA. War injuries of the chest. *Injury*. 1985;16:382–384.

a mini-thoracotomy when they carry out local wound management. Under general anesthesia, one or both wounds are extended so that it is possible to inspect the pleural space and lung and, if necessary, to repair accessible intrathoracic injuries.

Perhaps medical officers will need to reconsider the consensus that only a minority of thoracic casualties require a formal thoracotomy. The most compelling evidence stems from the experience of one civilian surgeon who treated 1,992 thoracic casualties of the civil war in Lebanon (1969–1982).[9] Of the casualties this surgeon treated, 282 had a cardiac injury, 1,251 had a noncardiac thoracic injury as the major treatment problem, and 456 had one or more injuries in addition to thoracic trauma. Of the noncardiac thoracic casualties, a formal thoracotomy

TABLE 19-3

THERAPEUTIC INTERVENTIONS IN THORACIC TRAUMA

Procedure	24th Evac. Hospital US Army, Vietnam[1]	Rambam Medical Center Haifa, Israel[2]	Basrah Teaching Hospital, Iraq[3]
Tube thoracostomy	448	38	113
Thoracotomy	78	6	11
Debridement of thoracic wounds		30	
Thoracentesis or no treatment	2	26	31
Major operation outside the thorax	~ 400	35	

Data sources: (1) McNamara JJ, Messersmith JK, Dunn RA, Molot MD, Stremple JF. Thoracic injuries in combat casualties in Vietnam. *Ann Thor Surg*. 1970;10:389–401. (2) Rosenblatt M, Lemer M, Best LA, Peleg H. Thoracic wounds in Israeli battle casualties during the 1982 evacuation of wounded from Lebanon. *J Trauma*. 1985;25:350–354. (3) Suleman ND, Rasoul HA. War injuries of the chest. *Injury*. 1985;16:382–384.

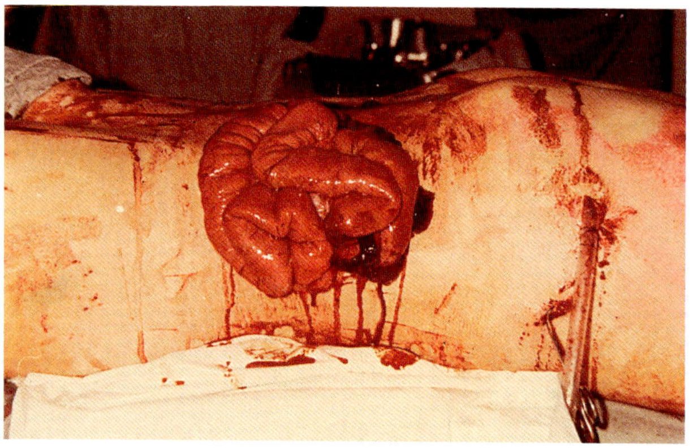

Fig. 19-2. A shell fragment entered this casualty's chest at the inferior-posterior portion of the left hemithorax at the site of the hemostat. It passed through the left lung, diaphragm, spleen, and small bowel before exiting through the left upper quadrant. The small bowel has eviscerated through the wound of exit. Notice that the chest tube is vented to the atmosphere. Suction applied to the tube would have caused ambient air to be sucked through the hole in the diaphragm into the thorax. Photograph: Wound Data and Munitions Effectiveness Team slide collection.

was performed in 818 (54.5% of the total procedures), and of these, an anatomical pulmonary resection was performed in 310. Although the U.S. Army Medical Department's experience during the Persian Gulf War was quite limited, anecdotal observations[10] from that war suggest that a greater fraction of thoracic casualties was treated by thoracotomy than during the Vietnam War. It is likely that in future wars, thoracotomy will increasingly be established as the standard of care for thoracic casualties.

Military trauma anesthesiologists need also to be aware of a variant of thoracic trauma: the thoracoabdominal injury (Figure 19-2). In about 10% of the casualties seen during World War II, the wounding missile was found to have passed from the chest through the diaphragm into the abdomen.[11] The vast experience of surgeons in World War II indicates that in most such casualties, the abdominal component was the more life threatening. This is probably because the casualties who had more-serious thoracic components died before they could be evacuated from the battlefield. The anesthetic management of the casualty with a thoracoabdominal wound will be similar to that of any abdominal casualty but with this important exception: unimpaired drainage of air and blood from the chest must be assured prior to the induction of anesthesia. Once the abdomen is opened, the hole in the diaphragm establishes a direct connection between the atmosphere and the left pleural space. Collapse of the left lung is prevented by positive-pressure ventilation through an endotracheal tube and a functioning chest tube.

GENERAL PRINCIPLES OF MANAGEMENT

Indications for Thoracotomy

Generally accepted indications for immediate or early thoracotomy are as follows[12]:

- an opacified hemothorax on the initial radiograph;
- initial drainage of 1,500 mL of blood, followed by 500 mL or more during the next hour;
- drainage of 200 to 300 mL of blood per hour for more than 4 hours;
- massive air leak with continuous bubbling throughout the respiratory cycle;
- radiographic evidence of massive pulmonary contusion or hematoma, with clinical and laboratory evidence of a life-threatening shunt or airway compromise secondary to bleeding into the airway; and
- physical signs of pericardial tamponade or suspicion of tamponade or shock, and radiographic evidence of a missile in proximity to the heart.

Most casualties with penetrating thoracic injuries will require some type of local wound management, which may or may not require general anesthesia. Casualties with large chest defects, such as would be associated with a sucking chest wound, will certainly require operative closure using general endotracheal anesthesia.

Preoperative Evaluation and Preparation

The U.S. Army Medical Department was one of the first supporters of the American College of

EXHIBIT 19-1

INITIAL MANAGEMENT OF TRAUMA VICTIMS

In the American College of Surgeons' Advanced Trauma Life Support (ATLS) approach, the initial management of the trauma victim is carried out in the following sequence, with the definitive-care phase being done later:

Primary Survey
- *A*irway management with cervical spine control
- *B*reathing and ventilation
- *C*irculation with hemorrhage control
- *N*eurological status
- *E*xposure

Resuscitation, including
- Inserting airways, chest tubes, and large-bore intravenous lines
- Infusing crystalloid fluid
- Obtaining blood samples
- Inserting urinary and gastric catheters
- Establishing vital-sign monitors
- Obtaining appropriate radiographic studies

Secondary Survey
- History
- Physical examination, including the following areas:
  - Head
  - Maxillae and face
  - Cervical spine and neck
  - Chest
  - Abdomen
  - Perineum/rectum/vagina
  - Musculoskeletal system
  - Neurological systems
- Additional laboratory and radiographic studies as needed

Source: Committee on Trauma, American College of Surgeons. Initial assessment and management. In: *Advanced Trauma Life Support Program for Physicians: Instructor Manual.* 5th ed. Chicago, Ill: American College of Surgeons; 1993: 17–37.

Surgeons' Advanced Trauma Life Support (ATLS) approach to the initial management of the trauma victim and has long emphasized such training—especially for medical personnel assigned to the field echelons. Military anesthesiologists serving at third- or fourth-echelon hospitals should, therefore, expect to find that the acute lifesaving interventions—the ATLS ABCs (airway, breathing, and circulation)—have already been performed before the casualty arrives at their hospital (Exhibit 19-1). Nevertheless, there are exceptions. In fact, during much of the Vietnam War, given the atrophy of the unit and division echelons of care, casualties commonly arrived at third-echelon hospitals without having received any care.[13] An equivalent situation—the lack of a mature field medical system—will likely exist in the future whenever the U.S. military becomes involved in peacekeeping or nation-building missions. As a member of the medical unit, the anesthesia provider should be involved in the resuscitation the moment the patient arrives to the receiving area.

After the initial management has been performed, the military anesthesiologist will be involved in the definitive care phase of management. Because the definitive-care phase may involve an emergency thoracotomy, the anesthesia provider should perform a specific preanesthesia evaluation only if time permits. In the conscious patient, a brief history and physical examination should be taken (Exhibit 19-2); laboratory investigation should include recent arterial blood-gas and hematocrit levels.

Because time is of the essence when dealing with trauma patients, it is important to have a resuscitation area and an operating room prepared to manage a trauma victim. The anesthesia machine and monitors should be ready for immediate use. Intravenous tubing and fluid warmers should be available for use, requiring only priming with the intravenous fluid when the patient arrives. Syringes should be labeled and cardiac drugs immediately available. A functioning defibrillator should also be ready.

The essential step that must be taken in preparing the casualty with thoracic injuries for general anesthesia, especially when the operation also involves another part of the body, is to assure that the potential for the development of an intraoperative hemothorax or pneumothorax is minimized by the placement of a functioning chest tube. Finally, it cannot be stressed too greatly that the military trauma anesthesiologist managing the casualty with a penetrating thoracic injury will constantly strive to keep the airway free of secretions.

Monitoring

In addition to the usual noninvasive monitors (electrocardiograph, pulse oximeter, end-tidal CO_2 monitor, automatic blood pressure cuff, precordial stethoscope), arterial, central venous pressure, and urinary output monitoring are essential. However, precious time should not be spent attempting to place these monitors in unstable, exsanguinating patients.

Induction of Anesthesia

Unconscious, moribund patients are intubated immediately without anesthesia, and surgery is performed without anesthesia until the patient's vital signs or state of consciousness indicate a need for anesthesia. The anesthesiologist is performing a resuscitation in this scenario, rather than an anesthetic. Concerns about possible intraoperative recall may be overstated: providing an ideal, complete anesthetic to a trauma patient at the risk of hemodynamic instability and possible cardiac arrest is inappropriate. Scopolamine may be administered as an amnestic agent, but valuable time should not be spent to locate or administer this drug when other, more-important lifesaving tasks need to be performed. Midazolam may be used but its hypotensive effect, particularly in the presence of hypovolemia or when given concurrently with narcotics, may preclude its use in the trauma patient. Patients in a state of shock are particularly susceptible to the adverse effects of thiobarbiturates, which should be administered only with extreme caution. To allow the surgeon to arrest hemorrhage, ketamine has been advocated as the drug of choice for induction of anesthesia in hypovolemic, hemorrhaging patients who require anesthesia (for further discussion, see Chapter 10, Intravenous Anesthesia). However, the direct myocardial-depressant effects of ketamine may be unmasked in the patient who is severely physically stressed and is relying on maximal intrinsic catecholamine secretion to maintain adequate vital signs. In most cases, though, the anesthesiologist will have had sufficient time to replace intravascular fluid deficits; therefore, thiobarbiturates or other induction agents can safely be used. Trauma is frequently associated with decreased gastric emptying, which places these patients at greater risk of aspiration pneumonitis; a rapid-sequence induction after preoxygenation is usually indicated. An awake intubation must certainly be considered in patients with obvious or suspected airway abnormalities.

EXHIBIT 19-2

HISTORY AND PHYSICAL EXAMINATION OF THE CONSCIOUS PATIENT

Brief history:

1. Review of systems
2. Past medical history
3. Past surgical history
4. Previous anesthesia difficulties
5. Family history of anesthetic complications
6. Current medications
7. Allergies
8. Time of last oral intake

Brief physical examination:

1. Global assessment
2. Evaluation of the airway
3. Respiratory and cardiovascular examinations
4. Vital signs

Maintenance of Anesthesia

Successful resuscitation of patients with major chest trauma requires teamwork; blood and fluid replacement must be prompt and given in appropriate quantities. If patients do not respond to volume replacement, then ongoing hemorrhage, tension pneumothorax, or pericardial tamponade must be suspected. Loss of infused fluid through an undiagnosed hole in the superior or inferior vena cava may explain why some patients fail to respond to fluid therapy. After the surgeon has entered the chest cavity, compression of the aorta above the site of bleeding may provide the valuable time needed to restore blood volume. Although patients in shock require little, if any, anesthesia, their consciousness rapidly returns when the blood volume is restored. At this point, anesthesia can be maintained with oxygen, narcotics, neuromuscular blocking drugs, amnestics, and small quantities of inhalational agents, if required. It is prudent to avoid nitrous oxide in patients with chest trauma because the gas tends to collect in the dependent areas of the lung. The risk is that nitrous oxide will expand in the closed chest and create a pneumothorax. (Nitrous oxide is not available in deployable hospitals.)

Special considerations with the use of neuromuscular blocking agents in the trauma patient deserve mention. Succinylcholine, the rapid-acting depolarizing relaxant often used for rapid-sequence inductions, is known to cause profound hyperkalemia in patients who have extensive muscle damage, particularly if the drug is given 24 to 36 hours after the traumatic insult. Alternatives include the nondepolarizing relaxants, such as vecuronium given at 0.28 mg/kg, for conditions requiring rapid intubation. This agent is useful during the maintenance of anesthesia because it has minimal hemodynamic effects. The vagolytic actions of pancuronium may be undesirable because the tachycardia may lead to further confusion in distinguishing drug effect from hypovolemia or inadequate levels of anesthesia. *d*-Tubocurarine and atracurium should probably be avoided because of their histamine-mediated hypotensive effects. It is important to remember that all neuromuscular blocking agents are subject to aberrant behavior in the presence of changing acid–base status, altered metabolism and excretion, hypothermia, and certain antibiotics. For this reason, it is mandatory to monitor the status of the neuromuscular blockade.

Hypothermia is a major problem in traumatized patients undergoing exploratory surgery, and every effort should be made to maintain a normal core body temperature. Heated humidifiers, low gas flows, warmed intravenous and irrigating fluids, and a warmed operating room can help maintain normothermia. Certainly, heating lamps, warming blankets, and plastic to wrap exposed body surfaces can also be used.

Positioning for Operation

The position of patients with thoracic injuries (whose major injury does not involve the thorax) will obviously depend on the location of that injury; the usual position will be with the trunk supine. The position of casualties who are to have an actual thoracic procedure will depend on the indication for the operation. Most thoracic surgeons use an anterolateral incision for the casualty who is *agonal* (ie, a casualty who exhibited one or more signs of life [motion, spontaneous respiration, palpable pulse] shortly before arrival at the hospital, but who is now lifeless) or in profound shock, although a few prefer a median sternotomy for the operative approach. Thus, the desired position for an emergency operation is supine. Because the needed operation is best done through a posterolateral thoracotomy incision with the patient in the right lateral decubitus position, there are two exceptions to this rule:

1. the unusual casualty who is known to have an injury to the proximal left subclavian artery, and
2. the casualty who has sustained blunt trauma to the chest and has radiographic evidence of a left hemothorax and a widened superior mediastinum, and who, therefore, may have a proximal descending aortic disruption.

Patients who are undergoing thoracic surgery in which the indications are less emergent (eg, control of nonexsanguinating hemorrhage, a large air leak, repair of a chest-wall defect, or simply to debride the wounds of entrance or exit) are placed in the decubitus position so that a posterolateral incision can be made. Care must be taken to ensure that there is no pressure on the brachial plexus of the dependent arm, and that the thorax and abdominal wall are free to move without restricting respirations. Endotracheal tube position and the position of all monitors must be checked for dislodgement following patient positioning. Patients with concurrent orthopedic injuries may be difficult to position because of pain and the potential for dislocation or worsening of the injury.

Postoperative Care

Most patients presenting for surgery secondary to battlefield chest trauma require postoperative care in an intensive care unit until an adequate level of physiological homeostasis can be achieved. The military trauma anesthesiologist is expected to play a significant role in the postoperative care of these patients, especially in the realm of acute pain and ventilatory management.[14]

DIAGNOSIS AND MANAGEMENT OF SPECIFIC INJURIES

Rib Fractures

The ribs are the most commonly injured component of the thoracic cage, and the incidence of serious complications increases with the number of ribs fractured. This increase is a reflection of the greater traumatic forces associated with multiple rib fractures. As a general rule, a young, otherwise healthy, active-duty recruit with a flexible chest wall is less likely to sustain a rib fracture than is a geriatric patient with thoracic trauma. With this in mind, the presence of multiple rib fractures in young patients implies a sizable transfer of force. Multiple rib fractures most commonly involve the seventh through tenth ribs and thus are often associated with hepatic or splenic lacerations. Acute gastric dilation commonly accompanies left-sided fractures and may increase the likelihood of acid aspiration. Fractures of the upper ribs (first through third) should be regarded as harbingers of serious blunt trauma to the chest. The bony framework of the upper limb and its muscular attachments provide a barrier to injury in this area. Therefore, severe maxillofacial, cervical, neurological, pulmonary, and vascular injuries may accompany upper-rib fractures.[15]

Rib fractures, even in the absence of underlying cardiopulmonary trauma, may contribute to serious pulmonary complications. The associated pain and reflex muscle splinting can exacerbate alveolar hypoventilation, resulting in retention of secretions, atelectasis, and respiratory failure. Taping or binding the ribs will cause even more splinting and further compromise. A tidal volume of less than 5 mL/kg or a forced vital capacity of less than 10 mL/kg indicates severe splinting.[16] Adequate analgesia is essential in the management of rib fractures. The use of intercostal nerve blocks is attractive because it avoids the respiratory depression associated with systemic narcotic administration. Comparable analgesia of longer duration and with less potential for systemic toxicity may be achieved with continuous thoracic epidural analgesia. Intrapleural injection of local anesthetics is another form of analgesia for rib fractures. The efficacy of this technique, however, is controversial at this time.

Flail Chest

Flail chest may be defined as an abnormal movement of the chest wall occurring as a result of fractures of three or more ribs in two places on the same side. This produces a segment of the chest wall that responds to changes in pleural pressure, as opposed to the muscular action of the chest wall, resulting in a paradoxical respiratory pattern. This injury is most commonly associated with blunt trauma to the chest wall and involves the anterolateral aspect of the chest. The posterior wall is rarely involved because it is heavily fortified with muscle. The flail chest injury is rarely isolated and is usually an ominous sign, indicating serious underlying injuries to intrathoracic or intraabdominal organs or both. This condition is often difficult to diagnose and may go unnoticed for extended periods, often overshadowed by more-overt injuries. Chest radiography may not reveal fractures unless the films are overpenetrated and oblique views are taken. Flail chest may not be apparent on simple inspection, as chest-wall muscular spasm may be able to splint the segment until the muscles become fatigued. Palpation is more likely to be diagnostic than inspection, with the presence of crepitus and abnormal respiratory motion aiding in the diagnosis. Serial blood-gas measurements can help establish the diagnosis, because the clinical hallmark of flail chest is *hypoxemia*.

Flail chest can cause hypoxemia by two mechanisms: (1) intrapulmonary shunting due to perfusion of the poorly ventilated, contused lung; and (2) atelectasis caused by compromised ventilatory mechanics. The pendelluft phenomenon, which is a to-and-fro movement of air from the damaged to the normal lung, was once thought to make a significant contribution to hypoxemia. However, it has been shown that there is an increase in ventilation and improved gas exchange on the injured side.[17]

The hypoxia observed in flail chest is now recognized to be caused by abnormalities in the contused lung underlying the flail segment.[18] Thus, the modern treatment of flail chest focuses on preventing the arterial desaturation (that results from the shunting) from reaching life-threatening proportions. Stabilization of the flail segment, maintenance of adequate ventilation, oxygen enrichment, physical therapy, and effective pain relief should all be tried; however, a period of intubation and ventilation may be necessary. The criteria for intubation, which should only serve as a guide, include:

- partial pressure of arterial oxygen (Pa_{O_2}) < 70 mm Hg with oxygen enrichment,

- partial pressure of arterial carbon dioxide ($Paco_2$) > 50 mm Hg,
- pH < 7.25,
- tachypnea > 30/min,
- vital capacity < 15 mL/kg, and
- negative inspiratory force < –20 cm water.

Both external stabilization of the flail segment by traction and internal fixation with intramedullary pinning of the fractured ribs have been described.[19,20] Continuous electrocardiographic monitoring is essential because flail chest can often be associated with cardiac contusions, from which arrhythmias may arise. Frequent arterial blood-gas analyses, along with other laboratory studies, justify placing an arterial line. Pulmonary artery catheterization, which may be available in deployable hospitals, may help with the evaluation of cardiac performance and guide fluid management. This is especially necessary because the injured lung underlying the flail segment is sensitive to both underresuscitation of shock and fluid overload, the latter condition leading to pulmonary edema in the injured lung tissue and a further impairment of gas exchange.[21] In intubated, ventilated patients, excessive airway pressure can also cause an iatrogenic injury by mechanically disrupting damaged alveolar capillary membranes in the lung underlying the flail segment. This may enlarge the volume of the contusion, but a more serious problem is the increased likelihood of systemic air embolism.[22]

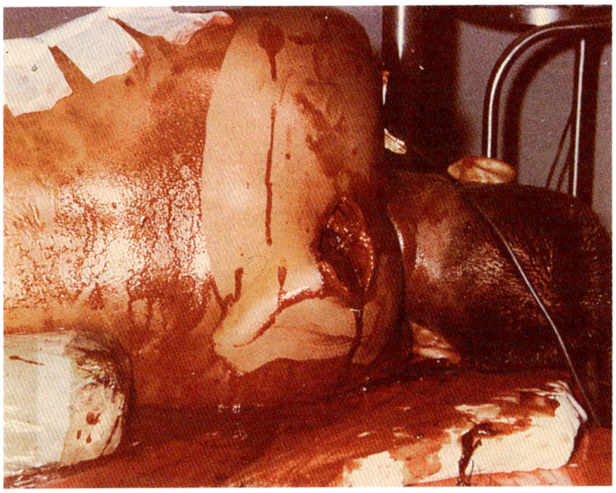

Fig. 19-3. This casualty had a sucking chest wound. A large fragment entered his back; frothy material can be seen in the base of the wound. Photograph: Wound Data and Munitions Effectiveness Team slide collection.

Sucking Chest Wound

An open, sucking, or blowing chest wound is a serious injury that is usually found at the site where a yawing or tumbling bullet has exited or where a large fragment from an explosive munition has entered. The most serious component of the wound is usually the injury to the underlying lung. The characteristic appearance is of bloody foam being alternately sucked into and blown from the wound (Figure 19-3). In this condition, intrapleural pressure equalizes with the atmosphere, resulting in a diminished movement of air on the affected side. The immediate treatment of this condition is to occlude the defect but provide for egress of air from the chest cavity by inserting a chest tube with a one-way valve. Sucking chest wounds are not especially common among combat casualties. In the Israeli series, they accounted for only seven (11%) of the total of the thoracic casualties.[2] The reason for their low prevalence is that the intrathoracic component of the injury is much more likely to be life-threatening than is the hole itself. Once the intrathoracic component has been treated, surgical treatment is directed toward achieving an air-tight closure of the chest wall defect.

Acute Traumatic Hemothorax

Hemothorax can occur with both penetrating and nonpenetrating thoracic trauma and is usually caused by blood emanating from injuries of the heart, great vessels, pulmonary parenchyma, or chest wall.[23] The diagnosis of hemothorax is made on the basis of history and clinical examination of the chest. When a significant quantity of blood has accumulated in the chest cavity, the trachea may be deviated, the chest wall is dull to percussion, and breath sounds are diminished on auscultation. A chest radiograph and an electrocardiogram should be obtained for all patients except those presenting in extremis. Approximately 500 mL of blood must accumulate in the chest cavity before it is radiologically detectable.

Because hypovolemia from blood loss is the most common problem in patients who present with significant chest injury, the immediate treatment should be directed toward restoring blood volume. Two large-bore intravenous cannulae should be inserted as soon as possible. Central venous pressure monitoring may be useful in both diagnosing and managing patients who have mechanical interference with ventilation, as the central venous pressure is low in the presence of severe hypovolemia but elevated in the presence of a chest cavity full of blood. Oxygen therapy is mandatory. Tube thoracostomy should be performed as soon as possible because it is not only therapeutic, it also provides an assessment of cumulative and ongoing blood loss, facilitates reexpansion of the lung, and simplifies autotransfusion when major bleeding is encountered. In most cases, the source of the bleeding is the pulmonary vessels, which normally have low perfusion pressures. On the other hand, bleeding from systemic vessels or the heart is usually more persistent and voluminous.

For casualties who have an indication for operative intervention but who are stable (ie, blood pressure > 100 mm Hg, pulse rate < 100, good peripheral perfusion and ventilation), the thoracotomy is performed in the operating room. Immediate thoracotomy in the admitting area of the hospital may be indicated in patients who become agonal on arrival. The best results have been obtained in casualties who have penetrating thoracic injuries, and the poorest results in those sustaining blunt trauma—especially when the abdomen is involved. Regardless of the etiology, survival in this group of casualties is poor. In one recent series,[24] survival was 6% in those with blunt trauma and 27% for casualties with penetrating wounds of the chest.

The reasons for performing a thoracotomy are to

- decompress a tension pneumothorax or pericardial tamponade, if present;
- perform open-chest cardiac massage; and
- stop bleeding if it arises within the thorax or, by occluding the descending aorta, to slow bleeding if it arises from the abdomen.

After the airway has been intubated, if necessary via cricothyroidotomy, an anterolateral incision is made on the side of injury, the pericardial sac opened, and cardiac compressions begun. Bleeding sites are controlled by direct pressure or by application of a clamp or Rommel tourniquet around the hilum of the lung. The military trauma anesthesiologist should anticipate the need to correct severe metabolic acidosis and to manage a variety of malignant cardiac arrhythmias. The patient is then transported to the operating room for definitive treatment.

The management of agonal casualties is very labor and resource intensive. The likely poor outcome, even with the best of care, has led some authorities[25] to argue that emergency thoracotomy for agonal victims of truncal trauma has no place in combat casualty care. The military trauma anesthesiologist, in consultation with the hospital thoracic or trauma surgeon and the hospital commander, should develop an agreed-upon triage policy for such casualties. By necessity, any such policy will have to take account of the existing tactical situation.

Cardiac Tamponade

Although cardiac tamponade is found in casualties who require emergency thoracotomy, its occurrence is not limited to this group. In some casualties, the presentation of cardiac tamponade may be quite subtle (Figure 19-4). Acute, traumatic pericardial tamponade is caused by the collection of blood or other fluid (eg, serous exudate) within an intact pericardial sac. This sac is composed of a fibrous, poorly compliant membrane. Rapid accumulation of 100 to 200 mL of fluid in this closed space restricts filling of the cardiac chambers during diastole, which produces a fixed, low, cardiac output. Positive-pressure ventilation will lower cardiac output even further, as will any cardiac depressant.

The diagnosis of cardiac tamponade requires a high degree of clinical suspicion. It should always be suspected in patients with wounds in the vicinity of the neck, precordium, or upper abdomen, and

Fig. 19-4. (**a**) This casualty was wounded when a grenade fragment penetrated his back. He was initially neither hypotensive nor in much distress but while being observed developed tachycardia, dyspnea, and distended neck veins. (**b**) The chest radiograph shows a fragment within the silhouette of a globular-shaped heart. A thoracotomy was performed because of the casualty's deteriorating clinical state and the appearance of the radiograph. (**c**) The pericardium has been opened and several blood clots have been extruded. (**d**) The removed clots. (**e**) A small defect, which was not then bleeding, in the free wall of the left ventricle. (**f**) The fragment after its removal from the myocardium. The tip of the hemostat serves as a reference for size. The left ventricular wall had not been perforated, possibly because of the fragment's small size. Other fragments lacerated the stomach and spleen; these were found during a subsequent laparotomy. Photographs: Swan Vietnam Surgical Slide Collection.

a

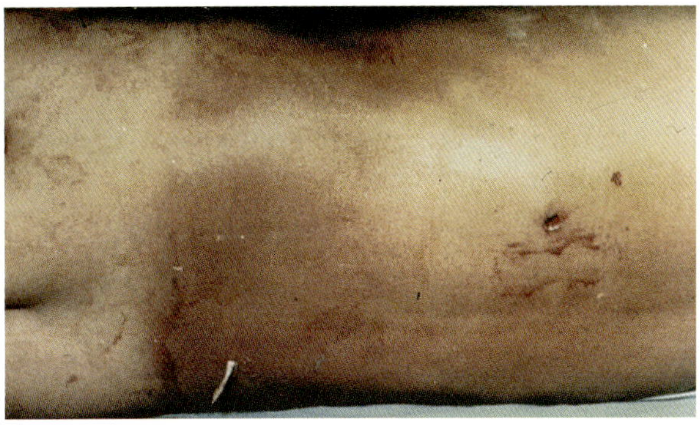

b

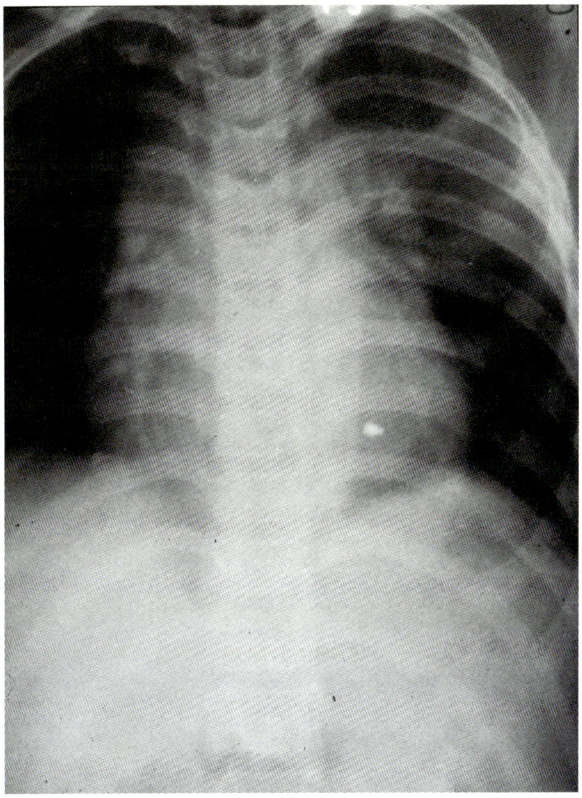

c

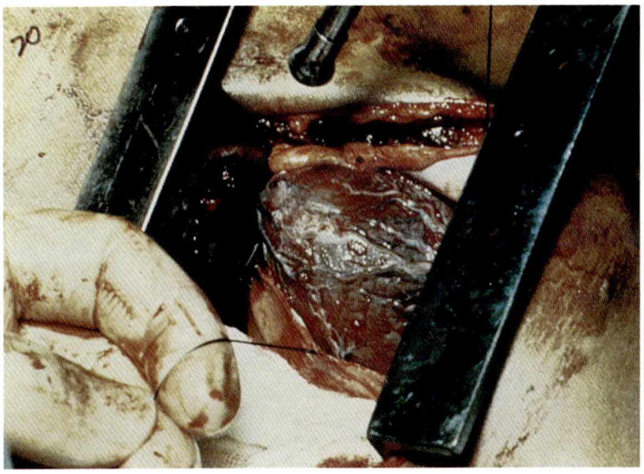

d

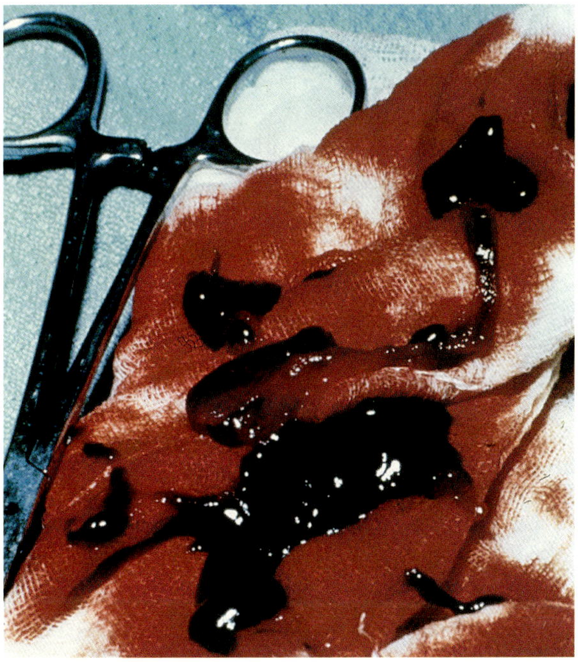

e

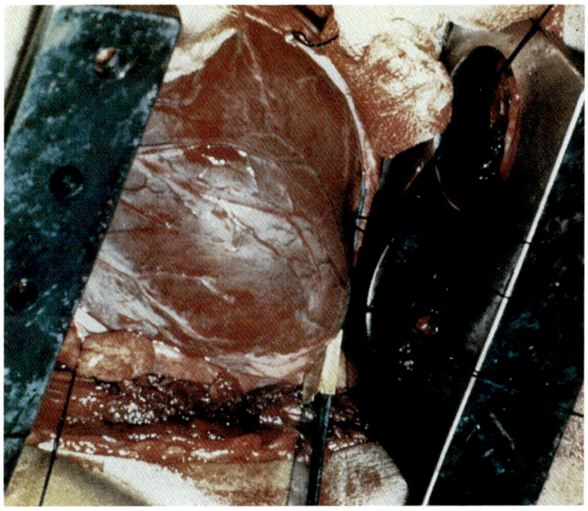

f

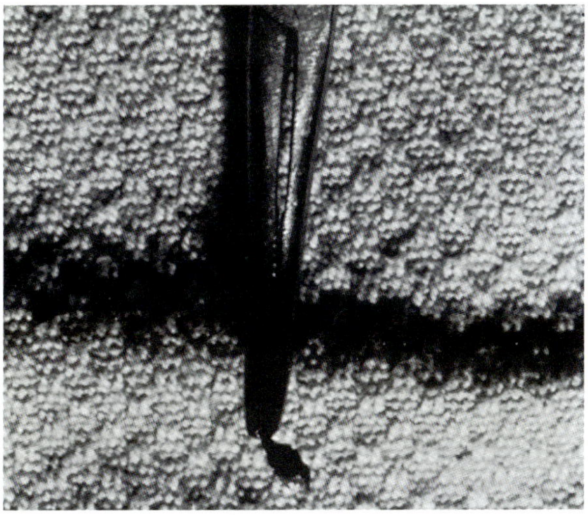

especially in patients who are in shock. The classic signs, although present in only 41% of patients with penetrating cardiac wounds,[26] include Beck's triad: hypotension, distended neck veins, and distant heart sounds. Other signs include pulsus paradoxus, which is a decline in systolic blood pressure of 10 mm Hg or more on inspiration. This is of limited value in the field, however, as continuous arterial pressure monitoring may not be possible.[27] Paradoxical filling of neck veins on inspiration (Kussmaul's sign) may be too subtle to detect in uncooperative, struggling patients. If significant blood loss has occurred, distension of neck veins may not occur. Equalization of pressures across the heart, measured by a pulmonary artery catheter, is very suggestive of tamponade. The chest radiograph may reveal a large, globular heart shadow, and the electrocardiogram will be either normal or show nonspecific ischemic changes. Occasionally, the electrocardiogram will show electrical alternans, which is usually diagnostic of tamponade.

Again, it should be emphasized that heavy reliance is placed on clinical impression in diagnosing patients on the battlefield with cardiac tamponade. *Shock and a wound in the anterior chest indicate cardiac tamponade until proven otherwise.* Elevation of the central venous pressure is strong confirmatory evidence of the diagnosis, and treatment should be started immediately. The definitive treatment of this condition is surgery as soon as possible. Pericardiocentesis may be used to relieve the tamponade in rapidly deteriorating patients. However, this is of limited value because blood rapidly reaccumulates in the pericardial sac.

The patient should be prepared and draped for surgery, and an arterial line should be inserted prior to the induction of anesthesia. *The administration of a general anesthetic to a patient with a significant tamponade is potentially lethal.*[28,29] Almost any maneuver, other than administration of 100% oxygen, including positive-pressure ventilation, causes deterioration.[30] Inhalational agents or thiopental cause further cardiac depression and impairment of diastolic filling. Peripheral vasodilation associated with these agents further impairs filling. Anesthetic goals include maintaining adequate preload with copious volume infusion (central venous pressure at least 15 cm H_2O), and avoiding vagotonic medications (eg, narcotics). It is important to maintain sinus tachycardia in the face of limited stroke volume to maximize cardiac output. The combination of ketamine and pancuronium is ideal for this purpose. The recommended dose of ketamine for patients with diminished cardiac output is 0.25 to 0.50 mg/kg. Despite careful anesthetic management, the patient's condition may deteriorate before the tamponade is relieved. If deterioration occurs, isoproterenol has been advocated,[31] infused at a rate of 0.1 µg/kg/min, and titrated to effect. When the pericardium is decompressed, the patient's vital signs usually improve instantaneously.

Cardiac Contusions

Myocardial contusion is the most common cardiac injury due to nonpenetrating trauma. Depending on the sophistication of the diagnostic armamentarium and the definition of the condition, cardiac contusions have been reported in approximately 15% to 70% of trauma patients who sustain blunt chest trauma. Rapid deceleration occurring during motor vehicle accidents is the most common cause of cardiac contusions. The heart is subjected to marked anteroposterior compression resulting in rupture of the intramyocardial vessels, which bleed into the myocardium. Subsequently, myocytes may die and undergo fragmentation. Iatrogenic trauma caused by closed-chest massage during cardiopulmonary resuscitation may also be responsible for myocardial contusion. The right ventricle is injured more frequently than the left during cardiopulmonary resuscitation, due to its proximity to the chest wall. However, the valves in the left side of the heart, especially the aortic valve, are more susceptible to injury than those in the right side of the heart.[16]

Symptoms of myocardial contusion may be similar to those of myocardial infarction or pericarditis, because anginal chest pain is the most common presenting complaint. However, contusion pain is not relieved by nitroglycerin. Many trauma patients with myocardial contusion report few or no symptoms from their cardiac injuries. Ventricular arrhythmias are the most common clinical sign of cardiac contusion. Conduction disturbances are more commonly associated with injuries to the right atrium and ventricle.[32] Other signs may be a current of injury on the electrocardiogram or a pericardial friction rub; there may be no change at all in cardiac examination. The diagnosis of cardiac contusion can be a real dilemma for the clinician, as most routine and sophisticated tests have proven unreliable.

Casualties presenting with myocardial contusion should be treated in the same manner as those presenting with myocardial infarctions. Many casualties with this condition need immediate surgery to treat their other injuries. Because the right ventricle is particularly vulnerable to contusion owing to its proximity to the anterior chest wall, right ventricular dysfunction and failure may complicate perioperative management. The right ventricle is sensitive to afterload; therefore, conditions that may increase pulmonary vascular resistance (ie, hypoxia, hypercarbia) should be avoided. Adequate preload is usually necessary in the setting of right ventricular dysfunction; intravascular volume resuscitation is therefore mandatory.

Cardiac Rupture

Rupture of the heart is a common cause of immediate death in victims of blunt trauma. In nonpenetrating injuries, severe compression may so raise cardiac chamber pressure and wall stress that the myocardium ruptures. Thus, the mechanism is similar to the process that gives rise to myocardial contusion. Puncture of the heart by ribs broken by blunt trauma has also been described. In combat casualties, penetrating injuries are a more frequent cause of cardiac perforations than is blunt trauma. Although right ventricular perforations may appear to predominate, a comparable incidence of left ventricular injuries has been described.[33] Because of the higher immediate mortality associated with ventricular trauma, patients with atrial perforations are more frequently encountered in the operating room.

The clinical presentation of cardiac rupture or perforation is determined by the status of the pericardium. With an open pericardial wound, blood extravasating from the heart drains freely into the pleural space, producing a rapidly fatal hemothorax. If the pericardial defect is small, or if it is occluded (as may happen on rare occasions by clotted blood or by the adjacent lung), the patient may not exsanguinate but live long enough to develop the signs of cardiac tamponade. The anesthetic management of cardiac rupture is similar to that for pericardial tamponade, except that exsanguination makes emergency thoracotomy more common.

Cardiopulmonary bypass, although usually not available in combat zone hospitals, may be required to repair some cardiac defects. Although traumatic ventricular septal defects may close spontaneously, most of them require surgical closure through the left ventricle, utilizing cardiopulmonary bypass.

Vasodilators often produce some degree of clinical and hemodynamic improvement. However, it should be emphasized that vasodilators are contraindicated in severely hypovolemic patients.

Injuries to the Coronary Arteries

The incidence of coronary artery laceration following penetrating cardiac injuries has been reported[34] to be about 4%. Division of a coronary artery invariably leads to hemorrhage and tamponade, and may cause myocardial infarction. Because the right coronary artery is protected by the sternum, most injuries involve the left coronary artery or its branches. Coronary artery occlusion after blunt chest trauma has been reported.[35] In these cases, myocardial infarctions evolved after the traumatic injury in patients without preexisting coronary atherosclerosis.

Several mechanisms may be involved in the pathogenesis of myocardial infarction after blunt chest trauma. In perhaps the simplest scenario, the forces accompanying an episode of blunt trauma could dislodge a previously adherent intramural plaque, resulting in intraluminal obstruction of the involved coronary artery.[36] Patients with preexisting atherosclerotic heart disease also may be at increased risk for infarction because of trauma-induced hemorrhage into a plaque, which is known to be richly vascularized with fragile, thin-walled capillaries.[37] A third possible mechanism of ischemic injury is trauma-induced coronary vasospasm. Although spasm also occurs in normal vessels, angiographically visualized spasm often occurs at a site of atherosclerotic narrowing.[38] Other etiologies of traumatic infarction include coronary thrombosis due to vascular trauma, direct transection of the coronary arteries, coronary embolization, and dissecting aneurysm.[39]

In the absence of cardiac tamponade, the anesthetic management of these casualties should be similar to that for patients with coronary artery disease with unstable angina. A variety of techniques are consistent with the hemodynamic goals of avoiding tachycardia and extremes of blood pressure. In young soldiers with good ventricular function, a combined technique with high-dose narcotics and an inhalational anesthetic agent is ideal: intraoperative sympathetic reflexes are reliably blunted, while myocardial contractility and oxygen consumption are appropriately depressed. Although there may be no ideal induction technique for the patient with ischemic heart disease and a full stomach, a moderate dose of narcotic (eg, 10–15 µg/kg fentanyl) combined with etomidate (0.1–0.2 mg/kg) and succinylcholine results in a stable induction, with adequate blunting of autonomic responses to laryngoscopy. In the setting of severe skeletal muscle injury, particularly if more than 24 to 36 hours have elapsed since the injury, nondepolarizing relaxants may be preferable because of the possibility of succinylcholine-induced hyperkalemia.

The common presentation of the casualty with a coronary artery injury caused by penetrating trauma is pericardial tamponade. Because direct repair of the arterial laceration in a beating heart is usually not feasible, and because the cardiopulmonary bypass apparatus that would allow the construction of an aortocoronary saphenous graph bypass is not likely to be available in field hospitals, the military surgeon has little option but to ligate the injured artery. Given this circumstance, the military trauma anesthesiologist should be prepared to treat potentially life-threatening cardiac arrhythmias and cardiogenic shock.

Injuries to the Great Vessels

The thoracic aorta can be injured as a result of penetrating or blunt trauma to the chest. The resulting hemorrhage is usually devastating, allowing only approximately 15% of patients to reach a field hospital alive.[40]

In the U.S. military, the great majority of aortic ruptures result from motor vehicle accidents and airplane crashes. Abrupt deceleration of the thorax (*a*) causes compression and displacement of the heart and (*b*) creates shearing and bending stresses in the aortic wall, which are greatest at the origin of the subclavian artery and, in the ascending aorta, at the level of the coronary arteries.[41] A minority of these patients (perhaps 10%) survive because of containment and tamponade of the hemorrhage by adjacent mediastinal structures. In the proximal descending aorta, the aortic adventitia may remain intact and temporarily prevent exsanguination. Sudden aortic rupture may develop in these patients at a later time.

Penetrating chest trauma may also involve the great vessels. Depending on whether the vessels are injured at an intrapericardial or an extrapericardial location, the clinical presentation is usually one of acute tamponade or massive hemothorax. These casualties may have sustained one or more penetrating cardiac injuries as well, but severe hypovolemia may account for the frequently atypical hemodynamic findings.

The clinical findings of aortic rupture include the diagnostic triad that is seen in more than 50% of cases[42]:

- increased arterial pressure and pulse amplitude in the upper extremities,
- decreased pressure and pulse amplitude in the lower extremities, and
- a widened superior mediastinum seen on the chest radiograph.

Other clinical and radiographic findings are included in Exhibit 19-3. An active search for these clinical and radiographic findings is important during evaluation because as many as one third of patients with aortic rupture have minimal or no external signs of chest trauma.[43,44]

When dealing with injuries to the major thoracic vessels, the foremost goal of the anesthesiologist is to simply maintain an adequate blood volume, which allows the surgeon the time needed to find the source of bleeding and, if possible, to repair the injured vessel. Ischemia of the abdominal viscera and spinal cord may occur during the period of proximal aortic clamping; the reported incidence of

EXHIBIT 19-3

CLINICAL AND RADIOGRAPHIC FINDINGS OF AORTIC RUPTURE

Clinical:

Increased arterial pressure and pulse amplitude of upper extremities
Decreased arterial pressure and pulse amplitude of lower extremities
Retrosternal or interscapular pain
Hoarseness
Systolic flow murmur over the precordium or medial to the left scapula
Neurological deficits in the lower extremities

Radiographic:

Widened mediastinum
Unsharp aortic contours
Widened paraspinal interfaces
Opacified pulmonary window
Broadened paratracheal stripe
Displacement of the left main-stem bronchus
Rightward deviation of the esophagus
Sternal or upper-rib fractures or both
Left hemothorax

paraplegia in survivors ranges from 1.0% to 11.7%.[41] Prophylactic measures for preserving spinal cord viability include partial cardiopulmonary bypass, heparin-coated shunts, partial bypass of the left side of the heart, draining the cerebrospinal fluid, and inducing systemic hypothermia.

The presumed mechanism of paraplegia in these patients is ischemia of the spinal cord caused by damage to the intercostal vessels that supply the spinal cord. Monitoring of somatosensory evoked potentials may be useful in heralding spinal cord ischemia but is not practicable in field hospitals.[45]

The kidney is the abdominal organ at greatest risk for ischemic injury during the period of aortic occlusion. Preserving distal perfusion with shunts or partial bypass is associated with a lower incidence of postoperative renal dysfunction; however, because the needed equipment is not available in the field, the military trauma anesthesiologist has no other recourse than to use mannitol, renal-dose dopamine, and/or diuretics as part of a strategy for renal protection similar to that used for abdominal aortic aneurysm surgery.[46]

Intraoperative monitoring should include placing a right radial arterial line and a lower-extremity arterial line for monitoring distal aortic pressure. The surgeon's possible clamping of the left subclavian artery would make monitoring the left radial arterial pressure impossible during that time. In all but the most emergent cases, pulmonary arterial catheterization is desirable because proximal aortic occlusion imposes a severe afterload stress on the left ventricle.

A double-lumen endotracheal tube is desirable because it allows the left lung to be collapsed to facilitate surgical exposure. Equally important, however, is the fact that the dependent right lung can be isolated from the parenchymal hemorrhage that may occur in the left lung as a result of pulmonary contusion.

Pneumothorax

Pneumothorax occurs secondary to blunt or penetrating trauma to the chest wall. Less obvious pneumothoraces occur as a result of penetration of the chest wall and lung by sharp objects, such as bullets, knives, or rib fragments. Pneumothoraces of less than 20% are usually not clinically detectable. Patients may complain of chest pain, which is accentuated by deep breathing. Cyanosis may be evident, and with larger pneumothoraces, the trachea can be deviated. Percussion of the chest reveals a tympanitic sound, and breath sounds may be diminished or absent. Conditions that can mimic pneumothorax include hemothorax or atelectasis. Radiological examination is the best diagnostic aid available, and all films should be exposed during expiration, if possible.[47] The presence of rib fractures or surgical emphysema should provide a clue to the diagnosis. In trauma patients, pneumothoraces with a volume greater than 10% should be treated by tube thoracostomy. Temporizing the treatment is inappropriate for the patient who may require intubation and positive-pressure ventilation during surgery for extrathoracic injuries, as the pneumothorax may enlarge under these conditions. Therefore, the prophylactic insertion of a chest tube is indicated.

A tension pneumothorax occurs when air enters the pleural cavity during inspiration but, owing to a ball-valve action, cannot escape during expiration. In conscious patients, rapid deterioration is noted. The cardinal signs of a tension pneumothorax are

- cyanosis,
- marked decrease in pulmonary compliance,
- rapid deterioration of vital signs,
- diminished or absent breath sounds, and
- tracheal deviation.

This condition can be easily confused with pericardial tamponade or shock, secondary to hypovolemia; however, the hypertympanic percussion note over the ipsilateral chest usually makes differentiation possible.

The casualty shown in Figure 19-5 is a particularly dramatic presentation of a tension pneumothorax. However, it is important to stress that a tension pneumothorax is a clinical rather than a radiological diagnosis. Two factors contribute to the hemodynamic deterioration: (1) hypoxia from decreased gas exchange and (2) increased impedance of venous return into the chest due to the mechanical distortion of the mediastinum that is caused by the expanding pneumothorax. During general anesthesia, a dramatic decrease in pulmonary compliance should alert the anesthesiologist to the problem. Nitrous oxide should be discontinued if it is being administered, as it accentuates the size of the pneumothorax.[48] As soon as a hemodynamically significant tension pneumothorax is suspected, the anesthesiologist might need to perform temporizing measures, including the immediate insertion of a large-bore needle into the second intercostal space along the midclavicular line. A "hissing" sound may be created by the escaping,

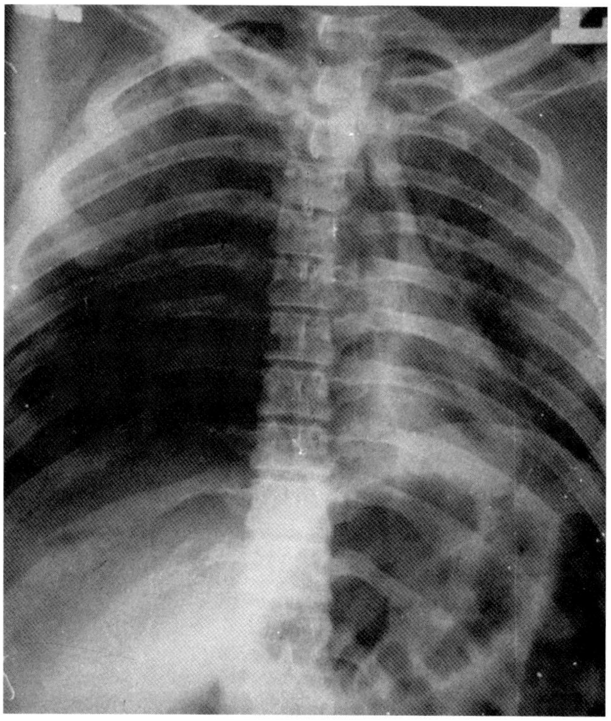

Fig. 19-5. This casualty was killed by a perforating gunshot wound of the right hemithorax. A radiograph was taken before the autopsy was performed. A tension pneumothorax with massive shift of the mediastinum is apparent. Photograph: Wound Data and Munitions Effectiveness Team slide collection.

pressurized air. Intravenous extension tubing can then be attached to the catheter and placed under water seal (ie, submerging it in a liter bottle of sterile water). Care must be taken to keep the water bottle lower than the patient; otherwise, the flow may be reversed, causing a hydrothorax. Temporizing measures should be replaced as soon as possible by the more definitive closed-system tube thoracostomy.

Tracheal and Bronchial Injuries

Tracheal and bronchial injuries are uncommon sequelae of thoracic trauma but are among the most serious encountered in thoracic surgery. Although most penetrating wounds to these structures are caused by fragments, these injuries also occur following blunt trauma associated with high-speed travel. A 2.8% incidence of tracheobronchial rupture has been reported[49] in patients who succumbed to blunt chest trauma. Approximately 80% of tracheobronchial disruptions occur within 2.5 cm of the carina. Three mechanisms may explain this finding[50]:

1. Sudden, forceful compression is the most common insult causing tracheobronchial injuries during blunt thoracic trauma. This anteroposterior compression combined with simultaneous lateral expansion of the lungs can result in severe traction on the pericarinal portion of the trachea.
2. Acute increase in intrabronchial pressure may be caused by reflex glottic closure at the moment of impact.
3. Shearing forces at points of fixation of the intrathoracic airways, caused by rapid deceleration, may account for the preponderance of disruptions near the carina.

Dyspnea, cough, painful hemoptysis, and subcutaneous emphysema are the most common clinical findings in patients with tracheobronchial disruption. However, 10% of patients are nearly asymptomatic,[51] which accounts for the frequent delays in diagnosis. Auscultation of the heart may reveal a crunching sound associated with pericardial air, also known as Hamman's sign. When the site of disruption freely communicates with the mediastinal pleura, pneumothorax results, and tube thoracostomy and suction often fail to reexpand the affected lung. When the pleural space and the site of disruption do not communicate, there is little or no pneumothorax, and mediastinal air may be the only radiographic abnormality. In addition to pneumothorax and pneumomediastinum, indicative radiographic findings include subcutaneous and deep cervical emphysema. With complete transection of a main bronchus, the superior margin of the affected lung drops below the level of the transection. This occurs because the lung is deprived of its normal bronchial tethering in the thoracic cage.

All patients with suspected tracheal or bronchial injury require diagnostic bronchoscopy as soon as they are stable. Blind endotracheal intubation without endoscopic visualization of the tracheobronchial tree is unlikely to be successful and may produce further trauma because the distal trachea is displaced posteriorly. In addition, acute airway obstruction may develop when the endotracheal tube enters a false passage and occludes the tracheal lumen. Both a surgically guided oral intubation of the distal tracheal segment and removal of the initial surgical airway are acceptable means of allowing surgical repair of the tracheal separation.

When the disruption and distal segment can be visualized clearly, a double-lumen tube can be inserted distal to the tracheal tear or, in the case of bronchial disruption, into the contralateral bronchus. Alternatively, the area of disruption can be visualized directly with a fiberoptic bronchoscope; then the instrument can be used as a guide over which an endotracheal tube can blindly be passed into the distal tracheal segment. This approach is equally acceptable for bronchial disruption, although it is preferable to intubate the uninjured bronchus selectively for ventilation during bronchial repairs. Therefore, the military trauma anesthesiologist must have available a variety of sterile endotracheal tubes that can be passed into the operative field and used to intubate the distal airway prior to and during its anastomosis to the proximal segment. Alternative techniques such as simply insufflating oxygen into the distal airway or employing high-frequency jet ventilation using uncuffed catheters in the contralateral bronchus have also been described.[52]

Parenchymal Lung Lacerations

Extensive laceration of the lung parenchyma—such as might occur when an assault-rifle bullet yaws and tumbles during its passage through the lung—can create one of the most difficult therapeutic problems for the military trauma anesthesiologist. Not only will there be massive leakage of air into the pleural space, which will make difficult the maintenance of an acceptable tidal volume, but the normal anatomical proximity of airways and blood vessels in the lungs potentiates (1) the passing of blood into airways and (2) the passing of air into the circulation. The first condition causes an airway obstruction as the casualty literally drowns in blood. The second causes rapidly fatal systemic air embolization. The simultaneous leakage of air into the pleural space and passage of blood into the tracheobronchial tree can best be managed by having the anesthesiologist pass a standard endotracheal tube into the bronchus of the uninjured lung. (The use of a double lung tube in this situation is too time consuming to be safe.) Once the injured lung has been isolated by the anesthesiologist, the surgeon, after exposing the injured lung, can then cross-clamp the pulmonary hilum. The appropriate surgical management may be to perform an anatomical pulmonary resection—a lobectomy or pneumonectomy—rather than to attempt a repair of the laceration (Figure 19-6).[53]

Systemic air embolism is a catastrophic complication that suddenly converts a previously stable patient into one who is agonal. Increasingly, evidence shows that cerebral and coronary air emboli are common causes of death in victims of penetrating lung injuries.[22] There is frequently a causal relation to the application of positive pressure to the airway. The treatment, insofar as there is one, consists of

- immediate performance of a thoracotomy,
- application of a large clamp or Rommel tourniquet around the hilum of the injured lung to prevent further embolization, and
- exposure of the heart to confirm the diagnosis (air bubbles should be visible in the coronary vessels).

If the diagnosis is confirmed, the surgeon manually occludes the ascending aorta and manually compresses the heart so as to drive the air bubbles through the coronary arteries and into the coronary sinus. The management of the cerebral component is a matter for conjecture.

Traumatic Rupture of the Diaphragm

Traumatic rupture of the diaphragm is a relatively uncommon injury, seen in 2% to 3% of patients with blunt chest trauma.[18] In the context of military operations, it is most frequently seen in casualties who are injured when the vehicle in which they are riding detonates a buried antitank mine. The soldier shown in Figure 19-7 was killed during the Vietnam War when the jeep in which he was riding was destroyed by a mine. The chest radiograph explains the scaphoid appearance of his abdomen: his stomach and much of his gut have herniated into the left hemithorax.

Rupture of the left hemidiaphragm accounts for 70% to 75% of these injuries, presumably because of the shielding effect of the underlying mass of the liver on the right.[54] Traumatic diaphragmatic hernia may be discovered at the casualty's initial evaluation or incidentally at thoracotomy or laparotomy performed for other reasons. The casualty may be asymptomatic or may present with respiratory distress. Patients with chronic rupture usually present with symptoms of intestinal obstruction.

Diaphragmatic hernia is caused by three factors in blunt trauma[55]:

1. The abdominothoracic pressure gradient may exceed the usual maximum value of 100 cm H_2O if the trauma patient gasps against a closed glottis at the instant that a large external force raises the intraabdominal pressure.

a

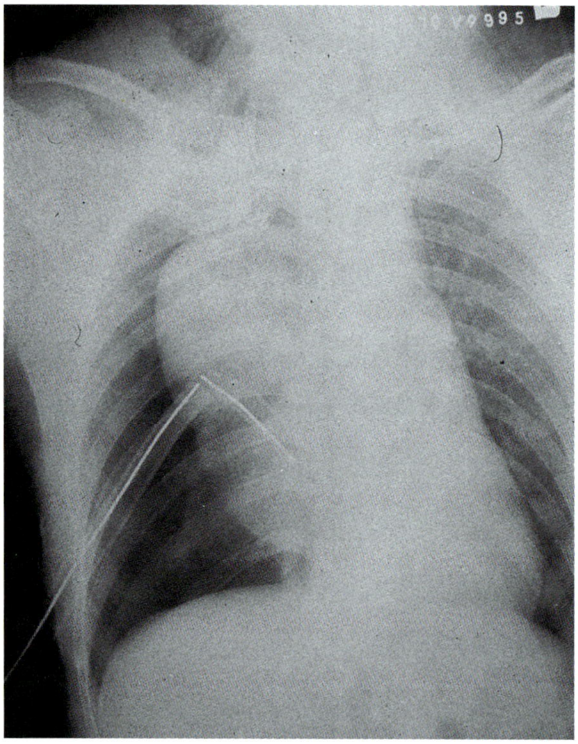

c

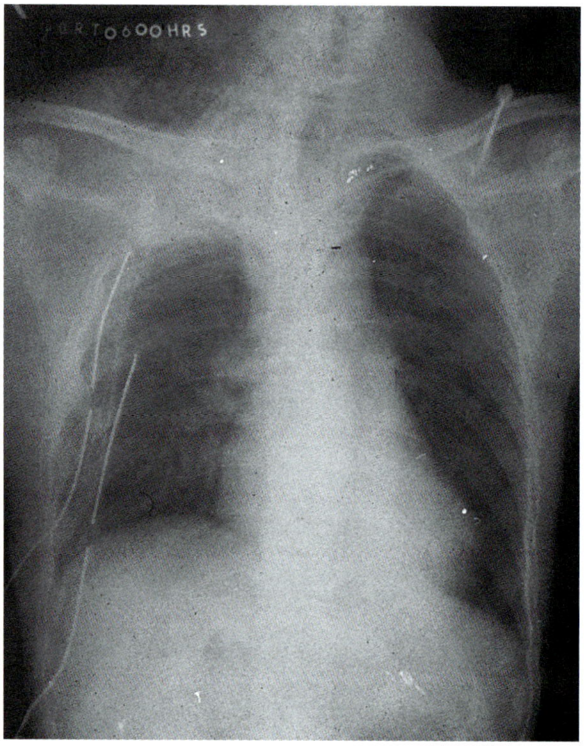

b

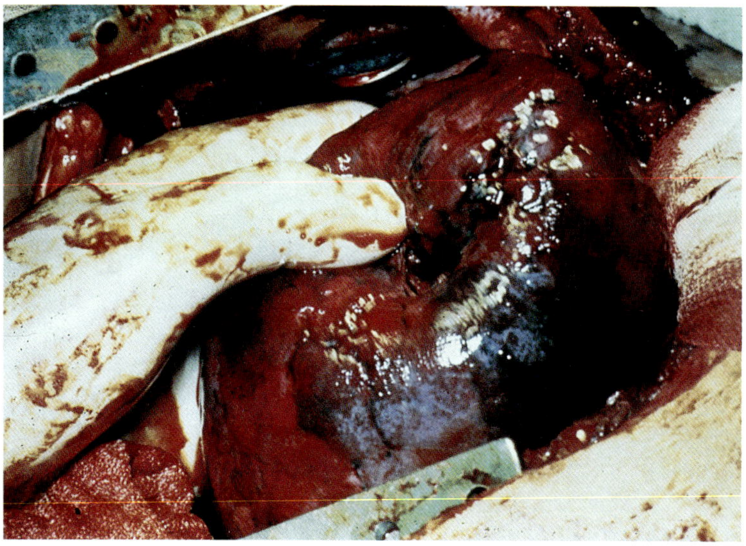

Fig. 19-6. This casualty presented with a parenchymal lung laceration due to a perforating gunshot wound of the chest. (**a**) The chest radiograph taken after insertion of a chest tube shows that the damaged lung remained collapsed. Although the chest tube kinked, it was patent. This finding, in addition to the magnitude of the air leak and the consequent difficulty of providing adequate ventilation, constituted an indication for thoracotomy. (**b**) A huge laceration was found in the right upper lobe of the lung. A lobectomy was performed. (**c**) The postoperative chest radiograph shows expansion of the residual lung. Photographs: Swan Vietnam Surgical Slide Collection.

2. Thoracic compression during blunt trauma distorts the anatomy of the diaphragm and tears it with large shearing forces.
3. The trauma patient may have a congenital weakness of the diaphragm.

The diagnosis of diaphragmatic trauma requires a high degree of clinical suspicion by the military anesthesiologist. Trauma to the diaphragm should be suspected in casualties who have (*a*) injuries below the fifth intercostal space and (*b*) injuries associated with high-energy impact (eg, fractures of the clavicles, upper ribs, scapulae, sternum, pelvis, or thoracolumbar spine). This condition must be suspected when unexplained changes in pulmonary compliance occur intraoperatively in patients who have sustained serious chest injury. Patients with significant migration of viscera into the chest cavity also appear to be at greater risk from aspiration pneumonitis. Postoperative difficulties in

a b

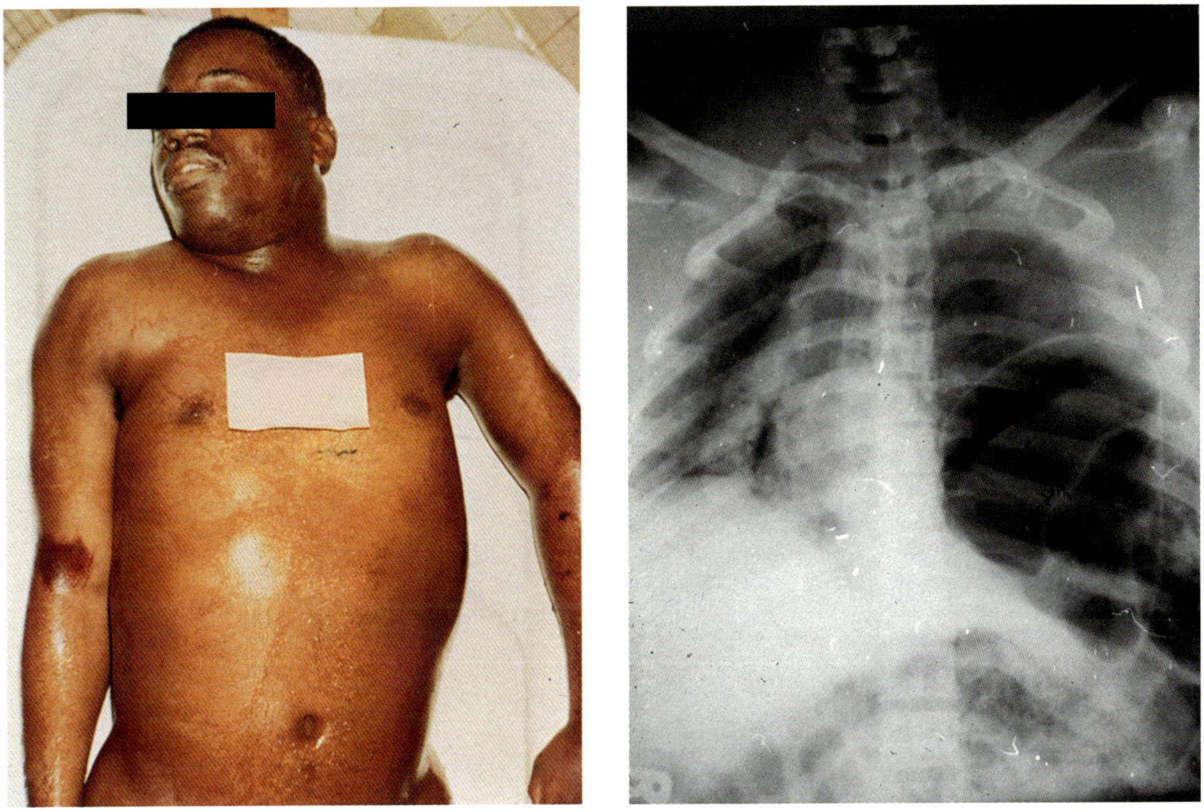

Fig. 19-7. (**a**) The external appearance of this dead soldier is notable for his scaphoid abdomen and his distended chest. (**b**) The chest radiograph shows several transverse lines in the left hemithorax, which are caused by the walls of hollow viscera that have herniated into the chest. The left diaphragm is not apparent. Massive displacement of the mediastinum into the right hemithorax has occurred. Photographs: Wound Data and Munitions Effectiveness Team slide collection.

weaning a patient with thoracic trauma from mechanical ventilation should arouse suspicion of a missed diaphragmatic hernia.

Operative positioning for the repair of a traumatic diaphragmatic hernia depends on the side of the injury and its chronicity. The more common left-side hernia is best repaired through a laparotomy when the diagnosis is made soon after the injury, and when there is no evidence of a significant intrathoracic injury. Chronic left-side hernias are best treated through a low posterolateral incision. Right-side hernias are nearly always repaired through a thoracotomy.

SUMMARY

Thoracic injuries in combat constitute 10% of the surgical workload in wartime. Most of these injuries are caused by penetrating missiles. In caring for soldiers with such injuries, the military trauma anesthesiologist will encounter a paradoxical situation: more often than not, it will be not the thoracic injury itself but an injury to another body part that will be the center of professional attention. The thoracic injury can usually be managed by such simple interventions as inserting a chest tube and debriding wounds.

In most cases in which thoracotomy is indicated, it will be performed for control of (*a*) bleeding from lacerated lung parenchyma or from the chest wall and (*b*) air leaks from lacerated lung parenchyma. Hemorrhage from a laceration, perforation, or rupture of the heart or great vessels will rarely be encountered: such injuries are so rapidly fatal that few casualties will survive long enough to reach a medical treatment facility. If such a casualty does arrive, the military trauma anesthesiologist may be confronted with the need to resuscitate an agonal patient; from the practical standpoint, this means being able to orchestrate an emergency thoracotomy.

Among the more severe intraoperative problems likely to be seen by the military trauma anesthesiologist are (*a*) an air leak that is so massive that tidal volume is inadequate, (*b*) airway obstruction due to accumulation of bloody secretions, and (*c*) systemic air embolism. These problems are best managed by selective intubation of the bronchus of the uninjured lung.

Pulmonary contusion and flail chest are the two treatment problems most likely to be seen in association with blunt trauma. Severe cases will require intubation and mechanical ventilation. As a general rule, the military trauma anesthesiologist will be most successful when treating a casualty with a thoracic injury if he or she prioritizes the many tasks at hand in terms of the elementary ATLS principles of airway, breathing, and circulation management.

REFERENCES

1. McNamara JJ, Messersmith JK, Dunn RA, Molot MD, Stremple JF. Thoracic injuries in combat casualties in Vietnam. *Ann Thor Surg*. 1970;10:389–401.

2. Rosenblatt M, Lemer J, Best LA, Peleg H. Thoracic wounds in Israeli battle casualties during the 1982 evacuation of wounded from Lebanon. *J Trauma*. 1985;25:350–354.

3. Beebe GW, DeBakey ME. *Battle Casualties*. Springfield, Ill: Charles C Thomas; 1952: 167, 181.

4. Bellamy RF, Zajtchuk R. The physics and biophysics of wound ballistics. In: Bellamy RF, Zajtchuk R, eds. *Conventional Warfare: Ballistic, Blast, and Burn Injuries*. Part 1, vol 5. In: Zajtchuk R, Jenkins DP, Bellamy RF, eds. *Textbook of Military Medicine*. Washington, DC: US Department of the Army, Office of The Surgeon General, and Borden Institute; 1991: Chap 4.

5. Berry FB. General considerations of thoracic wounds. In: Berry FB, ed. *Thoracic Surgery*. In: Coates JB Jr, ed. *Surgery in World War II*. Vol 1. Washington, DC: US Army Medical Department, Office of The Surgeon General; 1963: 59.

6. Viano DC, Lau IA. A viscous tolerance criterion for soft tissue injury assessment. *J Biomechanics*. 1988;21(5):387–399.

7. Viano DC. Live fire testing: Assessing blunt impact and acceleration injury vulnerabilities. *Milit Med*. 1991;156:589–595.

8. Suleman ND, Rasoul HA. War injuries of the chest. *Injury*. 1985;16:382–384.

9. Zakharia AT. Cardiovascular and thoracic battle injuries in the Lebanon War. *J Thorac Cardiovasc Surg*. 1985;89:723–733.

10. Thompson L. Former Lieutenant Colonel, Medical Corps, US Army. Personal communication, June 1991.

11. Brewer LA. Thoracoabdominal wounds. In: Berry FB, ed. *Thoracic Surgery*. In: Coates JB Jr, ed. *Surgery in World War II*. Vol 2. Washington, DC: US Army Medical Department, Office of The Surgeon General; 1963: 101–136.

12. Bowen TE, Bellamy RF, eds. *Emergency War Surgery NATO Handbook*. 2nd rev US ed. Washington, DC: US Department of Defense, Government Printing Office; 1988: 346–347.

13. Neal S. *Medical Support of the US Army in Vietnam 1965–1970*. Washington, DC: Department of the Army; 1973: 97–98.

14. Finucane BT. Thoracic trauma. In: Kaplan JA, ed. *Thoracic Anesthesia*. 2nd ed. New York, NY: Churchill Livingstone; 1991: 463–484.

15. Kirsh MM. Acute thoracic injuries. In: Siegel J, ed. *Trauma, Emergency Surgery and Critical Care*. New York, NY: Churchill Livingstone; 1987: 863.

16. Stene JK, Grande CM. *Trauma Anesthesia*. Baltimore, Md: Williams & Wilkins; 1991: 221, 226.

17. Duff JH, Goldstein M, McLean APH, et al. Flail chest: A clinical review and physiological study. *J Trauma.* 1968;8:63–74.

18. Symbas PN. *Cardiothoracic Trauma.* Philadelphia, Pa: WB Saunders; 1989: 344, 376–377.

19. Jones TB, Richardson EP. Traction on the sternum in the treatment of multiple fractured ribs. *Surg Gynecol Obstet.* 1926;42:283.

20. Moore BP. Operative stabilization of nonpenetrating chest injuries. *J Thorac Cardiovasc Surg.* 1975;70:619–630.

21. Fulton RL, Peters ET. Physiological effects of fluid therapy after pulmonary contusion. *Am J Surg.* 1973;126:773–778.

22. Meier GH, Symbas PN, Wood WJ. Systemic air embolism following penetrating lung injury. *Ann Thorac Surg.* 1979;27:161–169.

23. Symbas PN. Acute traumatic hemothorax. *Ann Thorac Surg.* 1978;26:195–196.

24. Kavolius J, Golocovsky M, Champion HR. Predictors of outcome in patients who have sustained trauma and who undergo emergency thoracotomy. *Arch Surg.* 1993;128:1158–1162.

25. DiGiacomo JC, Odom JW, Swan KG, Salant M. Resuscitative thoracotomy and combat casualty care. *Milit Med.* 1991;156(8):406.

26. Yao ST, Vanecko RM, Printen K, et al. Penetrating wounds of the heart: A review of 80 cases. *Ann Surg.* 1968;168:67–78.

27. Trinkle JK, Marcos J, Grover FL, et al. Management of the wounded heart. *Ann Thorac Surg.* 1973;17:230–236.

28. Cassell P, Cullum P. The management of cardiac tamponade: Drainage of pericardial effusions. *Br J Surg.* 1967;54:620–626.

29. Proudfit WL, Effler DB. Diagnosis and treatment of cardiac pericarditis by pericardial biopsy. *JAMA.* 1956;161:188–192.

30. Guntheroth WG, Morgan BC, Mullins GL. Effect of respiration on venous return and stroke volume in cardiac tamponade: Mechanism of pulsus paradoxus. *Circ Res.* 1967;20:381–390.

31. Fowler NO, Holmes JC. Hemodynamic effects of isoproterenol and norepinephrine in acute cardiac tamponade. *J Clin Invest.* 1969;48:502.

32. Moseley RE, Vernick JJ, Doty DB. Response to blunt chest injury: A new experimental model. *J Trauma.* 1970;10:673–683.

33. Symbas PN. Cardiac trauma. *Am Heart J.* 1976;92:387–396.

34. Rea WJ, Sugg WL, Wilson LC, et al. Coronary artery lacerations—an analysis of 22 patients. *Ann Thorac Surg.* 1969;7:518–528.

35. Parmley LF, Manion WC, Mattingly TW. Nonpenetrating traumatic injury of the heart. *Circulation.* 1958;18:371–393.

36. Roberts WC, Maron BJ. Sudden death while playing professional football. *Am Heart J.* 1981;102:1062–1063.

37. Moritz AR. Trauma, stress and coronary thrombosis. *JAMA.* 1954;156:1306–1309.

38. Hillis LD, Braunwald E. Coronary artery spasm. *N Engl J Med.* 1978;299:695–702.

39. Vlay SC, Blumenthal DS, Shoback D, et al. Delayed acute myocardial infarction after blunt chest trauma in a young woman. *Am Heart J*. 1980;100:907–916.

40. Parmley LF, Mattingly TW, Manion WC. Nonpenetrating traumatic injury of the aorta. *Circulation*. 1958;17: 1086–1101.

41. Mitchell RL, Enright LP. The surgical management of acute and chronic injuries of the thoracic aorta. *Surg Gynecol Obstet*. 1983;157:1–4.

42. Cohn PF, Braunwald E. Traumatic heart disease. In: Braunwald E, ed. *Heart Disease: A Textbook of Cardiovascular Medicine*. Philadelphia, Pa: WB Saunders; 1988: 1535.

43. Fleming AW, Green DC. Traumatic aneurysms of the thoracic aorta: Report of 43 patients. *Ann Thorac Surg*. 1974;18:91–101.

44. Kirsh MM, Behrendt DM, Arringer MB, et al. The treatment of acute traumatic rupture of the aorta: A ten year experience. *Ann Surg*. 1976;184:308–316.

45. Coles JG, Wilson GJ, Sima AF, et al. Intraoperative detection of spinal cord ischemia using somatosensory cortical evoked potentials during thoracic aortic occlusion. *Ann Thorac Surg*. 1982;34:299–306.

46. Sturm JT, Billiar TR, Luxenberg MG, Perry JF. Risk factors for the development of renal failure following the surgical treatment of traumatic aortic rupture. *Ann Thorac Surg*. 1987;43:425–427.

47. Murphy CH, Murphy MR. *Radiology for Anesthesia and Critical Care*. New York, NY: Churchill Livingstone; 1987: 67.

48. Eger EI II, Saidman LJ. Hazards of nitrous oxide anesthesia in bowel obstruction and pneumothorax. *Anesthesiology*. 1965;26:61–66.

49. Bertelsen S, Howitz P. Injuries of the trachea and bronchi. *Thorax*. 1972;27:188–194.

50. Kirsh MM, Orringer MB, Behrendt DB, Sloan H. Management of tracheobronchial disruption secondary to nonpenetrating trauma. *Ann Thorac Surg*. 1976;22:93–101.

51. Grover FL, Ellestad C, Arom KV, et al. Diagnosis and management of major tracheobronchial injuries. *Ann Thorac Surg*. 1979;28:384–391.

52. Pizov R, Shir Y, Eimerl D, et al. One-lung high frequency ventilation in the management of traumatic tear of bronchus in a child. *Crit Care Med*. 1987;15:1160–1161.

53. Fisher RP, Gieger JP, Guernsey JM. Pulmonary resections for severe pulmonary contusions secondary to high-velocity missile wounds. *J Trauma*. 1974;14:293–298.

54. Beal SL, McKennan M. Blunt diaphragm rupture: A morbid injury. *Arch Surg*. 1988;123:828–832.

55. Mulder DS, Shennib H, Angood P. Thoracic injuries. In: Maull KI, Cleveland HC, Strauch GO, Wolferth CC, eds. *Advances in Trauma*. Vol 1. Chicago, Ill: Year Book. 1986: 193–216.

Chapter 20

ABDOMINAL INJURIES

ROBERT G. KNIGHT, PH.D., M.D.*; AND RONALD F. BELLAMY, M.D.†

*Formerly, Major, Medical Corps, U.S. Army; Assistant Director, Cardiothoracic Anesthesia, and Director, Anesthesia Research, Walter Reed Army Medical Center, Washington, D. C. 20307-5001; currently, Chairman, Department of Anesthesiology, Floyd Medical Center, Rome, Georgia 30165

†Colonel, Medical Corps, U.S. Army; Managing Editor and Officer in Charge, Textbook of Military Medicine, Borden Institute, Walter Reed Army Medical Center, Washington, D. C. 20307-5001

INTRODUCTION

Abdominal trauma is a frequent indication for surgical exploration of the battlefield casualty. During one 16-month period (1966–1967) of the Vietnam War, 17,726 wounded American soldiers were admitted to U.S. Army hospitals in Vietnam. More than 70% of these injuries were due to small arms, mines, artillery, or mortar fire. Approximately 14% of these soldiers had abdominal wounds, which were frequently associated with wounds to the head, chest, or extremities. One authority[1] found that during the Vietnam War, hospital mortality was 4.5% in 2,454 casualties with abdominal wounds, which compares favorably with mortality rates of 21% in World War II and 12% in the Korean War. This reduction in mortality from abdominal wounds is due to many factors, but undoubtedly reflects the availability of rapid helicopter evacuation, improved understanding of the pathophysiology and treatment of hemorrhagic shock, improved antibiotic therapy, improved surgical technique, and the availability of trained anesthesia personnel.

ABDOMINAL TRAUMA AND WAR SURGERY

Battlefield casualties with abdominal trauma who reach the hospital level alive fall into two broad categories: (1) a smaller group, who have life-threatening, exsanguinating hemorrhage; and (2) a larger group, who are at risk of dying from sepsis due to intestinal spillage. The former group will frequently require urgent, if not emergent, surgery because of the high potential for death; medical personnel can take the time to perform thorough preoperative resuscitations and evaluations with the latter group. Israeli military surgeons made use of this distinction to treat abdominal casualties during the 1967 Yom Kippur War. Of 151 casualties who ultimately required a laparotomy, 30 who were in shock on arrival at the main field surgical hospital in the Sinai underwent immediate operation. The remaining 121 casualties, all of whom were hemodynamically stable, were given intravenous fluids and antibiotics and then evacuated by air to Israel for laparotomy. Mortality in the group who were operated on in the field was 20%, compared with 5% for those who were operated on in Israel.[2] By deploying far forward only enough medical assets to treat the nontransportable casualties, the Israeli army's medical commanders markedly simplified the logistics of medical support.

If they recognize that most casualties do not require immediate operation, medical officers can avoid hurried preoperative evaluations, which may overlook subtle findings indicative of serious internal injury. Thus, it is important to remember that apparent chest wounds may penetrate the abdominal cavity[3] and abdominal wounds may extend into the thoracic cavity (Figure 20-1). Close attention must be paid to unexplained hypotension in the apparently volume-resuscitated soldier undergoing thoracotomy, as it may reflect undiagnosed intraabdominal hemorrhage. Similarly, an exploratory laparotomy for an abdominal wound may be suddenly accompanied by wheezing, increased airway pressure, and arterial oxygen desaturation indicative of undiagnosed pneumothorax.

Myocardial laceration and cardiac tamponade may also be associated with abdominal wounds.

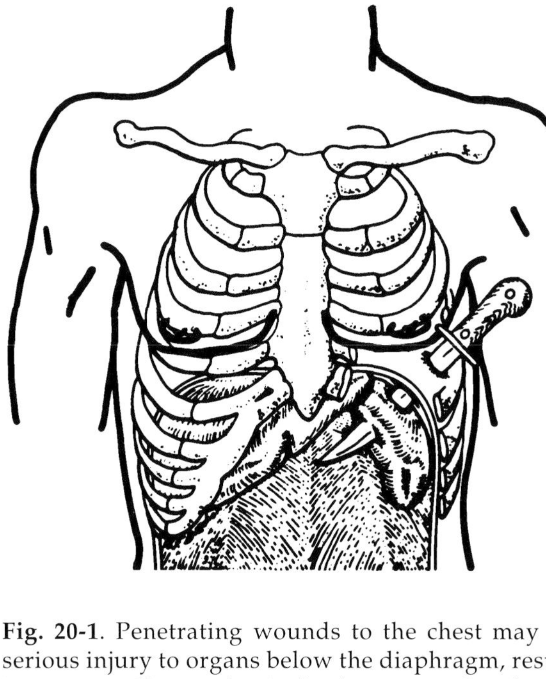

Fig. 20-1. Penetrating wounds to the chest may cause serious injury to organs below the diaphragm, resulting in a source of hemorrhagic shock not immediately apparent during thoracotomy. Penetrating abdominal wounds may similarly enter the thoracic cavity through small diaphragmatic perforations not readily seen during exploratory laparotomy.

The abdominal cavity is large and easily distended.[4] It may contain large quantities of blood with no readily apparent increase in circumference (Figure 20-2). A pelvic or retroperitoneal hematoma may also hold several liters of blood. Retroperitoneal and pelvic hemorrhage may not be immediately apparent during exploratory laparotomy, and should be considered when hypotension persists after volume resuscitation. Another potential cause of refractory hypotension is spinal shock: this diagnosis is suggested when hypotension is accompanied by bradycardia, strong pulses, and warm extremities in the presence of hemiplegia or quadriplegia.

Wound Ballistics

The intraabdominal organs can be injured by three mechanisms:

1. direct cutting and laceration, which are caused by a penetrating projectile;
2. radial stretching and displacement, which are caused by a penetrating projectile and are the result of cavitation within the organ; and
3. crushing, which is caused by blast or blunt trauma.

Most abdominal trauma in combat casualties is caused by penetrating projectiles. Penetrating injuries that enter the peritoneal cavity may require immediate exploration because of exsanguinating hemorrhage. The path followed by a projectile once it enters the abdomen generally follows a straight line, but injury involving multiple organs is common.

Projectiles with high kinetic energy can cause devastating injuries by the process of temporary cavitation (ie, stretch). Tissues around the wound tract are thrown aside with great force; the resultant radial stretching and displacement can cause gross disruption. Solid, friable organs such as the liver, kidney, and spleen are especially susceptible to injury by this mechanism (Figure 20-3).[5] Hollow organs such as the stomach, bowel, and bladder are resilient and resist temporary cavitation if empty but may be severely disrupted if distended with fluid at the time of injury. Muscle withstands temporary cavitation with little permanent effect. As might be expected, bone—markedly inelastic compared with muscle—may fracture when subjected

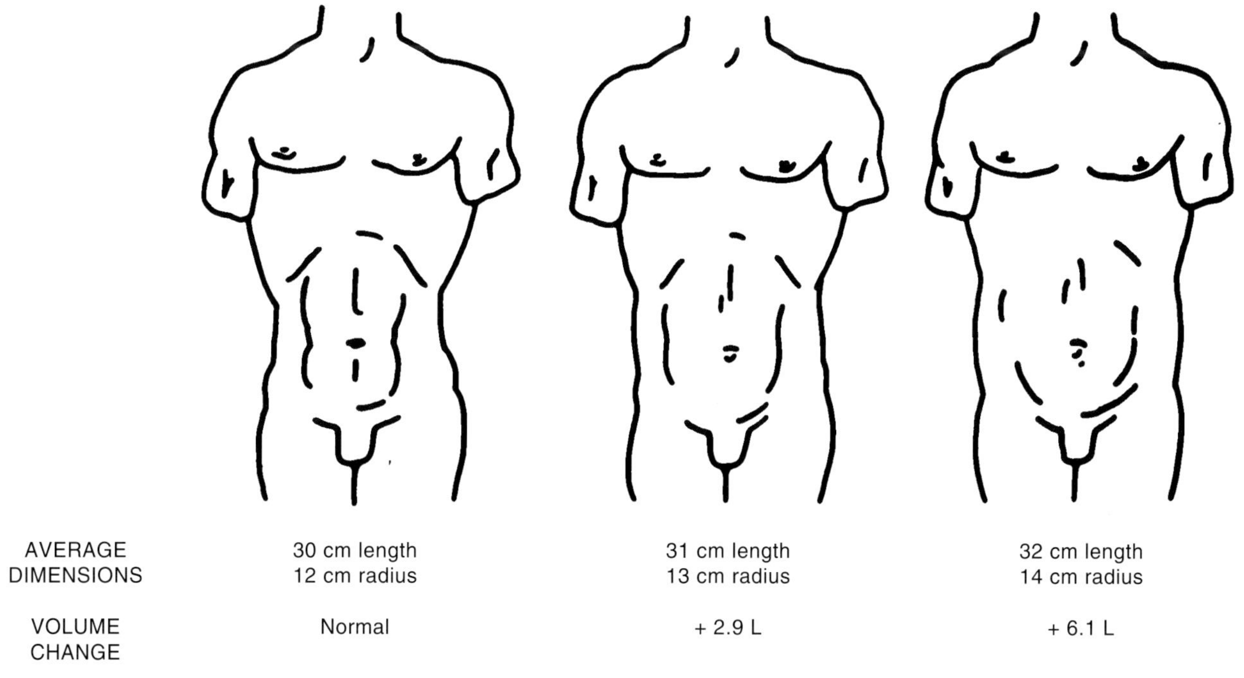

Fig. 20-2. The readily distensible abdominal cavity may hold large quantities of blood with minimal enlargement. Adapted with permission from Trunkey DD, Sheldon PF, Collins JA. The treatment of shock. In: Zuidemia PD, Rutherford RB, Ballinger WF, eds. *The Management of Trauma.* 4th ed. Philadelphia, Pa: WB Saunders; 1985: 107.

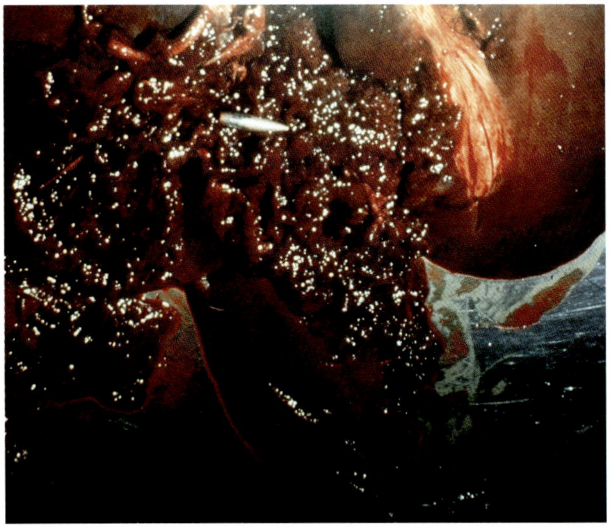

Fig. 20-3. An anesthetized swine was shot in the upper abdomen from a distance of 3 m with a Russian AK74 (5.45 mm). Massive disruption and laceration of the liver can be seen. The recovered, fired bullet was placed in the center of the disrupted liver for comparison. Reprinted from Fackler ML, Surinchak JS, Malinowski JA, Bowen RE. Wounding potential of the Russian AK-74 assault rifle. *J Trauma*. 1984;24(3):265.

to cavitation. (Weapons, the mechanisms of injury to bone and soft tissue, the behavior of projectiles in tissue, and cavitation phenomena are discussed in *Conventional Warfare: Ballistic, Blast, and Burn Injuries*, a volume in the *Textbook of Military Medicine* series.)[6]

The magnitude of temporary cavitation is greatly increased by certain features of bullet construction: fragmentation, as exemplified by rounds that are fired by the M16 series of assault rifles; deformation, as is common with soft-point or hollow-nose bullets; and the bullet's *yaw* and *tumbling*, which are related to the location of the bullet's center of mass and the rate of spin imparted by the rifling.[7]

Small, low-velocity fragments, in contrast to bullets fired by military small arms, do not produce damage by cavitation. The clinical corollary of this difference in behavior is that damage at a distance from the wound path is to be expected with cavitating bullets but not with certain fragments or knives. This is one of the reasons that some intraabdominal knife wounds do not require surgical intervention.[8,9]

Diagnosis

The diagnosis of penetrating abdominal trauma in combat casualties is quite straightforward, being made by the presence of one or more holes in the trunk. One of the principles of military surgery is that a laparotomy be performed whenever a penetrating projectile wound of the abdomen is found. However, a hole in the abdominal wall is not necessarily synonymous with an intraabdominal injury, and this principle—*always* operate—leads to the occasional laparotomy that finds no evidence of intraabdominal injury. The expected incidence is approximately 20%.[1]

Because solid organs such as the liver, spleen, and kidney are less able to dissipate kinetic energy (ie, they are displaced and distorted) and maintain their structural integrity, it is therefore not surprising that these organs are primary targets of injury in blunt trauma.[10–12] The decision to operate following blunt trauma is frequently based on the results of diagnostic peritoneal lavage (DPL).[13] An infraumbilical incision is made after local anesthesia is obtained, and 1 L of saline is introduced into the abdominal cavity through a catheter. The saline is then siphoned off. The following are indications for exploratory laparotomy:

- gross blood or enteric contents in the effluent,
- a red blood cell count greater than 100,000/mm^3,
- a white blood cell count greater than 500/mm^3,
- alkaline phosphatase greater than 3 international units,
- amylase greater than 20 international units, or
- bile or bacteria in the effluent.

However, a computed tomography scan may be needed for the preoperative diagnosis of retroperitoneal hematoma secondary to traumatic rupture of the aorta or vena cava. In general, the sensitivity, specificity, and predictive value of DPL is high in both blunt and penetrating trauma.[14] Computerized tomography complements the examination when DPL is equivocal. Magnetic resonance imaging is highly accurate in defining tissue disruption but is very time consuming; thus, it is impractical in both the acute trauma setting[15] and in third-echelon surgical hospitals, as such equipment is not yet fieldable.

Intraoperative Blood Salvage

Blood loss in combat casualties with intraabdominal trauma may be substantial. Data collected during the Vietnam War indicate that approximately 37% of casualties with abdominal wounds required blood transfusion, and the average amount of blood administered was 8.9 units.[16] In view of the extensive logistical demands posed by the transfusion requirements, an approach using interoperative blood salvage is clearly desirable. Equipment for intraoperative blood salvage is now available in some field hospitals and should be a valuable means of reducing the need for homologous blood transfusion. A typical blood-salvaging device includes a double-lumen tube that permits heparin to be added to the blood as it is aspirated. The blood is then pumped into a bowl, where it is washed with saline and then centrifuged. The wash solution contains surgical debris, white blood cells, platelets, and clotting factors; it is discarded. Intact red blood cells are concentrated to approximately 70% for transfusion. A dedicated operator is required to assemble the apparatus, select cycling parameters, match the rate of heparin flow to the rate of blood aspiration, and change solutions and waste collection bags. It is unlikely that a single anesthetist involved in the resuscitation of a hemorrhaging soldier will have the freedom from direct patient care needed to fulfill this role; therefore, someone other than an anesthesia provider will have to perform this procedure in field hospitals.

Intraoperative autotransfusion has been used effectively in open heart, vascular, orthopedic, and transplantation surgery.[17] Its use in trauma surgery has been limited.[18] The potential for intestinal soilage of free intraabdominal blood is the particular concern in abdominal surgery. Although the wash cycle removes many bacteria, significant numbers of anaerobes remain.[19] Nevertheless, in the presence of life-threatening hemorrhage, blood that was contaminated with intestinal contents, urine, and bile has been reinfused.[20] In deciding whether to reinfuse contaminated blood, trauma anesthesiologists must consider the source of the blood (small intestine vs. colon), the quantity of contamination, and the urgency of transfusion. Similar concerns arise when the wound has been irrigated with Betadine Solution (povidone-iodine, manufactured by Purdue Frederick, Norwalk, Conn.), antibiotics, or any other substance not appropriate for intravenous use.

PERIOPERATIVE CONSIDERATIONS

Once the decision is made to perform a laparotomy, the most important consideration regarding the casualty is whether there are injuries to other body parts that will be treated simultaneously by multiple operating teams. After this determination has been made, the following interventions must be considered.

Antibiotics

The military trauma anesthesiologist must ensure that the combat casualty with a penetrating intraabdominal injury receives antibiotics as soon as possible. In the past, appropriate therapy consisted of an aminoglycoside for Gram-negative coverage and one or two additional drugs to combat Gram-positive and anaerobic organisms. However, because of potential nephrotoxicity from aminoglycoside, interest has been shown in developing single-drug regimens, usually employing a semisynthetic penicillin or cephalosporin, to be administered to patients with penetrating abdominal trauma. No difference in the rate of infectious complications was found in one study in which a conventional regimen (clindamycin 600 mg, administered every 6 h, and gentamicin 80 mg, administered every 8 h, adjusted for body size and renal function) was compared to single-drug treatment using the semisynthetic penicillin mezlocillin (Mezlin, manufactured by Miles Pharmaceutical, West Haven, Conn.), given intravenously at a dose of 4 g every 6 hours.[21] Likewise, a meta-analysis in which aminoglycoside combinations were compared with single β-lactam antimicrobials showed no difference between the two therapies.[22] Military trauma anesthesiologists who are assigned to deployable hospitals should ascertain which available antibiotics are usable as single-drug prophylaxis in casualties who have penetrating abdominal trauma.

Intravenous Access

Perioperative considerations for the soldier with abdominal trauma are similar to those for any other type of trauma. Foremost is the need for adequate intravenous access. Multiunit transfusions are common; replacement of two to three blood volumes during the initial resuscitation is expected in 2% to 3% of patients.[1,23] Adequate intravenous access is thus imperative. During the Vietnam War, saphenous cutdowns were performed and intravenous tubing was sutured directly into the vein, permitting very high rates of flow.[24] Subclavian and internal jugular venous access has also found recent utility.[25] With these options available, little time should be spent searching for peripheral access in a patient with extreme vasoconstriction secondary to hemorrhagic shock.

Coexisting Disease and Monitoring

Unlike their civilian counterparts, the victims of battlefield trauma usually have no underlying disease. Although it is beneficial in hemorrhagic shock, invasive monitoring of arterial and central venous pressure contributes little to the eventual outcome of soldiers undergoing resuscitation and massive transfusion. Clinical signs of capillary perfusion, jugular distension, the quality of the pulse, urinary output, and the requirement for anesthetics are excellent indices of the adequacy of volume resuscitation of young, healthy soldiers.[26] If sufficient personnel and equipment are available, invasive monitoring is not contraindicated if it does not delay control of hemorrhage.

Induction of Anesthesia

Wounded soldiers with abdominal trauma may be intubated awake or with a rapid-sequence induction. In wartime, the rapid sequence is frequently performed—not because it is superior but because of the high demand for rapid turnover of the operating room. Either ketamine or sodium thiopental may be used for induction, but *using a dosage appropriate to the patient's condition* is of more importance than the particular anesthetic selected. A moribund patient requires no anesthetic, just succinylcholine to ensure muscle relaxation prior to intubation. An alert patient with a profound volume deficit requires correspondingly less anesthetic than an volume-replete patient. As little as 0.25 mg of ketamine or sodium thiopental per kilogram of body weight may be all that is necessary to produce unconsciousness in the hypovolemic patient. There are two reasons for this:

1. The anesthetic is diluted in a smaller total blood volume.
2. In the hypovolemic state, a much larger proportion of the cardiac output is delivered to the brain and heart.

Both these factors produce a higher content of anesthetic in these organs than might be expected from the reduced cardiac output characteristic of shock. The key to the successful anesthetic management of the trauma patient is the use of *reduced and fractionated dosages* of any medication given.

Maintenance of Anesthesia

Maintenance of anesthesia may consist of (*a*) continued incremental dosages of ketamine, (*b*) small dosages of narcotics, and (*c*) benzodiazepines or potent inhalational agents, as tolerated. The requirement for potent inhalational agents for nontraumatized euvolemic patients is usually described in terms of the minimal alveolar concentration (MAC), which prevents purposeful movement in response to a surgical stimulus in 50% of the patient population tested.[27] Several factors that reduce MAC may be present in the trauma patient, including hypothermia, hypoxia, severe anemia, and hypotension.[28] Hemorrhage ultimately produces all four of these conditions, so it is not surprising that the hemorrhaging patient will require less inhalational agent. The reason for this includes the previously discussed fact that with hemorrhage, a larger proportion of the cardiac output is delivered to the brain and the heart, and so the anesthetic partial pressures in these organs rise quickly. Additionally, blunting of sympathetic tone by anesthetics rapidly manifests as life-threatening hypotension. The trauma anesthesiologist can compensate for these responses by using fractional values of MAC as tolerated by the patient's blood pressure.

However, the tenuous balance between preserving an adequate blood pressure and ensuring anesthesia is difficult to maintain, as fluid and anesthetic requirements fluctuate widely during surgery. Lower partial pressures of anesthetic do not ensure lack of awareness; recall of intraoperative events is not uncommon in the trauma patient.[29]

The anesthetic partial pressure that prevents patient movement is not necessarily the same partial pressure that prevents intraoperative awareness or postoperative recall. For example, in a normovolemic patient, hypnosis is produced by fractions of MAC. The alveolar concentration of anesthetic at the time patients first open their eyes in response to verbal command during recovery from anesthesia is known as *MAC-awake*. For isoflurane, MAC-awake has been reported to be 0.19%, or 15% of MAC.[30] MAC-awake for other inhaled anesthetics has been reported to be 33% to 50% of MAC.[31] Most patients who are maintained on end-tidal concentrations of potent, inhaled anesthetics in this range do not recall intraoperative events. Conversely, there are case reports describing recall with apparent (but not measured) end-tidal concentrations exceeding these values.[32,33] The extent to which hemorrhage reduces MAC-awake has not been determined, but anesthesiologists can take some comfort from knowing that low concentrations of potent inhaled anesthetics produce amnesia in the normovolemic patient.

Nitrous Oxide

The use of nitrous oxide in the battlefield casualty with abdominal trauma deserves special mention. Since World War I, nitrous oxide has been an extremely valuable adjunct to the anesthetic care of the battlefield casualty.[23,25,34,35] Although nitrous oxide is not able to provide a complete anesthetic for the normovolemic patient undergoing elective surgery, it is excellent in preserving cardiovascular stability in many trauma patients. However, even nitrous oxide is not always tolerated by the most seriously wounded.[35]

Nitrous oxide is notorious for producing gaseous distention of the gut in the absence of bowel obstruction, and is therefore clearly contraindicated in the presence of a closed air space (eg, pneumothorax, pneumocephalus, bowel obstruction). That nitrous oxide diffuses into closed spaces more rapidly than relatively insoluble gases (eg, methane, hydrogen, nitrogen) diffuse out is unquestioned. Rather, the argument has been made that these gases are present in the gastrointestinal tract in small volumes and are thus insignificant even if their volume is increased 2- or 3-fold.[36] However, recent studies have demonstrated significant differences in qualitatively assessed gas content of the small and large bowel, and operating conditions of patients given nitrous oxide, compared with air, as part of their anesthetic for bowel surgery (Figure 20-4).[37] Additionally, return of bowel function and duration of hospital stay were shorter for patients not given nitrous oxide. Although not all patients given nitrous oxide had bothersome distention of the bowel by the end of surgery (the average duration of anesthesia was 282 ± 53 min), the evidence clearly favors the use of air rather than nitrous oxide during bowel surgery of this duration. When considered with the logistical demands of supplying compressed gases in the field environment, it may be that nitrous oxide is best avoided in the battlefield casualty undergoing abdominal surgery. For reasons such as these, nitrous oxide has been deleted from the U.S. Department of Defense's Deployable Medical Systems (DEPMEDS) list.

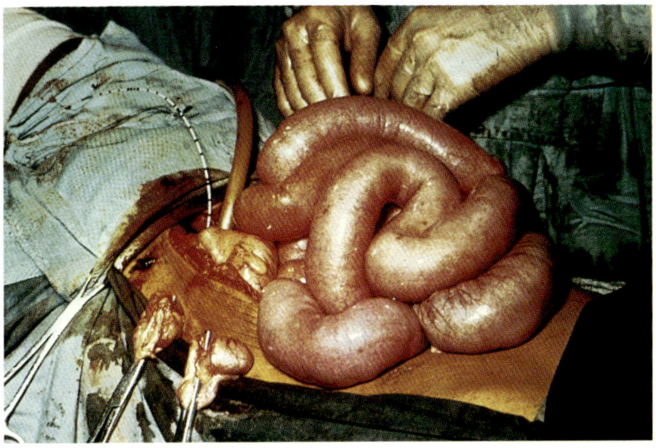

Fig. 20-4. A casualty's small bowel during a laparotomy for a fragment wound of the abdomen. The anesthetist ascribed the distension of the small bowel to the presence of nitrous oxide. Photograph: Swan Vietnam Surgical Slide Collection.

Positioning for Operation

Because a midline incision is the standard for a laparotomy on combat casualties, the supine position will be needed. Casualties in refractory shock may first be subjected to a thoracotomy, but this will usually be done through an anterolateral incision with the casualty in the supine position. Debridement should be performed prior to laparotomy in hemodynamically stable casualties who have multiple wounds, some of which involve the dorsum of the trunk, or a large wound of exit or entrance posteriorly. Thus, these casualties should initially be placed in either the prone or the lateral decubitus position.

SPECIFIC SITES OF ABDOMINAL INJURY

Data from the Wound Data and Munitions Effectiveness Team (WDMET) database, which was compiled during the Vietnam War, indicate that about 50% of casualties with an abdominal wound who survived long enough to reach a hospital had an injury to a single intraabdominal organ. The most commonly injured organs were large bowel including the rectum in 23% of these casualties, small bowel also in 23%, and liver in 14%. In casualties with injuries to multiple intraabdominal organs, 30% had an injury to two organs, 13% to three, 4% to four, and 3% to five or more organs.[38] The most common combinations in casualties with injuries to multiple organs were small bowel and colon; small bowel and liver; and small bowel, colon, and stomach.

Because casualties with injuries to multiple organs are common, a systematic approach is essential to avoid missing an important site. A wide range of severity will be encountered and the severity influences how the injury is managed. To bring clarity to discussions of abdominal trauma, the severity of injury has been scaled for each organ.[39,40] Although this system of injury severity classification has not yet been applied to combat casualties, military anesthesiologists need to know how to use it. In general, for any given organ, two broad classes of injuries are recognized: *hematoma* (more often than not indicating blunt trauma) and *laceration* (usually indicating penetrating trauma). For each type of injury, five or six grades of severity are recognized and in turn are correlated with the International Classification of Disease (ICD-9) and the Abbreviated Injury Scale (AIS). As an example, the scheme as it applies to the liver is reproduced in Table 20-1. Figure 20-5 shows a casualty from the Vietnam War with a grade III laceration caused by fragments from a Claymore mine.

Retroperitoneal Injuries

The retroperitoneum contains major blood vessels (aorta, inferior vena cava) as well as the kidneys, ureters, pancreas, and duodenum. Any of these sites may be involved in penetrating or blunt trauma if the vector of injury is of significant mag-

TABLE 20-1

CLASSIFICATION OF SEVERITY OF HEPATIC INJURY

Grade*		Injury Description†	ICD-9	AIS 90
I	Hematoma	Subcapsular, nonexpanding, < 10% surface area	864.01 864.11	2
	Laceration	Capsular tear, nonbleeding, < 1 cm parenchymal depth	864.02 864.12	2
II	Hematoma	Subcapsular, nonexpanding; 10%–50% surface area Intraparenchymal, nonexpanding; < 2 cm in diameter	864.01 864.11	2
	Laceration	Capsular tear, active bleeding; 1–3 cm parenchymal depth, < 10 cm in length	864.03 864.13	2
III	Hematoma	Subcapsular, < 50% surface area or expanding Ruptured subcapsular hematoma with active bleeding; Intraparenchymal hematoma > 2 cm or expanding		3
	Laceration	> 3 cm parenchymal depth	864.04 864.14	3
IV	Hematoma	Ruptured intraparenchymal hematoma with active bleeding	864.04	4
	Laceration	Parenchymal disruption involving 25%–50% of hepatic lobe	864.14	4
V	Laceration	Parenchymal disruption involving > 50% of hepatic lobe		5
	Vascular	Juxtahepatic venous injury (ie, retrocaval vena cava/major hepatic vein)		5
VI	Vascular	Hepatic avulsion		6

* Advance one grade for multiple injuries to the same organ
† Based on most accurate assessment at autopsy, laparotomy, or radiological study
ICD-9: International Classification of Disease, 9th revision; AIS 90: Abbreviated Injury Scale, 1990 revision
Adapted with permission from Moore EE, Shackford SR, Pachter HL, et al. Organ injury scaling: Spleen, liver, and kidney. *J Trauma.* 1989;29:1665.

a

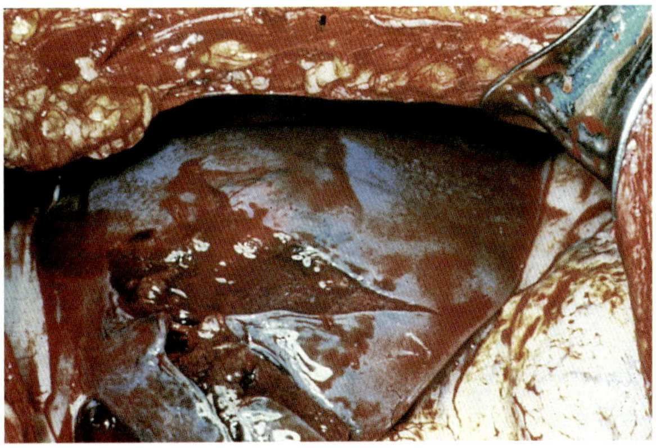

b

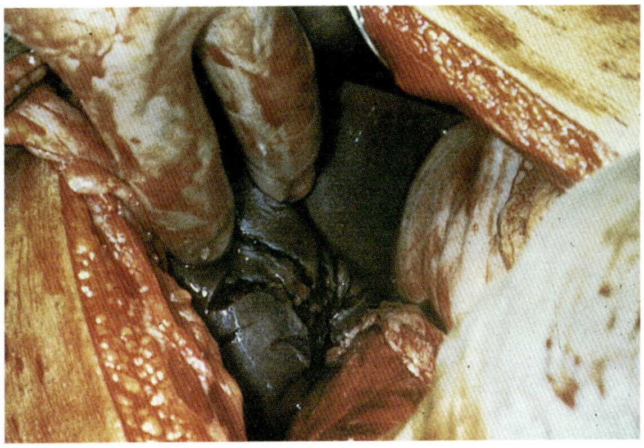

Fig. 20-5. This injury was caused by a fragment from an exploding munition. (**a**) The wound of entrance is in the dome of the lateral segment of the right lobe of the liver. This is a grade III laceration of the liver. (**b**) The wound of exit is in the *undersurface* of the right lobe of the liver. Photographs: Swan Vietnam Surgical Slide Collection.

nitude and direction. Isolated retroperitoneal injuries from penetrating missiles are unusual, because the missile usually passes from the retroperitoneal space into the abdominal cavity.

To assist in deciding on the optimal intraoperative intervention, it has become customary to divide the retroperitoneum into three zones[41]:

- Zone 1: midline to midclavicular lines (includes the great vessels and most of the duodenum and pancreas);
- Zone 2: from midclavicular lines laterally to the flanks (includes the kidneys); and
- Zone 3: below the iliac crests (includes the iliac vessels).

At the hospital level, Zone 3 injuries are encountered most commonly. Zone 1 injuries are least common, probably because injuries to Zone 1 frequently result in rapid exsanguination. Penetrating injuries are explored regardless of the zone. Blunt trauma involving Zone 1 is always explored, as is an enlarging hematoma in Zone 2. Exploration of a hematoma in Zone 3 should be avoided.

Great Vessels

Analysis of the WDMET database reveals that isolated injuries to the great vessels (the aorta, iliac arteries, and inferior vena cava) account for about one half of all deaths of combat casualties who were killed in action or died of intraabdominal injuries (see Chapter 1, Combat Trauma Overview, for a discussion of the WDMET database).[38] Intraabdominal injuries to the great vessels are very uncommon in combat casualties who survive; for example, there are only eight survivors of intraabdominal aortic injuries in the Vietnam Vascular Registry.[42] Nevertheless, the military anesthesiologist should be prepared for such a contingency. A midline retroperitoneal hematoma may reflect injury to the aorta or vena cava and should be explored. Although arterial injury is associated with more-rapid blood loss, venous injury, which is characterized by low-pressure but high-volume hemorrhage, frequently proves more difficult to control. Furthermore, attempts to define the anatomy of vena caval injury by occlusion may precipitate cardiac arrest in the hypovolemic patient. Atrial–caval or femoral–caval shunts have been suggested (but in fact are rarely employed) to maintain circulation while vascular clamps are applied to isolate the site of hemorrhage, but these techniques have not been demonstrated to improve survival. Injuries to the retroperitoneal vasculature carry a high mortality,[43,44] and lacerations of the retrohepatic vena cava are particularly lethal.[45]

Kidneys, Ureters, and Bladder

The kidneys, ureters, and bladder may be injured directly by projectiles or indirectly by blunt trauma. Blunt trauma, or the cavitary damage accompanying high-energy-transfer projectiles, may produce avulsion of the renal vascular pedicle, fracture of the renal parenchyma, or avulsion or disruption or both of the ureters. The elasticity of the bladder renders it less susceptible to disruption[46] and, more commonly, the injury results from direct cutting by the missile. These injuries may be revealed preoperatively by computed tomography scan, intravenous pyelogram, retrograde pyelogram, ultrasound, or, as is common in combat casualties, may be discovered incidentally during laparotomy.[47] In the latter situation, it is essential that an effort be made to demonstrate the presence of a functioning contralateral kidney before ablative renal surgery is undertaken. One way to do this is to clamp the ureter on the injured side and watch the Foley catheter for 5 minutes to see if urine continues to be formed. Ureteral injuries are difficult to diagnose except by direct visualization at the time of laparotomy.

Relatively minor degrees of renal trauma resulting from blunt trauma are managed nonsurgically. The diagnosis of renal injury associated with penetrating missiles is usually made at the time of laparotomy. Knowing exactly what to do about grade II (< 1-cm parenchymal depth of renal cortex without urinary extravasation) or grade III (> 1-cm parenchymal depth of renal cortex without collecting-system rupture or urinary extravasation) injuries is difficult and controversial. Treatment options are partial nephrectomy, debridement, and suture. Grade IV injuries (laceration extending through the cortex, medulla, and collecting system; or a major renal vessel injury) or grade V injuries (completely shattered kidney) are treated in combat zone hospitals by nephrectomy (Figure 20-6). Renal function declines more in patients who are managed operatively; whether this is due to the effects of surgery itself or the presence of more -underlying tissue destruction is unknown.[48,49]

Injuries to the dome of the bladder are often easy to repair because the remaining wall is usually sufficiently redundant to be closed primarily. Care must be taken to ensure that the ureteral orifices are not compromised during closure of the defect. The bladder is closed over a Foley catheter; ureteral injuries are closed over a ureteral catheter splint. Injuries to the trigone of the bladder that require reconstruction may require reconstruction of both the urethra and the ureteral orifices.

Pancreas and Duodenum

Blunt pancreatic injuries are difficult to detect with peritoneal lavage and may be missed by computed tomography scan. Elevated amylase in the lavage fluid from DPL raises suspicion but is neither sensitive nor specific: the absence of amylase does not exclude significant pancreatic injury, and its presence may only reflect small bowel or urinary tract injury.[50] Serum amylase should be measured serially if the site of injury leads to a suspicion of pancreatic damage. Severe pancreatitis will result if pancreatic enzymes are not contained within the pancreatic ducts, so careful, regular consideration must be given to this diagnosis when the physical examination and test results are equivocal.

Grades I or II pancreatic injuries (laceration without duct injury or tissue loss) resulting from penetrating trauma require only closed-suction drainage. More-severe pancreatic injuries such as a disrupted tail or distal ductal laceration (grade III) may be treated by distal pancreatectomy. Injuries of the head of the pancreas, especially when the ampulla or duodenum are involved (grades IV or V) may be treated with the Whipple procedure (pancreaticoduodenectomy with gastrojejunostomy and Roux-en-Y cholecystojejunostomy and Roux-en-Y pancreaticojejunostomy). Mortality is 30% to 40%.[51] The difficulty, complexity, and time-consuming nature of the Whipple procedure makes it unsuitable for performance in the combat zone except in unusual circumstances.

Isolated duodenal injuries are treated by closure of the defect, sometimes in conjunction with temporary defunctionalization of the duodenum brought about by closure of the pylorus with absorbable suture material. A gastrojejunostomy is constructed to reestablish gastrointestinal continuity. The pyloric suture can be expected to remain intact until the duodenal defect is securely healed. Severe injuries, especially when they involve the head of the pancreas, may require a Whipple procedure; however, an operation of such magnitude may severely disrupt the function of a forward surgical facility and should be performed only as a last resort. Dependent drainage is a necessary part of any duodenal or pancreatic operation.[52] Repeated surgeries are often required for treatment of pancreatic fistulas, abscesses, secondary hemorrhage, and pseudocysts. Catastrophic shock occurs in those few who develop hemorrhagic pancreatitis.

Intraperitoneal Injuries

For military anesthesia providers, the major treatment problems of casualties with abdominal injuries involve the intraabdominal organs, which contaminate the abdomen and give rise to peritonitis. To a lesser extent, hemorrhage is a threat; regrettably, however, most casualties who have significant intraabdominal vascular injuries will have exsanguinated before they reach the hospital. Two

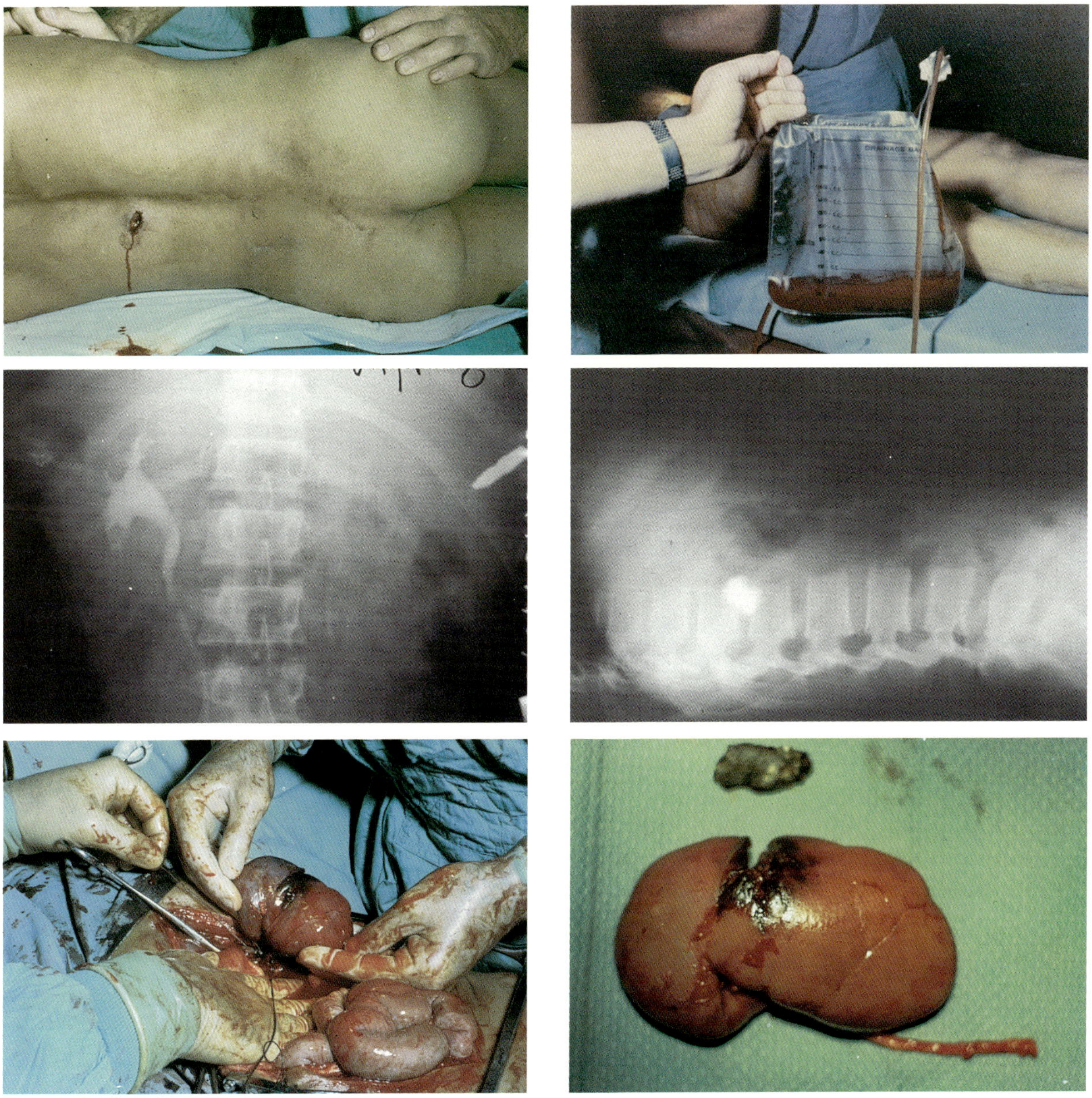

Fig. 20-6. (**a**) This grade IV kidney injury to a casualty during the Vietnam War was caused by a large mortar fragment and was treated by a nephrectomy. The wound of entrance is in the casualty's back. (**b**) Grossly bloody urine was found in the casualty's bladder, indicating a significant injury somewhere in the urinary tract. (**c**) Anteroposterior and (**d**) lateral radiographs taken during an intravenous pyelogram. A large metal fragment is seen in the left upper quadrant of the abdomen. There is no evidence of function by the left kidney. (**e**) The upper pole of the kidney appears cyanotic, a finding indicating a vascular injury. This was the indication for a nephrectomy, which is shown in progress. (**f**) The excised kidney and the fragment that caused the injury. Photographs: Swan Vietnam Surgical Slide Collection.

casualties of the Vietnam War who were seen at the hospital level of care illustrate the ramifications of penetrating abdominal trauma (Figures 20-7 and 20-8). Note that in both casualties, the retroperitoneal component of the injury is the less serious.

Stomach, Small Bowel, and Colon

Injuries to the stomach, small bowel, and colon are accompanied by hemorrhage and peritoneal contamination. Bacterial peritonitis may result from spillage of the stomach contents into the peritoneal

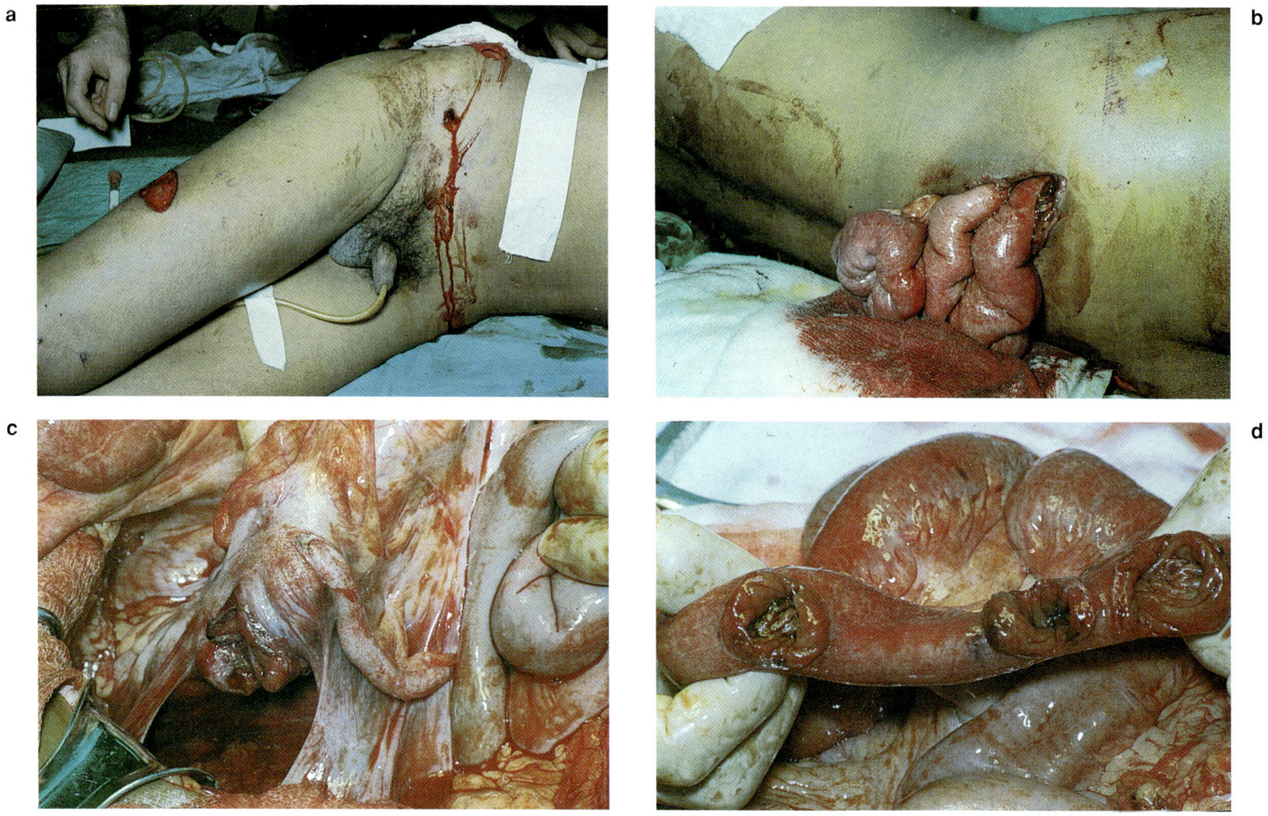

Fig. 20-7. (**a**) This soldier sustained a perforating AK47 (7.62-mm) bullet wound of the inferior portion of the right lower quadrant of his abdomen. The wound of entrance is shown. A second bullet wound in the thigh involved only soft tissue. (**b**) The bullet exited from the flank, causing an evisceration. (**c**) At laparotomy, the tip of the cecum was found to be perforated. The casualty underwent a cecostomy in lieu of an ileotransverse colostomy. (**d**) The casualty's multiple small bowel perforations were treated by small bowel resection and anastomosis. Photographs: Swan Vietnam Surgical Slide Collection.

cavity if a meal has recently been ingested, or, as is common in battle casualties, if stomach emptying is delayed. Salivary flora are ingested during a meal and bacterial counts rise rapidly as stomach acidity is neutralized. As the stomach empties, the hydrogen ion concentration again falls to bactericidal levels, rendering the stomach sterile.[53] Penetrating injury to the stomach is usually managed easily by primary suture. The stomach's good blood supply assures primary healing. With any wound of the

Fig. 20-8. This soldier sustained a perforating AK47 (7.62-mm) bullet wound of the lower abdomen. (**a**) The wound of entrance is seen in the right buttock. Proctoscopy demonstrated blood in the rectum, indicating an injury to the distal large intestine. (**b**) The wound of exit is in the left lower quadrant of the abdomen. The bullet apparently passed posterior to the right iliac vessels and anterior to the left iliac vessels, thereby sparing the casualty from death due to exsanguination. (**c**) The massive small bowel damage can be seen at laparotomy. (**d**) The shredded appearance of this resected specimen of small bowel is probably caused by temporary cavitation, which occurred as the bullet passed through the fluid- and gas-filled viscera. (**e**) The bladder was totally disrupted by the bullet. (**f**) Because of the proximity of the damage to the trigone of the bladder, safe reconstruction of the bladder required catheterization of both ureters and the urethra. The balloon of the urinary catheter is seen in the depth of the wound. (**g**) The rectosigmoid colon has been perforated by the bullet. A totally diverting end colostomy and a mucus fistula are being constructed. (**h**) The casualty is now in the prone position. The perirectal space is exposed for purposes of drainage. Photographs: Swan Vietnam Surgical Slide Collection.

a

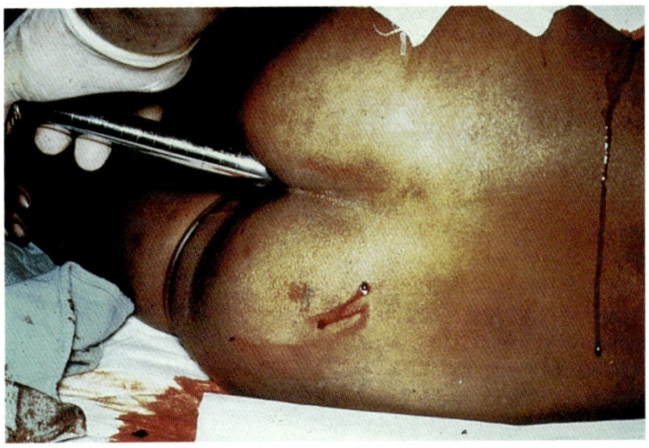

b

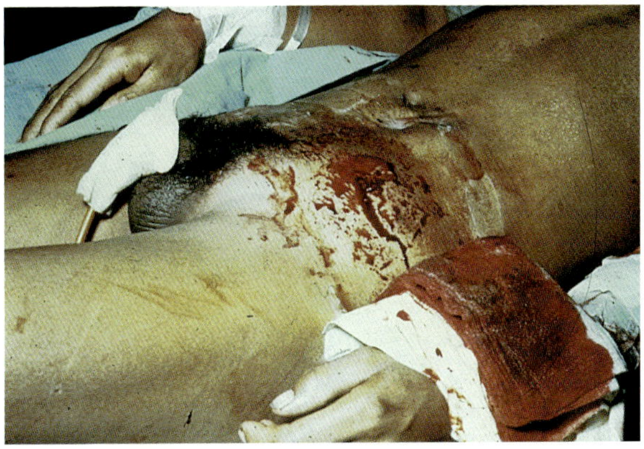

c

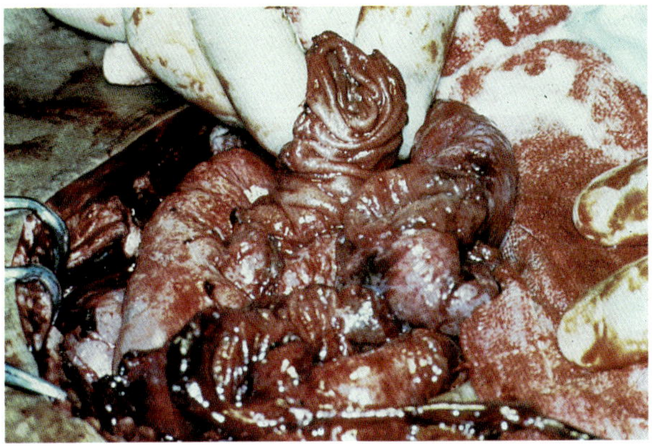

d

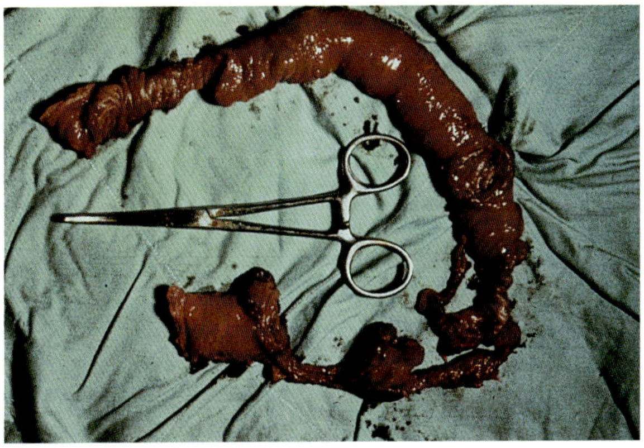

e

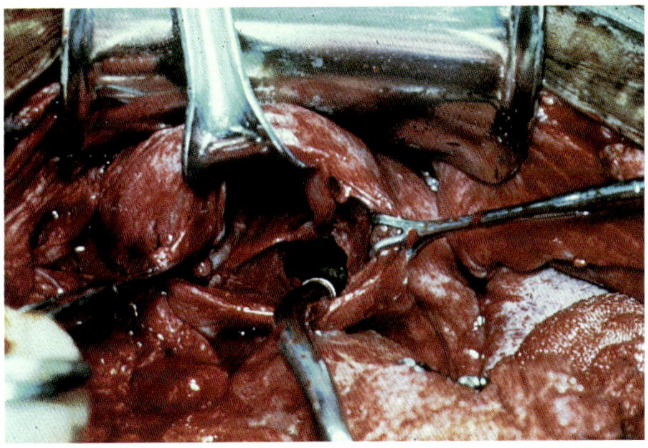

f

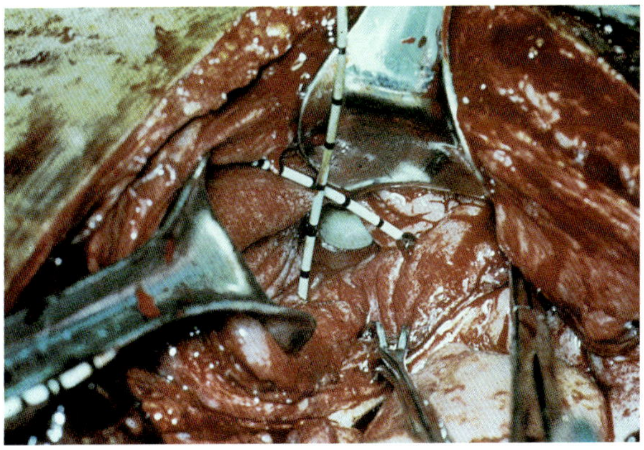

g

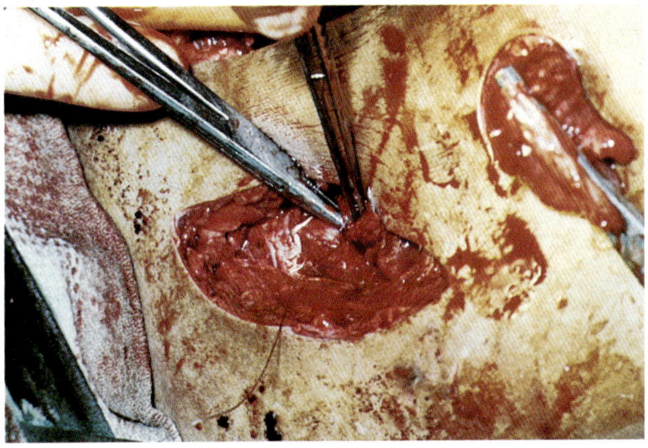

h

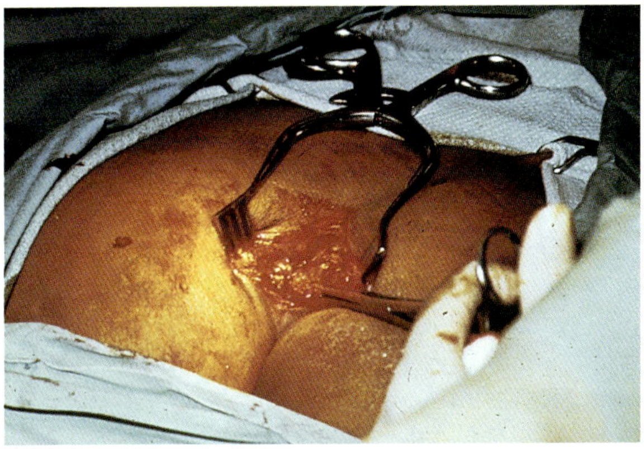

stomach, it is important to determine whether the projectile continued through the posterior wall into the lesser sac and the retroperitoneum.

The small bowel has a very low bacterial count, but peritonitis will eventually occur as the bacteria proliferate. Grades I and II injuries (partial-thickness and full-thickness wounds involving less than one half the bowel circumference) are managed by primary suture repair of the defect. Grade III injuries (defects of > 50%) and grade IV injuries (transection) are managed by resection and primary anastomosis. Multiple, contiguous grade II injuries are best managed by resection and anastomosis.

Colon wounds are difficult to manage: primary healing of a sutured colon wound, in contrast to a wound of the small bowel, has a disturbingly high rate of failure. The peritoneal cavity is capable of tolerating one episode of exposure to the vast bacterial population that resides in the colon, but continued contamination, as will occur with a suture-line breakdown, is rapidly lethal. The following scenario is much feared by military surgeons: a casualty's colonic wound is primarily repaired in a forward surgical hospital; the wound then dehisces during evacuation; and by the time the casualty reaches the next hospital, he is dying from fulminating peritonitis. To prevent this occurrence, military surgical doctrine dictates that a proximally diverting colostomy be constructed on all casualties with large bowel injuries. This practice is at variance with civilian trauma management, in which primary repair is frequently possible.

In grades I, II, or III colonic injuries, primary repair of the colonic wound may prove possible, but the colostomy will assure that the segment is defunctionalized so that leakage of colonic contents, if it occurs, will be inconsequential. Resection is indicated when the projectile transects the bowel (grade IV) or destroys a segment (grade V). The colon distal to the site of resection is mobilized so that it can be pulled through the abdominal wall as a mucous fistula.

Injuries to the rectum create special problems because of the need to both evacuate all feces from the retained bowel and drain the perirectal space in the perineum. Therefore, the casualty with a rectal wound will have a proximally diverting colostomy, a distal mucous fistula (or a closed intraabdominal segment known as a Hartmann's pouch), and an excised coccyx through which drainage of the perirectal space is established. To accomplish this sequence of procedures, the anesthesiologist must be prepared to turn the casualty from supine to prone.

Liver

Hepatic trauma is commonly encountered in abdominal wounds. Grades I and II injuries are rarely the sole cause of death and require no surgical intervention at the time of laparotomy.[54] Grades III and IV injuries are more difficult to treat: suture ligation of vessels will be necessary to control bleeding. Grade V injuries can be treated by formal right or left hepatic lobectomy, but not only is the mortality of this intervention extremely high (not a single casualty subjected to a right hepatic lobectomy in the Vietnam War is thought to have survived), the demands for blood and blood products will likely exhaust all but the largest blood bank. As an alternative to lobectomy, the practice dating from World War II of tamponading the bleeding liver by packing with large laparotomy pads has been proposed. The pack must be removed within 2 to 4 days.[55] The goal is to remove the packs safely after the casualty has reached a higher-echelon medical treatment facility that is capable of providing care of the needed sophistication.

The overwhelming problems that will encountered by the anesthesiologist caring for a casualty with a grade IV or V liver injury will be massive hemorrhage and its complications (hypothermia, acidosis, hypocalcemia, coagulopathy, and the adult respiratory distress syndrome). Intraoperative hemorrhage in these patients may be controlled by the Pringle maneuver (ie, manual compression of the porta hepatis at the epiploic foramen). If this fails, occlusion of the thoracic aorta or the proximal abdominal aorta may be attempted. The most difficult bleeding to control is from a vascular injury at the junction of the hepatic veins with the inferior vena cava. The problem arises from the fact that exposure of the site of injury is possible only when the inferior vena cava is occluded, but the resulting cessation of venous return usually precipitates a cardiac arrest in the already hypovolemic casualty. In rare circumstances, surgeons have been able to shunt blood from the infrahepatic vena cava to the heart, using a plastic tube with a large tangential port (an endotracheal tube can be so modified) inserted through the right atrial appendix and from there guided into the vena cava below the liver. Tourniquets are then tightened around the supradiaphragmatic and infrahepatic venae cava.[56] By isolating the liver and its blood supply, exposure is facilitated and transfusion requirements are reduced. An extension of the shunt may be passed to the anesthesiologist, who then uses it for transfusion. Blood glucose should be closely monitored, as hypoglycemia is not uncommon. Casualties with grades IV or V liver injuries will frequently need secondary operations for removal of a hepatic pack, further debridement, and drainage of hematomas or abscesses or both.[57]

Spleen

For many years, the spleen was considered to be a vestigial organ of no significance and was treated as such in abdominal trauma. Since the 1950s, however, the spleen has come to be recognized as a key component of the immune system. The risk of early or delayed infection is increased in asplenia. Overwhelming postsplenectomy infection occurs in about 0.6% of children and 0.3% of adults.[58] As a result, in civilian practice, the options for managing splenic injury emphasize conservation whenever possible. The options are (*a*) application of a topical hemostatic agent, (*b*) debridement and suturing, and (*c*) splenectomy, which is reserved as a last resort. Wrapping the spleen with an absorbable mesh bag has proven valuable in treatment of extensive capsular avulsion.[59] Grades I, II, and III injuries (ranging from slight capsular tear to parenchymal laceration not involving the hilum) in blunt trauma have been managed nonoperatively when hemodynamic instability and other organ involvement are absent (in the field, however, this can be established with certainty only at the time of laparotomy).[60]

Although splenic conservation is desirable, such an approach has little merit in the management of combat casualties: the essential condition for its application is time to observe the casualty, and this is precisely what cannot be guaranteed in a combat zone hospital. Furthermore, the specter of delayed hemorrhage during evacuation is too frightening to ignore. Accordingly, splenectomy remains the accepted treatment for combat casualties with all but grade I injuries. As is standard with civilian postoperative management of patients who have had splenectomy, antipneumococcal vaccine should be given, and the casualty should be warned of the possible implications of high fever in association with an infection.

Diaphragm

The diaphragm may be ruptured in blunt trauma or perforated in penetrating trauma. In either case, intraabdominal organs may herniate through the diaphragm and produce respiratory embarrassment or organ strangulation. Unless the diaphragm is carefully inspected at the time of laparotomy, a perforation can be missed until clinical symptoms or an abnormal chest radiograph provoke further study.[61–63] Even a small perforation needs to be closed because the defect will gradually enlarge and become the site of a potentialy fatal herniation. Holes in the diaphragm can also create problems for the anesthesiologist during the operation because air can pass from the open abdomen into the chest, creating a pneumothorax. A chest tube placed preoperatively will prevent this condition; however, the surgical team must remember that a missile wound in the area of the costal margin may first have passed through the pleural space and diaphragm before entering the abdomen.

The advent of endoscopic laparotomy is certainly the most significant development in modern gastrointestinal surgery, but the practicality of laparoscopy as a therapeutic modality for treating typical combat injuries in deployed hospitals is unclear. Both endoscopic thoracoscopy and laparoscopy in a diagnostic mode have been used to demonstrate penetrating diaphragmatic injury.[64] A thoracic endoscopic approach to diagnosing diaphragmatic injury (and by implication, a possible intraabdominal injury) following a missile wound to the lower thorax would appear to be a reasonable alternative to observation or an exploratory laparotomy. If a hole in the diaphragm is seen, a laparotomy is indicated both to close the hole and to treat any coexisting intraabdominal injuries.

Damage Control

The concept of staging the operative interventions in the severely injured to allow for optimizing the casualty's physiological status is known by a variety of names: "abbreviated laparotomy and planned reoperation,"[65] "staged celiotomy,"[66] and "delayed gastrointestinal reconstruction,"[67] among others. What these terms describe is the following sequence:

1. emergency laparotomy performed to stop exsanguinating hemorrhage and to prevent further peritoneal contamination;
2. a nonoperative resuscitative phase during which hypovolemia, hypothermia, acidosis, and coagulation defects are corrected; and
3. repeat laparotomy to definitively correct the injuries.

The essential feature of this regimen is the "damage control" of the life-threatening injuries that are found during the initial laparotomy: enteric injuries are ligated to prevent further peritoneal contamination, and exsanguinating hemorrhage is controlled by clamping or packing. Because of its staged nature, this regimen would appear to have much to offer military surgery, which is, after all, characterized by the provision of care by stages, or echelons. We can imagine a forward surgical team performing the initial laparotomy, and then the casualty's being immediately evacuated to a third-echelon hospital for resuscitation and definitive surgery. However, this regimen should be considered for use *only if rapid and reliable evacuation can be guaranteed*.

SUMMARY

Abdominal injuries are the most common life-threatening injuries that military anesthesia providers are likely to encounter. Casualties with abdominal injuries may present with exsanguinating hemorrhage, but more commonly, a stable patient will present with intraabdominal contamination as the major threat to life. with intraabdominal contamination. In the former circumstance, military anesthesia providers will strive for adequate oxygenation, with fluid resuscitation ongoing during surgical control of hemorrhage. In the latter circumstance, a more measured and thorough approach to preoperative preparation is usually possible. In the ideal circumstance, the casualty will receive adequate fluid resuscitation, intravenous antibiotics, and instrumentation for monitoring. Although operations have been done using regional anesthetic techniques, the overwhelming majority are best managed using endotracheal anesthesia.

REFERENCES

1. Hardaway RM. *Care of the Wounded in Vietnam*. Manhattan, Kan: Sunflower University Press; 1988: 39–59.

2. Pfeffermann R, Rozin R, Durst AL. Modern war surgery: Operations in an evacuation hospital during the October 1973 Arab–Israeli War. *J Trauma*. 1976;16:694–703.

3. Moore JB, Moore EE, Thompson JS. Abdominal injuries associated with penetrating trauma in the lower chest. *Am J Surg*. 1980;140:724–730.

4. Trunkey DD, Sheldon PF, Collins JA. The treatment of shock. In: Zuidemia PD, Rutherford RB, Ballinger WF, eds. *The Management of Trauma*. 4th ed. Philadelphia, Pa: WB Saunders; 1985: 105–125.

5. Fackler ML, Surinchak JS, Malinowski JA, Bowen RE. Wounding potential of the Russian AK-74 assault rifle. *J Trauma*. 1984;24:263–266.

6. Bellamy RF, Zajtchuk R. The physics and biophysics of wound ballistics. In: Bellamy RF, Zajtchuk R, eds. *Conventional Warfare: Ballistics, Blast, and Burn Injuries*. Vol 5. In: Zajtchuk R, Jenkins DP, Bellamy RF, eds. *Textbook of Military Medicine*. Washington, DC: US Department of the Army, Office of The Surgeon General, and Borden Institute; 1991: Chap 4.

7. Fackler ML. Wound ballistics: A review of common misconceptions. *JAMA*. 1988;259:2730–2736.

8. Demetriades D, Rabinowitz B. Indications for operation in abdominal stab wounds. *Ann Surg*. 1987;205:129–132.

9. Robin AP, Andrews JR, Lange DA, Roberts RR, Moskal M, Barrett JA. Selective management of anterior abdominal stab wounds. *J Trauma*. 1989;29:1684–1689.

10. Borman KR, Aurbakken CM, Weigelt JA. Treatment priorities in combined blunt abdominal and aortic trauma. *Am J Surg*. 1982;144:728–732.

11. Traub AC, Perry JF. Injuries associated with splenic trauma. *J Trauma*. 1981;21:840–847.

12. Carmona RH, Lim RC, Clark GC. Morbidity and mortality in hepatic trauma. *Am J Surg*. 1982;144:88–94.

13. Powell DC, Bivins BA, Bell RM. Diagnostic peritoneal lavage. *Surg Gynecol Obstet*. 1982;155:257–264.

14. Henneman PL, Marx JA, Moore EE, Cantrill SV, Ammons LA. Diagnostic peritoneal lavage: Accuracy in predicting necessary laparotomy following blunt and penetrating trauma. *J Trauma*. 1990;30:1345–1355.

15. Council on Scientific Affairs, Panel on Magnetic Resonance Imaging. Magnetic resonance imaging of the abdomen and pelvis. *JAMA*. 1989;261:420–433.

16. Hardaway RM. Viet Nam wound analysis. *J Trauma*. 1978;18:635–647.

17. Council on Scientific Affairs. Autologous blood transfusions. *JAMA*. 1986;256:2378–2380.

18. Popousky MA, Devine PA, Taswell HF. Intraoperative autologous transfusion. *Mayo Clin Proc*. 1985;60:125–134.

19. Stehling L. Autologous transfusion. *International Anes Clinics*. 1990;28:190–196.

20. Timberlake GA, McSwain E. Autotransfusion of blood contaminated by enteric contents: A potentially lifesaving measure in the massively hemorrhaging trauma patient? *J Trauma*. 1988;28:855–857.

21. Lou MA, Thadepalli H, Mandal AK. Safety and efficacy of mezlocillin: A single-drug therapy for penetrating abdominal trauma. *J Trauma*. 1988;28:1541–1547.

22. Hooker KD, DiPiro JT, Wynn JJ. Aminoglycoside combinations versus beta-lactams alone for penetrating abdominal trauma; a meta analysis. *J Trauma*. 1991;31:1155–1160.

23. Dripps RD. Anesthesia for combat casualties on the basic of experience in Korea. In: Howard JM. *Tools for Resuscitation*. In: Crosby WH. *Battle Casualties in Korea: Studies of the Surgical Research Team*. Vol 2. Washington, DC: Army Medical Service Graduate School, Walter Reed Army Medical Center; 1955: Chap 18: 241–255.

24. Noble MJ, Bryant T, Ing FYW. Casualty anesthesia experiences in Vietnam. *Anesth Anal*. 1968;47:5–11.

25. Davidson JT, Cotev S. Anesthesia in the Yom Kippur War. *Ann R Coll Surg Engl*. 1975;56:304–311.

26. Jowitt MD, Knight RJ. Anesthesia during the Falklands campaign. *Anesthesia*. 1983;38:776–783.

27. Markel G, Eger EI. A comparative study of halothane and halopropane anesthesia. *Anesthesiology*. 1963;24:346–357.

28. Cullen DJ. Anesthetic depth and MAC. In: Miller RD, ed. *Anesthesia*. New York, NY: Churchill Livingstone; 1986: 553–580.

29. Bogetz MS, Katz JA. Recall of surgery for major trauma. *Anesthesiology*. 1984;61:6–9.

30. Gross JB, Alexander CM. Awakening concentrations of isoflurane are not affected by analgesic doses of morphine. *Anesth Analg*. 1988;67:27–30.

31. Stoelting RK, Longnecker DE, Eger EI. Minimum alveolar concentrations in man on awakening from methoxyflurane, halothane, ether and fluroxene anesthesia. *Anesthesiology*. 1970;33:5–9.

32. Bahl CP, Wadwa S. Consciousness during apparent surgical anesthesia. *Brit J Anaesth*. 1968;40:289–291.

33. Saucier N, Walts LF, Moreland JR. Patient awareness during nitrous oxide, oxygen, and halothane anesthesia. *Anesth Analg*. 1983;62:239–240.

34. Courington FW, Calverley RK. Anesthesia on the western front: The Anglo-American experience of World War I. *Anesthesiology*. 1986;65:642–653.

35. Slocum HC. Anesthesia for combat casualties. In: Hardaway RM, ed. *Care of the Wounded in Vietnam*. Manhattan, Kan: Sunflower University Press; 1988: 121–138.

36. Eger EI II. Pharmacokinetics. In: Eger EI II, ed. *Nitrous Oxide*. New York, NY: Elsevier Science Publishing Company; 1985: 81–107.

37. Scheinin B, Lindgren L, Scheinin TM. Preoperative nitrous oxide delays bowel function after colonic surgery. *Brit J Anaesth.* 1990;64:154–158.

38. The single most useful database describing combat wounds and the circumstances of wounding is the Wound Data and Munitions Effectiveness Team (WDMET) study prepared by the U.S. Army Materiel Command during the Vietnam War. These data are stored at the National Naval Medical Center, Bethesda, Maryland. Access is controlled by the Uniformed Services University of the Health Sciences, Bethesda, Maryland 20814-4799; telephone (301) 295-6262. Three summary volumes contain extensive abstracts of the statistical data and can be obtained from Defense Documentation Center, Cameron Station, Alexandria, Virginia 22304-6145; telephone (703) 545-6700 and (703) 274-7633.

39. Moore EE, Shackford SR, Pachter HL, et al. Organ injury scaling, I: Spleen, liver, and kidney. *J Trauma.* 1989;29:1664–1666.

40. Moore EE, Cogbill TH, Malangoni MA, et al. Organ injury scaling, II: Pancreas, duodenum, small bowel, colon, and rectum. *J Trauma.* 1990;30:1427–1429.

41. Selivanov V, Chi HS, Alverdy JC, Morris JA Jr, Sheldon GF. Mortality in retroperitoneal hematoma. *J Trauma.* 1984;24:1022–1027.

42. Spencer F, Rich N. *Vascular Trauma.* Philadelphia, Pa: WB Saunders; 1978: 339.

43. Kudsk KA, Sheldon GF, Lim RC. Atrial–caval shunting (ACS) after trauma. *J Trauma.* 1982;22:81–85.

44. Collins PS, Golocovsky M, Salander JM, Champion H, Rich NM. Intra-abdominal vascular injury secondary to penetrating trauma. *J Trauma.* 1988;28:S165–170.

45. Buechter KJ, Sereda D, Gomez G, Zeppa R. Retrohepatic vein injuries: Experience with 20 cases. *J Trauma.* 1989;29:1698–1704.

46. O'Connell KJ, Clark M, Lewis RH, Christenson PJ. Comparison of low- and high-velocity ballistic trauma to genitourinary organs. *J Trauma.* 1988;28(suppl):139–144.

47. Bretan PN, McAninch JW, Federle MP, Jeffrey RB. Computerized tomographic staging of renal trauma: 85 consecutive cases. *J Urol.* 1986;136:561–565.

48. McGonigal MD, Lucas CE, Ledgerwood AM. The effects of treatment of renal trauma on renal function. *J Trauma.* 1987;27:471–476.

49. Carroll PR, Klosterman PW, McAninch JW. Surgical management of renal trauma: Analysis of risk factors, technique, and outcome. *J Trauma.* 1988;28:1071–1077.

50. Olsen WR. The serum amylase in blunt abdominal trauma. *J Trauma.* 1973;13:200–204.

51. Wynn M, Hill DM, Miller DR, Waxman K, Elsner ME, Gazzaniga AB. Management of pancreatic and duodenal trauma. *Am J Surg.* 1985;150:327–332.

52. Cogbill TH, Moore EE, Feliciano DV, et al. Conservative management of duodenal trauma: A multicenter perspective. *J Trauma.* 1990;30:1469–1475.

53. Drasar BS, Shiner M, McLeod GM. Studies on the intestinal flora. *Gastroenterology.* 1969;56:71–79.

54. Rivkind AI, Siegel JH, Dunham CM. Patterns of organ injury in blunt hepatic trauma and their significance for management and outcome. *J Trauma.* 1989;29:1398–1415.

55. Saifi J, Fortune JB, Graca L, Shah DM. Benefits of intra-abdominal pack placement for the management of nonmechanical bleeding. *Arch Surg.* 1990;125:119–122.

56. Beal SL, Ward RE. Successful atrial caval shunting in the management of retrohepatic venous injuries. *Am J Surg*. 1989;158:409–413.

57. Cogbill TH, Moore EE, Jurkovich GJ, Feliciano DV, Morris JA, Mucha P. Severe hepatic trauma: A multi-center experience with 1,335 liver injuries. *J Trauma*. 1988;28:1433–1438.

58. Lucas CE. Splenic trauma. *Ann Surg*. 1991;213:98–112.

59. Pickhardt B, Moore EE, Moore FA, McCroskey BL, Moore GE. Operative splenic salvage in adults: A decade perspective. *J Trauma*. 1989;29:1386–1391.

60. Cogbill TH, Moore EE, Jurkovich GJ, Morris JA, Mucha P, Shackford SR. Nonoperative management of blunt splenic trauma: A multicenter experience. *J Trauma*. 1989;29:1312–1317.

61. Feliciano DV, Cruse PA, Mattox KL, et al. Delayed diagnosis of injuries to the diaphragm after penetrating wounds. *J Trauma*. 1988;28:1135–1144.

62. Maddox PR, Mansel RE, Butchart EG. Traumatic rupture of the diaphragm: A difficult diagnosis. *Injury*. 1991;22:299–302.

63. Kaulesar-Sukul DMKS, Kats E, Johannes EJ. Sixty-three cases of traumatic injury of the diaphragm. *Injury*. 1991;22:303–306.

64. Ivatury RR, Simon RJ, Weksler B, Bayard V, Stahl WM. Laparoscopy in the evaluation of the intrathoracic abdomen after penetrating injury. *J Trauma*. 1992;33:101–109.

65. Burch JM, Ortiz VB, Richardson RJ, Martin RR, Mattox KL, Jordan GL Jr. Abbreviated laparotomy and planned reoperation for critically injured patients. *Ann Surg*. 1992;215:476–484.

66. Morris JA Jr, Eddy VA, Blinman TA, Rutherford EJ, Sharp KW. The staged celiotomy for trauma: Issues in packing and reconstruction. *Ann Surg*. 1993;217:576–586.

67. Carrillo C, Fogler RJ, Shaftan GW. Delayed gastrointestinal reconstruction following massive abdominal trauma. *J Trauma*. 1993;34:233–235.

Chapter 21

EXTREMITY INJURIES

RAYMOND R. LUPKAS, Jr., M.D.*; and RONALD F. BELLAMY, M.D.†

*Formerly, Major, Medical Corps, U.S. Army; Anesthesia and Operative Service, Walter Reed Army Medical Center, Washington, D. C. 20307-5001; currently, Staff Anesthesiologist, Moore Regional Hospital, Page Road, Pinehurst, North Carolina 28374
†Colonel, Medical Corps, U.S. Army; Managing Editor and Officer in Charge, Textbook of Military Medicine, Borden Institute, Walter Reed Army Medical Center, Washington, D. C. 20307-5001

INTRODUCTION

Combat casualties with orthopedic and soft-tissue injuries of the extremities constitute the majority of soldiers who require operative procedures in the corps and communications zones.[1] These injuries are usually not life threatening but are the major source of man-days lost by combat casualties. Extremity injuries are usually found in the secondary survey of the American College of Surgeons' Advanced Trauma Life Support (ATLS) examination unless the casualty has an obvious external hemorrhage associated with the injury.[2] In corps zone hospitals, casualties with extremity injuries undergo resuscitative surgery that is designed to control hemorrhage, decontaminate wounds, and stabilize fractures so the casualty can safely and comfortably be evacuated to hospitals in the communication zone or the continental United States (CONUS). Corrective surgery is undertaken in the higher-echelon hospitals for the purpose of closing wounds and restoring function. Providing anesthetic care in the corps support zone to casualties with extremity wounds may be difficult because such injuries commonly coexist with much more life-threatening injuries to the head or trunk. Multiple or simultaneous procedures that involve multiple surgical teams attending the casualty together or in succession may be required.

INJURY PATTERNS

The nature and severity of extremity injuries depend on the mechanism of injury. In general, the magnitude of injury depends on the magnitude of energy transferred to the tissue. High-energy blunt trauma (eg, a high-speed motor vehicle accident) is associated with extensive soft-tissue destruction and severely comminuted fractures.[3] These generally need to be reduced early to control bleeding and infection; early treatment also allows early mobilization to enhance pulmonary toilet. Frequently there are coexisting injuries to the cardiac, pulmonary, abdominal, and renal organ systems that complicate the injury. Fat emboli, thromboemboli, deep venous thrombosis, and adult respiratory distress syndrome often complicate the long-term care of the casualty.[3,4]

Low-energy blunt trauma (eg, skiing injuries and some falls) cause relatively simple fractures with minimal soft-tissue destruction. These usually require less-complex treatment and are not usually associated with severe coexisting injuries.

As with injuries caused by blunt trauma, the nature of penetrating injuries depends on the amount of kinetic energy transferred to the tissues. However, because the rate of energy transfer is much greater with penetrating injuries from, say, a bullet than it is with blunt trauma from, say, a vehicular bump, the same amount of energy transferred by the former mechanism will cause more damage.

With penetrating injuries, the kinetic energy is related to the mass of an object multiplied by its velocity squared. Therefore, doubling the velocity increases the kinetic energy 4-fold. The kinetic energy determines the maximum amount of energy that can be transferred, but whether the energy transfer actually occurs is determined by other factors, of which shape, stability, and construction of the missile are especially important. The small M16 bullet—even though its muzzle velocity is high—possesses less than half the kinetic energy of typical rifle bullets used during World War II; yet the M16 bullet is notorious for causing severe damage. Because of its propensity to fragment, a much greater fraction of the kinetic energy of the M16 bullet is usually transferred to the target tissue than occurred with bullets fired by earlier rifles. The surrounding tissue is damaged extensively by both the fragments and the temporary cavitation that is caused by the massive energy transfer. Skeletal muscle will be injured (*a*) by direct cutting and laceration caused by the bullet or fragments and (*b*) by being ripped apart by the stretch of cavitation. Several millimeters of necrotic muscle characteristically line the wound tract, although the major threat arises from infection in the surrounding tissue because it is both contused and contaminated with foreign material brought into the wound.[5]

In contrast, a low-velocity, penetrating injury (eg, a knife wound) is associated with only the local injury directly imposed by the object itself. A shotgun blast from a distance imparts only comparatively little energy to the body; when the wound is made at point-blank distance, however, all of the shell's energy—which is equal to that of an assault rifle bullet and is therefore much more dangerous—is imparted.

THE NATURE OF EXTREMITY INJURIES SEEN IN COMBAT CASUALTIES

The database compiled during the Vietnam War by the Wound Data and Munitions Effectiveness Team (WDMET) is a unique, underutilized repository of first-hand information on war wounds and the mechanisms of injury. (Chapter 1, Combat Trauma Overview, discusses WDMET data in some detail.) Analysis of the WDMET data reveals that about one half of combat casualties who survive long enough to be evacuated to the hospital level have injuries that involve only the extremities. In addition, a sizable number of the remaining casualties have injuries of the extremities in addition to more-serious injuries of the head or trunk (ie, combined injuries). About one third of extremity operations will be to treat injuries that involve only soft tissue (ie, skin, fat, and skeletal muscle). The remaining two thirds of extremity operations will be for injuries that involve soft tissue in addition to injuries to deeper structures such as long bones and neurovascular structures.[6] It is these latter injuries that may especially challenge the military anesthesiologist.

The prevalence of purely soft-tissue injuries has increased in recent wars due to the more frequent use of improved fragmentation munitions. These characteristically cause multiple, small fragment wounds (Figure 21-1). Another form of purely soft-

a b

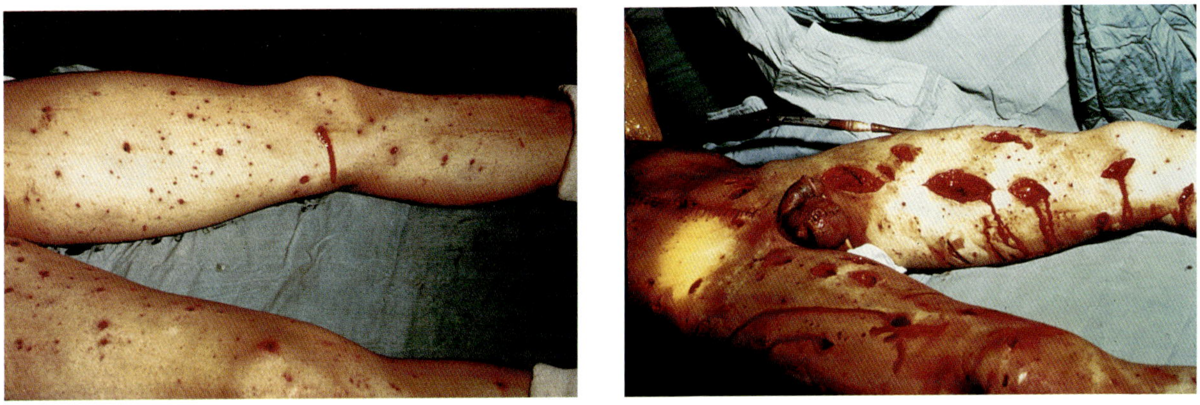

Fig. 21-1. (**a**) This casualty has multiple, tiny, fragment wounds of his lower extremities that were caused by hand-grenade fragments. (**b**) The surgeons have elected to excise some of the larger wounds, although there was probably little tissue damage or contamination. Photographs: Swan Vietnam Surgical Slide Collection.

a b

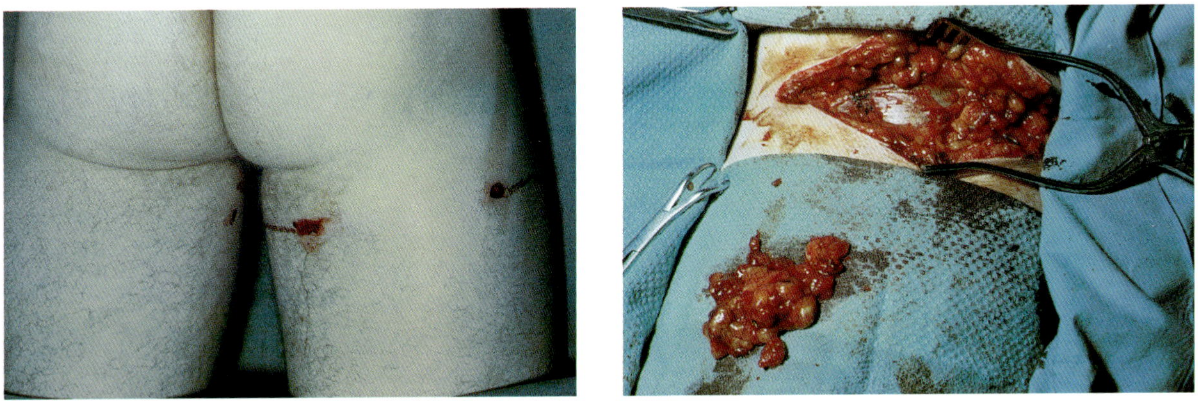

Fig. 21-2. (**a**) This casualty's through-and-through wound in the posterior thigh was made by a bullet fired by a .38-caliber pistol at close range. (**b**) The wound has been incised and the subcutaneous tissue superficial to the muscle fascia has been excised. It is possible that this wound could have been treated nonsurgically. Photographs: Swan Vietnam Surgical Slide Collection.

Fig. 21-3. This soldier was struck by several fragments from an exploding booby trap. (**a**) Wounds of entrance are seen in the left lateral thigh and just proximal to the right knee. There were no wounds of exit. (**b**) The radiograph shows a grossly comminuted fracture of the middle portion of the left femur. Several metallic foreign bodies are seen. (**c**) The radiograph shows intact bones in the casualty's right knee. Several small metallic foreign bodies are seen. (**d**) The casualty's appearance after wound debridement. The extensive nature of the operation carried out on the left thigh is justified by the need to excise injured soft tissue in proximity to the femur fracture. The extensive nature of the operation carried out on the casualty's right thigh is justified by the need to preclude an injury to the superficial femoral artery. (**e**) The casualty had delayed primary closure on the 6th day after the injury. Photographs: Swan Vietnam Surgical Slide Collection.

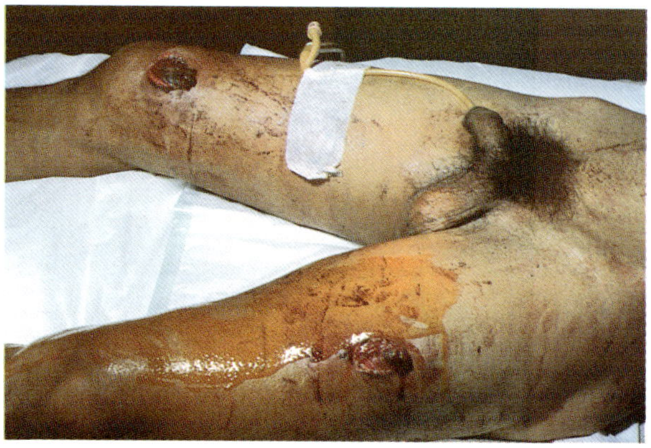
a

b
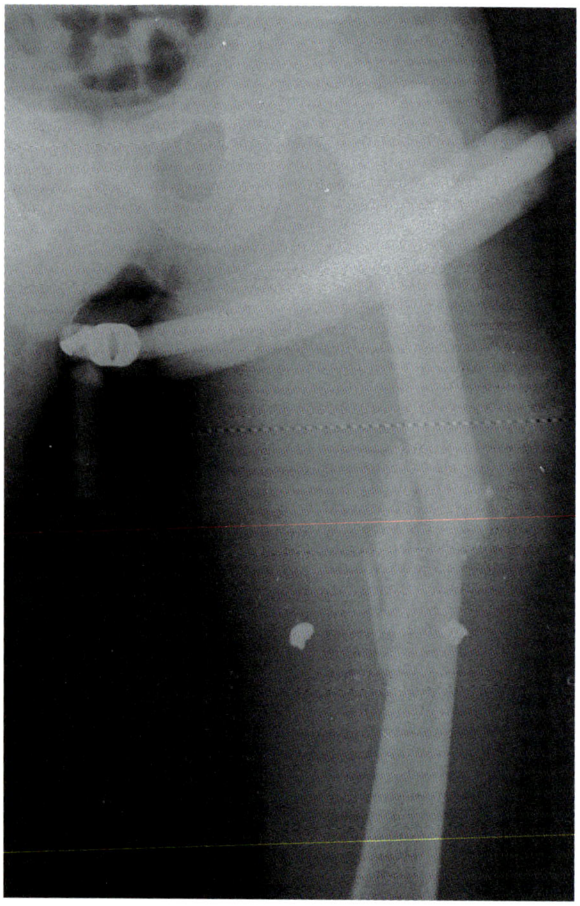

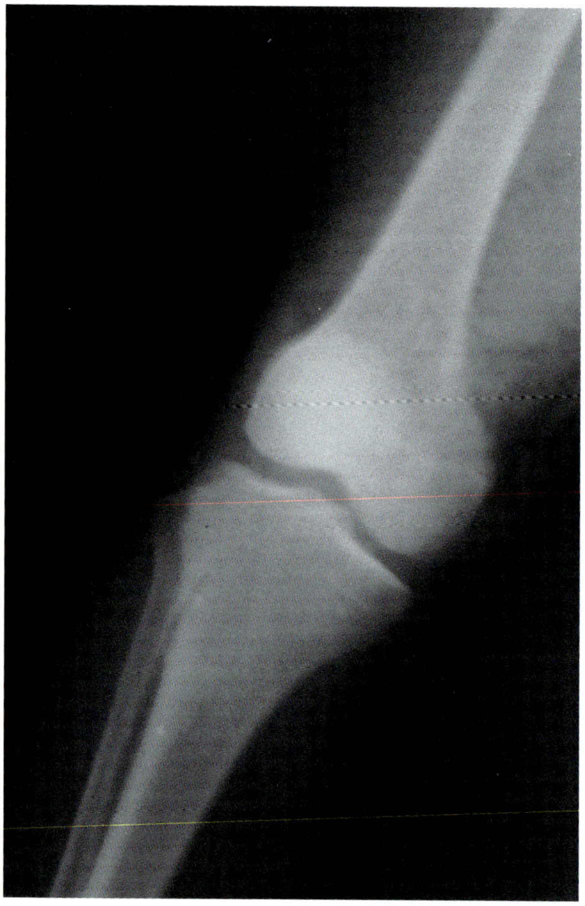
c

d
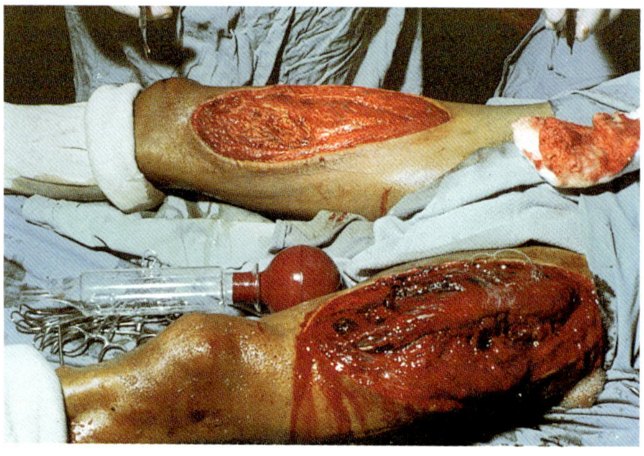

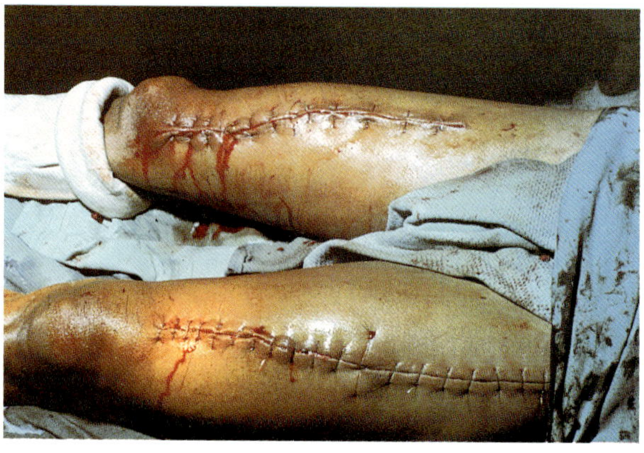
e

tissue injury is the *en seton* (ie, through-and-through) gunshot wound (Figure 21-2). Although en seton wounds may be made by high-velocity bullets, the tissue damage is surprisingly small because energy transfer has been minimized by the failure of the bullet to yaw, tumble, fragment, or deform. The treatment of an en seton wound should be no different from the treatment given to a casualty with a wound made by a low-velocity bullet fired from a civilian hand gun.

By way of contrast, very extensive soft-tissue wounds are frequently seen in conjunction with open, comminuted, long-bone fractures (Figures 21-3 and 21-4). In these wounds, the missile is stopped by the bone with consequent maximal energy transfer, which, together with secondary missiles arising from bone fragments, causes massive tissue damage.

Even more massive tissue damage to the extremities is found in casualties who detonate antipersonnel mines or who are injured by shaped-charge warheads. Such injuries almost always result in traumatic amputations (Figure 21-5).

The increasing likelihood of involvement by the U.S. military in operations other than war (OOTW) makes it likely that military anesthesiologists will be confronted by casualties, many of whom are civilians, who have neglected extremity injuries. Figure 21-6 shows such a patient.

In the WDMET database, about 35% of the extremity injuries involve an isolated fracture of an extremity long bone. Lower-extremity fractures were 2.5-fold more common than those of the upper extremity. About 12% of casualties with extremity wounds had fractures of the bones of the hands or feet. About 7% of casualties with extremity wounds had a major extremity amputation (arm or leg) and about 5% had amputations of the hands, feet, fingers, or toes. Of casualties with extremity wounds, 12% had an isolated vascular injury (the femoral artery the most common), and 5% had an isolated nerve injury (the sciatic nerve the most common).

Of casualties who survived to reach the hospital level, 6% had an injury that involved both a fractured bone and a vascular or nerve injury. The most common combinations were a fractured femur and a femoral arterial injury, and a fractured humerus with an injury to the radial nerve.

In summary, the most common extremity injuries—exclusive of those of soft tissue only—likely to be seen by the military anesthesiologist are

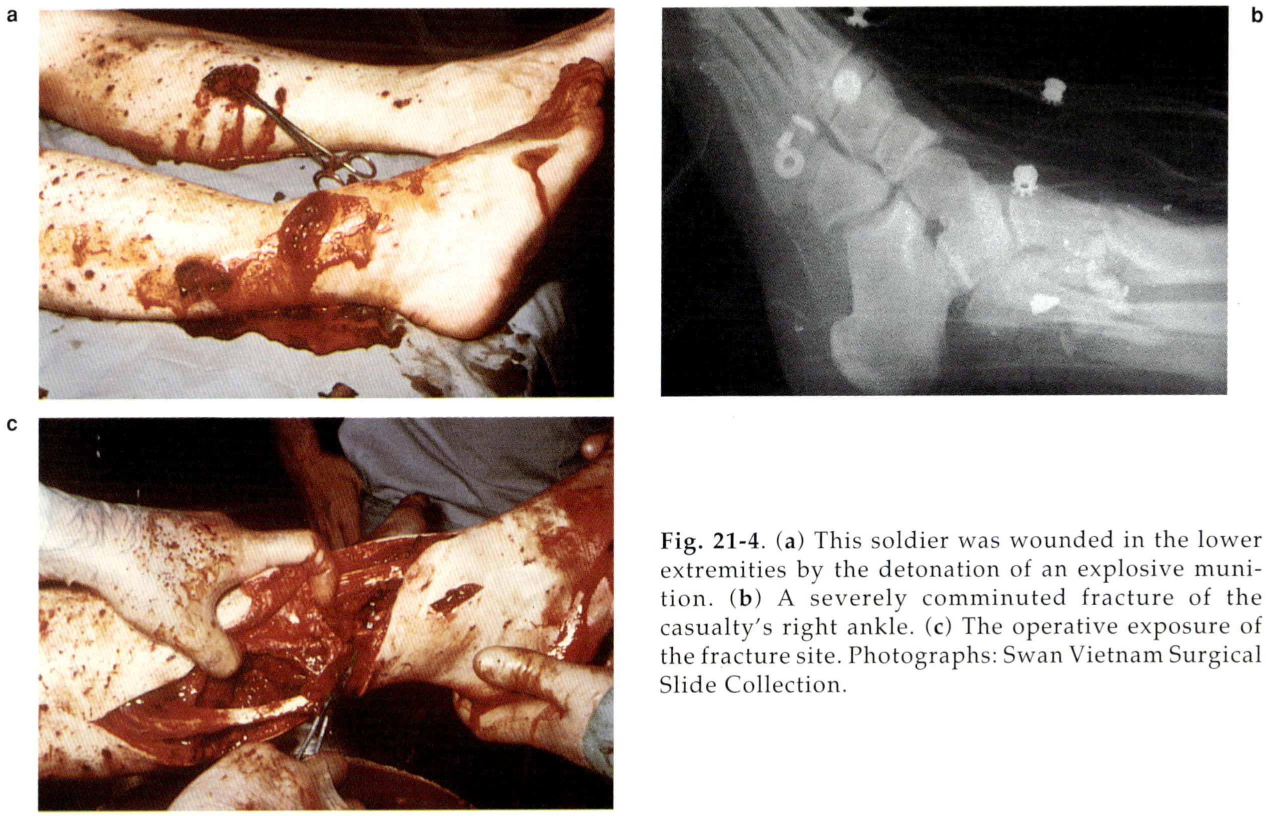

Fig. 21-4. (**a**) This soldier was wounded in the lower extremities by the detonation of an explosive munition. (**b**) A severely comminuted fracture of the casualty's right ankle. (**c**) The operative exposure of the fracture site. Photographs: Swan Vietnam Surgical Slide Collection.

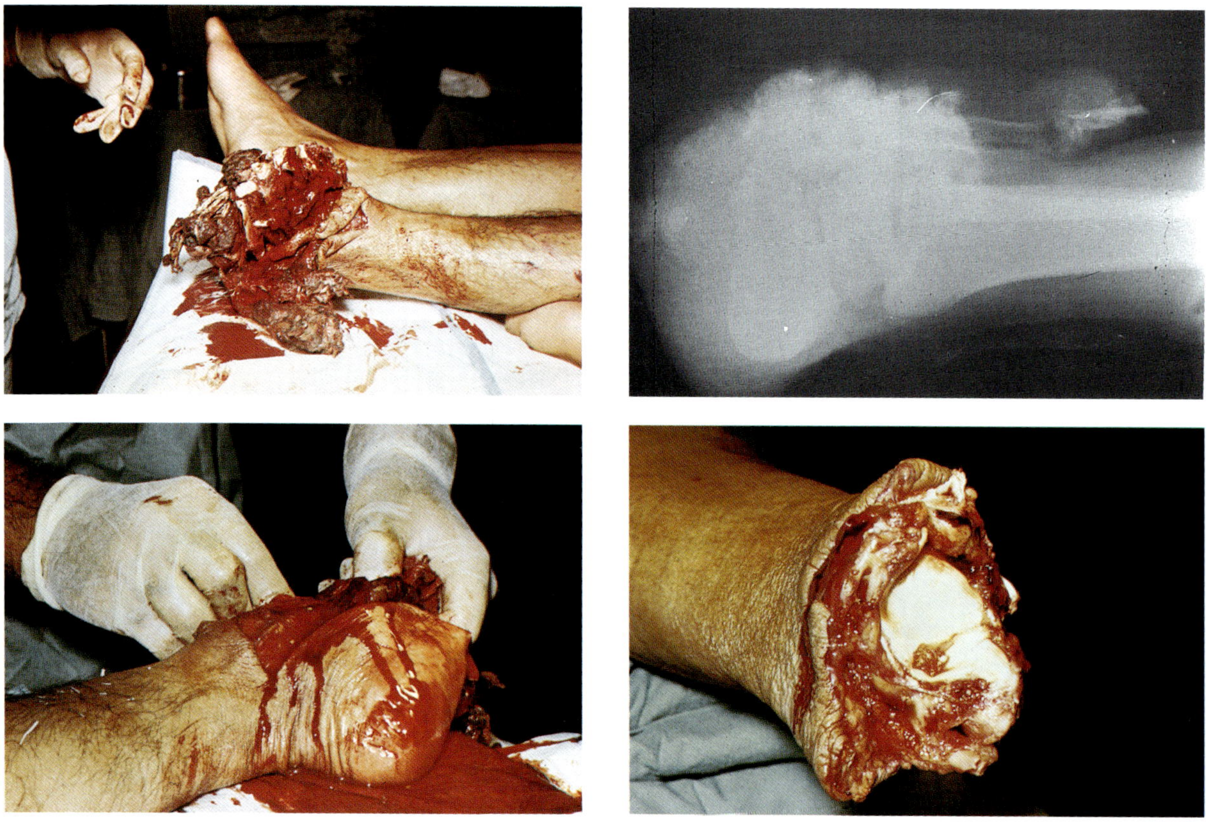

Fig. 21-5. (**a**) This soldier detonated an antipersonnel mine; a traumatic amputation of the distal portion of his foot (ie, the forefoot) has occurred. (**b**) The radiograph shows the extent of bony injury. (**c**) A formal forefoot amputation is in progress. (**d**) The finished amputation. Note that the forefoot has been removed at the talus. This is known as a Syme's amputation. Retaining sufficient skin to cover the stump is sometimes difficult to achieve with this procedure. Photographs: Swan Vietnam Surgical Slide Collection.

- an open, comminuted fracture of a long bone, the femoral shaft being the most common site;
- an amputation of the leg, arm, hand, or foot; and
- an isolated vascular injury, the superficial femoral artery being the most common site.

Management

Shock and sepsis are the two most serious medical treatment problems that may arise in combat casualties with extremity trauma. The relative importance of these two causes of death has been changed by modern military surgery. During World War I and earlier wars such as the American Civil War, sepsis in the injured extremity was the most frequent cause of death in hospitalized casualties. With the use of wound excision and antibiotics, life-threatening sepsis has become much less common.

Shock

Extremity wounds can be fatal. The WDMET database indicates that about 9% of casualties with extremity wounds that involved more than just soft-tissue damage died. Most casualties with injured extremities who were fatally wounded were killed in action; the most common cause of death was exsanguination—from amputation of an arm or a leg, or from lacerations of the femoral artery. The few casualties with extremity injuries who are at risk of dying at the hospital level have sustained either massive blood loss or have developed life-threatening sepsis, usually from an anaerobic wound infection.

Blunt injuries to the extremities may also be associated with hypovolemic shock secondary to hemorrhage, but this occurrence is due not to massive hemorrhage but to prolonged, slow bleeding secondary to rupture of intraosseous blood vessels or lacerations of blood vessels near the site of frac-a b c d

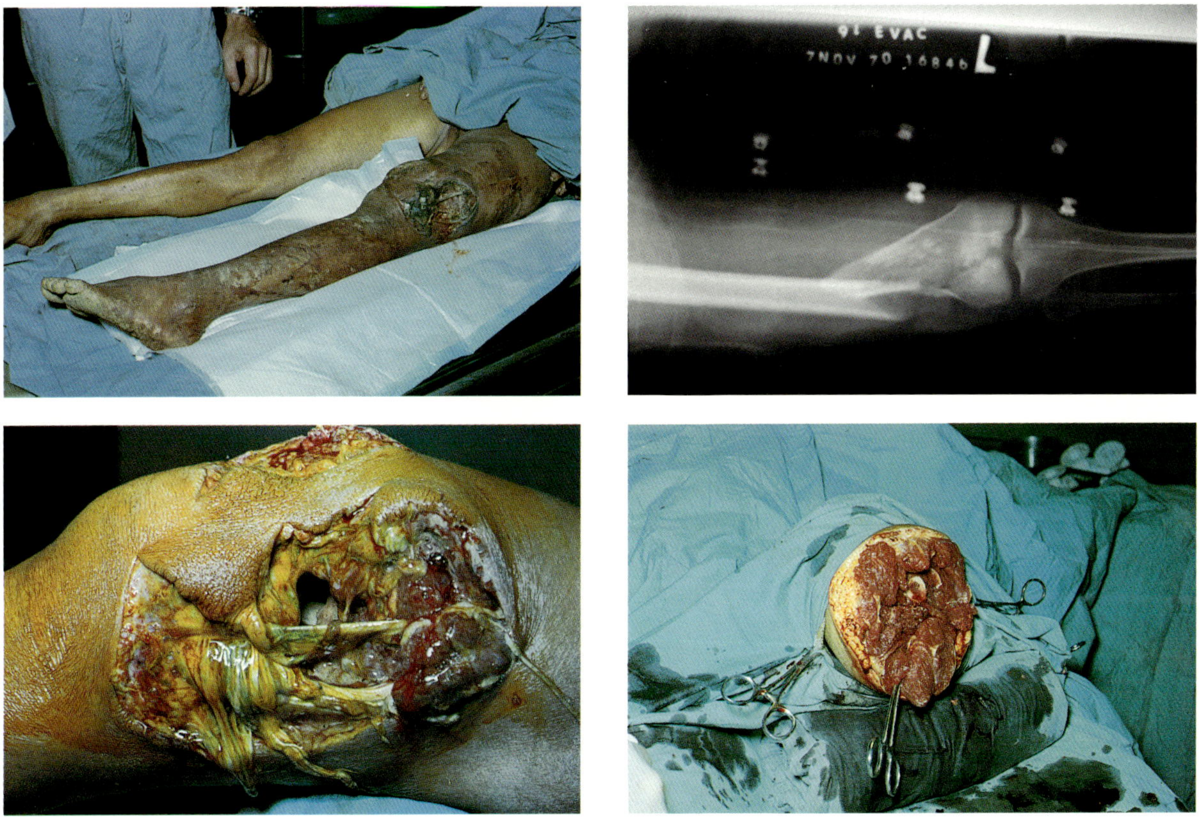

Fig. 21-6. (**a**) This woman has a 3-day-old open comminuted fracture of the left femur that was caused by a perforating gunshot wound. (**b**) The radiograph shows the comminuted fracture. (**c**) A close-up view of the wound of entrance. The wound shows signs of anaerobic sepsis. (**d**) An above-the-knee amputation of the guillotine type has been performed. Such an operation may be lifesaving when the patient has an infected open fracture. Photographs: Swan Vietnam Surgical Slide Collection.

ture.[4,7] Large volumes of blood can be sequestered in limbs even without significantly changing limb size.[8] Therefore, refractory shock in the casualty with blunt trauma to an extremity requires that a search be made for occult fractures. Large volumes of blood and blood products may be required, and coagulopathies should be anticipated (Table 21-1).

Pneumatic antishock garments can be beneficial in stabilizing fractures. These trousers have limited value in correcting hypovolemia, as the intravascular volume returned to the central circulation is minimal. They are beneficial in that they temporarily stabilize fractures of the pelvis and lower extremity and decrease the bleeding.[9]

Sepsis

The goal of military medical management is to return the injured soldier to full duty. This is accomplished by promoting rapid and complete

TABLE 21-1

POTENTIAL BLOOD LOSS FROM CLOSED FRACTURES

Expected Blood Loss (mL)	Bone Fractured
500	Forearm: radius and/or ulna
750	Elbow Tibia Ankle
1,000	Humerus Femoral shaft
1,250	Hip
> 1,500	Pelvis

Adapted with permission from Shumaik GM. Extremity trauma. In: Baxt WG, ed. *Trauma: The First Hour*. Norwalk, Conn: Appleton-Century-Crofts; 1985: 227.

healing of the wound. Sometimes, as in the case of an amputation, this is not possible. Return to duty is also unlikely for many casualties with severe fractures or nerve injuries. In most casualties, the major factor delaying wound healing and return to duty is sepsis, which occurs in about 5% of casualties with pure soft-tissue injuries but in as many as 30% or more of casualties with open, comminuted fractures of the femoral shaft.[10,11]

Wound sepsis is prevented by surgical excision of the contaminated and damaged tissue lining the wound tract. The operation is commonly known as *debridement*, although, strictly speaking, debridement means only wound incision. In general, the amount of tissue to be excised is related to the size of the wound. Tiny extremity wounds can be left alone, but this is rarely the case with the large wounds of exit that frequently accompany extremity fractures. Even in casualties with only soft-tissue wounds, debridement can be an extensive operation (see Figure 21-1). Perioperative administration of antibiotics—especially if they suppress the growth of clostridial bacteria and *Streptococcus pyogenes*—may be a useful adjunct. Wound sepsis that occurs weeks after injury is usually the result of the growth of staphylococci or Gram-negative organisms in open wounds that contain dead tissue. Such wounds require redebridement.

Surgical Treatment

The most common operative procedure performed by military surgeons is wound debridement, and the most common sites for this operation are the extremities. The goal of debridement is to decontaminate injured tissue so that healing is not impeded by local infection. Following debridement, a surgical intervention is usually required to bring about wound closure. In contrast to civilian practice, the military surgeon rarely closes the wound at the time of initial debridement. The most common approach, with the patient anesthetized, is to inspect the wound 4 to 6 days after wounding and to close the wound at that time if there is (*a*) no evidence of other than superficial infection and (*b*) little necrotic tissue that cannot be easily removed. This procedure is known as *delayed primary closure*. The delay in closure is a consequence of both the inability of the surgeon to be certain that all damaged and contaminated tissue has been removed and the provision of military medical care by echelons. Primary closure by a surgeon at one echelon, followed by the patient's evacuation to a higher echelon, would remove the casualty from observation just when the most lethal form of sepsis—gas gangrene—is most likely to appear.

Secondary closure is the name applied to the operation performed on extremity wounds that cannot undergo delayed primary closure but are closed after the appearance of granulation tissue—7 to 10 days after wounding. Some amputation stumps undergo secondary closure; however, most are not closed surgically but are allowed to close by scaring, a process known as healing by *secondary intention*. Reamputation of the stump is a common operation: the soft tissue retracts so much that the bone is relatively too long.

The most common vascular injuries involve the femoral artery, brachial artery, and femoral vein. Arterial reconstruction usually necessitates the insertion of a vein segment, which is usually taken from the saphenous vein of the opposite leg. Reoperation is a common occurrence following extremity arterial reconstructions in combat casualties: thrombosis, delayed hemorrhage, and wound sepsis seem to be more common than in civilian patients who have peripheral vascular operation. If the vascular injury coexists with a fracture, it is essential that the fracture first be stabilized. External fixation is especially useful for this purpose. It is desirable to reconstruct an injured femoral vein, especially when there is a coexisting injury to the femoral artery. In most venous reconstructions, thrombosis probably occurs in the repaired vein within 2 to 3 days; however, the vein stays open long enough to keep the arterial reconstruction open during the critical first 2 or 3 days. Venous ligations may be an acceptable alternative to reconstruction in the casualty with multiple injuries.

Immobilization

Because fractures are very common in soldiers with extremity wounds, immobilization is a necessary part of most extremity operations. In general, three approaches to fracture immobilization can be employed in preparing the casualty for evacuation from the combat or communication zones:

1. Internal fixation, wherein a metal rod is inserted longitudinally through the marrow cavity, or metal screws and plates are used to hold the fracture together. This approach is rarely desirable in combat casualties with open, comminuted fractures because of the strong possibility of sepsis.
2. External fixation, wherein long, threaded rods are inserted transversely into the bone

fragments above and below the fracture site and are held in place externally by an adjustable frame. This is an increasingly favored means of immobilizing fractures such as those of the tibia, but the approach depends on the availability of the necessary equipment.

3. Plaster of paris cast or splint, which is the traditional approach to immobilizing fractures, and is still the best approach to high femoral-shaft and hip fractures. The drawbacks to this approach are the discomfort of the casualty and the difficulty of exposing the soft-tissue component of the wound.

COMPLICATIONS

Injuries to other parts of the body frequently coexist with extremity injuries. The most common combinations are abdomen and legs, especially when the wounds are made by buried explosive munitions; and head, upper torso, and arms, when the wounds result from the detonation of a shaped-charge warhead. Wounds to the abdomen are discussed in Chapter 20, Abdominal Injuries; to the head in Chapter 16, Neurological Injuries; and to the upper torso in Chapter 19, Thoracic Injuries.

In addition to managing combined injuries, the military anesthesiologist needs to be prepared to manage complications that are unique to extremity injuries, of which compartment syndrome and thrombolic and embolic phenomena are the most serious.

Compartment Syndrome

Although compartment syndromes are not common in combat casualties for the simple reason that the wound tract usually decompresses the compartment via the wounds of entrance or exit, it may be seen following vascular reconstructions, especially when there has been a delay in operating.[12] Compartment syndromes are orthopedic emergencies that require early treatment to prevent long-term disability.[4,13] The myofascial compartments are of a fixed volume, and after injury, edema and hemorrhage cause increased pressure in this fixed space. The increased pressure causes decreased venous outflow and decreased microvascular perfusion of the tissues. As muscle dies, it losses its normal ability to regulate intracellular water and electrolyte concentrations. The result is a vicious cycle: swelling of the cells, further increase in compartment pressure, and decreased arterial flow.[3,14] If the cycle is not interrupted by early fasciotomy to decrease tissue pressure, severe muscle necrosis and peripheral nerve damage will follow, and a severely disabled, fibrotic myofascial compartment with severe disability will be the result (Figure 21-7).

Pain is the most frequent symptom of increased compartment pressures.[3] Decreased pulses distal to a fracture site should be a warning of an impending compartment syndrome or vascular injury. While full evaluations of motor and sensory function are difficult to perform early in the management of an extremity injury, function distal to a fracture site suggests that peripheral nerve damage, if any, is incomplete. Early diagnosis is important to decrease damage to the tissue. The clinical picture can be confusing, but pain on passive range of motion of the affected muscle and distal sensory deficits are the most reliable indicators. The patient will complain of subjective pain out of proportion to the degree of apparent injury, and may note a tense feeling in the tissue. Physical examination can reveal tense compartments with warm, tense skin overlying the area. Pain with passive range of motion of the joint is an important indicator, but can be confusing in the presence of other injuries.[15] Laboratory determinations are of little help in combat zone hospitals because the needed tests are not available, but elevated levels of creatine kinase and myoglobinuria are consistent with muscle destruction.

Compartment pressures can be evaluated in fractured limbs or in nonfractured limbs where the mechanism of injury suggests ischemia (ie, crush injury).[3] These pressure determinations can be helpful when the patient is unable to answer questions (eg, the patient is under anesthesia, uncooperative, or has proximal nerve injury and sensory nerve damage). The most common method of determining compartment pressure is to insert an 18-gauge needle into the compartment in question, and then connect the needle to a pressure transducer. There are no absolute pressure ranges to allow a definitive diagnosis. The normal intramuscular pressure is 0 to 8 mm Hg.[16] Various investigators recommend fasciotomy at various pressures: from 30 to 35 mm Hg,[17] to greater than 45 mm Hg,[18] to decompression when the intramuscular pressure is within 10 to 30 mm Hg of the diastolic pressure.[19]

Although the preceding discussion has emphasized the deleterious local effects of compression syndrome, dire systemic effects may also occur.

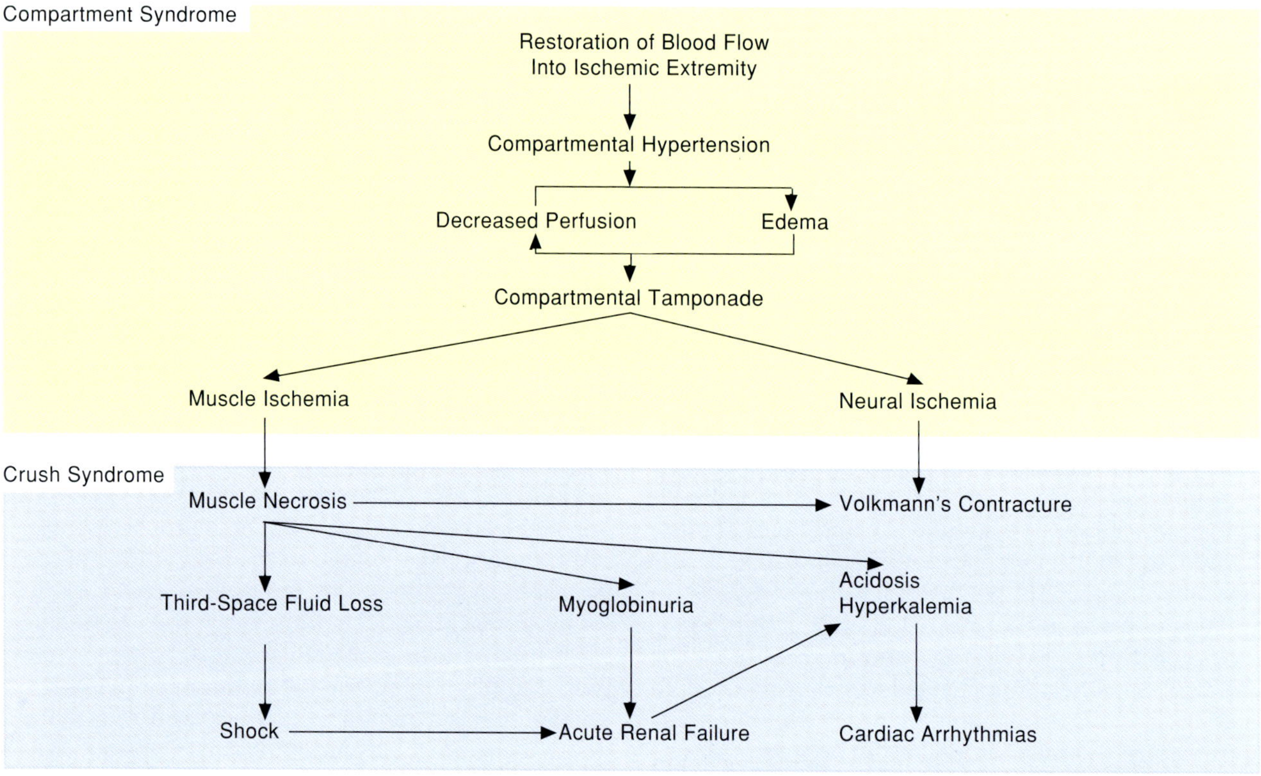

Fig. 21-7. The pathophysiology of compartment and crush syndromes. Adapted with permission from Kitka MJ, Meyer JP, Bishara RA, Goodson SF, Schuler JJ, Flanigan P. Crush syndrome due to limb compression. *Arch Surg*. 1987;122:1078–1081.

When systemic effects are present, the condition is known as crush syndrome. When the ischemic region is reperfused—either when arterial inflow is restored following a vascular reconstruction or when external compression is relieved, untreated or inadequately treated—the injured area may swell explosively due to fluid sequestered there. In addition, myoglobin from necrotic muscle is washed into the systemic circulation, which, in conjunction with hypovolemia, can cause acute renal failure. The prudent military anesthesiologist will see that a prophylactic approach is taken to prevent compartment syndrome by assuring that fasciotomies are performed in all casualties with extremity wounds whose arterial reconstruction has been delayed.

Thrombolic and Embolic Phenomena

Deep Venous Thrombosis and Pulmonary Embolism

The multiply injured combat casualty is at risk for deep venous thrombosis and pulmonary embolism. While soldiers usually have no underlying cardiopulmonary disease, those who have multiple injuries have multiple risk factors to develop a hypercoagulable state. Trauma to femoral or pelvic veins is associated with a high incidence of deep venous thrombosis and subsequent pulmonary embolism.[20,21] Additionally, surgery, venous stasis, trauma, immobilization, vascular damage, disseminated intravascular coagulation, thrombocytopenia, and the administration of heparin are associated with deep venous thrombosis.[22,23] Peripheral thrombosis below the knee is common in surgical patients, with an incidence approaching 45%, and with 10% of these patients having symptoms of pulmonary embolism.[24] Casualties having major lower-limb orthopedic reconstruction are at high risk for two reasons: (1) there is extensive vascular damage and (2) they will be immobilized for an extended time. It seems unlikely that combat casualties who have had extremity venous reconstructions are at a higher risk of deep venous thrombosis and pulmonary embolism than are casualties with isolated arterial reconstructions and casualties in whom the venous injury has been treated by ligation. Patients with thrombophlebitis and patients older than 40 years of age with extensive abdominal surgery have an incidence of calf-vein thrombosis of 40% to 80%, proximal vein thrombosis of 10% to 20%, and fatal pulmonary embolism of 1% to 5%.[25] Clearly, pulmonary embolism is a major risk factor in this surgical group, and recognition, treatment, and prophylaxis are mandatory.

Intraoperative presentations are quite dramatic and have been associated with leg manipulation, wrapping the leg with Esmarch bandage, and realigning of the proximal femoral fracture component; they have been seen days after the initial trauma.[26,27] The hemodynamic picture is one with increased central venous and pulmonary artery pressures, hypotension, and tachycardia.[28] The pulmonary capillary wedge pressure is unchanged unless there is underlying cardiac disease.[29] The cardiac output does not correlate to the degree of obstruction of the pulmonary vasculature.[28] The right ventricle is prone to failure, as it is a highly compliant ventricle that decompensates with acute increases in right ventricular afterload.[30–32] The degree of pulmonary hypertension correlates with the acute degree of obstruction. The mean pulmonary artery pressure never exceeds 40 mm Hg unless there is coexisting cardiac disease. A pulmonary artery pressure of 22 mm Hg correlates with a 30% obstruction of pulmonary vasculature, while 36 mm Hg correlates with 50% obstruction.[28] Further decompensation occurs when a coexisting patent foramen ovale allows right-to-left shunting of blood when pressure on the right side of the heart exceeds pressure on the left.[33]

Bilateral wheezing and arterial blood gas evidence of hypoxemia and hypercarbia, together with nonspecific roentgenographic chest findings, should alert the prudent practitioner to the possibility of pulmonary embolism.[34,35] As dead-space ventilation increases secondary to decreased perfusion, atelectasis ensues, with loss of surfactant in the involved alveoli. Platelet-mediated vasoconstriction and bronchospasm also contribute to the clinical picture.

Diagnosis. The diagnosis of pulmonary embolism needs to be made early because empirical treatment with heparin can lessen the disease process.[34] Pulmonary angiography is the standard for diagnosis but is very invasive and may be difficult to perform in combat zone hospitals. Ventilation–perfusion scans attempt to demonstrate lack of perfusion to ventilated lung; however, these are associated with a 25% to 40% false-negative rate in low-probability scans, and a 29% false-positive rate in high-probability scans. As most emboli arise in the proximal veins, impedance plethysmography is a highly specific, noninvasive test that can diminish the need for angiograms.[36] When needed, a pulmonary artery catheter can be used for pulmonary arteriography.

Treatment. The aim of treatment is to maximize the cardiac output and oxygen delivery to the body tissues. In the early treatment of the patient with right ventricular failure secondary to pulmonary embolism, the arterial partial pressure of oxygen decreases due to increased shunting of blood in the pulmonary bed. But oxygen delivery may actually be increased to tissues, since the mixed venous oxygen content is increased.[37]

Judicious volume infusion is indicated to increase central venous pressure to 12 to 15 mm Hg. Increasing the central venous pressure can shift the interventricular septum and compromise left ventricular filling because the noncompliant pericardium produces tamponade-like hemodynamics.[38]

Inotropic drugs are used to improve both the cardiac output and coronary perfusion. When the right ventricle is failing, there is a decrease in right ventricular perfusion and a loss of the continuous perfusion that is seen on the right side of the normal heart. This leads to a vicious cycle: decreased cardiac output leads to decreased perfusion, which leads to further decreased cardiac output, which leads to further decreased perfusion, and so on. Isoproterenol has been tried, but hypotension, tachycardia, and dysrhythmias have detracted from its usefulness.[39] After volume loading to central venous pressure of 12 to 15 mm Hg, dobutamine[40] and dopamine[39] have been used successfully to increase cardiac output, maintain blood pressure, and decrease pulmonary vascular resistance. In dog models, norepinephrine has increased cardiac output with improvement of right ventricle perfusion.[41]

Pulmonary vasodilators such as prostaglandin E_1 are nonspecific systemic vasodilators and can decrease right ventricular perfusion, and have been combined with norepinephrine.[34]

Heparin has been shown to reverse pulmonary vasoconstriction and bronchoconstriction from thrombin activation and platelet aggregation. Administering a bolus of heparin has been recommended when the clinical picture is highly suggestive of pulmonary embolus (even before definitive diagnosis).[33,42–45] The possibility of increasing a surgical patient's risk of hemorrhage must be weighed against heparin's vasodilating and bronchodilating actions.

Positive end-expiratory pressure (PEEP) needs to be used judiciously, if at all. Venous return to the heart is impeded, and stress to the right ventricular wall and oxygen consumption are increased. Small tidal volumes at rapid rates with no PEEP will help maximize cardiac output and mixed venous oxygen.[46–48]

Prophylaxis. Along with maintaining a high index of suspicion, military trauma anesthesiologists need to consider prophylaxis against deep venous thrombosis in all patients with orthopedic injuries. Low-dose heparin (5,000 units administered subcutaneously 2 h before surgery and every 8 h after, for several days) has been shown to decrease deep venous thrombosis, but it increases intraoperative bleeding, and there is no overall decrease in mortality.[49] Another concern with administering heparin is bleeding when regional anesthesia is used. External pneumatic compression stockings decrease venous stasis, induce fibrinolysis, are as effective as low-dose heparin,[50,51] and are especially effective when heparin is contraindicated. There may be decreased thrombosis when regional anesthesia has been used in hip and prostate surgery. The most effective prophylaxis is patient ambulation.

Fat Embolism Syndrome

Death as a result of fat embolism syndrome was first recognized in 1862. The syndrome has usually been diagnosed when there are fat globules demonstrated in the blood with predisposing conditions such as long-bone fracture. The classic triad (neurological dysfunction, respiratory insufficiency, and petechial skin rash) is only seen in 1% to 5% of patients with fat emboli. In contrast, respiratory insufficiency is seen in as many of 29% of patients with fat emboli, as demonstrated by arterial bloodgas monitoring.[52]

Pathophysiology. The pathophysiology of fat embolism syndrome is complex and not fully elucidated. The consensus is that fat globules gain access to the venous circulation through torn venules.[53] Long-bone fractures are commonly the source of fat emboli, but the syndrome is also seen with joint replacements, liposuction, bone marrow transplants, acute hemorrhagic pancreatitis, carbon tetrachloride poisoning, and external cardiac massage.[54]

An especially dramatic presentation of the fat embolism syndrome was reported in 1994, occurring in a patient who was undergoing intramedullary fixation of a femoral-shaft fracture. A two-dimensional transesophageal Doppler probe had been inserted as part of the patient's monitoring. Every time the femur was manipulated, a swarm of emboli appeared in the right side of the heart. Pulmonary hypertension soon developed and culminated in the opening of a probe patent foramen ovale, through which an ultimately fatal paradoxical embolization occurred.[55] It seems reasonable to speculate that fat emboli frequently occur when long-bone fractures are manipulated.

Studies with dogs have demonstrated that when the fat embolism syndrome is induced by fracturing the femurs, the fat found in the lung parenchyma has the same lipid profile as that seen in the bone marrow.[56] As there are only small quantities of femoral fat, other mechanisms must be at work to account for both the severe damage that is seen in the lung parenchyma and the neurological dysfunction, as they cannot be explained by simple vascular occlusion alone.[54]

Free fatty acids and platelet-mediated factors are postulated to increase the damage to the lung parenchyma. Multiple studies have demonstrated that free fatty acids damage lung tissue.[57–59] Because free fatty acids are increased as part of the stress response to injury, it is postulated that they work synergistically with the fat emboli to induce tissue damage (Figure 21-8).[60] This concept is difficult to demonstrate in the laboratory because free fatty acids caused by the trauma cannot be separated from those that are caused by local tissue injury.

Platelet aggregation around the fat microemboli can also cause lung damage. The platelets release a variety of mediators to cause vasospasm and

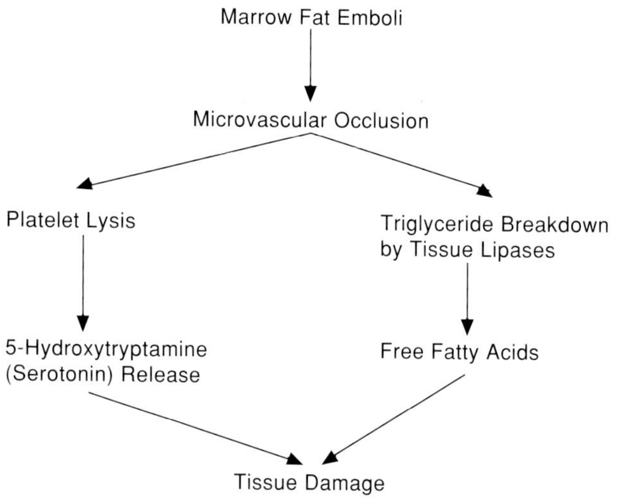

Fig. 21-8. Pathophysiology of the fat embolism syndrome. Reprinted with permission from Van Besouw J-P, Hinds CJ. Fat embolism syndrome. *Br J Hosp Med*. 1989:42:304.

EXHIBIT 21-1

DIAGNOSTIC FEATURES OF FAT EMBOLISM SYNDROME

Major Features

Respiratory insufficiency occurs 2 to 3 days after the injury in 75% of patients with fat emboli syndrome.[1] Tachypnea, dyspnea, and fine inspiratory rales are the usual clinical manifestations. Initial chest radiography is usually normal. As the disease progresses, bilateral, fluffy shadows and obliteration of the lung fields develop (appearing like adult respiratory distress syndrome). Respiratory failure occurs in 10% of cases.[2] Hypoxemia generally precedes respiratory distress by several hours and is considered to be a sensitive marker for the initiation of therapy.[3]

Central nervous system signs and symptoms can be early, often preceding respiratory symptoms by 6 to 12 hours and can be the primary cause of death.[4] Patients usually develop an encephalopathy manifested by a confused state that is exacerbated by hypoxia and not resolved by supplemental oxygen. Associated focal neurologic signs include hemiplegia, aphasia, apraxia, scotoma, and anisocoria.[3,5] These focal symptoms are secondary to the local effects of vascular occlusion. These are seen as widespread destruction in the white matter of the cortex, brainstem, and spinal cord and are secondary to platelet aggregation and free fatty acid mechanisms of injury.

Dermatological manifestations are seen as a petechial rash in the oral mucous membranes, conjunctiva, and skin folds of the upper half of the body (especially the neck and axilla). This rash, which is seen in 60% of those affected, is secondary to the occlusion by fat globules of the dermal capillary network.[1,6] The petechiae are seen on the nondependent body aspects, and are probably secondary to the embolization within the nondependent portions of the subclavian and carotid artery (analogous to oil floating on water). The rash is self-limited and resolves completely in 7 to 10 days.[7,8]

Minor Features

Pyrexia and tachycardia, which are related to the fat embolism itself or to secondary infection[9,10]

Electrocardiographic changes, which are associated with right ventricular strain (S wave in V1, Q wave in III, and nonspecific ST segment changes)

Retinal changes, which are manifested by soft, fluffy exudates; macular edema; retinal hemorrhages; and fat droplets

Renal changes of oliguria, lipuria, proteinuria, and hematuria, which are transient with the fat embolus syndrome and are unrelated to subsequent renal failure[4]

Hepatic changes, which are manifested by rare, self-limited jaundice[1]

(1) Gurd AR, Wilson RI. The fat embolism syndrome. *J Bone and Joint Surg*. 1974;56(B):408–416. (2) Guenter CA, Braun TE. Fat embolism syndrome: Changing prognosis. *Chest*. 1981;79:143–145. (3) Gosling HR, Donohue TA. The fat embolism syndrome. *JAMA*. 1979;241:2740–2742. (4) Sevitt S. The significance and pathology of fat embolism. *Ann Clin Res*. 1977;9:173–180. (5) Jacobson DM, Terrence CF, Reinmuth OM. The neurologic manifestations of fat embolism. *Neurology*. 1986;36:847–851. (6) Alho A. Fat embolism syndrome, etiology, pathogenesis and treatment. *Acta Chir Scand*. 1980;49:75–85. (7) Tachakra SS. Distribution of skin petechiae in fat embolism rash. *Lancet*. 1976;1:284–285. (8) Stephens JH, Fred HL. Petechiae associated with systemic fat embolism. *Arch Dermatol*. 1962;86:515–517. (9) Murray DG, Racz GB. Fat embolism syndrome (respiratory insufficiency syndrome). A rationale for treatment. *J Bone and Joint Surg*. 1974;56(A):1338–1349. (10) Wildsmith JAW, Masson AHB. Severe fat embolism: A review of 24 cases. *Scott Med J*. 1978;23:141–148.

bronchospasm with subsequent ventilation–perfusion mismatching.[61] Hypoperfusion causes secondary cellular disruption, which then causes the release of secondary tissue lipases. This then causes further increases in free fatty acids and further lung injury.[54]

Fat emboli that bypass the filtering capacity of the lung and gain access to the arterial circulation (ie, right-to-left shunt) are responsible for the dermatological and neurological manifestations of the syndrome. Normal shunting occurs through the bronchial and thebesian veins and allows small emboli to bypass the lung to the arterial circulation. As the amount of emboli increases and damage is occurring, the pulmonary artery pressure increases, and the opening of precapillary shunts increases the right-to-left shunt. This is associated with larger emboli and more-severe systemic manifestations.[62]

Diagnosis. Fat embolism syndrome is difficult to diagnose,[63–65] although respiratory insufficiency, central nervous system dysfunction, and dermatological manifestations are major diagnostic features; fever, tachycardia, and electrocardiographic, retinal, renal, and hepatic changes are minor, nonspecific diagnostic features not specific to the fat embolism syndrome per se (Exhibit 21-1). In 1987, four criteria (sustained $PaO_2 < 60$ mm Hg; $PaCO_2 > 55$ or pH <7.3; respiratory rate > 35; and increased work of breathing manifested by dyspnea, use of accessory muscles, and tachycardia) in the presence of a long-bone fracture were suggested as being diagnostic.[66] These criteria probably lead to overdiagnosis, which illustrates the difficulties of studying the syndrome, its pathophysiology, diagnosis, and treatment.

Laboratory Changes. The following hematological and biochemical changes can usually be seen in patients with fat embolism syndrome.

- Hematological changes:
  - Hematocrit usually decreases even in the face of adequate blood-loss replacement. This is usually due to intrapulmonary hemorrhage, lung parenchymal damage, and to increased blood aggregation and hemolysis.[54]
  - Platelet count is decreased secondary to the platelets' adherence to fat emboli and raw edges of bone. In addition, disseminated intravascular coagulation will consume platelets.[54]
  - Erythrocyte sedimentation rate is increased.
  - Coagulation times (prothrombin and thrombin) are increased.
- Biochemical changes:
  - Fat globules can be detected in blood, urine, and sputum but are not diagnostic in the absence of other clinical signs.[64]
  - Free fatty acids, cortisol, glucagon, and catechols increase as part of the stress response.[62]
  - Calcium is decreased secondary to binding to free fatty acids.[67]

Treatment. The fat embolism syndrome is difficult to diagnose because universal agreement on diagnostic criteria is lacking. This lack, coupled with the relatively low incidence of the syndrome, creates difficulties in prospectively evaluating treatment.

Treatment is supportive in nature. Because movement of the fracture increases the incidence of fat embolism syndrome, early immobilization is advocated.[68] Early immobilization will also allow early patient mobilization to increase pulmonary toilet, and decrease blood loss and platelet consumption by stopping the constant movement at the fracture site. Internal fixation decreases the incidence of the syndrome.[69,70]

Adequate fluid resuscitation and maintenance of colloid oncotic pressure with blood or colloid fluids help to absorb circulating free fatty acids. Studies with animals in hypovolemic shock have demonstrated their increased susceptibility to fat embolism syndrome.[71] Albumin is thought to bind free fatty acids, but this needs further investigation as to the appropriate levels of albumin required.[72] The patient should be given adequate analgesia to ablate the sympathetic responses that will cause increased free fatty acids and susceptibility to fat embolism syndrome.[54]

Respiratory care is of paramount importance in the treatment of fat embolism syndrome. Oxygen requirements range from supplemental oxygen provided via nasal catheter to intubation and PEEP required for frank respiratory failure. The pulse oximeter allows for noninvasive determination of saturation and permits continuous monitoring of pulmonary function.[52]

Neurological function must be evaluated serially to determine early deterioration of function. There is no information at present as to the incidence of increased intracerebral pressure, or if measures usually employed to control intracranial hypertension alter patient outcome.[54]

As alcohol is known to inhibit lipase, it was postulated, but never proven, that inhibiting lipase will limit the lipolysis of neutral fat emboli and decrease free fatty acid damage to the lung.[73] A resurgence of interest in alcohol has developed since researchers noted a decreased incidence of fat emboli in patients with femoral fractures and elevated blood alcohol levels.[74] However, no biochemical relationship has been demonstrated among blood alcohol levels, free fatty acid level, and fat embolism syndrome.[75]

Heparin, a stimulator of lipase, has been used to decrease the number of circulating fat globules, thereby preventing them from reaching the lung.[74,75] Heparin will also cause an increase in free fatty acids, which can cause increased damage. As expected, the data conflict.[76,77] Before administering heparin, the medical officer must weigh the concern of causing further bleeding against the continued circulation of fat.

Steroids, usually methylprednisolone, have been employed both prophylactically and therapeutically and may have beneficial effects, but all investigators in steroid studies note the need for adequate resuscitation and oxygen before using steroids.[54] The proposed mechanisms of action include stabilizing membranes, limiting the rise of free fatty acids, limiting complement, and inhibiting leukocyte aggregation. Steroids appear to attenuate the syndrome, and hypoxia has been shown to decrease after steroids were administered: in 1971, methylprednisolone in a first dose of 125 mg, then 80 mg every 6 hours for 3 days, was advocated[78]; in 1983, the dose was increased to 7.5 mg/kg every 6 hours for 12 doses (90 mg/kg total)[79]; and in 1987, 30 mg/kg was administered in one dose.[52]

Prognosis. The multiplicity of coexisting injuries makes the overall prognosis for patients with fat embolism syndrome difficult to assess; overall, the mortality is 5% to 15%, owing to the other injuries. As expected, if no mechanical ventilation is required to treat the patient, the mortality decreases.[52] Overall, the respiratory manifestations are self-limited, and if the physician maintains oxygenation, then the patient's respiratory function will return to normal.[80]

Neurological complications are responsible for most of the long-term morbidity and mortality, especially when focal deficits are present.[64,81]

ANESTHETIC MANAGEMENT OF COMBAT CASUALTIES

The anesthetic management of combat casualties with severe extremity wounds is demanding. The more common injuries, such as grossly comminuted femoral or tibial fractures, typically cause substantial blood loss before the casualty reaches the hospital level. By the time casualties with bilateral leg amputations have reached the hospital level, they have usually lost over half their blood volume and may be agonal. Even casualties who have multiple, small, soft-tissue extremity wounds may require extensive procedures, with consequent considerable blood loss. During the Vietnam War, 16% of casualties with extremity injuries received blood transfusions; the most common volume transfused ranged between two and five units.[82]

Depending on the severity of coexisting injuries, these procedures can be prolonged, and caring for the total patient, complex. Considerations include hypovolemia, shock, bleeding, and poor intravascular access. Medical officers must be aware that previously undiagnosed injuries may manifest intraoperatively (eg, pneumothorax and refractory hypovolemia secondary to occult fractures). Coexisting injuries include closed head injuries, cervical spine injuries, thoracoabdominal injuries, burns, and coagulopathies. Sepsis is always an impending risk, and patient transport requires expertise to avoid further injury.

Regional Anesthesia

Regional anesthesia is an attractive choice in the appropriate casualty whose injury is localized.[83,84] The advantages of regional anesthesia are (1) an awake patient is able to control his or her own airway; (2) the treatment team can perform sequential central nervous system examinations and further assess for occult injuries; and (3) the anesthesiologist can more accurately control the administered dose of postoperative analgesia. The disadvantages are (1) the patient may lose control of his or her airway and aspirate during surgery and (2) severe hypotension may develop in the intravascularly depleted patient secondary to the induced sympathectomy. Regional anesthesia is often not indicated for the initial surgery because the surgery tends to be prolonged and the patient will not tolerate the immobility required. In addition, many patients will require mechanical ventilation as part of their medical management.[85–89] A further consideration that applies to deployed hospitals (especially in OOTW when refugees are being treated) is the likelihood of a language barrier between the patient and the military anesthesiologist.

Intravenous regional anesthesia (ie, the Bier block) is acceptable for simple fractures and surgery to the forearm, wrist, and hand.[90–93] The simplicity of the technique, rapid onset, and minimal equipment needs make for an attractive field anesthetic. The disadvantages of brief duration and lack of postoperative analgesia detract from its use. Intravascular overdose can occur if the local anesthetic is injected too quickly near the tourniquet or if the tourniquet deflates prematurely.

Reduction of simple fractures can be facilitated by local infiltration of anesthetic into the hematoma.

This is technically easy to perform. Sterility is mandatory: the hematoma is an excellent culture medium for bacteria that may cause a subsequent osteomyelitis.

Axillary block is simple and offers prolonged anesthesia and postoperative analgesia. Inserting a catheter into the axillary sheath allows subsequent redosing to permit prolonged anesthesia. This technique is appropriate for procedures distal to the elbow. The musculocutaneous nerve and the intercostobrachial nerve diverge after the brachial plexus is formed in at least 50% of the population and, therefore, will need to be separately blocked if a tourniquet is used. In addition, axillary blockade has an effect beyond providing analgesia: by interfering with sympathetic nerve transmission, vasodilation and increased blood flow to the injured extremity may be induced.

The management of the hypovolemic patient is challenging in the face of continued bleeding that will only be controlled by surgical hemostasis. The use of ketamine can be considered while hemostasis is achieved, but the anesthesia provider needs to remember that ketamine is a potent myocardial depressant in the patient whose sympathetic system is already maximally stressed. Some experienced military trauma surgeons consider ketamine to be the anesthetic agent of choice for extremity operations, especially when combined with a benzodiazepine.[94] The uses and limitations of ketamine are discussed in Chapter 10, Intravenous Anesthesia.

General Anesthesia

Overall, the military trauma anesthesia provider needs to consider the casualty case load and balance general anesthesia's increased risk to the patient but shorter induction time against other anesthetic modalities that may be safer for the patient but take longer to induce. A well-conducted general anesthetic utilizing whatever airway protection is re-

EXHIBIT 21-2

PURPOSES OF PULMONARY ARTERY CATHETERIZATION IN CASUALTIES WITH EXTREMITY INJURIES

1. To measure cardiac output
2. To measure oxygen content of mixed venous blood
3. To assess hemodynamic indices:
   - mean arterial pressure, with an arterial line
   - cardiac index, with a pulmonary artery line
   - stroke volume
   - stroke volume index
   - systemic vascular resistance
   - left ventricular stroke work index
4. To measure derived indices in conjunction with other monitors such as oxygen consumption (Vo_2) by the Fick method: cardiac output • (arterial oxygen content – venous oxygen content)
5. To measure filling pressures in the right side of the heart (CVP) and the left side of the heart (PAWP) to assess for
   - shock
   - expected large volume shifts
   - myocardial dysfunction
6. To continuously monitor mixed venous oxygen saturation

CVP: central venous pressure; PAWP: pulmonary artery wedge pressure quired can be preferable to the potential complications of delaying surgery. The actual incidence of gastric aspiration is small compared to the potential risks of loss of function of an extremity.[95] Early fixation of severe fractures will decrease the incidence of fat embolism syndrome, deep venous thrombosis, and continuing hemorrhage. The incidence of morbidity and mortality following femoral fracture has been decreased after early fixation, allowing mobilization of the patient. Aggressive treatment of these patients is warranted, as the risk of deep venous thrombosis approaches 40% to 60% in the immobilized patient, with pulmonary embolism at 5% to 10%.[69,85,87,89,96]

INTRAOPERATIVE MONITORING

Trauma patients may benefit from invasive monitoring to optimize their hemodynamic performance (Exhibit 21-2). These patients require continuous vigilance to detect new injuries, with simultaneous monitoring of their arterial blood gases, hematocrit, urinary output, electrolytes, and coagulation status. The anesthesiologist needs to monitor the surgical field to estimate coagulation and blood loss. Temperature monitoring is vital as it is related to coagulation, cardiac output, shock, and so forth. A normothermic environment and warming fluids and gases will help to maintain the patient's temperature. Additionally, the anesthesiologist must rely on clinical skills, as there is frequently is not enough time to institute technologically advanced monitoring. Wartime and civilian mass casualty situations are examples where clinical skills are of paramount importance.

Prolonged surgery should not be terminated on the grounds that the patient has had too much surgery without objective evidence of refractory shock or hypothermia. The patient should not be taken to the intensive care unit until the life-threatening injuries are corrected. In addition, the military trauma anesthesiologist should consider that triage will be ongoing in mass casualty situations during war or disaster. This is important, considering the previously mentioned decreases in morbidity and mortality seen with early fixation of fractures.

SUMMARY

Extremity injuries in combat casualties are generally not immediately life threatening but are the major cause of morbidity as measured in man-days lost. In addition, extremity injuries are a frequent reason for disability separation or retirement of combat casualties. Most combat casualties with extremity injuries will have either a wound involving only soft tissues or a wound that involves soft tissue in addition to bone or, less commonly, neurovascular structures. The principles of management involve control of hemorrhage, excision of dead or contaminated tissue or both, and fixation of a fracture, if present, in a position likely to lead to restoration of normal function when union occurs. Wound sepsis is by far the most common complication that occurs with extremity injuries. Less common complications are fat embolism syndrome, deep venous thrombosis, compartment syndrome, and pulmonary embolism. Because wounds of the extremities constitute so large a fraction of the operative case load, expert and expeditious anesthetic care of these casualties is necessary to maximize the use of operating room resources.

REFERENCES

1. Nicholls BJ, Cullen BF. Anesthesia for trauma. *J Clin Anesth*. 1988;1:115–129.

2. Committee on Trauma, American College of Surgeons. *Advanced Trauma Life Support Program for Physicians: Instructor Manual*. Chicago, Ill: American College of Surgeons; 1989: Chap 8: 181–186.

3. Burgess AR, Brumback RJ. Early fracture stabilization. In: Cowley RA, Conn A, Dunham CM, eds. *Trauma Care*. Philadelphia, Pa: JB Lippincott; 1987: 182–203.

4. Bolhofer BR, Spiegel PG. Prevention of medical complications in orthopedic trauma. *Clin Orthop*. 1987; 222:105–113.

5. Bellamy RF, Zajtchuk R. The physics and biophysics of wound ballistics. In: Bellamy RF, Zajtchuk R, eds. *Conventional Warfare: Ballistic, Blast, and Burn Injuries*. Part 1, Vol 5. In: Zajtchuk R, Jenkins DP, Bellamy RF, eds. *Textbook of Military Medicine*. Washington, DC: Department of the Army, Office of The Surgeon General, and Borden Institute; 1991: Chap 4.

6. Bellamy RF. Colonel, Medical Corps, US Army, Walter Reed Army Medical Center, Washington, DC. Personal communication, April 1994. The single most useful database describing combat wounds and the circumstances of wounding is the Wound Data and Munitions Effectiveness Team (WDMET) study prepared by the U.S. Army Materiel Command during the Vietnam War. These data are stored at the National Naval Medical Center, Bethesda, Maryland. Access is controlled by the Uniformed Services University of the Health Sciences, Bethesda, Maryland 20814-4799; telephone (301) 295-6262. Three summary volumes contain extensive abstracts of the statistical data and can be obtained from Defense Documentation Center, Cameron Station, Alexandria, Virginia 22304-6145; telephone (703) 545-6700 and (703) 274-7633.

7. Coleman SS. Early care of the patient with multiple fractures. *Am J Surg*. 1959;97:43–48.

8. Trunkey DD, Sheldon GF, Collins JA. The treatment of shock. In: Zuidema GD, Rutherford RB, Ballinger WF, eds. *The Management of Trauma*. 4th ed. Philadelphia, Pa: WB Saunders; 1985: 105–125.

9. Flint LM, Brown A, Richardson JD, Polk HC. Definite control of bleeding from severe pelvic fractures. *Ann Surg*. 1979;189:709–716.

10. Simchen E, Sacks, T. Infection in war wounds. *Ann Surg*. 1975;182:754–761.

11. Klein RS, Berger SA, Yekutiel P. Wound infection during the Yom Kippur War. *Ann Surg*. 1975;182:15–20.

12. Bibi C, Nyska M, Howard C, Dekel S. Compartmental syndrome due to high velocity missile injury of the calf: Use of immediate mesh skin grafting. *Milit Med*. 1991;156:436–438.

13. Burgess AR, Mandlebaum BR. Acute orthopedic injuries. In: Siegel JH, ed. *Trauma: Emergency Surgery and Critical Care*. New York, NY: Churchill Livingstone; 1987: 1049–1074.

14. Sarokahn AJ, Eaton RG. Volkman's ischemia. *J Hand Surg*. 1983;8:806–809.

15. Hayden JW. Compartment syndromes: Early recognition and treatment. *Postgrad Med*. 1983;74:191–202.

16. Mubarek SJ, Hargens AR, Owen CA, et al. The wick catheter technique for measurement of intramuscular pressure: A new research and clinical tool. *J Bone Joint Surg*. 1976;58(A):1016–1021.

17. Rorabeck CH, Castle GSP, Hardie R, Logan J. Compartmental pressure measurements: An investigational investigation using the slit catheter. *J Trauma*. 1981;21:446–449.

18. Matsen FA. *Compartment Syndromes*. New York, NY: Grune and Stratton; 1980.

19. Whitesides TE, Haney TC, Morimoto K, Harade H. Tissue pressure measurements as a determinant for the need of fasciotomy. *Clin Orthop*. 1975;113:43.

20. Hull RD, Raskob GE. Prophylaxis of venous thromboembolic disease following hip and knee surgery. *J Bone Joint Surg*. 1986;68A:146–150.

21. Harris WH, Salzman EW, Athanasoulis C, et al. Comparison of warfarin, low-molecular weight dextran, aspirin, and subcutaneous heparin in prevention of venous thromboembolism following total hip replacement. *J Bone Joint Surg*. 1974;56(A):1552–1662.

22. Schafer AI. The hypercoagulable states. *Ann Intern Med*. 1985;102:814–828.

23. Kitchens CS. Concept of hypercoagulability: A review of its development, clinical application, and recent progress. *Semin Thromb Hemost*. 1985;102:293–315.

24. Kakkar W, Flanc C, Howe CT, Clarke MB. Natural history of postoperative deep-vein thrombosis. *Lancet*. 1969;2:230–233.

25. Hull RD, Raskob GE, Hirsch J. Prophylaxis of venous thromboembolism: An overview. *Chest*. 1986;89(suppl): 374–383.

26. Estrera AS, King RP, Platt MR. Massive pulmonary embolism: A complication of the technique of tourniquet ischemia. *J Trauma*. 1982;22:60–62.

27. Pollard BJ, Lovelock HA, Jones RM. Fatal pulmonary embolism secondary to limb exsanguination. *Anesthesiology*. 1983;5B:373–374.

28. McIntyre KM, Sasahara AA. The hemodynamic response to pulmonary embolism in patients without prior cardiopulmonary disease. *Am J Cardiol*. 1971;28:288–294.

29. Berry AJ. Pulmonary embolism during spinal anesthesia: Angiographic diagnosis via a flow directed pulmonary artery catheter. *Anesthesiology*. 1982;57:57–59.

30. Vlahakes GJ, Turley K, Hoffman JI. The pathophysiology of failure in acute right ventricular hypertension: Hemodynamic and biochemical correlations. *Circulation*. 1981;63:87–95.

31. Brooks H, Kirk ES, Vokonas S, et al. Performance of the right ventricle under stress: Relation to right coronary flow. *J Clin Invest*. 1971;50:2176–2183.

32. Guyton AC, Lindsey AW, Guilluly JJ. The limits of right ventricular compensation following acute increase in pulmonary circulatory resistance. *Circ Res*. 1954;2:326–332.

33. Ozier Y, Dubourg O, Farcot JC, et al. Circulatory failure in acute pulmonary embolism. *Intensive Care Med*. 1984;10:91–97.

34. McFadden ER, Braunwald E. Cor pulmonale and pulmonary thromboembolism. In: Braunwald E, ed. *Heart Disease*. 2nd ed. Philadelphia, Pa: WB Saunders; 1984: 1572–1604.

35. National Cooperative Study. The urokinase pulmonary embolism trial. *Circulation*. 1973;47(suppl):1–108.

36. Hull RD, Hirsch J, Carter CJ, et al. Diagnostic value of ventilation–perfusion lung scanning in patients with suspected pulmonary embolism. *Chest*. 1985;88:819–828.

37. Jardin F, Furdjian F, Desfonds P, et al. Hemodynamic factors influencing arterial hypoxemia in massive pulmonary embolism with circulatory failure. *Circulation*. 1979;59:909–912.

38. Wiedemann HP, Matthay RA. Acute right heart failure. *Crit Care Clin*. 1985;1:631–661.

39. Boudarias JP, Dubourg O, Gueret P, et al. Inotropic agents in the treatment of cardiogenic shock. *Pharmacol Ther*. 1983;22:53–79.

40. Jardin F, Genevray B, Brun-Ney D, Margairaz A. Dobutamine: A hemodynamic evaluation in pulmonary embolism shock. *Crit Care Med*. 1985;13:1009–1012.

41. Molloy WD, Lee KY, Girling L, et al. Treatment of shock in a canine model of pulmonary embolism. *Am Rev Respir Dis*. 1984;130:870–874.

42. D'Ambra MN, La Raia PJ, Philbin DM, et al. Prostaglandin E_1, a new therapy for refractory right heart failure and pulmonary hypertension after mitral valve replacement. *J Thorac Cardiovasc Surg*. 1985;89:567–572.

43. D'Alonzo GE, Bower JS, DeHart P, Dantzker DR. The mechanisms of abnormal gas exchange in acute massive pulmonary embolism. *Am Rev Respir Dis*. 1983;128:170–172.

44. Jamieson GG, Duranceau A, Hones RH. The influence of heparin and isoprenaline on the change produced by pulmonary embolism. *Aust N Z J Surg*. 1982;52:252–258.

45. Thomas D, Stein M, Tanabe G, Rege V, Wessler S. Mechanism of bronchoconstriction produced by thromboemboli in dogs. *Am J Physiol*. 1964;206:1207–1212.

46. Laver MB, Strauss HW, Pohost GM. Right and left ventricular geometry: Adjustments during acute respiratory failure. *Crit Care Med*. 1979;7:505–519.

47. Jardin F, Farcot JC, Boisante L, et al. Influence of positive end-expiratory pressure on left ventricular performance. *N Engl J Med*. 1981;304:387–392.

48. Fewe JF, Abedndschein DR, Carlson CJ, et al. Continuous positive-pressure ventilation decreases right and left ventricular end-diastolic volumes in the dog. *Circ Res*. 1980;46:125–132.

49. Kakkar W. Prevention of fatal postoperative pulmonary embolism by low doses of heparin. *Lancet*. 1975;2:45–51.

50. Nicolaides AN, Fernandes JF, Pollock AV. Intermittent sequential pneumatic compression of the legs in the prevention of venous stasis and postoperative deep venous thrombosis. *Surgery*. 1980;87:69–76.

51. Tarnay TJ, Rohr PR, Davidson AG, et al. Pneumatic calf compression fibrinolysis and the prevention of deep venous thrombosis. *Surgery*. 1980;88:489–496.

52. Lindeque BG, Schoeman HS, Domisse GF, Boeyens MC, Vlok AL. Fat embolism and the fat embolism syndrome: A double blind therapeutic study. *J Bone and Joint Surg*. 1987;69(B):128–131.

53. Raffer RK. Experimental production and recovery of pulmonary fat embolism in dogs: Origin of fats. *Surg Forum*. 1971;22:446–448.

54. Van Besouw J-P, Hinds CJ. Fat embolism syndrome. *Br J Hosp Med*. 1989;42:306–311.

55. Pell ACP, Hughes D, Keating J, Christie J, Busuttil A, Sutherland GR. Brief report: Fulminating fat embolism syndrome caused by paradoxical embolism through a patent foramen ovale. *New Engl J Med*. 1993;329:926–929.

56. Hallgren B, Kerstall J, Rudenstein CM, Swanborg A. A method for the isolation and chemical analysis of pulmonary fat emboli. *Acta Chir Scand*. 1966;132:613–617.

57. Peltier LF. Fat embolism: A current concept. *Clin Orthop*. 1969;60:241–253.

58. Kreis WR, Lindenaur SM, Dent TL. Corticosteroids in experimental fat embolism. *J Surg Res*. 1973;14:238–246.

59. Cahill JM, Daly BFT, Byrne J. Ventilatory response to oleic acid embolus. *J Trauma*. 1974;14:73–76.

60. McNamara JD, Molat M, Dunn R, Burran EL, Stremple EF. Lipid metabolism after trauma. *J Thorac Cardiovasc Surg*. 1972;60:968–972.

61. Peltier LF. Fat embolism, the toxic properties of neutral fat and free fatty acids. *Surgery*. 1956;40:665–666.

62. Sevitt S. The significance and pathology of fat embolism. *Ann Clin Res*. 1977;9:173–180.

63. Gurd AR. Fat embolism: An aid to diagnosis. *J Bone and Joint Surg*. 1970;52:732–737.

64. Gurd AR, Wilson RI. The fat embolism syndrome. *J Bone and Joint Surg*. 1974;56(B):408–416.

65. Murray DG, Racz GB. Fat embolism syndrome (respiratory insufficiency syndrome): A rationale for treatment. *J Bone and Joint Surg*. 1974;56(A):1338–1349.

66. Lindeque BG, Schoeman HS, Domisse GF, Boeyens MC, Vlok AL. Fat embolism and the fat embolism syndrome: A double blind therapeutic study. *J Bone and Joint Surg*. 1987;69(B):128–131.

67. Ross APJ. The fat embolism syndrome: with special reference to the importance of hypoxia in the syndrome. *Ann R Coll Surg Engl*. 1970;46:159.

68. Baker AB. The fat embolism syndrome: Results of a therapeutic regime. *Anaesth Intensive Care*. 1976;4:53–55.

69. Saikku LA. Fat embolism in connection with treatment of fractures. *Acta Chir Scand*. 1954;108:275–282.

70. Riska EB, Myllynen P. Fat embolism in patients with multiple injuries. *J Trauma*. 1982;2:891–894.

71. Watson AJ. Genesis of fat emboli. *J Clin Pathol*. 1970;23(suppl 4):132–142.

72. Moylan JA, Evenson ME. Diagnosis and treatment of fat embolism. *Annu Rev Med*. 1977;28:83–90.

73. Adler F, Lai SP, Peltier LF. Fat embolism: Prophylactic treatment with lipase inhibitors. *Surg Forum*. 1961; 12:453–455.

74. Schnaid E, Lamprey JM, Viljoen MJ, Joffe NI, Seftel HC. The early biochemical and hormonal profile of patients with long bone fractures at risk of fat embolism syndrome. *J Trauma*. 1987;27:309–311.

75. Myers R, Taljaard JJF. Blood alcohol and fat embolism syndrome. *J Bone Joint Surg*. 1977;59(A):878–880.

76. Korn ED. Clearing factor, a heparin activated lipoprotein lipase isolation and characterization of the enzyme from normal rat heart. *J Biol Chem*. 1955;215:1–14.

77. Corn D. The fat embolism syndrome. *Med Clin North Am*. 1964;48:1459–1466.

78. Fescher JE, Turner RH, Herndon JH, Riseborough EJ. Massive steroid therapy in severe fat embolism. *Surg Gynecol Obstet*. 1971;132:667–672.

79. Schoenfeld SA, Ploysongsang Y, DiLisio R, et al. Fat embolism prophylaxis with corticosteroids *Ann Int Med*. 1983;99:438–443.

80. Pepe EP, Potkin RT, Reus DH, Hudson LD, Carrico CJ. Clinical predictors of the adult respiratory distress syndrome. *Am J Surg*. 1982;144:124–130.

81. Sevitt S. The significance and pathology of fat embolism. *Ann Clin Res*. 1977;9:173–180.

82. Hardaway RM. Viet Nam wound analysis. *J Trauma*. 1978;18:635–643.

83. Desai SM, Bernard WN, McClary B. Regional anesthesia: Management considerations in the trauma patient. *Crit Care Clin*. 1990;6:85–101.

84. Gilbert R, Keighley JF. The arterial alveolar oxygen tension ratio, an index of gas exchange applicable to varying inspired oxygen concentrations. *Am Rev Respir Dis*. 1974;109:142–145.

85. Bone L, Bucholz R. The management of fractures in the patient with multiple trauma. *J Bone Joint Surg*. 1986; 68(A):945–949.

86. Peters RM. Fluid resuscitation and oxygen exchange in hypovolemia. In: Siegel JH, ed. *Trauma Emergency Surgery and Critical Care*. New York, NY: Churchill Livingstone; 1987: 157–179.

87. Bolhofer BR, Spiegel PG. Prevention of medical complications in orthopedic trauma. *Clin Orthop*. 1987;222:105–113.

88. Burgess AR, Brumback RJ. Early fracture stabilization. In: Cowley RA, Conn A, Dunham CM, eds. *Trauma Care*. Vol 1. In: *Surgical Management*. Philadelphia, Pa: JB Lippincott; 1987: 182–203.

89. Burgess AR, Mandlebaum BR. Acute orthopedic injuries. In: Siegel JH, ed. *Trauma: Emergency Surgery and Critical Care*. New York, NY: Churchill Livingstone; 1987: 1049–1074.

90. Zauder HL. Intravenous regional anesthesia. In: Zauder HL, ed. *Anesthesia for Orthopedic Surgery*. Philadelphia, Pa: FA Davis; 1980: 119–125.

91. Turner PL, Batten JB, Hjorth D, Ross ER, Eyres RL, Cole WG. Intravenous regional anaesthesia for the treatment of upper limb injuries in childhood. *Aust N Z J Surg*. 1986;56:153–155.

92. Olney BW, Lugg PC, Turner PL, Eyres RL, Cole WG. Outpatient treatment of upper extremity injuries in childhood using intravenous regional anaesthesia. *J Pediatr Orthop*. 1958;8:576–579.

93. Maletis GB, Watson RC, Scott S. Compartment syndrome: A complication of lower leg shaft fractures. *Orthopedics*. 1989;12:841–846.

94. Coupland RM. *War Wounds of Limbs*. Oxford, England: Butterworth-Heinemann, Ltd; 1993: 17.

95. Olsson GL, Hallen B, Hambraes-Jonzon K. Aspiration during anaesthesia: A computer-aided study of 185,358 anaesthetics. *Acta Anaesthesiol Scand*. 1986;30:84–92.

96. Keever JE, Rockwood CA Jr. Early mobilization of the severely injured patient. In: Zauder HL, ed. *Anesthesia for Orthopedic Surgery*. Philadelphia, Pa: FA Davis; 1980: 21–28.

Chapter 22

BURN INJURIES

ROGER L. WESLEY, M.D.*

*Formerly, Major, U.S. Army; Anesthesia and Operative Service, Department of Surgery, Brooke Army Medical Center, Fort Sam Houston, Texas 78234; currently, Staff Anesthesiologist, Lewis-Gale Clinic, 1802 Braeburn Drive, Salem, Virginia 24153

INTRODUCTION

Burn injury is both a predictable consequence of modern combat and a challenge for military medical personnel. For several reasons, thermal injuries will comprise a not-insignificant fraction of the casualties of modern warfare, not only in the army but even more so in the navy and air force[1]:

- The very nature of existing antipersonnel and antitank explosive munitions such as shaped-charge warheads makes thermal injury likely.
- Secondary explosions and fires from the fuels required for air and ground mobility due to battle damage make thermal injury a real possibility.
- Other weapons used in conventional warfare, such as fuel-air explosive bombs, which are designed to injure by blast overpressure, can cause thermal injuries.
- Nuclear weapons produce extremely high temperatures capable of producing severe thermal burns at a great distance.

In fact, thermal burns will constitute a major portion of the injuries in nuclear warfare.[2]

Throughout this chapter, the term *burn injury* refers to thermal injury caused by fire except when chemical or electrical burns are specified. Combat casualties with burns present challenges to those caring for them: some unique to thermal injury, and some common to severe trauma of other types. One of the major distinctions between burned soldiers and civilians is the propensity for soldiers to have additional injures. Data from a World War II study of tank casualties show that of the 50% of casualties who were injured while in the tank and who survived to reach medical care, one half had penetrating injuries in addition to having been burned.[3]

Combat action is neither the only nor necessarily the most important source of thermal trauma for soldiers. Historically, nonbattle injuries resulting from fires from vehicular accidents or aircraft crashes have generated more burns than have combat action. Data from the Korean War illustrate this point: 1% of total admissions for combat injuries (766 soldiers) were for treatment of burns, while 7.3% of admissions for with nonbattle-related injuries (5,510 soldiers) were for treatment of burns.[4]

Besides the immediate concerns of narrowing of the upper airway, respiratory compromise, and hemodynamic instability, the burn casualty can also present with a host of problems including altered fluid requirements, limited intravenous access and monitoring sites, altered thermoregulatory response, hypermetabolism, and immunosuppression. Other physiological perturbations affecting intensive care and anesthetic management include altered drug response, deranged pulmonary dynamics, altered hematological profile, malnutrition, sepsis, and multiple organ failure.

Large numbers of burn casualties will place heavy demands on both the medical personnel and the logistics of the military medical system. A clear understanding of the unique challenges presented by such casualties is necessary for us most efficiently and effectively to use existing medical resources and capabilities through each echelon of combat medical care.

The first step in battlefield burn care is to stop the burning process by removing the source of the burn injury: extricate the casualty from the burning armored fighting vehicle, ship, or aircraft; extinguish the flame; remove the smoldering clothing; break contact with the electrical current source; flush off the offending caustic chemical. Immediate assessment of airway adequacy, respiratory exchange, and hemodynamic stability follows. Then basic life-support measures are begun, including cardiopulmonary resuscitation if indicated. Supplemental oxygen should be administered if available and if the burn occurred in a closed space, as carbon monoxide poisoning is likely.[5] Extensive upper-airway burns with resultant edema, obtundation, inadequate ventilation, or associated severe facial or chest trauma necessitate endotracheal intubation and ventilatory support.

After cardiopulmonary stabilization, gross estimation of all injuries including extent and depth of burn injury is made, and a clean dressing is placed over the burns. If associated injuries are extensive, blood loss is brisk, or time until definitive treatment will exceed 30 minutes, intravenous access should be secured, preferably via a large-bore peripheral percutaneous cannulation, and a balanced salt solution administered.[6] The casualty is then transported to a location for more definitive examination and treatment.

At the level of the medical company or battalion, decisions will be made as to the further disposition of the burn casualty. Because subsequent treatment is based on the extent and severity of the burn and associated injuries, a careful physical exam and assessment of burn depth and percentage of body surface involved should be performed at this echelon of care. Burn severity is described as *partial* thickness or *full* thickness, based on the depth of injury. Initially, burn depth may be difficult to estimate correctly and the depth may even progress over time from partial to full thickness.[7] Superficial, partial-thickness burns range from erythematous sunburn to a devitalization of the superficial layers of the epidermis with blister formation overlying a wet, red, hypersensitive, edematous skin bed; this injury will heal spontaneously. Deeper partial-thickness burns appear dry, waxy, and white beneath the devitalized epidermis. These injuries are sensitive only to deep pressure and will heal with hypertrophic scarring if protected well. Full-thickness burns involve complete destruction of the skin and appendages, and appear dry, leathery, and somewhat translucent.[8] Eventual excision and grafting are required for wound closure.

The extent of body surface area burned is an important variable in delivering adequate fluid resuscitation, and is estimated by the "Rule of Nines" (Figure 22-1). This involves assigning percentages of total body surface area (TBSA) to various body parts.[1] Major burn injuries are considered to be those consisting of partial-thickness burns of greater than 25% of TBSA, full-thickness burns of greater than 10% TBSA, or smaller burns (of hands, face, feet, perineum) with complicating features (eg, inhalation injury, extremes of age, significant preexisting disease, or associated trauma).[9]

Current conventional burn care dictates that major thermal injuries be managed in a specialized burn treatment facility. Moderate, uncomplicated burn injuries (ie, 15%–25% TBSA partial-thickness burn or 2%–10% TBSA full-thickness burn) will usually require hospitalization in a general hospital that has some experience in burn care.[7] Minor burn injuries (ie, < 15% TBSA partial-thickness burn or < 2% TBSA full-thickness burn) may be treated on an outpatient basis. The *Emergency War Surgery NATO Handbook* modifies these recommendations and suggests that, to conserve medical resources in times of mass casualties, casualties with burns of less than 20% TBSA be treated either as outpatients or via self-care in a minimal care facility. In addition, these casualties are removed from active combat. Those with burns of the head and neck, hands, or feet, however, require hospitalization. Casualties with burns of 20% to 50% TBSA; or smaller burns with associated blunt, blast, or penetrating trauma, require hospitalization for definitive care and ultimate surgical closure. Casualties with very severe burns (ie, > 50% TBSA) are given minimal care, based on their increasingly poor chances for survival as the TBSA involved increases. They are treated as time and resources allow.[2]

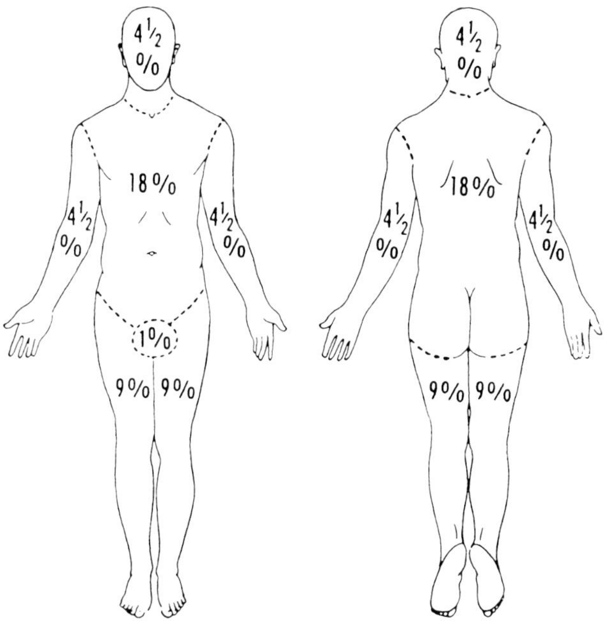

Fig. 22-1. The "Rule Of Nines" for calculating total body surface area burned: head and neck, 9%; anterior trunk, 18%; posterior trunk, 18%; upper extremity, 9%; lower extremity, 18%; and genitalia and perineum, 1%. Reprinted with permission from Moylan JA. First aid and transportation of burned patients. In: Artz CP, Moncrief JA, Pruitt BA, eds. *Burns—A Team Approach.* Philadelphia, Pa: WB Saunders; 1979: 153.

EARLY CARE

At the second or third echelon of care, and before evacuation to a definitive burn care facility or general hospital with burn care experience, several steps should be initiated: some important data collected, fluid resuscitation established and monitored, peripheral perfusion maintained, tetanus prophylaxis provided, gastrointestinal precautions initiated, analgesics administered, and burn wound care initiated.

Data Collection

When the capability to do so exists, several data need to be procured. These include the casualty's weight (for calculating resuscitation fluid requirements), followed by daily weights; baseline chemistry and arterial blood-gas studies; and a chest radiograph to assess pulmonary status, and as a baseline for comparison with subsequent radiographs during the resuscitation and postresuscitation phases. When thermal injury is complicated by other nonthermal trauma (eg, blunt, blast, or penetrating trauma), other data should be accumulated. These may include cervical spine or inhalation/exhalation radiographs, hematocrit, gross urinalysis, or diagnostic peritoneal lavage cell count, when indicated.

Fluid Resuscitation

Fluid management of the burn casualty presents a particular challenge to the medical officer. Thermal injury necessitates aggressive, early fluid resuscitation. Burn patients exhibit a dramatic, early intravascular/extravascular disequilibrium resulting from the loss of functional capillary integrity, extravasation of intravascular fluid, resultant edema formation, and loss of circulating blood volume. Fluids are administered to restore blood and plasma volume, and organ and tissue blood flow; increase cardiac output; and decrease peripheral vascular resistance.[10] A number of resuscitation formulas exist (Table 22-1), each consisting of crystalloid and colloid volume guidelines for the first 48 hours after the burn.

The widely used Modified Brooke Formula calls for 2 to 4 mL of lactated Ringer's solution to be infused per kilogram of body weight per percentage of the total body surface area burned (2–4 mL/kg/% TBSA) during the first 24 hours after the burn. The rate of infusion of resuscitation fluid is increased or decreased within this range based on clinical response. Occasionally with massive burns exceeding 50% TBSA, the rate of 4 mL/kg/% TBSA burned is not sufficient, and higher infusion rates (to 6 mL/kg/% TBSA burned) may be required. A colloid-containing fluid equivalent to plasma may be initiated at a rate of 0.3 to 0.5 mL/kg/% TBSA burned during the second 24-hour period, along with 5% dextrose in water at a rate sufficient to maintain desired urinary output (which is discussed later in this chapter).

Including colloids during the second 24-hour resuscitation period may provide some oncotic benefit and allow more-effective restoration and maintenance of intravascular volume, since most pulmonary capillary integrity is reestablished by this time. Five percent dextrose in water makes up the balance of the second 24-hour resuscitation fluids because a high sodium intake typically occurs during initial resuscitation.

Monitoring of Resuscitation

Assessing the adequacy of resuscitation is accomplished by monitoring urinary output, blood

TABLE 22-1

RESUSCITATION FORMULAS FOR ADULT BURN CASUALTIES

Component	Modified Brooke	Parkland
First 24 Hours		
Ringer's lactate	2–4 mL/kg/% TBSA	4 mL/kg/% TBSA
Colloid	—	—
$D5H_2O$	—	—
Second 24 Hours		
Colloid	0.3–0.5 mL/kg/%TBSA	20%–60% of plasma volume
$D5H_2O$	Volume sufficient to maintain urinary output	Volume sufficient to maintain urinary output

$D5H_2O$: 5% dextrose in water; TBSA: total body surface area.
Data sources: (1) Pruitt BA Jr. Advances in fluid therapy and the early care of the burn patient. *World J Surg.* 1978;2:139–150. (2) Baxter CR, Shires T. Physiologic response to crystalloid resuscitation of severe burns. *Ann NY Acad Sci.* 1968;150:874–894. (3) Baxter CR. Fluid and electrolyte changes of the early postburn period. *Clin Plast Surg.* 1974;1(4):693.

pressure, mental status, and, occasionally, cardiac filling pressures. A Foley catheter has been described as the single best monitor of the adequacy of resuscitation in patients with normal renal function and an absence of congestive heart failure, pulmonary dysfunction, or history of shock. These criteria probably describe the majority of burn combat casualties *if* the burn occurs without associated blast, blunt, or penetrating injury. The target urinary output is 0.5 mL/kg/h in adults and 1 mL/kg/h in children who weigh less than 30 kg.[11] Hypotension, cardiovascular collapse, renal failure, progression of burn depth, or mental status changes may result from inadequate resuscitation. Overzealous fluid administration can result in increased morbidity and mortality from pulmonary edema and increased peripheral edema, which can impair wound healing and convert a partial-thickness burn into a full-thickness injury.[12]

Several groups of patients have been shown to require more than the standard amounts of resuscitation fluid. These include patients with inhalation injuries, intoxicated patients, those with electrical injuries, and those undergoing delayed resuscitation.[10,13] The Parkland Formula (see Table 22-1) was originally developed for patients with inhalation injuries and may also be more appropriate for these other subsets of patients. Also, because pediatric patients may have fluid needs not accurately predicted by most of the weight-based formulas, their fluid resuscitation should be individualized.[9] In every case, the adequacy of resuscitation should be closely monitored, and fluids added or withheld based on the desired response of adequate peripheral perfusion rather than strict adherence to a standard formula.

Maintenance of Peripheral Perfusion

Because full-thickness, circumferential burns of the thorax, upper abdomen, or extremities can lead to loss of life or limb, early, aggressive care is mandatory. Any item of clothing or jewelry must be removed if it could potentially constrict and contribute to subsequent edema formation. Similarly, escharotomy is necessary to prevent life-threatening ventilatory compromise, limb loss, or permanent damage to underlying neurovascular structures.[14] Escharotomy is performed by incising linearly at the midmedial and midlateral lines, down to and just through the subdermal fascial attachments. Anesthesia is not usually required since these deep burns are insensate.[9]

In other large burn injuries, peripheral pulses should be checked at least hourly to assess perfusion as edema worsens. A Doppler flow detector is useful to detect blood flow.

Antibiotics

As a general rule, prophylactic, systemic antibiotics are of no value in the management of burns. However, the chapter on burn injuries in *Emergency War Surgery* recommends the administration of penicillin to *all* thermally injured combat casualties (unless contraindicated) to prevent β-hemolytic streptococcal burn wound infections.[1] This recommendation, differing as it does from civilian standards of practice, reflects both the different milieu in which combat injuries occur vis à vis civilian trauma and the likely delay that will be encountered in evacuating the casualty from the battlefield to a fourth- or fifth-echelon burn center.

Penicillin is to be given for up to 5 days, after which antibiotics are administered only if there are signs of clinical infection or if burn sepsis is thought to be present. When burn sepsis is thought to be present, incisional biopsy is necessary to identify the origin of the infection. Appropriate antibiotics (eg, penicillin against β-hemolytic streptococcal bacteria) are instituted when the causative organism has been verified by culture or there is a high degree of clinical suspicion. In contrast to systemic antibiotics,

> [t]opical antimicrobial agents decrease the incidence of invasive infections in burns. Three effective chemotherapeutic agents that are frequently used to treat burn infections are [mafenide acetate], [silver sulfadiazine], and silver nitrate.[15(p357)]

Tetanus Precautions

Since all burn injuries are considered contaminated, tetanus prophylaxis is indicated except in casualties who have been actively immunized within the preceding 12 months. If a booster dose was administered within the preceding 10 years, an injection of 0.5 mL of adsorbed tetanus toxoid will provide prophylaxis. If active immunization was not done within 10 years before the burn, 250 to 500 units of tetanus immunoglobulin (human) should simultaneously be administered at another site.[16]

Gastrointestinal Precautions

Since most patients with burns of more than 20% TBSA develop a paralytic ileus during the first 24 hours after the injury, all oral intake is withheld and a nasogastric tube is inserted for gastric decompression if not contraindicated by associated injury. In addition, gastroduodenal ulceration is a frequent complication of burn injury. First described by Curling in 1842,[17] these stress ulcers appear within 72 hours of the burn,[18] have the potential to hemorrhage or perforate, and are associated with high mortality rates.[19] Curling's ulcers occur with increasing frequency as burn size increases and, if not prevented, appear in 40% of burns of 70% TBSA.[20] Presumptive diagnosis is made on evidence of gastrointestinal bleeding, while definitive diagnosis is by gastroduodenoscopy. Proper preventive treatment, which greatly reduces the incidence, involves early control of gastric pH (to > pH 5) with antacids or histamine 2 receptor antagonists (ie, H_2 blocking agents). Accordingly, antacids or H_2 blocking agents should be instituted via the nasogastric tube, or H_2 blocking agents can be given intravenously.

Analgesia

Although full-thickness burns are insensate, partial-thickness burns or associated injuries can cause marked pain, which further intensifies the neurohumoral stress response and may worsen morbidity and mortality. Administering small amounts of intravenous narcotics such as morphine sulfate, or partial narcotic agonists such as nalbuphine or butorphanol, will lessen patient discomfort and apprehension, as well as facilitate intravenous line placement and early wound care.

Wound Care

Several objectives are important in early care of combat burn wounds. Perfusion to the wound must be maintained to supply needed tissue-oxygen levels.[21] This is accomplished by providing hemodynamic stability, restoring circulating blood volume, and performing escharotomy as needed. Remaining viable dermis must be protected in partial-thickness burns by initially leaving large blisters intact.[22,23] Debris and devitalized tissue should be removed from full-thickness burns[21] and the wound should be cleaned with soap and water. Since all burn wounds are invariably contaminated, topical antibiotics should be applied to the surface to temporarily retard bacterial growth and to help prevent burn wound infection.[22–24] Topical chemotherapy may consist of sulfonamide cream, 0.5% silver nitrate solution, or mafenide acetate cream. Due to its solubility in water, mafenide acetate burn cream diffuses well into the burn eschar and may be the best choice for limiting bacterial proliferation.[6]

PATHOPHYSIOLOGY OF BURN INJURY

Pulmonary Pathophysiology

Derangements in pulmonary physiology accompany all major burns, even in the absence of inhalation injury. These pulmonary manifestations are a major cause of morbidity and mortality, and also clearly worsen the manifestations of inhalation injury. Early in the course of injury, pulmonary derangement is manifested by changes in lung capillary permeability, vasoreactivity, and ventilation. Surface burns cause an increase in pulmonary vascular resistance, paralleling the increase in systemic vascular resistance that occurs with hypovolemia. Subsequently, vasoactive mediators such as histamine, serotonin, and thromboxane A_2 are liberated from the burn wounds and further increase pulmonary artery pressures.[21] Concomitant hypoproteinemia and complement activation, with subsequent white blood cell aggregation and deposition in the lung vasculature and release of proteolytic enzymes and oxygen free radicals, produce dramatic increases in lung vascular permeability. This may produce the classic radiological and hypoxemic condition known as adult respiratory distress syndrome.[25] Hypoxemia is worsened by elevation of the closing volume (ie, the alveoli become unstable and collapse) and subsequent atelectasis.[21]

Ventilation is initially unchanged or decreased as a result of hypovolemia, concomitant increase in small-airway resistance, pain-induced splinting, or narcotic-induced hypoventilation.[21] Ventilation may be severely depressed by electrical injury as a consequence of central nervous system depression or from large increases in total lung compliance from chest wall edema. If necessary, endotracheal intubation and mechanical ventilation should be instituted.

When adequate hemodynamics are restored, hyperventilation begins, with an increase in both tidal volume and respiratory rate. This increase in ventilation, which is secondary to the demands of hypermetabolism, peaks at the second week after the burn, subsequently declines to a level 2- to 3-fold greater than normal, and then persists until wound closure has been effected. Hyperventilation is accentuated by several factors including the presence of topical mafenide acetate cream (which inhibits carbonic anhydrase activity), sepsis, fever, anemia, pulmonary parenchymal disease, pain, and anxiety.[5]

Hemodynamic Derangements

Early hemodynamic changes are due to deficits in blood volume that are related to transvascular loss of fluid, electrolytes, and protein. This hypovolemia causes tachycardia and, when pronounced, reduction of cardiac output. Both systemic and pulmonary vascular resistance rise in response to neurohumoral mediators, including catecholamines. Cardiac filling pressures decrease, which may further decrease the cardiac output. Perfusion to the periphery is ultimately decreased, but output to the viscera is maintained. A circulating myocardial depressant factor was previously thought to be liberated in burn patients but has not been definitively characterized to date. Positive pressure ventilation can superimpose a further reduction in cardiac output. With adequate fluid resuscitation, the cardiac output returns to normal by the end of the first 24 hours after the burn and then to supranormal levels thereafter. Hyperdynamic changes persist until the wound is closed.

Hematological Derangements

Hematological changes are manifested by early destruction, injury, and loss of red blood cells. As much as 8% to 19% of the red blood cell pool may be destroyed by heat. Subsequent loss secondary to wound debridement (as much as one unit every 3–4 d), phlebotomy for frequent laboratory studies, clearance of damaged red blood cells by the reticuloendothelial system, and decrease in hematopoiesis cause anemia that persists until the wound is closed.[11] In addition, free plasma hemoglobin and hemoglobinuria can be seen shortly after the burn.[21] Early anemia is often masked by plasma-volume deficits that are proportionally greater than red blood cell losses. Maintenance of blood volume is important to minimize catecholamine release and subsequent catabolic stress,[11] since the hypermetabolic cardiovascular system is already stressed in attempts to provide oxygen delivery.

Other hematological changes include early leukocytosis and development of a hypercoagulable state, probably secondary to activation of clotting factors in the burn wound.[21] Platelet count and platelet adhesiveness increase for about 3 weeks.[26] Factors V and VIII increase to levels 4- to 8-fold greater than normal and remain elevated for 2 to 3 months. Fibrinogen levels are initially reduced, then return to normal within 36 hours, and finally remain elevated for as long as there is an open wound (eg, 3 mo[26]). Fibrin split products may be elevated for the first 3 to 5 days. A massive burn may also be complicated by consumption of clotting factors, leading to a hypocoagulable state.[21]

Metabolism and Nutrition

After hemodynamic stability has been afforded by adequate resuscitation, a period of hypermetabolism ensues, with increased utilization of substrate, accelerated tissue breakdown, and depletion of lean body mass.[27] The metabolic rate rises in proportion to the extent of the injury and may be twice normal. In addition, heat production and skin and core temperatures rise secondary to central thermoregulatory changes. Protein stores are utilized via hepatic gluconeogenesis pathways to provide glucose for burn wound metabolism. Thus, increased energy substrate and nitrogen requirements must be met if large reductions in lean body mass are to be avoided. Energy requirements may exceed 2,000 kcal/m^2 body surface area, while nitrogen requirements may exceed 15 g/m^2.[10] The goal should be to meet these nutritional demands as soon as possible, preferably as soon as the gastrointestinal tract is functioning normally. Providing carbohydrate needs will minimize the nitrogen losses. Fat, vitamins, minerals, and nitrogen will be required. The enteral route is preferred for feeding, as it is less expensive, physiologically closer to normal, and may be associated with fewer complications than parenteral nutrition.[28]

Immunological Changes

The burn casualty's immune function is globally impaired. The mechanical barrier of the skin is destroyed and humoral factors are decreased, as are cellular immune responses including lymphocyte and neutrophil activity, and the reticuloendothelial system is impaired.[5] In addition, casualties with thermonuclear burns exhibit bone marrow depression with variable leukopenia, particularly of lymphocytes.[2] Burn casualties, then, are particularly susceptible to infectious complications.

INHALATION INJURY

Deranged respiratory physiology is both the result of inhalation injury and the end-organ response to the generalized systemic insult. Inhalation injury is a major source of morbidity and mortality: 50% to 60% of all burn-related deaths are related to inhalation injury, with most being due to carbon monoxide intoxication.[29] Two important facts are associated with inhalation injury:

1. it is the single most important associated injury that contributes to thermal burn mortality,[11] and
2. the casualty may or may not have an associated thermal burn.

A high suspicion of inhalation injury should exist if the burn occurred in a closed space such as a vehicle or bunker, or if there are burns on the casualty's face or within the mouth or throat. Difficulty breathing, singed facial or nasal hair, changes in the voice, brassy cough, sooty or bloody sputum, or circumferential burns of the chest should alert the medical officer that inhalation injury is likely.[30] A radiograph of the chest is an insensitive, and sometimes a misleading, indicator of inhalation injury. Confirmatory diagnostic studies including fiberoptic bronchoscopy and xenon 131 lung scans are performed when available.

Inhalation injury has three components, each of which may occur independently or concurrently: (1) carbon monoxide intoxication, which is a consequence of incomplete combustion; (2) upper-airway injuries, which are caused by heat; and (3) lower-airway injuries, which are caused by chemical vapors or fumes.

Carbon Monoxide Intoxication

Carbon monoxide intoxication produces severe hypoxemia because carbon monoxide avidly binds to the hemoglobin molecule, forming carboxyhemoglobin, which displaces oxygen, resulting in decreased blood oxygen saturation. This desaturation is worse at the scene of injury as fire consumes much of the available oxygen. Carboxyhemoglobin also shifts the oxyhemoglobin dissociation curve to the left. The result is decreased oxygen delivery to the tissues, causing tissue hypoxia.[31,32] Initial symptoms of carbon monoxide intoxication include palpitations, headache, dizziness, and confusion. Higher carboxyhemoglobin levels result in restlessness, excitement, and even unconsciousness when the carboxyhemoglobin level rises above 40%.

Early administration of a high concentration of inspired oxygen is important in treating carbon monoxide intoxication. The half-life of carboxyhemoglobin is reduced from about 4 hours when breathing room air to 30 minutes when 100% oxygen is administered.[11] Treatment in a hyperbaric chamber has been reported[33] to be efficacious for severe carbon monoxide poisoning.

Upper-Airway Injury

Because the heat-carrying capacity of air is quite low, and hot vapors are rapidly cooled to body temperature as they pass through the nasopharyngeal area and upper airway, direct heat injury usually only affects the upper airway.[34] Heat injury below the level of the upper trachea is rare except with steam injury. Moreover, reflex closure of the glottis often protects the trachea and lung parenchyma.[35] Marked edema occurs in the mucosa within minutes to hours after the burn; ulceration and hemorrhage are also found in the mucosa. The edema may be worsened by large amounts of fluid given during resuscitation.[36] The airways of patients with these conditions should be protected immediately by intubation, even if only prophylactically, since the edema lasts several days and may make late intubation difficult or impossible. Orotracheal or nasotracheal intubation is preferable to tracheostomy because surgical airway manipulation is associated with high mortality.[37]

Lower-Airway Injury

Damage to the lower airway is usually in the form of chemical tracheobronchitis resulting from the liberation of water-soluble gases from burning plastics and rubber. These gases—ammonia, phosgene, sulfur dioxide, and chlorine—cause epithelial damage when converted to acids and alkali on contact with airway mucosa. Lipid-soluble toxins—nitrogen oxides and aldehydes—are produced from burning wood and destroy lipid cell membranes and denature proteins. These toxins damage both alveolar and capillary endothelium, which causes increased permeability and pulmonary edema even at normal capillary filling pressures. Ciliary paralysis and severe bronchospasm also occur. The end result is plugged airways, obstructive and secondary atelectasis, relative hypoxemia, postobstructive emphysema, and occasionally complete lobar collapse.[35]

Depending on the severity of the initial insult, patients with lower-airway injury progress through three clinical stages of injury. During the first 36 hours after the burn, acute pulmonary insufficiency occurs, characterized by hypoxemia, tracheobronchitis, bronchospasm, cough, atelectasis, and pronounced upper airway swelling. The second stage is pulmonary edema, which develops 6 to 72 hours after injury. Pulmonary edema is seen in 5% to 30% of patients and is associated with high mortality. The third stage is bronchopneumonia, seen in 15% to 60% of casualties, beginning 3 to 10 days after the burn. Bronchopneumonia is associated with 50% to 80% mortality.[38]

Treatment

Treatment of severe inhalation injury involves endotracheal intubation, mechanical ventilatory support, supplemental oxygen, and aggressive tracheobronchial toilet including humidification, frequent suctioning, postural drainage, and repeated bronchoscopy. Antibiotics are instituted for culture-proven pneumonia. Systemic steroids have been found to be of no value except to treat bronchospasm unresponsive to parenteral and inhaled bronchodilators.[35] These patients' high minute ventilation requirements and reduced pulmonary compliance increase their susceptibility to the complications of mechanical ventilators and place added stress on conventional ventilators. Ventilators that are capable of generating high minute volumes are invaluable for intensive care and operating room use for these patients. In addition, it appears that high-frequency percussive ventilation is effective in the treatment of patients with severe inhalation injury.[39]

Increasing evidence indicates that oxygen-derived free radicals contribute to the pathophysiology of inhalation injury, especially in the period beginning 24 hours after exposure. Studies[40] carried out in a laboratory model of inhalation injury show that airway injury was markedly reduced by instillation of the iron-chelating agent deferoxamine complexed with pentastarch. Free iron, which is removed by deferoxamine, is known to catalyze the formation of such reactive species as the hydroxyl radical. Interventions based on these observations may have important therapeutic implications in human victims of smoke inhalation.[41]

CHEMICAL AND ELECTRICAL BURNS

Chemical burns to the skin and lungs, and the serious respiratory problems that arise when chemical warfare agents such as mustard and phosgene are inhaled, are described in Chapter 30, Anesthesia for Casualties of Chemical Warfare Agents. Chemical burns caused by acid or alkali have a component of injury caused by heat that is released when the chemical contacts the tissue. The severity of the burn is related to both the duration of exposure and the concentration of the chemical.[14] In general, burns from strong alkalis are more severe than those from strong acids, since the alkalis bind more avidly to the tissues and are therefore more difficult to remove. Initial treatment lies in expedient removal of the chemical by copious water lavage of all exposed surfaces, after all the casualty's clothing has been removed. The prolonged use of cold water and subsequent hypothermia should be avoided, as this increases morbidity. Neutralizing agents should be avoided since their use may liberate more-intense heat. Severe chemical burns may appear deceptively superficial in the initial stages.[5]

Although electrical burns are uncommon among combat casualties, military anesthesiologists need to know about this entity, with its distinctive appearance and unique associated injuries, fluid requirements, wound care, and complications. Electrical injury is arbitrarily categorized into burns caused by low-voltage sources (< 1,000 volts) or high-voltage sources (> 1,000 volts). High-voltage burns are associated with substantial morbidity and mortality: of patients who survive to reach the hospital, mortality may approach 3% to 15%.[42]

The tissue's resistance converts electromagnetic energy to thermal energy, which damages tissue.[6] In addition, electrical injury may cause cardiac irritability or even asystole. Associated injuries are common, including bone fractures (from falls or severe, sudden muscular contraction); neurological damage, which may be progressive (since electrical current may flow through low-resistance neurovascular bundles); ruptured organs; or unexpected and widespread destruction of any soft-tissue structure.[11,26] In fact, an unimpressive wound may overlie large areas of devitalized tissue; this may lead to underestimating the required resuscitation fluid. Muscle burned by electricity may progress to myoglobinuria and acute renal failure if additional fluids and diuretics are not administered to induce a brisk diuresis. This type of injury may cause edema to occur beneath the investing fascia, which requires fasciotomy rather than escharotomy.[6]

Initial wound care involves removal of the patient from the electrical source. Unconsciousness, which necessitates intubation and mechanical ventilation, may result from high-voltage injury, as can seizure activity. Along with the thermal damage, electrical injury may cause cardiac arrest, requiring cardiopulmonary resuscitation at the scene. Further treatment involves hemodynamic stabilization; close monitoring; and early tissue exploration for debridement, assessment of tissue viability, and determining the need for amputation.[6]

Complications, which may be unpredictable, include cataracts; recurrent gastrointestinal dysfunction with a high incidence of cholelithiasis, hemorrhage, or prolonged ileus; immediate or delayed spinal cord damage; peripheral nerve deficits; delayed hemorrhage from large vessels; and causalgia.[6,26] The most common complication in the hospital is the need for major amputation, which occurs in 25% to 68% of patients.[42]

FLUID ADMINISTRATION AFTER RESUSCITATION

Vigorous fluid resuscitation causes abnormal expansion of total body water and salt. Thus, the postresuscitation burn casualty's weight may substantially exceed his or her normal weight. A gradual loss of the perhaps 15% to 20% gain in body weight should be accomplished by a 2% to 3% weight loss per day, so as to reach preburn weight by the 10th day after the burn. This is accomplished by reducing the fluid rate by 25% per hour for patients who maintain adequate urinary output.[10] Initial salt loading and subsequent high evaporative losses may predispose the burn patient to hypernatremia, so 5% dextrose in water is used to maintain serum sodium at 140 mEq/L.

Hypertonic Saline

The use of hypertonic saline as a component of the resuscitation fluid may be efficacious for patients in whom it is desirable to limit the total volume of resuscitation fluid. Hypertonic saline may cause less wound edema and may be particularly useful in patients with inhalation injury, circumferential full-thickness burns of the extremities, or intracranial injuries where massive fluid accumulation could be catastrophic.[9] In addition, hypertonic saline may be desirable for patients with limited cardiopulmonary reserves (ie, the very old or the very young) and those with cardiopulmonary disease.[10] However, no study has demonstrated that any particular sodium concentration is superior for improving survival in burn patients.[9] Moreover, the critical factor in administering hypertonic saline is the development of hypernatremia; serious complications may result if serum sodium concentration rises above 160 mEq/L. Only very experienced clinicians should use hypertonic saline.[11]

Colloids

During the first 12 to 24 hours after the burn, the diffuse capillary leakage allows colloid fluid to extravasate through the endothelial junction, preventing any demonstrable oncotic benefit over crystalloid fluid.[11] Thereafter, capillary integrity is reestablished, and most resuscitation formulae include colloidal solutions as integral components of fluid therapy.

Diuretics

Diuretics are not included in burn resuscitation, except for a few special classes of patients. These include patients who have large, high-voltage electrical injuries; burns involving muscle; burns associated with large, soft-tissue injuries; and massive burns, who remain oliguric despite adequate fluids. Patients in this last category may be predisposed to acute renal failure secondary to large amounts of hemochromogens in the urine. A brisk diuresis is desirable in these patients.

EVACUATION OF THE BURN CASUALTY

Despite the implementation of Medical Force 2000, which focuses on enhancing far-forward surgical care, increasing intensive-care capability in the combat zone, and returning soldiers to duty as soon as possible, a large proportion of burn patients will be evacuated and transported. Forward surgical teams, field hospitals, combat support hospitals, and mobile army surgical hospitals will not be equipped to handle definitive surgical burn care. The extensive blood loss, larger surgical manpower requirements, and lengthy period required for skin-graft maturation would place too great a burden on

EXHIBIT 22-1

BURN INJURY EVACUATION CHECKLIST

Patient Data

_____ Preburn weight
_____ Preevacuation weight
_____ Allergies
_____ Medical history
_____ Medications
_____ Time of last oral intake
_____ Vital signs chart

Laboratory Values

_____ ABG   _____ Blood type
_____ UOP   _____ Electrolytes
_____ CXR   _____ Other

Burn Data

_____ % TBSA burn
_____ Facial burn?
_____ Airway: intubated/nonintubated?
_____ Inhalation injury suspected?
_____ Summary of early care
_____ Locations, types of catheters and IV lines

Equipment

_____ Fluids: Ringer's lactate, D5H_2O, albumin
_____ Airway management: ET tubes, masks, laryngoscopes, O_2, positive-pressure breathing circuit or mask-valve-bag device
_____ Analgesics
_____ IV administration sets

ABG: arterial blood gases; CXR: chest X ray; D5H_2O: 5% dextrose in water; IV: intravenous; ET: endotracheal; UOP: urinary output; TBSA: total body surface area

these military healthcare resources. Therefore, casualties will be evacuated to a general hospital with burn care capability and experienced personnel, or to a specialized burn care center. However, there are several associated risks and challenges.

The evacuation process may be accomplished very early in the course of injury, be lengthy, and occur when only minimal medical care can be provided. All these factors have particular impact on the burn casualty, since evacuation may occur while critical fluid requirements must be met, when tissue edema may compromise the airway or associated complicating factors (eg, inhalation injury; preexisting cardiorespiratory disease; blunt, penetrating, or blast trauma) may impact heavily on the burn casualty's medical management and survivability. The anesthesiologist, who may be the last healthcare provider to see the casualty before the lengthy evacuation, can play a key role in reducing the burn casualty's morbidity and mortality.

The anesthesiologist must ensure adequate preparation and communication before evacuation. Preparation involves ensuring that all patient data and records are clearly documented and that adequate airway equipment, resuscitation drugs, and intravenous fluids are assembled. Communication must be clear to both the evacuation team and the receiving burn care team. These objectives are most efficiently accomplished by using a burn injury–evacuation checklist (Exhibit 22-1), which must be completed and included with the casualty.

PERIOPERATIVE CONSIDERATIONS

Early excision and grafting of small burn wounds is considered the norm. Since early excision and grafting of large burns (> 30% TBSA) have been shown to decrease mortality in patients aged 17 to

30 years,[43] these surgical procedures are being accomplished earlier and earlier in the postinjury course. This may pose several challenges for the anesthesiologist, particularly if surgery is planned during the resuscitative phase or if associated injuries are present.

Preoperative Assessment

Preoperatively, the military trauma anesthesiologist should review the history of the current injury, including the amount of associated TBSA burn, elapsed time since injury, and associated traumatic injuries. Concomitant medical problems, chronic and recently instituted medications, family history, postsurgical and postanesthetic history, drug allergies, transfusion history, time since last oral intake, and presence of intravenous lines and invasive monitors should also be assessed. Current vital signs, including hemodynamic data from invasive monitors, should be noted along with present and preburn weight and laboratory data, including hematology, acid–base status, coagulation profile, liver function tests, and electrolytes. The casualty's electrocardiogram and a recent chest radiograph should be reviewed. A physical exam with emphasis on airway, pulmonary, and cardiovascular assessment is important. Evaluation of any concomitant trauma should proceed as indicated.

Preoperative Medications

While an individualized approach to each casualty should be used for preoperative medication, several goals should be met: anxiolysis, sedation, analgesia, amnesia, antisialagogue effect, elevation of gastric-fluid pH, and reduction of gastric volume.[44] Based on the patient's hemodynamic stability, degree of apprehension, discomfort, personal preference, and planned procedure, rational choices for premedications can be made.

With few exceptions, medications that are being administered before surgery are continued. In particular, medications that support hemodynamics (eg, inotropics, vasodilators, and antidysrhythmics) are continued, as are antibiotics and hyperalimentation fluid. In terms of sedation, critically ill patients may not tolerate depressant medications. An amnestic agent such as scopolamine may be given to these patients. Other seriously ill and intubated patients may be receiving narcotics, sedatives, and nondepolarizing muscle relaxants. If so, intravenous narcotics or benzodiazepines can be administered to facilitate patient comfort during transfer and transport.

Patients who are more stable may be given small amounts of intravenous narcotics or benzodiazepines, or, for patients who prefer an oral premedicant, diazepam or lorazepam orally 1 to 2 hours before induction. For patients being given a ketamine-based anesthetic, a deeper level of sedation is provided in the form of oral diazepam 1 to 2 hours before induction, followed by intravenous diazepam or midazolam on induction. This reduces the incidence of undesirable reactions when the patient emerges from anesthesia. Glycopyrrolate is given for its potent antisialagogue effects if a ketamine anesthetic is planned, or if airway manipulation dictates a secretion-free field. The use of other antisialagogues is discouraged; owing to the crossing of the blood–brain barrier, they interact poorly with ketamine.

Owing to their tendency to form Curling's ulcers, most burn patients will be given an H_2 blocking agent or a sucralfate regimen. If so, this is continued perioperatively. If not, oral or intravenous ranitidine, famotidine, or cimetidine is administered. If the patient has been on particulate antacids, these are discontinued 6 to 8 hours before induction. For emergent surgery, an oral, nonparticulate antacid such as Bicitra (sodium citrate and citric acid, manufactured by Baker Norton Pharmaceuticals, Miami, Fla.) administered 15 to 30 minutes before induction is nearly 100% effective in elevating the gastric fluid pH above 2.5.[44] Metoclopramide speeds gastric emptying and is effective if given orally 30 to 60 minutes before induction; the effect is seen much quicker if administered intravenously.

Monitoring

Burn casualties can pose major challenges in placing and maintaining appropriate monitors. Adequate intraoperative monitoring is especially important considering the potential for extensive blood loss, the frequent changes of position, and the duration of surgery. The monitors that are considered essential for burn casualties are those that ensure the adequacy of oxygenation and ventilation, including continuous pulse oximetry, end-tidal carbon dioxide monitoring, peak airway pressure, and frequent arterial blood-gas analysis. Other routine intraoperative monitors should include a continuous electrocardiograph (ECG); an automated blood pressure cuff; esophageal, nasopharyngeal or rectal temperature-monitoring devices; inspired oxygen tension–monitoring devices; a peripheral nerve stimulator; and precordial or esophageal stethoscopes. Lack of unburned tissue may necessitate placement of needle ECG electrodes, use of a "backpack" ECG pad, or even an esophageal ECG lead. Pulse oximetry probes can be placed on any finger, toe, lip, tongue, ear lobe or helix, or ala nasi. Blood pressure cuffs may be placed on the upper arm, thigh, or calf, and may be sterilized and placed over burned or grafted skin intraoperatively, as needed.

For more critically injured patients and those with preexisting severe systemic disease, more-invasive intravenous lines or monitors are placed. A Foley catheter, arterial line, central venous catheter, or pulmonary artery catheter may be placed as indicated. Frequent arterial blood-gas and hematocrit determinations must be made.

Adequate intravenous access must be established before a major excision. This should include two large-bore peripheral intravenous lines or one peripheral and one central line. If lack of access necessitates placing an intravenous line through burned or grafted tissue, a meticulous sterile field must be maintained. Equipment for rapid infusion of crystalloid resuscitation fluid and blood should be at hand. Anesthesia providers may utilize a pneumatic pressure infuser powered by a pipeline oxygen source that can be regulated to achieve flow rates up to 250 mL/min. If pressure devices are used for intravenous infusions, care must be taken to ensure that air is not infused inadvertently.

Transport

Monitoring and therapy must not be compromised while critically ill, burn casualties are transported to and from the operating room. Appropriate preparation includes notifying the intensive care nurse well in advance of the need for organizing lines and tubes. The casualty is counselled again, reassured, and given additional premedication as the level of apprehension warrants. A mechanical lifting device can be used to move the patient from the bed to a stretcher. A portable oxygen tank and a disposable positive-pressure breathing circuit are used for ventilation, except when precluded by extremely high minute ventilation or elevated peak airway pressures. In these cases, a portable transport ventilator is used, accompanied by a respiratory therapist. A portable suction device should be available for casualties who require frequent suctioning.

The monitors considered routine for transport are a precordial stethoscope and a portable pulse oximeter. A portable ECG monitor with an arterial line channel should be available for more unstable patients. Care must be taken with all lines and invasive monitors, which, if tenuous, should be sutured into place. A free-flowing intravenous line is imperative, since resuscitative drugs might be given during transport. Continuous-infusion devices are attached to the delivery pole on the stretcher, so that any cardioactive medications or hyperalimentation fluids can be continued.

Anesthetic Technique

The choices for the optimum anesthetic technique to use for the burn casualty are varied; however, rational decisions can be made based on known physiological responses to our interventions. Regional anesthesia, although desirable in certain cases, generally is avoided in burn casualties for several reasons:

- The burn may cover the site of anesthetic block placement, and it is undesirable to expose the patient to the risk of central neuraxis infection from colonized burn wounds via spinal or epidural needle placement.
- Excision or grafting procedures are accompanied by large fluid shifts and blood loss, and the loss of sympathetic tone resulting from a regional block may be undesirable.
- These casualties will likely undergo procedures at multiple excision and donor sites, including both upper and lower body sites at a single operation.
- In addition, an awake patient's comfort is frequently difficult to maintain during lengthy excision and grafting procedures.

Induction and the Compromised Airway

Induction of general anesthesia is accomplished on the operating room table, except when the initial excision or graft harvest is on the patient's posterior surface. In that case, induction proceeds on the stretcher, with subsequent positioning of the patient in the prone position. Choices for induction of general anesthesia depend on associated hemodynamic instability, presence or absence of intravenous access, and airway status. For the nonintubated patient, a combination of preoxygenation, midazolam, a narcotic, sodium thiopental, and a large dose of nondepolarizing muscle relaxant is frequently used. Although ketamine has been advocated as a better induction choice in hypovolemic patients, this impression has not been proven. Etomidate is an effective induction agent that offers substantial hemodynamic stability, and is a good choice for patients when cardiac depression would be undesirable. While both ketamine and etomidate both support hemodynamics well, military anesthesiologists must be aware that maximally stressed patients may exhibit hemodynamic deterioration on induction due to some degree of myocardial depression or loss of sympathetic tone. Propofol is a satisfactory induction agent in young, physiologically stable burn patients.

Inhalation induction using halothane, isoflurane, or enflurane, with oxygen and nitrous oxide is another option. Small doses of sodium thiopental (1–2 mg/kg) may provide better tolerance for the irritating vapor. After induction, the ability to ventilate by bag is demonstrated. An intubating dose of a nondepolarizing muscle relaxant may be given at this time to improve conditions for airway instrumentation.

The burn casualty may well have a compromised upper airway, secondary to airway burns or to massive peripheral edema secondary to burns elsewhere. Upper-airway obstruction is a life-threatening complication that appears in the first 36 hours after injury.[45] Large volumes of resuscitation fluid may accentuate supraglottic edema, and concomitant facial and neck burns, constricting dressings, and edema make mask ventilation and airway instrumentation difficult. Later in the course of hospitalization, airway management may be compromised by limited neck extension or mandibular mobility. Lastly, airway management in the burn casualty, both early on and later in the course of treatment, may be difficult and be dictated by concomitant nonthermal trauma (eg, mandibular or facial fractures) that will require individualized approaches.

Several options exist for patients with a compromised airway. An awake intubation may be performed before anesthetic induction using topical airway anesthesia via a blind nasal approach, direct oral laryngoscopy, fiberoptic laryngoscopy, or a lighted stylet (light wand) technique. If airway difficulty is not anticipated, and a full stomach or predisposition to gastroesophageal reflux exists, a modified rapid-sequence induction using preoxygenation, intravenous induction using a large dose of nondepolarizing muscle relaxant, ventilation through cricoid pressure, and rapid intubation via direct laryngoscopy or light wand technique is used. If the patient's airway is not compromised, and if the patient's stomach is empty, then an inhalation induction can be followed by the airway instrumentation of the anesthesia provider's choice. In situations where anatomical alterations suggest difficulty, alternate measures should be at hand, including the ability to perform emergent cricothyroidotomy, tracheostomy, or retrograde translaryngeal guidewire technique.

Maintenance of Anesthesia

No specific anesthetic agent is contraindicated in the burn patient except succinylcholine, which can trigger a potentially fatal hyperkalemic response and is discussed later in this chapter. A wide variety of anesthetic agents can be used satisfactorily. The burn patient's altered pharmacokinetic and pharmacodynamic responses, combined with the nature of the physiological insult and the type of surgery planned, dictate the choice of maintenance drugs.

Intravenous Anesthesia. Ketamine, a popular anesthetic for patients with thermal burns, produces sedation, profound analgesia, and a dissociative anesthetic state resulting from functional and electrophysiological disruption of the association between the thalamocortical and limbic systems.[46–49] (The use of ketamine is also discussed in Chapter 10, Intravenous Anesthesia.) This drug has been described as the only available intravenous agent that can function as a sole anesthetic, without requiring adjunctive agents, owing to its unique combination of amnestic, analgesic, and anesthetic properties. Ketamine has particular application in the critically ill patient, where a period of hypotension or apnea could be life threatening.[50] Ketamine produces a dose-related rise in the heart rate–blood pressure product and supports hemodynamics through direct stimulation of central nervous system structures.[51] Although ketamine does have some direct myocardial depressant and vasodilatory effects, it will help maintain blood pressure in hemorrhagic and septic shock.[52] Ketamine maintains respiratory response to carbon dioxide (ie, the respiratory rate is proportional to the carbon dioxide level), precluding significant respiratory depression except when given in a rapid intravenous bolus of more than 3 to 4 mg/kg. Similarly, ketamine effects an increase in pulmonary compliance with a decrease in airway resistance and bronchospasm. This effect is probably mediated by vagolytic and direct, smooth-muscle, relaxant effects rather than through beta receptors. Oral and bronchial secretions are stimulated by ketamine, necessitating pretreatment with an anticholinergic agent. While pharyngeal and laryngeal reflexes are preserved to some degree,[53] pulmonary aspiration of gastric contents can occur,[54,55] and careful airway management is necessary.

Ketamine has been associated with anesthetic-emergence delirium, which occurs after 5% to 30% of surgeries performed under ketamine anesthesia.[50] This delirium is characterized by vivid dreams, hallucinations, dysphoria, and a sensation of floating in space. The incidence of this reaction can be decreased by (*a*) preoperative counselling concerning the expected side effects and (*b*) pretreatment with benzodiazepines. Oral diazepam, 0.15 mg/kg, administered 1 hour before induction, followed by 0.2 to 0.3 mg/kg intravenous diazepam, or 0.05 to 0.14 mg/kg intravenous midazolam, administered just before induction, is effective. Tolerance to the analgesic effects of ketamine occurs with repeated exposure to the drug.[56]

Balanced Anesthesia. A narcotic-based, balanced anesthetic technique is an option for stable intraoperative hemodynamics, smooth emergence, and easily titratable levels of postoperative analgesia. The technique most commonly used at the U.S. Army Institute of Surgical Research Burn Unit consists of fentanyl, sufentanil, or alfentanil administered either in incremental boluses or by continuous infusion, in combination with oxygen, nitrous oxide, and low concentrations of inhaled vapor. Burn patients may have increased narcotic requirements.[57,58] This may be due to both pharmacokinetic and pharmacodynamic factors,[59] but perhaps is due specifically to altered responses to the endogenous opioids that are actively released during the stress of thermal injury.[60,61] In selected patients, morphine is also an attractive choice for use before emergence, because its slower elimination will effect longer postoperative analgesia. Respiratory depression, skeletal-muscle rigidity, and the development of tolerance with repeated use must all be considered with any narcotic.

Inhalational Anesthesia. The four currently used volatile inhalational anesthetics—halothane, isoflurane, enflurane, and desflurane—produce satisfactory anesthesia for burn casualties, and may have particular efficacy in those with inhalation injuries. The inhalation agents all act at various sites to prevent or reverse the bronchoconstriction that may accompany inhalation injury. The mechanisms of action are probably (*a*) suppression of airway reflexes and (*b*) direct, smooth-muscle relaxation (through action on the calcium flux in tracheal smooth-muscle cells, which interferes with excitation–contraction coupling).[62] To some extent, inhalational anesthetics reverse the hypermetabolic and hyperdynamic state of burn patients.[63] Both halothane and enflurane tend to decrease cardiac output and oxygen demand to approximately an equal degree, thus maintaining the oxygen supply-and-demand balance.[64] To date, halothane hepatitis has not been described in patients with burns, even after repeated exposure.[65]

Some investigators have voiced their concern over the suppression of the immune response by the combination of major surgery and inhalational agents: bone marrow suppression by nitrous oxide[66]; reduced phagocytic function by halothane; and reduction of lymphocyte reactions to antigens.[67] However, most researchers believe that depressed immunocompetence is not caused by the anesthetics but is the effect of the stress of the surgery itself.[63]

The potential exists that volatile anesthetics will interact with topical epinephrine that has been applied to the exposed capillary bed following burn wound excision to help achieve hemostasis. Halothane, and to a lesser extent isoflurane and enflurane, do sensitize the myocardium to both endogenous and exogenous catecholamines.[68–70] In fact, plasma catecholamine levels up to 10-fold higher than normal have been measured in such circumstances.[71] However, various studies show minimal changes in cardiovascular parameters and an absence of arrhythmias after topical epinephrine during burn surgery.[72,73] This apparent normalcy may be due to the preexisting, injury-induced, elevated level of circulating catecholamines that burn patients have, which leads to a decrease in the number of receptors and a downregulation of the receptor affinity.[71,74–76]

The burn patient's response to neuromuscular blocking agents is perhaps the most striking of all altered drug responses, and is the most familiar to anesthesiologists. As was mentioned earlier, these patients can have a potentially fatal hyperkalemic response to depolarizing muscle relaxants (ie, succinylcholine). The release of massive amounts of potassium by muscle cells is related to the dose, the extent of burn injury, and the time elapsed after the burn.[77] Succinylcholine, then, may be used safely in the first 24 hours after the burn but, in a patient with a burn exceeding 10% TBSA, *should be avoided for the subsequent 18 months.*[78] The mechanism of action is an increased sensitivity of the muscle membrane secondary to a proliferation of extrajunctional receptors, similar to that seen in patients with degenerative neurological disorders.[78]

This response begins within days of the burn and may persist for as long as 18 months after the burn.[79] If succinylcholine is inadvertently administered, then calcium chloride, a therapeutic mixture of glucose and insulin, and sodium bicarbonate should be administered, along with cardiopulmonary resuscitation, if cardiac arrest results. Calcium chloride should be subsequently continued until peaked T waves in the electrocardiographic tracing return to normal.[59]

Resistance to nondepolarizing muscle relaxants has been well documented with respect to anesthetics such as metocurine,[79,80] pancuronium,[81,82] alcuronium,[83] *d*-Tubocurarine,[84,85] and atracurium,[86,87] and is likely to be encountered with all competitive agents.[86] (This topic is also discussed in Chapter 11, Neuromuscular Blocking Agents.) The mechanism of this resistance may be alterations both in the pharmacokinetics of the relaxant and at the neuromuscular junction. Pharmacokinetic factors may involve increased plasma-protein binding, depressed hepatic metabolism, and changes in blood flow that cause lengthened equilibration time between the relaxant in the plasma and in the neuromuscular junction, causing an artifactual rightward shift in the dose-response curve. Possible alterations at the neuromuscular junction include an increase in the number of acetylcholine receptors, decreased cholinesterase levels, or some type of prejunctional pathology. Clinically, this resistance is manifested as an increase of 2- to 5-fold in the requirements for both dosage and serum concentration over that of patients who are not burned. Despite this resistance, there appears to be no prolongation of recovery time or difficulty with reversal of the relaxants.[88] The altered response to nondepolarizing agents has been shown to persist for as long as 463 days.[81]

Intraoperative Fluid Management

Casualties with burns pose particular challenges with respect to fluid management. Thermal injury necessitates aggressive, early fluid resuscitation, and, for reasons unconnected to the burn, the casualty may require surgery and anesthesia at any phase of resuscitation. Continued derangements in fluid and electrolyte balance continue in the postresuscitative phase.

Intraoperative fluid therapy for excision and grafting procedures involves very rapid infusion of crystalloid, colloid, and packed red blood cells. The loss of one or more blood volumes is not unusual in a major tangential excision. Pressure infusion devices are necessary, as are efficient blood- and fluid-warming devices.

Thermally injured patients frequently present for anesthesia and surgery with anemia that is caused by heat-induced lysis of red blood cells, reduced erythropoiesis, or frequent blood drawing. Early in thermal injury, anemia may be masked by a loss of plasma volume that exceeds the loss of red blood cells. Transfusion of red blood cells may therefore begin before excision if extensive blood loss is anticipated. Moreover, the adequacy of tangential excision is demonstrated by a briskly bleeding capillary bed. Large amounts of blood may be lost before hemostasis, and estimating this loss is difficult because surface oozing is difficult to collect in a suction device and the blood ends up in soaked gauze; on the drapes; or on the floor, sometimes under the operating room table. Visual estimation, heart rate and blood pressure, urinary output, and perhaps central venous pressure or cardiac filling pressures, all help guide the need for blood replacement. Hematocrit measurement made while blood loss is ongoing is of questionable value.

Because of associated potential risks, including disease transmission and the risk of transfusion reaction, homologous blood transfusion today should be justified only by the need for increased oxygen delivery. However, the burn patient may require a higher hematocrit than a patient who is not burned, secondary to elevated oxygen delivery requirement in the face of hypermetabolism, inability of an already stressed cardiovascular system to compensate for anemia, and reduced hematopoiesis.[89] While maintenance of hematocrit values in the low to mid twenties may be adequate for an otherwise physiologically healthy burn patient, the presence of concomitant physiological impairment may effect a need for a somewhat higher target hematocrit (ie, in the range of 0.30–0.35).

Temperature Regulation

Paradoxically, hypermetabolic patients whose central thermoregulatory set point is elevated are especially susceptible to hypothermia during anesthesia and surgery. Thermally injured patients have a propensity for abnormal heat loss secondary to the burn itself, the nature of the surgical procedure, the temperature of the operating room, and general anesthesia. Burn injury accentuates heat loss of all kinds, especially evaporative loss, which accounts for most of the difference in heat loss between burned and unburned patients.[90] Losses from conduction and convection are also increased[90] since considerably large areas of body surface are often excised or prepared for donor sites, and large areas of body surface are exposed in the operating room.

General anesthetics cause increased heat loss via several mechanisms. Dry anesthetic gases cause evaporative water and heat loss from airways. Anesthetics cause a loss of ability to preserve core temperature through cutaneous vasoconstriction and shivering. Specifically, inhalational agents cause a 15% decrease in the basal metabolic rate,[90] promote surface blood flow, and promote hypothermia through effects on central thermoregulatory centers.[91] A narcotic–nitrous oxide anesthetic decreases metabolic oxygen uptake (VO_2) by 50%, while ketamine has been shown not to alter VO_2.[92] In addition, neuromuscular blocking agents prevent shivering and lower the metabolic rate.

Decreases in core temperature produce several intraoperative and postoperative problems. Hypothermia can depress cardiac output, induce dysrhythmias, abolish hypoxic pulmonary vasoconstriction, shift the oxyhemoglobin dissociation curve to the left, and depress hepatic and renal functions.[93] A clinical impression is that increased intraoperative blood loss occurs secondary to poor hemostasis from exposed vascular beds following excision or donor harvesting if core temperature is less than 36°C. Hypothermia also causes postoperative shivering, which increases VO_2 to 300% to 400% of normal, may cause graft shearing, and can make the patient very uncomfortable.

To prevent intraoperative hypothermia, the patient should be covered with a space blanket while being transported. The operating room is warmed to 25°C to 30°C and humidified to 50% to 60% relative humidity. All solutions for preparation of the skin are warmed, as are all crystalloid and colloid solutions for infusion. Anesthetic gases are warmed and humidified. A warming blanket is placed under the patient, all nonoperative sites are draped, and portable warming lights are used.

Postanesthetic Considerations

Major postanesthetic considerations include the need for a smooth emergence from anesthesia, the decision whether to extubate, the provision of comfort in the postoperative period, and the need for adequate physiological monitoring. A smooth emergence from anesthesia is desirable, since patient movement causes shearing of freshly placed grafts. Adequate pain control is necessary for this, and extubation while the patient is deeply anesthetized, followed by gradual emergence in the intensive care unit or recovery room, may be appropriate in selected patients.

Many burn patients will remain intubated postoperatively secondary to the need for continued mechanical ventilation, continued airway protection, or pulmonary toilet. Others may be extubated, provided that they are awake, able to follow commands, have adequate ventilation and oxygenation, have had adequate reversal from neuromuscular blockade, and are warm.

Transport to the recovery room should be undertaken with the precautions discussed previously. Adequate analgesia should be afforded via intravenous narcotics. If the anesthetic was ketamine-based, a quiet recovery area and adequate reassurance may reduce the incidence of undesirable emergence delirium.

SUMMARY

Combat casualties with burns are likely to have, in addition, penetrating missile wounds. This fact is a consequence of modern warfare, in which most soldiers who sustain burn injuries are wounded within armored fighting vehicles and are therefore subject to injury from fragments arising from the antiarmor warhead, in addition to the secondary explosives that may accompany battle damage. Thus, military anesthesia providers are frequently faced with the problem of treating casualties with multiple traumas, one of which is a cutaneous burn. In addition, we must maintain heightened vigilance for the possibility of coexisting inhalation injury in casualties who have sustained burn injuries within the closed confines of tanks and warships. Assuming that there is no evidence of airway compromise, initial care of the burn casualty focuses on fluid resuscitation. During the first 24 hours, the essential component of fluid resuscitation is the Modified Brooke Formula (ie, the intravenous infusion of 2–4 mL Ringer's lactate/kg body weight/% TBSA burned). The adequacy of fluid resuscitation must be monitored frequently by observing such indicators of the normalcy of peripheral perfusion as the urinary output.

Anesthesia may be required during several different phases of burn wound care. Casualties with full-thickness burns of the extremities in which the peripheral circulation is compromised, or in whom thoracic excursion is hindered, will require escharotomy. This procedure can usually be performed without anesthesia. When a substantial cutaneous burn is present (> 30% TBSA), the initial wound care is best carried out with a narcotic-based, balanced anesthesia using a low concentration of inhaled vapor. Initial wound care of lesser burns can be carried out with intravenous ketamine. Ketamine can also be used for subsequent wound management in some casualties. Those casualties who require general endotracheal anesthesia at 24 hours or more after the burn injury should not receive succinylcholine because of its recognized propensity to cause massive release of potassium and possible sudden death from hyperkalemia.

REFERENCES

1. Bowen TE, Bellamy RF, eds. Burn injury. In: *Emergency War Surgery NATO Handbook.* 2nd rev US ed. Washington, DC: Department of Defense, Government Printing Office; 1988: 35–56.

2. Bowen TE, Bellamy RF, eds. Mass casualties in thermonuclear warfare. In: *Emergency War Surgery NATO Handbook.* 2nd rev US ed. Washington, DC: Department of Defense, Government Printing Office; 1988: 95–119.

3. Wright HB, Harkness RD. A Survey of Casualties Amongst Armored Units in North West Europe: Survey of Casualties in Tank Crew—21st Army Group, Jan 1946. Medical Research Council Team. Wright Patterson Air Force Base, Ohio: SURVIAC Co; 1946. Document 1862.

4. Reister FA. Battle casualties and medical statistics. In: *US Army Experience in the Korean War.* Washington DC: Department of the Army, The Surgeon General; 1973: p 7; Figure 2, p 8; Table 7, p 9.

5. Pruitt BA Jr, Goodwin CW. Thermal injuries. In: Davis JH, Drucker WR, Foster RS Jr, eds. *Clinical Surgery.* St. Louis, Mo: CV Mosby; 1987: 2823–2909.

6. Pruitt BA Jr. The burn patient, I: Initial care. *Curr Probl Surg.* 1979;16:1–62.

7. Punch JD, Smith DJ, Robson MC. Hospital care of major burns. *Postgrad Med.* 1989;85:205–215.

8. Moncrief JA. Burns, I: Assessment. *JAMA.* 1979;242:72–74.

9. Goodwin CW. Current burn treatment. *Adv Surg.* 1984;18:145–176.

10. Pruitt BA Jr, Goodwin CW. Current treatment of the extensively burned patient. *Surg Annu.* 1983;15:331–364.

11. Herndon DN, Curreri PW, Abston S, Rutan TC, Barrow RE. Treatment of burns. *Curr Probl Surg.* 1987;24:341–397.

12. Graves TA, Cioffi WG, McManus WF, Mason AD, Bruitt BA Jr. Fluid resuscitation of infants and children with massive thermal injury. *J Trauma.* 1988;28:1656–1659.

13. Merrell SW, Saffle JR, Sullivan JJ, Navar PD, Kravitz M, Warden GD. Fluid resuscitation in thermally injured children. *Am J Surg.* 1986;152:664–669.

14. Briggs SE. First aid, transportation, and immediate care of thermal injuries. In: Martyn JAJ, ed. *Acute Management of the Burned Patient.* Philadelphia, Pa: WB Saunders; 1990: 1–11.

15. Cioffi WG, Rue LW III, Buescher TM, Pruitt BA Jr. The management of burn injury. In: Bellamy RF, Zajtchuk R, eds. *Conventional Warfare: Ballistic, Blast, and Burn Injuries.* In: Zajtchuk R, Jenkins DP, Bellamy RF, eds. *Textbook of Military Medicine.* Washington, DC: US Department of the Army, Office of The Surgeon General, and Borden Institute; 1991: 357.

16. Pruitt BA Jr, Goodwin CW. Burns. In: Sabiston DC Jr. *Textbook of Surgery.* Philadelphia, Pa: WB Saunders; 1981: 287–316.

17. Curling TB. On acute ulceration of the duodenum in cases of burns. *Med Chir Trans (London).* 1842;25:260.

18. Cuono CB. Early management of severe thermal injury. *Surg Clin North Am.* 1980;60:1021–1033.

19. Czaja AJ, McAlhany JC, Andes WA, Pruitt BA Jr. Acute gastric disease after cutaneous thermal injury. *Arch Surg.* 1975;110:600–605.

20. Pruitt BA Jr, Foley FD, Moncrief JA. Curling's ulcer: A clinical pathology study of 323 cases. *Ann Surg.* 1970;172:523–539.

21. Demling RH. Pathophysiological changes after cutaneous burns and approach to initial resuscitation. In: Martyn JAJ, ed. *Acute Management of the Burned Patient.* Philadelphia, Pa: WB Saunders; 1990: 12–24.

22. Alvarez A, Mertz P, Eaglstern W. The effect of occlusive dressings on collagen synthesis and re-epithelialization in superficial wounds. *J Surg Res.* 1983;35:142–148.

23. Wilson J, Moncreif J. Vapor pressure of normal and burned skin. *Ann Surg.* 1965;162:130–136.

24. Lamke L. Evaporative water loss from normal and burnt skin. *Scand J Plast Reconstr Surg Hand Surg.* 1971;5:17–22.

25. Strongin J, Hales C. Pulmonary disorders in the burn patient. In: Martyn JAJ, ed. *Acute Management of the Burned Patient.* Philadelphia, Pa: WB Saunders; 1990: 23–45.

26. Szyfelbein SK. Anesthetic considerations for major burn surgery. In: Hershey SG, ed. *Refresher Courses in Anesthesiology.* Vol 8. Philadelphia, Pa: JB Lippincott; 1980: 201–216.

27. Wechtel TL. Nutritional support of the burn patient. In: Bostwick JA, ed. *The Art and Science of Burn Care.* Rockville, Md: Aspen Publishers; 1987: 203–220.

28. Bell SJ, Blackburn GL. Nutritional support of the burn patient. In: Martyn JAJ, ed. *Acute Management of the Burned Patient.* Philadelphia, Pa: WB Saunders; 1990: 138–158.

29. Lamb JD. Anaesthetic considerations for major thermal injury. *Can Anaesth Soc J.* 1985;32:84–92.

30. Jelenko C, Mckinley JC. Postburn respiratory injury. *Journal American College of Emergency Physicians.* 1976;5:455–458.

31. Larkin JM, Brahos GJ, Moylan JA. Treatment of carbon monoxide poisoning: Prognostic factors. *J Trauma.* 1976;16:111–114.

32. Moylan JA. Smoke inhalation and burn injury. *Surg Clin North Am.* 1980;60:1533–1540.

33. Smith G, Ledingham IM, Sharp GR, Norman JN, Bates EH. Treatment of coal gas poisoning with oxygen at 2 atmospheres pressure. *Lancet.* 1962;1:816–818.

34. Madden MR, Finkelstein JL, Goodwin CW. Respiratory care of the burn patient. *Clin Plast Surg.* 1986;13:29–38.

35. Robinson L, Miller RH. Smoke inhalation injuries. *Am J Otolaryngol.* 1986;7:375–380.

36. Yoshioka T, Maemura K, Ohhashi Y. Effect of intravenously administered fluid on hemodynamic change and respiratory function in extensive thermal injury. *Surg Gynecol Obstet.* 1980;151:503–507.

37. Eckhauser FE, Billote J, Burke JF, Quinby WC. Tracheostomy complicating massive burn injury—a plea for conservatism. *Am J Surg.* 1974;127:418–422.

38. Herndon DN, Langner F, Thompson P, Linares HA, Stein M, Traber DC. Pulmonary injury in burned patients. *Surg Clin North Am.* 1987;67:31–46.

39. Cioffi WG, Graves TA, McManus WF, Pruitt BA Jr. High-frequency percussive ventilation in patients with inhalation injury. *J Trauma.* 1989;29:350–354.

40. LaLonde C, Ikegami K, Demling R. Aerosolized deferoxamine prevents lung and systemic injury caused by smoke inhalation. *J Appl Physiol.* 1994;77(5):2057–2064.

41. Crapo JD. Invited Editorial On "Aerosolized deferoxamine prevents lung and systemic injury caused by smoke inhalation." *J Appl Physiol*. 1994;77(5):2055–2056.

42. Remensnyder JP. Acute electrical injuries. In: Martyn JAJ, ed. *Acute Management of the Burned Patient*. Philadelphia, Pa: WB Saunders; 1990: 66–86.

43. Herndon DN, Barrow RE, Rutan RL, Rutan TC, Desai MH, Abston S. A comparison of conservative versus early excision: Therapies in severely burned patients. *Ann Surg*. 1989;209:547–553.

44. Stoelting RK. Psychological preparation and preoperative medication. In: Miller RD, ed. *Anesthesia*. 2nd ed. New York: Churchill Livingstone; 1986: 381–397.

45. Haponik EF, Meyers DA, Munster AM. Acute upper airway injury in burn patients. Serial changes of flow-volume curves and nasopharyngoscopy. *Am Rev Respir Dis*. 1987;135:360–366.

46. Roberts FW. A new intramuscular anesthetic for small children. *Anaesthesia*. 1967;22:23–28.

47. Corssen G, Oget S. Dissociative anesthesia for the severely burned child. *Anesth Analg*. 1971;50:95–102.

48. Bjarnesen W, Corssen G. CI-581: A new nonbarbiturate short-acting anesthetic for surgery in burns. *Mich Med*. 1967;66:177–181.

49. Corssen G, Miyasaka M, Domino EF. Changing concepts in pain control during surgery: Dissociative anesthesia with CI-58. *Anesth Analg*. 1968;47:746–759.

50. White PF, Way WL, Trevor AJ. Ketamine—its pharmacology and therapeutic uses. *Anesthesiology*. 1982;56:119–136.

51. Ivankovich AD, Miletich DJ, Reimann C, Albrecht RF, Behrooz Z. Cardiovascular effects of centrally administered ketamine in goats. *Anesth Analg*. 1974;53:924–933.

52. Wong DHW, Jenkins LC. The cardiovascular effects of ketamine in hypotensive states. *Can Anaesth Soc J*. 1975;22:339–348.

53. Lanning CF, Harmel MH. Ketamine anesthesia. *Ann Rev Med*. 1975;26:137–141.

54. Taylor PA, Towey RM. Depression of laryngeal reflexes during ketamine anesthesia. *Br Med J*. 1971;2:688–689.

55. Penrose BH. Aspiration pneumonitis following ketamine induction for a general anesthetic. *Anesth Analg*. 1972;51:41–43.

56. Slogoff S, Allen GW, Wessels JV, Cheney DH. Clinical experience with subanesthetic ketamine. *Anesth Analg*. 1974;53:354–358.

57. Perry S, Heidrich G. Management of pain during debridement: A survey of US burn units. *Pain*. 1982;13:267–280.

58. Perry S. Pain and anxiety in the burned child. *J Trauma*. 1984;24:S191–S195.

59. Martyn J. Clinical pharmacology and drug therapy in the burned patient. *Anesthesiology*. 1986;65:67–75.

60. Szyfelbein SK, Osgood PF, Carr DB. The assessment of pain and plasma beta-endorphin immunoreactivity in burned children. *Pain*. 1985;22:173–182.

61. Levine J. What are the functions of endorphins following thermal injury? *J Trauma*. 1984;24:S168–S172.

62. Korenaga S, Tekeda K, Ho Y. Differential effects of halothane on airway nerves and muscle. *Anesthesiology*. 1984;60:309–318.

63. Martyn JAJ. Clinical pharmacology and therapeutics in burns. In: Martyn JAJ, ed. *Acute Management of the Burned Patient*. Philadelphia, Pa: WB Saunders; 1990: 180–200.

64. Gregoretti S, Gelman S, Dimick AR. Total body oxygen supply-demand balance in burned patients under enflurane anesthesia. *J Trauma*. 1986;27:158–160.

65. Gronert GA, Schaner PJ, Gunther RC. Multiple halothane anesthesia in burn patients. *JAMA*. 1968;205:878–880.

66. Amos RJ, Amess JAL, Hinds CJ. Incidence and pathogenesis of acute megaloblastic bone marrow change in patients receiving intensive care. *Lancet*. 1982;2:835–838.

67. Koenig A, Koenig UD, Binhold B. Differences in lymphocyte mitogenic stimulation pattern depending on anesthesia and operative trauma. *Eur J Anaesthesiology*. 1987;4:17–24.

68. Joas TA, Stevens WC. Comparison of the arrhythmic dose of epinephrine during Forane, halothane, and fluroxene anesthesia in dogs. *Anesthesiology*. 1971;35:48–53.

69. Johnston RR, Eger EI, Wilson C. A comparative interaction of epinephrine with enflurane, isoflurane, and halothane in man. *Anesth Analg*. 1976;55:709–712.

70. Horrigan RW, Eger EI, Wilson CB. Epinephrine-induced arrhythmias during enflurane anesthesia in man: A nonlinear dose-response relationship and dose-dependent protection from lidocaine. *Anesth Analg*. 1978;57:547–550.

71. Timonen RM, Pavlin GG, Haschke RH, Heimbach DM. Epinephrine level pre and post application of topical epinephrine during burn surgery. *Anesthesiology*. 1982;57:A138. Abstract.

72. Snelling CFT, Shaw K. Effect of topical epinephrine hydrochloride in saline on blood loss following tangential excision of burn wounds. *Plast Reconstr Surg*. 1983;72:830–836.

73. Glasson DW. Topical adrenaline as a hemostatic agent. *Plast Reconstr Surg*. 1984;74:451–452.

74. Wilmore DW, Long JA, Mason AD, Skreen RW, Pruitt BA Jr. Catecholamines: Mediator of hypermetabolic response to thermal injury. *Ann Surg*. 1974;180:653–668.

75. Goodall MC. Sympatho-adrenal medullary response to thermal burn. *Ann N Y Acad Sci*. 1968;150:685–689.

76. Fozzard HA. Myocardial injury in burn shock. *Ann Surg*. 1961;151:113–119.

77. Schaner PJ, Brown RL, Kirksey TD, Gunther RC, Ritchey CA, Gronert GA. Succinylcholine hyperkalemia in burned patients. *Anesth Analg*. 1969;48:764–770.

78. Gronert GA, Theye RA. Pathophysiology of hyperkalemia in burned patients. *Anesthesiology*. 1975;43:89–99.

79. Martyn JAJ, Matteo RS, Szyfelbein SK. Unprecedented resistance to neuromuscular blocking effects of metocurine with persistence after complete recovery in a burned patient. *Anesth Analg*. 1982;61:614–617.

80. Martyn JAJ, Goudsouzian NG, Liu LMP, Szyfelbein SK, Kaplan RF. Metocurine requirements and plasma concentration in burned pediatric patients. *Br J Anaesth*. 1983;55:263–268.

81. Martyn JAJ, Liu LMP, Szyfelbein SK, Ambalavanar ES, Goudsouzian NG. Neuromuscular effects of pancuronium in burned children. *Anesthesiology*. 1983;59:561–564.

82. Yamashita M, Shiga T, Matsuki A. Unusual resistance to pancuronium in severely burned patients: Case reports. *Can Anaesth Soc J*. 1982;29:630–631.

83. Sarubin J. Increased requirement of alcuronium in burned patients. *Anesthetist*. 1982;31:392–395.

84. Martyn JAJ, Szyfelbein SK, Ali HH. Increased *d*-Tubocurarine requirement following major thermal injury. *Anesthesiology*. 1980;52:352–355.

85. Martyn JAJ, Greenblatt DJ, Lebowitz PW, Savarese JJ. Pharmacokinetics of *d*-Tubocurarine in patients with thermal injury. *Anesth Analg*. 1982;61:241–246.

86. Dwersteg JF, Pavlin EG, Heimbach D. Burn patients are resistant to atracurium. *Anesthesiology*. 1985;63:A338. Abstract.

87. Mills A, Martyn JAJ, Szyfelbein SK. Evaluation of atracurium neuromuscular blockade in burned children. *Anesthesiology*. 1985;63:A339. Abstract.

88. Owen RT. Resistance to competitive neuromuscular blocking agents in burn patients: A review. *Methods Find Exp Clin Pharmacol*. 1985;7:203–207.

89. Pavlin EG. Perioperative fluid requirements in the thermally injured patient. In: Martyn JAJ, ed. *Acute Management of the Burned Patient*. Philadelphia, Pa: WB Saunders; 1990: 231–238.

90. Pavlin EG, Strakeljahn C. Operating room considerations in care of the burn patient. In: Boswick JA, ed. *The Art and Science of Burn Care*. Rockville, Md: Aspen Publishers; 1987: 82–91.

91. Martyn JAJ, Szyfelbein SK. Anesthetic management of the burned patient. In: Martyn JAJ, ed. *Acute Management of the Burned Patient*. Philadelphia, Pa: WB Saunders; 1990: 217–230.

92. Pavlin EG, Yazaki S, Heimbach DM. The effects of ketamine and neurolept anesthesia on oxygen consumption (V_{O_2}) and cardiac output in the hypermetabolic burned patient. *Anesthesiol*. 1981;56(suppl):A190. Abstract.

93. Morley-Foster PK. Unintentional hypothermia in the operating room. *Can Anaesth Soc J*. 1986;33:515–528.

Chapter 23

METABOLIC DERANGEMENTS AND NUTRITIONAL SUPPORT

DOUGLAS N. WHATMORE, M.D.*

*Lieutenant Colonel, Medical Corps, U.S. Army (ret); formerly, Chief, Critical Care Medicine Service, Walter Reed Army Medical Center, Washington, D. C. 20307-5001, and Consultant in Critical Care Medicine to The Surgeon General, U.S. Army; currently, private practice of critical care medicine, 2860 Channing Way, Suite 214, Idaho Falls, Idaho 83404

INTRODUCTION

A detailed review of the biochemistry of normal metabolism is beyond the scope of this chapter but a brief review of the more fundamental processes is not inappropriate. Greater emphasis will be placed on recording the gross perversions of normal metabolism that occur during life-threatening trauma—especially when accompanied by sepsis. The remainder of the chapter will describe practical aspects of the nutritional interventions at the disposal of military critical care specialists.

The energy to drive all cellular processes is stored in high-energy phosphate compounds, either adenosine 5′-triphosphate (ATP) or phosphocreatine. These are generated by (*a*) glycolysis, which occurs within the Embden-Meyerhof pathway, and (*b*) oxidative phosphorylation, which takes place in the tricarboxylic acid (TCA) cycle in conjunction with the proteins that constitute the respiratory chain. In glycolysis, glucose is broken down into pyruvate or lactate, while the TCA cycle produces carbon dioxide and metabolic intermediates that carry electrons and protons to the chain of respiratory proteins located in the inner membrane of the mitochondria (Figure 23-1). In contrast to glycolysis, in which the enzymatic machinery is found distributed throughout the cytoplasm of cells and can function without oxygen, the complete complement of enzymes needed for the TCA cycle is found exclusively within mitochondria and functions only in the presence of oxygen. As the electrons are passed along the respiratory chain, protons are driven into the space between the inner and outer membranes of the mitochondria, resulting in the development of a proton gradient across the inner membrane. Under the influence of the gradient, protons flow back through the inner membrane, passing through specialized proteins that generate ATP. The electrons combine with oxygen and protons to form water. Oxidative phosphorylation produces the vast majority of the body's metabolic energy: in the presence of oxygen, 1 molecule of glucose can be made to generate as many as 38

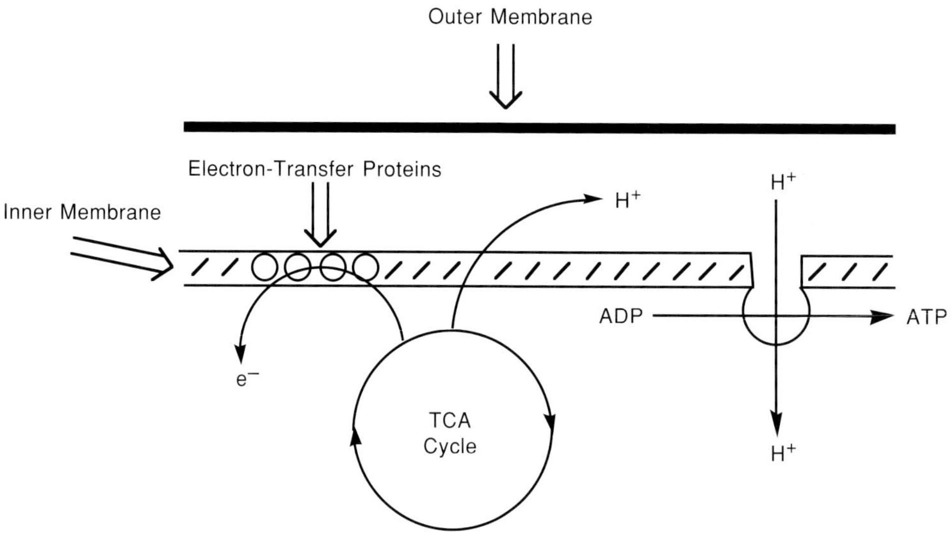

Fig. 23-1. The *chemiosmotic* theory, illustrated here, is the accepted explanation of how oxidative phosphorylation produces high-energy phosphate compounds. The schematic shows a portion of the wall of a mitochondrium. A characteristic feature of this organelle is a wall formed by an outer and an inner membrane that are separated by a space. The cytochrome oxidation-reduction proteins are located in the inner membrane. The tricarboxylic acid (TCA) cycle produces protons (H^+), which are extruded through the inner membrane, and electrons (e^-), which are passed along the cytochrome system until they react with oxygen. The protons, which have collected in the space between the membranes, ultimately pass back into the interior of the mitochondrium through specialized proteins embedded in the inner membrane. Here they cause adenosine 5′-triphosphate (ATP) to form from adenosine diphosphate (ADP) and inorganic phosphate. The protons subsequently react with oxygen to form water.

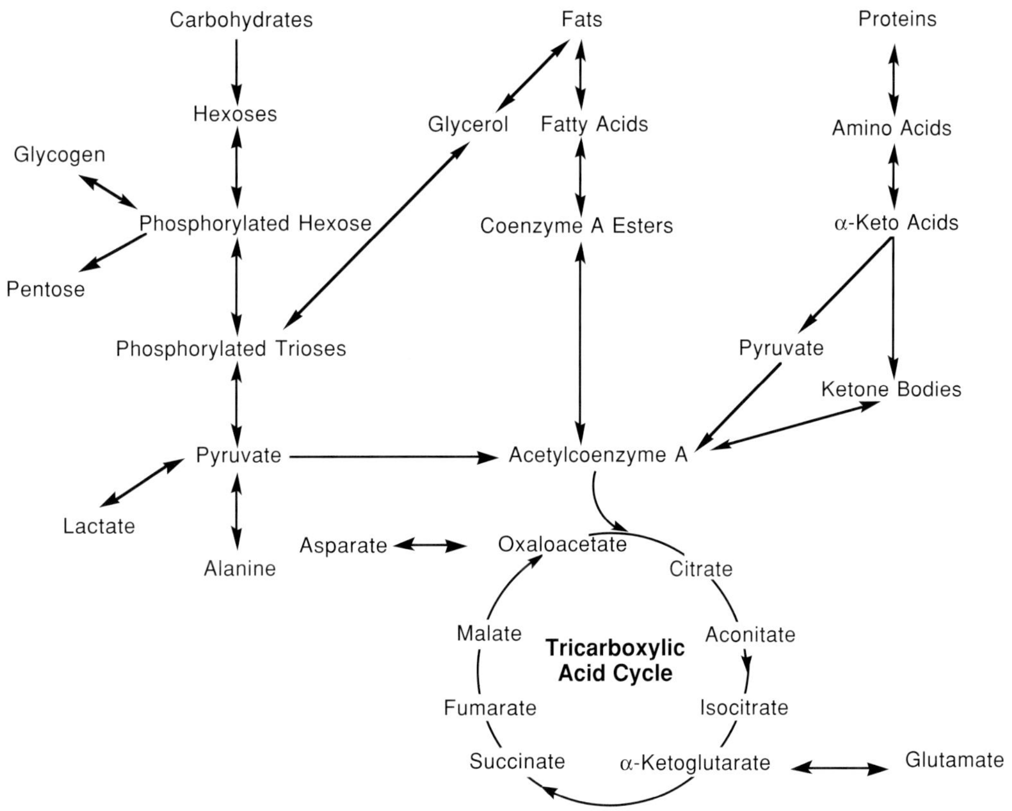

Fig. 23-2. The interrelation of the principal classes of metabolites that serve as the source of energy for human activity: carbohydrates, fats, and proteins. The central process is that of the tricarboxylic acid (TCA) cycle, entrance into which is by means of acetylcoenzyme A (acetyl-CoA). The latter substance is made from pyruvate, which comes from the metabolism of carbohydrates and certain amino acids, and from coenzyme A esters formed from fats. Most of the reactions shown are reversible (double-ended arrows) except for the one linking pyruvate and acetyl-CoA. This fact has important implications for understanding the metabolic derangements that occur during severe trauma. Although carbohydrates can be converted into fats, fats cannot be converted directly into carbohydrates. When the supply of carbohydrates to individual cells is inhibited, such as during starvation and when insulin resistance exists, fat catabolism is accelerated to supply acetyl-CoA for use by the TCA cycle. However, an alternative source of glucose is needed to meet the needs of organs that use glucose as the obligatory substrate. The glucose cannot be obtained from fat because the the pyruvate–acetyl-CoA reaction is irreversible. The needed glucose is obtained by a process in which alanine is converted into pyruvate. There will also be accelerated entry of amino acids such as aspartate and glutamate into the TCA cycle. In this metabolic state, which is commonly seen following severe trauma, the amino acids needed to form glucose are obtained from the catabolism of protein—but not from fat because of the irreversibility of the pyruvate–acetyl-CoA reaction.

molecules of ATP. By way of contrast, the metabolism of 1 molecule of glucose in the absence of oxygen produces only 2 molecules of ATP.[1]

The ultimate metabolic precursors of high-energy phosphate compounds are complex carbohydrates, which are, for the most part, polymers of six-carbon molecules known as hexoses; fats, which are glycerol–fatty acid esters; and proteins, which are polymers of amino acids (Figure 23-2). The initial steps leading to the formation of ATP involve the breaking down of the complex carbohydrate, fat, and protein molecules into their constituents, which then form the substrates for oxidative phosphorylation. Hexoses, of which glucose is the most important, are converted to pyruvate, which, depending on the availability of oxygen, is converted either to lactate or to acetylcoenzyme A (acetyl-CoA). Fatty acids as well as the nitrogen-free residue of amino acids also form acetyl-CoA. Acetyl-CoA is the point of entrance into the TCA cycle, where metabolic intermediates derived from carbohydrates, fats, and proteins interact. Amino acids derived from protein in skeletal muscles can be converted to glucose, and excessive dietary ingestion of glucose can lead to the formation of fatty acids, which are then stored as fat in adipose tissue. Fat, however, cannot be converted directly to glucose unless the constituent fatty acids either contain an odd number of carbon atoms or have branching chains.

Glucose is the most immediately available energy source and the one in highest demand by the body. A number of tissues, the central nervous system particularly, are obligate glucose users and must have a continuous supply. Fibroblasts and formed elements of the blood such as erythrocytes, as well as the renal medulla, all depend on glucose. Six hundred to 1,000 kcal/d must be provided to these tissues, and glucose is preferentially made available even if the rest of the body must shift to another energy source such as lipid. However, glucose reserves are sharply limited and consist of about 20 g within the body at any given time. More important are the 300 to 400 g glycogen (a polymer of glucose) that are stored in the liver and skeletal muscle. Although the synthesis of glycogen from glucose is easily reversed by the process of glycogenolysis, glycogen is not an optimally efficient storage medium because both its formation and its degradation require the expenditure of energy. In fact, when the synthesis of glycogen stems from noncarbohydrate sources, instead of the usual 3.4 kcal/g obtained from the oxidation of glucose to water and carbon dioxide, a net increase of as little as 1 to 2 kcal additional energy may be produced by the complete oxidation of 1 g of glycogen.

The availability and utilization of carbohydrate are controlled by a complex interplay of hormones, with insulin and glucagon the major factors. Insulin is an anabolic hormone; it reduces plasma glucose levels by (*a*) increasing glucose transport into cells, whereby glycolysis is stimulated, and (*b*) increasing glycogen synthesis in liver and muscle. Insulin also blocks gluconeogenesis (wherein amino acids derived from the catabolism of body proteins are converted into glucose) and promotes protein synthesis. Glucagon counters these effects of insulin by promoting glycogenolysis and gluconeogenesis in the liver and lipolysis in the adipose stores. (The latter effect is opposite of that of insulin, which causes fat synthesis.) The ratio of insulin to glucagon controls the balance and is a major determinant of the ability to mobilize energy stores. A high ratio defines an *anabolic* state (ie, more-complex molecules are synthesized from simpler molecules); a low ratio, a *catabolic* state (ie, complex molecules are degraded to simpler molecules).

As previously indicated, the body has the biochemical machinery to use triglycerides and proteins for oxidative phosphorylation once glucose and glycogen reserves are used up (see Figure 23-2). The relative importance of the body's reserves of carbohydrates, fat, and protein as sources of energy is shown in Table 23-1. At any given time, the actual contribution of the carbohydrates, fats, and proteins to overall energy production can be estimated by measuring the respiratory quotient (RQ), which is discussed in Exhibit 23-1 and in greater detail later in this chapter.

Lipids are the most abundant, although not the most readily available, energy source. The average 70-kg soldier has 100,000 kcal stored as lipid (9 kcal/g),[2] and this reserve becomes the principal fuel source during starvation. Fats are broken down into their constituent fatty acids and glycerol, a process known as lipolysis. Two types of lipases act to convert stored lipid to the more readily available fuels glycerol and fatty acid. Hormone-sensitive lipase (activated by adenosine 3′,5′-cyclic monophosphate [cAMP], which, in turn, is triggered by catecholamine receptors on the adipocyte membrane) degrades lipids to fatty acids and glycerol. The fatty acids enter the TCA cycle as acetyl-CoA, and the glycerol is either transformed to pyruvate or esterified to triglyceride in the liver. The second lipase, lipoprotein lipase, catalyzes the release of triglycerides from low-density lipoproteins and chylomicrons, an effect that is *inhibited* by catecholamines. The presence of glucose and insulin tends to enhance the effects of lipoprotein lipase.

TABLE 23-1

ENERGY STORES IN A 70-KG MAN

		Energy Stores	
Energy Source	**Tissue**	**(g)**	**(kcal)**
Triglycerides	Fat	15,000	100,000
Protein	Muscle	6,000	25,000
Glycogen	Liver	70	280
	Muscle	120	480
Glucose	Throughout body	20	80

Adapted with permission from Linder MC. Energy metabolism, intake, and expenditure. In: Linder MC, ed. *Nutritional Biochemistry and Metabolism with Clinical Applications*. New York, NY: Elsevier; 1985: 290.

EXHIBIT 23-1

METABOLIC TERMINOLOGY

Respiratory Quotient (RQ): The molar ratio of CO_2 produced for O_2 consumed, or $\dot{V}CO_2/\dot{V}O_2$. For carbohydrates, this is 1.0 (ie, one mole of CO_2 is generated for each mole of O_2 consumed). For the oxidation of fats, the ratio is 0.7; for protein, 0.82. *The conversion of carbohydrate to fat (ie, lipogenesis) can theoretically have an RQ > 8.0.* Whenever the respiratory quotient is > 1.0, lipogenesis (and therefore overfeeding) is occurring. Remember that changes in the respiratory quotient directly affect PO_2 and PCO_2. Alveolar PO_2 will fall with a decreasing RQ, for any given level of PCO_2. PCO_2 will rise with an increasing RQ, and will require a higher minute ventilation to normalize.

O_2 Consumption ($\dot{V}O_2$): The amount of oxygen consumed by metabolic processes in 1 min, given as

$$\text{Minute Ventilation (L/min)} \bullet (FIO_2 - FEO_2)$$

when the RQ is 1.0.

CO_2 Production ($\dot{V}CO_2$): The amount of CO_2 generated by metabolic processes in 1 min, given as

$$\text{Minute Ventilation (L/min)} \bullet FECO_2$$

O_2 Delivery (DO_2): The amount of O_2 carried to the tissues each minute, calculated as

$$\text{C.O. (L/min)} \bullet CaO_2\text{, or}$$

$$\text{C.O.} \bullet [(1.39 \bullet SaO_2 \bullet Hb) + (0.003 \bullet PO_2)]$$

DO_2 is given in mL/kg/min; about 16 mL/kg/min is normal for adults. Normal $\dot{V}O_2$ is about 4 mL/kg/min.

O_2 Extraction Ratio (OER) The percentage of the delivered O_2 actually consumed in metabolic processes, or $\dot{V}O_2/DO_2$. This is about 25% in normal adults, and *normally* decreases as O_2 delivery increases.

Resting Energy Expenditure (REE): The energy expenditure measured at rest or lying down. REE can be calculated from $\dot{V}O_2$, $\dot{V}CO_2$, and a measurement of metabolized nitrogen (eg, Nu, nitrogen excreted in the urine)*:

$$\text{REE (in kcal/min)} = 3.581 \text{ (kcal/L)} \bullet \dot{V}O_2 \text{ (in L/min)} + 1.448 \text{ (kcal/L)} \bullet \dot{V}CO_2 \text{ (in L/min)} - 1.773 \text{ (kcal/g)} \bullet \text{Nu (in g/min)}$$

*REE may be normalized for body surface area or mass by dividing by area in square meters, or mass in kilograms, respectively. Since the contribution of the term 1.773 Nu is small, Bursztein has calculated that a 100% error in measured Nu will be associated with only a 1% error in REE. Therefore, from the practical standpoint, the last term in the REE equation can be ignored, since determination of nitrogen excretion is not necessary to estimate energy expenditure. Source for REE definition and equation: Bursztein S, Elwyn DH, Askanazi J, Kinney JM. *Energy Metabolism, Indirect Calorimetry, and Nutrition.* Baltimore, Md: Williams & Wilkins; 1989: 30, 59, 62.

CaO_2: arterial oxygen contents; C.O.: cardiac output; FEO_2: fraction of expired oxygen; FIO_2: fraction of inspired oxygen; Hb: hemoglobin; PCO_2: partial pressure of carbon dioxide; PO_2: partial pressure of oxygen; SaO_2: oxygen saturation of arterial blood

Insulin inhibits lipolysis; in fact, a high ratio of insulin to glucagon will promote storage of fuel as lipid. Catecholamines, glucagon, and somatotropin (ie, growth hormone) all promote the breakdown of the lipid stores for energy. Steroids will enhance the lipolytic effects of catecholamines and glucagon.

An additional option that the body has to supply glucose or substrates for oxidative phosphorylation is to utilize amino acids, from either ingested or structural proteins, as fuel. There are five points where the carbon skeletons of amino acids can enter the glucose oxidation pathway: as pyruvate, acetyl-CoA, α-ketoglutarate, fumarate, and succinylcoenzyme A (succinyl-CoA). Protein may be diverted for use as a fuel source, normally as excess dietary protein, or as catabolized structural protein in stress states. Protein yields 4.1 kcal/g.

Normal protein turnover—breakdown and synthesis—is approximately 300 g/d.[3,4] Normal daily protein turnover in skeletal muscle is 100 g/d. Roughly 50 g, which is used to produce digestive juices, and another 20 g of small intestinal lining cells are lost daily in digestion. Eighty to one hundred grams of protein is ingested daily in a typical Western diet. Excess is converted to fuel, and the nitrogen is excreted as urea. Enzymes are continually made, used, and broken down; structural proteins are continually modified; and cells are continually replaced. In normal adults, 15% to 20% of the basal metabolic rate (BMR) is due to metabolism of protein.

Amino acids are transported by a membrane carrier system,[3,4] often against a steep concentration gradient (as opposed to the glucose carrier system). There are seven carriers, specific for different amino acids but with some overlap. Amino acids are constantly being cycled into and out of the cells and transaminated or deaminated for use in cellular processes. Different processes feed these substrates into the cellular plants—hydrolysis of dietary (or structural, in starvation) protein, amination of keto acids, conversion of amino acids and ketoacids to other compounds, use of amino acids for protein synthesis, oxidation of ketoacids—to balance the supply of amino acids with the demand. Most processes involve transamination to glutamate as the common path for transfer.

Metabolism of carbohydrates, fats, and proteins is regulated by a complex neural and hormonal feedback system. The hypothalamus controls both the normal function of the system and the response of the organism to starvation and stress. Stimulation of the ventromedial hypothalamic nucleus by concentrations of metabolic substrates (eg, carbohydrate, lipid, and amino acids), along with input from aortic baroreceptors, renal nerves, and the carotid sinuses, as well as changes in the concentration of hormones are all feedback elements that guide the orchestration of the system by the hypothalamus. When the nucleus is stimulated, sympathetic and parasympathetic outflow increase. The adrenal medulla is stimulated via the great splanchnic nerve. This increase in sympathetic outflow mobilizes substrate (from glycogen stores, lipid pools, and skeletal muscle), increases cardiac output and minute ventilation, and releases insulin and glucagon from the pancreas. Parasympathetic outflow increases absorption of nutrients by the gut. Pituitary hormones—adrenocorticotropic hormone (ACTH), somatotropic hormone (STH), thyroid-stimulating hormone (TSH), prolactin (PRL), luteinizing hormone (LH) and follicle-stimulating hormone (FSH) from the anterior pituitary, and antidiuretic hormone (ADH) from the posterior pituitary—control utilization of substrate and fluid balance and osmolarity. Insulin is stimulated by the release of β-adrenergic catecholamines, while glucagon is stimulated and insulin is inhibited by α-adrenergic catecholamines and increased adrenal hormones. Portal blood levels of both insulin and glucagon are significantly higher than systemic levels, as is their utilization by the liver. The ratio of insulin to glucagon concentration dictates whether the response is anabolic or catabolic.

The mobilization of free fatty acids is controlled by an interplay among ACTH, corticosteroids, catecholamines, and glucagon. ACTH also controls the secretion of beta endorphin and melanocyte-stimulating hormone (MSH). This corticotrophin-releasing hormone (CRH)–ACTH–cortisol axis plays a crucial role in our ability to respond to a stressful stimulus. The patterns of response are nearly uniform; only the degrees differ.

The critical importance of the relative ratio of insulin to glucagon cannot be overemphasized. The ratio is one of the chief determinants of catabolism versus anabolism and is responsible for maintaining normal glucose levels in all tissues, particularly the obligate glucose users. Depletion of glycogen stores triggers a shift in the ratio: a fall in insulin levels and an increase in glucagon. The liver responds to this change by increasing gluconeogenesis: amino acids from skeletal muscle protein are stripped of their carbon skeleton to make more glucose. Glucagon activates catecholamine-sensitive lipase in adipose tissues; triglycerides are broken down and the circulating free fatty acids and glycerol are fed to the liver, which catabolizes them to ketones to be used as an oxidative fuel source. When the ratio is reversed, carbohydrate is converted to glycogen and fat for storage of chemical energy, and protein synthesis is stimulated.

Before we move on to specific metabolic derangements and nutritional support, the reader should review the metabolic terms and their descriptions in Exhibit 23-1.

METABOLIC DERANGEMENTS IN COMBAT CASUALTIES

Most patients seen by medical officers in field medical facilities will be members of the armed forces: young, well developed, predominantly male, and with no significant medical history. The typical soldier in the U.S. Army will have entered the combat zone with a large muscle mass and greater-than-normal glycogen stores, but many factors are likely to modify the picture of this healthy, muscular soldier. Of these factors, the most important are starvation, exercise and stress and, in the event of a combat injury, the wound itself. Major W. J. Phillips, Medical Corps, U.S. Army, has published an excellent introduction to this subject.[5]

Starvation

How does starvation affect metabolism? Glucose is no longer available either from glycogen or from externally supplied carbohydrates, yet several organs such as the brain will not tolerate an interruption in their supply of glucose. After only 8 hours without intake, the body begins to use its glycogen reserves to support the obligate glucose-utilizing tissues—the central nervous system, renal medulla, formed blood elements, and fibroblasts—while the metabolic economy shifts to fatty acid oxidation. Even though energy expenditure may be minimized by a decrease in resting energy expenditure (REE, which is discussed later in this chapter), the available glycogen stores will be depleted within 24 hours. A starved, stressed patient will rapidly catabolize nonvital structural proteins to fuel metabolic processes.

The initial adjustment to an inadequate intake of nutrients is to form glucose from amino acids derived from skeletal muscle protein. Branched-chain amino acids are transaminated to alanine and glutamine, which are "stripped" in the liver for their carbon skeletons to make glucose, or they are used as intermediates in the TCA cycle. A starved patient loses roughly 75 g of muscle protein, or 200 to 300 g of structural muscle tissue, each day. The urea and ammonia generated by this process are excreted by the kidney. The energy for gluconeogenesis comes from catabolism of fatty acids supplied by the lipolysis of adipose tissues.[3,6,7]

Within 1 week, metabolism of fatty acids becomes the principal source of fuel to meet the body's needs. The activation of catechol-sensitive lipase in adipose tissue causes the release of free fatty acids and glycerol. Glycerol is converted to glucose or to pyruvate, which enters the TCA cycle. A consequence of the accelerated metabolism of fatty acids during starvation is the production of ketone bodies and their increasing use by organs such as the heart and brain in place of glucose. The adaptation of the heart and brain to utilize ketone bodies is of critical importance in prolonging survival during starvation, since it allows for a marked reduction in the glucose needs of the body (perhaps 5% of normal) that otherwise could not be meet by gluconeogenesis beyond about 2 weeks (Figure 23-3).

Fats become the primary fuel, with the utilization of lipid becoming a major adaptive response, conserving protein. Protein catabolism declines as the body's energy needs are increasingly met by catabolism of fat. As simple starvation continues, the rate of catabolism decreases from roughly 300 g of muscle tissue per day to 150 g/d. In simple starvation, the intake of carbohydrate can spare protein to some extent. How are these responses to starvation brought about? The fall in glucose causes a fall in insulin, with a consequent, although lesser, inhibition of lipolysis. Glucagon rises as insulin falls, accelerating both lipolysis and glycogenolysis.

What are the systemic medical effects of starvation for a significant period (ie, longer than several days)? All organs are affected by the loss of structural, and often of functional, proteins. The lungs lose the ability to clear bacteria, connective tissues degenerate, and emphysematous changes are the result. Respiratory muscles atrophy. The heart dilates, and, after a time, focal necrosis and fibrosis appears, with myofibrillar degeneration. Red and white blood cell counts fall with decreased production of erythropoietin (ie, erythropoietic hormone) and stem cells. The gut, which has more rapidly dividing cells than any other organ, loses mass out of all proportion to its size as it atrophies. The liver and kidneys lose mass, and the liver begins to accumulate fat. The immune system becomes less and less able to respond to infection, as the number of T helper cells declines and polymorphonucleocytes lose their chemotactic abilities. If hypermetabolism is added to simple starvation, then the catabolism of protein predominates, and the changes discussed are far more profound.

Exercise

The metabolic consequences of exercise depend on both the duration and the intensity of the exer-

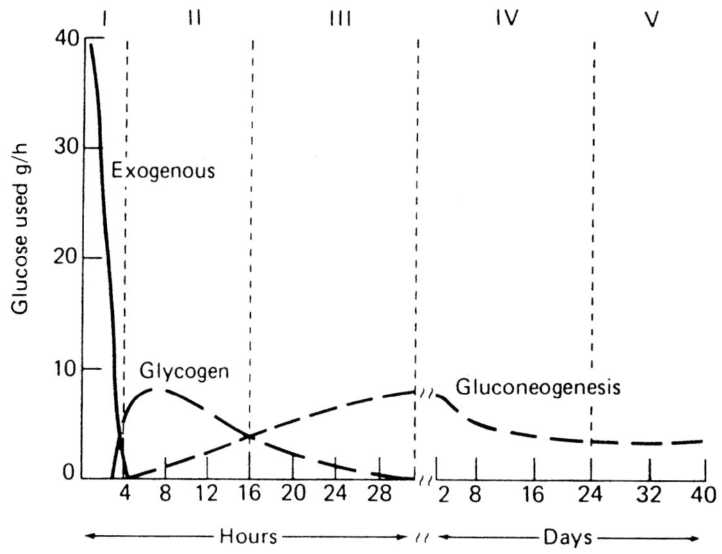

The Five Phases of Glucose Homeostasis

	I	II	III	IV	V
Origin of blood glucose	Exogenous	Glycogen Hepatic gluconeogenesis	Hepatic gluconeogenesis Glycogen	Gluconeogenesis, hepatic and renal	Gluconeogenesis, hepatic and renal
Tissues using glucose	All	All except liver Muscle and adipose tissue at diminished rates	All except liver Muscle and adipose tissue at rates intermediate between II and IV	Brain, red blood cells, renal medulla; small amount by muscle	Brain at a diminished rate, red blood cells, renal medulla
Major fuel of the brain	Glucose	Glucose	Glucose	Glucose, ketone bodies	Ketone bodies, glucose

Fig. 23-3. The amount of glucose consumed and its source depend on the phase of alimentation. In the immediate postabsorptive phase, exogenous glucose forms the major source and is consumed by all tissues (I). Within 3 to 4 hours of eating, glycolysis of liver glycogen is the major source of glucose (II). The major source of glucose after 24 hours is gluconeogenesis from amino acids released by the catabolism of skeletal muscle protein (III). When fasting progresses to starvation, glucose consumption is increasingly restricted to red blood cells and the renal medulla (IV). During starvation, glucose consumption by the brain progressively falls, as the brain increasingly uses ketone bodies as its major source of energy (V). Whatever glucose is produced comes from gluconeogenesis. Reprinted with permission from Linder MC. Energy metabolism, intake, and expenditure. In: Linder MC, ed. *Nutritional Biochemistry and Metabolism with Clinical Applications*. New York, NY: Elsevier; 1985: 291.

cise. The most intense exercise (eg, running at maximum speed carrying full combat gear) causes muscle ATP and phosphocreatine to be totally consumed in less than 1 minute. If the exertion, albeit at a reduced rate, is prolonged beyond 10 seconds, muscle glycogen stores begin to be broken down to glucose, which, in turn, is metabolized to lactic acid. Anaerobic metabolic pathways—and especially the breakdown of muscle glycogen—are the primary energy source for maximum-intensity exercise that lasts less than several minutes. The amount of glycogen available in muscle is the major metabolic determinant of performance during short, high-intensity exertion. In normal circumstances, about 80% of the lactic acid formed during anaerobic exercise is converted rapidly back to glucose; the remainder enters the TCA cycle where it will be metabolized to carbon dioxide.

Only when the duration of high-intensity exercise exceeds 3 or 4 minutes does aerobic metabolism become the predominant source of high-energy phosphates. During prolonged exercise under aerobic conditions, the initial major source of energy is liver glycogen, followed by fatty acids. Neverthe-

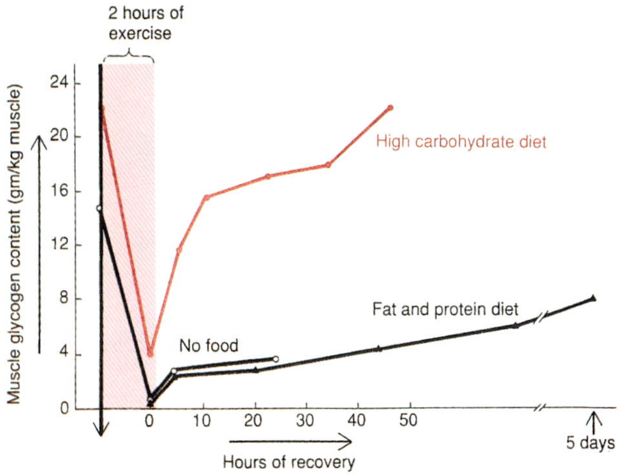

Fig. 23-4. Restoration of muscle glycogen levels after vigorous exercise very much depends on the consumption of a diet high in carbohydrates. A similar degree of glycogen repletion will not occur when most of the calories are provided by a diet rich in fats and proteins. Reprinted with permission from Fox EL. *Sports Physiology*. Dubuque, IA: Times Mirror Higher Education Group; 1984: 69.

less, glycogen depletion occurs with long-distance running or prolonged marching with a full combat load, even given the steady-state conditions of aerobic energy production. Reconstitution of depleted glycogen becomes an important determinant of further exercise performance. Restoring muscle and liver glycogen stores to normal greatly depends on the types of food consumed after the exercise (Figure 23-4). Thus, the combination of prolonged exercise and nutritional deprivation may seriously degrade exercise performance.

Starvation, Exercise, and Stress

Starvation is simply the lack of nutrient intake. Few inflammatory mediators are released, and the body responds to exogenous replacement. But now we add moderate stress in the forms of sleep deprivation, anxiety or even fear, cold or heat, and arduous physical exertion—a combination especially likely to occur during military operations. Starvation puts humans into glycogenolytic and gluconeogenetic metabolic modes, the latter being ultimately suppressed by the development of lipolysis and the formation of ketone bodies. Unfortunately, exercise and stress interfere with this adaptation. Stress increases glucose utilization out of proportion to total energy expenditure, while it also increases energy expenditure. Glycogen stores are depleted more rapidly. Increased levels of glucagon, catecholamines, and cortisol—hormones that characterize the human response to stress—accentuate gluconeogenesis. Fat is no longer the primary energy source; the body utilizes protein stores instead. Each day, 250 g of fat and 3- to 4-fold that amount of muscle tissue are catabolized to produce new glucose.

Actual measurements of these derangements during combat operations are next to impossible to make for obvious reasons. Fortunately, however, the U.S. Army Research Institute of Environmental Medicine (USARIEM) has studied the effects of starvation, exercise, and stress during the U.S. Army's Ranger Training Course.[8] This is the training exercise that most closely mimics real combat. The training course is extremely arduous; typically, only 40% to 50% of its students pass. The course lasts 62 days and is carried out in four phases in geographically and climatically diverse settings: at Fort Benning, Georgia, and in mountain, jungle, and desert environments in Georgia and elsewhere in the United States.

In the USARIEM study, which was published in 1992, the mean weight loss of Rangers in training over the 62-day course was 12.1 ± 3.4 kg (range 6.5–20.6 kg), which corresponded to a median weight loss of 15.6% of initial body weight. Body fat fell from about 15% of body weight at the beginning of the training to about 6% at the end. Fat-free mass (an index of muscle tissue) fell an average of 4.6 kg. These reductions in body mass were clearly due to the marked imbalance between total body energy expenditure (which averaged 4,010 ± 830 kcal/d) and estimated food energy intake (which averaged 3,930 ± 290 kcal/d) (Figure 23-5). Peak energy expenditures during the mountain phase were estimated to exceed 6,000 kcal/d. By way of contrast, an average, unstressed man requires about 2,000 kcal/d, and an unstressed woman about 1,800 kcal/d.

The combination of inadequate caloric intake, stress, and exercise caused profound endocrine disturbances (Figure 23-6). As expected, the level of insulin and insulinlike growth factor (IGF-1) showed significant decreases, which suggest the magnitude of the ongoing protein catabolism. The cortisol level increased and although glucagon was not measured, we may assume that it also increased since glucagon's role, like cortisol's, is to mobilize the body's noncarbohydrate energy reserves. Not shown on the graph, but of considerable interest, is the nearly 1,000% increase in growth hormone (ie, somatotrophin). The homeostatic importance of

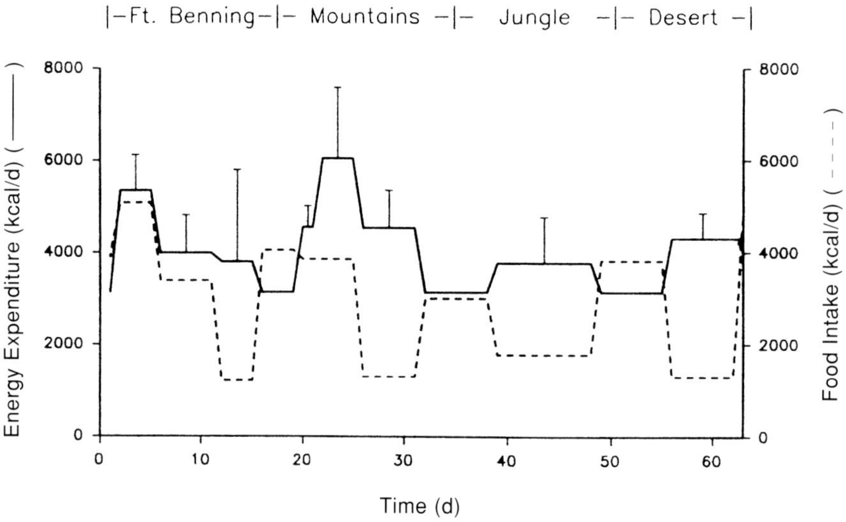

Fig. 23-5. Energy balance during the 2 months of the U.S. Army Ranger training course. Solid lines represent estimated energy expenditure, while broken lines represent estimated energy intake. Except for the brief periods of transition between the training phases, the Rangers ate fewer calories than they expended. Reprinted from Moore RJ, Friedl KE, Kramer TR, et al. *Changes in Soldier Nutritional Status and Immune Function During the Ranger Training Course.* Natick, Mass: US Army Research Institute of Environmental Medicine; 1992: 51. USARIEM Report T13-92.

this alteration is unclear, since growth hormone has anabolic effects and, in fact, is increasingly used for that purpose in nutritionally depleted catabolic surgical patients.[9]

Other consequences of the combined starvation, exercise, and stress that characterize the Ranger Training Course, and military operations in general, are loss of strength in large muscle masses such as the thighs (no doubt due to the generalized loss of lean body mass) and dramatic evidence of a loss of cell-mediated immune function. Such indices of T lymphocyte function as phytohemagglutinin-stimulated proliferation and interleukin-2 (IL-2) production were reduced by one half. Production of IL-6 fell to a similar extent. These derangements are clinically relevant: 50% of the population studied were treated with antibiotics for infection. The cumulative effects of starvation, exercise, and stress can have tragic, unintended consequences. On 15 February 1995, four Ranger students at Fort Benning died from hypothermia after a water-immersion portion of their training. Ironically, the official recommendations that had been prepared on the basis of the USARIEM study had emphasized that

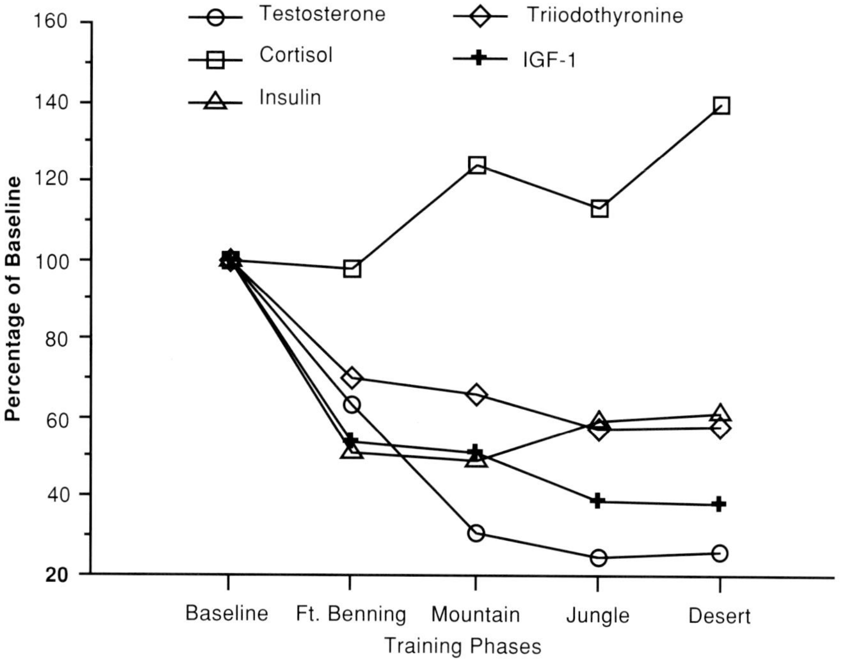

Fig. 23-6. Measured changes in the levels of various hormones during the 62-day U.S. Army Ranger training course. Data are given as percentages of the baseline values. The elevation of cortisol and the depression of insulin are consistent with stress and starvation. The actual concentration of testosterone approached the level found in castrated men. However, the cause in the Rangers is not testicular dysfunction but rather a profound suppression of the elaboration of pituitary gonadotropin. Data source: Moore RJ, Friedl KE, Kramer TR, et al. *Changes in Soldier Nutritional Status and Immune Function During the Ranger Training Course.* Natick, Mass: US Army Research Institute of Environmental Medicine; 1992: Table 23, p 68. USARIEM Technical Report T13-92.

the normal thermogenic response to mild cold is impaired during massive weight loss.

Given the extreme psychological and physical stresses and the less-than-ideal circumstances for eating and resting associated with prolonged exposure to combat—or even just living in the combat zone—the metabolic, endocrine, and immune derangements found in USARIEM's Ranger study are to be expected. The importance of weight loss in soldiers should not be underestimated. The extensive slide collection of the Wound Data Munition Effectiveness Team (WDMET) database that was compiled during the Vietnam War contains few photographs of combat casualties who show either significant obesity or who have a muscular mesomorph body habitus. Many of the soldiers portrayed in the WDMET database appear to be significantly malnourished (Figure 23-7).[10] Medical officers must expect to treat soldiers who are not in optimal nutritional status when wounded. Furthermore, in every war in which the United States has been a combatant, U.S. forces have cared for children, the elderly, and prisoners of war. This must be kept in mind when nutritional support is planned, because such potential casualties are likely to manifest some degree of starvation.

The Effect of Injury

When even a peripheral injury of an arm or leg is added to starvation, mediators are released, catecholamines levels increase further, thyroid hormone is elevated, and cardiac output, oxygen delivery, and oxygen extraction all increase. If the injured soldier is not resuscitated adequately, oxygen delivery may fall and anaerobic metabolism be initiated. Further inflammatory mediators will be released. Should the wound be of the trunk, the metabolic stresses would be the same, but with this larger body compartment will come more tissue damage; greater blood loss; higher levels of inflammatory mediators; and greater risks of inadequate resuscitation, infection, and organ failure.[11–13]

The chain of metabolic events set in motion by injury is complex. Not only are there direct effects of the injury on tissue, but the body responds with a cascade of direct effects (the immediate response to the injury, including the steps the body takes to protect itself from further injury) and indirect effects (those effects on metabolism resulting from the injury and the direct effects the injury sets in motion).

The body's immediate responses to an injury are (*a*) the activation of the sympathetic nervous system and (*b*) a secondary discharge of catecholamines from the adrenal medulla. Cardiac output, and thus the delivery of oxygen to the tissues, increases, and the oxygen extraction ratio also rises as tissue metabolism increases. The release of thyroid hormones, in response to the catecholamine surge, is responsible for 50% to 60% of this increase in metabolism. As the rate of biochemical reactions increases, the core body temperature increases—but owing to homeothermic compensatory changes, not to the extent predicted by the inverse of van't Hoff's law (ie, a reaction rate increases 7.2% for each 1°F rise in temperature). The extent to which the temperature rises is proportional to the severity of the illness.[13,14] An increase in motor activity, whether due to running, shivering, thrashing secondary to pain, seizures, and so forth, usually accompanies these responses and further increases both metabolism and temperature.

The indirect effects of stress and injury on the body are more subtle but play as great a role in altering metabolism. Stress acutely suppresses

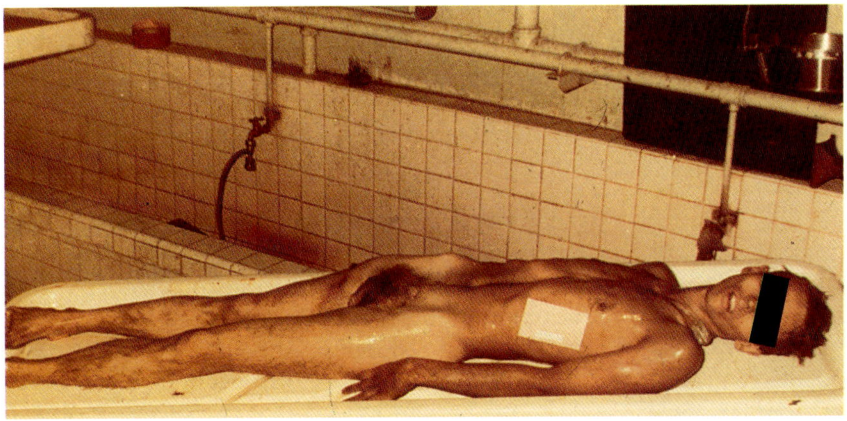

Fig. 23-7. Five months after he arrived in Vietnam, this soldier was killed by a bullet that transected his upper spinal cord. His degree of malnutrition was not unusual. Photograph: Wound Data and Munitions Effectiveness Team slide collection.

pyruvate dehydrogenase, decreasing the amount of pyruvate available for formation of acetyl-CoA, and eventually of ATP. Glycogen stores are depleted quickly. Oxidation and phosphorylation may uncouple, resulting in a markedly less-efficient metabolism. ATP production decreases, but the production of heat rises as the efficiency of the TCA cycle decreases. Futile cycling of substrate via the Cori cycle occurs; at the site of the injury, glucose is metabolized to lactate, which is then transported back to the liver, where it is converted back to glucose. This process produces heat but no net gain of ATP. Oxygen consumption increases, and the body appears to enter a state of hypermetabolism.[13,14]

The release of the counterregulatory hormones—glucagon, cortisol, and ACTH—further promotes the situation. Cortisol increases gluconeogenesis to 6- to 10-fold higher than the baseline. Peripheral proteins are catabolized, and the amino acids are taken up by the liver. Free fatty acids are mobilized from lipid pools and transported to the liver, where glucagon stimulates the use of the carbon skeletons of amino and fatty acids for gluconeogenesis. Release of inflammatory mediators, such as IL-1, IL-6, and the tumor necrosis factor (TNF), further drives the breakdown of protein and lipid while promoting the waste of fuel resources in futile paths such as the Cori cycle.[11,13,14]

So what do we find when we consider the casualty? A young, previously healthy patient, whose higher-than-normal physiological reserves have been affected not only by his recent health and nutrition but also by complicating stresses such as cold or heat, anxiety, pain, volume loss, and infection. In general, heat is tolerated better than cold, and a warmer environment is a better one for the casualty. The presence or absence of military air superiority will determine evacuation times, and in many cases, the adequacy of resuscitation. The length of time to evacuation, continued pain, volume depletion, and so forth, all effect the production of catecholamines, thyroid hormones, cortisol glucagon and ACTH, and the inflammatory mediators, all of which, in turn, affect the metabolism of the patient.

"Fatigue poisons" (ie, elevated levels of catecholamines, counterregulatory hormones, and inflammatory mediators brought on by the stress of combat or the prolonged stress of waiting for combat) take their toll. Metabolism becomes less efficient, receptors for catecholamines and thyroid hormones down-regulate, glycogen stores *slowly* deplete, and gluconeogenesis and ketosis are present at continual low levels. Catecholamines initially increase both oxygen consumption and delivery, although inflammatory mediators, as well as the catecholamines themselves, may interfere with both cardiac output and the peripheral distribution of blood flow. Arteriovenous shunting may actually decrease oxygen delivery to the tissues. The key to metabolic control is adequate and continuing resuscitation to prevent both damage to enzyme systems and cells and the formation of free-radical oxidation of tissues.[15]

Other factors (predominant among them volume depletion and concomitant hypoperfusion of tissues) trigger or amplify a hypermetabolic response to stress and injury. The initial state of the injured patient, and the adequacy of initial and continuing resuscitation at the first and second echelons and during evacuation rearward, will determine the efficiency of organ function, the generation of inflammatory mediators, and the subsequent medical course of the patient. Cold and high glucose loads may each promote a subtle diuresis that may be overlooked during extended transport or if there are large numbers of casualties. A significant limb injury, delayed evacuation, and volume depletion worsened by hypothermia may combine to create a hypermetabolic state that will result in multiple organ failure and death weeks after the injury.

Stages in the Response to Stress

Stress, whether emotional or physical (from illness, injury, or infection), induces specific patterns of metabolic response in the body. The patterns presumably evolved as a survival advantage, a means to deal with overwhelming stimuli. They work reasonably well most of the time but often at great expense to the patient, as Shakespeare knew: "Diseases desperate grown by desperate appliance are reliev'd, or not at all."[16]

The Immediate Response

The immediate response to stress is modulated by the sympathetic nervous system, hypothalamus, pituitary, and adrenals. The hypothalamus orchestrates the activation of the sympathetic nervous system and stimulates the release of pituitary hormone and the production of glucagon by the pancreas. ACTH released by the pituitary increases the production of cortisol and other steroids; these, in turn, increase the breakdown of skeletal muscle protein and the turnover of protein in the liver, as well as the breakdown of hepatic glycogen for glucose release. Catecholamines increase available glucose by acting on skeletal muscle to increase protein turnover, on lipid storage cells to release free fatty acids, on the pancreas to increase output of both glucagon and insulin, and on the liver by promoting glycogenolysis and gluconeogenesis. Steroids and glucagon also act to promote gluconeogenesis.[12–14]

Trauma causes a mobilization of resources to deal with the injury, inducing a hypermetabolic state in which oxygen and substrate consumption are greater than normal the availability of ATP does not necessarily increase correspondingly. Oxidative phosphorylation makes available, in the form of ATP, about 40% of the energy that is available in glucose. The remainder appears as heat. Unfortunately, the normal efficiency can be reduced by the uncoupling of oxidation and phosphorylation as well as by the appearance of futile cycles, which consume oxygen and substrate but yield little net gain in energy except for the production of heat necessary for thermostasis.[17] It is apparent that this state will often be induced when the casualty is in a preexisting stressed state and has limited reserves for the new demands. The changes are different from those of starvation but are similar to those seen in the stressed state, although of a much greater magnitude.

The state of hypermetabolism has been known by a variety of names, including sepsis, sepsis syndrome, autocatabolism, and most recently as the systemic inflammatory response syndrome (SIRS). This syndrome is discussed in detail in Chapter 24, The Syndromes of Systemic Inflammatory Response and Multiple Organ Dysfunction, but a brief description of mediators and hormone responses is in order here. The hypermetabolic response to stress, especially trauma and infection, is orchestrated by the activation of the neuroendocrine and cytokine systems. The appearance and magnitude of the mediator response depends directly on the severity of trauma, the amount of inflammatory tissue present, and the presence or absence of infection. Mediators (peptide regulatory factors) are produced by macrophages, lymphocytes, and other cells that are reacting to a stress stimulus, and have both paracrine and autocrine effects on other cells, inducing the expression of a variety of genes and the synthesis of several proteins that mediate the inflammatory response. Two of the most important in terms of metabolism are TNF and IL-1.

In addition to its role as an immune modulator, TNF modulates a great deal of the metabolic response of the organism. Circulating levels of TNF-α and TNF-β increase with stress and increase markedly with infection. Bacterial toxins are one of many kinds of stimuli that activate production of TNF in hepatic macrophages and lymphocytes. TNF activates T and B lymphocytes and the production of interleukins (specifically, IL-1 and IL-6), growth factors, and eicosanoids—especially the lipoxygenase and cyclooxygenase pathways of the arachidonic acid cascade.[11,12,15] The production and output of corticotropin, adrenal cortisol, glucagon, and catecholamine are all increased in response. Fever, a fall in white blood cell count, and hypotension are the immediate results, followed by an increase in white blood cells with a relative lymphopenia, an increase in lactoferrin, and a fall in iron stores. Collagenase synthesis increases, with reabsorption of bone and cartilage. Formation of structural proteins other than at the wound site, albumin production, and the synthesis of nonessential proteins all slow dramatically, while acute-phase protein synthesis in the liver, prostaglandin production, and proliferation of fibroblasts at the site of injury all markedly increase. Serum lipids increase as fat stores are catabolized, and amino acid turnover accelerates.[3,11,13,15] Cytotoxic effects on certain cells—the beta cells of the islets of Langerhans, for example—decrease the availability of the anabolic hormones.[3]

IL-1 also has a broad spectrum of activity, from acting as an inflammatory and immune mediator to affecting metabolic, hematopoietic, and physiological functions. IL-1, the "endogenous pyrogen," is also responsible for fever, elevation of the white blood cell count, increase in the level of colony stimulating factors and other interleukins, and the marked increase in acute-phase protein synthesis by the liver. IL-1 also decreases iron levels; this may be a protective mechanism, as bacteria deprived of iron are less cytotoxic than those with easy access to iron stores. Serum albumin and serum zinc levels drop as zinc (as well as iron) is taken up by the liver.[3] A decrease in appetite is common, possibly due to the decreased serum zinc. The release of ACTH increases the production of adrenal steroids. IL-1, like TNF, is cytotoxic to pancreatic beta cells. Proteolysis is accelerated, as is hepatic uptake of amino acids for gluconeogenesis and acute-phase protein synthesis. IL-1 and TNF act synergistically to produce acute-phase protein synthesis, the immune response, shock, and hypermetabolism as a response to stress, injury, and bacterial invasion. Other interleukins and eicosanoids amplify the response that the phrase "metabolic tide" describes.

Catecholamines, as well, respond to circulating mediators and the urging of the ventromedial nucleus of the hypothalamus. Epinephrine and norepinephrine levels increase within 5 minutes of injury, from both sympathetic nervous system stimulation and adrenal output. The degree of response correlates directly with the degree of stress.[13] The catecholamines orchestrate the neuroendocrine response: glucose is released from the breakdown of glycogen, and insulin release is inhibited at the same time glucagon production increases. Serum osmolality rises, which temporarily augments blood volume (although to a lesser extent in the starving or fasting patient). It is unclear to what extent the decrease in insulin affects cellular glucose entry early on, as glucose can enter hypoxic cells without the need for insulin. Certainly, in a hypovolemic, hypotensive patient, many tissues will have some degree of hypoxia. Glucose will also move down a concentration gradient, and as the serum glucose concentration rises, more will enter cells; however, the cells may not be able to utilize the glucose effectively. In addition to the initial decrease in insulin output, the peripheral tissues become less responsive to insulin over time as insulin receptors down-regulate. The shift to a catabolic state brought on by the high levels of TNF, interleukins, catecholamines, steroids, and glucagon causes proteolysis and the release of amino acids from muscle tissue. TNF directly inhibits lipoprotein lipase, decreasing the availability of lipid fuel stores for energy production. Both $\dot{V}O_2$ and the metabolic rate increase, an increase that is directly linked to catechol production.[12,13]

Other hormonal balances change, as well. Thyroxine (3,5,3´,5´-tetraiodothyronine, known as T_4) production does not change, but the conversion of T_4 to 3,5,3´-triiodothyronine (T_3) decreases markedly as T_4 breaks down not to T_3 but to the metabolically inactive *reverse* T_3 (3,3´,5´-triiodothyronine).[14] This decrease in metabolically active T_3 is one of the causes of the hyperglycemia common to the hypermetabolic state.[18,19] The production of growth hormone increases during stress, which promotes protein synthesis; the increase is enhanced if two stressors occur in a short period, such as a high physical or emotional stress state followed by injury, or injury followed by infection. Arginine vasopressin is released by the posterior pituitary and acts to retain fluid. The adrenal glands pour out corticosteroid in response to ACTH, catecholamines, antidiuretic hormone, and growth hormone, increasing glucose intolerance. Erythropoietin production by the kidney increases, and the renin-angiotensin axis becomes activated.

Once again, the ratio of insulin to glucagon plays a major role. After an initial decrease following stress, insulin levels may rise to far above normal, but they never catch up with the rise in glucagon production and release. The ratio of the hormones is altered to favor catabolism, promoting glycogenolysis and gluconeogenesis. The counter-regulatory hormones, glucagon, growth hormone, catecholamine, and steroids keep glucose levels elevated. It is often difficult to control hyperglycemia even with massive doses of exogenous insulin. Triglycerides are being converted to free fatty acids and glycerol by high insulin levels, increasing lipase activity. This action is overridden to large extent by the counterregulatory hormones but still provides fatty acids to fuel metabolic processes.[13,14]

Immediately after an injury, when blood flow is directed to vital organs in an attempt to preserve oxygen delivery, the insulin response to hyperglycemia is blunted: the beta cells of the pancreas are delayed in responding to hyperglycemia, and the response is less than normal for the level of hyperglycemia. This is due in part to hypoperfusion, and in part to the direct effects of catecholamines and IL-1 and TNF on the beta cells.[13] After resuscitation and stabilization, the insulin response to glucose is normal to increased, occasionally markedly increased. Glucagon, however, has also increased, and the ratio determines catabolism or anabolism. Even when the rise in insulin production outstrips glucagon output, the cells are less responsive to the insulin. Cell-surface insulin receptors down-regulate in response to alterations in growth hormone and cortisol, and there may well be a postreceptor defect similar to that seen in non–insulin-dependent diabetes mellitus.[13,15]

The physiological response of the body to trauma and sepsis has been classically described as having two phases, an *ebb* and a *flow*.[13–15] The ebb phase occurs during the first 24 to 48 hours after the stress event, including the initial resuscitation, and is characterized by hypodynamic circulatory and metabolic responses. Cardiac output, temperature, blood volume, and metabolic rate all decrease, as though the tissues are stunned. Lactate levels and body weight (from third-spacing of resuscitation fluids) increase, often dramatically. Data for this phase come from only a small number of patients, and not all experts agree on the presence or importance of the ebb phase. While oxygen delivery does decrease, recent data[20,21] show this to be offset by a rise in the oxygen extraction ratio of some tissues. There is general agreement on the flow phase, however. Massive release of epinephrine and norepinephrine push hypercatabolism and the maximum mobilization of nutrients. While the severity of the trauma or sepsis dictates the course, the adequacy of resuscitation dictates the duration of the active phase and the eventual outcome. The shift to an acute-phase response markedly increases the energy needs of the organism, and a massive mobilization of fuels, as well as of structural elements for wound repair, occurs.[15] The flow of substrate generally exceeds the requirements for energy. Tissues adapt to the oxidation of other fuels. These processes will either shift to an adaptive response—anabolism and repair—as the stimulus for inflammation is removed, or will continue to multiple organ failure and death.

Changes in Organ Beds and Blood Flow

The response to stress is an adaptive mechanism that makes substrates available to meet the body's metabolic needs. The substrates, however, may not always go where they are needed. Microcirculatory dysfunction is present in many organ beds and may last days to weeks in some. Normal hepatic perfusion is not restored for 2 to 3 days after adequate resuscitation. Both heat production and oxygen consumption of injured tissue rise in the flow phase, due to increased energy expenditure by the heart and breakdown and recycling of lipid and protein—in some cases futile recycling. Oxygen delivery increases and total body oxygen consumption rises, owing to the oxidation of mixed fuels. Carbon dioxide production increases concomitantly, and minute ventilation follows. The increase in total oxygen consumption, however, may not reflect regional blood flow. While in most regions blood flow rises, in some it remains depressed. Both the renal and the splanchnic beds increase their oxygen consumption, generally in proportion to the severity of injury, but changes in the microcirculation may prevent an increase in oxygen delivery. Anaerobic means of ATP production ensue, with increase in tissue lactate. "Adequate" blood pressure does not necessarily mean adequate perfusion. Hypoperfusion is expected in the ebb phase and is vigorously treated. Epinephrine and norepinephrine output rise rapidly in the first 5 minutes after trauma, with elevation of vascular resistance and increased shunting of blood. When this is superseded by the flow phase, the metabolic rate increases and protein catabolism begins. This usually maximizes at 4 to 8 days but persists until the stress stimulus resolves or the injury is repaired. Hepatic blood flow and oxygen consumption increase shortly after a stress stimulus to allow the liver to meet the increase in metabolic demand. In trauma with inadequate resuscitation, however, or with any combination of sepsis, general anesthesia, or abdominal surgery, hepatic blood flow decreases, limiting delivery of both oxygen and nutrients. Renal blood flow changes in much the same fashion, with a normal increase in glomerular filtration rate to aid in the excretion of toxins and urea. Daily loss of body water generally increases, not only from insensible losses due to fever but also due to this increased glomerular filtration rate and the osmotic load resulting from hyperglycemia and the products of tissue breakdown. While insulin output falls early due to inhibited production in the pancreas, the elevated catecholamines, cortisol, and growth hormone stimulate the alpha cells of the islets of Langerhans to release glucagon in large amounts. High levels of their accustomed fuel, glucose, are made available to all tissues, and the increased serum osmolality helps to augment blood volume. As levels of these catabolic hormones continue to rise after resuscitation, insulin levels rise as well, often to levels severalfold higher than normal. Cell-membrane insulin receptors down-regulate in response, and the hyperglycemia needed for cellular operations under adverse conditions persists. Hepatic adenyl cyclase activates, acute-phase proteins are produced, and both glycogenolysis and gluconeogenesis rapidly maximize.

Metabolic Changes in Trauma with Sepsis

Consider for a moment the massive energy expenditure as the body responds to the stress of trauma or sepsis or both. Some cells must acutely perform many times the normal work of the body by

- producing hormones, inflammatory mediators, and acute phase proteins;
- mobilizing host defenses and producing new neutrophils, lymphocytes and antibodies;
- destroying invading bacteria;
- circulating greater-than-normal amounts of oxygen and nutrients to all parts of the body while removing increased volumes of carbon dioxide; and
- directing nutrients to the wound and producing new protein for granulation tissue, performing repair, and restructuring.

Protein synthesis continues in the face of catabolism, although at a reduced rate; the resources merely shift.

Add to these the metabolic cost of processes necessary to simply obtain fuel when the normal logistics break down—glycogenolysis, proteolysis, lipolysis and gluconeogenesis, generation of urea—and we realize just how *much* energy production is actually necessary, once the "hormonal tide" sweeps in. Add to this the loss in efficiency of glucose utilization. Although clearance of glucose by muscle tissue rises, a lower fraction of the maximum potential energy available from glucose actually appears as useful work, probably because the inhibition of enzymes causes a decrease in the ability of pyruvate to enter the TCA cycle. The increasing amount of pyruvate and increased amounts of lactate, alanine, and glutamine, are carried to the liver, where glucose recycles futilely in the Cori cycle. The high levels of catechols and other mediators support this recycling. Because of the abnormal glucose metabolism, many tissues switch from glucose to fatty acids for fuel, and lipid becomes the primary energy source. Lipolysis occurs despite elevated levels of glucose and insulin. The actual utilization of lipid varies, however, and appears not to be as extensive as would be thought given the elevated metabolic rate. Many tissues cannot utilize lipid effectively, either, and futile cycling of fatty acids to triglycerides and back occurs, at a net energy cost as well as the penalty of fatty deposition in the liver.

Hormone- and mediator-driven muscle breakdown releases amino acids into the circulation, both to increase the precursor pool for visceral protein synthesis and to provide a ready fuel source. Branched-chain amino acids, from structural proteins (skeletal muscle, connective tissues, unstimulated gut mucosa), donate their carbon skeletons for conversion to glucose to support the increased metabolic rate of the liver. Glutamine, alanine, and the aromatic amino acids are readily available for protein synthesis, while the availability of the branched-chain amino acids falls as they are used for fuel. Leucine, released by the catabolism of skeletal muscle, is in large part irreversibly oxidized in muscle. This amino acid is essential to the utilization of other amino acids by the liver; if levels of leucine fall, the liver can no longer efficiently utilize other amino acids. These are broken down and excreted. Total body protein synthesis is reduced, although hepatic protein synthesis rises.[15] Alanine stimulates hepatic protein synthesis, with the synthesis of nonacute-phase proteins (ie, albumin and transferrin) held in check by mediator release from hepatic macrophages. Structural protein, however, was never intended as an intrinsic energy source except over the briefest time. Trauma initiates an obligatory, normal catabolism over 24 to 48 hours, to provide glucose when glycogen stores are depleted. Further stress stimuli—sepsis, for example—will perpetuate and magnify this response. Lean body mass becomes significantly depleted after 7 to 10 days, placing the patient in a poorer risk group for survival.

Shifts in Oxidative Metabolism

Glucose is the preferred fuel for many tissues, particularly the central nervous system and granulation tissue. The maximum rate of glucose oxidation for most tissues, however, is 3 to 6 mg/kg/min, inadequate for cellular needs under these conditions. Ready supply of glucose is also limited, and new glucose must be slowly mobilized from noncarbohydrate sources. If exogenous calories are provided, with the bulk from carbohydrate, then nitrogen sparing will occur to a much lesser degree than is seen in starvation. The RQ will remain below 1.0, indicating a failure to use glucose as a fuel, or may climb to much greater than 1.0 as exogenous glucose is used to make fat deposits in the liver. Some tissues change over to other fuel sources in an effort to keep up with the demand of the metabolic rate. An RQ of 0.75 to 0.85 generally indicates the use of mixed fuel, most often lipid and protein.

Early response—prior to adequate resuscitation—of oxidative metabolism to trauma or sepsis generally results in an oxygen debt, which itself results from the sum of individual organ decrements in oxygen consumption. Low levels of oxygen consumption are often due to hypoperfusion due to hypovolemia, sepsis, or both; however, hypothermia, malnutrition, and sedation may all contribute and should be considered. Total body oxidative metabolism increases as the hypermetabolic response to a stress state develops. The increase in oxygen consumption in the flow phase represents the increase in total body consumption, and is directly proportional to the severity of injury and adequacy of resuscitation. It peaks between days 3 and 10. Oxygen consumption of individual tissues or organ beds may actually decrease, depending on the state of their perfusion, so the total body oxygen consumption does not necessarily reflect adequate blood flow to all tissues.

As glucose stores are consumed, a shift to lipolysis and proteolysis provides free fatty acids, alanine, and glutamine for the TCA cycle. Unfortunately, a significant portion of the lipid is squandered to make additional triglycerides, driven by high insulin and glucose levels.[3] Amino acids become the chief fuels for the TCA cycle. While there is an absolute increase in the oxidation of lipid and glucose, the percentage of calories derived from these two sources declines steadily. The rate of endogenous glucose production from all sources increases, but glucose concentrations remain stable, although elevated, because of a matching rise in glucose uptake. Glucose turnover is proportional to total body oxygen consumption, which, in turn, is proportional to the severity of injury or infection. Regional uptake of glucose, though, is related to regional blood flow, and is generally matched by regional lactate release, but is not directly related to regional oxygen consumption. It is the combination of a steep glucose gradient and the diversion of blood flow to regions of inflammation that drives regional glucose uptake. The glucose is often converted to lactate via glycolysis in areas of inflammation, even if oxygen delivery is adequate. As a result, regional oxygen consumption is not predictive of regional glucose utilization.

Serum lactate rises as a consequence of hypoperfusion, but it is a late indicator of that state. Most tissues will tolerate a partial pressure of oxygen as low as 30 torr before excessive lactate generation occurs. Both (*a*) catecholamines driving gluconeogenesis and glycolysis and (*b*) decreased hepatic perfusion will raise lactate levels significantly: the first by generation of lactate; the second by limiting clearance.

Endogenous glucose is produced by the liver from a number of precursors. Lactate, alanine, glutamine, glycine, serine, and glycerol are all substrates that can be used to produce glucose, although several of the mechanisms are futile pathways. Since gluconeogenesis consumes energy, the limited ATP generated at the tissue level from the new glucose is balanced by the loss in the liver. The net energy gain for the total body is zero, although the heat produced may be necessary for maintaining thermal neutrality.[17] The site of the wound or inflammation does, however, gain 2 moles of ATP for each mole of glucose consumed, and a few tissues, such as myocardial cells, can utilize lactate directly via the mitochondrial malate shuttle. Alanine can also be converted to glucose and, in fact, is the major source of new glucose. The conversion of alanine to glucose requires the use of ATP and generates urea, the excretion of which requires that further energy be expended. The high-energy phosphate pool gradually shrinks through losses of TCA cycle efficiency and the loss of labile proteins.

Because of the increased lipolysis that develops a few days after injury, fatty acid deficiencies can occur early. Following trauma, there is a 55% increase in the rate of lipid oxidation; following infection, a 25% increase.[22] The lesser increase in lipid utilization during infection is thought to be due to the impaired activity of lipoprotein lipase by TNF, IL-1, and IL-2.[23] These are not suppressed by carbohydrate feeding, a difference from the oxidation in simple starvation; nor is there an increase in ketones, which are used as fuel under these circumstances. Long-chain, essential fatty acids, linoleic and arachidonic in particular, rapidly decrease after injury. Essential fatty acid deficiency can develop after 2 to 3 weeks, and requires a minimum of 10% of exogenous calories in the form of lipid to prevent.

Protein Turnover and Preferential Amino Acid Utilization

Protein turnover increases with stress, and increases dramatically with trauma or sepsis (Figure 23-8). The level may be taken as a measure of the severity of the stress event. As we discussed earlier, glucose stores are used early, leaving the body to depend on lipid calories and, for those obligate glucose-using tissues, on amino acids and glycerol to generate additional glucose. Protein turnover is also increased to free amino acids for production of acute-phase proteins, including TNF and the interleukins, and for wound repair. Both proteolysis and hypermetabolism peak shortly after the onset of the stress state, gradually returning to normal as recovery progresses. The catabolism results in early and rapid muscle wasting.

Branched-chain amino acids from muscle tissue are deaminated and their carbon skeletons oxidized in the TCA cycle for the vastly increased metabolic processes. The rate of protein catabolism can surpass 300 g/d of muscle protein, or nearly 50 g/d of nitrogen lost.[24] Skeletal muscle makes up as much as 80% of the free amino acid pool,[13] with the bulk of this intracellular. A 70-kg man has roughly 87 g of free amino acids in the intracellular space but less than 2 g extracellularly. Protein catabolism is largely an intracellular event, with the changes in skeletal muscle tissue due to changes in the intracellular pools. Breakdown of body protein stores and urinary loss of nitrogen parallels the REE. Hepatic blood flow increases dramatically to meet the hypermetabolic demand. Those amino acids not used to form new protein are deaminated in the liver for their carbon skeletons and their amino groups used

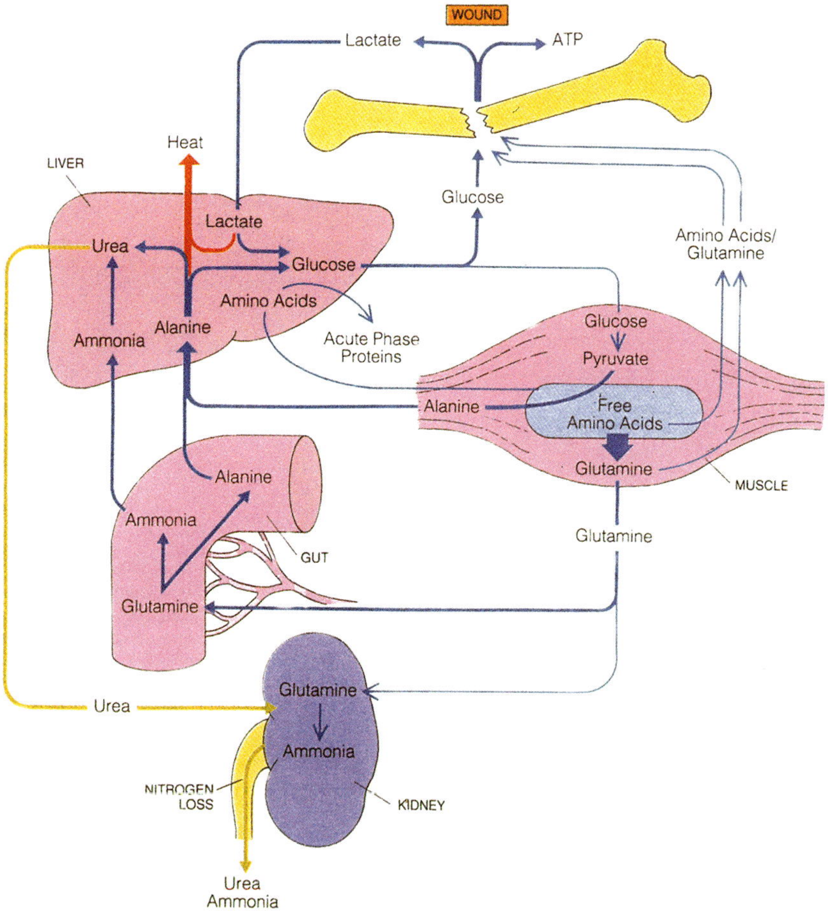

Fig. 23-8. Metabolic interrelationships in the wounded casualty. The wound is an obligatory user of glucose, which, for the most part, is derived from amino acids by the process of gluconeogenesis. Glucose is metabolized by glycolysis in the wound, forming lactate. The lactate is then transported back to the liver where it is reconverted to glucose. This process is known as the Cori cycle and, being energy demanding, is one of the determinants of the hypermetabolic state that characterizes trauma. Two amino acids released by the catabolism of skeletal muscle are of special importance: alanine, which is transported to the liver to form glucose; and glutamine, which forms the primary substrate of the intestines. Reprinted with permission from Bessey PQ. Metabolic response to critical illness. Chap 11. In: Part 2. Care in the ICU. In: Wilmore DW, Brennan MF, Harken AH, Holcroft JW, Meakins JM, eds. Vol 1. *Critical Care*. In: *Care of the Surgical Patient.* New York, NY: Scientific American, Inc; 1989: 11-11.

for the synthesis of glutamine and alanine. The concentrations of glutamine and alanine in blood are greater than would be expected from their concentrations in muscle protein, indicating both synthesis in and net release from myocytes. Glutamine has two essential functions: (1) it is the preferred substrate for oxidative phosphorylation in the gut, and (2) ammonium ions from glutamine are used in the kidney to buffer metabolic acids.

Glutamine makes up a large part of the "buffer pool" of amino acids. This nonessential amino acid makes up 5% to 6% of the total body protein, and 60% of the total intracellular free amino acid pool[25] (the eight essential amino acids together make up only 8.4 % of the intracellular pool). Body proteins are not intended to be a long-term energy source. They are structural components, and their loss interferes with a broad spectrum of body functions (eg, locomotion, immunological competence). The level of intracellular glutamine falls rapidly with stress, starvation, and after surgery or trauma, as glutamine is transported to the gut and converted to alanine to be fed into the TCA cycle in the liver.[4,26,27] The extent of the fall in glutamine levels seen with sepsis parallels the severity of the sepsis. Intracellular concentrations of other amino acids—leucine, isoleucine, valine, alanine, phenylalanine, and tyrosine—rise in stress, trauma, and sepsis, reflecting the catabolism present in the muscle. As they are used to fuel the metabolic engines, levels fall. As the branched-chain amino acid levels decline in sepsis or after severe trauma, the level of aromatic amino acids rises, and the ratio between the two shifts.[4]

Protein synthesis continues even as proteins are catabolized. New cells are built; antibodies, coagulation factors, cytokines, and so forth are elaborated: the shift is from maintenance of general structural elements to defense and wound healing. Probably even more than the neurohormonal controls, the inflammatory mediators are responsible for the degree of hypermetabolic response. When more than 20% of the lean body mass has been lost—generally after 7 to 10 days without nutritional support—insufficient substrate remains to support synthetic function. After 14 days, the wound will be catabolized and is likely to dehisce. What is left is used as fuel, with decreasing efficiency, until the patient dies.[14,15] Lean body mass cannot be regained so long as the inflammatory mediators are present, although loss of nitrogen can be countered with aggressive feeding. Feeding with a formula high in branched-chain amino acids—leucine, isoleucine, and valine—may ameliorate the protein loss to a greater degree than with standard amino acid formulas. These are preferentially oxidized by muscle, providing nitrogen and energy for skeletal muscle synthetic processes, as well as carbon skeletons for glucose-requiring tissues. Indeed, in the face of insulin resistance and lipase dysfunction, branched-chain amino acids may be the single best source of fuel for a hypercatabolic patient with organ dysfunction.[4,28,29]

As the structural proteins redistribute to areas of increased metabolic need (ie, the visceral organs, macrophages, and wounds) to support acute-phase protein synthesis, nonacute-phase protein synthesis (albumin and transferrin) declines. Hepatic cells release mediators such as nitric oxide, IL-6, and granulocyte-macrophage colony stimulating factor,[11,13,15,30] which maintain the release of inflammatory mediators from the Kupffer cells in an autoamplifying cascade. The effects can persist for days after the initial stress stimulus has been removed, driving the hypermetabolic response. Tissue repair does not begin until late in the flow phase, during the *adaptive* phase, when the metabolic processes organize and regularize. This is the phase when nutritional support is the most effective for rebuilding structural proteins; the body is at last able to respond to exogenous nutrition by increasing cell mass rather than by merely minimizing losses.

Energy Requirements of Patients With Injuries or Infections

All stress states increase the metabolic requirements of the patient to some degree, which can be estimated by a rule of thumb (Table 23-2). A simple, uncomplicated surgery will increase energy requirements by 5% to 10% over the REE. Multiple trauma or sepsis increases requirements by 30% to 55%; a mechanically ventilated patient with sepsis or trauma has energy requirements 50% to 75% over REE. As a comparison, while doing manual labor, a normal person has energy requirements approximately 100% to 400% above REE. For example, if basal metabolism equals 1 kcal/kg/h, and if intense manual labor requires 5 kcal/kg/h (400% above normal), but this level of activity persists for only one fourth or one third of the day, then the manual laborer's energy requirements are approximately 100% higher than normal.

TABLE 23-2

PREDICTION OF CALORIC REQUIREMENTS IN STRESSED PATIENTS*

Patient Status	Correction Factor
Confined to bed	1.2 • REE
Ambulatory	1.3 • REE
Fever	(1.0 + 0.13 per °C) • REE
Peritonitis	1.2–1.37 • REE
Soft-tissue trauma	1.14–1.37 • REE
Multiple fractures	1.2–1.37 • REE
Sepsis	1.4–1.8 • REE
Burns (as % TBSA)	
0–20	1–1.5 • REE
10–40	1.5–1.85 • REE
40–100	1.5–2.05 • REE

*Based on alterations in their metabolic rate
REE: resting energy expenditure; TBSA: total body surface area
Data source: Zimmerman JE. Nutritional support in the ICU. Lecture presented at Update in Critical Care—1993; April 1993; Washington, DC.

Oxygen consumption rises to match the increase in REE. Normal resting V_{O_2} averages 100 to 125 mL/min/m^2; consumption in a severely stressed patient may be greater than 170 mL/min/m^2 (in general, the higher the consumption can be raised—by altering the available partial pressure of oxygen, available hemoglobin, and cardiac output—the greater the chance for survival). Failure to alter D_{O_2} and thereby successfully raise V_{O_2} generally ends with a poor outcome.[31]

Energy requirements can be estimated for individual patients in a number of ways; unfortunately, many of the techniques do not lend themselves to battlefield application. Nutritional assessment by intake and weight history is valuable but difficult to obtain in the field. Indirect calorimetry is a moderately useful tool but requires special equipment, a stringent metabolic steady state during measurement, and will only give a "snapshot"—the require-

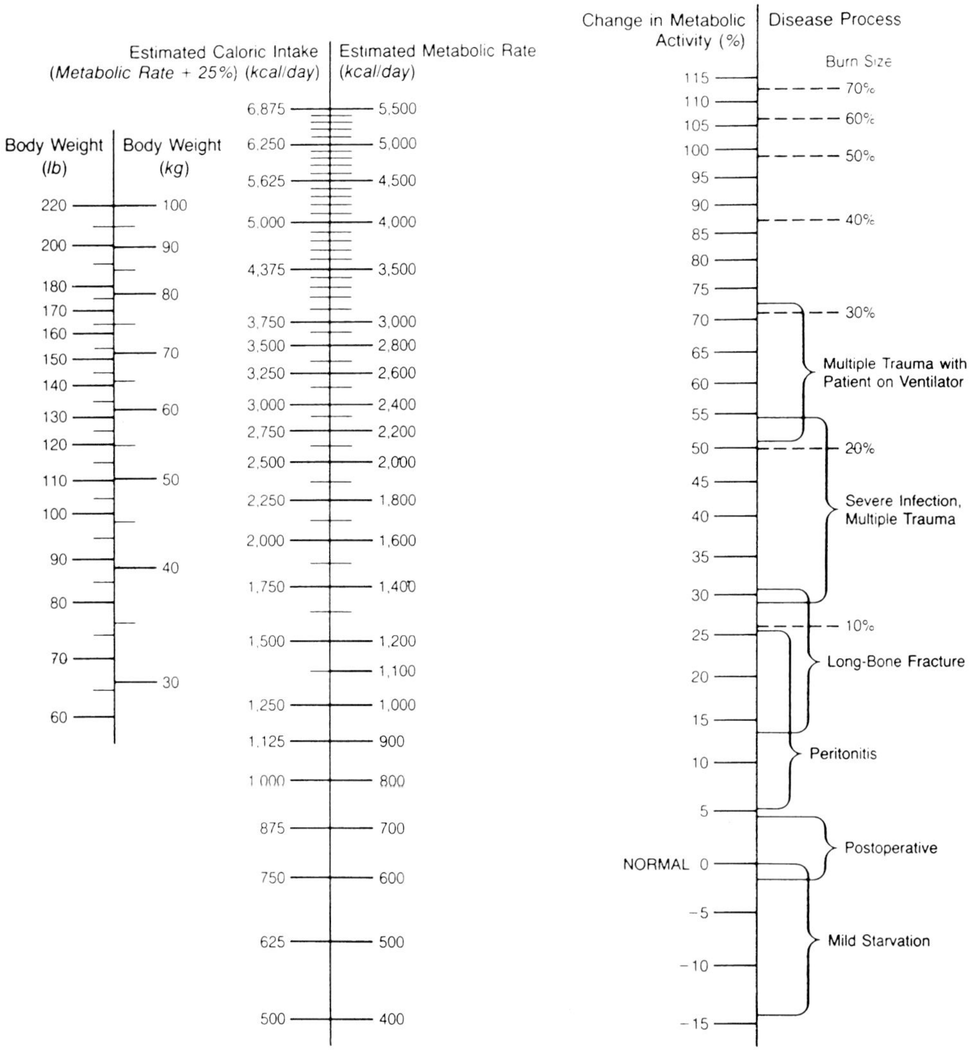

Fig. 23-9. This nomogram provides estimates of the caloric intake required for weight maintenance in patients with various disease processes. If the point that represents the patient's body weight on the scale at left is connected by a straight line to the point that represents the patient's disease process on the scale at right, then estimates for the patient's caloric requirement and metabolic rate can be read off the left and right sides of the middle scale, respectively. This nomogram should be used only for patients from 15 to 45 years of age whose height is normal. Reprinted with permission from Wilmore DW. *Metabolic Management of the Critically Ill.* New York: Plenum Press; 1977: 36.

ments at the time of measurement. Linear-regression formulas frequently overestimate energy requirements. Any of these may be used, so long as the shortcomings of each are borne in mind. Probably the best method of estimating nutritional state and energy requirements, whether in the field or at a fourth- or fifth-echelon hospital, is by a combination of the physical exam and tables that define REE or BMR based on a combination of body weight and disease process (Figure 23-9). Other specialized tests for nutritional assessment are discussed below.

Medical officers must keep in mind that *REE will change with feeding*. A casualty with a burn to less than 10% of his body surface area will have an increase in REE of 6% to 7% if unfed. Feeding will increase this by a factor of 5; overfeeding will result in an even greater increase. It requires energy to process fuel and building material. This is known as the specific dynamic effect. A mixed-fuel diet (carbohydrate and fat) will be less costly in terms of energy than an all-carbohydrate or an all-fat diet, and the energy expended to process enteral feeding is significantly less than that used to process parenteral nutrition.

The RQ changes with injury or sepsis. In the stressed state, the RQ is initially between 0.75 and 0.85, reflecting the mixed oxidation of carbohydrates, fats, and proteins in aerobic glycolysis and the TCA cycle. Lipolysis increases, as does release of lactate and pyruvate from muscle tissues, wound tissue, and macrophages and monocytes. The ratio of lactate to pyruvate remains normal, and the redox potential of the mitochondria is unchanged. As SIRS develops, the mitochondria increase their capacity to oxidize the two-carbon fragments being fed to them, and the RQ rises slightly. As organs become less functional, the RQ continues to rise, indicating a net lipogenesis, often aided by overfeeding total calories or carbohydrate.

Oxygen Consumption and Oxygen Delivery

Both oxygen consumption and delivery increase with sepsis or injury, modulated by the elevation of catecholamines. Should sepsis/SIRS progress to shock, both oxygen consumption and REE fall sequentially.[15,21] This progressive decrement in the metabolic response reflects both the maldistribution of blood flow and the impairment of oxygen extraction that are characteristic of the state, as well as an enzymatic failure at the mitochondrial level that inhibits the TCA cycle. The rise of endotoxin levels matches the fall in metabolic rate. As oxygen delivery falls further, an oxygen debt is incurred and lactate accumulates, shifting the ratio of lactate to pyruvate, with a resultant metabolic acidosis.[31] Reversal of the shock state restores the hypermetabolism, driven by catecholamines and inflammatory mediators, but only restoration of adequate oxygen delivery will reverse the oxygen debt and the lactic acidosis.

Patterns of Response

The pattern of response to stress—injury or infection—is standard regardless of the inciting insult, presumably because of a survival advantage to the pattern. The response involves the liver, skeletal muscle, gut, kidneys, and heart, and the wound or focus of inflammation. The neuroendocrine system and the cytokine-mediator system act interdependently to bring about the characteristic changes, with the neuroendocrine stress response amplified many times by cytokine mediators, and vice versa. Norepinephrine increases endotoxin-induced TNF production, while TNF pushes ACTH and growth hormone production and alters thyroxine conversion, and glucocorticoids feed back to decrease transcription and posttranslational processing of TNF and IL-1.[11,13] The focus of the inflammatory response acts as a physiological arteriovenous shunt, increasing cardiovascular work and restructuring oxygen delivery. It is often a site of tremendous metabolic activity, with killing of bacteria, removal of dead bacteria and necrotic material, and wound repair continuously going on. The focus may be relatively hypoxic and depend on glycolysis for energy, with production of lactate and heat. Lactate and catabolized proteins are transported to the liver, where lactate, glutamine, and alanine are converted to glucose, which is returned to the focus of inflammation. Creatinine, creatine, potassium, and magnesium are all released. The ammonia produced by the catabolism of amino acids helps to neutralize acid loads, which must be excreted by the kidney.[13] Skeletal muscle and the mucosa and smooth muscle cells of the gut are also catabolized for fuel and amino acids. The gut loses its normal immunological function soon after injury, and after that, the ability to mechanically block bacteria and bacterial products from the bloodstream. Stimuli from intestinal bacteria now add to the inflammatory burden. This catabolism cannot be stopped by feeding, but exogenous amino acids can be utilized for both fuel and protein synthesis. (For further discussion of this process, see Chapter 24, The Syndromes of Systemic Inflammatory Response and Multiple Organ Dysfunction).

Should the inflammatory stimulus be removed at this time (by antibiotic treatment, removal of necrotic tissue, wound healing, etc), metabolism enters an *adaptive* phase, where output from the paraventricular nuclei of the hypothalamus decreases, sympathetic activity follows, cortisol and glucose levels fall, and the ratio of insulin to glucagon becomes more appropriate, although still less than normal. Fluids are mobilized, the urinary urea nitrogen decreases and ketones are spilled into the urine. The trend is toward a positive nitrogen balance, although the metabolic rate is still high. Caloric intake may need to be 1.5- to 2-fold higher than the REE to stop protein catabolism, even at this point. The metabolism gradually becomes anabolic.

If the inflammatory stimulus is excessive or prolonged or both, the neuroendocrine and cytokine responses to injury gradually erode the metabolic and immunological reserves. The transition to organ dysfunction comes about from a combination of microcirculatory hypoxia, mediator-induced injury, and toxin-induced injury to cells. Four classic phases have been identified: shock, resuscitation, persistent hypermetabolism (ie, SIRS), and organ dysfunction.[15] Shock and resuscitation affect primarily the microcirculation and the endothelial cells; the success or failure of the initial therapy sets the course for subsequent events. Four to six days after injury or infection, systemic inflammation and altered organ function are seen. Oxygen consumption increases. Oxygen delivery must match for the patient to survive, so cardiac output and minute ventilation follow the rise in oxygen consumption. The RQ is now between 0.78 and 0.82, and the proportion of calories from glucose and fat has dropped. This hypermetabolic pattern will peak in 3 to 4 days, and if the inciting stimulus—infection, persistent perfusion deficit (ie, inadequate resuscitation), local inflammation, or necrotic tissue—is corrected, it should resolve in 7 to 10 days. A portion of these patients, particularly those with prolonged SIRS with shock, will develop a hypermetabolic state that will persist for 14 to 21 days, even if the cause is corrected. If the inciting stimulus remains, the condition will progress to organ dysfunction.

The transition from hypermetabolism to multiple organ dysfunction syndrome (MODS) is usually due to a persistent, often unrecognized, perfusion deficit; a new or resistant focus of infection; or a persistent focus of inflammation. The actual death of a certain mass of cells is probably not the explanation for progressive organ dysfunction; rather, an increasing dysfunction of cellular subsystems to a certain critical point is the likely mechanism.[12,15] Microbial toxins directly inhibit intracellular glycolytic enzymes and intracellular hepatic protein synthesis; mediators such as TNF and IL-1 inhibit lipoprotein lipase, cytochrome P450, and albumin and thyroglobulin production; and products of metabolism in one region (eg, arachidonic acid metabolites) adversely alter metabolism in others. Hydrogen ion shuttles, electron transport systems, and gating proteins are all parts of the clockwork mechanism that enters a state of metabolic dysregulation.

Oxygen consumption becomes flow dependent as the ability to extract oxygen decreases and lactate production rises. A state of subclinical flow-dependent (inadequate) oxygen consumption may be present in SIRS even without shock, or in the adult respiratory distress syndrome, or pancreatitis, leading to MODS.

If refeeding has not begun by 7 to 10 days, then metabolic failure based on loss of a critical amount of body mass becomes a factor. As the breakdown and redistribution of lean body mass continues and approaches 20%, acute-phase protein synthesis begins to fail. The combination of (*a*) the loss of structural protein and (*b*) dysfunction of the remaining systems due to continuing catabolism will in itself cause organ dysfunction, and will also greatly amplify toxin- and mediator-induced organ failure. The transition from a hypermetabolic state to MODS is a significant prognostic event, raising the probability of death from 25% to 40% to 40% to 60% in the early stages of organ dysfunction,[15] to 90% to 100% in the later stages.[15,32] Wound healing and immune function suffer early in organ dysfunction, but impairments of the kidney and liver have the greatest impact on the deranged metabolism. Metabolic requirements are especially increased in uremia. Potassium, phosphates, and magnesium all rise; pH falls; and the patient becomes both volume and protein intolerant. Naturally, hypermetabolism accelerates these processes. Hepatic failure means that the liver no longer efficiently deaminates and transaminates amino acids. Branched-chain amino acids are still used, leading to an imbalance in the ratio between branched-chain and aromatic amino acids. False neurotransmitters are generated, leading to encephalopathy. Effects on lipid metabolism vary, with some patients able to metabolize large amounts of exogenous lipid and others developing severe hypertriglyceridemia (Zieve's syndrome) and, occasionally, pancreatitis.

Treatment of the metabolic derangements—with early, aggressive feeding; correction of flow-dependent oxygen consumption (or maximizing oxygen consumption where it cannot be corrected); and improving perfusion of all organ beds, as measured by tissue pH (ideally) or serum lactate (practically)—assure that morbidity and mortality are markedly reduced. The goal is to overcome the catabolic state, or, where this is impossible, to allow (*a*) protein synthesis to continue in the face of catabolism and (*b*) the cellular mechanisms to repair themselves and correct the hypermetabolic state. Enteral feeding, in particular, restores the mucosa of the gut and alters translocation of bacteria and bacterial products.

NUTRITIONAL SUPPORT

In general, it is easier to feed a malnourished patient—with the proviso that we carefully observe for hypophosphatemia—than a hypermetabolic patient. The results are also more clearly beneficial in the former case. Some recommendations for nutritional support suggest that "nutritional support should be considered if the patient has been without nutrition for 5 to 7 days"[27(p3)] and that "deficits occur in critically ill patients after 7 to 10 days of starvation."[27(p3)] However, "starvation rarely assists recovery from critical illness."[33] Most intensive care specialists would begin support 24 to 48 hours after the ebb phase. Nutritional support should be formulated according to the type and severity of the injury or illness, the presence and degree of organ dysfunction, electrolyte abnormalities, and glucose tolerance. Energy requirements are primarily related to age, gender, body size, and activity. In hospitalized, physically intact patients, the REE is the major caloric expenditure (see Figure 23-9).

The magnitude of the increase in the REE in an injured or septic patient is proportional to the degree of injury and the amount of support given. The total energy expenditure (TEE) is the REE plus the thermic effect of food (TEF) and the energy expenditure of activity (EEA). The goal in feeding the patient is weight maintenance, corrected for fluid gains and losses. Generally, 1,800 to 2,200 kcal/d is required for this. Baseline protein requirements are 0.8 grams of protein (or 0.128 g of nitrogen) per kilogram of body weight per day, increasing with the degree of catabolism as established by the severity of trauma. The ratio of nitrogen to calories is roughly 1:150, but may be as low as 1:200 or as high as 1:100. The gut is the preferred route for providing nutritional support, but many times it cannot be used.

Nutritional Assessment

Several methods are used to assess caloric needs. Indirect calorimetry is in common use and may be easily performed with only a metabolic cart and a trained operator. Unfortunately, it requires that the patient remain in a strict steady-state condition during the period of measurement (eg, no changes can be made in ventilator settings, the patient is not allowed to move). Caloric requirements are based on calculation of oxygen consumption using the Fick method:

$$V_{O_2} = (Ca_{O_2} - Cv_{O_2}) \bullet C.O.$$

$$V_{CO_2} = (Cv_{CO_2} - Ca_{CO_2}) \bullet C.O.$$

where V_{O_2} represents oxygen consumption per unit time, Ca_{O_2} represents arterial oxygen contents, Cv_{O_2} represents venous oxygen contents, C.O. represents cardiac output, V_{CO_2} represents carbon dioxide consumption per unit time, Ca_{CO_2} represents arterial carbon dioxide contents, and Cv_{CO_2} represents venous carbon dioxide contents.

When calculated by gas exchange in indirect calorimetry, these become:

$$V_{O_2} = (V_I \bullet F_{IO_2}) - (V_E \bullet F_{EO_2})$$

$$V_{CO_2} = V_E \bullet F_{ECO_2}$$

where V_I represents the inspired volume per unit time, F_{IO_2} represents the fraction of inspired oxygen, V_E represents the expired volume per unit time, F_{EO_2} represents the fraction of expired oxygen, V_{CO_2} represents carbon dioxide consumption per unit time, and F_{ECO_2} represents the fraction of expired carbon dioxide.

The required caloric input can be written as follows[34]:

$$\text{REE (in kcal/min)} = 3.581 \text{ (kcal/L)} \bullet V_{O_2} \text{ in L/min} + 1.448 \text{ (kcal/L)} \bullet V_{CO_2} \text{ in L/min} - 1.773 \text{ (kcal/g)} \bullet Nu \text{ in g/min}$$

where *Nu* represents nitrogen excreted in the urine.

Even small fluctuations in F_{IO_2} or V_{O_2} can alter the value for oxygen consumption. If properly measured, oxygen consumption is quite accurate over the period of measurement, but it is difficult to extrapolate to a 24-hour period in an unstable patient or a patient with varying levels of activity.

Linear-regression–derived "standard" equations generally overestimate caloric needs but may be useful under field conditions. The Harris-Benedict equation,[35] the one most commonly used at military teaching hospitals, uses separate formulas for men:

$$\text{REE (kcal/d)} = 66.47 + (13.75 \bullet \text{kg body wt}) + (5.0 \bullet \text{height in centimeters}) - (6.76 \bullet \text{age in years})$$

and women:

$$\text{REE (kcal/d)} = 65.51 + (9.56 \bullet \text{kg body wt}) + (1.85 \bullet \text{height in centimeters}) - (4.68 \bullet \text{age in years})$$

Probably the simplest, and often the most accurate, method for field use is a combination of standard tables based on body surface area and gender, and a physical examination of the patient. (An even quicker rough estimate: at rest, men consume roughly 25 kcal/kg/d; women, 20 kcal/kg/d.) All caloric estimates are for *nonprotein* calories.

The severity of the trauma or degree of stress increases the requirement for calories. Most critically ill patients require 25 to 35 kcal/kg/d. Patients with severe burns and trauma may require 35 to 45 kcal/kg/d, as may those patients who were severely calorie- and protein-depleted prior to injury. Patients on ventilators—at least those whose ventilation is adequately controlled—have a generally lower requirement, often less than 25 kcal/kg/d (30% of caloric input may be required for ventilation in a nonintubated, critically ill patient).

Protein requirements are initially determined by energy requirements, degree of malnutrition, and severity of injury, then adjusted by following the amounts of urinary urea nitrogen. Generally, the urinary urea nitrogen plus unmeasured nitrogen in the stool (approximately 3 g/d) are taken to be the daily protein requirement. Protein replacement can be guided somewhat more closely by calculating the catabolic index (Exhibit 23-2); the goal is to obtain a low number (< 0 is ideal).[36]

The goals of nutritional therapy are commonsense goals:

EXHIBIT 23-2

CATABOLIC INDEX

Catabolic Index = 24-h urinary urea nitrogen (UUN) excretion – (0.5 • dietary nitrogen intake + 3 g)

< 0	No stress
0–5	Moderate stress
> 5	Severe stress

The catabolic index makes two important assumptions:

1. obligatory UUN excretion is 3 g/d, and
2. 50% of ingested protein is utilized.

Data source: Bistrian BR. A simple technique to estimate the severity of stress. *Surg Gynecol Obstet*. 1979;5:54–61.

- to restore nitrogen balance;
- to provide the appropriate amount of fuel to maintain lean body mass;
- to provide appropriate vitamins, minerals, and trace elements; and
- to avoid overfeeding with any nutrient, but particularly to avoid overfeeding calories.

Excessive calories are converted to fat, particularly in the liver; this shifts the RQ to much greater than 1.0, increasing oxygen consumption and minute ventilation requirements markedly. Caloric overfeeding also depletes potassium and stimulates the release of catecholamines and the formation of lactate, while failing to suppress gluconeogenesis or to alter catabolic or synthetic rates. Overfeeding enterally can result in increased bacterial growth, gas production, and bowel distention.

In general, the sicker the patient, the poorer the accuracy of any of the means of estimating the metabolic rate. Remember also that before any benefits are derived, feeding imposes its own metabolic demands on the patient: increasing oxygen consumption, carbon dioxide production, and ventilatory drive, as well as increasing the workload of the cardiovascular system. A number of empirical correction factors have evolved to improve our ability to estimate calorie and protein requirements of the severely ill. Energy requirements increase 10% to 20% with fever; 30% to 50% with the perioperative state, sepsis, multiple trauma, head injury, or acute renal failure; and 50% to 100% with severe burns or seizures. Energy requirements *decrease* with paralysis, mechanical ventilation, hypotension, and unstressed malnutrition (see Figure 23-9).

As a general guideline, a critically ill patient will consume 25 to 35 kcal/kg/d; this is often useful as a starting point for nutritional replacement. Protein requirements are somewhat simpler to estimate. The nitrogen to calorie ratio should be roughly 1:150, although with severe trauma this may rise to 1:100 (1 g nitrogen is equivalent to 6.25 g protein). In ongoing protein catabolism with a rising blood urea nitrogen (BUN) and increasing ratio of BUN to creatinine, increased calories may ameliorate catabolism to some degree, and a nitrogen-to-calorie ratio of 1:200 may be more appropriate. A greater caloric intake will also be necessary to maintain a positive nitrogen balance at a lower level of protein intake. In general, protein requirements may be estimated by severity of stress.

Acute renal failure, hepatic failure, and MODS all restrict the body's ability to meet its protein requirements. Bear in mind that *catabolism* is not sensitive to exogenous amino acids, but *synthesis* is. Protein feeding will not reverse catabolism but will increase the synthetic rate until it catches the catabolic rate and restores the nitrogen balance.

What nutrients are essential in formulating a nutritional support plan? The standard total parenteral nutrition (TPN) formula used at Walter Reed Army Medical Center, Washington, D. C., includes carbohydrate sufficient to provide 50% to 70% of the estimated caloric need (3.4 kcal/g); lipid to provide a minimum of 10% of calories (9 kcal/g) and to prevent fatty acid deficiency (essential fatty acids, chiefly linoleic acid, must make up 1%–2% of total calories, roughly 2–4 g/d); essential amino acids; electrolytes; vitamins; and trace elements (Figure 23-10).

Parenteral Nutrition

The parenteral route is not the best way to provide nutritional support but is often the only route available when delay would compromise the patient. Standard TPN uses hypertonic glucose—25% or 50%—as a primary source of calories, with a 10% lipid solution to provide additional calories and essential fatty acids. The carbohydrate is oxidized directly, with an RQ of 1.0, while the exogenous lipid is generally added to the fat stores and mobilized as needed to be processed into fatty acids and glycerol. A combination of the two sources provides essential fatty acids, avoids hyperglycemia, stimulates insulin production, and decreases carbon dioxide production. A 6.9% to 10% amino acid solution is added, depending on the formulation, and the resulting mixture diluted to a tonicity of 1,900 to 2,000 mOsm/L. As this solution is administered, via a central line in the superior or inferior vena cava, it is rapidly diluted to a nearly isotonic osmolality. The solution provides 0.85 to 1.1 kcal/mL, and 2 to 2.5 L/d will generally provide adequate protein and calories for any degree of stress.

Standard amino acid formulations have 19% to 25% branched-chain amino acids in a balanced mix with other amino acids. Because catabolism of protein in muscle is the primary source of the branched-chain amino acids used by the liver for gluconeogenesis (branched-chain amino acid aminotransferases are primarily found in skeletal muscle), and leucine, in particular, seems to have anticatabolic properties (a dose-dependent ability to decrease catabolism and possibly increase synthesis of muscle proteins as well as improving the synthetic efficiency of the liver), many intensive care specialists recommend using an amino acid formula that is higher in branched-chain amino acids. These modified amino acid formulations contain roughly 45% branched-chain amino acids. While nitrogen balance, and possibly immunocompetence, are improved, a clear improvement in outcome has yet to be shown.[4]

Replacement Minerals

Minerals must be added to the TPN solution, both to replace those lost during hypercatabolism and owing to the osmotic load of feeding. Magnesium, calcium, potassium, and phosphorus are all used in increased amounts during hypermetabolism. Rather large amounts of magnesium ($\geq$ 30 mEq/d), potassium ($\geq$ 100 mEq/d), and phosphorus (as phosphate, 20–30 mmol/d) are often required. Injury and carbohydrate loads both increase the loss of potassium, as does the fall in plasma magnesium seen after trauma or even elective surgery. Cell membranes become "leaky" after trauma or sepsis, and the intracellular concentration of sodium rises while potassium dips. When the patient improves, extracellular potassium loss accentuates because anabolism drives the uptake of potassium. Hypokalemia can easily result, especially if the patient is diuresing by this time. Seventy to one hundred milliequivalents of a potassium salt is required each day—more if the patient is either hypercatabolic or actively diuresing. Sodium is generally less problematic. One-half to two-thirds normal saline (75–100 mEq/L) is generally adequate to keep plasma sodium in the 135 to 145 mEq/L range. Patients who have received a large sodium load during resuscitation or surgery may more appropriately be given one-third normal saline (50 mEq/L) as a maintenance dose to avert hypernatremia. Sodium input should also be reduced in patients who are actively diuresing, because more free water than solute is lost and these patients can easily become hypernatremic. If frequent adjustments to the sodium or potassium content of the TPN are necessary, it is more practical to establish a lower, fixed amount of each cation for the TPN and to administer additional salt as short-run piggyback intravenous infusions.

Phosphorus is a vital electrolyte, and costly in terms of lessons learned. Feeding the survivors of concentration camps after World War II resulted in an unexpectedly high number of deaths.[37] It took a

MEDICAL RECORD—SUPPLEMENTAL MEDICAL DATA

For Use of this form, see AR 40-66; the proponent agency is the Office of The Surgeon General.

REPORT TITLE
ADULT TOTAL PARENTERAL NUTRITION (TPN) & PERIPHERAL PARENTERAL NUTRITION (PPN) ORDER FORM

OTSG APPROVED (*Date*)

Wt: _____ kg/lb
Ht: _____ cm/in
Age: _____ yr
Ward: _____

	[ ] STANDARD CENTRAL	[ ] STANDARD PERIPHERAL
	Very concentrated solution for the average patient with perioperative needs (has no free water).	Limited time use via peripheral vein while NPO/advancing enteral nutrition or in perioperative status
	(AMOUNT/LITER)	(AMOUNT/LITER)
PROTEIN	46 gm	30 gm
PROTEIN SOURCE	Travasol 10%	Travasol 10%
DEXTROSE	195 gm	55 gm
FAT	38 gm	35 gm
CALORIES	1,005 cal	520 cal
Dextrose cal	663 (66%)	195 (39%)
Fat cal	342 (34%)	324 (61%)
Sodium chloride	15 mEq	15 mEq
Sodium acetate	35 mEq	35 mEq
Potassium chloride	20 mEq	20 mEq
Potassium acetate	0 mEq	0 mEq
Calcium gluconate	4.8 mEq	4.8 mEq
Magnesium sulfate	8 mEq	8 mEq
Sodium phosphate	0 mM	0 mM
Potassium phosphate	12 mM	8 mM
	[ ] LITERS/DAY	[ ] LITERS/DAY

* Above standard solutions help expedite initiation of TPN/PPN.
* Determine protein and calorie needs using guidelines page, select solution and indicate # liters which is closest to patient's needs.

[ ] 'INDIVIDUALIZED CENTRAL/PERIPHERAL'		
For patients not able to tolerate any of the standard formulations (Indicate Amount/Day)		
PROTEIN	gm	
PROTEIN SOURCE	[ ] Travasol 10% [ ] FreAmine HBC 6.9% [ ] Hepatamine 8%	Suggested
DEXTROSE	gm	Initial
FAT	gm	Amounts
CALORIES	cal	per Day:
Sodium chloride	mEq	(30 mEq)
Sodium acetate	mEq	(70 mEq)
Potassium chloride	mEq	(40 mEq)
Potassium acetate	mEq	(0 mEq)
Calcium gluconate	mEq	(9.6 mEq)
Magnesium sulfate	mEq	(16 mEq)
Sodium phosphate	mM	(0 mM)
Potassium phosphate	mM	(24 mM)
[ ] MINIMAL VOLUME OR [ ] LITERS/DAY		
Give: [ ] CENTRALLY OR [ ] PERIPHERALLY		

* Above option requires physician determine amounts and volume needed per day and route of administration.
* All orders must reach 4th floor pharmacy by 1300 hours.

ADDITIVES/INSTRUCTIONS

[ ] Multi-Vitamins 10 mL or____ per day [ ] Cimetidine 900 mg or____ mg per day [ ] Reg. Human Insulin____ units per day
[ ] Multi-Trace-5 4 mL or____ per day [ ] Famotidine 40 mg or____ mg per day [ ] Other:
[ ] Additional Zinc 2 mg or____ mg per day [ ] Other: ______
[ ] Hydrocortisone 5 mg/L Peripheral Soln. [ ] Other: ______

(*Continues on reverse*)

PREPARED BY (*Signature & Title*)	DEPARTMENT/SERVICE/CLINIC NUTRITION SUPPORT SERVICE	DATE

PATIENT'S IDENTIFICATION (*For typed or written entries give: Name—last, first, middle; grade; date; hospital or medical facility*)

☐ HISTORY/PHYSICAL ☐ FLOW CHART
☐ OTHER EXAMINATION OR EVALUATION ☐ OTHER (*Specify*)
☐ DIAGNOSTIC STUDIES
☐ TREATMENT

DA FORM 1 MAY 78 4700

WRAMC OVERPRINT 257
1 NOV 91

Fig. 23-10. The standard forms used when ordering parenteral nutrition at Walter Reed Army Medical Center, Washington, DC.

ADULT PARENTERAL NUTRITION GUIDELINES

(Central vein total parenteral nutrition (TPN) and Peripheral vein parenteral nutrition (PPN))

ADMINISTRATIVE INFORMATION

*The Standard Formulas specified on the order sheet meet the requirements of the vast majority of patients who do not have significant renal/liver dysfunction.
*Peripheral Solutions (PPN) are initiated full volume on the first day.
*One-half of the amount of Central TPN ordered is normally sent on 1st day.

*Pharmacy sends one 24 hr solution bag at 2000 hr.
*Orders must be in the 4th Floor Pharmacy by 1300 hr.
*The last TPN bag is used to discontinue TPN.
*For assistance call Pharmacy (1421/22), or page: Nutrition Support Pharmacist (#1352), Dietitian (#580), Nurse (#272 or #697), or Physician (#1654).

1. DAILY NON-PROTEIN CALORIE (NPC) GUIDELINES: ◆Give: 25–35 Non-Protein Calories /kg of body weight.

◆Most patients: 25–30 Cal/kg (30% from Fat) ◆Hypermetabolic/hypercatabolic patients: 30–35 cal/kg (up to 50% from Fat)

◆1 gm Dextrose = 3.4 Cal ◆1 gm Fat = 9 Cal ◆Avoid giving > 5 mg Dextrose/kg/min or > 2 gm Fat/kg/day

◆gm Dextrose needed: ________ cal/kg [desired total cal/kg] X ________ kg [patient's wt.] X ________ [% desired Dextrose cal] ÷ 3.4 = [____] [gm DEXTROSE/DAY]

◆ GM Fat needed: ________ cal/kg [desired total cal/kg] X ________ kg [patient's wt.] X ________ % [% desired Fat cal] ÷ 9 = [____] [gm FAT/DAY]

— OR USE —

Energy expenditure = The Harris Benedict Equation X Stress Factor X Activity Factor

MALES = [66 + (13.7 X ____wt in kg) + (5 X ____ ht in cm) – (6.8 X ____ age)] X (____SF) X (____ AF)

FEMALES = [655 + (9.7 X ____wt in kg) + (1.8 X ____ ht in cm) – (4.7 X ____ age)] X (____SF) X (____ AF)

Stress Factor (SF):
1.0 to 1.3 (maintenance) Up to 1.5 (for weight gain)

Activity Factor (AF)
Non-ambulatory patient = 1.2
Ambulatory patient = 1.3

PERIPHERAL NUTRITION SOLUTIONS:

◆Dextrose: 50–60 gm/Liter (Should provide not less than 150 gm/day)
◆Fat: 50–62% of cal from Fat ◆Osmolarity should be < 800 ◆5 mg of Hydrocortisone/Liter helps reduce phlebitis
◆Approximately osmolarity (mOsm) of a PPN solution = 50 X final % of protein + 100 X final % of dextrose + 150

2. DAILY PROTEIN GUIDELINES:

◆Total Protein needs: ______gm/kg [No. of gm/kg] X ______kg [patient's wt] = [____] [gm PROTEIN/DAY]
◆Most patients need: 1 – 1.4 gm/kg (via Central or Peripheral vein)
◆Hypermetabolic/hypercatabolic patients need: 1.5 – 2 gm/kg
◆Non-dialyzed renal failure patients need: 0.8 – 1 gm/kg
◆Dialyzed renal failure patients need: 1.0 – 1.5 gm/kg

3. AMINO ACID SOLUTIONS: per 100 mL

Have:	Protein	Essential Amino Acids	Branch Chain Amino Acids	mEq Sodium	mEq Chloride	mEq Acetate	mM Phosphate
◆Travasol 10%: A general purpose amino acid	10 gm	45.3%	19%	0	4	8.7	0
◆FreAmine HBC 6.9%: For severely compromised patients	6.1 gm	66.7%	45%	1	0	5.7	0
◆Hepatamine 8%: For hepatic encephalopathy patients	8 gm	55%	36%	1	0	6.2	1

WRAMC OVERPRINT 257
1 NOV 91

Fig. 23-10 (continued)

ADULT PARENTERAL NUTRITION GUIDELINES

4. DAILY MACRONUTRIENT GUIDELINES:

Sodium:	60–180 mEq/day, or 40–60 mEq per liter of TPN	
Potassium	80–120 mEq/day, or 40–60 mEq per liter of TPN	
Chloride:	60–180 mEq/day, or 30–60 mEq per liter of TPN	
Magnesium:	12–30 mEq/day, or 8–12 mEq per liter of TPN (0.3–0.45 mEq/kg)	
Calcium:	5–15 mEq/day, or 2–5 mEq per liter of TPN (0.2–0.3 mEq/kg)	
Phosphorus:	10–15 mM /1,000 cal, or approximately: 8–12 mM per liter of TPN	

Note: 3 mM of K Phosphate has 4.4 mEq K, and 3 mM of Na Phosphate has 4 mEq Na

Acetate: Balances cations and anions, adjusts acid-base balance of the solution. One mEq of Acetate through intermediary metabolism equates to administration of 1 mEq of Bicarbonate

5. DAILY MICRONUTRIENT GUIDELINES:

◆Daily dose 4 mL, reduce by 50% in non-dialysis renal failure patients

METAL	IV DAILY ADULT DOSE	MULTI-TRACE-5 /4mL
Zinc:	*2.5–4.0 mg	4.0 mg
Copper:	0.5–1.5 mg	1.6 mg
Manganese:	0.15–0.8 mg	0.4 mg
Chromium:	10.0–15.0 mcg	16.0 mcg
Selenium:	20.0–60.0 mcg	80.0 mcg

* An additional 2 mg per day is suggested for highly catabolic states
* Significant G.I. fluid loss requires an additional 12 mg Zinc/L of TPN

6. DAILY FLUID GUIDELINES:

◆Normal TPN patient requires approximately 1 mL per cal

7. DAILY ADULT MULTIPLE VITAMINS:

◆Provide a minimum of 10 mL/day

◆10 mg of Vitamin K should be given intramuscularly q Monday for patients not receiving anticoagulants.

8. INSULIN IN ADULT PARENTERAL NUTRITION:

◆If adding insulin to nutrition soln., add a max of 50% of previous days total insulin usage

◆Suggested Insulin Sliding Scale:

Finger Stick:	Insulin Dose (q 6 hr)
150–249 mg%	2 Units Reg. Human Insulin
250–300 mg%	4 Units Reg. Human Insulin
301–350 mg%	6 Units Reg. Human Insulin
351–400 mg%	8 Units Reg. Human Insulin
> 401 mg%	draw STAT Serum Glucose and NOTIFY PHYSICIAN

9. NUTRITIONAL STATUS INDICATORS:

◆Degree of malnutrition:	Mild	Moderate	Severe	Notes:
Albumin (mg/dL)	3.0–3.5	2.1–3.0	< 2.1	half-life 18 days, affected by hydration status, blood loss, etc
Transferin (mg/dL)	150–200	100–150	< 100	half-life 8 days, affected by iron deficiency, chronic infection
Prealbumin (mg/dL) Males: 19–39 mg/dL and Females: 19–30 mg/dL				half-life 1.9 days, indicator of catabolism, synthesis, and liver function. Obtain a baseline value before initiating TPN/PPN

Steady state nitrogen balance = [nitrogen in (gm protein ÷ 6.25)] – [24 hr Urinary Urea Nitrogen (UUN) in gm + 4 gm]

WRAMC OVERPRINT 257
1 NOV 91

Fig. 23-10 (end)

while to realize that these patients were already phosphorus depleted, and had adjusted to a low-calorie, low-protein diet. Feeding with a high-calorie, high-protein diet consumed what phosphate they had left: ATP levels fell; 2,3-diphosphoglycerate levels fell; red blood cells could no longer unload oxygen; glucose-dependent organs could no longer effectively uptake glucose; and the patients died. Thirty years later, phosphate depletion was rediscovered when critically ill, catabolic patients were placed on TPN before the vital role of phosphorus was appreciated.[38,39]

Increased amounts of phosphorus are lost in the urine after trauma and sepsis, and even after routine surgery. Levels decrease further with early postoperative feeding, as glucose enters cells as glucose-6-phosphate, and as ATP levels fall in hypercatabolism. Phosphorus is the major intracellular anion; the normal intracellular concentration of phosphorus is 75 mEq/L. The plasma concentration is far less, 1.0 to 1.5 mEq/L, or 2.3 to 4.5 mg/dL (or 1–1.4 mmol/L; there is considerable lack of consistency in reporting results with this anion).

An extracellular phosphorus level of less than 1.0 to 1.2 mg/dL will cause respiratory weakness and usually cardiac arrest when it reaches 0.8 μg. Intravascular hemolysis, white blood cell and platelet dysfunction, myocardial dysfunction, and central nervous system dysfunction (including ataxia, seizures, and coma) all result from phosphorus depletion. Unfortunately, the serum phosphate levels do not accurately reflect intracellular depletion and are not a perfect guide for replacement. In addition, the phosphorus content of lipid solutions, or of phosphate in lipid solutions, may not be bioavailable, and the replacement therefore is less than predicted.

The phosphorus content of salts (sodium or potassium) is expressed in millimoles: 15 mmol of potassium phosphate provides 15 mmol of phosphate. The cations in the salt are, however, expressed as milliequivalents: 15 mmol of potassium contains 22 mEq of potassium. The fact that the cation and phosphate have different valences must be borne in mind when replacing phosphorus. Generally, 15 to 30 mmol of the salt per day mixed with the TPN provides adequate maintenance phosphorus. Sodium or potassium phosphate may be given as a piggyback intravenous infusion, at a rate of 15 to 30 mmol over 2 to 4 hours. Infusion rates more rapid than this may cause intravenous precipitation of calcium phosphate and hypocalcemia, and, if potassium phosphate is used, hyperkalemia.

Trace Elements

Trace elements are the catalysts and cofactors that drive the cellular machinery; defects in these impair protein synthesis and cellular energetics. More than nine elements are considered essential, but deficiencies in only five are likely to present problems in the intensive care setting (see Figure 23-10). Little is known of the changes that levels of these undergo in metabolic stress due to trauma or sepsis.

Iron is one trace element that is generally not replaced.[27] Inflammation, fever, and intravascular endotoxin are associated with a fall in serum iron levels. Lactoferrin and transferrin both bind iron when release of inflammatory mediators occurs, activating granulocytes. This binding of iron is essential for normal immune function, at least partly because the body makes iron unavailable to invading bacteria.[40] Peritoneal or retroperitoneal blood, intravascular hemolysis, and other conditions that make hemoglobin available to bacteria are all associated with an increased incidence of sepsis.

More than 200 enzymes essential to metabolic function depend on the availability of zinc. Carbohydrate, lipid, protein, and nucleic acid metabolism all depend on an adequate level of zinc, although "adequate" may be difficult to define in the critically ill. Inadequate amounts of tissue and plasma zinc can impair normal wound healing, platelet aggregation, neutrophil chemotaxis, and transformation of lymphocytes. Obvious signs of deficiency (eg, poor appetite, malabsorption with diarrhea, mental depression) are not uncommon in the critically ill, and not specific. The scaly, hyperpigmented dermatitis may be a late finding and may be misdiagnosed. Normal oral zinc intake is 10 to 20 mg/d, of which 20% to 30% is absorbed. Normal losses are 0.5 mg/d in urine, at least 0.5 mg/d in perspiration, and 2 to 3 mg/d in the gastrointestinal tract. Loss of zinc accelerates in bowel disorders, as absorption depends on intact enterocytes; malabsorption, inflammatory bowel disease, massive small-bowel resection, and pancreatitis all are associated with higher losses and decreased absorption. Alcohol abuse and chronic (or massive) diuretic use also accelerate zinc loss, and patients may present with already low or low-normal zinc stores. Patients with burns and acute renal failure also show increased zinc loss. Urinary zinc losses increase in critical illness, in association with the increased nitrogen losses, and IL-1 release causes a rapid decline in serum zinc as the liver takes up large amounts of the mineral. Zinc accumulates in the liver as metallothionein, which is used to produce α_2-macroglobulin, a protease inhibitor, as a check on the inflammatory reaction. The maintenance dose of zinc is 2 to 4 mg/d added to the TPN solution. In patients who are highly stressed or catabolic or both, however, an additional 2 mg/d should be added. There is some suggestion[41] that nitrogen balance may improve with zinc repletion.

Copper is another mineral that is depleted by bowel disorders. Short-bowel syndrome, jejunoileal bypass, malabsorption, enterocutaneous fistulae, and biliary obstruction all lose copper. An increased hepatic synthesis of ceruloplasmin in infection or inflammatory states, mediated by IL-1, acutely drops serum copper levels. Prolonged administration of zinc, because of the increase in metallothionein, also lowers copper levels. Copper is required for the normal function of cytochrome oxidase and superoxide dismutase, two vital enzyme systems in our patient population. Normal daily replacement dose is 0.5 to 1.5 mg/d.

Manganese is also required for a number of enzyme reactions, and is generally added to trace element formulas. This element should be avoided in biliary obstruction.

Chromium improves glucose tolerance in the critically ill and allows maximum enhancement of the initial reaction of insulin with its receptor. Adding chromium has little effect on glucose tolerance in patients who are not chromium deficient, but improves it in those who are. Chromium, like zinc, decreases in acute renal failure.

Selenium is required at the catalytic site of glutathione reductase. Its role is to help reduce organic hydroperoxides and lipoperoxides resulting from stress, sepsis, and ischemia. Selenium deficiency impairs immune function by (*a*) impairing the ability of granulocytes to kill bacteria and (*b*) damaging granulocytes by the excess accumulation of hydrogen peroxide, which damages the free radical–generating system in those cells. The functioning of T helper cells is also impaired by selenium deficiency. In the lungs, glutathione reductase scavenges oxygen-derived free radicals, offering some protection against damage from these radicals, particularly in patients who require high F_{IO_2}. Selenium is excreted renally, and is also lost in burn and wound exudates, bowel fluids, and enterostomy fluids or enterocutaneous fistulae. The daily requirement is 20.0 to 60.0 µg. Higher doses are generally required for higher stress states; however, ingestion of more than 1 mg/d may cause toxicity. Replacement of 50 to 200 µg/d is considered adequate.

Vitamins

Vitamins are small, organic molecules that are needed in tiny amounts for the normal function of metabolic processes. In general, the metabolic machinery needed for their synthesis is lacking in humans, and a prolonged, deficient intake of a given vitamin will ultimately result in a characteristic and sometimes dramatic clinical syndrome such as scurvy due to a lack of ascorbic acid (vitamin C) and beriberi due to a lack of thiamine (vitamin B_1). Members of the U.S. military who are deployed to a combat zone are most unlikely to manifest evidence of vitamin deficiencies. However, some degree of vitamin intake is indicated. Without *any* intake, body stores of water-soluble vitamins (C and the B group) will disappear within 4 to 5 months.[42] Fortunately, data from the Ranger Training Study indicate that consumption of the U.S. Army's meals ready to eat (MREs) maintained normal serum levels of vitamins A, C, B_1, B_6, and B_{12} over a 2-month period.[8(Fig 20, Fig 21)]

Nevertheless, the normal daily requirement of certain vitamins (eg, vitamins A, certain members of the B group, and especially C) may be increased by as much as 3 to 10 fold in the severely injured.[43] In addition, vitamin supplementations have subtle effects that may possibly be beneficial, such as the increased mobility of polymorphonuclear neutrophils in trauma patients brought about by high doses of either α-tocopherol or vitamin C.[44] Recommended vitamin doses are given in Table 23-3.

Care should be taken to prevent overdosing, especially when administering fat-soluble vitamins such as A and D. Large doses—10-fold greater than the recommended dietary allowances—of the water-soluble vitamins such the B complex and C appear not to be associated with toxicity.

Both fat- and water-soluble vitamins must be regularly replaced during TPN. Commercial preparations are usually available, and one 10-mL ampule per day of a multivitamin mix added to the TPN will suffice. Vitamin K, 10 µg/wk, should be given intravenously, but slowly.

Delivery of Total Parenteral Nutrition

TPN should be thought of as "preenteral" feeding. It lacks the gut stimulation necessary to decrease bacterial translocation and preserve mucosal structure, but it is often the only way to feed a patient. TPN requires a *dedicated* line. This means that *nothing* else goes through that line, not even a little (including withdrawing blood at 3 AM). When

TABLE 23-3

VITAMIN REQUIREMENTS

Vitamin	Units	RDA for Daily Oral Intake[1]	Daily, for the Moderately Injured	Daily, for the Severely Injured	Amount Provided by One Vitamin Pill	Daily Amount Provided by Standard IV Preparations[2]
Vitamin A (retinol)	IU	1,760 (females) 3,300 (males)	5,000	5,000	10,000	3,000 (retinal)
Vitamin D (ergocalciferol)	IU	200	400	400	400	200
Vitamin E (tocopherol)	mg TE	8–10	unknown	unknown	15	10 IU*
Vitamin K (phylloquinone)	µg	20–40†	20	20	0	0‡
Vitamin C (ascorbic acid)	mg	60	75	300	100	100
Thiamine (vitamin B_1)	mg	1.0–1.5	2	10	10	3.0
Riboflavin (vitamin B_2)	mg	1.2–1.7	2	10	10	3.6
Niacin	mg	13–19	20	100	100	40
Pyridoxine (vitamin B_6)	mg	2.0–2.2	2	40	5	4
Pantothenic acid	mg	4–7 (adults)	18	40	20	15
Folic acid	mg	0.4	1.5	2.5	0	0.4
Vitamin B_{12} (cobalamin)	µg	3.0	2	4	5	5
Biotin	µg	100–200†	unknown	unknown	0	60

*Equivalent to RDA
†Estimated to be safe and adequate dietary intakes
‡Must be supplemented in peripheral venous solutions
IU: international units; RDA: recommended dietary allowance; TE: α-tocopherol equivalent; IV: intravenous
Sources for these values: (1) *Food and Nutrition Board. Recommended Dietary Allowances.* 9th ed. Washington, DC: National Academy of Sciences, National Academy Press; 1990. (2) Nutrition Advisory Group. Multivitamin preparations for parenteral use: A statement by the Nutrition Advisory Group, American Medical Association Department of Foods and Nutrition, 1975. *JPEN.* 1979;3:258.
Reprinted with permission from Rombeau JL, Rolandelli RH, Wilmore DW. Nutritional support. Chap 10. In: Part 2. Care in the ICU. In: Wilmore DW, Brennan MF, Harken AH, Holcroft JW, Meakins JM, eds. Vol 1. *Critical Care.* In: *Care of the Surgical Patient.* New York, NY: Scientific American, Inc; 1988: 10-6.

protocol is violated, lines become infected. Strict asepsis—cap, mask, gloves, and *sterile* gown—is required to insert and care for the intravenous line. Insertion is into the subclavian vein where possible, using a modified Seldinger technique (Figure 23-11).

A TPN line may also be inserted using the internal jugular vein or the femoral vein. These sites have slightly higher rates of infection, but as long as no gross soiling of the catheter is probable and strict aseptic technique is used, any difference in infection rate will be minimal. The antecubital fossa veins should be avoided for a number of reasons, among them a high rate of infection.

Single-lumen catheters may be used but are often impractical in the intensive care unit. Most intensive care specialists favor using a triple-lumen catheter, with one port dedicated to TPN. As another alternative, a dedicated infusion port—not the central venous pressure port and *under no circumstances* the pacing port of a Paceport pulmonary artery catheter (manufactured by Edwards/Baxter, Irvine, Calif.), which opens directly into the right ventricle—may be used, with the same protocol as for a single or multilumen central line. The position of the catheter *must* be verified by chest X-ray examination prior to infusion of TPN. Relative contra-

a

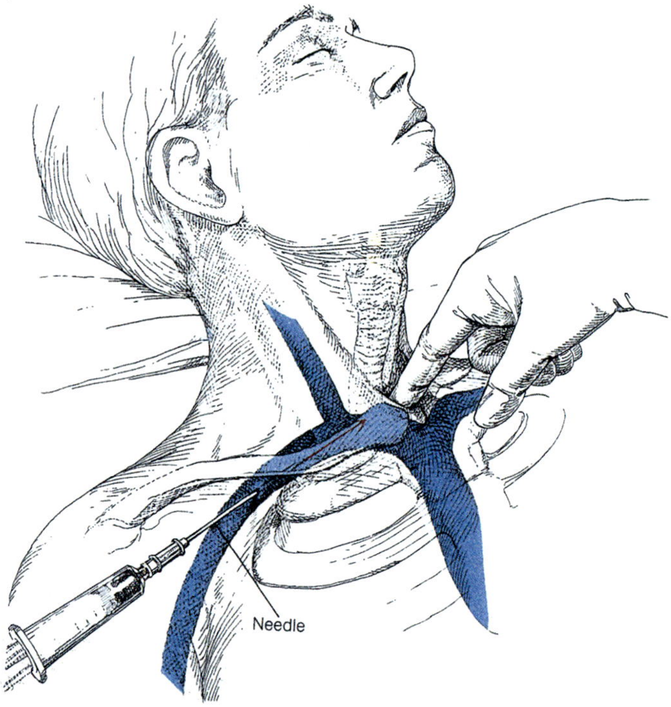

b

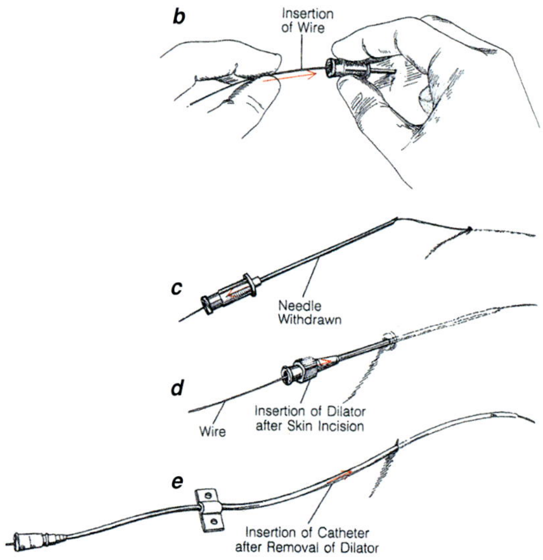

c

d

e

f

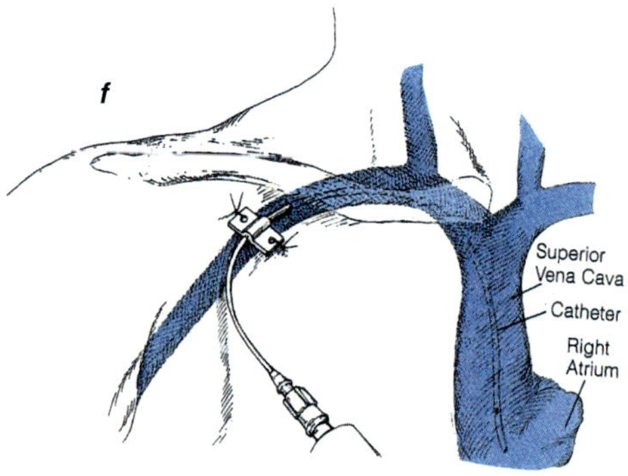

Fig. 23-11. The subclavian approach to central venous catheterization. The patient is placed in Trendelenburg's position to allow filling and dilation of the subclavian vein (**a**). The shoulders are thrown back maximally (a small sheet roll may even be placed beneath the spinal column), and the head is rotated to the side opposite the insertion site. The upper chest and neck are prepared and draped using aseptic technique (the operator should wear hat, mask, gown, and gloves). Local anesthetic is infiltrated into the skin and underlying tissue along the inferior border of the clavicle at or slightly lateral to its midpoint. The needle found in a standard subclavian catheter insertion kit is attached to a syringe and advanced through the anesthetized area parallel to and beneath the clavicle, but over the first rib. The tip of the needle is aimed at a fingertip pressed firmly into the suprasternal notch. With the needle shaft parallel to the frontal plane of the patient (ie, parallel to the bed), the needle will enter the subclavian vein after advancing about 1.5 to 2.0 in. beneath the skin. Slight negative pressure applied to the syringe will allow the prompt inflow of blood when the vein is entered. The needle is advanced a few millimeters after venous blood is obtained to ensure that the entire beveled tip is within the vein lumen.

As the patient performs the Valsalva maneuver to prevent air embolism, the syringe is removed and the guide wire inserted (**b**). The wire should advance into the venous system without resistance or pain to the patient. After at least one half of the wire has been advanced into the vein, the needle is removed over the guide wire (**c**). A small incision is made at the entrance site into the skin, and a dilator is passed over the wire and into the soft tissue (**d**). In a well-muscled person, some resistance may be met; the fascia is best traversed by using a screwlike motion and firm, constant pressure on the dilator. As the dilator is advanced, the wire should always remain freely movable within the dilator's lumen. The dilator is then removed over the wire and replaced by the catheter, an approximate length of which is advanced over the wire into the patient (**e**). This length can be approximated before insertion by measuring the distance between the insertion site and the point on the sternum at the level of the second intercostal space. The wire is then removed, and the catheter lumen is aspirated free of all air and flushed with saline. The catheter is sutured into position (**f**), the exit site cleaned, and a dressing applied. Reprinted with permission from Rombeau JL, Rolandelli RH, Wilmore DW. Nutritional support. Chap 10. In: Part 2. Care in the ICU. In: Wilmore DW, Brennan MF, Harken AH, Holcroft JW, Meakins JM, eds. Vol 1. *Critical Care*. In: *Care of the Surgical Patient*. New York, NY: Scientific American, Inc; 1988: 10-15.

indications are those for insertion of any central line: high intrathoracic pressures, platelets less than 50,000, prolonged bleeding time, or elevated prothrombin time/partial thromboplastin time. Under these circumstances, the femoral vein or a surgical cutdown should be considered.

The question of how often to change intravenous TPN lines is controversial. At Walter Reed Army Medical Center, if proper technique is used, we find little difference in infection rates—whether the lines are changed every 3 days or every 5 days. Double-gloving or double-operator techniques give equally low colonization and infection rates regardless of whether the line change is performed over the wire or the catheter is removed to a new location. We use over-the-wire changes every 5 days and culture all catheter tips. We change to a new site only if a line tip is colonized (> 15 colonies). Line dressings are aseptically changed daily. While the practice of leaving lines in until the site is inflamed may have a low incidence of infection under normal peacetime conditions on hospital wards, during wartime, patient care in intensive care units will require regular changes of all central lines, with culture of all catheter tips whenever possible.

At a minimum, glucose and electrolytes must be monitored daily. In unstable or highly catabolic patients, electrolytes, and especially glucose, must be followed more closely, occasionally as often as every 3 hours. Protein, glucose, lipids (therefore total calories), and electrolytes must be reviewed and adjusted daily to fit the needs of the patient. If insulin or potassium requirements grow out of proportion to caloric load or normal daily losses, it is far better to use a baseline amount in the TPN and give additional amounts of hormone or electrolyte as a separate intravenous infusion, than it is to alter the TPN mixture continually.

Complications of Total Parenteral Nutrition

Complications of parenteral feeding may be grouped into three categories: (1) injury to contiguous anatomical structures during catheter insertion, (2) catheter-related sepsis, and (3) metabolic complications caused by parenteral nutrition. The likelihood of catheter-related complications such as pneumothorax and laceration of vessels in the root of the neck is, to a high degree, determined by the experience of the practitioner and meticulous attention to detail during catheter insertion. Expertise in inserting central lines is *the* essential prerequisite for a low incidence of iatrogenic injuries.

Measures to minimize sepsis arising from a parenteral line depend primarily on the adequacy of nursing care. An excerpt from the *Infection Control Policy and Procedure Guide* developed at Walter Reed Army Medical Center in 1991 is reprinted at the end of this chapter for the benefit of interested readers. The complexity of the control measures serves to remind us why parenteral nutrition is not always feasible in the field echelons of care.

A multitude of metabolic derangements occur during parenteral nutrition. For the sake of completeness, they are listed in Table 23-4, although many are not likely to occur in combat casualties receiving parenteral nutrition. It should be noted that the diagnosis of metabolic complications is somewhat dependent on the availability of an extensive array of laboratory tests, not all of which will be available in deployable medical facilities. Among the more common metabolic derangements are

- hyperglycemia due to too-rapid infusion of glucose, which, if not corrected, can give rise to hyperosmotic nonketotic coma; and
- hypoglycemia due to excessive endogenous or exogenous insulin.

Modifications of Total Parenteral Nutrition

Certain preexisting medical conditions such as renal, hepatic, and respiratory failure are known to complicate the application of parenteral nutrition. Experience has shown us that modifications in standard protocols for parenteral nutrition are indicated whenever these conditions are present.

Modifications for Renal Failure. Acute renal failure prevents the excretion of the end products of nitrogen metabolism. Urea accumulates from both dietary proteins and endogenous protein catabolism, the measured BUN representing the balance between the increased urea production and the limited ability of the kidney to excrete nitrogenous wastes. Gastrointestinal bleeding and reabsorption of blood nitrogen can markedly elevate BUN in a short time, and this situation is not uncommon in the critically ill.

Protein intake can be decreased in renal failure by reducing exogenously provided amino acids and by providing amino acids of high biological value (Table 23-5). Protein should be reduced to 0.5 g/kg/d when the BUN reaches 60 to 80. Additional carbohydrate calories are supplied, to allow utilization of the elevated nitrogen pool as well as to take advantage of the relative protein sparing provided

TABLE 23-4

METABOLIC COMPLICATIONS OF TOTAL PARENTERAL NUTRITION

Problems	Possible Causes	Corrective Measures
Glucose		
Hyperglycemia, glycosuria osmotic, diuresis, hyperosmolar nonketotic dehydration and coma	Excessive total dose or rate of infusion of glucose; inadequate endogenous insulin; increased glucocorticoids; sepsis	Reduce amount of glucose infused; increase insulin; administer a portion of calories as fat emulsion
Ketoacidosis in diabetes	Inadequate endogenous insulin response; inadequate exogenous insulin therapy	Give insulin; reduce glucose input
Postinfusion (rebound) hypoglycemia	Persistence of endogenous insulin production secondary to prolonged stimulation of islet cells by high-carbohydrate infusion	Administer 5%–10% glucose before infusion is discontinued
Fat		
Pyrogenic reaction	Fat emulsion, other solutions	Exclude other causes of fever
Altered coagulation	Hyperlipidemia	Restudy after fat has cleared bloodstream
Hypertriglyceridemia	Rapid infusion, decreased clearance	Decrease rate of infusion; allow clearance before blood tests
Impaired liver function test results	May be caused by fat emulsion or by an underlying disease process	Exclude other causes of hepatic dysfunction
Cyanosis	Altered pulmonary diffusion capacity	Discontinue fat infusion
Essential fatty acid deficiency	Inadequate essential fatty acid administration	Administer essential fatty acids in the form of one 500-mL bottle of fat emulsion every 2–3 d
Amino Acids		
Hyperchloremic metabolic acidosis	Excessive chloride and monohydrochloride content of crystalline amino acid solutions	Administer Na^+ and K^+ as acetate salts
Serum amino acid imbalance	Unphysiological amino acid profile of the nutrient solution; differential amino acid utilization with various disorders	Use experimental solutions if indicated
Hyperammonemia	Excessive ammonia in protein hydrolysate solutions; deficiency of arginine, ornithine, aspartic acid, or glutamic acid, or a combination of these deficiencies in amino acid solutions; primary hepatic disorder	Reduce amino acid intake
Prerenal azotemia	Excessive amino acid infusion with inadequate administration	Reduce amino acid intake;calorie increase glucose calories
Calcium and Phosphorus		
Hypophosphatemia	Inadequate calcium administration; reciprocal response to phosphorus repletion without simultaneous calcium infusion; hypoalbuminemia	Administer phosphorus ($\geq$ 20 mEq potassium dihydrogen phosphate/1,000 IV calories); evaluate antacid or calcium administration or both
Hypocalcemia	Inadequate calcium administration; reciprocal response to phosphorus repletion without simultaneous calcium infusion; hypoalbuminemia	Administer calcium
Hypercalcemia	Excessive calcium administration with or without high doses of albumin; excessive vitamin D administration	Decrease calcium or vitamin D
Vitamin D deficiency; hypervitaminosis D	Inadequate or excessive vitamin D	Alter vitamin D administration
Miscellaneous		
Hypokalemia	Potassium intake inadequate relative to increased requirements for protein anabolism; diuresis	Alter nutrient administration
Hyperkalemia	Excessive potassium administration, especially in metabolic acidosis; renal failure	Alter nutrient administration
Hypomagnesemia	Inadequate magnesium administration relative to increased requirements for protein anabolism and glucose metabolism; diuresis; cisplatin administration	Alter nutrient administration
Hypermagnesemia	Excessive magnesium administration; renal failure	Alter nutrient administration
Anemia	Iron deficiency; folic acid deficiency; vitamin B_{12} deficiency; copper deficiency; other deficiencies	Alter nutrient administration
Bleeding	Vitamin K deficiency	Alter nutrient administration
Hypervitaminosis A	Excessive vitamin A administration	Alter nutrient administration
Elevations in SGOT, SGPT, and serum alkaline phosphatase	Enzyme induction secondary to amino acid imbalance or to excessive deposition of glycogen or fat, or both, in the liver	Reevaluate status of patient

SGOT: serum glutamic-oxaloacetic transaminase; SGPT: serum glutamic-pyruvic transaminase

Reprinted with permission from Rombeau JL, Rolandelli RH, Wilmore DW. Nutritional support. Chap 10. In: Part 2. Care in the ICU. In: Wilmore DW, Brennan MF, Harken AH, Holcroft JW, Meakins JM, eds. Vol 1. *Critical Care*. In: *Care of the Surgical Patient*. New York, NY: Scientific American, Inc; 1988: 10-23.

TABLE 23-5

COMPOSITION OF AMINO ACID SOLUTIONS FOR PATIENTS WITH RENAL FAILURE

	BUN 40–60 mg/dL		BUN 60–80 mg/dL		BUN 80–100 mg/dL	
	Moderate Calories	High Calories	Moderate Calories	High Calories	Moderate Calories	High Calories
Volume						
Amino acids (mL)	500 (mixture high in essential amino acids*)	500 (mixture high in essential amino acids*)	250 (mixture high in essential amino acids*)	250 (mixture high in essential amino acids*)	400 (essential amino acids only)	400 (essential amino acids only)
Dextrose (mL)	500 (50%)	500 (70%)	500 (50%)	500 (70%)	500 (50%)	500 (70%)
Total (mL)	1,000	1,000	750	750	900	900
Contents						
Amino acids (g)	32.5 (3.2%)	32.5 (3.2%)	16.3 (2.1%)	16.3 (2.1%)	20.8 (2.3%)	20.8 (2.3%)
Dextrose (g)	250 (25%)	350 (35%)	250 (33%)	350 (47%)	250 (28%)	350 (39%)
Total nitrogen (g)	5	5	2.5	2.5	3.3	3.3
Nonprotein kcal/g N	170	238	340	476	258	360
Total kcal	875	1,315	913	1,253	932	1,273
kcal/mL	0.9	1.3	1.2	1.7	1.0	1.4

*70% essential amino acids and 30% nonessential amino acids
Reprinted with permission from Rombeau JL, Rolandelli RH, Wilmore DW. Nutritional support. Chap 10. In: Part 2. Care in the ICU. In: Wilmore DW, Brennan MF, Harken AH, Holcroft JW, Meakins JM, eds. Vol 1. *Critical Care*. In: *Care of the Surgical Patient*. New York, NY: Scientific American, Inc; 1988: 10-18.

by an increased carbohydrate load in the catabolic patient. Total volume is decreased, to 1 to 1.5 L/d in the anuric or significantly oliguric patient. Parenteral formulations must be modified to decrease phosphorus, magnesium, and, usually, potassium. Electrolyte supplementation must be recalculated daily, based on close monitoring of the patient's electrolytes, as carbohydrate loading and glucose intolerance will produce electrolyte shifts. Chloride intake should be reduced, and the acetate salts of sodium and potassium utilized to a greater extent, to counter the metabolic acidosis that accompanies uremia. Caloric input from fat is reduced, as fats do not have as great a protein-sparing effect as do carbohydrates, and fats contain 15 mmol of phosphate per liter. Trace elements should be decreased, or withheld for 1 to 2 weeks, unless the patient requires dialysis. If the BUN rises to the 80 to 100 range or above, replacing the standard amino acid mixture with a specialized renal failure formulation is justified. These renal failure–specific formulations generally have a higher proportion of essential amino acids.

Patients receiving hemodialysis regularly, or those on continuous arteriovenous hemofiltration (CAVH) or continuous arteriovenous hemodiafiltration (CAVH-D), will not need the severe restrictions in volume, protein, and fat that patients with renal failure who are not undergoing dialysis receive. Volume is generally liberalized to 2 to 2.5 L/d in patients undergoing dialysis. In noncatabolic patients, protein requirements are 1.0 to 1.5 g/kg/d. Higher protein intake will be required in patients who remain catabolic or are on CAVH or CAVH-D. Caloric requirements also increase for hemodialysis patients and those on CAVH. Patients receiving CAVH-D, however, absorb some glucose from the countercurrent dialysate solution, and caloric input from TPN is often reduced slightly to compensate. In patients on hemodialysis or CAVH-D, folate and the B vitamins must be replaced in greater-than-normal amounts. Increased replacement should be considered in patients in the diuretic phase of acute tubular necrosis, as well.

This late phase of acute tubular necrosis is often marked by hypokalemia and hypomagnesemia, as these electrolytes "wash out" while sodium is, relatively, retained. Close monitoring of electrolytes and frequent adjustments to TPN and maintenance fluids are required during this period.

Modifications for Hepatic Failure. The nutritional requirements in severe hepatic dysfunction or hepatic failure depend primarily on the primary disease or trauma, rather than on the hepatic failure per se. The only exception is acute, fulminant hepatitis, where metabolic demands on the liver must be severely restricted. Protein is often limited in hepatic encephalopathy, but has not been shown to alter outcome in severe hepatic dysfunction or multiorgan failure. Similarly, formulations specific for hepatic dysfunction or failure or both (ie, those high in branched-chain amino acids and low in aromatic amino acids) are often used to offset the elevated levels of aromatic amino acids found in hepatic dysfunction. Like protein limitation, these specific formulations have not effected significant improvements in outcome, although patients remain responsive longer and are somewhat easier to manage metabolically. A reasonable strategy is to provide 1.0 to 1.5 g/kg/d to patients with hepatic failure, until their ammonia levels rise to the point where the encephalopathy worsens, and then to switch to a formula low in aromatic amino acids and high in branched-chain amino acids.

Hepatic failure formulations generally contain no trace elements (see the hepatic amino acid section of Figure 23-10). These must be individually added, based on the needs of the particular patient. Nearly all critically ill patients will require the addition of zinc, but certain trace elements may actually be harmful. Copper, in particular, is best avoided in patients with hepatic failure. Folate and the B vitamins must be supplemented in these patients, as they must also in patients with renal failure.

Modifications for Respiratory Failure. Modification of TPN for patients with respiratory failure is somewhat easier. Glucose is oxidized to carbon dioxide and excreted via the lungs. Since the rate of gas exchange is altered by the administration of carbohydrate, changes in minute ventilation requirements with feeding should be noted. Patients with inadequate pulmonary reserve, or with a fixed rate of carbon dioxide excretion (ie, those on mechanical ventilation) are particularly susceptible, as they cannot vary the rate of gas exchange with feeding. While overfeeding calories should be avoided in all patients, those with respiratory insufficiency are particularly sensitive to carbohydrate calories. Fortunately, probably fewer than 10% of mechanically ventilated patients need modification of standard nutritional formulae. In those few who do, a 50:50 division of calories between carbohydrate and fat, with 1 g of protein per kilogram of body weight per day and a 150:1 ratio of calories to nitrogen, is usually adequate. If this is unsuccessful in allowing the patient to wean from the ventilator, a reduction in total calories to 60% to 70% of calculated requirements may be tried briefly.

Peripheral Parenteral Nutrition

In patients who do not require complete nutritional support but who need a brief period of supplementation, peripheral parenteral nutrition (PPN) may be used. The most significant advantage of PPN is that a peripheral intravenous catheter—albeit a dedicated, single-purpose line—may be used instead of a central catheter. The feeding is necessarily of lower caloric density, generally 0.3 to 0.6 kcal/mL, but 1,200 to 2,300 kcal can be delivered daily.

The singular disadvantage of PPN is that it requires a large volume of fluid, often 2 to 4 L/d. The fluid has an osmolarity between 600 and 800 mOsm/L and should not be given peripherally if greater than 800 mOsm/L. Osmolarity can be approximated as follows:

$$(50 \bullet \%\ \text{protein in final mix}) \\ + (100 \bullet \%\ \text{glucose in final mix}) + 150$$

Intravenous catheter sites must be changed every 48 to 72 hours, both because of the risk of infection and because of the irritation that a hyperosmolar fluid causes in small veins. A small amount of hydrocortisone (5–10 µg/L) added to the infusion may help to reduce phlebitis. Fat emulsions are given separately, every day or every other day, and should provide 50% to 60% of the calories.

Insulin

Insulin may be added to both TPN and PPN, generally to a maximum of 50% of the insulin used the previous day. This will never provide—and should not provide—complete insulin coverage. Some of the added insulin will be adsorbed onto the intravenous catheter tubing. Insulin will have to be supplemented by either an intravenous insulin infusion (often the easiest route of administration to use in critically ill patients) or by injecting intermittent boluses of insulin according to a sliding scale (see part 8 of Figure 23-10). An intravenous infusion can be prepared by adding 125 units of insulin to 250 mL of 5% dextrose in water, running 100 mL through the tubing to saturate the tubing and prevent further adsorption, and then beginning the infusion at 0.5 to 1.0 unit per hour. The insulin infusion can be titrated to a blood glucose between 180 and 220 µg/dL. Alternatively, a sliding scale may be based on glucose determinations from finger sticks, with laboratory confirmation every 4 hours. Insulin given according to a sliding scale must be administered subcutaneously because the half-life of regular insulin is too short when given intravenously, and hourly injections would be required.

Sliding-scale dosages of insulin often must be adjusted and often have to be imposed on top of a baseline insulin infusion, particularly in hypercatabolic patients who are refractory to the action of exogenous insulin.

Enteral Nutrition

Enteral feeding has recently come to be accepted as the preferred route for providing nutritional support after trauma or during infection. While there are often reasons that the parenteral route must be used, enteral feeding is the more physiological, and provides several advantages. The gut is an active organ, deeply involved in the processing and regulation of a large number of nutrients, peptides, inflammatory mediators, hormones, and immunoglobulins. It is a major component of host defense against invading microorganisms, both as a mechanical barrier and as a major immune organ, especially during periods of stress. During starvation and the catabolic state induced by trauma or sepsis, the health of the gut relates directly to the health of the organism.

The cells of the intestinal mucosa, the enterocytes, are the most rapidly proliferating cells in the body. Feeding is the primary stimulus—both direct and indirect—for the growth of these cells. Feeding directly stimulates desquamation of the gut lining and enhanced renewal of the enterocytes, while enteroglucagon, gastrin, and other gut hormones indirectly stimulate cell renewal and growth. The gut, in turn, regulates circulating nutrients through mechanisms more complex than the simple digestion and absorption of feedings. Amino acids and glucose released from catabolized muscle are processed by the gut before they are transported to the liver. Glutamine, a "nonessential" amino acid that makes up a large percentage of the amino acids released from skeletal muscle during stress, is the principal oxidizable fuel for the small bowel. Half the glutamine extracted by the small bowel is oxidized to ammonia, which is, in turn, passed on to the liver for processing to new proteins, and which represents a good part of total body protein turnover. During the catabolism that follows trauma or infection, amino acid uptake by the gut accelerates. This acceleration is, to some extent, matched by the increased release of glutamine by catabolized skeletal muscle. During stress, however, consumption outstrips production, glutamine concentrations fall, and the small intestine finally runs short of fuel and substrate.

Mucosal epithelial cells of the colon use glutamine to a lesser extent. The large bowel depends on short-chain fatty acids—chiefly butyric, acetic, and propionic—and keto acids for fuels. The short-chain fatty acids are vital for sodium and water reabsorption by the colon and for cell growth and proliferation. Short-chain fatty acids are produced by bacterial fermentation of polysaccharides. The gut bacteria use less than 10% of the energy of the polysaccharides themselves. The rest of the energy goes to produce large amounts of short-chain fatty acids, with acetate, propionate, and butyrate comprising 83% of the product in a ratio of 1:0.3:0.25. These energy-carrying compounds can then either be absorbed (> 500 kcal/d in a fed gut) or excreted.

Release of inflammatory mediators, the use of antibiotics and histamine type 2 (H_2) blocking agents, and inadequate provision of enteral calories will each alter the functions and mechanical integrity of the intestine. An intact mucosal barrier and intact immunological function reduce both transmigration of bacterial endotoxin and translocation of enteric bacteria. Endotoxin is normally absorbed across the cell barrier in a controlled fashion and presented to the Kupffer cells for detoxification. Production of stress hormones and the normal catabolic response to injury are modulated. Loss of cell mass because of starvation or increased catabolism diminishes this normal modulation. Continued loss of cell mass or the introduction of hypotension result in cell edema and loss of function, and physically disrupt the barrier by (*a*) decreasing antibody and mucous production and (*b*) allowing the tight junctions between cells to open as cells swell or necrose. Both endotoxin and bacteria can move across the barrier unchallenged. A vicious cycle is set in motion: with the decrease of cell mass, concomitant loss of mucosal villi decreases the bowel's ability to absorb nutrients, which then decreases the production of immunologically and oncotically active proteins, which then further reduces the ability of the bowel—as well as the rest of the body—to function.

Most of the alterations in intestinal function with stress are not inevitable; they can be prevented by enteral feeding. Enteral feeding provides the best means of maintaining the integrity of the intestinal mucosa. Even so simple a measure as exposing the mucosa to a continuous normal saline infusion decreases villous atrophy.[45] Stimulation of enteroglucagon and gastrin by feeding has a trophic effect on stomach and intestinal mucosa. Feeding enterally decreases the elaboration of stress hormones

TABLE 23-6

ENTERAL FORMULAS AND ORAL SUPPLEMENTS USED AT WALTER REED ARMY MEDICAL CENTER*

Product Name	Citrotein	Shakeup	Instant Breakfast (with 8 oz whole milk)	Sustacal	Ultracal	Nutren 1.5
Features	Clear liquid High protein Low-fat orange and punch flavors	High calorie Moderate protein Vanilla, chocolate, and strawberry flavors	High protein Vanilla, chocolate, and strawberry flavors	High protein Vanilla, chocolate, and strawberry flavors	14 g fiber/L; suitable for most tube-fed patients	Calorie-dense to limit volume Vanilla, chocolate, and unflavored
Calories/mL	0.66	1.4	1.06	1	1.06	1.5
Protein g/L (% Cal)	41 (25)	50 g	53 (22)	61 (24)	44 (17)	60 (16)
Carbohydrate g/L (% Cal)	120 (73)	226 g	126 (51)	140 (55)	123 (46)	170 (45)
Fat g/L (% Cal)	1.6 (2)	33 g	30 (27)	23 (21)	45 (37)	68 (39)
Fat Source	Soy oil	Milk fat	Milk fat	Soy oil	40% MCT; 60% soy oil	50% corn oil; 50% MCT oil
Free Water (%)	93		81	84	85	78
mOsm/kg Water	480		670–715	650	310	410–590
Na mg/L†	710		950–1,200	940	930	750
K mg/L‡	710		2,150–3,000	2,100	1,620	1,875
P mg/L	1,100		965	930	850	1,050
Ca mg/L	1,100		1,240	1,010	850	1,050
Mg mg/L	420		302	380	340	500
Cal/100% Vit. RDA	1,000		1,200	1,080	1,250	1,500
Our Cost/L	$3.26		1 pkg = $0.36	$2.36	$3.88	$3.88
Source	Sandoz		Nestle	Mead Johnson	Mead Johnson	Clintec

*All WRAMC enteral products contain vitamin K except Citrotein and Instant Breakfast
†1 mEq Na = 23 mg
‡1 mEq K = 39 mg
MCT: medium-chain triglycerides; LCT: long-chain triglycerides

and the catabolic response to trauma and infection. Glutamine and alanine both improve nitrogen balance. In studies with animals,[27,46] administration of glutamine alone has been shown to increase mucosal cellularity, improve nitrogen balance, and improve outcome; however, glutamine is unstable in solution and is not added to amino acid preparations used in TPN. Glutamine is in some enteral products, but often not in sufficient amount.[46,47]

Enteral Formulations

Enteral formulations may be balanced or disease specific. The latter are, generally speaking, not

Osmolite HN	Isocal	Nepro	Amin-Aid	Peptamen	Lipisorb	Vivonex T.E.N.
Suitable for most tube-fed patients Unflavored	Moderate in protein and electrolytes OK for > 3 years of age Unflavored	Renal. High calorie, high protein For oral or tube feeding	Renal. No electrolytes Essential amino acids	Semielemental Small and large peptides and amino acids Flavor packs available	For fat malabsorption Whole protein Palatable	Elemental Amino acids Very low fat Usually unpalatable
1.06	1.06	2	2	1	1	1
44 (17)	34 (13)	70 (14)	19 (4)	40 (16)	35 (14)	38 (15)
141 (53)	133 (50)	216 (43)	366 (75)	141 (51)	117 (46)	206 (82)
37 (30)	44 (37)	96 (43)	46 (21)	39 (33)	48 (40)	3 (2.5)
50% MCT; 50% corn and soy oils	80% soy oil; 20% MCT oil	Safflower oil; Soy oil	Soy oil	70% MCT oil; 30% LCT oil	86% MCT; 14% LCT	Safflower oil
84	84	71	74	85	83	84
300	270	635	700	270	320	630
930	530	835	< 345	500	734	460
1,561	1,320	1,060	< 117	1,250	1,251	782
758	530	690	0	700	701	500
758	630	1,380	0	800	701	500
304	210	215	0	400	200	200
1,320	2,000	1,900	No vitamins	1,500	2,000	2,000
$5.20	$2.00	$12.33	$18.00	$19.11	$7.96	$15.82
Ross	Mead Johnson	Ross	McGaw	Clintec	Mead Johnson	Sandoz

balanced, with nutrients often in their simplest form: amino acids rather than intact proteins of high biological value, or dipeptides and tripeptides; an emphasis on carbohydrate, often as simple sugars, for calories; and essential fatty acids or medium-chain triglycerides for fats. Often, these ingredients are not as easily absorbed or utilized as those in balanced diets. The formulations are for a single, specific purpose. Renal formulations, for example, contain no nonessential amino acids, the intent being to promote the reuse of the nitrogen in urea. Hepatic formulations are often deficient in aromatic amino acids (phenylalanine, tyrosine, and tryptophan) and contain high concentrations of the branched-chain amino acids, the opposite of the condition we normally find in the patient with hepatic failure.

Balanced formulations, on the other hand, usually contain carbohydrate and fat in a ratio of 70:30, and provide 1 to 2 kcal/mL. They are generally isotonic, although formulations with a higher proportion of their calories from carbohydrate have a higher osmolarity. Carbohydrates are usually provided as oligosaccharides and polysaccharides or maltodextrins, with fats in the form of medium-chain or long-chain triglycerides. Balanced formulations are often lactose free—as much as possible—since lactase is often markedly decreased in an injured or unused gut. The diarrhea (which is not infrequently seen when enteral feeding is started) more often is caused by bowel-wall edema from a low serum albumin, abnormal bowel flora from long-term antibiotic use, lactase deficiency, or any combination of the three, rather than a "hypertonic" formulation. Since there is some variation between formulations, often the substitution of one balanced formula for another will resolve a problem: feeding a formula higher in carbohydrate, often via the stomach, may help patients with steatorrhea; a formula with a higher percentage of calories from fat may help if diarrhea is secondary to a hyperosmolar (eg, a high-carbohydrate) product. Protein is usually provided at a fixed ratio of calories to nitrogen, often 150:1. The proteins most easily absorbed in a balanced formulation are the intact proteins of high biological value (eg, egg albumin) and dipeptides and tripeptides. Amino acids are *not* easily absorbed.

Electrolytes, vitamins, and trace elements are added to both balanced and disease-specific formulations; the amounts obviously vary with specific requirements in the latter. Formulations offer a wide range of caloric, protein, and electrolyte options (Table 23-6).

Delivery

Before enteral feeding can be initiated, the patient's readiness for such feeding must be assessed. Does the patient have a history of gastroesophageal reflux? Prior aspiration? Is the patient on medication that might promote reflux? The list is a long one and includes a broad range of drug types: theophylline, anticholinergics, calcium channel–blocking agents, catecholamines, vasodilators; in other words, any agent that decreases contraction of the lower esophageal sphincter. Is the patient conscious; if not, does the patient have an intact gag reflex? Is the gut functional? Does the stomach empty normally, or does ileus or obstruction interfere? How recently has the patient had surgery involving the bowel? Unfortunately, bowel sounds and the passage of flatus are not specific indicators of gut health. If gastrointestinal output from all sources (nasogastric tube, ostomies, and rectum) exceeds 600 mL/24 h, then enteral feeding is less likely to be successful. Gastroparesis, bowel obstruction, ileus, pancreatitis, high-output enteric fistulae, and gastrointestinal bleeding are all relative contraindications to enteral alimentation. The decision to feed enterally or parenterally (or both) will be based on not only the presence of one or more of the above, but also on the extent to which they are present.

The serum albumin level and the extent of bowel edema also play major roles in how well enteral nutrients are absorbed by the bowel. A serum albumin level of less than 2.7 g/dL will often allow enough interstitial fluid to remain in the bowel wall to diminish uptake of enterally provided nutrients, particularly amino acids and hydrolyzed proteins, which may require functional enterocytes for absorption. Similarly, an edematous or dysfunctional colon cannot reabsorb sodium and water properly.

Surgical Access. Two surgical procedures can be used to gain access to enteral feeding. First, surgical insertion of a gastrostomy tube may be accomplished either during the initial operative procedure, or may be done percutaneously (via esophagogastroscopy) a few days after surgery. Once the insertion wound has healed sufficiently—usually 24 hours[48]—gastric feeding can begin. Second, a feeding jejunostomy may be placed surgically, either as a separate procedure or through the gastrostomy tube, and jejunal feeding instituted. The gastrostomy tube may then be used to decompress the stomach, administer medication, and measure gastric residual volumes if gastroparesis is a postoperative problem.

Access Via a Feeding Tube. More commonly, however, nasogastric tubes are used. Nasogastric tubes are usually made of polyurethane and are relatively inflexible. They were designed for, and are commonly used for, gastric decompression, but are often used for feeding as a matter of convenience. While feeding into the stomach does have a theoretical advantage in neutralizing gastric pH, this advantage is offset by the wicklike action of the nasogastric tube, which prevents competent functioning of the lower esophageal sphincter and allows gastric contents to reflux into the esophagus. This problem is compounded by gastroparesis or ileus, although use of a nasogastric tube will allow residual gastric volumes to be followed in these conditions.

One of the simplest and best-tolerated means of providing enteral nutrition is by use of a duodenal feeding tube, inserted either orally or nasally, and passed into the second portion of the duodenum. These tubes are made of polyurethane or silicone rubber and are thin walled and highly flexible. They come with a wire stylet to stiffen them enough to insert, and a combination of the stylet, the patient's position, gravity, and twisting and turning of the catheter as it is inserted will get the tube to the proper position in the duodenum. Duodenal feeding tubes are often designed to be self-passing, with a weighted tip, and once in the stomach and left to their own devices, will pass nicely into the duodenum, provided that the tube has not been taped onto the patient. Always leave some "play" in the tubing (a loop that will allow the feeding tube to traverse the pyloric sphincter). It is often helpful to place the patient with his right side down for several hours. Sometimes, increasing gastrointestinal peristalsis by using a cholinergic drug like Reglan (metoclopramide, manufactured by A. H. Robins, Richmond, Va.), will facilitate placement. However, the medical officer must ensure that the patient does not have a bowel obstruction before Reglan is administered.

Tube Placement. An easy method of tube placement, which seems to work most of the time, has been described.[49] After the feeding tube is passed to the stomach with the patient sitting, the head of the bed is lowered and the patient is placed on his right side. The feeding tube is then twisted in a corkscrew motion while it is advanced a distance sufficient to pass into the duodenum. Passage through the pyloric sphincter can often be felt. If resistance is encountered, the feeding tube, with a loop, should be taped to the patient. The feeding tube, now free to advance on its own, passes more often than not. Initial tube placement may be checked by auscultation; however, the position of the tube is always verified by X-ray examination before feedings are instituted.

Tolerance to Feeding

Tolerance to feeding should be assessed by beginning the infusion at a low rate (eg, 30 mL/h) for the first 24 hours. The patient should be closely monitored for abdominal distention or cramping, and for the onset of nausea, vomiting, or diarrhea. Residual volumes may be assessed if a nasogastric tube is used for feeding, or if a nasogastric tube was left in place when the feeding tube was placed. The relative position of both tubes is important in assessing residual volume. If the feeding tube has slipped back to the duodenal bulb or stomach, or if the nasogastric tube is at the pylorus, then large residual volumes may not accurately reflect the function of the stomach and the bowel.

Monitoring

In general, enteral nutrition requires at least as careful monitoring as parenteral. Tubing must be changed daily, and formula at least every 8 hours, to prevent bacterial overgrowth. Intake and output must be followed as closely as they are in parenteral nutrition. Residual volumes should be checked every 4 hours, initially. The risk of aspiration is significant in enteral feeding; even the presence of two sphincters (pyloric and lower esophageal) between the feeding-tube outlet and the lungs does not completely remove the risk. The head of the bed should be elevated 30° during enteral alimentation, with feeding interrupted, if necessary, to allow for sleeping.

Diarrhea

Diarrhea (passage of more than 300 g or 300 mL of liquid or semisoft stool per day) can develop in up to three fourths of critically ill patients who receive enteral alimentation. As stated before, this is usually due to atrophy of villi, bowel-wall edema, and the use of multiple antibiotics, with consequent disruption of the normal intestinal flora. Pseudomembranous colitis due to *Clostridium difficile* must always be considered. Therapeutic response to diarrhea includes replacement of lost fluid and electrolytes, decreasing the rate of feeding, changing to a different product, and adding Kaopectate (manufactured by Upjohn, Kalamazoo, Mich.; the active ingredients are kaolin and pectin) to the formula. Fifteen to 30 mL of Kaopectate administered every 2 to 6 hours will often slow diarrhea. Kaopectate binds bacterial toxins and is often useful in diarrhea due to bacterial overgrowth. It also apparently stimulates villous trophism (soluble fiber polysaccharides have a similar effect on mucosal growth and function, and have been shown[50] to improve recovery from inflammation). Remember to *flush the feeding tube* afterwards; frequent flushing ensures the tube's continued patency and reduces the need for replacement. Opiates should be avoided, as they may worsen or induce ileus and allow further bacterial overgrowth. Water may be added if the patient has a free-water deficit (eg, large insensible losses, hypernatremia due to diuresis), but enteral formulae for diarrhea rarely require dilution, as most are isotonic. Decreasing the osmolarity to 150 mOsm may be tried, but if a decrease in rate and osmolarity and the addition of Kaopectate do not solve the problem, then fat and carbohydrate malabsorption should be assessed with stool fat, D-xylose, and finally breath hydrogen laboratory tests, looking for bacterial overgrowth. Stool specimens should be sent to the laboratory early to be tested for *Clostridium difficile* toxin; if the test is negative but diarrhea persists, then consider evaluation with a flexible sigmoidoscope.

Maintaining the Feeding Tube

Clogging of feeding tubes can be minimized by flushing the tube with water after use (eg, after administering medication, when feeding bags are changed). Medications in pill form should never be crushed and given through a feeding tube. Pills and tablets should be dissolved in 15 to 30 mL of water, injected into the tube by Toomey syringe, and flushed. Should a clog develop, a small amount of a carbonated cola soft drink injected into the feeding tube may dissolve it.

Feeding tubes tend to migrate and should be adequately secured. They should be taped (always with a loop) to the patient's forehead or cheek; take care not to put pressure on the nares. The tubes may also be more firmly hobbled should their wandering become a problem.

Assessment of Nutritional Repletion

The assessment and consequences of nutritional depletion are well described: a loss of 40% of total body weight is usually fatal; there are generally accepted "panic values" for electrolytes and micronutrients; and the value of nutritional support is widely accepted. Assessment of nutritional repletion is not so clear cut. The question of *how* to monitor nutritional repletion has been asked by a number of authorities: there is a difference between monitoring structural repletion versus monitoring cell function. Nutritional repletion alters the performance of cells before it restores mass, by altering membrane ion transport and by returning enzyme function to normal. Nuclear magnetic resonance studies using phosphorous 31 labeling have shown a fall in oxidative phosphorylation in malnutrition, implying a decrement in mitochondrial function. Cell energetics return to a more normal function before protein synthesis restores cell mass but still require 2 to 4 weeks of nutritional repletion in a severely malnourished patient. Three fourths of the energy liberated by the hydrolysis of ATP is used to maintain ion gradients across cell membranes, even at the expense of protein synthesis, in a malnourished patient. Protein synthesis is a metabolically expensive cell function, requiring five molecules of ATP for each amino acid incorporated into a protein. It should come as no surprise that cells take care of their basic requirements first.[51]

As an index of nutritional repletion, serum albumin has a sensitivity of only about 10%. While the half-life of albumin in normal individuals is 18 days, it is much shorter in catabolic patients. Albumin levels fall before significant malnutrition occurs in patients who are starved, stressed, or both, because of ongoing catabolism of nonessential proteins. In the stressed patient, protein production is shifted to acute-phase proteins. Large-scale volume expansion, not uncommon in critically ill patients, also lowers albumin levels significantly. Generally, a level of 2.5 to 3.0 g/dL reflects a mild-to-moderate depletion of the albumin pool, 2.0 to 2.5 g/dL a moderate depletion, and less than 2.0 g/dL a severe depletion, but this assessment may not accurately reflect the patient's overall nutritional status. Albumin rises slowly following nutritional repletion, usually taking weeks to rise in patients receiving TPN. Any earlier rise may be artifactual and due to contraction of the extracellular water pool, rather than to an actual increase in albumin mass. Albumin may actually rise more rapidly with enteral feeding than with TPN, although bowel-wall edema may preclude this route until adequate oncotic pressure is established and tissue edema reduced. Because albumin is necessary to maintain intravascular oncotic pressure, supplementation may be accomplished by continuous infusion at 4, 8, or 12 mL/h to increase serum osmolarity and decrease bowel-wall edema in preparation for enteral feeding. Bolus supplementation of serum albumin is not effective in mobilizing fluid.

Transferrin is also a nonsensitive indicator of nutritional repletion, even though the half-life of transferrin (8 d) is shorter than that of albumin, and therefore turnover is faster. Transferrin is a necessary component of the white blood cell response to infection and inflammation. Levels tend to increase earlier than serum albumin levels with feeding, partly as a reflection of this function. Transferrin levels also increase with iron deficiency, as the protein is no longer bound. Levels between 100 and

150 mg/dL reflect a moderate depletion of the pool; less than 100 mg/dL, a severe depletion.

Thyroxine-binding prealbumin is more sensitive than either albumin or transferrin to nutritional repletion. It has a half-life of 1.9 days and is a fairly useful indicator of catabolism and protein synthesis. The fall in this protein in critical illness may be related to changes in thyroxine levels rather than to malnutrition, however, making clinical application difficult. Normal levels in men are between 19 and 39 mg/dL; in women, 19 and 30 mg/dL.

Similarly, retinol-binding protein is a more sensitive indicator of nutritional repletion than is either albumin or transferrin, but the use of this plasma protein as an indicator has limited utility outside academic medical centers.

Fibronectin levels provide a very sensitive barometer of nutritional depletion and repletion. Fibronectin is rapidly consumed during critical illness, with a corresponding fall in serum levels. Levels peak early with adequate repletion, but after 1 to 2 weeks become relatively useless in assessing nitrogen balance. Most other indices have problems as well.

The Creatinine-Height Index[3] overestimates muscle mass in critical illness, and is sensitive to renal dysfunction. Cutaneous reactivity and lymphocyte counts are nonsensitive and nonspecific indices of nutrition, as immune function is affected by multiple factors: infection, uremia, cirrhosis, hepatitis, steroids, burns, hemorrhage, trauma, general anesthesia, and others.

The urinary urea nitrogen test is extremely useful in assessing the catabolic rate, and therefore the physician's ability to balance protein breakdown with nutrition repletion. While it is a gross measure, the nitrogen balance is still the best indicator of the adequacy of repletion of protein. Adequacy of caloric repletion is best assessed by indirect calorimetry.

The problem of providing nutritional support to casualties in the theater of operations has recently been addressed.[52] At present, the limitations of deployed resources may not allow either enteral or parenteral forms of nutritional support; however, both forms should be available in fourth-echelon hospitals. Although parenteral nutrition is probably not possible in the third echelon during a major war, enteral nutrition—being much more feasible logistically—is certainly an acceptable alternative. For this reason, surgeons should be encouraged to insert feeding tubes during resuscitative surgery on all casualties who are likely to require nutritional support.

SUMMARY

Metabolic interventions are important in the treatment of wounded casualties because the common perception of the soldier as a vigorous, muscular mesomorph obscures reality: combat casualties are frequently nutritionally depleted or even frankly malnourished. Unfortunately, however, the applicability of nutritional therapy for combat casualties is a function of the nature of the deployment. In short but intense conventional wars and in operations other than war, only limited medical assets will be deployed in the combat zone, and they will be used primarily for resuscitative surgery. Casualties who require nutritional support will probably be evacuated for the needed treatment to hospitals at the fourth echelon or in the continental United States. Ideally, however, nutritional support would begin prior to evacuation.

The primary constituents of ingested food—carbohydrates (hexoses, of which glucose is preeminent), fats (triglycerides), and proteins (amino acids)—are interconverted by the TCA cycle found within mitochondria. Metabolic intermediates are formed within the mitochondria, which store chemical energy in molecular bonds to be used in a variety of essential, life-sustaining processes. Metabolic intermediates in excess of the body's immediate energy needs are converted into fatty acids for storage in fat cells, or into glucose, which is stored as glycogen in liver and muscle. Although at any given moment the metabolism of glucose is the major source of the body's energy-supplying intermediates, lipids are the major form of nutrient storage. Proteins can serve as storage deposits for amino acids; their primary role, however, is structural, and protein metabolism results in functional impairment. Interconversion of glucose, fatty acids, and amino acids is not perfect; although glucose can be converted into fat and certain amino acids can be converted into glucose, fatty acids are not easily converted into glucose. During uncomplicated starvation, when glucose is in short supply, free fatty acids (or ketone bodies formed from their partial metabolism) are used by most organs in place of glucose. Low circulating insulin levels are necessary for the metabolic adaptation to starvation.

When stress and physical exertion are superimposed on starvation, not only are overall metabolic demands increased, but mobilization of fatty acids is also impeded by elevated levels of stress hormones such as catecholamines, cortisol, and glucagon. Hence, when physical stress occurs with starvation, there is an increased need for glucose, which (because of the lack of metabolic machinery allowing free conversion of fatty acids to glucose) can only be obtained through the process of gluconeogenesis: amino acids derived from the catabolism of body proteins are converted into glucose. The need for glucose and the associated accelerated catabolism of protein are even greater when a wound is present, because healing tissue is an obligate consumer of glucose. Protein catabolism is further accelerated when the wound is septic, owing to the formation of mediators of inflammation such as IL-1 and the eicosanoids. Thus, the combat casualty with severe wounds that have become septic is both hypermetabolic (ie, the REE is 30%–60% greater than normal) and hypercatabolic with a negative nitrogen balance (ie, more than 10 g of urea nitrogen is excreted via the urine per day). Paradoxically, both hyperglycemia and hyperinsulinemia are frequently present, indicating that the hormonal milieu associated with injury and sepsis has induced a state of resistance to the normal biological effects of insulin.

Ideally, optimal metabolic management of the hypermetabolic and hypercatabolic combat casualty requires knowledge of both the REE and the nitrogen balance. Caloric intake can then be set at 30% to 40% of measured energy expenditure, and the amount of nitrogen at 1g/150 kcal of caloric intake. Since the equipment for indirect calorimetry is not likely to be available in deployable hospitals, a more empirical approach will be necessary there (eg, giving 40 kcal/kg/d, with nitrogen being given in the ratio of 1 g/200 kcal. At least half the total caloric intake should be in the form of carbohydrates. The route of administration will depend on whether the gastrointestinal tract is functional. If it is, the enteral route is preferable since it is safer, cheaper, and, perhaps most importantly, it helps to preserve the integrity of the intestinal mucosa.

REFERENCES

1. Murray RK, Granner DK, Mayes PA, Rodwell VW, eds. *Harper's Biochemistry*. 23rd ed. Norwalk, Conn: Appleton & Lange; 1993: 180.
2. Linder MC. Energy metabolism, intake, and expenditure. In: Linder MC, ed. *Nutritional Biochemistry and Metabolism with Clinical Applications*. New York, NY: Elsevier; 1985: Chap 8: 290.
3. Schlichtig R, Ayres SM. *Nutritional Support of the Critically Ill*. Chicago, Ill: Year Book Medical Publishers, Inc; 1988: 571.
4. Skeie B, Kvetan V, Gil KM, Rothkopf MM, Newsholme EA, Askanazi J. Branch-chain amino acids: Their metabolism and clinical utility. *Crit Care Med*. 1990;18(5):549–571.
5. Phillips WJ. Starvation and survival: Some military considerations. *Milit Med*. 1994;159:513–516.
6. Lemoyne M, Jeejeebhoy KN. Total parenteral nutrition in the critically ill patient. *Chest*. 1986;89:568–575.
7. Cahill GF. Starvation in man. *N Engl J Med*. 1970;282:668–675.
8. Moore RJ, Friedl KE, Kramer TR, et al. *Changes in Soldier Nutritional Status and Immune Function During the Ranger Training Course*. Natick, Mass: US Army Research Institute of Environmental Medicine; 1992. USARIEM Technical Report T13-19.
9. Byrne TA, Morrissey TB, Gatzen C, et al. Anabolic therapy with growth hormone accelerates protein gain in surgical patients requiring nutritional rehabilitation. *Ann Surg*. 1993;218:400–418.
10. Bellamy RF. Colonel, Medical Corps, US Army. Personal communication, December 1994.
11. Cipolle MD, Pasquale MD, Cerra FB. Secondary organ dysfunction: From clinical perspectives to molecular mediators. *Crit Care Clin*. 1993;9(2):261–298.
12. Baue AE. Nutrition and metabolism in sepsis and multisystem failure. *Surg Clin North Am*. 1991;71(3):549–565.

13. Bessey PQ. Metabolic response to critical illness. Chap 11. In: Part 2. Care in the ICU. In: Wilmore DW, Brennan MF, Harken AH, Holcroft JW, Meakins JM, eds. Vol 1. *Critical Care*. In: *Care of the Surgical Patient*. New York, NY: Scientific American, Inc; 1989.

14. Douglas RG, Shaw JHF. Metabolic response to sepsis and trauma. *Br J Surg*. 1989;76:115–122.

15. Cerra FB. Multiple organ failure syndrome. *Dis Mon*. 1992;Dec:846–895.

16. Shakespeare W. *Hamlet*. Act IV; scene iii; line 9.

17. Hers GH. The usefulness of "futile cycles." *Biochem Soc Trans*. 1976;4:985–988.

18. Dahn MS, Jacobs LA, Lange MP, Smith S, Mitchell RA. Endocrine mediators of metabolism associated with injury and sepsis. *JPEN*. 1986;10:253–257.

19. Wilmore DW. Are the metabolic alterations associated with critical illness related to the hormonal environment? *Clin Nutrit*. 1986;5:9–20. The Sir David Cuthbertson Lecture, 1985.

20. Wysocki M, Besbes M, Roupie E, Brun-Buisson C. Modification of oxygen extraction ratio by change in oxygen transport in septic shock. *Chest*. 1992;102:221–226.

21. Tuchschmidt J, Fried J, Astor M, Rackow B. Elevation of cardiac output and oxygen delivery improve outcome in septic shock. *Chest*. 1992;102;216–220.

22. Nordenström J, Carpentier YA, Askanazi J, et al. Free fatty acid mobilization and oxidation during total parenteral nutrition in trauma and infection. *Ann Surg*. 1983;(198):725–735.

23. Kinney JM. Metabolic responses of the critically ill patient. *Crit Care Clin*. 1995;11:(3)569–585.

24. Shaw JMF, Wolfe RR. An integrated analysis of glucose, fat and protein metabolism in severely injured patients. *Ann Surg*. 1989;209:63–72.

25. Bergström J, Fürst P, Norée L-O, Vinnars E. Intracellular free amino acid concentration in human muscle tissue. *J Appl Physiol*. 1974;36:693–697.

26. Dudrick PS, Souba WW. Amino acids in surgical nutrition: Principles and practice. *Surg Clin North Am*. 1991;71(3):459–476.

27. Rombeau JL, Rolandelli RH, Wilmore DW. Nutritional support. Chap 10. In: Part 2. Care in the ICU. In: Wilmore DW, Brennan MF, Harken AH, Holcroft JW, Meakins JM, eds. Vol 1. *Critical Care*. In: *Care of the Surgical Patient*. New York, NY: Scientific American, Inc; 1988.

28. Baticci F, Bozzetti F. Anticatabolic properties of branched chain amino acids in post-operative patients: A prospective study. *Clinical Nutrition*. 1990;9:246–252.

29. Jiménez Jiménez FJ, Ortiz Leyba C, Morales Méndez S, Barros Pérez M, Muñoz García J. Prospective study on the efficacy of branched-chain amino acids in septic patients. *JPEN*. 1991;15:252–261.

30. Dinarello CA. Role of interleukin-1 and tumor necrosis factor in systemic responses to infection and inflammation. In: Gallin JI, Goldstein IM, Snyderman R, eds. *Inflammation: Basic Principles and Clinical Correlates*. 2nd ed. New York, NY: Raven Press; 1992: Chap 12.

31. Shoemaker WC, Appel PL, Koum HB. Role of oxygen debt in the development of organ failure, sepsis and death in high-risk surgical patients. *Chest*. 1992;102:208–221.

32. Knaus WA, Draper EA, Wagner DP, Zimmerman JE. APACHE II: A severity of disease classification system. *Crit Care Med*. 1985;13:818–829.

33. Zimmerman JE. Nutritional support in the ICU. Lecture presented at Update in Critical Care—1993; April 1993; Washington, DC.

34. Bursztein S, Elwyn DH, Askanazi J, Kinney JM. *Energy Metabolism, Indirect Calorimetry, and Nutrition*. Baltimore, Md: Williams & Wilkins; 1989: 30, 59, 62.

35. Harris JA, Benedict G. Standard basal metabolism constants for physiologists and clinicians. In: Carnegie Institute of Washington. *A Biometric Study of Basal Metabolism*. Philadelphia, Pa: JB Lippincott; 1919: 233–250. Publication 279.

36. Bistrian BR. A simple technique to estimate the severity of stress. *Surg Gynecol Obstet*. 1979;5:54–61.

37. Knochel JP. The pathophysiology and clinical characteristics of severe hypophosphatemia. *Arch Int Med*. 1977;137:203–220.

38. Ritz E, principal discussant. Acute hypophosphatemia. *Kidney Int*. 1982;22:84–94. Nephrology forum. Cohen JJ, Harrington JT, Kassirer JP, eds.

39. Thompson JS, Hodges RE. Preventing hypophosphatemia during total parenteral nutrition. *JPEN*. 1984;8(2): 137–139

40. Bullen JJ. The significance of iron in infection. *Rev Infect Dis*. 1981;3:1127–1138.

41. Wolman SL, Anderson H, Marliss EB, Jeejeebhoy KN. Zinc in total parenteral nutrition: Requirements and metabolic effects. *Gastroenterology*. 1979;76:458–467.

42. Guyton AC. *Textbook of Medical Physiology*. 8th ed. Philadelphia, Pa: WB Saunders; 1991: 944.

43. Crandon JH, Lennihan R Jr, Mikal S, Reis AE. Ascorbic acid economy in surgical patients. *Ann NY Acad Sci*. 1961;92:246–267.

44. Maderazo EG, Woronick CL, Hickingbotham N, Jacobs L, Bhagavan HN. A randomized trial of replacement antioxidant vitamin therapy for neutrophil locomotory dysfunction in blunt trauma. *J Trauma*. 1991;31:1142–1150.

45. Zaloga GP, Knowles R, Black KW, Prielipp R. Total parenteral nutrition increases mortality after hemorrhage. *Crit Care Med*. 1991;19:54–59.

46. Zaloga GP. Enteral versus parenteral nutrition in the critically ill patient. Lecture presented at American College of Chest Physicians; November 1993; Orlando, Fla.

47. Meredith JW, Ditesheim JA, Zaloga GP. Visceral protein levels in trauma patients are greater with peptide diet than with intact protein diet. *J Trauma*. 1990;30(7):825–828.

48. Daly JM. Malnutrition. Chap 12. In: Part 7. Special problems in perioperative care. In: Wilmore DW, Brennan MF, Harken AH, Holcroft JW, Meakins JM, eds. Vol 2. *Elective Care*. In: *Care of the Surgical Patient*. New York, NY: Scientific American, Inc; 1991: 12-6.

49. Zaloga GP. Bedside method for placing small bowel feeding tubes in critically ill patients: A prospective study. *Chest*. 1991;100:1643–1646.

50. Rolandelli RH, Saul SH, Settle RG, Jacobs DO, Trerotola SO, Rombeau JL. Comparison of parenteral nutrition and enteral feeding with pectin in experimental colitis in the rat. *Am J Clin Nutr*. 1988;47:715.

51. Jeejeebhoy KN. How should we monitor nutritional support: Structure or function? *New Horizons*. 1994;2(2):131–135.

52. Shikora SA. Approaches to nutritional support for battle casualties and trauma: Current military practice and lessons learned from the civilian sector. *Milit Med*. 1995;160(6):312–317.

EXCERPT FROM WALTER REED ARMY MEDICAL CENTER INFECTION CONTROL POLICY AND PROCEDURE GUIDE

For the benefit of the interested reader, the following excerpt is reprinted from Roup BJ, ed. Lieutenant Colonel, Army Nurse; Chief, Infection Control Service, Department Of Nursing. *Walter Reed Army Medical Center Infection Control Policy and Procedure Guide*. 3rd ed. Washington, DC: Walter Reed Army Medical Center; November 1991; previous editions February 1987, June 1989.

PERIPHERAL AND INTERMITTENT INTRAVENOUS THERAPY

I. GENERAL

This SOP establishes WRAMC policy for the insertion and maintenance of peripheral intravascular devices, fluids, delivery systems, and the procedure to be followed in the event of suspected infection.

II. SPECIFIC

A. IV Insertion

1. Equipment
   a. IV solution
   b. IV tubing set, primary
   c. Steel needle or plastic catheter

(NOTE: Steel needles, eg, butterfly or scalp vein, are recommended over plastic catheters as they appear to cause less phlebitis. Plastic catheters should be used when a secure route for vascular access is imperative or when administered drugs may tissue damage if they infiltrate.)

   d. Iodophor or alcohol for skin prep
   e. Tourniquet
   f. Tape
   g. IV stand
   h. Waste container
   i. Sterile dressing (2 x 2 gauze pad or semi-permeable plastic membrane)
   j. Chux (blue pad)
   k. Gloves

2. Procedure
   a. Wash hands with antiseptic soap and water for at least 30 seconds.
   b. Visually inspect IV container for cloudiness or particulate matter. Check glass bottles for cracks; squeeze plastic bags for air leaks. DO NOT USE IF STERILITY IS SUSPECT.
   c. Connect tubing to solution container using aseptic technique. Glass bottles require vented tubing; plastic bags require non-vented tubing.

(NOTE: Use of extension tubing, especially 3-way stopcocks is discouraged. Frequent manipulation and open stopcocks provide microorganisms direct access to the blood stream. If 3-way stopcocks are used, the cap covering the unused port should be a Luer-Lok cap or taped in place.)

   d. Fill entire length of tubing with solution and close tubing clamp.
   e. Select venipuncture site in an upper extremity.

(NOTE: The risk of infection with lower extremity cannulation is extremely high. Cannulae inserted into lower extremities should be removed as soon as venous access in an upper extremity is established.)

   f. DO NOT SHAVE insertion site. Remove excess hair by clipping with scissors.
   g. Place Chux under extremity to protect bed linen.
   h. Apply tourniquet and palpate blood vessel. (A tourniquet that is too tight will not allow the vein to distend.)
   i. Cleanse site with prep solution, using friction from center to periphery in a 2" diameter spiral.
      1) PREFERRED PREP: Cleanse site with iodophor, eg, Betadine. Allow to dry. DO NOT remove with alcohol. The antimicrobial action depends in part on the continued release of free iodine.
      2) ALTERNATE PREP: Cleanse site with isopropyl alcohol for AT LEAST ONE MINUTE and allow to air dry. (Alcohol contact time is the kill factor.)

j. After the venipuncture site has been prepped, DO NOT touch the skin with your finger unless wearing a sterile glove.
k. Put on gloves.
l. Holding the skin taut, insert the needle/catheter along-side the vein, bevel up, about ½ inch from the site of vein puncture. Carefully puncture the vein and thread the needle into it. Observe for blood return. If blood return is present, continue with procedure.

(NOTE: If no blood return is obtained, manipulate the needle carefully to gain entry into vein. If unsuccessful, withdraw the needle, obtain fresh needle, prep skin again, and make another attempt. DO NOT MAKE REPEATED ATTEMPTS USING THE SAME NEEDLE.

m. If using plastic catheter, withdraw the needle.

(NOTE: Once the catheter has been withdrawn, do not reinsert it into the catheter as it may sever the catheter and cause it to "float" through the circulatory system.)

n. Connect filled tubing to needle/catheter hub, release tourniquet, open tubing clamp and adjust flow to appropriate rate of infusion.
o. Secure needle/catheter with small piece of tape (chevron style). DO NOT place tape directly over venipuncture site.
p. Apply sterile dressing. Two methods are acceptable:
   1) Apply dry, sterile 2 x 2 gauze pad. Secure with tape. Avoid bulky dressing.
   2) Apply semi-permeable transparent dressing following manufacturer's guidelines.
q. Anchor tubing securely to patient's extremity.
r. Record date, time of insertion, type of device and initials of person performing venipuncture on a piece of tape. Attach to IV dressing. Record same information in the clinical record.
s. Label IV tubing with appropriate dated label (per Department of Nursing/Department of Nursing Administrative Policy guidelines) and record date, time and initials on the label.
t. Instruct patient to report signs and symptoms of phlebitis, infection or infiltration (pain, burning, redness, swelling, numbness or fluid/blood seepage).
u. Remove all excess/used supplies and equipment from the patient's room. Dispose of needles and syringes into plastic sharps container; trash into the waste basket.

B. IV Maintenance

1. Inspect IV insertion sites for evidence of phlebitis, pain, infiltration, leakage or blockage at least daily and every time a new IV solution container is hung. If the patient has unexplained fever, pain, or tenderness at the site, the gauze dressing should be removed and the site visually inspected.
2. Change the IV tubing and dressing at the same time the IV site is rotated: EVERY 72 HOURS. Start the IV at another site BEFORE the old set is removed.

(NOTE: This procedure should be accomplished as one maneuver to reduce the amount of manipulation of the system.)

3. When the patient's physician has determined that sites cannot be changed every 72 hours:
   a. Meticulous site care should be performed every 72 hours; more often if indicated.
   b. Document in the clinical records the reason(s) for not rotating the sites, and observations of the site.
4. 250 ml container should be used for "TKO" or "KVO" infusions.
5. Fluid containers must be clearly labeled with patient's name, added medications, and time-stripped for easy monitoring of fluid volume infused.
6. Fluid container must be changed at least every 24 hours.

C. Site Care

1. Remove dressing down to, but not including, chevron tape.
2. Remove old iodophor with alcohol.
3. Cleanse site thoroughly with iodophor solution.

(NOTE: Alcohol may be used for iodophor-sensitive individuals.)

4. Allow to dry. DO NOT remove with alcohol.
5. Redress with sterile dressing.

(NOTE: Site care is to be performed when cannulae are left in longer than 72 hours or when dressing becomes wet or soiled.)

6. Record date of dressing change, date of insertion, type of device, and initials on piece of tape; attach to dressing. Record dressing change in the clinical record with observations of site appearance.

D. Administration of IV Piggyback Medications

1. All piggyback medications should be mixed in the pharmacy.
2. Connect the secondary (piggyback) tubing to the medication container using aseptic technique.
3. Attach secondary tubing to the primary tubing with a needleless connector. Ascertain that connection is secure.
4. Lower the primary infusion container to a level lower than the piggyback container, using the hook provided with the tubing.
5. Set flow rate for proper infusion period.

(NOTE: Infusion periods are listed on the label of all IV piggybacks prepared in the pharmacy.)

6. After infusion of the medication, clamp the secondary tubing, raise the primary container to its original height and leave the secondary tubing connected to the primary tubing.

(NOTE: Secondary tubing can be flushed by lowering the piggyback below the level of the primary bag, flush and drain back into primary tubing.)

7. When ready to administer the next dose, remove the empty bag and replace it with the new one. Fill secondary tubing by lowering the secondary container and opening the clamp on the secondary tubing. Close the clamp and proceed as in 4. and 5. above.
8. When administering more than one medication, and the medications are compatible, follow the procedure outlined in 7. above.
9. When administering incompatible medications, lower the secondary set WITH THE EMPTY MEDICATION CONTAINER ATTACHED and open the clamp on the secondary set. Fluid will flow through the tubing into the previously empty medication container and proceed with steps 4–6 above.

(NOTE: Piggyback tubing is changed every 72 hours, the same as primary tubing.)

E. Administration of Intermittent Infusions

1. Ascertain that the "Heparin Lock" has the appropriate needleless connector component attached.
2. Using a needleless connector component attached to a syringe containing sterile normal saline for injection, connect the syringe to the Heparin Lock and aspirate slightly. If blood return is noted, inject 2–3 cc of normal saline solution to assure patency of the device and to clear device of residual heparin.
3. Attach infusion to heparin lock using a needless connector component.
4. Infuse medication as ordered.
5. At completion of the infusion, unhook the tubing from the heparin lock.
6. Using a needleless connector component attached to a syringe containing heparin solution, connect the syringe to the heparin lock and flush the lock.
7. Discard tubing. A new set of IV tubing will be used for each infusion.

F. IV Infusion Pumps

1. One piece administration sets are recommended. Follow the manufacturer's guidelines for set-up and line flushing procedure.
2. IMPORTANT: Check under site dressing for swelling frequently. Use of a pump increases the risk of extensive infiltration if a needle or catheter becomes dislodged.
3. All surfaces of the pump must be thoroughly cleaned when soiled, and between patients, using a housekeeping disinfectant detergent or product recommended by the manufacturer.

G. If IV-Associated Sepsis Is Suspected

1. Culture any purulent drainage around catheter site prior to cleansing the skin.
2. Cleanse skin around catheter with antiseptic to remove skin organisms.
3. Clip off catheter tip with sterile scissors, dropping catheter into DRY, STERILE specimen cup. Request quantitative cultures of the tip. Send to laboratory IMMEDIATELY to prevent drying and death of organisms.

(NOTE: In addition to routine identification data, culture request should include type of specimen (catheter tip), site of catheter (R forearm), signs and symptoms.)

4. A blood culture should be drawn from the opposite arm after carefully prepping the venipuncture site with iodophor.
5. If IV solution contamination is suspected:
   a. Cap end of IV tubing with a capped, sterile needle.
   b. Send ENTIRE IV set-up and solution container to the laboratory for culture. DO NOT disconnect any part of the set-up.
   c. Call Infection Control IMMEDIATELY (phone 782-4350/4351) to alert them of the problem.

(NOTE: The laboratory will NOT culture IV systems without coordination with Infection Control.)

6. Record observations and actions in the clinical record.
7. Complete WRAMC Form 1811, Quality Control and Risk Management Report, and submit through proper channels.

RECOMMENDATIONS FOR CENTRAL INTRAVASCULAR LINE INSERTION

I. GENERAL

A. Purpose: To provide guidelines to all personnel involved in performing or assisting with the insertion of a central intravascular catheter.

B. References:

1. Miller, S., Sampson, L.K., Soukup, S.M. AACN Procedure Manual for Critical Care, Philadelphia: W.B. Saunders Co., 1985, pp. 47–53.
2. Hospital Infections Program, Center for Infectious Diseases, CDC, Atlanta, Ga., 1985.
3. Nutrition Support Core Curriculum 2nd ed., C. Kennedy Caldwell, P. Guenter, eds., American Society for Parenteral and Enteral Nutrition, 1988.

II. SPECIFIC

A. Equipment

*Caps
*Masks
*Sterile gown(s) for physician(s)
**Sterile gloves (appropriate size)
*Sterile drapes
*Acetone (10%)/alcohol (70%) swabsticks (2 packs of 3)
*Povidone/iodine scrub swabsticks (2 packs of 3)
*Alcohol (70%) swabsticks (2 packs of 3)
*Povidone/iodine solution swabsticks (2 packs of 3)
*1% Lidocaine
*4 x 4s
*2 x 2s
*4-0 silk suture on cutting needle
*22g needle (1)
*10 cc syringes (2)
*20g needle (1)
*25g needle (1)
*Scissors
*Hemostats
Heparin Solution (100 units per cc)
Catheter kit for insertion
Tape
Alcohol wipes

*All items contained in Central Venous Insertion Tray
**Size 7½ gloves in Central Venous Insertion Tray

Also need Central Venous Dressing Tray which contains:
2 prs sterile gloves (size 7½)
Acetone (10%)/alcohol (70%) swabsticks (pack of 3)

Povidone/iodine scrub swabsticks (pack of 3)
Alcohol (70%) swabsticks (pack of 3)
Povidone/iodine solution swabsticks (pack of 3)
Skin prep swabstick
2 x 2 gauze
Sterile cotton tip applicator
Scissors
Masks (2)
Cap
Elastoplast dressing

B. Procedure

1. Explain procedure to patient to promote understanding and minimize anxiety. Obtain written consent (Physician).
2. Organize and assemble supplies and equipment at bedside.
3. Wash hands; turn off faucet with paper towel.
4. Place patient in supine and Trendelenburg position of at least 15 degrees. Place a rolled towel between scapulae with head turned away from insertion site. This positioning promotes maximum filling and distention of the subclavian vein to the angle between the clavicle and the first rib. The increased pressure created in the upper thorax also decreases the possibility of air embolism.
5. Place a mask over patient's mouth and nose (and trach). If patient is unable to tolerate a mask, use a towel or drape as a barrier between patient's mouth/nose/trach and insertion site.
6. Don gown, cap, and mask to avoid contamination of site and equipment. Open and prepare insertion tray.
7. Don sterile gloves and begin preparation of skin for insertion. The area to be prepped should extend from above the clavicle to the nipple line and from the shoulder to just beyond the sternal notch. Cleanse with friction using a circular motion from center to periphery. The following order should be observed.
   a. Start with the acetone/alcohol swabsticks to remove skin fats and oils which may harbor pathogens. It is also effective in removing old tape and glue from previous dressings.
   b. Cleanse area with povidone/iodine SCRUB swabsticks using same friction and circular motion from center to periphery.
   c. Remove povidone/iodine with alcohol swabsticks. The povidone/iodine scrub solution is now contami nated with organisms. If left on skin, it will cause irritation because it contains soap. Again, use a circular motion from center to periphery.
   d. Paint area just prepped with povidone/iodine solution swabsticks. This provides a protective barrier against skin organisms.
8. Apply sterile drapes so that only area not covered is the prepped area.
9. Assist physician in donning mask, cap, sterile gown and sterile gloves.
10. Open catheter kit and drop in sterile tray or allow physician to remove contents.
11. Clean top of heparin flush solution with alcohol wipe and hold for physician to draw up sufficient solution to flush catheter prior to insertion.
12. Physician will insert catheter. Monitor patient during catheter insertion. Assist patient to remain immobile. Notify physician if breaks in aseptic technique are noted. Assist physician as necessary.
13. Catheter should be secured to skin by 4 separate sutures by the physician. This is necessary to minimize movement of the catheter and prevent accidental dislodgement. Line should be sutured in the vertical position. Avoid suturing line horizontally toward the shoulder because of extra stress on the sutures as the patient ambulates.
14. The area around the insertion site and sutures should be reprepped and an occlusive dressing applied using the following steps:
   a. Open Central Venous Dressing Tray.
   b. Don sterile gloves (and cap and mask if not already wearing them).
   c. Using acetone/alcohol swabsticks remove all blood from around the insertion site and sutures. Blood left on the skin may provide medium for bacterial growth.
   d. Reprep the skin by using povidone/iodine scrub swabsticks. Use a circular motion and start at the insertion site, then around the sutures.
   e. Remove povidone/iodine scrub with the alcohol swabsticks starting at the insertion site using a circular motion.
   f. Paint the area with povidone/iodine solution and blot dry with 2 x 2s. Use the cotton tip applicator to remove any extra solution from under the line.
   g. Place folded 2 x 2 over the insertion site and line down to and including the sutures. This is to prevent the occlusive dressing from sticking to the line and sutures.

h. Cut the Elastoplast to fit over the insertion site and sutures. Round all corners and be sure 2 x 2s are completely covered.

15. Remove mask from self and patient. Also remove rolled towel from patient's scapula. Apply skin prep around edge of Elastoplast and tape around the edges of the dressing.
16. Label the dressing with date, time and initials of person doing the dressing.
17. Remove all supplies and wash hands.
18. Ensure that a STAT portable chest X-ray is obtained before ANY infusion is started. The patient is to remain in bed until confirmation of line placement is obtained.
19. Chart the procedure, any problems encountered, patient's tolerance of the procedure, and verification of line placement.
20. Infusions may begin only after verification of line placement. If patient has a triple lumen catheter and is to receive TPN, do not infuse anything through the DISTAL port except TPN. The other two ports may be used to draw blood or infuse other solutions.

III. RELATED CARE

A. Assess and monitor the patient and IV site q2h for complications:

1. Pneumothorax
2. Hemothorax due to subclavian or innominate artery puncture
3. Hematoma at the puncture site
4. Myocardial perforation related to the catheter advancement
5. Infection
6. Phlebitis
7. Thrombosis
8. Air embolism
9. Mediastinal fluid infusion (hydrothorax)
10. Catheter shearing or embolism
11. Brachial plexus injury durıng subclavian catheter placement
12. Osteomyelitis related to subclavian insertion.

B. Maintain catheter asepsis:

1. Change central line dressing every 48–72 hours, or whenever the catheter is changed. If a fever occurs, obtain culture of site and blood cultures.
2. If dressing becomes soiled, disrupted, or non-occlusive, it must be changed.

C. The patient is to remain supine until line placement is confirmed. Reposition the patient following catheter insertion; elevate the head of the bed. Place the patient in the recumbent position when the IV tubing is disconnected from the catheter to minimize the risk of air embolus.

D. Monitor the IV flow rate at frequent intervals; all TPN and IV solutions with medications must be infused via an infusion pump (IMED).

E. Removal of catheter:

1. The recommended duration of a central line is 72 to 96 hours; however, under certain circumstances, a patient's clinical condition may necessitate a central line remaining in a site for a longer period. This is acceptable if proper documentation by the physician is in the Doctor's Progress Note (SF 509) regarding the circumstances, clinical need and the condition of the central line site, and is accomplished on a daily basis.
2. At the earliest sign of sepsis, the central line site should be changed in conjunction with other therapeutic measures.
3. Procedure for removal of catheter when appropriate:
   a. Apply non-sterile gloves. Remove dressing.
   b. Remove the sutures, using a suture removal kit.
   c. Have the patient take a deep breath and hold. Withdraw the catheter out and upward away from the skin.
   d. Inspect the catheter to make sure it is intact.
   e. Using a second sterile suture removal kit, culture the catheter tip if infection is suspected.
   f. Apply pressure to the area to prevent bleeding.
   g. Apply a sterile occlusive dressing.
   h. Assess the patient and monitor for complications after catheter removal.

RECOMMENDATIONS FOR CENTRAL VENOUS CATHETER DRESSING CHANGES

I. GENERAL

A. This procedure guideline applies to all personnel involved in performing or assisting with central venous catheter dressing changes and is the procedure used by the Nutrition Support Service, WRAMC.

B. Frequent use of central lines for monitoring and IV administration of fluids, medications, and/or total parenteral nutrition (TPN) requires a standard and meticulous method of care to minimize the risk of contamination and sepsis. In support of the current literature and national standards, central line dressings will be changed every 24 to 72 hours (depending upon local protocols), whenever the catheter is changed, or when there is drainage and/or sign of infection at the site.

II. SPECIFIC

A. Equipment

1 cap
2 masks
1 clean gown
1 roll of tape
Central Line Dressing Kit Containing:
- 2 pairs of gloves
- 1 triple pack acetone-alcohol swabsticks
- 1 triple pack povidone-iodine scrub swabsticks
- 1 triple pack isopropyl alcohol swabsticks
- 1 triple pack povidone-iodine solution swabsticks
- 1 protective dressing swabstick (skin prep)
- 1 4 x 5 Elastoplast dressing
- 2 2 x 2 cotton gauze sponges
- 1 cotton tip applicator
- 1 pair scissors

B. Procedure

1. Wash hands. Explain the procedure to the patient and/or significant others. Check for povidone-iodine or tape allergy.
2. Organize supplies and equipment at the bedside to decrease the amount of time that the site is open to the air.
3. Don gown, mask and cap. Place the patient in a supine with head turned away from catheter insertion site to decrease potential for contamination by nursing personnel and by patient secretions. Place a mask over patient's mouth and nose (and trach) if patient is able to tolerate. If patient is unable to tolerate the mask, use a towel as a barrier between patient's mouth/nose and insertion site.
4. Open central line dressing kit and don a pair of gloves.
5. Remove present dressing carefully to minimize trauma and prevent accidental dislodgement of catheter. Place soiled dressing in proper trash receptacle.
6. Inspect the skin and catheter site infection, leakage, or other mechanical problems.
7. Don sterile gloves.
8. Cleanse the insertion site with acetone/alcohol swabsticks, working in a circular motion from the insertion site outward to the edge of the dressing border. This removes adhesive material and defats the skin. Repeat 3 times. Do not apply over broken skin.
9. Working in a circular motion from site outward, cleanse the insertion site and distal portion of the catheter with the povidone-iodine scrub swabsticks 3 times to remove bacteria and fungi from the skin and catheter.
10. Working in a circular motion as before, cleanse the site of the povidone-iodine scrub with alcohol swabsticks 3 times to remove the povidone-iodine scrub.
11. Paint a 3 x 6 area from site to periphery with povidone iodine solution swabsticks 3 times. Blot excess or pooled solution. Allow to dry. This provides a protective barrier against pathogens.
12. Place a folded 2 x 2 over the insertion site and line down to and including the sutures. This is to prevent the occlusive dressing from sticking to the line and sutures.
13. Cut the Elastoplast to fit over the insertion site and sutures. Round all corners and be sure 2 x 2s are completely covered.

14. Apply Elastoplast. Paint around edges of Elastoplast with skin prep and tape all around dressing.
15. Tape all connections or ensure that all Luer lock connections are tight. This prevents dislodgement of the tubing from the catheter and reduces the potential for air embolism. Tape edges of dressing, if necessary.
16. Write the date and time of dressing change, and your initials on the dressing. This allows for easy identification and documentation of the interval to change the line and the dressing.
17. Document the dressing change and the condition of the insertion site, the patient's tolerance of the procedure, and any problems encountered in the nursing notes.

C. Related Care

1. Inspect site frequently for signs of infection, inflammation, drainage, and infiltration.
2. Whenever the catheter is changed, the dressing must be changed.
3. IV tubing for TPN must be changed every 24 hours —or every bag change. Dressing should be changed every Monday, Wednesday, Friday or according to local protocol (ie, ICU).

SUMMARY TABLE FOR SITE, DRESSING, AND TUBING CHANGES

I. GENERAL

A. Change all IV fluid containers every 24 hours.
B. Handle all intravascular devices with aseptic technique.

II. SPECIFIC

Duration of Site/Needle	Dressing Change	Tubing Change	Documentation of Appearance of Site
Central (Short Term) According to Protocol	48–72 h	24*–72 h	With dressing change
Central (Long Term) N/A	48–72 h	24*–72 h	24 h
Implanted Devices 6–7 d	48–72 h	24*–72 h	24 h
Peripheral, Arterial 72–96 h	48–72 h	48–72 h	24 h
Peripheral, Intravenous 72 h	72 h	72 h	24 h
Piggyback Meds, Continual Infusion 72 h	N/A	72 h	N/A
Piggyback Meds, "Heparin Lock" 72 h	N/A	Each infusion	N/A

*With every new bag of TPN or every 72 h for all other fluids

Chapter 24

THE SYNDROMES OF SYSTEMIC INFLAMMATORY RESPONSE AND MULTIPLE ORGAN DYSFUNCTION

DANIEL P. STOLTZFUS, M.D.*; AND JAMES A. GEILING, M.D.†

*Formerly, Major, Medical Corps, U.S. Army; Staff Anesthesiologist, Staff Intensivist, Anesthesia and Operative Services, Walter Reed Army Medical Center, Washington, D. C. 20307-5001; currently, Assistant Professor of Anesthesiology, University of Florida College of Medicine, Gainesville, Florida 32608-1197; Co-director, Surgical Intensive Care Unit, Veterans Affairs Medical Center, P. O. Box 100254, Gainesville, Florida 32610-0254

†Lieutenant Colonel, Medical Corps, U.S. Army; Chairman, Pulmonary and Critical Care Service, Landstuhl Regional Medical Center (Landstuhl, Germany), APO, AE 09180

INTRODUCTION

Sepsis is a systemic response to an infectious process. An infection, usually caused by Gram-negative enteric bacilli, initially provokes a localized beneficial inflammatory response. However, if bacteria invade the surrounding tissue (thus gaining access to the bloodstream) and elicit an acute systemic inflammatory response by the host, myriad organ and systemic dysfunctions, possibly culminating in death, can ensue. Gram-positive organisms usually associated with suppuration, viruses, fungi, rickettsiae, and protozoa can also cause this systemic response. It is the systemic response—especially when it is manifested by cardiovascular shock and progressive, sequential dysfunction of multiple organs—that differentiates bacteremia or localized infection from sepsis. Diagnosis of an infection, however, may not be easy, as fever, leukocytosis, and a hyperdynamic "septic" state may naturally occur soon after injury.[1] Furthermore, everyday clinical use of words such as "infection" and "sepsis" does not always make this distinction.

Compounding this semantic imprecision is the confusion that the signs and symptoms themselves introduce. The signs and symptoms seen when sepsis is associated with bacterial infection are indistinguishable from those seen with noninfectious inflammatory states. Clinical conditions that mimic sepsis include pulmonary atelectasis, pulmonary emboli, hematomas, tissue necrosis, transfusion reactions, myocardial infarction, hypotension or hypovolemia from an ongoing occult hemorrhage, spinal shock, central fever, or drug fever.[1] Although infection often occurs in patients with these conditions, the conditions themselves must be considered as possible causes for a patient's deteriorating condition. Therefore, paradoxically, some patients seem to have sepsis but no microorganisms can be cultured.

In an attempt to both address the paradox and clarify the meaning of the constellation of terms revolving around "sepsis," the American College of Chest Physicians and the Society of Critical Care Medicine held a joint consensus conference in August 1991. The *Textbook of Military Medicine* uses their recommended definitions and guidelines (Exhibit 24-1).[2] The Consensus Conference introduced a new term that provides an overall conceptual and practical rubric: the systemic inflammatory response syndrome (SIRS).

The relationship of SIRS to sepsis can be demonstrated in a Venn diagram that comprises three overlapping populations (Figure 24-1): (*a*) infection, in which most of the population has neither sepsis nor SIRS; (*b*) sepsis, which is a subgroup of the infection population that by definition also has SIRS; and (*c*) SIRS, which comprises both those with sepsis and those in whom there is no apparent infectious process. The Consensus Conference recommended that sepsis be defined as the clinical condition that exists when the systemic inflammatory response state is due to *infection*, the most common cause for SIRS. For this reason, the term sepsis/SIRS will be used in this chapter.

The two most severe pathophysiological consequences of SIRS are septic shock (the most severe circulatory derangement caused by sepsis) and multiple organ dysfunction syndrome (MODS, the sequential and progressive failure of two or more organ systems). Although the terms "multiple system organ failure" and "multiorgan failure" are also to be found in the literature, this chapter uses MODS, the terminology adopted by the Consensus Conference.[2] The term SIRS/MODS, which reflects the intense relation of SIRS and MODS, will also be used.[3] MODS is most often associated with sepsis (any diffuse inflammatory stimulus may act as the initiating event), with a temporal relation to septic shock (Exhibit 24-2 and Figure 24-2).

This definition and description of MODS should not be applied to the casualty with multiple trauma who has concomitant injuries to more than one organ system. Such *primary* MODS should be distinguished from MODS that is *secondary* to sepsis/SIRS with the concomitant release of endogenous vasoactive mediator substances and is associated with such systemic manifestations of sepsis as hypotension and hypermetabolism.

EPIDEMIOLOGY

To understand the etiology and treatment of SIRS/MODS, it is first necessary to understand the circumstances in which it arises (ie, its epidemiology). The most extensive experience with this syndrome has been in civilian medicine, for not only is that patient population much larger than the population encountered by military medicine, but the conditions for providing care are much more suitable for making clinical observations. Furthermore, the military experience with SIRS/MODS is epi-

EXHIBIT 24-1

DEFINITIONS OF TERMS

Infection	Microbial phenomenon characterized by an inflammatory response to the presence of microorganisms or the invasion or normally sterile host tissue by those organisms.
Bacteremia	The presence of viable bacteria in the blood.
SIRS	*Systemic inflammatory response syndrome*; the systemic inflammatory response to a *variety* of severe clinical insults. The response is manifested by two or more of the following conditions: (1) temperature > 38°C or < 36°C, (2) heart rate > 90 beats per minute, (3) respiratory rate > 20 breaths per minute or Pa_{CO_2}< 32 mm Hg, or (4) leukocyte count > 12,000 mm^3, < 4,000/mm^3, or > 10% immature (band) forms.
Sepsis	The systemic response to infection; manifested by two or more of the following conditions as a result of *infection*: (1) temperature > 38°C or < 36°C, (2) heart rate 90 beats per minute, (3) respiratory rate > 20 breaths per minute or Pa_{CO_2} < 32 mm Hg, or (4) leukocyte count > 12,000 mm^3, < 4,000/mm^3, or > 10% immature (band) forms.
Severe Sepsis	Sepsis associated with organ dysfunction, hypoperfusion, or hypotension. Hypoperfusion and perfusion abnormalities may include, but are not limited to, lactic acidosis, oliguria, or an acute alteration in mental status.
Septic Shock	Sepsis-induced, with hypotension despite adequate fluid resuscitation, along with the presence of perfusion abnormalities that may include, but are not limited to, lactic acidosis, oliguria, or an acute alteration in mental status. Patients who are receiving inotropic or vasopressor agents may not be hypotensive at the time that perfusion abnormalities are measured.
Sepsis-Induced Hypotension	A systolic blood pressure < 90 mm Hg or a reduction of ≥ 40 mm Hg from baseline in the absence of other causes for hypotension.
MODS	*Multiple organ dysfunction syndrome*; the presence of altered organ function in an acutely ill patient such that homeostasis cannot be maintained without intervention.

Data source: Bone RC, Balk RA, Cerra FB, et al. The American College of Chest Physicians/Society of Critical Care Medicine Consensus Conference Committee. Definitions for sepsis and organ failure and guidelines for the use of innovative therapies in sepsis. *Chest*. 1992;101:1644–1655.

sodic, depending on the random occurrence of wars. Nevertheless, the military experience with sepsis/SIRS has been of disproportionately great importance to understanding this syndrome: observations made by military physicians led to the initial concepts of the renal and pulmonary components of MODS.[4,5]

The Civilian Experience

Sepsis/SIRS and the related pathological conditions of septic shock and MODS occur in 5 to 10 of every 1,000 hospitalized patients; the rate for patients admitted to intensive care units (ICUs) is increased by 10-fold.[6,7] This equates to 100,000 to 500,000 new cases per year in the United States, with 70,000 to 300,000 cases per year arising from Gram-negative infections alone.[6,8] Of these, approximately 200,000 will develop septic shock with a mortality rate of about 50%.[8] The prevalence of SIRS/MODS appears to be increasing as a consequence of (*a*) the population of patients now receiving treatment and (*b*) advances in medicine; for example,[6]

- the care being given to an ever-increasing aged population with their associated chronic diseases;

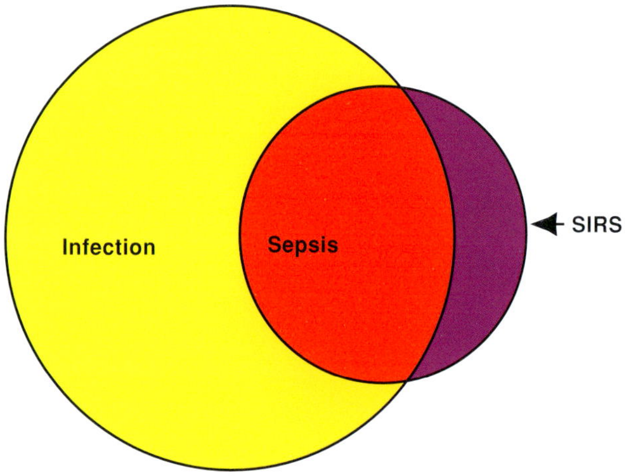

Fig. 24-1. In this Venn diagram showing the interrelation of infection, sepsis, and the systemic inflammatory response syndrome (SIRS), the large circle represents the population with infection and the small circle represents the population with SIRS. The intercept—sepsis—represents the subpopulation who have both infection and SIRS. Note that some patients with SIRS do not have sepsis. Data source: Bone RC, Balk RA, Cerra FB, et al. The American College of Chest Physicians/Society of Critical Care Medicine Consensus Conference Committee. Definitions for sepsis and organ failure and guidelines for the use of innovative therapies in sepsis. *Chest*. 1992;101:1645.

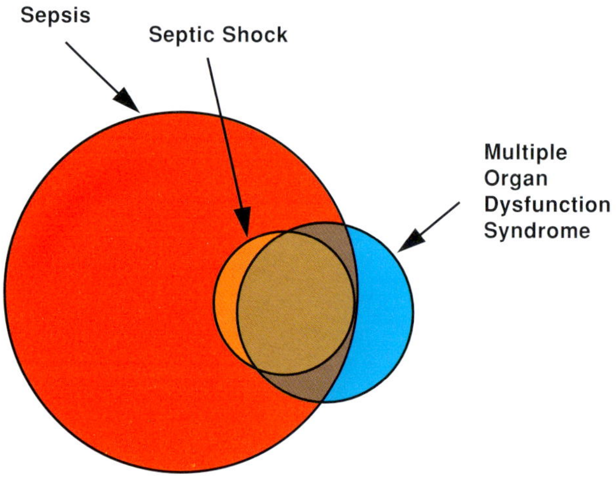

Fig. 24-2. This Venn diagram represents the interrelation of sepsis, septic shock, and multiple organ dysfunction syndrome (MODS). By definition, all patients with septic shock have sepsis, but not all patients who develop MODS have sepsis as the etiology.

- the numbers of immunocompromised patients (steroidal or chemotherapy, transplantation, human immunodeficiency virus [HIV] disease) now receiving care;
- the widespread use of antibiotics with subsequent development of resistant bacterial strains,
- an increased number of patients surviving severe trauma; and perhaps
- the sophistication, increased invasiveness, and aggressive use of current medical diagnostic procedures, interventions, and treatments.

EXHIBIT 24-2

KNOWN ETIOLOGY OF SEPSIS/SIRS

Microbial Agents
- Bacteria
- Viruses
- Fungi, protozoa, rickettsiae, etc

Gram-Negative Bacterial Component
- Endotoxin

Tissue Inflammation Caused by
- Multiple trauma
- Pancreatitis
- Long-bone or pelvic fractures
- Aspiration pneumonitis
- Adult respiratory distress syndrome

Tissue Hypoperfusion
- Distributive shock

The Military Experience

During peacetime, the epidemiology of sepsis and its related conditions is the same in the civilian and military healthcare systems with the important distinction that the military population consists of young, healthy individuals who are less likely to become ill compared to the civilian population as a whole. During wartime, injuries and diseases that may predispose to the development of sepsis have a high prevalence. In U.S. Army, attrition (as assessed by hospital admissions) has been due predominantly to disease and nonbattle injury and not due to injury that resulted from combat. The ratio of admissions to admissions for combat-related injuries ranged from 16:1 during World War I to 88:1 during World War II.[9] Most of these admissions were for relatively minor illnesses and injuries that occurred outside the combat zone and rarely progressed to a septic state.

In contrast to the 18th and 19th centuries, death due to septic consequences of disease and nonbattle injuries has been less common during the 20th century. However, given special circumstances such as the influenza pandemic of 1917 to 1919, sepsis can be the leading cause of mortality. For example, of the 3,264,694 enlisted personnel who were admitted to the hospital for disease from April 1917 through December 1919 in the United States and Europe, 51,447 died of disease compared with 50,385 deaths caused by combat.[10–12] The most common sepsis-related disorders causing death during this period (1917–1919) included general septicemia, broncho- and lobar pneumonia, and suppurative pleurisy.[11] Although disease-related death rates have decreased in subsequent wars, diseases accounted for a large proportion of all U.S. Army hospital admissions during the Vietnam War (1965–1970): from a high of 74% in 1965 (when diseases accounted for 5,697 of 7,682 hospitalizations) to a low of 56% in 1968 (when diseases accounted for 51,082 of 91,417 hospitalizations).[12,13]

Traumatic Injury

Traumatic battle injuries pose a major threat to combat forces—vastly greater than anything seen in the civilian experience. Severe injuries often result in death. On the basis of the civilian experience with trauma, it is possible to categorize deaths from injury into three categories, based on the time of death in relation to the time of injury. *Immediate* deaths are caused by massive trauma, aortic rupture, decapitation, and so forth. These can only be prevented by measures designed to prevent trauma (eg, public safety measures, safer cars and airplanes). *Early* deaths occur during the first hour following injury and are caused by posttraumatic conditions such as hypovolemic shock or tension pneumothorax. These conditions can be effectively managed only by individuals or institutions capable of providing early interventions and therapy. (It is this category of deaths that has been the focus of the Advanced Trauma Life Support Course sponsored by the American College of Surgeons.) *Late* deaths occur during the first week after traumatic injury. Two major causes are irreversible brain injury and sepsis.[14,15] The civilian experience has been that from one third to one half of all trauma deaths fall in the *late* category. SIRS/MODS progressing to organ failure is important for anesthesiologists and critical care specialists to understand because

- the syndrome is a major cause of death from civilian trauma,
- the potential for live-saving intervention is real, and
- the need to develop effective means of prevention and treatment cannot be overemphasized.

The potential that combat-related deaths can be reduced through improved prevention and management of SIRS/MODS is less favorable. In contrast to the civilian experience, most combat-related deaths (70%–80%) are early (this is the category called *killed in action*) and only about 10% of the total fatalities occur during treatment in a hospital (*died of wounds*). By far most combat deaths are due to hemorrhage or mutilating brain injury.[16] This population does not live long enough to develop sepsis. SIRS/MODS is the cause of death in about one third of those who die while being treated (or perhaps 5% of all fatally wounded soldiers).

Trauma-Related Sepsis and Septic Shock

The traumatized combat victim is at great risk for developing sepsis. A civilian study of 437 trauma patients who sustained both blunt and penetrating injuries revealed that more than three fourths of deaths that occurred after 7 days resulted from sepsis and MODS.[15] In another study, almost 90% of deaths after 7 days in patients sustaining blunt trauma were shown to be related to sepsis.[17] And in patients sustaining thermal injury or trauma, at least 75% of deaths may, in part, be due to sepsis.[18]

Military data on posttraumatic sepsis are best delineated in statistics describing the U.S. Army's experience in World War II and the Korean and Vietnam Wars. The decrease in the died-of-wounds rate—from 8% in World War I to the overall 4.5% recorded in World War II—has been attributed to the prevention of sepsis in extremity wounds by earlier and more extensive surgery. As expected, shock and hemorrhage were the major causes of death among the hospitalized wounded, followed by infection (especially in the peritoneal cavity). Other cases of unrecognized sepsis may well have occurred in those patients whose cause of death was described as myocardial failure, anuria, pulmonary edema, or atelectasis.[19]

The incidence of true septic shock was not described outside these categories. However, in 1944 in the Fifth U.S. Army, the deaths of 1,273 hospitalized soldiers were attributed to shock. Of these, 34% resulted from trauma and hemorrhage in association with documented sepsis. An additional 22% might appropriately be included: those patients without recognized sepsis but who had, in addition to trauma and hemorrhage, what was then called cardiorespiratory embarrassment.[19] The severity and complexity of combat-related wounds, then, portends a particularly significant risk for the development of infection and sepsis. MODS and eventual death are common among those who sustain severe war wounds and who survive long enough to reach a medical treatment facility. The U.S. Army's most recent extensive experience was during the Vietnam War. Data on the causes of hospital deaths show that sepsis and its complications probably caused about one third of the deaths (Figure 24-3).[20]

Most individuals deployed for possible combat are relatively young and healthy. Thus, soldiers generally do not have the medical illnesses that predispose to the development of sepsis (eg, diabetes mellitus, hepatic cirrhosis, chronic renal insufficiency, underlying malignancies, and inherited or acquired immunological defects).[21,22] But larger mobilizations that employ personnel not on active duty will most certainly include individuals whose underlying illnesses will become manifest. Illnesses acquired during military operations, principally infectious diseases such as malaria, will alter the host's immunoregulatory function in such a way that bacterial sepsis may be likely to occur. The fatigue, stress, and loss of sleep associated with combat maneuvers may also be associated with an increased incidence of infection.[23]

As trauma management continues to improve, more patients remain alive 2 or 3 days after injury. Infection during these first several days is rare, but increases in prevalence thereafter. Most cases of SIRS/MODS in the military will occur in casualties with multiple injuries whose infectious complications are caused by some or any of the following predisposing factors:

1. contaminated, open injuries (ie, penetrating thoracic or abdominal wounds, open fractures, or burns), which have a high propensity for infection and the subsequent systemic responses; for example, penetrating abdominal trauma results in an infection rate of 14% in patients without hemorrhagic shock (among patients with hemorrhagic shock, the infection rate increases 2- to 2.5-fold)[24];
2. depression of both the humoral and the cell-mediated immune systems, which traumatic injury causes[1];
3. compromised host defenses, which can be caused by medications such as steroids and the use of parenteral nutrition[1]; and
4. transfused blood products, which can spread such viral infections as hepatitis B and C, as well as HIV.[1]

Prolonged stay in an ICU increases the incidence of nosocomial infections as a consequence of the use of endotracheal tubes, intravascular and in-dwelling urinary catheters, and other monitoring and support systems. Therapies including hyperalimentation, antibiotics, and dialysis also contribute to the development of infection because normal

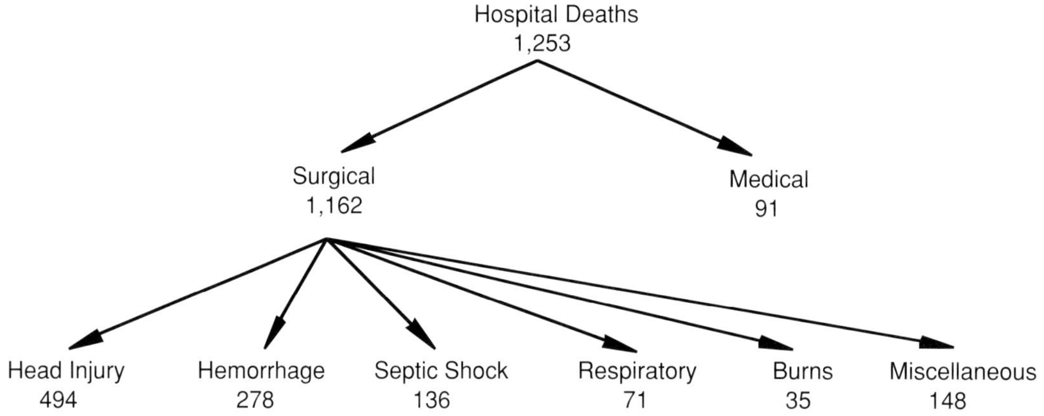

Fig. 24-3. The causes of death for 1,253 casualties who were hospitalized in Vietnam in 1969. The "miscellaneous" category includes entries such as fat embolism, 24; acute renal failure, 15; quadriplegia, 15. Data source: Arnold K, Cutting RT. Causes of death in United States military personnel hospitalized in Vietnam. *Milit Med*. 1978;143:161–164.

skin and mucosal physical barriers to infection are broken by these devices. Contamination of these devices during insertion or use can also result in superinfection.[25]

As a consequence, after 3 days in a surgical ICU, 50% of patients become colonized with potentially pathogenic bacteria, and by 10 days, 95% of patients acquire new flora.[26] In a study done between 1977 and 1984 at the Shock Trauma Center, Maryland Institute for Emergency Medical Services Systems (MIEMSS) in Baltimore, Maryland, 1,407 patients (14% of total admissions) developed 2,310 documented infections.[1] Among trauma patients who survived their initial injury, 22% to 63% developed one or more infections, with a 41% to 65% mortality. Once the patient contracted an infection, the duration of stay in the ICU increased from 7.4 to 13.5 days. The five leading infections in this study were, in order of frequency, urinary tract infections, pneumonia, surgical-wound infections, phlebitis, and intraabdominal infections. Patients with pneumonia or intraabdominal infection had mortality rates of 29% and 25%, respectively.[1] Most nosocomial infections in surgical patients occur in the urinary tract, the surgical wound and skin, and the respiratory tract.[27] Tabulated data from 82 hospitals show the frequencies of these infections to be 39%, 32%, and 16%, respectively.[28] The causative organisms vary somewhat with the location. Across all services (medical and surgical), *Escherichia coli* is the most prevalent pathogen and *Staphylococcus aureus* the second most common. The second most prevalent pathogen on medical and general surgical services alone is *Pseudomonas aeruginosa*. (*Enterococcus* is the second most common on gynecological and obstetrical services.[25])

Infections in trauma patients were well described in the MIEMSS study. The most frequent pathogens were *S aureus* (25%), *E coli* (13%), *P aeruginosa* (10%), *Enterobacter* species (10%), and *Klebsiella* species (9%). Gram-positive cocci were causative alone or partially involved in 43.9% of the infections, Gram-negative bacilli in 66.8%, anaerobic bacteria in 9.3%, and yeast in 1.5%. Nationwide, the pathogen most frequently found in the traumatized patient is *S aureus*.[1]

The true incidence of sepsis resulting from trauma is difficult to glean from the literature. At MIEMSS, of the more than 10,000 patients admitted during the study period, 1,407 developed 2,310 infections, 900 (39%) of which were documented cases of bacteremia.[1] The mortality rate of patients with bacteremia was 21%. Additional studies reported an 8.3% incidence of sepsis with bacteremia in 300 trauma patients,[29] and a 17% incidence in 200 patients.[30] Thus among trauma patients, the incidence of bacteremia with subsequent sepsis is 10% to 20%.[1]

Other sources of bacteremia in trauma patients in the MIEMSS study include vascular infections (22%), pneumonias (14%), intraabdominal infections (10%), empyemas (9%), and wound infections (8%). The vascular infection rate may have been underestimated, as it is only a recent practice to culture the tips of intravenous lines. An additional 21% of cases were without a definite source.[1]

The organisms resulting in bacteremia were similar to those causing all diagnosed infections. *Staphylococcus aureus* was the most common, resulting in 35% of the cases of bacteremia. Others were *Klebsiella* (12%), *Enterobacter* (10%), *Pseudomonas aeruginosa* (8%), and *Escherichia coli* (9%).[1]

Microbes in the bloodstream are the consequence of, or perhaps lead to the development of, overwhelming infection. Two separate complications arise from the systemic circulation of microorganisms[31]:

1. Organisms are seeded throughout the body, with subsequent formation of microscopic or even macroscopic abscesses.
2. A systemic effect occurs as a consequence of the mere presence of the organism or organism components (eg, the cell wall) in the bloodstream. This activates a cascade of inflammatory and endocrinological events that produce the systemic deterioration seen in sepsis, the final stage of which is septic shock.

Cellular and Subcellular Mechanisms Leading to SIRS/MODS

SIRS/MODS is now believed to result from the patient's systemic response to the growth of microorganisms at what is initially a localized site of infection (the *nidus*). Various components of microorganisms (eg, the cell wall), or substances elaborated by microorganisms (eg, toxins) are now thought to provoke the cellular components of blood (eg, monocytes and neutrophils) that are responsible for the normal immune response. The normal immune response results in the formation of endogenous mediators, which, if overproduced, have many deleterious pathophysiological effects (eg, myocardial depression and peripheral vascular vasodilation). Shock, MODS, and possible death then ensue.[32] Figure 24-4 is a schematic representation of this sequence of events.

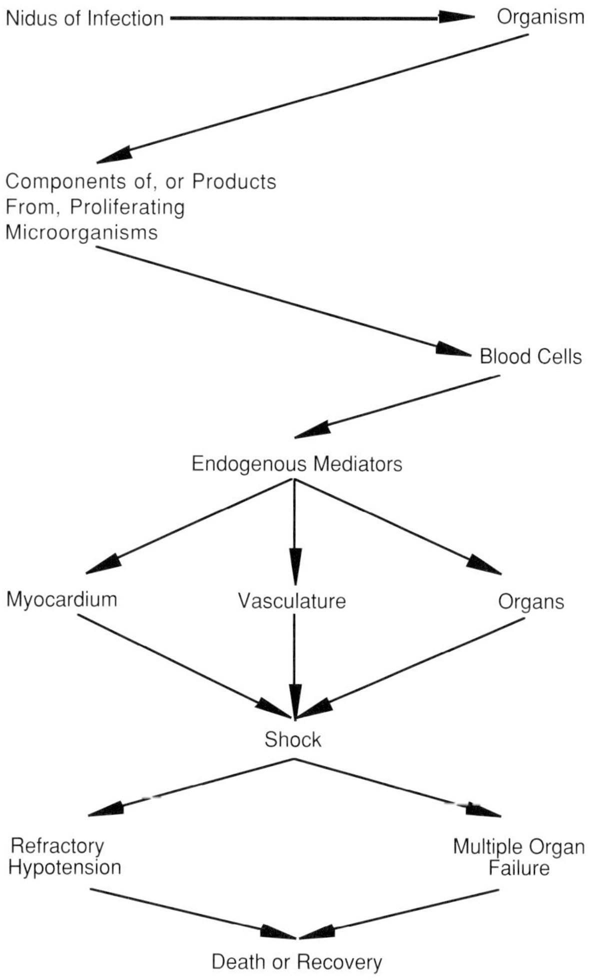

Fig. 24-4. Schematic showing important steps by which infection can cause shock, multiple organ failure, and death. Endogenous mediators released from normal cellular constituents of the blood play a crucial role. Adapted with permission from Parrillo JE. Pathogenetic mechanisms of septic shock. *N Engl J Med*. 1993;328:1472.

By emphasizing the primacy of the host response, this paradigm advances our understanding of the origins of the deleterious consequences of sepsis. The immune system, which normally protects the host, releases endogenous mediators as part of its "normal" inflammatory response to infection. Such detrimental phenomena as cell and organ damage and death seem to result from the immune system's hyperresponsiveness to the insult.

Components and Products From Microorganisms Giving Rise to SIRS/MODS

The most notorious toxins produced by microorganisms include the neurotoxin of food-borne botulism, the neurotoxin that causes tetanus, the cardiotoxin of diphtheria, and the various histotoxins produced by species of *Clostridium*. These toxins, which are secreted by Gram-positive bacteria, are polypeptides with specific tissue targets. In contrast, *endotoxins* (literally, toxins from within) are normal constituents of the cell wall of Gram-negative bacteria; they are injurious to humans in the clinical setting that we now recognize as sepsis/SIRS. In fact, the most widely studied triggering event for sepsis/SIRS is the presence of endotoxin.

Endotoxin, from inside to outside the cell wall, comprises Lipid A, the core polysaccharide, and the O Antigen (Figure 24-5). In addition, endotoxin has one chemically unique constituent, the strange sugar molecule *Kdo* (3-deoxy-D-manno-2-octulosonic acid), which is found in all endotoxins and links the core polysaccharide to lipid A.[33] It is important to recognize that the peptidoglycan/teichoic acid complex of the cell wall of Gram-positive organisms, as well as the polysaccharide constituents of certain yeasts, have toxicity similar to that of endotoxin. As Lewis Thomas described in 1974, endotoxin is not only a strange substance chemically, it also provokes a violent and frequently self-destructive response in humans and other animals:

> Our arsenals for fighting off bacteria are so powerful, and involve so many different defense mechanisms, that we are in more danger from them than from invaders. We live in the midst of explosive devices; we are mined.
>
> It is the information carried by the bacteria that we cannot abide.
>
> The gram-negative bacteria are the best examples of this. They display lipopolysaccharide endotoxin in their walls, and these macromolecules are read by our tissues as the very worst of bad news. When we sense lipopolysaccharides, we are likely to turn on every defense at our disposal; we will bomb, defoliate, blockade, seal off, and destroy all tissues in the area. Leukocytes become more actively phagocytic, release lysosomal enzymes, turn sticky, and aggregate together in dense masses, occluding capillaries and shutting off the blood supply. Complement is switched on at the right point in its sequence to release chemotactic signals, calling in leukocytes from everywhere. Vessels become hyperreactive to epinephrine so that physiologic concentrations suddenly possess necrotizing properties. Pyrogen is released from leukocytes, adding fever to hemorrhage, necrosis, and shock. It is a shambles.
>
> All of this seems unnecessary, panic-driven. There is nothing intrinsically poisonous about endotoxin, but it must look awful, or feel awful, when sensed by cells. Cells believe that it signifies the presence of gram-negative bacteria, and they will stop at nothing to avoid this threat.[34(p92)]

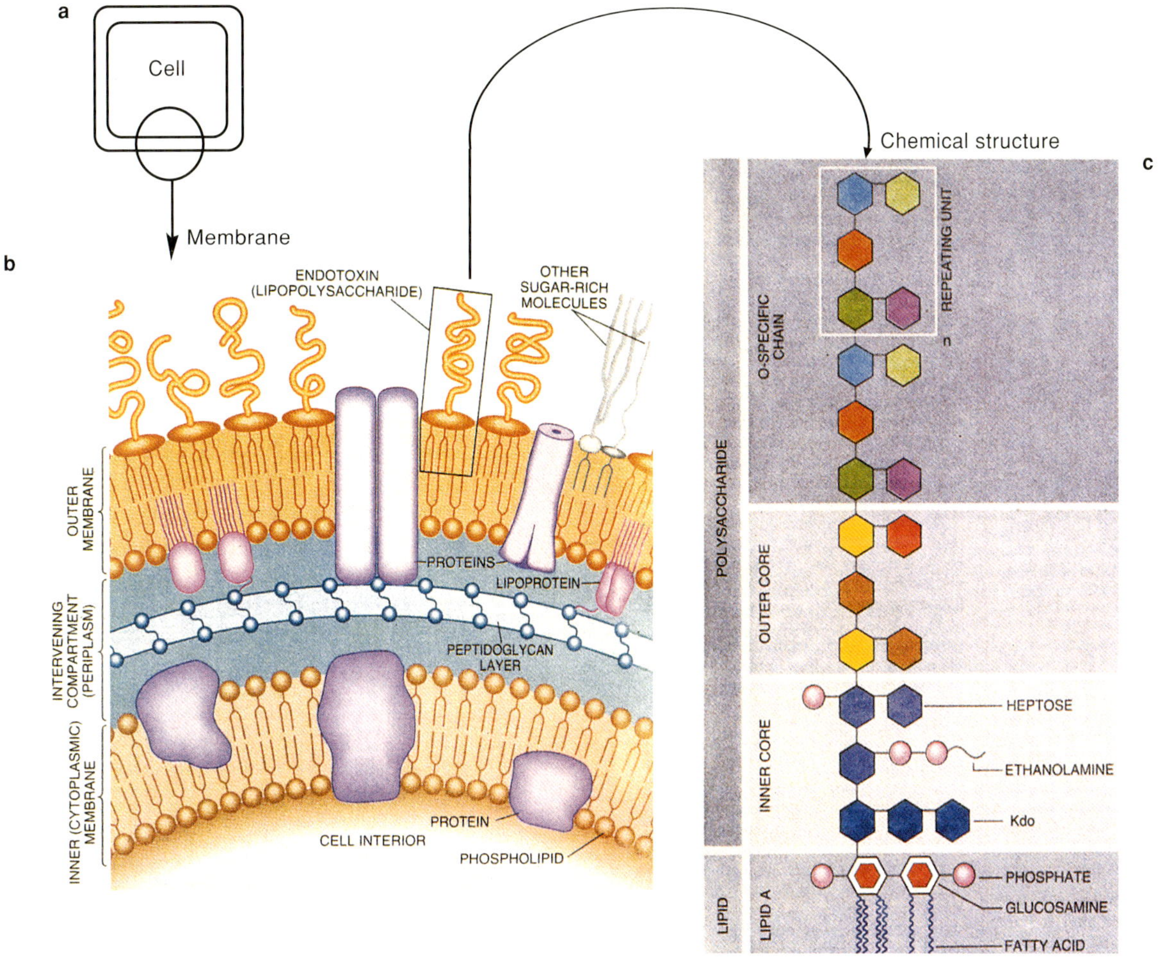

Fig. 24-5. The cell membrane of a Gram-negative bacterium, diagrammed at successively higher magnifications. (**a**) The cell wall, composed of two layers of lipids. (**b**) Endotoxin in its normal position in the outer membrane. (**c**) The chemical composition of the endotoxin. There are two important moieties: (1) a polysaccharide known as the O-chain and (2) a fat called lipid A. Several sugar molecules of unusual composition are found at the polysaccharide–lipid A junction. Lipid A, together with the sugar 3-deoxy-D-manno-2-octulosonic acid, is the portion of the endotoxin molecule that is responsible for its pathophysiological effects. Reprinted with permission from Rietschel ET, Brade H. Bacterial endotoxins. *Sci Am*. 1992;August:56, 57.

Until recently, data had been accumulated only from animal studies, but prospective assays reported in 110 patients with shock show a 43% incidence of endotoxemia in septic shock, compared with a 10% incidence in shock from other causes.[35] Patients who had endotoxemia developed organ failure 10-fold more frequently than other patients, indicating that the damaging role of this compound is significant.

Cellular Components Contributing to SIRS/MODS

It is now generally agreed that endotoxin by itself is not the direct cause of the pathophysiology of sepsis/SIRS. Rather, its effect is mediated through a variety of cells both in the blood and in tissue.

Mononuclear Cells

The mononuclear phagocyte system is composed of (*a*) bone marrow–derived monocytes that circulate in the blood stream and (*b*) tissue macrophages such as the hepatic Kupffer cells and pulmonary alveolar macrophages.[36,37] These blood and tissue macrophages appear to be the essential cellular components required for the development of sepsis and SIRS/MODS. As part of the inflammatory process, resting macrophages exposed to stimuli such as T cell–produced interferon gamma (IFN-γ) or lipopolysaccharide (endotoxin) from Gram-negative–organism cell walls are activated into larger, more metabolically active cells. These activated macrophages secrete lysozyme, proteases (collagenase and elastase), plasminogen activator, interleukin-1 (IL-1), various leukotrienes, and cytokines such as tumor necrosis factor (TNF).[34]

Polymorphonuclear Cells

An interaction occurs between activated macrophages and polymorphonuclear leukocytes (PMNs). Human alveolar macrophages, and perhaps others, secrete a neutrophil activating factor that appears to enhance the PMNs' bactericidal activity by causing a greater release of superoxide. This interaction likely contributes to further host-tissue damage and inflammation.[36]

Protection of the host against many infections depends greatly on both the absolute number and the functions of PMNs, including chemotaxis, adherence, phagocytosis, and the eventual destruction of the ingested microorganism.[36] It is during the killing of the phagocytized organisms that the neutrophil may release substances that are toxic to the host, resulting in injury to the host (the patient).

Polymorphonuclear adherence to vascular endothelial sites (leukostasis) contributes to vascular injury in inflammation, particularly in the lung, and may also explain the initial neutropenia noted in some patients with sepsis.[36,38–40] To be effective, the PMNs must act at the site of microbial invasion. Chemotaxis or directed migration to the inflammatory nidus occurs in response to many agents, including oligopeptides produced by the invading organism, complement factor C5a induced by both the organism and the accumulated neutrophils, and leukotriene B_4 produced by on-site neutrophils.[37] After the neutrophil's phagocytosis, a respiratory burst within the PMN contributes to the inflammatory response in the following three ways:

1. The increased oxygen consumption of this respiratory burst is associated with the increased production of lethal oxidants (superoxide anion, hydrogen peroxide, hypochlorous acid, the hydroxyl radical, and the hydroxyl anion).
2. Lipid metabolism results in the production of thromboxane, leukotrienes, platelet activating factor, and leukotoxin.
3. The PMN degranulates.

The inflammatory process in the host is activated and propagated by these mechanisms. The various mediators released by the neutrophil, in particular the oxygen radicals, are not specific for foreign antigens. Thus the host tissues are susceptible to the toxic effects of these substances. This is a major factor in the adverse response to infection.

In the adult respiratory distress syndrome (ARDS), the abundance of neutrophils retrieved from a bronchoalveolar-lavage sample is evidence for the central role that neutrophils play.[41] In contrast, few neutrophils are recovered from bronchoalveolar lavage in patients with non-ARDS respiratory failure. Abundant neutrophils are a component of syndromes other than ARDS, however: ARDS can also occur in neutropenic patients. Neutrophils in the pulmonary circulation have been shown to release several harmful byproducts (eg, collagenase, myeloperoxidase, and elastase) that may cause systemic injury.

Lymphocytes

Specifying the host's immunological response to invading pathogens is the role of the lymphocyte. The full response requires an extensive interaction between these lymphocytes and macrophages. Lymphocytes are subdivided into T lymphocytes, which make up 70% of all mononuclear cells, and B lymphocytes, which, along with natural killer cells and monocytes, comprise the remaining 30%.[42]

T lymphocytes direct cell-mediated immunity in the host and exist in two forms:

1. helper/inducer or cluster of differentiation (CD) 4+ cells, which enhance the host's immunological response by supporting T-T cell, T-B cell, and lymphocyte–macrophage interactions; and
2. suppressor or CD8+ cells, which inhibit B cell–antibody production and, hence, diminish immunological function.

Antibody-mediated (humoral) immunity is governed by the differentiation of B lymphocytes into plasma cells that are capable of secreting antibodies. Antigens processed by the macrophage are presented to B cells specific for that particular antigen, based on the antigen binding site (Fab segment) on the B lymphocyte's membrane-bound immunoglobulin. The degree of B cell and plasma-cell clonal expansion is controlled by helper and suppressor T cells.[43]

Macrophages are known to interact with both T and B cells at inflammatory sites. An interaction between T cells and the macrophage causes the T cell to secrete lymphokines (eg, IFN-γ, macrophage inhibitory factor, monocyte chemotactic factor, IL-2) and the macrophage to release monokines (including IL-1 and TNF).[37] These lymphokines also modulate the host's immunological response by their effects on other lymphocytes, macrophages, neutrophils, and invading organisms.[43]

Endogenous Mediators

Much of the current experimental and clinical research is directed toward finding the endogenous mediators produced by cells that link such pathophysiological derangements as septic shock and MODS to microorganisms and their endotoxins. The two leading candidates at present are a group of small-molecular-weight proteins known as cytokines and the eicosanoid metabolites of arachidonic acid.

Cytokines: Tumor Necrosis Factor and the Interleukins

TNF (also called *cachectin*)—a small polypeptide protein with a molecular weight about 17,000—is released when endotoxin stimulates blood or tissue macrophages, endothelial cells, and lymphocytes. Its effects include

- enhancement of the immune system,
- hypotension due to a decrease in peripheral vascular resistance,
- loss of fluid from the vascular bed (caused by an increase in both the systemic and pulmonary capillary permeability),
- a variety of metabolic changes (eg, lipolysis and increased amino acid loss from skeletal muscle), and
- the long-term acceleration of wound healing.

Many of these changes are virtually identical to those observed with endotoxin, including fever, shock, and lactic acidosis. Several studies have identified a prime role for TNF in clinical sepsis or MODS:

- Intravenous injection of human recombinant TNF into laboratory rats[44] and dogs[45] results in hypotension, shock, metabolic acidosis, and death due to respiratory arrest within hours. Autopsy showed many of the same findings seen in patients who had died of MODS.[46]
- The administration of monoclonal antibodies to TNF almost completely prevents obvious organ injury in most animal models of septic shock including those in which endotoxin is also administered.[47]
- TNF produces myocardial cell dysfunction in an animal model[48] and may be the substance responsible for myocardial depression in human sepsis/SIRS.[49]

Studies on humans with sepsis have begun to provide support for the paradigm that views TNF as the proximate cause of SIRS:

- Serum levels of TNF are significantly higher in patients with sepsis who ultimately developed septic shock, compared with patients who did not develop shock.[50]
- Patients who died of sepsis within 25 hours of starting treatment for septic shock had TNF levels nearly 20-fold greater than those who die later.[50]
- TNF production from monocytes taken from trauma victims correlated with septic episodes.[51]

Interleukin-1 and Interleukin-2

IL-1, which can be thought of as an endogenous pyrogen, is classified as a *monokine*, which is produced when a macrophage is stimulated by bacteria. The effects of this mediator include hypothalamic stimulation, producing fever, leukocytosis, an increase in the hepatic acute-phase reactants (eg, C-reactive protein), and an increase in muscle proteolysis. An intravenous infusion of IL-1 in laboratory animals results in the hemodynamic appearance of septic shock. The exact contribution of IL-1 in the pathophysiology of MODS is unknown.

IL-2 is a macrophage product that has been administered to patients with metastatic cancer as part of immunotherapy. Administration of IL-2 causes hemodynamic changes that mimic the sepsis syndrome. Furthermore, case reports have described patients who developed organ failure during immunotherapy with IL-2.[52,53]

Eicosanoids: The Arachidonic Acid Metabolites

Eicosanoid is the generic term for the leukotriene, prostaglandin, and thromboxane metabolites of arachidonic acid (a polyunsaturated fatty acid). For the most part, they are potent but short-lived molecules produced by all nucleated cells anywhere in the body. Endothelial cells, macrophages, and platelets produce eicosanoids in areas where microorganisms have invaded tissue, a feature that is of special importance to the study of sepsis.

Given any number of stimuli such as hypoxia, damaged vascular endothelium, and especially the liberation of cytokines, free arachidonic acid is liberated from the phospholipid component of the cell membrane, from which it diffuses into the cytosol. Depending on the cell type, arachidonic acid becomes the substrate for one of two enzymes: lipoxygenase or cyclooxygenase (Figure 24-6). Lipoxygenase catalyses the formation of the leukotriene eicosanoids, while cyclooxygenase forms multiple eicosanoids, of which the most important are thromboxane A_2, prostacyclin (prostaglandin I_2), and prostaglandin E_2.

Of the myriad biological effects associated with eicosanoids, the effects most likely to be relevant to our understanding of sepsis/SIRS are those caused by

- the leukotrienes, which cause alterations of neutrophil function leading to increased chemotaxis, synthesis of the superoxide anion radical, increased microvascular permeability, vasoconstriction, and bronchoconstriction;
- thromboxane, which causes platelet aggregation and vasoconstriction;
- prostacyclin, which causes platelet disaggregation and vasodilation; and
- prostaglandin E_2, which causes intensive pulmonary and systemic vasodilation, hyperalgesia, and fever.

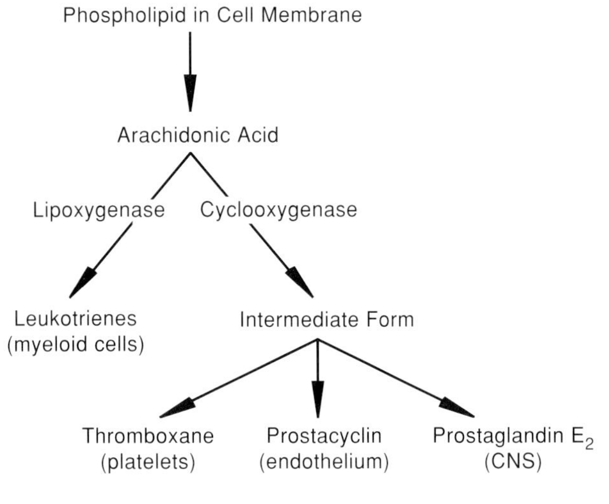

Fig. 24-6. The origin and partition of several biologically important eicosanoids. Note that arachidonic acid can be acted on by two enzymes: (1) lipoxygenase, which gives rise to the leukotrienes, and (2) cyclooxygenase, which gives rise to thromboxane, prostacyclin, and prostaglandin E_2, which have markedly different physiological effects.

The leukotrienes have the ability to cause many of the pathophysiological changes that are seen in sepsis/SIRS. However, there are two reasons why the eicosanoids produced by the lipoxygenase pathway are less likely to be important than those produced by cyclooxygenase:

1. The enzyme lipoxygenase is present only in myeloid cells, whereas cyclooxygenase is present in all cells.
2. Lipoxygenase, in contrast to cyclooxygenase, is normally inactive and needs to be "turned on" before any eicosanoids are produced.

Several lines of evidence support the role of the cyclooxygenase metabolic products of arachadonic acid in the development of sepsis/SIRS. Putative reasons for the involvement of phospholipids as endogenous mediators of sepsis/SIRS have been the subject of considerable research.[54] Many of the signs and symptoms of sepsis/SIRS such as fever and shock can be replicated by eicosanoids. For example, elevated levels of thromboxane B_2 have been measured in patients with sepsis, but whether a cause-and-effect relationship exists is unclear at present. Some of these findings include the following:

- There is less hemodynamic compromise and increased survival when thromboxane is inhibited.[55]
- In human volunteers, ibuprofen lessens the signs and symptoms associated with endotoxin administration.[56]
- Ibuprofen normalizes hemodynamic indices in dogs with experimental sepsis.[57]
- Pulmonary permeability edema decreases in a large-animal sepsis model using ibuprofen to inhibit the cyclooxygenase pathway.[58]

Prostacyclin, because of its strong vasodilator properties, may be the mediator of the peripheral vasodilation seen in most cases of human septic shock—although why its effect should predominate over that of its antagonist, thromboxane, is unclear.

The ability of prostaglandin E_2 to cause hyperpyrexia relates to its direct effect on the thermoregulatory center in the hypothalamus. The activity of the enzyme cyclooxygenase is decreased by drugs that contain or are metabolized to salicylic acid (eg, aspirin). The antipyretic action of aspirin depends on its ability to decrease the formation of prostaglandin E_2. The same mechanism—inhibition of cyclooxygenase—explains the analgesic effects of aspirin: prostaglandin E_2, which is known to sensitize nerve endings to noxious stimuli, is not produced.

Unfortunately, the most recent and methodologically valid study of the role of eicosanoids in humans with severe sepsis failed to show a clear-cut advantage from pharmacologically blocking the formation of eicosanoids with the nonsteroidal antiinflammatory drug ibuprofen. Although fever, blood pressure, heart rate, and oxygen transport were at least partially normalized in the treated patients, the researchers found no decrease in mortality compared with control patients.[59] These negative findings suggest that the cascade of mediators causing systemic response and sepsis is so complex that blockade of only one component will not result in improved patient survival.

Endorphins

A role in the pathogenesis of sepsis/SIRS for endogenous opioids, of which β endorphin is the best known, was first proposed in 1977 by researchers at Walter Reed Army Institute of Research, Walter Reed Army Medical Center, Washington, D. C. Naloxone, an antagonist of β endorphin, was shown in a rat model to reverse the hypotension that was caused by endotoxin.[60] Significant species differences exist; in baboons, for example, hypotension from endotoxin is not reversed by naloxone.[61] Studies in which naloxone is given to humans with septic shock have shown transient reversal of hypotension but no effect on survival.[62,63] Even though β endorphin levels rise with trauma,[64] the attention paid to endogenous opioids in the pathogenesis of septic shock should probably be minimized, because these substances do not give rise to the hyperdynamic and vasodilated state that characterizes human septic shock.

Free Radicals

Free radicals are chemical entities that contain one or more unpaired electrons in their outermost molecular orbitals. Their chemical activity is markedly heightened compared with molecules with paired outermost electrons. Most free radicals are derived from oxygen (a not-unsurprising situation given the prominence of oxygen in our environment and our dependence on oxygen for the energy-producing processes necessary for life). Nearly all the oxygen that enters into the normal mitochondrial production of adenosine triphosphate is converted to water by the near-simultaneous addition of four electrons. However, in a process known as the *univalent leak*, about 1% of the oxygen molecules normally undergo a four-step reduction that involves the addition of one electron at a time. Each time an electron is added, a different type of oxygen-derived free radical is formed. These are, in order of their generation: the superoxide anion radical ($O_2^{\bar{\bullet}}$), the hydroperoxyl radical ($HO_2\bullet$), hydrogen peroxide (H_2O_2), and the hydroxyl radical ($OH\bullet$). Although hydrogen peroxide itself is not a free radical, it is rapidly converted into the hydroperoxyl and hydroxyl radicals.

Mammalian cells normally contain substances with strong antioxidant properties, of which the enzymes *superoxide dismutase* and *catalase* are best known; these enzymes prevent the intracellular accumulation of the toxic free radicals. Superoxide dismutase catalyzes the conversion of the superoxide anion radical to hydrogen peroxide, while catalase catalyzes the conversion of hydrogen peroxide to water. When these antioxidants function properly, they prevent the generation of the hydroperoxyl and hydroxyl radicals and thereby minimize the potential for oxygen-derived free-radical injury.

Superoxide dismutase and catalase effectively minimize oxygen-derived free-radical injury except in two circumstances: the first is during the reperfusion phase, when blood flow is normalized following shock, ischemia, or hypoxia; the second, paradoxically, is when neutrophils are activated as part of their normal function (ie, they display their respiratory burst). The generation of free radicals presumably evolved for a beneficial purpose: the destruction of foreign objects such as bacteria by phagocytic cells. Neutrophils and macrophages have on their cell membranes a liberal amount of the enzyme *nicotinic acid diphosphohydrogen oxidase*, which, when activated by any of several endogenous mediators such as TNF, generates superoxide anion radicals and hydrogen peroxide. At the same time, the enzyme *myeloperoxidase* is released by the cell and catalyses the formation of hypochlorous acid from hydrogen peroxide and chloride ions in the cell's neighborhood. Hypochlorous acid kills bacteria. The effect is twofold: not only does the neutrophil's respiratory burst produce lethal oxidants, but it also contributes to the inflammatory response by generating thromboxane, leukotrienes, platelet activating factor, and leukotoxin.

Increasingly, the generation of oxygen-derived free radicals in shock, ischemia, and hypoxia is believed to be a major source of the injury that characterizes these conditions. Although all constituents of a cell are at risk, the lipid-containing membranes appear to be especially sensitive to destruction because of the self-propagating nature of free-radical attack on the polyunsaturated fatty acid portion of the cell wall. Reaction of a free radical with a polyunsaturated fatty acid not only chemically alters the fatty acid but also generates new free radicals—lipid peroxides—that incorporate into parts of the original fatty acid. Two different free-radical attacks are possible. First, the *hydroperoxide* pathway generates two free radicals for every lipid molecule destroyed. Second, the *endoperoxide* pathway generates three free radicals. Thus, rapid dissolution of cell membranes occurs in a process reminiscent of the chain reaction that characterizes atomic fission.

Nonoxygen-derived free radicals may also play a role in the pathophysiology of sepsis/SIRS. One of the most significant recent advances in vascular physiology is the recognition that normal vascular endothelium produces a potent vasodilator. This was subsequently shown to be nitrogen monoxide in one or more of its three forms: the free radical nitric oxide (NO•), the nitrosonium cation (NO^+) or the nitroxyl anion (NO^-).[65] The vasodilator property of TNF has been shown to be dependent on the presence of normal vascular endothelial cells, suggesting that nitric oxide may be the proximate cause of the hypotension associated with sepsis.[66] In fact, high concentrations of the metabolites of nitric oxide have been described in patients with clinically apparent sepsis, but not in trauma patients or controls who did not have sepsis. Furthermore, the concentrations of these metabolites was inversely related to the peripheral vascular resistance.[67] These data suggest that increased production of nitric oxide may be a causative factor in the development of septic shock. Specific blockers of the generation of nitric oxide have been tried in patients in septic shock.[68] Although the patients' hypotension was ameliorated, their survival was not enhanced (which is not too surprising given that hypotension by itself is one of the several derangements that occur in septic shock).

Additional Mediators

Complement. The alternate pathway of complement is known to be activated by endotoxin and other bacterial products. The resultant release of C3a and C5a leads to neutrophil stimulation and the following adverse effects, which are seen in patients with sepsis/SIRS:

- increased vascular permeability,
- histamine release,
- release of tissue proteases leading to autocatabolism, and
- development of oxygen free radicals.

Fibronectin. Fibronectin is an endogenous compound that functions like an opsonin (ie, it enhances phagocytosis). In concert with the reticuloendothelial system, fibronectin helps to clear particulate matter from the circulation. Many studies have shown that depletion of fibronectin occurs in a state of multiple trauma, shock, or sepsis. Fibronectin, in the form of cryoprecipitate, has been administered to patients who then demonstrate a slight improvement in their hemodynamic status. Because cryoprecipitate is a multidonor product, carrying with it a significant risk for the transmission of infectious agents, great skepticism surrounds the advisability of using it in the treatment of SIRS/MODS.

Platelet Activating Factor. Platelet activating factor can be released from leukocytes, macrophages, or the vascular endothelium. The two effects of this agent are (1) the induction of platelet and neutrophil aggregation and (2) stimulation of the arachidonic acid pathway, causing the release of eicosanoid compounds.

Stress Hormones. Several hormones are released during a state of physical stress, which characterizes the "fight or flight" survival response. These include glucagon, hydrocortisone, epinephrine, growth hormone, and thyroid hormone. One hypothesis concerning this neuroendocrine secretion is that vascular or organ damage may occur when states of hypermetabolism and negative nitrogen balance are created.

Cascade of Events Leading to SIRS/MODS

For SIRS to become fully developed, multiple endogenous mediators and several different types of cells interact in ways that result in a continuous amplification of the original stimulus provided by

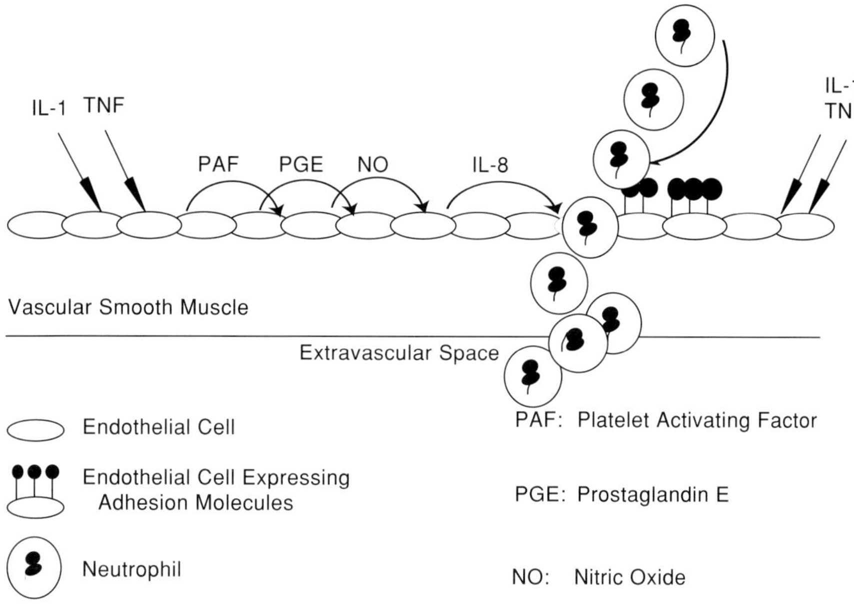

Fig. 24-7. Schematic showing the putative interaction of several endogenous mediators (interleukin-1 [IL-1] and tumor necrosis factor [TNF]) and the vascular endothelium. The mediators cause the endothelium to generate the potent vasodilators nitric oxide (NO) and prostaglandin E (PGE), as well as platelet activating factors (PAF). The mediators also cause a substance (endothelial adhesion molecule) to be formed that attracts circulating neutrophils. The neutrophils become activated and generate oxygen-derived free radicals and other substances that damage the microcirculation and contiguious cells. Reprinted with permission from Dinarello CA, Gefland JA, Wolff, SM. Anticytokine strategies in the treatment of the systemic inflammatory response syndrome. *JAMA.* 1993;269(14):1830.

endotoxin. This cascade of events (Figure 24-7) appears to follow this sequence[69]:

- TNF and IL-1 stimulate endothelial cells to produce nitric oxide, prostaglandin E_2, IL-8, and the platelet activating factor.
- Nitric oxide and prostaglandin E_2 produce vasodilation and hypotension.
- IL-8 and the platelet activating factor cause neutrophils to adhere to the endothelial cells and then to migrate to the extravascular space.
- Cells are damaged by the release of oxygen-derived free radical from the extravascular neutrophils. If the cellular damage is sufficiently extensive, organ dysfunction will occur.

ORGAN-SPECIFIC RESPONSES

If the effects of this cascade are confined to the local area of microorganism growth and tissue invasion, it is probably advantageous to the patient. However, if the endogenous mediators and their effects become systemic, as may occur in human bacteremia and sepsis/SIRS, then functional impairment of one or more organs can be expected, a process that may culminate in a perpetuating organ injury.

Cardiovascular Response

Cardiovascular and hemodynamic dysfunction in septic shock have been the subjects of much interest and debate since the 1950s. Two subsets of patients were initially described in the setting of Gram-negative bacteremia. The differentiating factor was postulated to be their *cardiac index* (the amount of blood ejected by the heart in a unit of time, divided by the body surface area, and usually expressed in liters per minute per square meter). Patients presumed to have a low cardiac index had cold, clammy skin with weak and thready pulses, while warm, dry skin and bounding pulses were attributed to a high cardiac index.[70] In 1956, an animal model of intravenously administered endotoxin elicited a syndrome similar to that ascribed to low cardiac index (hypotension with a depressed cardiac index). Most early studies with animals and humans reported a characteristic hemodynamic profile of septic shock, particularly in those cases with a poor prognosis: one of depressed cardiac output with associated increased systemic vascular resistance.[71]

By the mid-1960s, however, the usual hemodynamic pattern seen in septic shock in humans was reported to be one of normal or increased cardiac index with an associated low systemic vascular resistance.[72] Subsequent studies have confirmed that this pattern is the usual cardiac profile seen early in patients in septic shock.

In retrospect, the occurrence of these two hemodynamic patterns is probably iatrogenic; specifically, the therapy affected ventricular preload. Therapy during the early 1960s was likely to be associated with an inadequate restoration of ventricular preload, which therefore led to an inadequate cardiac index. It was thought then that fluid therapy in septic shock had to be judicious, for vigorous fluid resuscitation resulted in pulmonary edema. In reality, much of the lung fluid may have been related to ARDS, a phenomenon of increased pulmonary capillary leakage that is most often a consequence of sepsis. With greater understanding of ARDS and with the introduction of the pulmonary artery catheter (also called the Swan-Ganz catheter), patients with depressed cardiac indices were found to have low left ventricular preload, as estimated by pulmonary capillary wedge pressure (PCWP). Thus, in attempting to prevent the development of pulmonary edema, too little volume or preload was utilized, thereby depressing the cardiac index.[73,74] With the PCWP as a guide to left ventricular preload, infusion of large amounts of fluids to compensate for the septic shock–induced vasodilation and capillary leakage results in a pattern of elevated cardiac index in more than 90% of patients in septic shock.[73]

Hemodynamic Data Derived From Clinical Investigation

Despite the hemodynamic pattern described above, patients who die in septic shock were thought by many to manifest a falling cardiac index and progressive acidosis before they die.[71] Although this mechanism of death appears plausible, whether systemic hypoperfusion was the cause or the effect remained to be proven.[73]

To more thoroughly investigate serial cardiovascular variables, 48 consecutive patients with hypotension and blood cultures positive for bacteria were evaluated.[75] With a pulmonary artery catheter in place, hypotension was managed with fluids, then dopamine, and finally levarterenol (norepinephrine) as needed to maintain a mean arterial pressure of at least 60 mm Hg. Hemodynamic variables were recorded for any change within the first 24 hours, and at least daily until the patient either recovered or died. Of the 60% of patients who died, three fourths had irreversible hypotension. Eighty percent of this hypotensive group died with a persistently elevated cardiac index and decreased systemic vascular resistance. The remaining patients died of continued worsening cardiac index and heart failure. All these hypotensive patients died within 7 days of the onset of shock. The remaining patient (who died after the 7th d), died as a consequence of MODS. Thus, death from refractory hypotension due primarily to a low cardiac index is not common. The more likely cause of early death in patients with sepsis is refractory hypotension associated with a low systemic vascular resistance.

Early studies that predicted the outcome of patients in septic shock were conflicting, with some showing a progressive fall in cardiac index and worsening of a metabolic acidosis prior to death, others showing no difference from the initial hemodynamic profile between survivors and nonsurvivors. One study[71] showed that patients with an extreme elevation in cardiac index (> 7.0 L/min/m^2) had a very poor prognosis. Another[75] revealed that an initial heart rate less than 106 beats per minute, and a rate at 24 hours of less than 95 beats per minute predicted survival. An initial hyperdynamic response was found in both survivors and nonsurvivors, although survivors tended to return toward a more normal hemodynamic state over the first 24 hours, with a decrease in heart rate of at least 18 beats per minute or a decrease in cardiac index of at least 0.5 L/min/m^2. Nonsurvivors tended to have a persistently low systemic vascular resistance and an elevated cardiac index and heart rate.[75] Persistent vasodilation may be the result of systemic absorption of previously mentioned mediators.

Myocardial Dysfunction

Early studies of myocardial dysfunction correlated a low cardiac index, particularly in the setting of an elevated central venous pressure, with myocardial depression. More sophisticated monitoring has added other means of evaluating ventricular function (ie, left ventricular stroke work index

[LVSWI] in response to volume infusion). Further calculation of oxygen delivery and consumption data has been proposed by some as a more accurate reflection of the adequacy of cardiac function.[71]

Radionuclide cineangiography was first introduced in the evaluation of patients with sepsis in 1981.[76] This technique was used in patients with septic shock and was reported in 1984.[77] Of the 20 patients evaluated, 13 survived. Survivors and nonsurvivors alike were found to have the characteristic hemodynamic profile seen in septic shock: an elevated cardiac index with a decreased systemic vascular resistance. The left ventricular end diastolic volume index (LVEDVI) was also evaluated (stroke volume index determined from thermodilution cardiac index divided by the radionuclide-determined ejection fraction); this is a more accurate indicator of left ventricular preload than is PCWP, because the real determinant of left ventricular ejection is *volume* (myocyte stretch) not intraventricular *pressure*. Survivors were noted initially to have a depressed ejection fraction, which returned to normal in 7 to 10 days. This reduced ejection fraction was associated with an increased end diastolic volume index, which also returned to normal in 7 to 10 days. Thus, in survivors, the initial decrease in ejection fraction was associated with left ventricular dilation. This pattern of depressed ejection fraction with increased LVEDVI has been subsequently confirmed in other studies using two-dimensional echocardiography.[73] Thus, the increased cardiac index that occurs despite myocardial depression is the result of both an increased heart rate and a normal or slightly elevated stroke volume. Gross dilation of the left ventricle, which is usually considered to be a pathological process, can be considered to be a compensatory mechanism in septic shock, for it allows the maintenance of a more normal stroke volume and, hence, cardiac output. Interestingly, nonsurvivors maintained a normal ejection fraction and left ventricular end diastolic indices because the left ventricle ejects against the pathologically low afterload of a dilated systemic vascular bed.

An increased cardiac index in sepsis requires adequate preload. In 1977, researchers demonstrated that compared with survivors of septic shock, nonsurvivors of septic shock had significantly depressed ventricular performance curves. That is, LVSWI in nonsurvivors was depressed in response to volume infusion as monitored by the PCWP.[78] More recently, ventricular performance curves using LVEDVI, rather than PCWP, as a measure of preload were studied in three groups of patients—controls, hemodynamically stable patients with sepsis, and patients in septic shock.[79] In response to volume infusion, both groups of patients with sepsis had decreased LVSWIs compared with controls, and demonstrated no further increase in ventricular performance when the PCWP exceeded 18 mm Hg. Volume administration with PCWP as a guideline may not achieve the expected improvement in left ventricular performance because left ventricular end diastolic pressure (LVEDP) is not related to LVEDVI by a simple linear relation.

Left ventricular diastolic dysfunction also appears in sepsis. Compared with normal controls, patients with sepsis, both with and without shock, were shown to have abnormal diastolic filling (Figure 24-8).[80] Echocardiographic and pulsed-wave Doppler studies were characterized by an increase in peak atrial velocity, increased atrial filling fraction, and prolongation of the atrial filling period as a function of the diastolic filling period. Septic patients may have an increased dependence on atrial systole for diastolic filling.

Right ventricular dysfunction also occurs in patients with sepsis and appears to be independent of right ventricular afterload. In a study of right ventricular function in 25 patients in septic shock, utilizing radionuclide ventriculography as well as catheterization of the right side of the heart, 13 had a depressed right ventricular ejection fraction.[81] As expected, right ventricular dysfunction occurred in patients with respiratory failure or increased pul-

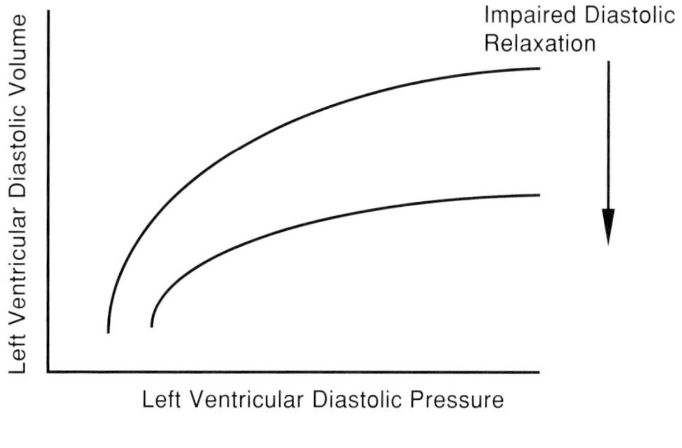

Fig. 24-8. This schematic drawing shows the relation between left ventricular diastolic pressure and volume for two different states of left ventricular compliance. The upper curve represents normal diastolic relaxation, while the lower curve represents impaired diastolic relaxation. Note that for any given filling pressure, the ventricle with impaired relaxation has a smaller filling volume. The arrow shows the direction of increasing impaired relaxation.

monary arterial pressures. However, in many of the patients, the degree of dysfunction was out of proportion to right ventricular afterload. While 8 of the 13 patients had concomitant decreases in left ventricular performance, the ejection fraction was normal in 5 patients.

In one study,[82] significant right ventricular systolic dysfunction, as defined by decreased ejection fraction and right ventricular dilation, was seen in all patients in septic shock. Nonsurvivors appeared to have depressed right ventricular performance because of a decrease in contractility, as manifested by a marked increase in end-systolic volume without significant change in right ventricular afterload. Apparent diastolic dysfunction of the right ventricle was also suggested by the downward displacement of the pressure–volume curves.

Depressed biventricular function and biventricular dilation was noted in another study[83] of 38 patients in septic shock; these abnormalities returned to normal within 7 to 14 days. In this study, 31 patients (82%) with depressed right ventricular function had simultaneous left ventricular dysfunction. Thus, the myocardial depression seen in septic shock is a biventricular phenomenon.[71]

The mechanism of myocardial dysfunction has been attributed to either ischemia secondary to inadequate coronary perfusion or the presence of a circulating humoral factor that depresses myocardial contractility.[84] Studies that evaluate coronary sinus blood flow and myocardial metabolism have demonstrated neither decreased coronary blood flow nor increased myocardial lactate production. High coronary sinus oxygen saturation with a low myocardial oxygen extraction is similar to the arteriovenous shunting seen peripherally in septic shock. Thus, septic shock does not appear to cause myocardial dysfunction by decreasing cardiac perfusion.[71]

Myocardial Depressant Factor

A circulating humoral substance that results in myocardial depression has been proposed for many years. This myocardial depressant factor has been reported in animal models and in a number of bioassays that utilize plasma or serum from patients in septic shock. In 1985, using a bioassay of beating newborn rat heart-cell cultures, researchers[85] described a circulating myocardial depressant substance or factor in patients with septic shock. To accomplish this, the researchers imaged and analyzed the leading edge of the beating rat myocardial cells, and recorded the extent and velocity of shortening. The cells were bathed in sera from 20 patients with septic shock. The sera were then assayed for evidence of a depressant factor. In a comparison study[71] with sera from three different groups of patients, sera from the patients in the acute phase of septic shock caused the least myocardial cell shortening. Of note, there was a significant correlation between this decrement in vitro and the measured left ventricular ejection fraction in vivo. This temporal and quantitative association between the in vitro results and the clinical myocardial depression noted in vivo appears to validate the presence of a circulating myocardial depressant factor in patients with septic shock.[71] Revisions in this assay and subsequent studies have confirmed the association between myocardial depression in these patients and a circulating substance that decreases myocardial contraction in vitro.[84]

A plethora of septic shock mediators has been evaluated for myocardial depressant activity, of which TNF and endotoxin have been found to be the most potent.[35,48] Other mediators that may contribute, determined from both animal models and humans, include prostaglandins, histamine, IL-1 and IL-2, and platelet activating factor. No one substance appears to be the universal myocardial depressant substance. Rather, myocardial depression probably occurs as a consequence of many mediators that may work synergistically.[71]

Regardless of the actual etiology, survival of septic shock appears improved when the patient's left ventricle dilates sufficient to maintain cardiac output in the presence of decreased contractility, due to the circulating myocardial depressant substance. Presumably, the ventricles of nonsurvivors could not dilate sufficiently to compensate for the decrease in contractility caused by the circulating myocardial depressant substance.

Pulmonary Response

The best known clinical manifestations of sepsis/SIRS are arterial hypoxemia and respiratory failure. As the lung is probably the first organ to manifest physiological derangement from sepsis, the astute clinician will be alerted early to the onset of sepsis, ideally *before* shock occurs. Why should the lung be injured so frequently during sepsis? The following statements are among the possible explanations[86]:

- The lung is a source of marginated polymorphonuclear leukocytes.

- All of the body's venous return passes through the lung.
- The lung is exposed to blood-borne mediators and endotoxin.

Clinical Features

The association between lung injury and sepsis is perhaps best typified by ARDS, a frequently fatal pulmonary condition. This association has been known since 1967, when this constellation of clinical signs resulting from a variety of pulmonary insults was first described.[87] In the proper clinical setting, the presence of ARDS can be inferred from tachypnea and dyspnea, a decrease in pulmonary compliance, and refractory hypoxemia and diffuse alveolar radiological densities. The full-blown syndrome does not always develop; lesser degrees of impairment of pulmonary function can occur. Hypoxemia during sepsis is frequent and occurs prior to the onset of pulmonary edema or other changes characteristic of ARDS. Minimally, most patients will manifest both an increased intrapulmonary shunt, resulting in mild-to-moderate hypoxemia, and an increased physiological deadspace, resulting in an elevated minute ventilation.

Pathophysiology

Most of the data presented here are the results of experiments on animals. Studies on humans are difficult or impossible to conduct for the following reasons:

- Pulmonary dysfunction in patients is frequently not recognized early.
- There are no laboratory markers to chart the course of impending pulmonary injury during sepsis.
- When ARDS does develop, it frequently occurs quickly following the onset of sepsis.
- Histological examination of the lung in the early phases of sepsis is only possible in the animal model.

Although the exact incidence of pulmonary dysfunction during sepsis in humans is unknown, the incidence is probably higher than was reported previously.[86] As is true for other conditions in the critically ill patient, the reported incidence depends on the diagnostic criteria. This is particularly important because the terms "sepsis," "sepsis syndrome," "septic shock," and "hypermetabolism" have been used imprecisely and have been confusing to many clinicians.

The clinical situation of sepsis-induced pulmonary dysfunction is complex and is not due simply to the presence of a single endogenous mediator or an inflammatory response. Many factors may contribute to the development of hypoxemia during sepsis (Exhibit 24-3).

Perhaps the earliest demonstration of pulmonary dysfunction in the septic animal model is an increase in airway resistance.[88] Decreased dynamic compliance occurs within hours and precedes both radiographic and clinical evidence of pulmonary parenchymal disease. Increases in airway reactivity have been demonstrated in humans even during the recovery phase of ARDS. Bronchoconstriction is likely the result of release, either locally or systemically, of endogenous mediator substances in response to endotoxin (in the Gram-negative sepsis models).

Prominent among these mediators are the byproducts of arachidonic acid metabolism, including the well-described vasoconstrictor thromboxane A_2 and the leukotrienes. Other mediators include complement and the proteolytic enzymes and superoxide radicals generated locally by pulmonary neutrophilic sequestration. This leukocytic sequestration occurs within minutes of an endotoxin infusion.[88] Supporting evidence for the role of these compounds in the development of increased airway reactivity is (*a*) the presence of eicosanoids in lung lymph flow and (*b*) the partial attenuation of abnormal mechanics when prostaglandin antagonists, or nonsteroidal antiinflammatory drugs are administered. The polymorphonuclear leukocyte is not, however, an absolute prerequisite for the development of ARDS; this syndrome has also been described in neutropenic oncology patients.[89]

In animal models, pulmonary hypertension also occurs early after endotoxin infusion.[88] Clinical experience in patients with existing pulmonary artery catheters at the time sepsis develops supports the frequency with which this physiological alteration also occurs in humans. Once again, the most likely etiology for pulmonary vasoconstriction is the arachidonic acid metabolites. Increased amounts of thromboxane has been recovered from animals' pulmonary lymph flow following endotoxin administration. The origin of the release of thromboxane is unclear as the depletion of both neutrophils and platelets does not prevent the onset of pulmonary hypertension.

An increase in the pulmonary capillary permeability is probably the most widely recognized pul-

EXHIBIT 24-3

CAUSES OF HYPOXEMIA DURING SEPSIS

Endogenous mediator-induced bronchoconstriction[1]

Ventilation–perfusion mismatch due to maldistribution of ventilation, exacerbated by positive-pressure ventilation[2]

Increased shunting due to loss of regional hypoxic pulmonary vasoconstriction[3]

Increased pulmonary vascular permeability leading to interstitial and alveolar pulmonary edema[3]

Pulmonary hypertension and increased cardiac output leading to an increased gas exchange surface area in the presence of poor ventilation[3]

Increased oxygen consumption, both systemically and in respiratory muscles[4]

Respiratory muscle fatigue[5]

Alveolar collapse due to decreased surfactant[6,7]

Sources: (1) Esbenshade AM, Newman JH, Lams PM. Respiratory failure after endotoxin infusion in sleep: Lung mechanics and lung fluid balance. *J Appl Physiol.* 1982;54:967–976. (2) Norwood S. Physiologic principles of conventional mechanical ventilation. In: Kirby RK, Banner MJ, Downs JB, eds. *Clinical Applications of Ventilatory Support.* New York, NY: Churchill Livingston; 1990: 145–171. (3) Brighman KL. Specific organ function/dysfunction in sepsis: Pulmonary. In: Sibbald WJ, Spung CL, eds. *Perspective and Sepsis and Septic Shock.* Fullerton, Calif: The Society of Critical Care Medicine; 1986: 147–156. (4) Griffel MI, Asiz ME, Rackow EC, Weil MH. Effect of mechanical ventilation on systemic oxygen extraction and lactic acidosis during early septic shock in rats. *Crit Care Med.* 1990;18(1):72–76. (5) Hussain SN. Respiratory muscle fatigue: A cause of ventilatory failure in septic shock. *J Appl Physiol.* 1985;58:2031–2033. (6) Pison V, Obertacke U, Brand M, et al. Altered pulmonary surfactant in uncomplicated and septicemia-complicated courses of acute respiratory failure. *J Trauma.* 1990;30(1):19–26. (7) Oldham KT, Guice KS, Stetson PS, Wolfe RR. Bacteremia-induced suppression of alveolar surfactant production. *J Surg Res.* 1989;47(5):397–402.

monary injury that occurs during sepsis. Lymph-flow analysis that demonstrates increases in both volume and protein content supports the existence of increased capillary permeability in many septic animal models. The pathophysiology of this capillary "leak" appears to be largely the result of leukocytic-directed injury to the endothelial lining (ie, production of superoxide radicals and elastase); perhaps endothelial gaps are a direct cytotoxic effect of endotoxin.

Although pulmonary edema clearly may worsen gas exchange, this is not the only cause of hypoxia during sepsis. Both animal and human measurements have shown a lack of correlation between calculated variables of the efficiency of oxygenation, (eg, the alveolar-to-arterial oxygen difference, $ADo_2 - aDo_2$) and the amount of extravascular lung water.[88] Despite the development of pulmonary hypertension, experimental evidence shows that within hours of an endotoxin infusion the regional ability of the lung for hypoxic vasoconstriction is lost.[86] Thus, blood flow continues to areas of the lung that are poorly ventilated; the result is poor gas exchange and hypoxemia.

Renal Dysfunction

The incidence and significance of acute renal failure in hospitalized patients were documented in 1983, when 2,216 consecutive hospital admissions were analyzed, revealing 129 episodes, in 109 patients (4.9%) of newly developed renal insufficiency.[90] (Impairment in renal function was defined as an increase of the serum creatinine of 0.5 mg/dL when the admission serum creatinine was less than 1.9 mg/dL, or an increase of 1.0 mg/dL for patients with a baseline serum creatinine of 2.0 to 4.9 mg/dL). This study concluded that decreased renal perfusion caused new-onset renal insufficiency in 54 episodes (42%), and 10 episodes (19%) were associated with septic shock. An important finding was the marked increase in patient mortality, 16 of 25 (64%) when the increase in serum creatinine exceeded 3.0 mg/dL, compared with 6 of 104 (6.5%) mortality when the rise in serum creatinine was less than 3.0 mg/dL.

Consecutive admissions to medical and surgical ICUs in 13 different medical institutions were evaluated in 1985.[91] Definitions for clinically significant renal failure were drafted and validated by the observed rate for survival. In this study, renal failure was identified by the occurrence of any of the following measures:

- urinary output < 480 mL/24 h or <160 mL/8 h,
- serum creatinine > 3.5 mg/dL, or
- serum blood urea nitrogen (BUN) >100 mg/dL.

Another study[92] (N = 315) used a stricter definition: a rise in serum creatinine of 20% above the hospital admission level. Twenty-nine of 47 (62%) patients who developed acute renal insufficiency died.

Two studies[93,94] addressed the significance of renal failure occurring during sepsis. The first, published in 1980, studied 612 patients with Gram-negative bacteremia and found that the development of azotemia increased the fatality rate and the subsequent incidence of shock.[93] The second, published in 1987, studied 250 consecutive cases of severe, acute renal failure (defined as a serum creatinine > 5.5 mg/dL) that occurred at a single hospital.[94] Of the new cases, 125 (50%) occurred in medical patients, and 118 (47%) in surgical patients. Within the surgical group, major vascular surgery was the most common association (42 of 118). Renal failure associated with sepsis resulted in a greater need for dialysis (23 of 24), compared with renal failure following vascular surgery (33 of 42). Recovery of renal function occurred more frequently following vascular surgery (22 of 42), compared with sepsis (5 of 24). In the group of medical patients, the most common cause of renal failure was sepsis (29 of 65 patients), which was also associated with a nearly uniform requirement for dialysis (24 of 29) and a low recovery rate (11 of 29). The mortality rate for sepsis-induced renal failure was significantly higher than the overall group mortality (62%–78% compared with 44.4%).

Literature revealing the pathophysiological mechanisms of sepsis-induced renal failure is sparse. Because sepsis and septic shock cause clinical events that may be injurious to the kidney, the pathophysiology is certain to be multifactorial (Exhibit 24-4).

EXHIBIT 24-4

PATHOPHYSIOLOGICAL MECHANISMS IN SEPSIS-INDUCED ACUTE RENAL FAILURE

Decreased effective intravascular volume

Decreased cardiac output

Decreased renal blood flow secondary to decreased renal perfusion pressure

Positive pressure ventilation,[1] resulting in decreased cardiac output

Alterations in renal afferent and efferent arterial vasodilation from sympathetic or neurohumoral effects[2,3]

Tubular obstruction and renal tubular cellular swelling

Concomitant trauma or extremity ischemia resulting in the release of heme pigment

Sepsis-induced disseminated intravascular coagulation

Reperfusion injury (no reflow phenomenon and the release of oxygen free radicals)

Direct effect of substances such as endotoxin[4]

Nephrotoxic antibiotics used to treat a focus of infection

Intrarenal redistribution of blood flow away from the cortical nephrons[5]

Sources: (1) Rosenthal MH. Hemodynamic effects of pulmonary insufficiency. *Int Anesthesiol Clin*. 1986;24:145–148. (2) Turnquest PE, Rosenthal MH. Acute renal failure in trauma and critically ill patients. *Sem Anesth*. 1989;8(4)338–346. (3) Cumming AD, Kline R, Linton AL. Association between renal and sympathetic responses to nonhypotensive systemic sepsis. *Crit Care Med*. 1988;16(11):1132–1137. (4) Wardle N. Acute renal failure in the 1980s: The importance of septic shock and of endotoxemia. *Nephron*. 1982;30:193. (5) Lucas CE. The renal response to acute injury and sepsis. *Surg Clin North Am*. 1976;56:953–975.

Neurological Manifestations

Dysfunction of the nervous system, particularly the central nervous system, is of paramount importance, for the degree of recovery determines the functional status of the patient who leaves the ICU or hospital. Brain dysfunction may appear early in sepsis without an infectious agent present in the central nervous system. Acutely altered mental status due to sepsis alone has been reported to occur in approximately 23% of patients with sepsis.[95]

Clinical Features

Encephalopathy associated with sepsis is usually nonfocal, with mental-status changes ranging from mild disorientation and confusion through lethargy, agitation, and confusion, to deep coma.[96] Elderly patients appear to be at particularly high risk; agitation or subtle mental-status changes may be the only clinical signs of early sepsis in this group. Metabolic or septic encephalopathy typically presents with a constellation of signs, including normal pupils and eye movements, tremor, asterixis, and multifocal myoclonus.[97] Also, generalized seizures, focal seizures, and other focal signs such as hemiparesis and gaze paresis have been seen.[98] Thus, the presence of focal findings does not exclude the clinical presentation of sepsis.

Patients with sepsis may have a multitude of physiological derangements that may contribute to encephalopathy. These include not only hypotension, hypoxia, and uremia, but also electrolyte, endocrinological, or metabolic abnormalities. Nevertheless, sepsis-associated central nervous system depression can occur in the absence of these factors. Direct microbial invasion or their products such as endotoxin have been implicated, and diffuse microabscesses appear to be common in patients with sepsis.[97,98] Patients in septic shock may develop vascular lesions that include cerebral purpura or microinfarctions.[98] Decreases in cerebral blood flow in these patients may not correlate with mean arterial blood pressure or perfusion pressure.[99] Lastly, administered therapies can also cause encephalopathy. Common causes include sedative medications and hyperosmolality or other metabolic derangements from total parenteral nutrition.

Diagnosis and Prognosis

Diagnosis of septic encephalopathy is based initially on diagnosing a central nervous system infection. Computerized tomography scan will show a mass lesion such as an abscess, hemorrhage, or infarction, but not cerebral microabscesses, hemorrhages, or microinfarctions. Further resolution may be sought with magnetic resonance imaging. Cerebrospinal fluid examination is also necessary to rule out meningitis. Clearly, etiologies for encephalopathies other than meningitis must be entertained, for the majority of patients with sepsis do not have a central nervous system infection.[96]

Although many electroencephalogram changes occur in septic encephalopathy, they are not specific and may be seen in many toxic and metabolic encephalopathies. Electroencephalogram changes include diffuse slow-wave abnormalities, generalized suppression, burst suppression, triphasic waves, and focal or generalized seizures.[97]

Prognosis varies with the course of sepsis, failures of other organ systems, associated central nervous system trauma, and the initial Glasgow coma score. Of patients with nontraumatic coma, 68% of those whose coma was caused by metabolic disease or sepsis were either dead or comatose when reevaluated at 2 weeks.[100] Patients with acutely altered mental status due to sepsis have a higher mortality than those who have no mental-status changes.[95]

Peripheral Neuropathy

Peripheral nerve dysfunction also appears in patients with sepsis. This critical-illness polyneuropathy occurs in at least 50% of patients who remain septic or critically ill for longer than 2 weeks.[97] In a study[101] of patients with sepsis/SIRS who were admitted to an ICU for longer than 5 days, electrophysiological studies revealed that 70% developed some form of polyneuropathy; 30% developed primary axonal degeneration of both motor and sensory fibers. This disorder may present as difficulty in weaning from the ventilator, with severely ill patients showing no diaphragmatic responses to phrenic nerve stimulation.[97] Limb weakness and depressed or absent deep-tendon reflexes occur in mild cases. In severe cases, the absence of any voluntary or reflex-induced movement in all four limbs has been reported.[101]

This polyneuropathy occurred primarily in older patients (mean age 64 y) and affected males and females equally.[101] The etiology of this polyneuropathy remains unclear. The factors that most closely correlated with the development of polyneuropathy were

- the number of invasive procedures performed,

- elevated glucose,
- low serum albumin, and
- the duration of stay in the ICU (mean onset was 28 d).

All patients had concomitant evidence of septic encephalopathy. Complete recovery occurred only in patients whose illness was mild to moderately severe. Patients with a severe peripheral nerve dysfunction, in which diaphragmatic and limb paralysis occurred, failed to improve and eventually died. Thus, critical-illness polyneuropathy can have a significant impact on the course or the eventual recovery of the patient with sepsis.

Metabolic and Endocrinological Responses

Acute illness or injury results in a hypermetabolic state that is characterized by increased gluconeogenesis, mobilization of fat stores, and rapid nitrogen metabolism. Oxygen consumption increases and epinephrine, cortisol, and glucagon levels are increased.[93] Newly manifested hyperglycemia in a critically ill patient should always raise the differential diagnosis of early sepsis. The severity of this increased metabolic demand relates in part to the severity of the illness or injury, with the resting energy expenditure increasing by 10% to 20% with multiple fractures, 12.9% with respiratory failure, and 40% to 100% with extensive thermal injury.[102]

Immunological Aberrations

Cellular and subcellular interactions, the mediators that are released by these cells, and the response to infection and sepsis were discussed previously in this chapter. The immunological changes and defects related to trauma, infection, and critical illness are the focus of this section. Inadequacy or decrements in immune function predispose the patient to overwhelming sepsis, MODS, and death.

Immunosuppression and Critical Illness

Serious injury or illness primarily affects T cell function, as reflected by anergy on skin testing. B cell dysfunction is less common but can appear in individuals who are ill for a prolonged time period, are inadequately nourished, or are subjected to severe burns.[43] B cell function is generally assessed by measuring total serum immunoglobulin levels or the amounts of the individual immunoglobulin subclasses. Tetanus toxoid in vivo and pokeweed mitogen in vitro test the B cell's recall or secondary immune function.

Infections. Primary infectious disease processes often predispose individuals to further infection. Bacterial pneumonia following viral infection or bacterial sepsis associated with malaria are common examples. Much of the predisposition may relate to the breakdown of natural host defenses from the primary infection. One example is the tracheobronchial mucous membrane derangements secondary to the local effects of viral infections. Infectious diseases that depress cell-mediated immunity can potentially complicate the course of an already compromised host. Several infections that have been associated with depressed cell-mediated immunity in humans include influenza, measles, infectious mononucleosis, herpes simplex virus, cytomegalovirus, tuberculosis, histoplasmosis, leprosy, syphilis, pertussis, and streptococcal infections. Malaria has been shown to depress the humoral immune system as well.[103] These common infections, particularly among deployed forces (soldiers are stressed because they have been removed from their normal immunological milieu), then may compromise the individual's immunological response to other insults, such as wound infections or trauma.

Trauma. Major trauma has a profound effect on the patient's immunological function. Total T cell counts and T cell function are markedly depressed in response to injury. The T cell count decreases within hours of injury and may remain depressed for up to 10 days.[1,43] The percentage of T cells in the peripheral blood remains normal, although it may decrease to less than 40% of normal 6 to 8 days following severe burns.[1,43,104] The suppressor/helper T cell ratio increases from 0.55 to 1.04 after trauma.[1]

Testing of cell-mediated immunity with delayed cutaneous hypersensitivity testing has found patients to be anergic following major trauma, a condition that usually persists 4 to 7 days.[104,105] Persistent anergy is associated with an increase in septic complications. Up to 59% of trauma victims with complete anergy to delayed cutaneous hypersensitivity testing develop a significant infectious or septic process.[104,106] Anergy early in a patient's course may predict infectious complications, although later anergy may result from a septic focus.[43]

B cell counts also fall after trauma, although their percentage of the total lymphocyte count remains unchanged.[1] Total immunoglobulin levels fall. Immunoglobulin (Ig) G levels have been shown to be severely depressed for 1 to 2 months after thermal injury.[1,104] However, most of the decrease in the levels of IgG and other immunoglobulins appears to be dilutional.[104]

B cell dysfunction does not appear to be a major factor leading toward increased infection. A study of burn patients who were immunized with a polyvalent *Pseudomonas* vaccine reported effective humoral immune responsiveness; the incidence of *Pseudomonas* bacteremia decreased from 16% to 6%.[107]

Trauma activates the complement pathways, affecting primarily the alternate pathway. The classic pathway becomes active prior to and during the appearance of sepsis.[1] As a result, serum levels of complement as well as fibronectin are depressed, with C3 levels inversely related to the severity of injury.[1,104,108] Fibronectin levels, falling within 4 hours of injury, return to normal within 3 days barring complications.[104]

Malnutrition. Most soldiers injured in combat should be relatively well nourished when injured, unless they have been involved in an arduous or protracted campaign. Without adequate nutrition, immunological dysfunction occurs within days. T cell numbers decrease and the function of T-helper cells is impaired. Evaluations of cell-mediated immunity have revealed a relationship between malnutrition, anergy, and humoral immunological impairment. In response to new antigens, these patients' immunoglobulin generation is impaired, leading to an increased infection rate.[43,109]

Surgery in the Immunocompromised Patient With Sepsis/SIRS

Wounded casualties frequently require surgery, and anesthetic agents can contribute to significant perioperative immunological aberrations. Halothane, nitrous oxide, and pentothal decrease total lymphocytic counts and the number of antibody-forming cells in the spleen.[110] Polymorphonuclear leukocyte chemotaxis and phagocytosis is also impaired.[109]

The immunological abnormalities that occur in accidental trauma also appear in patients who undergo the more controlled traumatic injury performed in the operative suite. For example, the phagocytic capacity of reticuloendothelial cells is depressed following surgery and trauma in proportion to the severity of the insult. Opsonization of bacteria, which enhances these cells' function, is depressed, perhaps as a result of decreased levels of the major opsonic protein, fibronectin.[109] Administering cryoprecipitate that contains high levels of fibronectin to surgical and traumatized patients with sepsis has been shown to improve physiological variables (cardiac index, oxygen consumption, oxygen delivery, and pulmonary shunt fraction); however, improved survival has yet to be shown definitively.[111]

Cell-mediated immunity is the immunological function most affected in the postoperative patient. T cell changes parallel those described above in the traumatized patient. In 46 otherwise healthy, nontraumatized patients who were studied, minor surgical procedures under general anesthesia did not appear to alter skin test results significantly (ie, these patients did not become anergic).[112] However, of patients who underwent major cardiovascular procedures (such as coronary artery bypass grafting or abdominal aortic aneurysm repair), 42% became anergic by postoperative day 3. Compared with patients who retained their immunocompetence, these anergic patients had more infectious complications and were hospitalized longer. Restoration to normal, reactive skin tests may take as long as 28 days.

Perioperative hemorrhage that requires the transfusion of 10 or more units of blood in 24 hours has a mortality rate of approximately 50%. Young, otherwise-healthy trauma victims who require 25 or more units of blood have a 71% mortality rate.[104] Transfusion of blood appears to contribute to the immunological depression seen in trauma victims, even allowing the prediction of subsequent infection.[113] Only 10% of patients who received no transfusion developed an infectious complication, whereas 80% of patients who required more than 15 units of blood did.

Persistent anergy has been seen in postoperative patients with sepsis. The prompt return of normal skin tests follows surgical drainage of an intraperitoneal abscess, an infected common bile duct, or another inflammatory process.[114]

Immunological depression in the battlefield casualty may occur in response to many factors. The severity of these defects clearly dictates the patient's eventual outcome and survival. As no specific therapy has yet been proven to correct these immunological defects, meticulous patient care is important to prevent compounding immunological depression.[43]

Hematological and Coagulation Defects

Sepsis adversely affects the hematopoietic system, resulting in a variety of clinical maladies that can complicate an already seriously ill patient's course. Pancytopenia, which may occur in a variety of medical illnesses, clearly predisposes a patient to develop significant infections. On the other hand, pancytopenia has also been *caused* by infections such as *Mycobacterium tuberculosis*, atypical mycobacteria—especially *Mycobacterium kansasii*, *Histoplasma capsulatum*, *Salmonella typhi*, *Mucor* species, and *Brucella* species.[115] Isolated infections (eg, localized pulmonary infections) do not typically cause this significant hematological insult. Rather, overwhelming infection (during which these organisms are frequently recovered on bone marrow culture) is the typical clinical scenario leading to pancytopenia.

Leukocyte Interactions

Neutrophilia. The degree of neutrophilia varies among patients and the severity of their infections. Mild, localized infections may be associated with neutrophil cell counts of 12,000 to 14,000/mm^3, while severe, pyogenic infections may have cell counts reaching 50,000 to 75,000/mm^3. Leukemoid reactions with cell counts of 50,000 to 100,000/mm^3 are exaggerated responses to these phenomena and, although uncommon, they do occur in a substantial number of infections (eg, pneumonia, meningitis, diphtheria, and tuberculosis).[115]

Neutrophil-releasing factor is stimulated by endotoxin and may, in fact, be the activated complement component C3a.[96] IL-1 also plays a role in the release of neutrophils from the bone marrow.[115] Neutrophilia that persists with chronic infection is probably mediated by colony-stimulating factors, which increase the cell division and turnover of granulocyte precursors.

Although most bacterial infections result in a leukocytosis, this is not universal. In a study of medical patients with sepsis whose blood cultures were positive for bacteria, only 69% had leukocytosis on the first day of septicemia.[116] Neutrophilia is uncommonly seen in infections caused by *Chlamydia* species, *Mycoplasma* species, *Rickettsia*, *Mycobacteria*, and fungal infections.[115]

Neutropenia. Neutropenia is characteristically seen in infections such as typhoid fever, brucellosis, salmonellosis, pertussis, rickettsial infections, disseminated histoplasmosis, and disseminated tuberculosis. However, development of neutropenia in a patient with sepsis may portend a bad prognosis and may result from splenic sequestration, altered immunity, complement-induced neutrophil aggregation,[96] or increased neutrophil consumption in the setting of depleted bone marrow. This condition can be seen in infants, the elderly, and patients with alcoholism, diabetes, malnutrition, or shock.

Neutrophil Morphology. In a study[116] of medical patients with sepsis, 38% had toxic granulations noted on the initial day of sepsis and over one half developed them at some time during their septic course. Another study[117] of patients with bacteremia and fungemia found toxic granulations in 75%. Döhle bodies, Pelger-Huët anomaly (bilobed neutrophils), and vacuolation were also found, the latter being touted as a sensitive and specific marker for bacteremia.[96] However, although they are suggestive, none of these findings are pathognomonic for infection.

Eosinophils. Eosinophilia is rare in bacterial and fungal infections, though in adults it is common in bronchopulmonary aspergillosis and coccidioidomycosis.[115] It classically occurs in invasive helminth infections. Eosinopenia (50 cells/mm^3), on the other hand, commonly heralds the onset of severe bacterial infections. Causes include margination or migration of these cells from the vascular space, inhibition of bone marrow release, and lastly, a decrease in bone marrow production.[96] The absence of eosinopenia when a febrile patient is evaluated is thought by some to question the diagnosis of severe infection.[118] Counts greater than 5% may suggest a nonbacterial etiology such as drug fever, Addison's disease, myeloproliferative disease, or a parasitic infection.[96] Although without defined sensitivity and specificity, eosinopenia is commonly associated with the acute onset of sepsis.

Monocytes and Lymphocytes. Monocytosis (> 800 cells/mm^3) has been associated with a variety of infections, though usually in those of a subacute or chronic course. It is found in approximately 15% to 20% of patients with disseminated tuberculosis, and similarly in those with subacute bacterial endocarditis.[115] Because there is no bone marrow reserve of monocytes, an increased turnover in association with exudates may result in a monocytopenia.[118]

Lymphocytosis (> 4,000 cells/mm^3) is not usually seen in traumatized patients with sepsis. Lymphocytosis occurs commonly in pertussis, rarely with other bacterial or fungal infections, and occasionally in tuberculosis, syphilis, brucellosis, rickettsial, and viral infections. More commonly, however, lymphocytopenia (< 1,000 cells/mm^3) is associated with acute bacterial infections.

The Effect of Sepsis on Erythrocytes

The principal erythrocytic response to infection is anemia, which can arise after several days in an acute, severe infection but is more typically associated with chronic bacterial or fungal infections. The rapid appearance of anemia in an acute infection is the result of one of four processes[118]:

1. hemorrhage,
2. erythrocyte destruction secondary to the infection itself (eg, malaria),
3. microangiopathic hemolysis in association with disseminated intravascular coagulation (DIC), or
4. activation of an underlying, preexisting hemolytic process.

Although most patients are anemic when they are admitted to a medical ICU, 85% demonstrate a further drop in hematocrit in association with sepsis.[116] A reticulocytopenia as well as a shortened erythrocyte survival time persist for approximately 2 weeks in these patients. Occasionally, hypochromic and microcytic indices occur when iron metabolism is disturbed, resulting in low values for serum iron and transferrin. Two possible causative factors are IL-l and TNF. Of particular significance is IL-1's ability to induce the release and activation of lactoferrin from neutrophils and to decrease hepatic transferrin synthesis, both of which contribute to the decrease in serum iron. Decrease in serum iron levels may, in part, be a host-defense mechanism, for free iron contributes to microbial virulence. Chronic anemia that develops during the first month of an illness is typically normochromic and normocytic. Anemia may result from chronic, suppurative infections such as meningitis, empyema, cavitary pulmonary disease, endocarditis, or occult intraabdominal abscesses. Although a variety of bacterial and fungal agents have been reported to cause hemolytic anemia, it actually occurs only rarely. Although three fourths of patients infected with *Mycoplasma pneumoniae* develop cold agglutinins, Coombs-positive hemolytic anemia is exceedingly rare.[115]

Sepsis-Induced Platelet Dyscrasia

Thrombocytopenia (platelet counts < 150,000/mm^3) is present in 33% of medical patients with sepsis and blood cultures that are positive for bacteria.[116] In 65% of these patients, the thrombocytopenia is recognized prior to the onset of sepsis. Most of these patients experience further declines in their platelet counts. The incidence of thrombocytopenia in patients with sepsis ranges from 30% to 100%.[115,119] Approximately two thirds of patients with bacteremia have platelet counts lower than 150,000/mm^3, while one third have platelet counts lower than 50,000/mm^3.[120] Thus, thrombocytopenia is a common finding in patients with sepsis, particularly when associated with DIC (88%–100% incidence).[115]

Thrombocytopenia may occur in critically ill patients prior to the onset of severe infections. Many etiologies for depressed platelet counts are present in this patient population and have been reviewed elsewhere.[119] Briefly, low platelet counts can be due to clumping and therefore spurious, thus warranting close evaluation of the peripheral blood smear. Platelet production can be depressed from the use of alcohol or drugs, toxins, infection-induced aplastic anemia, and nutritional deficiencies, particularly vitamin B_{12} or folate. Distribution and dilution problems also result in thrombocytopenia, as occurs in hypersplenism, hypothermia, and massive transfusion or fluid therapy.

Another category of causes of thrombocytopenia is platelet consumption or destruction. This is the most common reason for thrombocytopenia found in the critically ill patient, and it occurs via two mechanisms: *nonimmune* (mediated by thrombin or surface interactions) and *immune-mediated*. Either mechanism—alone, or in concert with the other—contributes to thrombocytopenia in many settings, only one of which is infection. The most common means of increased platelet destruction during bacterial infections is consumption during DIC. The organisms most commonly implicated are *Neisseria meningitidis*, *Escherichia coli*, *Pseudomonas aeruginosa*, and *Klebsiella pneumoniae*.[119]

Bacterial, viral, fungal, rickettsial, and protozoal infections all may cause thrombocytopenia. Although usually associated with blood-borne organisms, thrombocytopenia can develop in severe infections with blood cultures that are negative for bacteria (eg, pneumonia, peritonitis, or abscesses).[115]

Platelet aggregation, particularly as induced by *Staphylococcus aureus* or endotoxemia, is a major cause of increased platelet turnover. An immunologically mediated destruction is also seen, particularly in Gram-negative infections. Platelet-associated IgG has been found to be elevated in almost three fourths of patients with Gram-negative sepsis and thrombocytopenia, and in 80% of patients with Gram-positive sepsis.[121] Damage to vascular endothelial cells by *Rickettsia* species and perhaps *Neisseria meningitidis* may result in increased platelet adherence.[119,120]

Viral-induced thrombocytopenia is probably as common as that associated with bacterial infections.[119] Viral infections commonly implicated include mumps, varicella, disseminated herpes simplex, cytomegalovirus, infectious mononucleosis, rubeola, and rubella.[120] Thrombocytopenia is also common in HIV infections, whether it be based solely on serologic evidence or in association with acquired immunodeficiency syndrome (AIDS).[120] Although usually mild, the thrombocytopenia seen in these infections can at times be life threatening.[119]

Finally, protozoal infections that can be seen in deploying forces can cause thrombocytopenia. A chronic disorder is seen with toxoplasmosis, whereas more-acute thrombocytopenia, often in conjunction with DIC, is seen in malaria or trypanosomiasis.[120]

Disseminated Intravascular Coagulation

The development of DIC in patients with sepsis, particularly sepsis from Gram-negative organisms, has been well described.[118,122] Endothelial cells become damaged, activated, or are shed as a consequence of the onset of sepsis. Contributory factors include endotoxin, cellular hormones such as TNF, and tissue hypoxia. Tissue thromboplastin is released and, with exposed collagen, causes platelet adhesion and activation. Diffuse coagulation ensues and overwhelms normal compensatory mechanisms. Fibrinogen, platelets, and coagulation factors are consumed. The formation of fibrin and fibrin monomers activate the fibrinolytic system, which then produces fibrin degradation products. These products then inhibit coagulation, impair platelet function, and can cause pulmonary vascular constriction.[118] The predominant clinical findings in DIC, whether they may be thrombosis or hemorrhage, depend upon the balance of pathological processes or the competing compensatory mechanisms.

Dermatological and Ophthalmological Manifestations

Outward cutaneous manifestations of sepsis are often present and may be overlooked in the evaluation of the patient with sepsis. Three patterns of cutaneous lesions appear in these patients.[96] The first is a consequence of bacterial invasion directly into the skin or subcutaneous tissues. Both the nature of the invading organism and the host's response determine the appearance of the lesion. The second occurs as a result of the septic picture, such as hypotension or DIC, without direct cutaneous involvement of the infection. And third, signs of immune-mediated vasculitis or microinfarctions from infective endocarditis may appear.

Gram-negative sepsis from *Campylobacter fetus*, *Vibrio* species, *Aeromonas hydrophila*, *Bacteroides* species, *Yersinia enterocolitica*, and *Serratia marcescens* cause cellulitis, erysipelas, and fasciitis.[96] The lower extremities are at particular risk, with *C fetus* causing lesions that may appear similar to deep venous thrombosis.[123]

Bacterial involvement of the skin and subcutaneous tissues can occur without much associated inflammation and can therefore appear in the granulocytopenic host. The invading organisms are usually Gram negative, particularly *Pseudomonas aeruginosa*, and initially form vesicles or erythema multiforme. These later progress to necrotizing bullous lesions, termed ecthyma gangrenosum.[124]

In sepsis, DIC is associated with acrocyanosis of peripheral tissues such as the fingertips, toes, ears, and nose.[96] Subsequent necrosis may occur and is termed *symmetrical peripheral gangrene*. Although typically associated with Gram-negative infections, these findings can also occur in sepsis associated with Gram-positive organisms.

In patients who have ophthalmological complications of sepsis/SIRS, fundoscopic examination can often aid in the diagnosis of the causative organism. Common, nonspecific retinal changes include retinal hemorrhages, cotton wool spots, and subconjunctival hemorrhages. Roth's spots secondary to infective endocarditis can also appear. Other nonbacterial organisms can present with retinal findings. These include viruses such as cytomegalovirus, parasites such as toxoplasmosis, and fungi such as *Candida* species.[71] Ophthalmological consultation for diagnosis and management is usually necessary for many of these disorders.

DIAGNOSIS AND MONITORING

The physician's senses of vision, hearing, and touch, accompanied by a high index of suspicion, remain the most valuable monitors for the early detection of sepsis. No other diagnostic tool can replace the clinical acumen of an experienced physician. However, regardless of the physician's clinical experience, various laboratory analyses should be made to confirm the diagnosis. The microbiologic diagnosis of the potential cause of sepsis in a patient requires proper submission and handling of the specimens. Close coordination between the clinician and the microbiology laboratory is indicated.

Hematological Evaluation

The clinical and laboratory diagnosis of sepsis and septic shock were reviewed earlier in this chapter. Typical findings include: leukocytosis with a left shift or leukopenia, thrombocytopenia, and prolonged prothrombin time or activated partial thromboplastin time.[125] Most hematological and chemistry studies are routinely performed on critically ill patients, based on a thorough history and physical examination. The patient's clinical condition and course should then dictate the diagnostic laboratory studies to be performed.

Microbiologic Evaluation

Diagnosis of the infection responsible for the septic picture in the critically ill patient requires that adequate, appropriate, and representative samples be collected for laboratory and microbiologic processing. Specimens of blood and respiratory-tract exudates are the most frequent submissions for evaluation. Urine samples obtained from clean-catch, mid-stream, catheter, or suprapubic specimens are also usually submitted for evaluation. Significant values are more than 10^6 organisms per milliliter, although any growth in newly catheterized or suprapubic specimens is significant. Other specimens from body fluids, exudates, pus, and mucous membranes also require submission for study.

Ideally, specimens should be collected from normally sterile body sites and not be contaminated by the usual skin or mucous-membrane flora. Whenever possible, tissue specimens are preferred over specimens obtained via swabs. Specimens also require prompt transport to the laboratory for proper processing to ensure optimal recovery of the causative organisms. If possible, the specimens should be obtained before antimicrobial therapy is initiated.[125]

Specimens should initially be examined directly. The test that should be performed most commonly is the Gram's stain, to evaluate the bacterial population in the specimen. Wet mounts are useful in demonstrating protozoa; india ink or potassium hydroxide is added to look for *Cryptococcus neoformans* or fungi, respectively. Acid-fast stains identify *Mycobacteria* species and fluorescent stains can identify *Legionella*. Silver stains are useful for fungi and *Pneumocystis*, and malarial parasites can be seen with a Giemsa stain.[126]

Cultures are performed on all suitably submitted specimens. Different isolation techniques are required for the wide variety of bacteria, fungi, viruses, and protozoa. Once an organism is identified, the susceptibility of the isolated pathogen to various antimicrobial agents is performed. Susceptibility or resistance to the agent is expressed as the minimal inhibitory concentration of the antimicrobial agent required to prevent the growth of a specific inoculum of organisms. The therapeutic goal in choosing an antimicrobial agent is to achieve a mean drug concentration in the affected tissue that is 2- to 4-fold greater than the minimal inhibitory concentration.[126]

Blood Cultures

Bacteremia, particularly with Gram-negative organisms, is the prototypical infection that causes sepsis and septic shock. Blood cultures obtained from sterile venipunctures are the primary means of detecting bacteremia. In untreated patients who eventually develop bacteremia, a single blood culture will be positive approximately 75% of the time; if three blood cultures are drawn, this rate increases to 98%. Most of these cultures turn positive during incubation within 72 hours. Thus, three sets of blood cultures observed for 3 days will detect Gram-negative bacteremia in more than 90% of patients who will eventually become bacteremic.[127]

Respiratory-Tract Cultures

Specimens from the respiratory tract are usually obtained from sputum samples taken via an endotracheal tube. (Obtaining pulmonary specimens is complicated by the inevitable contamination by upper-airway flora. Gram-negative organisms that colonize the upper airways of patients in the ICU may or may not be pathogenic.) Examination of the sputum is necessary to ensure an adequate sample. In the nonintubated patient, finding a single dominant type of organism in the presence of polymorphonuclear cells is useful in determining the pathogenic organism of a lower-respiratory-tract infection. The reliability of these criteria is less well known in intubated patients.[126] Potential complications and the lack of clinically useful data have caused the use of transtracheal aspiration to decline.

Specimens obtained via bronchoscopy may be useful for microbiologic study of the respiratory tract. Simple bronchial washings for bacterial flora are difficult to interpret; the reliability of these specimens to diagnose lower-tract infections is similar to that of sputum cultures. Protected brush specimens may improve the diagnostic yield; the sensitivity and specificity for properly diagnosing the etiologic bacteria normally ranges from 59% to 70%, although some report 90%.[126]

Bronchoalveolar lavage has also proven to be a beneficial means of obtaining specimens and is particularly efficacious in patients with AIDS. Yields of nearly 100% for *Pneumocystis carinii* have been reported, with yields for other pathogens ranging from 60% to 85%.[126] Bronchoalveolar lavage makes it possible to diagnose infections by means of both rapid-staining techniques and cultures. Rapid stains for *Pneumocystis*, viral inclusions, *Legionella*, fungi, *Mycobacteria*, and bacteria have been beneficial in aiding early, appropriate antimicrobial therapy.

Additional Tests

Diagnostic tests other than culturing can be performed to determine the potential cause of sepsis in a patient. Capsular polysaccharide antigens can be detected for *Hemophilus influenza*, *Streptococcus pneumoniae*, *Neisseria meningitidis*, or *Cryptococcus neoformans*. Enzyme-linked immunosorbent assays (ELISAs) to detect bacterial antigens have been useful in diagnosing infections by *N gonorrhea* and *Legionella* species. And lastly, serologic evidence for antibody detection has been used to diagnose typhoid fever, brucellosis, tularemia, Legionnaires' disease, acute viral diseases, histoplasmosis, rickettsial typhus and spotted fevers, toxoplasmosis, and amebiasis.[126] Other organisms are being detected and other diagnostic measures are continually being developed.

Sophisticated Bedside Monitors

Because significant cardiovascular dysfunction occurs in sepsis/SIRS, accurate assessment of hemodynamic function is imperative to successfully manage these critically ill patients. Clinical assessment and observation often fail to accurately determine the hemodynamic status, and, hence, the optimal therapy for these patients. Hemodynamic monitoring can be invasive and noninvasive.

Pulmonary Artery Catheter

The development of the flow-directed pulmonary artery catheter has enabled us to more accurately assess the hemodynamic status of patients with sepsis. Newer catheters now allow the physician to measure and calculate intracardiac and pulmonary arterial pressures, cardiac output and cardiac index, intracardiac and mixed venous oxygen saturation, right ventricular ejection fraction, right ventricular end diastolic and end systolic volumes, and "continuous" cardiac output.[128] With this information at hand, the clinician can obtain a more accurate assessment of the patient's intravascular volume status and ventricular performance, calculate hemodynamic and respiratory indices to aid management, and determine oxygen delivery and tissue oxygen consumption.

Many indications for the use of the pulmonary artery catheter have evolved since its introduction.[129,130] If ARDS develops in the patient with sepsis, it can be more readily diagnosed and managed with a pulmonary artery catheter that distinguishes cardiogenic from noncardiogenic pulmonary edema. Particularly in the traumatized or postoperative patient, intravascular volume status can be more accurately assessed.

Insertion techniques have been described in detail elsewhere.[131] Catheterization of the pulmonary circulation can be performed by inserting the pulmonary artery catheter into the internal jugular, subclavian, femoral, or antecubital veins. Minor and major complications can occur with the placement and use of these catheters, however.[128,132] Insertion complications include bleeding, vessel perforation, pneumothorax or hemothorax, and ventricular dysrhythmias. Maintaining the catheter in the pulmonary artery has complications, as well. These include local vascular thrombosis, pulmonary arterial rupture, pulmonary infarction, or catheter-related sepsis. So, although a pulmonary artery catheter is beneficial in the management of patients with sepsis, further injury is possible and warrants consideration before the catheter is inserted.

Two major assumptions must be made before the data obtained from the pulmonary artery catheter can be interpreted correctly:

1. The equipment must be properly functioning and calibrated, and the transducer zeroed at the mid-left atrial level. The function of the pulmonary artery catheter is to obtain an estimate of left ventricular preload, which is determined by left ventricular end diastolic volume.
2. A direct relationship is assumed between the left ventricular end diastolic volume, which is difficult to measure, and the more easily obtained left ventricular end diastolic pressure. Changes in left ventricular compliance, however, alter this volume-to-pressure relationship.

Under conditions of a normal pulmonary vascular bed, mitral valve, and left ventricular function or compliance, PCWP measured at end expiration in pulmonary zone III is equal to both the mean left atrial pressure and left ventricular end diastolic pressure. The second major assumption is altered by changes in any of these factors or catheter placement.[129] Other factors, such as the application of positive end-expiratory pressure to mechanical ventilation, also alter this assumption.

Pulmonary artery catheters also provide a means of obtaining an estimate of cardiac output by thermodilution. Using the proper volume and temperature of injectate required by the specific catheter and cardiac computer is of utmost importance in obtaining an accurate estimate. Timing the injections for cardiac output measurement within the same period in the respiratory cycle may improve the reproducibility of the results. However, indiscriminate timing of injections for cardiac output throughout the respiratory cycle more accurately determines the clinical status of the patient. Cardiac output divided by body surface area yields cardiac index, a figure that can then easily be compared between individuals. Obtaining these figures is necessary to determine systemic vascular resistance (SVR), pulmonary vascular resistance (PVR), stroke work index (SWI), and oxygen delivery (Do_2).

One measurement that can be obtained only from a pulmonary artery catheter is a mixed venous blood gas. This measurement can be (*a*) obtained intermittently or, via a specially designed catheter that uses reflectance oximetry, (*b*) monitored continuously. The measurement of venous oxygen saturation (Svo_2) is necessary to determine oxygen consumption ($\dot{V}o_2$).

Svo_2 varies directly with cardiac output, hemoglobin, and arterial oxygen saturation. Decreasing Svo_2 may result from increased metabolic rate, with concomitant tissue extraction of oxygen or decreased oxygen delivery as a result of cardiac dysfunction, anemia, or arterial hypoxemia. Increases in Svo_2 occur where less oxygen is either utilized or extracted, as in arterial-venous fistulae, cirrhosis, left-to-right cardiac shunts, peripheral shunts, cyanide poisoning, hypothermia, inadvertent sampling of blood from the pulmonary artery (taken when the catheter is improperly inflated or wedged), and sepsis.[128]

Sepsis causes an increase in measured Svo_2 as a result of decreased tissue oxygen extraction when

1. a disproportionately high percentage of cardiac output is distributed to the skin, where oxygen consumption is minimal, and
2. microvascular occlusion occurs from leukocyte aggregates, microthrombi, vasoconstriction, and platelet aggregates.

Additional findings that typically occur in patients with sepsis with a pulmonary artery catheter in place include

3. a moderate-to-high cardiac output in the presence of
4. a low systemic vascular resistance.

These findings are necessarily contingent on other determining factors such as adequate hemoglobin, arterial oxygen saturation, and intravascular volume. Any reduction in these determining factors could lead to misinterpretation of the data. Using a pulmonary artery catheter has aided the diagnosis of unsuspected sepsis. One study revealed that unsuspected septic shock was diagnosed in 38% of patients only after a pulmonary artery catheter was inserted.[133] Whether the use of pulmonary artery catheters improves outcome from septic shock remains to be definitively determined. Proponents have advocated its use to optimize oxygen delivery to tissues in an attempt to maintain adequate tissue oxygen consumption and hence, improve survivability.

Echocardiography

The major noninvasive means of evaluating cardiac performance is the echocardiogram. Through the use of the traditional M-mode echocardiograph, two-dimensional echocardiography, and the recently developed Doppler color-flow mapping, echocardiography can be used to assess left ventricular function both quantitatively and qualitatively, diagnose ischemic heart disease, to include infarction, evaluate pathological lesions in and around the heart in the great vessels, and observe intracardiac blood flow through the valves and intracardiac shunts.[134] The effectiveness of these studies has been further improved through the development of transesophageal imaging. Placing the transducer within the chest cavity can eliminate many of the artifacts of chest-wall deformities, subcutaneous tissue, emphysematous lungs, or even surgical bandages, and thus provide a more accurate, detailed study.

In addition to these diagnostic capabilities, echocardiography can now be used as a noninvasive monitor of cardiac output via a continuous-wave

Doppler cardiac-output computer. This technique depends on measuring blood flow velocity through the aortic valve and accurately measuring the cross-sectional area of the valve.[134] Two transducers are used, one in the suprasternal notch and the other on an esophageal stethoscope. Cardiac output is determined by the formula:

$$C.O. = SVI \bullet Ao\ area \bullet HR$$

where *C.O.* represents cardiac output, *SVI* (systolic velocity integral) represents the integral of the area under the velocity curve measured by the transducer aimed at the aortic valve, *Ao area* represents the cross-sectional area of the aortic valve (usually measured by M-mode or two-dimensional echocardiography), and *HR* represents heart rate.

The accuracy of Doppler-measured cardiac output depends on both the patient and the operator. Comparisons with standard thermodilution techniques have been in conflict, although a correlation between $r = 0.88$ and 0.97 has been reported.[134]

Echocardiography has proven useful in the evaluation of patients with sepsis. Two-dimensional echocardiography has been used to monitor myocardial failure and ventricular dilation, as well as the recovery from septic shock.[135] Segmental myocardial dysfunction in septic shock can be seen by echocardiography. Typically associated with ischemic heart disease, this abnormality has also been seen in patients with sepsis who have no evidence of either coronary artery disease or myocardial injury.[136]

Echocardiography may not at this stage replace invasive pulmonary arterial catheterization in the evaluation and management of patients with sepsis. It is, however, complementary, as it is able to monitor chamber size in sepsis and during therapeutic interventions.[137] Improvements in equipment and the development of other noninvasive techniques such as bioimpedance cardiography will further increase our ability to obtain information about the hemodynamic status of patients with sepsis.[138]

Radiological Procedures

Many radiological procedures may be beneficial in the diagnosis and management of patients with sepsis. All procedures and tests must be performed while keeping in mind the potential complications inherent in preparing and transporting the patient, and weighing these potential complications against the potential benefit from obtaining useful information. Suboptimal patient preparation, such as the inability to administer oral contrast solution prior to an abdominal computed tomography (CT) scan, impairs the adequacy of the results and may warrant delaying the study.

Chest Radiography

The principal radiographic study utilized in the evaluation and management of the critically ill patient with sepsis is a chest roentgenogram made by a portable X-ray apparatus. The roentgenogram must be reviewed in a systematic fashion, examining from the peripheral soft tissues to the mediastinum and including all structures, including those iatrogenically placed.

Evaluation of the pulmonary parenchyma is usually the focus of attention in the patient with sepsis. In these patients, loss of alveolar space is commonly in the form of atelectasis (loss of lung volume), which appears rapidly and occurs commonly in the postoperative setting.

Pneumonia can present as a wide variety of radiographic appearances. It can be interstitial and diffuse or localized with dense, airspace consolidation. Combinations and variations are common. The definitive diagnosis requires information other than that obtained on the roentgenogram, as atelectasis or pulmonary edema may be indistinguishable from pneumonia.[139]

Patients with ARDS usually present with a diffuse interstitial and alveolar infiltrate, which many diffuse pulmonic processes can mimic. These other processes include pulmonary edema, fat embolism syndrome, diffuse pneumonia, or massive aspiration pneumonitis.[139] The definitive diagnosis requires further clinical and hemodynamic data and cannot be made solely on the basis of its radiographic appearance.

Pleural-based disease must also be evaluated. Pleural fluid is not specific and can occur in a wide variety of disorders in the septic patient, including congestive heart failure, empyema or parapneumonic inflammation, and pancreatitis. The pleural space must also be evaluated for evidence of barotrauma, as pneumothorax is common in mechanically ventilated patients (with an incidence of approximately 10%). Pleural air is usually seen without difficulty in an upright film. However, in the supine patient, air may collect in the anteromedial portion of the hemithorax, producing a medial pneumothorax, or dissect over the hemidiaphragm, producing an abnormally deep costophrenic sulcus (the *deep sulcus* sign).[139]

Sinus Evaluation

Critically ill patients frequently require nasotracheal intubation, nasogastric suctioning, or nasogastric feeding, all of which may cause iatrogenic sinusitis. Sinusitis should be considered in the differential diagnosis in the seriously ill, febrile patient. Physical exam and bedside routine sinus roentgenograms frequently miss the diagnosis. CT is useful in making the diagnosis of occult sinusitis-induced sepsis.[140]

Ultrasonography

Ultrasonography has proven beneficial in the diagnosis of clinical dilemmas in critically ill patients with sepsis. Improved imaging and portability have made bedside evaluations possible. The bedside procedure is safer for the patient as well, as it obviates the need to transport the patient to the radiology department (which, for critically ill patients, is potentially complicated and dangerous).

Ultrasound can now be used in the initial evaluation of acute renal failure to screen for obstruction, with a 93% to 98% sensitivity in the detection of hydronephrosis.[141] Intrinsic renal disease and renovascular disease can also be evaluated, the latter aided by Doppler analysis. Acute pancreatitis, which can accompany or mimic sepsis, can also be evaluated by ultrasound. Diagnosis of the complications of pancreatitis, such as hemorrhage, pseudocysts, or biliary tract obstruction can all be confirmed by sonography.

Biliary tract evaluation can help determine the etiology of jaundice that may appear in the septic patient. By identifying and measuring the common hepatic duct, obstructive jaundice can be diagnosed with 90% accuracy.[141] Hepatocellular disease is evaluated with much less sensitivity. Using ultrasonography to exclude intraabdominal fluid collection is particularly useful. Those areas most amenable for study are the right upper quadrant (liver, subhepatic space, subphrenic space, and right kidney), abdominal wall, pelvis, and left upper quadrant for splenic pathology. Abscesses can be seen in these areas, including within the liver, spleen, and kidney, with a 90% to 98% accuracy.[141] Ultrasonographic signs of acalculus cholecystitis in a patient with sepsis/SIRS include pericholecystic fluid, gall bladder distension and wall thickening, and intrahepatic duct dilation and the absence of stones.[142]

Other abdominal areas are less well seen because of bowel gas and surgical dressings; other patient variables such as obesity can also limit the study. Depending on accessibility, ultrasound-guided percutaneous drainage of a fluid collection can be performed to determine its composition, or can at times be used as an alternative to surgical drainage of an abscess.

Computerized Tomography

Imaging of the patient with sepsis, particularly if the patient also has had trauma, is probably best performed with CT. Inherent in this study is the need to transport the patient with all accompanying life support equipment to the machine in other areas of the hospital. Transporting for elective procedures—to the CT scanner in particular—have a high incidence of mishaps.[143]

In a study[144] of 20 patients in the ICU who received routine, portable chest roentgenograms, researchers found that in 15 (75%) of them, a thoracic CT scan was helpful in determining treatment plans. Another study[145] found clinically significant lesions such as pneumothorax and pulmonary or mediastinal abscesses. The overall accuracy of radiographic studies in diagnosing intraabdominal pathology has been shown to be about 76%. The most accurate diagnostic study appears to be the CT scan, with sensitivity and specificity in diagnosing an abdominal source of infection reported at approximately 90%.[145] The accuracy of diagnosis by ultrasound and radioactive gallium scan is lower than with CT scanning.[146] Diagnostic accuracy with CT scanning improves with the addition of oral and perhaps intravenous contrast.

Abdominal examinations should include the pelvis because fluid collects in the cul-de-sac or the retrovesicular spaces. CT scans have proven beneficial in diagnosing empyema and abdominal abscesses, postoperative pancreatitis, bile leakage, or delayed hemorrhage from trauma or surgical procedures.[139] The CT has been used in a similar—and at times, more successful—fashion than ultrasound in guiding needle aspiration or percutaneous drainage of fluid collections. With the exception of case reports, there is no literature indicating that magnetic resonance imaging (MRI) is a useful diagnostic tool in the patient with sepsis/SIRS.

Surgical Reexploration

Abdominal injuries are frequent in combat casualties. Thus, abdominal infections are a significant possibility during the recovery phase following the initial laparotomy. Reoperation or intervention after abdominal surgery during the same hospitalization may be the only therapeutic intervention that can successfully treat a patient with sepsis whose condition is deteriorating. The indications for reoperation have changed little over the past 60 years and include the need to eliminate or remove the source of infection, remove infectious exudative material, perform intraperitoneal lavage to attempt to reduce the infective organism load, and drain an abscess sufficiently. Most reoperations are performed for peritonitis (45%), mechanical ileus (29%), postoperative bleeding (17%), and miscellaneous causes (9%), including a second acute process such as gangrenous cholecystitis, wound dehiscence, or acute bowel ischemia.[147] The mortality of patients undergoing reexploration is approximately 43%: the lowest mortality in one series[146] was found in trauma patients; the highest, in the patients undergoing evaluation for MODS who did not have a treatable finding at the time of laparotomy.

Evaluation of the patient prior to reoperation requires a thorough physical examination. More than 85% of patients who prove to have an abnormality at laparotomy have tenderness, fever, and absent bowel sounds.[146] These findings can be misleading in the sedated patient or the patient with mental status changes. The decision to reexplore can be made in most patients solely on clinical grounds. In addition to the clinical examination, radiographic studies can be beneficial when deciding whether to reexplore a patient with sepsis. A 1985 review[148] of the indications and results of reoperation for sepsis found that no patient without organ failure died, and that the risk associated with a normal exploration was outweighed by the potential of finding drainable intraperitoneal pus.

The etiology of postoperative peritonitis is most commonly (54%) secondary to an abdominal abscess.[146] The second most frequent cause (16%–39%) is a suture leak.[146,147] Other causes include necrotic bowel and technical error at the first operation.

The need for reexploration depends largely on the patient's clinical examination and hospital course. Additional beneficial information can be gleaned from radiographic evaluation, principally the CT scan. Although mortality rates from reexploration have not dropped significantly, current critical-care management has allowed more patients to tolerate such a procedure.[146,147] Early intervention in a surgically reparable disease process will perhaps lead to lower reoperative morbidity and mortality.

THERAPEUTIC MODALITIES

The primary issue in resuscitation for shock of any type, including septic shock, is to preserve adequate oxygen delivery to the tissues. Simple fluid administration may accomplish this in the volume-depleted patient as a result of increasing venous preload and thus optimizing the cardiac stroke volume.

Although the patient's clinical condition should be monitored (eg, mental status, mucous membranes, and urinary output), a more accurate means, particularly with a pulmonary artery catheter, may be desirable. However, the limitations of both the use and the interpretation of these data must be considered.

Fluid Resuscitation

Intravascular volume is decreased in patients with septic shock for the many reasons previously discussed. Increased vascular permeability markedly increases fluid and protein transport into the interstitium.[149] This absolute intravascular fluid loss, coupled with any additional loss from trauma or surgery, is aggravated by a redistributive loss due to the systemic vasodilation of septic shock.

Volume resuscitation, ideally with the aid of hemodynamic monitoring, should be the initial therapeutic intervention in the unstable patient in septic shock. However, the following facts must be kept in mind:

- Sepsis alters the normal response to volume infusion.
- Myocardial function is depressed in septic shock.

In these patients, volume infusion has been shown to result in only a minor increase in left ventricular end diastolic volume and stroke work when compared to other critically ill patients who do not have sepsis.[79] Thus, many patients with sepsis have a blunted ability to either dilate or increase ventricular contractility in response to volume infusion. One therapeutic strategy is to increase the PCWP, using 250-mL fluid boluses, until the cardiac index fails to increase further. In patients with septic shock, the PCWP associated with this maximal preload is approximately 10 to 14 mm Hg.[150] It is the choice of resuscitation fluid in the bolus—crystalloid or colloid—that remains controversial (Table 24-1).

TABLE 24-1

FACTORS IN FLUID SELECTION

Factor	Crystalloid	Colloid
Cost	Inexpensive	Expensive
Peripheral edema	Significant	Minimal
Anaphlyactoid reaction	Absent	Small risk (< 2%)
Colloid osmotic pressure	Decreases	Increases
Amount needed to maintain intravascular volume	Large	Small

Crystalloid Solutions

Crystalloid solutions can pass through a semipermeable membrane; colloid solutions cannot. The cheapest and most commonly used crystalloid resuscitation fluids are isotonic saline solutions, principally normal saline (0.9% sodium chloride) and Ringer's lactate (Table 24-2). These fluids distribute throughout the extracellular space. In normal, healthy adults, only 25% of the volume infused remains in the intravascular space after 1 hour. In the critically ill patient, however, less than 20% remains intravascular.[150] (Because 5% dextrose in water distributes throughout the total body water space, it is not effective in increasing intravascular volume.)

Isotonic saline and Ringer's lactate can be used interchangeably if the electrolyte differences are kept in mind. The theoretical concern of a hyperchloremic acidosis from the administration of large volumes of normal saline is not of clinical significance except in patients with severe renal insufficiency. Also, the administration of lactate in Ringer's solution does not potentiate an existing lactic acidosis or alter blood lactate measurements.[151,152] The rare exception is a patient with severe hepatic insufficiency who cannot metabolize lactate.

Colloid Solutions

Albumin. Albumin is the primary colloid used in the volume resuscitation of patients with sepsis. It is a natural protein of 584 amino acids synthesized in the liver at a rate of 130 to 200 mg/kg/d in healthy adults.[151] Albumin synthesis is regulated in part by colloid osmoreceptors located in the interstitial spaces near the sites of hepatic synthesis.[152] This may be of therapeutic significance when exogenous albumin or other colloids are administered. Its molecular mass ranges from 66,000 to 69,000 daltons and has a strong negative charge at physiological pH levels. Albumin is a major transport protein for metals, drugs, hormones, enzymes, fatty acids, amino acids, and bilirubin.[151,152]

Albumin is the major oncotically active protein in plasma, providing approximately 80% of the colloid osmotic pressure. The normal serum albumin is approximately 3.5 to 5.0 g/dL, with 40% of the body's albumin located in the intravascular space.[152] Extravascular stores are largest in the skin, but are also located in muscle and viscera. Only free, non-tissue-bound, interstitial-space albumin is able to return to the intravascular compartment via the lymphatic system in response to hypovolemia.[151]

In response to hemorrhage, albumin synthesis increases and its degradation or metabolism decreases. Mobilization of extravascular stores helps to minimize the loss in oncotic pressure. However, under severe stress, as in sepsis, albumin synthesis falls and the colloid osmotic pressure subsequently follows.

Exogenous albumin can be administered as either a 5% or a 25% solution. The 5% solution contains 50 g of albumin per liter of physiological saline and is isooncotic. The 25% solution contains 12.5 g of albumin in 50 mL of a buffered diluent that contains 130 to 160 mEq of sodium per liter.[152] When 100 mL of the hyperoncotic 25% solution is administered, the intravascular volume increases during the next 30 to 60 minutes to a maximum of 450 mL through the translocation of 350 mL of interstitial fluids. Hence the use of the hyperoncotic solution may be most beneficial in the intravascularly de-

TABLE 24-2

COMPOSITION OF CRYSTALLOID SOLUTIONS

Component	Normal Saline	Lactated Ringer's
Sodium	154 mEq/L	130 mEq/L
Chloride	154 mEq/L	109 mEq/L
Potassium	0	4 mEq/L
Calcium	0	3 mEq/L
Lactate	0	28 mEq/L
Osmolality	308 mOsm/L	275 mOsm/L
pH	6.0	5.1

pleted patient with elevated total body water or edema. The 5% solution is often used in initial volume resuscitation of the hypovolemic patient without edema.

Albumin is safe when used properly. Albumin-induced anaphylaxis occurs at a rate of only 0.47% to 1.53%; the reactions are generally mild, consisting of fever, chills, and urticaria. No infectious risk of hepatitis or human immunodeficiency virus is associated with its use secondary to prolonged heat-killing processing.[151] One major drawback to the use of albumin is its cost, which is approximately 30-fold greater than that of crystalloid fluids.

***Hetastarch*.** Hydroxyethyl starch (hetastarch) is another colloid commonly used to treat hemorrhagic shock. This compound is a synthetic colloid composed of amylopectin that resembles glycogen. It is available in 500-mL containers of a 6% solution with an average molecular mass of 69,000 daltons (range 10,000–1,000,000) and an osmolarity of 310 mOsm/L.[151] After administration, smaller-molecular-weight molecules are cleared rapidly in the urine, whereas larger molecules require amylase hydrolysis before they can be excreted in the urine or bile.[152] Delayed excretion occurs because of (*a*) the necessary breakdown of the larger molecules and (*b*) tissue absorption, most notably in the reticuloendothelial system. In normal volunteers, approximately one half the hetastarch is eliminated in the urine within 2 days.[151]

The plasma-volume expansion that occurs with hetastarch is roughly equivalent to that of 5% albumin.[151] Hetastarch is not immunogenic and does not cause a histamine release, although minor anaphylactic reactions can occur with an incidence of less than 0.085%.[151,152] Minor alterations in coagulation studies appear to be dose dependent and are not associated with clinical bleeding, in patients without a bleeding diathesis, in a dose less than 1,500 mL/d. Transient thrombocytopenia and prolonged prothrombin and activated partial thromboplastin times are the three abnormalities that have been noted.[151]

Because its major route of elimination is via the kidney, patients with renal impairment are at increased risk of volume overload and tissue accumulation if hetastarch is used for volume resuscitation. Amylase levels will rise, commonly to 2-fold higher than normal values, after its administration. These raised levels may persist for 5 days, although no change in pancreatic function occurs.[151]

Despite these few side effects, hetastarch remains a safe and viable option for colloid volume resuscitation in the patient with sepsis. Its major advantage over albumin is that it costs approximately one fourth as much as an equivalent amount of 5% albumin (Table 24-3).

TABLE 24-3

COMPARISON OF COMMERCIAL COLLOID SOLUTIONS

Factor	Albumin 5%/25%	Hetastarch
Cost	Expensive	¼ cost
Infectious risk	None	None
Anaphylactoid reaction	0.5%–1.5%	< 0.08%*
Half-life	< 24 h	2 d (assuming normal renal function)

*Source for this value: Rainey TG, English JF. Pharmacology of colloids and crystalloids. In: Chernow B, ed. *The Pharmacologic Approach to the Critically Ill Patient*. Baltimore, Md: Williams & Wilkins; 1988: 235.

Selection of Resuscitation Fluid

Which of the two classes of fluid should be used for volume resuscitation remains controversial. However, proponents of either agree on several points[153]:

- Colloid solutions more efficiently replace blood volume than crystalloids.
- Colloid solutions are more expensive.
- Crystalloid solutions cause no anaphylactoid reactions.
- Both types of fluid are more readily available than blood, and should be used initially in the management of hemorrhagic shock as the patient will tolerate anemia better than hypovolemia.
- Colloid therapy provides a more effective maintenance of colloid osmotic pressure.
- Regardless of the fluid selected, fluid overload is to be avoided.

It seems quite clear that patients with septic shock have a heightened potential for extracellular fluid sequestration, compared with trauma patients who are not septic. No doubt this is caused by the capillary membrane damage that results from the sequential interaction of endogenous mediators and cells in SIRS.[154] The circumstances under which these pathophysiological differences may become clinically relevant are not the only factors that need to be considered when the choice of fluid is discussed. Additional areas of debate in the use of these two fluids are whether there is a significant difference in their effects on the patient's coagulation, renal function, pulmonary interstitial water, development of ARDS, length of stay in the hospital or ICU, and survival.[153] The answers to these clinical questions should determine whether continued use of colloid fluids is warranted in light of the cost and potential side effects.

The main reason for using colloids is to prevent pulmonary edema. The amount of pulmonary edema that forms depends on (*a*) microvascular hydrostatic pressure (estimated by the PCWP), (*b*) colloid osmotic pressure, and (*c*) permeability of the alveolar-capillary membranes. The role played by hydrostatic pressure is more important than that of colloid osmotic pressure. The low colloid osmotic pressure seen with hypoalbuminemia does not, in and of itself, lead to pulmonary edema. The development of pulmonary edema is encouraged when capillary permeability is altered, for increased hydrostatic pressure results in increased transudation of fluid into the interstitial space. One concern with colloid infusions in this setting is that increasing protein, and hence oncotic pressure in the interstitium, will worsen edema. This hypothesis, however, remains to be definitively confirmed.[155]

Most studies comparing colloids and crystalloids have occurred in the setting of surgery, thermal burns, or trauma. One study compared the cardiorespiratory effects of treating patients in circulatory shock with 5% albumin, 6% hetastarch, or 0.9% saline.[156] Over two thirds of the patients studied were in septic shock; the remainder were in hypovolemic shock. Their median age was 79 years. All three solutions were found to provide the same cardiac function and hemodynamic stability. Neither albumin nor hetastarch depressed myocardial function. Hetastarch and albumin were of equivalent efficacy in treating circulatory shock. To attain the same physiological end points, 2- to 4-fold more crystalloid solution was required. Saline administration decreased the colloid osmotic pressure as expected. When the patients were resuscitated to the same physiological end points, the crystalloid solution caused an increased incidence of pulmonary edema compared with the two colloids.[155]

These results were, however, a summation of the effects seen in patients with sepsis and patients in hypovolemic shock. In studies of patients who do not have sepsis, alterations in capillary, microvascular membrane permeability are relatively minor, an aberration that occurs early in sepsis.[155] Nevertheless, a study that used the technique of meta-analysis concluded that, in the trauma patient with sepsis, better survival and better resuscitation are achieved with crystalloid solution.[157]

Which fluid is to be used varies with the clinical setting. Those clinical conditions associated with both intravascular hypovolemia and extracellular fluid deficit are best replenished with crystalloids. These fluids are more plentiful, less expensive, and without anaphylactoid side effects. More volume must be administered when compared with colloids, a condition easily tolerated in patients with trauma and perhaps surgical patients, particularly if they are young. Older individuals, and possibly patients with sepsis, are at greater risk of developing pulmonary edema. However, inadvertent volume overload with crystalloid solutions is relatively short lived, due to equilibration with the extravascular space.

A lesser volume of colloid solution is needed to obtain the same hemodynamic parameters as crystalloids; a greater percentage remains in the intravascular space for a longer time period.

Hetastarch is cheaper than albumin and increases colloid osmotic pressure over 3-fold that of an equivalent volume of albumin,[158] although its use has other potential effects (discussed above). The concern that colloid molecules pass through membranes of increased permeability, as is seen in sepsis, thereby increasing interstitial oncotic pressure and edema, remains speculative. Some authorities[151,159] recommend using only crystalloid solutions in this setting until the "leak" has sealed. The following are general guidelines for the use of crystalloid and colloid solutions:

- Colloids may be used for prompt volume expansion, and should be used in conjunction with crystalloids when more than 30% of the intravascular volume requires replacement.
- The total volume of crystalloid used and perhaps the subsequent development of interstitial edema may be minimized by concomitant administration of albumin or hetastarch to maintain colloid oncotic pressure.
- In the setting of increased total body water or edema, 25% albumin should be used.
- Volume overload must be monitored because colloids remain for a prolonged time within the intravascular space.

- Little additional benefit is gained in intravascular colloid osmotic pressure when the pressure is greater than or equal to 20 mm Hg, the serum albumin is greater than or equal to 2.5 g/dL, or the total serum protein is greater than or equal to 5.0 g/dL.

Tissue Oxygen Delivery and Consumption

Tissue oxygen delivery (Do_2) is a function of cardiac output (C.O.) and arterial oxygen content (Cao_2):

$$Do_2 = C.O. \bullet Cao_2$$

Arterial oxygen content is a function of hemoglobin (Hb) concentration and the degree of oxygen saturation of the blood (Sao_2), the latter being determined by the partial pressure of oxygen (Po_2):

$$Cao_2 = 1.34 \bullet \text{grams of Hb} \bullet Sao_2 + 0.003 \bullet Po_2$$

Tissue oxygen consumption (Vo_2) can be calculated as the difference between the arterial (Cao_2) and venous (Cvo_2) oxygen contents multiplied by the cardiac output (C.O.):

$$Vo_2 = C.O. \bullet (Cao_2 - Cvo_2)$$

If tissue oxygen delivery is inadequate or if tissue oxygen extraction is abnormal, all three factors—cardiac output, hemoglobin, and oxygen saturation—must be optimized.

Cardiac Index

Optimal left ventricular preload has been described previously in this chapter. Less is known concerning the optimal cardiac index for patients with sepsis or septic shock. Most patients with sepsis or septic shock manifest an elevated cardiac index as the principal compensatory mechanism by which tissue oxygen delivery is increased to meet demand.

Increased survival in patients with sepsis whose cardiac outputs are higher than normal has been demonstrated.[160–162] In a study[160] comparing critically ill patients after surgery, the variables that showed the greatest statistical discrimination between survivors and nonsurvivors were left ventricular stroke work, oxygen delivery, and oxygen consumption.

Hemoglobin

Hemoglobin is the major determinant of the oxygen content of arterial blood. One gram of hemoglobin increases arterial oxygen as much as increasing the partial pressure of arterial oxygen (Pao_2) from 100 to 400 torr. This is because hemoglobin oxygen saturation is close to 100% at a Po_2 of 100 torr. A higher Po_2 increases oxygen content only slightly because the added oxygen is carried dissolved in the plasma and constitutes only about 2% of the total oxygen being carried. The optimal hematocrit for patients with sepsis is not known. The conventional wisdom has been than a hematocrit between 0.30 and 0.40 provides the maximum oxygen delivery if all other factors are held constant. This is based on clinical studies that show increased viscosity, decreased cerebral blood flow, and increased incidence of vascular occlusive episodes when the hematocrit exceeds 0.45. Despite a calculated increase in the arterial oxygen content that would result from transfusion of packed erythrocytes, in patients with septic shock, significant increases in systemic oxygen consumption are not apparent.[162] The explanation may be a reflexive decrease in cardiac output.

A clinical study that was published in 1993 also showed that transfusion of packed red cells did not cause an increase in systemic oxygen consumption, even though cardiac index did not change.[163] As part of this study, gastric intramucosal pH was also measured. The pH fell after the transfusion, and the magnitude of the decrease was directly related to the age of the blood. The researchers suggest that (*a*) the ability of erythrocytes to *deform* (ie, to fold, which enables them to pass more easily through capillaries—a capacity that is known to be decreased in aged blood) was reduced in aged blood, and (*b*) this factor depressed tissue oxygen availability.

Arterial Saturation

Arterial oxygen saturation depends on the partial pressure of dissolved oxygen and the position of the oxyhemoglobin dissociation curve; specifically, the point on the dissociation curve where the hemoglobin is 50% saturated (P_{50}). Fresh red blood cells have a higher P_{50} than bank blood that has been stored for several weeks, and therefore might be expected to display more-favorable oxygen-unloading characteristics.[164] Nevertheless, although shifts of the hemoglobin saturation curve occur under many clinical situations (eg, P_{50} is decreased by hypothermia or alkalosis but is increased by hyperthermia or acidosis), there is virtually no evidence in the literature that this results in a clinically significant change in tissue oxygen delivery.

Critical Oxygen Delivery

In well individuals, a biphasic relation exists such that when oxygen delivery is decreased to a critical point (approximately 8–10 mL/kg/min), oxygen consumption falls. Above this critical level, oxygen consumption remains constant and independent of oxygen delivery. However, this relation may not be true for patients with sepsis/SIRS or MODS. Many studies[150,165–167] indicate that in these patients, either the critical level of oxygen delivery is much higher or a definable critical level is lost (Figure 24-9). As a result of this change in physiology, tissue oxygen utilization may become "supply dependent" and, although the utilization is greater than normal, it may actually be associated with cellular hypoxia. This is suggested by the frequent presence of elevated plasma lactate levels. A number of explanations have been proposed for the paradoxical coexistence of elevated oxygen delivery and apparent hypoxia (Exhibit 24-5). These explanations fall into two categories: (1) abnormalities in blood flow at the level of the microcirculation and (2) deranged cellular metabolism.

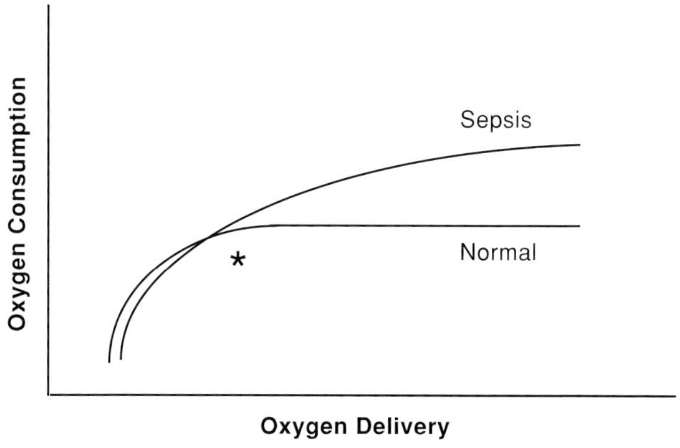

Fig. 24-9. This schematic drawing shows the relation between oxygen consumption and oxygen delivery in normal humans and in patients with sepsis. In normal humans, oxygen consumption does not increase once a certain level of delivery is reached; it remains essentially constant and independent of delivery. This phenomenon is indicated by (*). In patients with sepsis, however, a similar phenomenon is not seen: oxygen consumption continues to increase as oxygen delivery increases.

EXHIBIT 24-5

FACTORS CONTRIBUTING TO SUPPLY-DEPENDENT TISSUE OXYGEN UTILIZATION

1. Mitochondrial cellular respiration is inhibited (there are no clinical human data).
2. Decreased VO_2 is a protective mechanism to prevent organ damage (this has been disproved in cerebral ischemia model).
3. The phenomenon is simply the result of mathematical coupling (this is probably not true because the correlation between VO_2, as measured directly by gas analysis, is well correlated with the value calculated by the Fick equation, and the VO_2–DO_2 correlation appears "linked" in septic patients but not in control groups).
4. A disproportionate percentage of the cardiac output may be delivered to organs with low metabolic demands and oxygen extraction (eg, skin and muscle).
5. Arteriovenous shunts may occur in the precapillary tissue beds.
6. There is a maldistribution of microcirculatory flow as a result of the following factors:
   - microembolization or microthrombi blocking the peripheral vascular bed,
   - endothelial injury and tissue edema increasing the membrane thickness through which oxygen must diffuse,
   - leukocyte aggregation blocking the peripheral vascular bed,
   - altered erythrocyte deformability,[1] and
   - endogenous mediator-induced vasoconstriction reducing flow of the tissue vascular beds.

[1]Hud TC, Dasmahapatia KS, Rush BF, Machiodo GW. Red blood cells deformability in human and experimental sepsis. *Arch Surg*. 1988;123:217–220.

Most animal studies support the concept that shunting blood flow past tissue beds is frequently secondary to the factors listed in Exhibit 24-5. Shunting of blood from the visceral organs to the skin is evident in patients with sepsis, who have vasodilated and warm skin in the presence of oliguria. Because the skin has very little metabolic need and thus extracts little oxygen, the saturation of venous blood returning to the heart (mixed venous oxygen saturation) remains higher than normal.

Many important questions remain unanswered. What causes shunts to open in the skin? Why is the increased cardiac index that characterizes septic shock in humans not adequate to simultaneously perfuse *both* the skin and the visceral organs? Furthermore, although open shunts at the microcirculatory level in viscera would allow blood to bypass nutrient pathways at the cellular level, there is little evidence that such shunts open. However, it is possible that blood flow at the microcirculatory level in a given organ might be maldistributed in a manner similar to that seen when ventilation and perfusion are mismatched in the lung.

The metabolic abnormalities that occur in sepsis/SIRS may arise at the cellular level. Perhaps endogenous mediators impair metabolic pathways in the Krebs cycle, leading to the need for augmented formation of adenosine triphosphate through glycolysis. Experimental and clinical evidence does not provide convincing support for this explanation, for neither the cellular high-energy phosphate levels nor the ratio of the concentrations of pyruvate and lactate are consistently abnormal in either humans or experimental animals with severe sepsis.[168]

A number of studies (some of which confirm, others which do not) demonstrate the presence of abnormal oxygen-supply dependency during septic shock. The reason for the conflict in results is not known; however, this difference may be the result of the heterogeneous population of patients who develop septic shock and the great variety of metabolic demands that may be associated with the septic shock syndrome. If a defect in oxygen utilization does exist, it probably results from tissue hypoperfusion secondary to microcirculatory flow abnormalities.

Lactic Acidosis

The usual cellular response to hypoperfusion is anaerobic metabolism; lactic acidosis may develop as a consequence. However, it is important to recognize that lactate, not lactic acid, is the product of anaerobic glycolysis, and it is the breakdown of adenosine triphosphate, not its formation, that generates hydrogen ions.

Lactate levels are most accurately assessed through an arterial sample so that focal limb hypoperfusion does not affect the sample. Frequent monitoring of the lactate level in the patient with sepsis may yield information regarding the severity of disease,[169] the possible presence of oxygen-supply dependency, the response to therapy (particularly volume administration),[170] and the patient's prognosis.[170,171] Decreased survival has been documented in critically ill patients who have arterial lactate levels greater than 2.0 mmol/L.[172] Both the initial and the subsequent degree of reduction of the lactate levels have been used as prognostic indicators: a study[170] published in 1991 of 48 patients in septic shock documented the superiority of blood lactate levels over oxygen-derived variables in estimating the patient's prognosis.

The monitored variables discussed above (Do_2, Vo_2, and lactate level) are probably best used in complement to aid the physician's decision making regarding therapeutic responses and ultimate prognosis.

Inotropic and Vasopressor Drugs

Not infrequently, the profound vasodilation that occurs in sepsis causes refractory hypotension despite adequate volume resuscitation. Inadequate tissue perfusion that occurs as a result of hypotension will exacerbate organ damage and thus must be corrected. Although inotropic and vasopressor medications are commonly used, few studies compare the efficacy of these agents in the treatment of septic shock. In contrast to cardiogenic shock, for which the selection of a drug with α-agonist properties is undesirable, sepsis-induced vasodilation often demands the use of a drug with significant effect on vascular tone. For example, amrinone lactate causes vasodilation predominantly, making this agent a poor choice for sepsis-induced hypotension unless the patient also has myocardial depression. Table 24-4 lists the characteristics of several commonly used vasopressor/inotropic drugs.

At one time, the use of norepinephrine was shunned because physicians feared that peripheral vasoconstriction, digital ischemia, and renal insufficiency would ensue. Using a canine septic model, researchers demonstrated that the addition of low-dose dopamine (4 µg/kg/min) caused an increased level of renal blood flow whenever norepinephrine was used.[173] The use of norepinephrine has recently been reappraised, particularly in patients with shock refractory to dopamine. One study[174] reported a

TABLE 24-4

CHARACTERISTICS OF USEFUL INTROPES AND VASOPRESSORS

	DOP	DOB	EPI	NOR	AMI
Alpha selectivity	++	–	+++	++++	–
Renal vasodilation	++	–	–	–	–
Tachycardia	++	+	+++	–	+
Dysrhythmias	++	+	+++	–	+
Dosage (μg/kg/min)*	2–20	4–20	0.01–1.0	0.01–1.0	5–20

*Dosages listed are the standard range for patient treatment, and do not infer a maximum safe dosage
DOP: dopamine in moderate dose range (5–10 μg/kg/min); DOB: dobutamine; EPI: epinephrine; NOR: norepinephrine; AMI: amrinone

40% incidence of dopamine resistance in 29 patients in septic shock. The addition of norepinephrine infusion reversed the shock in 10 of 12 (83%) patients. Another study[175] reported a 100% success rate in reversing hypotension in 10 patients with intractable septic shock.

The fear that potential renal insufficiency and decreased tissue blood flow will result from using norepinephrine has been shown to be unfounded. Five studies[175–179] evaluating renal function following the use of norepinephrine for refractory hypotension and oliguria in septic shock are reviewed in Table 24-5. One notable study[179] indicates that patients with a persistent perfusion deficit, as evidenced by lactic acidemia, did not demonstrate an improvement in renal function following the administration of norepinephrine.

Support of the Respiratory System

As discussed earlier in this chapter, respiratory insufficiency is common in patients with sepsis. Although the patient may be able to maintain an adequate level of arterial oxygenation, the increased

TABLE 24-5

NOREPINEPHRINE IN REFRACTORY SEPTIC SHOCK

No. of Patients	Success Rate	Urinary Output*	Creatine Clearance*	Survival
25[1]	100%	I (100%)	I (100%)	16/25 (64%)
5[2]	100%	I (100%)	N/A	2/5 (40%)
6[3] (elevated lactate)	100%	NC	D (100%)	0
9[3] (normal lactate)	100%	I (100%)	NC	4/9 (44%)
24[4]	100%	I (83%)	I (83%)	16/24 (67%)
10[5]	100%	I (100%)	N/A	4/10 (40%)

*The incidence in which the target blood pressure was achieved with norepinephrine
NC: no change; N/A: not measured; I: increased; D: decreased
Data sources: (1) Desjars P, Pinaud M, Bugnon D, Tasseau F. Norepinephrine therapy has no deleterious renal effects in human septic shock. *Crit Care Med.* 1989;17(5):426–429. (2) Hesselvik JF, Brodin B. Low-dose norepinephrine in patients with septic shock and oliguria: Effects on afterload, urine flow, and oxygen transport. *Crit Care Med.* 1989;17(2):179–180. (3) Fukuoka T, Nishimura M, Imanaka H, Taenaka N, Yoshiya I, Takezawa J. Effects of norepinephrine on renal function in septic patients with normal and elevated serum lactate levels. *Crit Care Med.* 1989;17(11):1104–1107. (4) Martin C, Eon B, Saux P, Aknin P, Gouin F. Renal effects of norepinephrine used to treat septic shock patients. *Crit Care Med.* 1990;18(3):282–285. (5) Meadows D, Edwards JD, Wilkins RG, Nightingale P. Reversal of intractable septic shock with norepinephrine therapy. *Crit Care Med.* 1988;16(7):663–666.

work of breathing and the corresponding increased oxygen consumption may be harmful. Earlier studies have shown that during respiratory failure, blood flow to the diaphragm may approach 20% of the total cardiac output, compared with the normal 3% to 5%, potentially depriving other tissues of necessary oxygen delivery. Additionally, oxygen utilization of the respiratory muscles alone may account for up to 25% of the total oxygen consumption.[180] Although it remains unproven, the institution of mechanical ventilation may reduce systemic oxygen consumption and thus aid in clearing lactic acidosis. The clinician must ensure that hypovolemia has been treated because the institution of positive pressure ventilation may cause a decrease in both venous return and cardiac output.

Antimicrobial Therapy

Although the diagnosis of sepsis may be elusive, once considered, therapy must begin early and decisively. This treatment includes excision, debridement and drainage of abscesses or focal sites of infection, and the restoration of a volume deficit. Adequate tissue oxygen delivery, support of organ dysfunction, and the initiation of antimicrobials[181] are the primary therapeutic goals.

The most common category of wound sustained in combat involves only the soft tissue of the body (skin, fat, and skeletal muscle)—wounds that are infrequent sources of fatal sepsis when treated following the established principles of military surgery. However, wounds that involve deeper structures such as bones and especially intraabdominal viscera, even given state-of-the-art surgical care, have a high likelihood becoming infected, with the possibility of inducing sepsis (45% of open comminuted fractures of the femur become infected,[182] as did 45% of open comminuted fractures of the tibia,[183] and 50% of colonic wounds[184]).

Nosocomial infections, though, are common in traumatized patients and are significant potential causes of sepsis.[181] In these instances, antimicrobial therapy can be directed at the identified or presumed pathogens. However, in those cases of generalized sepsis without an identified source, or those with several possible sources, antimicrobials—particularly antibiotics—must be initiated early and broadly enough to cover a variety of potential pathogens.

Selection of Antimicrobial Therapy

Ideally, the infecting pathogen should be identified before antibiotic therapy is started. This requires identification through culture, a process that delays initiating therapy. Specific clues as to the organisms may be gleaned from the physical examination and Gram's stain of material from potential pathogenic sites. Examination of the skin may be of significant benefit, as it allows infections in surgical wounds, venipuncture sites, or intravenous catheter sites to be identified. Pathognomonic lesions from meningococcemia, toxic shock syndrome, or infectious endocarditis may also be identified.[185] All potentially infected materials such as blood, urine, sputum, wound exudate, and cerebrospinal fluid should be examined and cultured based on the patient's condition.[186] Cultures and Gram's stains require proper handling to prevent contamination and potential misinterpretation. Additional diagnostic studies such as CT scan may help identify a potential source of infection. Not uncommonly, though, critically ill patients cannot undergo the optimal diagnostic procedure. They may be too hypoxic for a bronchoscopy, too thrombocytopenic for a tissue biopsy, or too unstable for transport to the radiology department or operating room.[187]

After all diagnostic measures have been completed, specific treatment aimed at the isolated pathogen should begin. Often, however, the initial therapy is nonspecific, pending identification of the responsible pathogen. When selecting an antibiotic, some of the many factors that must be considered include the following[185,186]:

- onset of infection (traumatic, community-acquired, or nosocomial),
- assumed infective focus,
- immunological status of the patient,
- underlying diseases,
- accompanying organ failure,
- previous antibiotic treatment,
- pharmacokinetics and toxicities of the antibiotics, and
- epidemiology of isolated organisms at the institution, including patterns of resistance.

Ideally, the chosen antibiotic regimen is well tolerated by the patient, is bactericidal, has minimal side effects, and covers all potential pathogens for the particular patient. Antibiotics must be given early, in sufficient dosages, and usually parenterally[186] in the critically ill patient.

Bacterial Infections. Although Gram-negative infections are well known for producing sepsis/SIRS, Gram-positive organisms can also cause it. Immunocompetent patients are often infected with a single pathogen. Immunocompromised patients, however, are frequently infected with many different organisms; hence, they require broad antibiotic coverage. Broad, initial antibiotic coverage is ideally narrowed to more-specific, less-toxic antibiotics after culture results are obtained. Such measures minimize drug toxicity, lower costs, reduce the incidence of superinfection, and lower the development of antibiotic resistance.[185]

After a thorough diagnostic evaluation, empirical treatment is usually based on the presumed site of infection. Nosocomial pneumonias are usually caused by resistant, aerobic, Gram-negative rods, particularly *Pseudomonas* species. Treatment includes an antipseudomonal penicillin (mezlocillin, ticarcillin, or piperacillin) or an effective cephalosporin (ceftazidime) in combination with an aminoglycoside. Cephalosporins with activity against Enterobacteriaceae from the lung and other sites include cefotaxime, ceftizoxime, and ceftriaxone.[151] Other bacterial causes of nosocomial pneumonia are *Legionella,* which is treated with erythromycin; *Staphylococcus aureus,* which, depending on whether the microorganism is methicillin-resistant or penicillinase-producing, can be treated with methicillin, vancomycin, or a cephalosporin such as cephalothin or cefazolin; and the anaerobic organisms, which are treated with clindamycin or metronidazole. However, imipenem/cilastatin, a combination of a carbapenem and a metabolic inhibitor (Primaxin, manufactured by Merck, Sharp and Dohme, West Point, Pa.), is a more recent and possibly a better choice.

Urosepsis is usually caused by Gram-negative rods or enterococci and can be treated with ampicillin (or vancomycin in the penicillin-allergic patient) and an aminoglycoside. Enterobacteriaceae can be treated as above.

Peritonitis or intraabdominal infections are polymicrobial and include enteric Gram-negative rods and anaerobes. Initial treatment includes an aminoglycoside and metronidazole or clindamycin, with the addition of ampicillin or vancomycin for enterococci.

Cellulitis is caused by streptococci or staphylococci and can be treated with a first-generation cephalosporin (such as cefazolin), oxacillin, or vancomycin. Sepsis associated with an intravenous catheter is caused by *Staphylococcus aureus, Staphylococcus epidermidis* or Gram-negative rods and will respond to treatment with vancomycin, an appropriate cephalosporin or, in the case of Gram-negative rods, an aminoglycoside.

Outpatient meningitis, which is often seen in troop populations that are in close confines (eg, in barracks), is caused by *Streptococcus pneumoniae* or *Neisseria meningitidis,* and can be effectively treated with high-dose penicillin. Meningitis seen after trauma requires treatment for (*a*) Gram-negative infections, with a third-generation cephalosporin such as cefotaxime or ceftriaxone, or (*b*) *Staphylococcus aureus,* with vancomycin.

Usually the initial therapy of sepsis consists of a β-lactam antibiotic and an aminoglycoside. The β-lactams include the penicillins and cephalosporins as well as the newer carbapenems and monobactams. These agents may be combined with β-lactamase inhibitors such as clavulanic acid or sulbactam.[186] Quinolones are also potentially beneficial. The antibiotics with the broadest aerobic Gram-negative, Gram-positive, and some anaerobic coverage are imipenem/cilastatin and ticarcillin/clavulanate (Timentin, manufactured by SmithKline Beecham, Pittsburgh, Pa.). These are often held in reserve for severe septic infections or in those cases where the etiologic septic focus is unclear and a simplified, less-toxic antibiotic regimen is required. Aztreonam is a monobactam active only against Gram-negative strains and at times may provide an alternative to aminoglycosides.

Lastly, the quinolones are emerging as a potential complement to the regimen in treating patients with sepsis, particularly as resistance to other antibiotics appears. Ciprofloxacin from this group has displayed activity against Enterobacteriaceae, *Legionella* species, *Campylobacter* species, *Yersinia* species, *Staphylococcus aureus, Hemophilus* species, and *Pseudomonas aeruginosa.*[186]

Appropriately chosen antibiotics should be expected to result in patient improvement within approximately 48 hours. The patient's failure to improve may suggest one or more of the following problems[185]:

- inappropriate antibiotic selection, due either to inactivity against the pathogen or to poor penetration into the infected site,
- inadequate dosing,
- an antibiotic-induced toxicity such as drug fever,
- an undrained focus of infection,
- an infection such as infective endocarditis that requires a longer time to show a clinical response, or
- infection with another pathogen not covered by the chosen antibiotic.

Nonbacterial Infections. Nonbacterial infections can occur in the immunocompromised, septic patient, particularly those on antibiotics. Fungal infections are becoming more prevalent in the compromised host. The most common pathogenic fungus is *Candida*, particularly *C albicans*. Superficial mucosal infections are common as normal bacterial flora are inhibited by antibiotics. Local visceral involvement of the kidneys, lung, and central nervous system can also occur. Finally, disseminated candidiasis with candidemia, *Candida* endophthalmitis, or multiorgan involvement can occur in the seriously ill patient who is being treated with antibiotics.

The source of *Candida* is usually the patient's own gastrointestinal tract. Overgrowth occurs when bacterial flora are reduced, and invasion occurs via surgery, intravenous devices, or translocation across the gastrointestinal wall.[188] Disseminated disease is notoriously difficult to diagnose, with less than one half the patients having documented candidemia or candiduria. Treatment of disseminated candidiasis is with high-dose amphotericin B. Empirical amphotericin B may become justified when adequate antibacterial therapy fails to elicit an appropriate clinical response and candidiasis is suspected.[189]

Infections with viruses such as herpes simplex, varicella-zoster, and cytomegalovirus are common in medical patients with primary or secondary immunodeficiencies, although these may also appear in patients with sepsis or other severe illnesses. For example, reactivation of latent herpes infections may appear in many patients, particularly those with burns or skin breakdown.[189] Lastly, occult tropical or parasitic diseases endemic to the theater of operations may complicate a seriously ill patient's course (eg, by causing persistent fever).

Proposed Therapies

Although the high mortality for sepsis/SIRS and septic shock is widely recognized, the disparate definitions for sepsis and septic shock that were used prior to the American College of Chest Physicians–Society of Critical Care Medicine Consensus Conference contribute to the difficulty of scientific analysis of therapeutic trials. Fluid therapy, optimization of oxygen delivery and consumption, inotropic support, and antimicrobial therapy are the mainstay treatments for sepsis/SIRS. As we learn more about the derangements of this syndrome and the consequences of the disease state itself, and its treatments, newer therapies are being discovered. Investigational therapies have suggested evidence of success, but their validity is not yet established; therefore, this chapter will treat these as proposed therapies.

Prevention of Nosocomial Pneumonia

Nosocomial pneumonia is a significant cause of morbidity and mortality in hospitalized patients and is particularly prevalent in mechanically ventilated patients. In the past, four causes of pneumonia have been theorized[190]:

1. bacterial inoculation by hematogenous spread,
2. direct extension into the lung from a contiguous site,
3. contamination of hospital equipment, and
4. aspiration of bacteria from the stomach and oropharynx.

Of these, the first two are thought to be rare, the third has been implicated, and the fourth appears to be the most common.

Bacterial overgrowth of Gram-negative organisms occurs in the stomach when the pH is increased (> 3.5–4.0).[191] This occurs in patients treated with antacids or histamine type 2 (H_2) blocking agents that are used as prophylaxis against stress-induced gastrointestinal bleeding. With this bacterial overgrowth, reflux of bacteria with subsequent aspiration predisposes to the development of Gram-negative pneumonia.[190]

Sucralfate is a nonabsorbable, cytoprotective agent that minimally neutralizes stomach acid, although it is as protective as antacids and H_2 blocking agents in preventing stress ulceration.[191] In 1987, researchers reported that, when compared with gastrointestinal prophylaxis with sucralfate, the use of antacids or H_2 blocking agents or both resulted in a 2-fold increase in the incidence of pneumonia and a 6-fold increase in the mortality.[192] These data suggest, then, that elevating gastric pH increases the risk of nosocomial pneumonias through increased bacterial overgrowth.

This information, however, remains controversial. Further review of these data suggest that other factors may play a role in the development of nosocomial pneumonias. When the use of antacids was separated from the use of H_2 blocking agents, only the groups using antacids had the high incidence of pneumonias, whereas the patients who received H_2 blocking agents alone did not. One suggestion is that antacids increase gastric volume, leading to more reflux, whereas H_2 blocking agents reduce gastric volume.[190] Differences in the kinds of organisms found colonizing the stomach and the lung have also been reported. One study[193] reported that different pathogens were found in these two locations 28% of the time, and 22% of the time the organisms appeared in the trachea before they appeared in the stomach. These data throw the pathophysiological mechanism previously reported into question. Thus, prophylactic gastric protection, and its relationship to nosocomial pneumonias, remains controversial.

Selective Gut Decontamination

After 1 week in an ICU, 70% to 90% of mechanically ventilated patients become colonized with hospital-acquired bacteria in the oropharynx, with subsequent infection occurring in more than 60%.[194] Most infections are endogenous, in the sense that they are caused by potentially pathogenic organisms that are normal constituents of the oral or intestinal flora at the time of the patient's admission to the ICU (primary endogenous infections); others are acquired from the environment while in the ICU (exogenous infections).[195] The organisms primarily involved in the colonization and subsequent infection are the Enterobacteriaceae, *Pseudomonas* species, *Acinetobacter* species, and *Candida* species.[194,195]

Infection occurs when normal host defenses break down. Normal colonization defenses include mucous membrane integrity, normal physiology and motility (swallowing, peristalsis, and salivation), secretions (saliva, mucous, gastric acid, and bile), secretory IgA, normal mucosal-cell turnover, and indigenous anaerobic flora. The causes of the breakdown in critically ill patients include instrumentation, anesthetics and muscle relaxants, antacids and H_2 blocking agents, and antibiotics.[195]

Attempts to prevent infection from colonizing organisms were first introduced in the ICU following a 1981 study involving patients undergoing colorectal surgery, and patients who were immunocompromised, granulocytopenic, or victims of a burn injury.[196] The antimicrobial regimen most commonly used covers all potential pathogens, avoids indigenous (mostly anaerobic) flora, is nonabsorbable, has minimal bactericidal concentrations for most potential pathogens, and is not degraded by food or enzymes within the gut lumen.[195] One example of selective gut decontamination by antibiotics is the following[194,195,197]:

- a 10-mL suspension of 100 to 200 mg of polymyxin E, 80 mg of tobramycin, and 500 mg of amphotericin B is administered through a gastric tube four times daily;
- a paste containing 2% each of polymyxin E, tobramycin, and amphotericin B is applied to the oral mucosa every 6 hours; then
- an intravenous antibiotic is usually given as prophylaxis for 4 days after the patient is admitted to the ICU until most colonizing potential pathogens are eliminated, to prevent early pulmonary infections caused by community-acquired pathogens (the antibiotic is usually cefotaxime, 1 g administered intravenously every 6 h).

The reported results are varied. Most studies have been performed in Europe and their results have been reviewed and summarized recently.[195] Many studies included patients who were already infected when they were admitted, although some studies included noninfected, traumatized patients. Nevertheless, all studies confirmed a significant reduction in secondary colonization and infection of the respiratory tract. Among the general surgical patients, although selective gut decontamination significantly reduced the incidence of acquired infections, it did not reduce mortality. The mortality of trauma patients was reduced, particularly among those who were severely injured. In this population, mortality from sepsis or MODS was almost completely prevented. The emergence of organisms resistant to the antimicrobials used did not occur.

The enteric flora controlled by this regimen may be responsible for much of the sepsis seen in the control population (ie, those who did not receive the gut decontamination). Potential enteric pathogens may, theoretically, contribute to the patient's illness (known as "gut-origin sepsis") through one of three mechanisms[195]:

1. direct spread to contiguous organs or through aspiration of oral or stomach flora;
2. absorption of endotoxin from enteric, aerobic Gram-negative organisms; and,
3. as demonstrated in animal studies, translocation of potential pathogens through a permeable gut mucosa that has been impaired as a result of ischemia, shock, burns, trauma, or endotoxin.

Although the results published to date appear to support these theories, many questions remain to be answered. In a study of patients with combined acute renal and respiratory failure who received selective gut decontamination, 10 of 12 (83%) control patients developed defined infections, compared with 5 of 15 (33%) patients who received the regimen. However, no significant difference in survival between the groups was seen.[197] Infections appear to be controlled with this technique, although further evaluation is necessary to determine its indications.

Immunotherapy

As noted throughout this chapter, conventional therapy with antimicrobials and supportive measures in the treatment of sepsis/SIRS has not appreciably reduced morbidity and mortality, particularly in the case of Gram-negative sepsis. Immunotherapy directed at causative organisms has been evaluated as a means to improve survival. Specific immunotherapy directed at causative organisms is not simple, for the three common Gram-negative organisms often implicated in sepsis have many serotypes: *Escherichia coli*, approximately 150; *Klebsiella* species, approximately 80; and *Pseudomonas aeruginosa*, approximately 17.[198] Thus, less-complicated schemes have been devised and are being investigated. It is the invasion of Gram-negative organisms that usually initiates the series of events that ultimately produces the sepsis/SIRS syndrome. Immunomodulation of several of these steps has been evaluated in an attempt to abate the septic process at whatever stage it has reached. The areas studied have been therapies directed against the common pathogens; endotoxin; and the cytokines, the end products of the sepsis process.

The use of intravenous IgG in patients with sepsis remains controversial. Generally, in the absence of a functional hypogammaglobulinemia, intravenous IgG does not significantly mitigate the infectious process.[198] Some studies in patients with impaired defense mechanisms (such as occurs in multiple trauma or major surgery) suggest a possible therapeutic role for the use of intravenous IgG in combination with antibiotics.[191,199,200] More specific anti-*Pseudomonas* immunoglobulins are being prepared and tested.

Sepsis caused by *Pseudomonas*, *Klebsiella*, and *Escherichia coli* has been found to be caused by relatively few of their many serotypes. With this information, in an attempt to target Gram-negative pathogens more specifically, vaccines against these predominant serotypes have been developed and are being tested both as active vaccines and for use in the induction of type-specific antibodies that could then be used to prepare a hyperimmune intravenous immunoglobulin for passive immunotherapy. Some progress has been made with these vaccines and they may, at some future time, be given prophylactically to patients at risk for infection (eg, prior to elective bowel surgery) or to populations at risk for trauma (eg, soldiers).[198]

The most intriguing data on immunotherapy published during the 1980s is that directed against the lipopolysaccharide moiety of endotoxin. In 1982, researchers prepared an antiserum to endotoxin by vaccinating healthy men with the J5 mutant *Escherichia coli*.[201] Lacking the oligosaccharide side chain, the lipopolysaccharide core—known as lipid A—of this mutant, which is nearly identical to that of most other Gram-negative bacteria, was exposed to promote antibody formation. In a controlled trial, patients with bacteremia and those in profound shock had improved survival when treated with the J5 antiserum, when compared with controls. Whether the factor responsible for these patients' improvement was an immunoglobulin has not been validated. One study that used intravenous immunoglobulin from donors immunized with a J5 vaccine failed to replicate these results.[202]

More recently, a human monoclonal IgM antibody that binds specifically to the lipid A domain of endotoxin (HA-1A) has been produced, alleviating the need to further pursue the active factor in the J5 antiserum.[203] In a study of 197 patients with documented Gram-negative bacteremia, treatment with HA-1A resulted in a lower mortality in 32 of 105 patients (30%), compared with 45 of 92 patients (49%) in the control group. A similar benefit was seen in those patients who were admitted to the hospital with a diagnosis of Gram-negative bacteremia and shock (33% mortality with treatment, compared with 57% in the control group). Although mortality was lowered as a whole for patients who received the antibody, the 63% of study patients who did not have documented Gram-negative bacteremia showed no significant improvement in survival with the treatment.

Despite the apparent improvement that occurred in the group of treated patients in this study, a significant number of the patients with sepsis died, including approximately one third of patients with demonstrated Gram-negative bacteremia. The final common pathway in the septic process is the release of cytokines from macrophages in response to infections. These compounds may be the source of many of the adverse effects seen in those patients in this study with documented Gram-negative bacteremia who died, as well as in that group of patients who had sepsis/SIRS but did not have a Gram-negative infection. If the septic process has progressed beyond the endotoxin interaction with macrophages, or if it is caused by a non-Gram-negative organism, treatment with the HA-1A antibody would not be expected to cause significant improvement.

Immunological or pharmacological modulation of the cytokine release may be of additional benefit in patients with sepsis. Antibodies directed at TNF have proven beneficial in animal studies and are now beginning to be investigated in human studies. Antagonists against platelet activating factor and the use of pentoxifylline against TNF and IL-1 are also being studied.[191,198]

Hence, immunotherapy directed at different steps in the septic process is being developed. Combination therapy with antibiotics, other pharmacological agents, and immunomodulation of sequential stages of sepsis is being investigated intensively and may prove to be the most effective. This combined approach may be beneficial because the stage in the sepsis continuum in which a given patient lies is not easily determined.[198]

Immunoglobulins cannot, however, be administered with impunity. An upper limit may exist beyond which host-defense mechanisms, such as decreased production of immunoglobulin, are impaired.[204] One researcher states this concern regarding immunotherapy:

> A word of caution is warranted regarding the use of inhibitors of the mediators of septic shock. The pathogenetic mechanisms of septic shock are complex and interdependent, and many of them represent the body's compensatory response to sepsis and therefore have salutary effects.[32(p1476)]

Also of practical concern is the enormous costs involved in immunotherapy.[198] Nevertheless, the promise of an effective management tool against sepsis makes this form of therapy worth ongoing evaluation.

Corticosteroids

The use of glucocorticoids in sepsis/SIRS has been theorized to be beneficial by preventing the release of mediators of tissue damage and hemodynamic instability, improving cardiac performance, inhibiting inflammation and complement activation, stabilizing cell membranes, and preventing lysosomal release.[191] Impaired immune responses such as leukocyte chemotaxis that occurs with their use may, however, be harmful. Animal studies done in 1976 suggested some benefit, although usually only when administered before or soon after experimentally induced sepsis. In 1976, a prospective, randomized, controlled study[205] of patients with sepsis who were treated with infusions of high-dose glucocorticoids reported a reduction in mortality with treatment (10% vs 38%). The results of this study have not been replicated, but have prompted several evaluations of the possible role of glucocorticoids in both sepsis and septic shock as well as in the treatment and prevention of ARDS.

Studies of Adult Respiratory Distress Syndrome

At least two studies have failed to demonstrate a significant benefit when corticosteroids were used in the management of ARDS. In one study[206] of 99 patients with established ARDS from several causes, treatment with methylprednisolone (30 mg per kg body weight given every 6 h for 24 h) was evaluated. The study reported no difference in mortality or in the reversal of ARDS with treatment. A similar study[207] of patients admitted to an ICU with fever and hypotension, using methylprednisolone in an identical fashion, failed to demonstrate any reduction in the subsequent development of ARDS or of mortality. One recent uncontrolled study[208] of patients with established ARDS reported that a sustained course of steroids resulted in improvement of ARDS; however, these results have yet to be verified in a controlled fashion.

Studies of Human Sepsis

Other studies have attempted to confirm the previously reported benefits of steroids in the treatment of sepsis. In one study[209] investigating the effects of high-dose corticosteroids in patients with septic shock, patients were treated an average of 18 hours after the onset of sepsis with methylprednisolone (30 mg/kg), dexamethasone (6 mg/kg), or no therapy. A one-time second dose was administered 4 hours later if shock persisted. Patients who received steroids within 4 hours after the onset of shock had a higher incidence of shock reversal. Similarly at 24 hours after drug administration, more patients who received treatment had reversal of shock than those who did not. However, over the course of the study, the reversal of shock disappeared and no improvement in survival was apparent. These researchers concluded that steroids were not beneficial, although they may be helpful early in the septic course in a select group of patients.

Two other controlled studies that followed reached similar conclusions. In 1987, the Veterans

Administration Systemic Sepsis Cooperative Group[210] reported a study of patients with sepsis who received a high-dose corticosteroid bolus (30 mg/kg methylprednisolone) followed by an infusion (5 mg/kg/h for 9 h) within an average of 2.8 hours after the diagnosis of sepsis had been made. Again, no statistical improvement in survival was noted at 14 days. Also in 1987, another group[211] published the results of their controlled multicenter study, in which patients received 30 mg/kg of methylprednisolone every 6 hours for four doses beginning within 2 hours of the diagnosis of sepsis or septic shock. They found no significant improvement in the treatment group with regard to the prevention of shock, reversal of shock, or overall mortality; however, the incidence of secondary infections was increased.

So despite the improvement noted in a 1976 animal study,[205] the conclusions of more-recent studies in sepsis are that high-dose corticosteroids have no place in the management of sepsis. And also, despite the recent, uncontrolled report[208] of the use of a sustained course of corticosteroids in established ARDS, most controlled data suggest that steroids neither prevent nor reverse ARDS.

Naloxone

Endogenous opioid peptides have been reported to be involved in the pathophysiology of septic shock. Animal studies that utilize the opioid antagonist naloxone have demonstrated some improvement in the treated animals' conditions.[191] Clinical responses in humans have been varied, however. Most often cited is a 1981 study[212] in which blood pressure increased in 8 of 13 patients with hypotension and shock following the infusion of 0.4 to 1.2 mg of naloxone, although only 3 of the 13 treated patients survived. Most of the nonresponders in this study were adrenally insufficient; hence, it has been postulated that naloxone therapy requires intact adrenocortical function. Prolonged infusions of naloxone have been shown to reduce inotropic and vasopressor requirements and improve stroke volume and heart rate.[213] One uncontrolled study[214] reported an increase in systolic and mean arterial pressure in patients with sepsis with a naloxone bolus followed by an infusion, although no overall effect on mortality was observed. Naloxone may provide a temporizing means to improve the hemodynamics or cardiovascular status of a patient in septic shock. But without a randomized, prospective, controlled study, its use to improve survival remains unproven.

Cyclooxygenase Inhibitors

Cyclooxygenase inhibitors and thromboxane synthetase inhibitors have also been shown to have some benefit in animal models of sepsis.[191] Many of the mediators of sepsis activate enzymes that release fatty acids, such as arachidonic acid, from cell membranes. Cyclooxygenase inhibitors such as indomethacin may help ameliorate some of the hypotension and organ damage reported to be associated with arachidonic acid metabolites. Administration of ibuprofen decreases extravascular lung water in septic animals.[58]

Metabolic Manipulations

Bacterial translocation from the bowel has been discussed as a potential endogenous source of enteric, Gram-negative sepsis. Total parenteral nutrition and the absence of enteral feeding have been associated with gut mucosal atrophy, bacterial and fungal invasion, and increased mortality.[191] As demonstrated in animal models, bacterial translocation from the gut is increased in animals fed parenterally versus those receiving enteral feeding.[215] Early enteral feeding stimulates gut function and protects the gut barrier. The early institution of enteral feeding may prove to be a major therapeutic modality in the prevention of sepsis. This was the case in trauma victims who had fewer infections and lower mortality when fed enterally.[216]

Calcium abnormalities are common in the septic state. The hypocalcemia seen appears to result from aberrations in the parathyroid hormone–vitamin D axis, perhaps aggravated by endotoxin.[217] Although hypocalcemia is usually mild, it can be severe. Only ionized calcium levels can accurately reflect true hypocalcemia. Replacement, though, is not always indicated, for intracellular calcium overload results in activation of protease and other digestive enzymes and the uncoupling of oxidative phosphorylation, with the end result being cellular death.[218] Sepsis itself may increase intracellular calcium by diminishing adenosine 5′-triphosphate (ATP), by interfering with calcium transport systems, or increasing calcium entry into the cell, or both.[191] In this regard, the calcium channel–blocking agents have been shown to improve hemodynamics, cardiovascular function, and survival in a dog model of sepsis.[219] Further study is warranted before widespread use of calcium channel–blocking agents in sepsis is recommended.

Other investigational therapies for sepsis are also being explored.[191] Toxic oxygen radicals have been implicated in many clinical disorders including sepsis/SIRS. Enzymes such as superoxide dismutase, catalase, and peroxidase are being evaluated for their ability to remove free radicals. Xanthine oxidase, which is involved in free-radical formation, is inhibited by allopurinol; iron chelators such as desferrioxamine limit the availability of iron and therefore also limit the subsequent free-radical formation. Many other theoretical modes of therapy are being investigated. Most of these require more animal testing before clinical trials can be initiated. As is the case with the corticosteroids, widespread acceptance or rejection of a new therapy requires proven clinical efficacy through a well-designed, randomized, controlled, and preferably double-blind study.

ESTABLISHED MULTIPLE ORGAN FAILURE

Multiple, sequential, progressive organ failure as a syndrome is relatively newly described. Other nomenclature used in the literature of the past include the syndromes of hypermetabolism[220] and malignant intravascular inflammation.[221] The initial descriptions of an organ-failure syndrome were written near the end of the Vietnam War.[4,5] Since then, the United States has been involved in no major conflict or war resulting in a large number of casualties, and most of the military medical experience in recognizing and treating the syndrome results from the peacetime care of military members, their dependents, and retirees.

Sequential or progressive organ failure following an initial injury or illness was described in 1973.[222] The syndrome was defined in 1975.[52] In 1980, Fry and associates[223] reported the principal predisposing factors for the development of MODS: (*a*) resuscitation with a large volume of fluid or (*b*) the presence of infection. This paper was also the first to report the mortality rate for multiple, sequential organ failure. The development of multiple organ failure became an accepted indication for an exploratory laparotomy to search for an unrecognized source of sepsis. Also in 1980, infection was observed to be not the only preceding factor for the development of multiple organ failure, as only 50% of patients were found to have positive blood cultures.[224] The term "non-bacteremic sepsis" was coined to describe this phenomenon. By 1985, other researchers[225] wrote that multiple organ failure could be produced by any process initiating an inflammatory response.

Multiple organ failure is now the major cause of death in patients surviving longer than 48 hours following severe trauma, and is also the most common cause of death in patients in surgical ICUs.[220]

Before we can discuss the importance or prevalence of this medical condition, we must clearly define the syndrome. Much of the earlier research regarding this condition was hampered by the lack of a uniform description or definition. Again, Fry and associates[223] were the first to carefully define organ-system dysfunction in the postoperative patient. The frequency of multiple-system organ failure was retrospectively examined in 1,200 patients. The criteria used for sepsis were the most strict; thus, these patients were quite seriously ill.

In 1985, using a large database, the Critical Care Medicine group at George Washington University Hospital, Washington, D. C., developed a uniform set of definitions of organ system failure (Exhibit 24-6).[91] Their goal—to use criteria that were not only objective but also independent of therapy—was intended to facilitate an analysis of patient therapy and outcome. The definition for respiratory failure was the exception to these stringent criteria; respiratory failure is increasingly difficult to define when the clinical signs are masked by mechanical ventilatory support.

Prevalence

The George Washington University team used the definitions in Exhibit 24-6 to evaluate more than 2,800 patients admitted to ICUs in 13 medical centers within the United States and more than 2,400 patients admitted to ICUs in hospitals in France. The resultant combined database contained 5,248 randomly selected admissions to ICUs. The prevalence of organ-system failure on admission was not published in the 1985 study, but, "49% [of the patients met] at least one of the definitions prior to discharge from the ICU or death."[226(p224)] Furthermore, if multiple organ failure is literally the presence of more than one failed organ system, then this occurred in approximately 15%, or one of every seven patients. Three principal factors that would aid in predicting subsequent development of multiple-system organ failure in patients cared for in combined medical–surgical ICUs were identified[226]:

- the severity-of-disease score (as measured by the Apache II test),
- the admission diagnosis, and
- age greater than 65 years.

EXHIBIT 24-6

DEFINITIONS OF ORGAN SYSTEM FAILURE

One of the following criteria needs to be met during a 24-hour period:

Cardiovascular Failure[1]

Heart rate $\leq$ 54/min

Mean blood pressure $\leq$ 49 mm Hg

Ventricular tachycardia or fibrillation

Serum pH $\leq$ 7.24 with a $Paco_2$ of $\leq$ 49 mm Hg

Respiratory Failure[1]

Respiratory rate $\leq$ 5/min or $\geq$ 49/min

$Paco_2 \geq$ 50 mm Hg

$A\text{–}aDo_2 \geq$ 350 mm Hg, with $A\text{–}aDo_2$ calculated as $(713 \bullet Fio_2) - Paco_2 - Pao_2$

Dependent on ventilator on the 4th d of organ system failure

Renal Failure[1]

Urinary output < 480 mL/24 h or < 20 mL/h/8 h

Serum blood urea nitrogen $\geq$ 100 mg/dL

Serum creatinine $\geq$ 3.5 mg/dL

Hematological Failure[1]

White blood cells $\leq$ 1,000 mm^3

Platelets $\leq$ 20,000 mm^3

Hematocrit $\leq$ 0.20

Neurological Failure[1]

Glasgow coma score $\leq$ 6 in the absence of sedative drugs

Hepatic Failure[2]

The patient must have *both*:

Bilirubin > 6 mg/dL

Prothrombin time > 4 s over control, in the absence of systemic coagulation defect or anticoagulant medication

$A\text{–}aDo_2$: alveolar – arterial difference in partial pressure of oxygen; Fio_2: fraction of inspired oxygen; $Paco_2$: arterial partial pressure of carbon dioxide; Pao_2: arterial partial pressure of oxygen
Data sources: (1) Knaus WA, Draper EA, Wagner DP, Zimmerman JE. Prognosis in acute organ-system failure. *Ann Surg.* 1985;202:685–693. (2) Knaus WA, Wagner DP. Multiple systems organ failure: Epidemiology and prognosis. *Crit Care Clin.* 1989;5(2):221–232.

Additional authorities have reported the subsequent development of multiple organ failure in surgical patients (Table 24-6).

TABLE 24-6

INCIDENCE OF MULTIPLE SYSTEM ORGAN FAILURE

Date	Patient Characteristic	Prevalance (%)
1985	Medical/surgical intensive care unit[1]	15
1986	Multiple trauma[2]	5–12
1986	Emergency surgery[3]	7–22
1986	Intraabdominal abscess[3]	30–50
1988	Emergency surgery[2]	7

Data sources: (1) Knaus WA, Draper EA, Wagner DP, Zimmerman JE. Prognosis in acute organ-system failure. *Ann Surg*. 1985;202:685–693. (2) Fry DE. Multiple system organ failure. *Surg Clin N Am*. 1988;68(10):107–122. (3) Carrico CJ, Meakins JL, Marshall JC, Fry D, Maier RV. Multiple-organ-failure syndrome. *Arch Surg*. 1986;121:196–208.

Prognosis

Several researchers have investigated the risk of death from MODS (Tables 24-7 and 24-8).[91,223,227,228] Their data demonstrate two main points regarding the prognosis following the onset of organ failure. First, patient age greater than 65 years increases the risk of death by 10% to 20%. The outcome for elderly patients is also affected to a greater degree by the length of time during which organ failure continued. Second, the mortality rate is so high for patients with three or more organ-system failures that youthful age is no longer a protective factor. By the second day of failure of three or more organ systems, the mortality rate exceeds 90%.

It appears that not all organ-system failures affect mortality equally. In particular, neurological

TABLE 24-7

PROGNOSIS FOLLOWING THE ONSET OF MULTIPLE ORGAN FAILURE

Patient Characteristics	Mortality (%)	Patient Characteristics	Mortality (%)
ARDS alone (n = 13)[1]	31	Emergency surgery/MOF[3]	74
ARDS with MOF (n = 38)[1]	74	Medical-surgical ICU/MOF admissions[4]	64–98
ARDS with MOF[2]	50		

ARDS: adult respiratory distress syndrome
ICU: intensive care unit
MOF: multiple organ failure (≥ two organ failures)
Data sources: (1) Richardson JD. Adult respiratory distress syndrome. *Surg Profiles*. 1988;10–15. (2) Bell R, Coalsu J, Smith J. Multiple organ system failure and infection and the adult respiratory distress syndrome. *Ann Intern Med*. 1983;99:293–298. (3) Fry DE, Pearlstein L, Fulton RL, Polk HC. Multiple system organ failure. *Arch Surg*. 1980;115:136–140. (4) Knaus WA, Draper EA, Wagner DP, Zimmerman JE. Prognosis in acute organ-system failure. *Ann Surg*. 1985;202:685–693.

TABLE 24-8

AGE-RELATED RISK OF DEATH FROM MULTIPLE SYSTEM ORGAN FAILURE

Day of Failure	No. of Failed Organ Systems	64 Years Old and Younger			65 Years Old and Older			All Ages		
		Deaths	Patients	%	Deaths	Patients	%	Deaths	Patients	%
1	1	440	2,297	19	488	1,323	37			
	2	313	718	44	267	419	64			
	3 or more							404	491	82
2	1	294	1,291	23	347	842	41			
	2	262	561	47	221	302	73			
	3 or more							302	322	94
3	1	248	1,036	24	309	672	46			
	2	219	415	53	153	214	71			
	3 or more							208	223	93
4	1	221	846	26	264	561	47			
	2	185	350	53	139	191	73			
	3 or more							152	159	95
5	1	198	729	27	235	491	48			
	2	160	311	51	128	178	72			
	3 or more							127	131	97
6	1	170	615	28	222	441	50			
	2	146	270	54	111	138	80			
	3 or more							103	105	98
7	1	145	542	27	179	353	51			
	2	126	217	58	87	105	83			
	3 or more							103	105	98

Adapted with permission from Knaus WA, Wagner DP. Multiple systems organ failure: Epidemiology and prognosis. *Crit Care Clin*. 1989;5(2):228.

failure has been associated with an independent mortality rate of nearly 40%. All other organ-system failures are accompanied by approximately a 30% risk of death. However, the researchers at George Washington University Hospital concluded in 1989:

> Indeed it can be argued that virtually all patients who die in intensive care units, unless they have sudden death, die with some degree of multiple system organ failure.[226(p224)]

Etiology and Pathophysiology

A brief review of the medical literature published only during the 1980s will help the reader understand the pathophysiology of this condition. (In view of the still-evolving descriptions of this syndrome and our incomplete understanding of it, hereinafter we will use the term MODS when discussing this syndrome in its historical context, regardless of the extant terminology.) During 1980, MODS was believed to be the result of either an inadequate circulatory state or unresolved sepsis. Fry's research revealed four pathological conditions, each of which was associated with a 24% to 28% incidence of MODS: (1) oligemic shock, (2) septicemia, (3) massive crystalloid therapy (> 6 L) and (4) massive blood therapy(> 6 units).[223] The latter two conditions were associated with the development of MODS independent of the initial disease state.

In further support of the role of infection during this syndrome, Fry demonstrated that 34 of 38 (89%) emergency surgery patients with two or more organ-system failures had sepsis. Furthermore, 100% of patients with three or more organ-system failures had sepsis, and infection was considered to be the cause of death in 58% of all fatalities.[223]

Fry believed that abnormal oxygen utilization secondary to infection was common and in 1980 supported that view with the following observation:

> The failure of organ function in tissues anatomically and functionally different suggests that a common cellular insult may be the fundamental pathophysiologic event in patients with uncontrolled systemic infection.[223(p139)]

By 1982, while reviewing enterococcal bacteremia, Garrison and Fry[229] reported that 48 of 114 patients (42%) had no identifiable primary focus of infection and did not respond to the usual antibiotic regimen. They believed that these bacteremic episodes were the result of bacteria translocated across the gastrointestinal tract. In order for this event to occur, the authors postulated that there must be a break in the gastrointestinal tract mucosal barrier, which is followed by either perihepatic shunting or an overwhelming of the hepatic reticuloendothelial system, as previously demonstrated in states of starvation, excessive alcohol use, or use of corticosteroids. Many studies have been published since that support the translocation of bacteria across the gastrointestinal lumen (Table 24-9).

In 1985, the interaction of endotoxin (also called lipopolysaccharide) with hepatic Kupffer cells was reported in an animal model.[230] The result was a marked decrease in hepatic protein synthesis and subsequent liver failure. Endotoxin that was administered systemically did not have the same effect. Much of the adverse effects appeared to be mediated through the macrophage (Kupffer cell), and its secretory products including complement, IL-1, the prostaglandins, and oxygen free radicals. The report suggests that

> [because lipopolysaccharide] is known to activate Kupffer cells and other macrophages, and [lipopolysaccharide] had no effect on isolated hepatocytes, all combine to support the idea that endotoxin may stimulate Kupffer cells to release mediators, which impair hepatocyte function.[230(p93)]

Thus, new information revealed that bacteria alone may not be responsible for all of the effects on organ systems, and that the presence of live bacteria are not necessary to initiate the cascade. This observation further supports the existence of "culture-negative" sepsis.

In 1985, a retrospective review[225] comparing patient groups of multiple trauma to those with intraabdominal infections and sepsis was published. The incidence of patients with a blood culture positive for bacteria was 40% in the trauma group compared with 73% in patients with intraabdominal sepsis. However, the sequence and severity of organ failure were the same in both groups. Pulmonary failure occurred within 3 days, followed by hepatic, and finally, cardiovascular. Of patients with MODS, 34% had negative blood cultures. The theoretical pathophysiological explanation is that complement is activated, which stimulates polymorphonuclear cells to aggregate, which, in turn, releases prostaglandins and oxygen free radicals, setting in motion a vicious circle:

TABLE 24-9

EVIDENCE OF BACTERIAL TRANSLOCATION IN THE GASTROINTESTINAL TRACT

Date	Model	Significant Findings
1969[1]	Human shock	Histological changes in the gastrointestinal tract were observed after shock
1974[2]	Animal	*Candida* organisms were found to cross from the gastrointestinal tract to the portal venous system
1982[3]	Human sepsis	Description of focus enterococcal bacteremia
1988[4]	Animal	Translocation of bacteria into the mesenteric nodes was proven at autopsy, yet fewer than one third had positive blood cultures
1988[5]	Animal, nontraumatized and on total parenteral nutrition	Higher incidence of bacteria in mesenteric lymph nodes was seen in the group receiving nothing by mouth
1989[6]	Animal, in hemorrhagic shock	Mesenteric lymph nodes, liver, and blood were all positive for bacteria

Data sources: (1) Sorenson FH, Vetner M. Hemorrhagic mucosal necrosis of the gastrointestinal tract without vascular occlusion. *Acta Chir Scan.* 1969;135:439–448. (2) Stone HH, Kolb LD, Currie CA. *Candida* sepsis: Pathogenesis and principles of treatment. *Ann Surg.* 1974;179:697–711. (3) Garrison RN, Fry DE. Enterococcal bacteremial clinical implications and determinants of death. *Ann Surg.* 1982;196:43–47. (4) Baker JW, Deitch EA, Berg RD, Specian RD. Hemorrhagic shock induces bacterial translocation from the gut. *J Trauma.* 1988;28(7):896–906. (5) Alverdy JC, Aoys E, Moss GS. Total parenteral nutrition promotes bacterial translocation from the gut. *Surgery.* 1988;104:185–190. (6) Deitch EA, Bridges W, Ma L, Berg R, Specian RD, Granger DN. Hemorrhagic shock-induced bacterial translocation: The role of neutrophils and hydroxy radicals. *J Trauma.* 1990;30(8):942–951.

> [I]t should be realized that after appropriate surgery the vicious circle of activated complement, permeability edema, and tissue anoxia is in itself able to perpetuate severe generalized inflammation and has the potential to kill the patient.[225(pp1114–1115)]

Clinical Manifestations

One of the features that distinguishes MODS is the usual *sequential* failure of organ systems, as opposed to the immediate failure of many organs that is seen with trauma. An inciting injury or event is followed initially by successful resuscitation. This may be followed by a period of 2 to 3 days of relative stability. Following this is a period of hypermetabolism (manifested by a near doubling of the patient's metabolic rate and carbon dioxide production). The mortality during this phase alone is approximately 25% to 40%.[21] If the patient's metabolic needs are not abated by resolution of infection, inflammation, or circulatory compromise, then progressive organ failure will develop in approximately 7 to 21 days. This occurs in approximately 40% of patients who develop the hypermetabolic state.[220]

Thus, although the an initiating injury may have been localized to a single organ (eg, the lung), the physiological response can be thought of as a "global circulatory injury."[231(p888)] While established MODS is nearly always manifested by hepatic failure, one study reveals two separate clinical courses for the development of this condition[220]:

- One subset of patients has lung injury as the predominant clinical feature with other organ failure developing shortly before death.
- A second, more-common clinical course is early lung injury followed by a stable period of 10 to 14 days, after which progressive organ failure occurs.

Metabolic Changes

In addition to a greatly increased metabolic rate and oxygen requirement, the body's handling of cellular substrate changes. The metabolic mechanism that normally promotes the entry of pyruvate into the Krebs cycle decreases. Despite the fact that glucose cannot be utilized properly, a relative insulin deficiency exists, which results in hyperglycemia as a result of increased glucagon, increased hepatic gluconeogenesis, and increased glycolysis. Increased lactate production is an additional result of the changed metabolism of pyruvate. The body's tissues must receive their substrate needs from other sources (eg, fat and protein). This results in increased lipolysis and decreased peripheral lipoprotein lipase activity, and leads to hypertriglyceridemia. Administration of excess lipid via nutrients can lead to hypoxemia and immunosuppression.[220]

Perhaps the most injurious metabolic feature of this syndrome is the extreme catabolism resulting from muscle breakdown: urinary nitrogen excretion exceeds 20 g/d.[220] A marked decrease in the normal hepatic synthesis of albumin and other proteins compounds this protein loss.

Pulmonary Failure

The lung is usually the first organ to fail in the sequence of MODS.[223] Pulmonary injury may occur directly (eg, via aspiration or infectious pneumonia) or secondarily (eg, via sepsis). Why does the lung so frequently become injured in patients who have distant foci of infection or injury? The answer probably can be found in two pathophysiological mechanisms:

1. Inflammatory mediators and toxic byproducts are released.
2. Cellular aggregates comprising leukocytes, platelets, and fibrin may block pulmonary capillaries leading to an elevation of the pulmonary vascular resistance and ventilation–perfusion abnormalities. (This mechanism is inherent to the normal function of the lung as a component of the reticuloendothelial system.)

Patients in an early state of MODS may present with "soft" clinical signs and symptoms of distress (ie, a slight increase in respiratory rate and a subjective feeling of dyspnea at rest). This frequently progresses rapidly to respiratory failure accompanied by marked tachypnea, the use of accessory muscles of respiration, and hypoxemia. Patients in early MODS require mechanical ventilatory support for hypoxemia, which requires that supplemental oxygen be administered to an elevated concentration, and to provide relief from the work of breathing. In models of respiratory failure, blood flow to the diaphragmatic musculature alone may use up to 30% to 40% of the entire cardiac output.[232]

The pathophysiological changes include decreases in both (*a*) pulmonary compliance associated with interstitial fluid accumulation and (*b*) the functional residual capacity (ie, the volume that ensures normal oxygenation of the continuous blood flow adjacent to the alveoli). Positive end-expiratory pressure functions mainly to increase this volume, which, in turn, generally decreases the shunted fraction.

Despite the problem that hypoxemia presents, these patients generally do not die of hypoxia. Maintaining a Po_2 greater than 60 mm Hg is usually not difficult. The clinical situation is more complicated; Po_2 represents only the dissolved oxygen carried in the blood. In ARDS and MODS, it appears that some tissue beds do not utilize oxygen. Much of the current literature supports the contention that this is caused by the shunting of blood flow past tissue or organ beds, particularly in the splanchnic circulation.[150,233]

Once mechanical ventilatory support is required, additional risks include a significant incidence of nosocomial pneumonia, oxygen toxicity, and a state of lung inflammation that acts as a self-perpetuating cause of further organ damage.

The lung also functions as a metabolic organ, clearing vasoactive substances such as the prostanoids and bradykinin from the circulation. When this lung function fails, elevated plasma levels of certain mediator substances may also play a role in the hemodynamics of sepsis, manifesting as refractory vasodilation.

Cardiovascular Failure

The hemodynamic responses are the best-studied clinical signs in patients with either sepsis/SIRS or MODS. Most clinicians are aware that high cardiac output and low systemic vascular resistance measurements are characteristic. However, not all patients who demonstrate these values, as measured by the pulmonary artery catheter, should be labeled septic, for the following reasons:

1. Systemic vascular resistance is a *calculated* variable, so if an elevated cardiac output occurs, the systemic vascular resistance value will be calculated as low. This may not match the patient's actual physical state.
2. High cardiac output and decreased systemic vascular resistance have other causes, including severe anemia, cirrhosis, excessive volume resuscitation, thryotoxicosis, and arteriovenous malformation or shunt.

Despite the consistent measurements of high cardiac output, there is still considerable myocardial dysfunction observed in sepsis or MODS.[77] Myocardial depression, as evidenced by a global cardiomyopathy or dilation of the left ventricle, has been documented. Patients who are unable to develop this dilation, usually viewed as an abnormal state, have a higher mortality than patients who do. In patients with ARDS, improved survival has been observed to be associated with an elevated left ventricular end diastolic volume. This compensatory response allows for the development of an increased stroke volume, cardiac index, and oxygen delivery. Increasing evidence has demonstrated dysfunction of the right ventricle as well, particularly if there are high pulmonary arterial pressures.[82,83]

The most obvious hemodynamic change is the profound degree of vasodilation, which results in hypotension. This low perfusion pressure at the time of increased metabolic needs may further contribute to organ damage. Despite a high cardiac output, blood flow does not appear to be properly distributed among tissues, leading to an inappropriately high, mixed venous-oxygen content, reflecting a decreased tissue-organ oxygen uptake.[234]

The degree of oxygen debt may reflect the elevated arterial lactate level and is correlated with decreased survival.[235,236] A low cardiac output is observed only in the final stages of sepsis or MODS, with this caveat: some patients with a previous history of myocardial infarction, particularly the elderly, are unable to mount a hyperdynamic response. This compensatory response—hyperdynamic circulation—appears to increase the probability of survival.[160]

Other possible explanations for an abnormal relationship between oxygen delivery and consumption include the following:

- The tissues may not be able to extract oxygen.
- There may be areas of underperfused capillary beds (unrecruited).
- A disproportionate percentage of the cardiac output may be delivered to organs with low metabolic demands and oxygen extraction (eg, skin and muscle).
- Arteriovenous shunts may occur in the precapillary tissue beds.
- Endothelial injury may result in tissue edema, thereby increasing the distance across which oxygen must diffuse.
- Microthrombi may block the peripheral vascular bed.
- Mediator-induced vasoconstriction may reduce flow through tissue vascular beds.

Hepatic and Gastrointestinal Failure

The liver and other components of the gastrointestinal tract comprise another organ system that fails in MODS. This organ system's role in the pathophysiology and clinical features of MODS was ignored for many years, but interest has been renewed. Some authorities view the gastrointestinal tract as a target organ, while others see it as the motor that drives the entire MODS process.[220,237,238] Primary among the clinical signs seen are those involving hepatic injury. The liver is directly downstream from the gastrointestinal tract, and thus may be exposed to a large number of bacteria translocated into the portal venous system.[239] Functioning as a component of the reticuloendothelial system, the liver filters out bacteria and particulate matter. Hepatic Kupffer cells comprise nearly 70% of the body's entire macrophage population.

The gastrointestinal tract appears to play a significant role in the perpetuation of MODS, usually manifesting injury concomitantly with the lungs:

> [T]he important role played by the reticuloendothelial system is suggested by the fact that the liver and lungs, two large reticuloendothelial organs, are in series and can, therefore, filter particulate matter from blood draining from the [gastrointestinal] tract, preventing their passage to the systemic circulation.[240(p199)]

Thus the liver may become injured, mechanically blocked, or it may completely fail.[241] The clinical signs are jaundice, altered protein handling, and immunosuppression from a decreased secretion of IgA antibodies.

The stomach is also known to be affected in these syndromes. Endotoxin decreases mucosal blood flow, increases mucosal permeability, and increases total acid production.[242] The result may be stress ulceration or gastritis and gastrointestinal hemorrhage. This is much less frequent than it was even as recently as the 1980s, as antacids, histamine blocking agents, or sucralfate (Carafate, manufactured by Marion Merrell Dow, Kansas City, Mo.) are now routinely administered to seriously ill patients. This may come with a price, though, as bacterial overgrowth in the stomach occurs when the normal acidic environment is changed to alkaline. The same bacteria were found in the stomach and upper airway in 52 of 60 (87%) surgical ICU patients.[243]

Small-bowel dysfunction frequently occurs, presenting as abdominal distention, ileus, or intolerance to enteral feeding.[240] This occurs secondary to edema of the small-bowel wall and a decrease of the villous absorptive area. Animal models of shock show that these changes may occur within hours of the inciting injury.[191]

The gallbladder is not infrequently involved, with a pattern of cholecystitis different than usual. Patients who are critically ill as a result of trauma, burn injury, or medical illness may not tolerate enteral feeding. The lack of enteral nutrition or the use of total parenteral nutrition has been associated with acalculus cholecystitis. The importance of this condition is the high incidence of gallbladder gangrene (approximately 50%), and perforation (10%).[244] Thus, despite their degree of illness, these patients must have drainage. Recent practice has been to drain these abscesses percutaneously at the bedside under ultrasound guidance, rather than to perform an open cholecystotomy in the operating room.

Renal Failure

Renal failure occurs frequently as a component of MODS (45%–65% incidence).[225] Anecdotally, the kidneys appear to be injured more from uncontrolled sepsis than they are from the use of relatively toxic antibiotics (eg, gentamicin or tobramycin). Renal failure is discussed as a consequence of sepsis earlier in this chapter, and is the subject of Chapter 26, Acute Renal Failure; therefore, it will not be discussed further here.

Coagulation Failure

The most controversial issue regarding DIC is the therapy for it. Clearly, the most effective management tool is effective treatment of the underlying or precipitating infection or disorder and associated factors such as shock. The use of heparin in an attempt to block enhanced clotting activity has not proven to be efficacious in treating DIC that is associated with sepsis/SIRS.[118] Heparin should be reserved for use in patients exhibiting thrombotic complications.[122] Replacement therapy with platelets and fibrinogen is likewise controversial but may be prudent in the patient who is hemorrhaging.[96] Antifibrinolytic agents such as ε-aminocaproic acid are probably contraindicated due to an increased incidence of significant thrombotic events.[118]

Current Treatment Modalities

The current treatment of MODS centers around four modalities. First and foremost is the prevention, control, or elimination of any known inciting or promoting condition. This includes the drainage of abscesses, excision of a burn wound, control of hemorrhage, and aggressive hemodynamic support during shock.

The second approach is additional circulatory resuscitation, the proper end point of which has not yet been elucidated. The parameters that have been considered normal are not normal for the critically ill patient with sepsis.[245,246] Previously, conventional wisdom had recommended increasing the patient's hemodynamic state only if it fell below the individual's baseline preoperative value. More recently, researchers have recommended increasing oxygen delivery until a supranormal level has been reached, or until the consumption no longer increases and the arterial lactate level decreases.[160,244,247,248] General criteria to ensure optimal tissue perfusion include the following:

- minimal or absent acidosis and an *arterial* lactate level less than 2 mmol/L, and
- urinary output maintained above 0.5 mL/kg/h (polyuria may sometimes occur in sepsis as a result of a concentration defect).

In states of oxygen-supply dependency, use Shoemaker's therapeutic goals:

- cardiac index > 4.5 L/min/m^2,
- oxygen delivery > 650 mL/min/m^2, and
- oxygen consumption > 160 to 170 mL/min/m^2.

An alteration in cardiac function and ventricular dilation results in right atrial pressure and PCWP, which do not accurately reflect the intracardiac volumes. This has been recently confirmed in patients with ARDS.[248] The PCWP may help in guiding fluid therapy to avoid further increases in the extravascular lung water and subsequent pulmonary edema.

The third modality in therapeutic support for MODS is nutritional or metabolic modification. The subject, particularly as it applies to combat casualties, is well described in Chapter 23, Metabolic Derangements and Nutritional Support, and therefore will be mentioned only briefly here. As previously discussed, these patients become markedly catabolic. Malnutrition results in a decreased function of both humoral and cellular immunity. Specifically, achieving a positive nitrogen balance appears to improve survival. Nutritional formulae with higher concentrations of the branched-chain amino acids appear to better increase hepatic synthesis of protein and result in lower urea production. However, use of high-branched-chain amino acid formulae does not appear to lessen mortality.[246] Most authorities recommend between 1.5 and 2.0 grams of protein per kilogram of body weight per day. The total caloric supplement should not exceed 30 to 35 nonprotein kilocalories per kilogram of body weight per day to avoid the development of fatty liver. The calorie-to-nitrogen ratio should be low, as near 100 as possible.[220]

A controversy has arisen recently regarding whether enteral nutrition is superior to parenteral nutrition for critically ill patients. A prospective randomized trial[248] of enteral versus parenteral nutrition, beginning within 6 days after the onset of sepsis, demonstrated no difference in the overall incidence of MODS or mortality. A retrospective study[249] published in 1987 found that patients given total parenteral nutrition developed higher septic-severity scores than patients fed enterally.

In a prospective study[250] done in 1988 that evaluated early enteral feeding following laparotomy for trauma, patients who received enteral feeding within 12 to 18 hours of admission to the ICU had fewer infections and improved survival. Animal models of *Escherichia coli* peritonitis[251] or hemorrhagic shock[252] have demonstrated a marked decrease in the mortality in groups fed enterally. Specifically, the peptide-based diets, compared with total parenteral nutrition for metabolic support, led to increased survival. Other nutritional therapies are also being studied:

- Tailored nutritional therapy, including the administration of fish oil high in omega 3 polyunsaturated fatty acids. These fatty acids are incorporated into cellular membranes and competitively inhibit the cyclooxygenase and lipoxygenase pathways. This has been shown to decreases the production of prostaglandins and leukotrienes (such as TNF and IL-1) by hepatic macrophages.
- Increased glutamine diet. Glutamine is a trophic factor and increases the small-bowel villous absorptive area. Glutamine is also thought to be involved in maintaining the mucosal-barrier function of the gastrointestinal tract.

The fourth modality in treating renal failure in patients with sepsis/SIRS or MODS is hemodialysis. Because supporting renal failure with hemodialysis is the subject of Chapter 26, Acute Renal Failure, it will not be discussed in this chapter.

SUMMARY

Although the etiologies of the syndromes of systemic inflammatory response and multiple organ dysfunction are varied, the pathophysiological mechanisms leading to their clinical manifestations are remarkably similar. The current state of our understanding reveals this to be the result of the activation of the patient's endogenous cellular and humoral defense systems with the subsequent release, activation, or synergistic stimulation of endogenous mediator substances. The multiplicity of these mediator-induced cell-to-cell and tissue interactions reveals the extreme complexity of the human response to foreign material (ie, endotoxin released from Gram-negative bacteria). Good medical supportive care remains a cornerstone of therapy for patients with sepsis/SIRS to prevent progression to MODS. Early recognition and aggressive treatment of (*a*) persistent foci of infection or inflammation and (*b*) residual microcirculatory shock cannot be overemphasized: appropriate treatment by the vigilant clinician can alter the outcome of these patients before the abnormalities of these syndromes become irreversible.

The body's initial, local, tissue response to infection or inflammation is beneficial. If, however, the response becomes generalized, the body becomes flooded with a multitude of complex mediators; this initiates an unrestrained, perpetuating, systemic response. The nature of some of the mediators (ie, the endotoxin moiety) and the subsequent antigen–antibody formation suggest that immunotherapy might be useful in obviating the effects. Immunotherapy may become an effective treatment in the future.

Sepsis/SIRS and MODS have particular relevance for medical officers. Although the actual number of soldiers who die of these syndromes is small, the potential that this population may benefit from lifesaving intervention is great.

REFERENCES

1. Stillwell M, Caplan ES. The septic multiple-trauma patient. *Crit Care Clin.* 1988;4:345–373.

2. Bone RC, Balk RA, Cerra FB, et al. The American College of Chest Physicians/Society of Critical Care Medicine Consensus Conference Committee. Definitions for sepsis and organ failure and guidelines for the use of innovative therapies in sepsis. *Chest.* 1992;101:1645.

3. Beal AL, Cerra FB. Multiple organ failure syndrome in the 1990s: Systemic inflammatory response and organ dysfunction. *JAMA.* 1994;271(3)226–233.

4. Teschan PE, Post RS, Smith LH, et al. Post traumatic renal insufficiency in military casualties. *Am J Med.* 1955;18:172–186.

5. Whelan TJ, Burkhalter WE, Gomez A. Management of war wounds. *Curr Prob Surg.* 1965;5:297–298.

6. Parker MM, Parrillo JE. Septic shock: Hemodynamics and pathogenesis. *JAMA.* 1983;250:2324–2327.

7. Schuster HP. Sepsis: Clinical definition and incidence. In: Reinhart K, Eyrich K, eds. *Sepsis, An Interdisciplinary Challenge.* Berlin, Germany: Springer-Verlag; 1989: 1–6.

8. Parrillo JE. Septic shock in humans. *Ann Intern Med.* 1990;113:227–242.

9. Palinkas LA, Coben P. Disease and non-battle injuries among US Marines in Vietnam. *Milit Med.* 1988;153:150–155.

10. Love AG. *Statistics: Medical and Casualty Statistics.* Vol 15, Part 2. In: Ireland MW. *The Medical Department of the United States Army in the World War.* Washington, DC: Government Printing Office; 1925.

11. Reister FA, ed. *Medical Statistics in World War II.* Washington, DC: Department of the Army, Office of The Surgeon General; 1975: 11.

12. Ognibene AJ. Full-scale operations. In: Ognibene AJ, Barrett O'N Jr, eds. *General Medicine and Infectious Diseases.* Vol 2. In: Ognibene AJ, Barrett O'N Jr, eds. *Internal Medicine in Vietnam.* Washington, DC: US Army, Medical Department, Office of The Surgeon General, Center of Military History; 1982: 64.

13. Ognibene AJ. Medical and infectious diseases in the theater of operations. *Milit Med.* 1987;152:14–18.

14. McGuire GP, Pearl RG. Sepsis and the trauma patient. *Crit Care Clin.* 1990;6:121–146.

15. Baker CC, Oppenheimer L, Stephens B, Lewis FR, Trunkey DO. Epidemiology of trauma deaths. *Am J Surg.* 1980;140:144–150.

16. Bellamy RF. The causes of death in conventional land warfare. *Milit Med.* 1984;149:55–62.

17. Goris RJA, Draaisma J. Causes of death after blunt trauma. *J Trauma.* 1982;22:141–146.

18. Polk HC. Consensus summary on infections. *J Trauma.* 1979;19(suppl 11):894–896.

19. Beebe GW, DeBakey ME. *Battle Casualties: Incidence, Mortality, and Logistic Considerations.* Springfield, Ill: Charles C Thomas; 1952.

20. Arnold K, Cutting RT. Causes of death in United States military personnel hospitalized in Vietnam. *Milit Med.* 1978;143:161–164.

21. Rackow EC. Clinical definition of sepsis and septic shock. In: Sibbald WJ, Sprung CL, eds. *Perspectives on Sepsis and Septic Shock*. Fullerton, Calif: Society of Critical Care Medicine; 1986: 1–9.

22. Lode H, Wagner J, Mueller F, Hund M, Fangmann B, Loehr A. Epidemiology, clinical course, and prognosis of sepsis in 691 patients. In: Reinhart K, Eyrich K, eds. *Sepsis, An Interdisciplinary Challenge*. Berlin, Germany: Springer-Verlag; 1989: 7–11.

23. Meakins JL. Predisposing factors and host defense response to sepsis and septic shock. In: Reinhart K, Eyrich K, eds. *Sepsis, An Interdisciplinary Challenge*. Berlin, Germany: Springer-Verlag; 1989: 12–22.

24. Machiedo GW. Systemic infection and the trauma patient. *Infections in Med*. 1990;Nov(suppl):13–17.

25. Segreti J. Nosocomial infections and secondary infections in sepsis. *Crit Care Clin*. 1989;5:177–189.

26. Northey D, Adess ML, Hartsuck JM, Rhoades ER. Microbial surveillance in a surgical intensive care unit. *Surg Gynecol Obstet*. 1974;139:321–325.

27. Horan TC, White JW, Jarvis WR, et al. Nosocomial infection surveillance, 1984. *MMWR*. 1986;35(1SS):17SS–29SS.

28. Brachman PS, Dan BB, Haley RW, Hooten TM, Garner JS, Allen JR. Nosocomial surgical infections: Incidence and cost. *Surg Clin North Am*. 1980;60:15–25.

29. Allgoewer M, Duerig M, Wolff G. Infection and trauma. *Surg Clin North Am*. 1980;60:133–144.

30. Fry DE. Infection in the trauma patient: The major deterrent to a good recovery. *Heart Lung*. 1978;7:257–261.

31. Sheagren JN. Pathophysiology of sepsis and septic shock. In: Reinhart K, Eyrich K, eds. *Sepsis, An Interdisciplinary Challenge*. Berlin, Germany: Springer-Verlag; 1989: 23–24.

32. Parrillo JE. Pathogenetic mechanisms of septic shock. *N Engl J Med*. 1993;328:1471–1477.

33. Rietschel ET, Brade H. Bacterial endotoxins. *Sci Am*. 1992;Aug:54–61.

34. Thomas L. *The Lives of a Cell: Notes of a Biology Watcher*. New York, NY: Viking (Bantam Books, Inc); 1974: 92.

35. Danner RL, Elin RJ, Hosseine JM, Wesley RA, Reilly JM, Parrillo JE. Endotoxemia in human septic shock. *Chest*. 1991;99(1):169–184.

36. Jacobs RF, Tabor DR. Immune cellular interactions during sepsis and septic injury. *Crit Care Clin*. 1989;5:9–26.

37. Babior BM. Function of neutrophils and mononuclear phagocytes. In: Shoemaker WC, Ayres S, Grenvik A, Holbrook PR, Thompson WL, eds. *Textbook of Critical Care*. Philadelphia, Pa: WB Saunders; 1989: 951–957.

38. Zimmerman JJ. Polymorphonuclear leukocytes—Agents of host defense and autoinjury. In: Shoemaker WC, Ayres S, Grenvik A, Holbrook PR, Thompson WL, eds. *Textbook of Critical Care*. Philadelphia, Pa: WB Saunders; 1989: 969–976.

39. Harlan JM. Leukocyte–endothelial interactions. *Blood*. 1985;65:513–525.

40. Tate RM, Repine JE. Neutrophils and the adult respiratory distress syndrome. *Am Rev Respir Dis*. 1983;128:552–559.

41. Weiland JE, Davis WB, Holter JF, Mohammed JR, Dorinsky PM, Gadel JE. Lung neutrophils in the adult respiratory distress syndrome. *Am Rev Respir Dis*. 1986;133:218–225.

42. Zimmerman JJ. Sepsis and leukocyte function: Harm and benefit. In: Reinhart K, Eyrich K, eds. *Sepsis, An Interdisciplinary Challenge*. Berlin, Germany: Springer-Verlag; 1989: 180–201.

43. Abraham E. Cellular and humoral immunity in the critically ill patient. In: Shoemaker WC, Ayres S, Grenvik A, Holbrook PR, Thompson WL, eds. *Textbook of Critical Care*. Philadelphia, Pa: WB Saunders; 1989: 1024–1028.

44. Tracey KJ. Shock and tissue injury induced by recombinant human cachectin. *Science*. 1986;234:470–474.

45. Tracey KJ. Cachectin/tumor necrosis factor induces lethal shock and stress hormone responses in the dog. *Surg Gynecol Obstet*. 1987;164:415–422.

46. Tracey KJ, Beutler B, Lowry SF. Shock and tissue injury induced by recombinant human cachectin. *Science*. 1986;234:470.

47. Tracey KJ, Fong Y, Hesse DG. Anti-cachectic/TNF monoclonal antibiotics prevent septic shock during lethal bacteremia. *Nature*. 1987;330:662.

48. Kumar A, Dimou C, Hollenberg SM. Tumor necrosis factor produces a concentration-dependent depression of myocardial cell contraction in vitro. *Clin Res*. 1991;39:321A. Abstract.

49. Vincent J-L, Bakker J, Marécaux G, Schondene L, Kahn RJ. Dupont E. Administration of anti-TNF antibody improves left ventricular function in septic shock patients: Results of a pilot study. *Chest*. 1992:101:810–815.

50. Offner F, Philippe J, Vogelaries D, et al. Serum tumor necrosis factor levels in patients with infectious disease and septic shock. *J Lab Clin Med*. 1990;116:100–105.

51. Takayama TK, Miller C, Szabo G. Elevated tumor necrosis factor a production concomitant to elevated prostaglandin E_2 production by trauma patients' monocytes. *Arch Surg*. 1990;125:29–35.

52. Baue AE. Multiple progressive or sequential systems failure. *Ann Surg*. 1975;110:779–781.

53. Shalmi CL, Dutcher JP, Feinfeld DA, et al. Acute renal dysfunction during interleukin-2 treatment: Suggestion of an intensive renal lesion. *J Clin Oncol*. 1990;8(11):1839–1845.

54. Lefer AM. Significances of lipid mediators in shock states. *Circ Shock*. 1989;27:3–12.

55. Wise WC, Cook JA, Eller T. Ibuprofen improves survival from endotoxin shock in the rat. *J Pharmacol Exp Ther*. 1980;215:160.

56. Revhaug A, Michie HR, Manson JM. Inhibition of cyclooxygenase attenuates the metabolic response to endotoxin in humans. *Arch Surg*. 1988;123:162–168.

57. Fink MP, MacVittie TJ, Casey LC. Inhibition of prostaglandin synthesis restores normal hemodynamics in canine hyperdynamic sepsis. *Ann Surg*. 1984;200:619–624.

58. Gnidec AG, Sibbold WJ, Cheung H, Metz CA. Ibuprofen reduces the progression of permeability edema in an animal model of hyperdynamic sepsis. *J Appl Physiol*. 1988;65(3):1024–1032.

59. Haupt MT, Jastremski MS, Clemmer TP, Metz CA, Goris GB. Effect of ibuprofen in patients with severe sepsis: A randomized double-blind multicenter study. *Crit Care Med*. 1991;19:1339–1347.

60. Holaday JW, Faden AI. Naloxone reversal of endotoxin by potensin suggests role of endorphins in shock. *Nature*. 1978;275:450–451.

61. Hinshaw LB, Beller BK, Chang ACK, et al. Evaluation of naloxone for therapy of *Escherichia coli* shock: Species differences. *Arch Surg*. 1984;119:1410–1418.

62. DeMaria A, Craven DE, Heffernan JJ, McIntosh TK, Grindlinger GA, McCabe WR. Naloxone versus placebo in treatment of septic shock. *Lancet*. 1985;1:1363–1365.

63. Safani M, Blair J, Ross D, Waki R, Li C, Libby G. Prospective, controlled, randomized trial of naloxone infusion in early hyperdynamic septic shock. *Crit Care Med.* 1989;17:1004–1009.

64. Shatney CH, Cohen RM, Cohen MR, Imagawa DK. Endogenous opioid activity in clinical hemorrhagic shock. *Surg Gynecol Obstet.* 1985;160:547–551.

65. Stamler JS, Singel DJ, Loscalzo J. Biochemistry of nitric oxide and its redox-activated forms. *Science.* 1992; 258:1898–1902.

66. Hoolenberg SM, Cunnion RE, Parrillo JE. The effect of tumor necrosis factor on vascular smooth muscle: In vitro studies using rat aortic rings. *Chest.* 1991;100:1133–1137.

67. Ochoa JB, Udekwu AO, Billiar TR, et al. Nitrogen oxide levels in patients after trauma and during sepsis. *Ann Surg.* 1991;214:621–626.

68. Petros A, Bennett D, Vallance P. Effect of nitric oxide synthase inhibitors on hypotension in patients with septic shock. *Lancet.* 1991;1(338):1557–1558.

69. Dinarello CA, Gefland JA, Wolff, SM. Anticytokine strategies in the treatment of the Systemic Inflammatory Response Syndrome. *JAMA.* 1933;269(14):1829–1835.

70. Waisbren BA. Bacteremia due to Gram-negative bacilli other than *Salmonella. Arch Intern Med.* 1951;88:467–488.

71. Parker MM, Parrillo JE. Myocardial function in septic shock. *J Crit Care.* 1990;5:47–61.

72. Wilson RF, Thal AP, Kindling PH, Grifka T, Ackerman E. Hemodynamic measurements in septic shock. *Arch Surg.* 1965;91:121–129.

73. Parrillo JE. Septic shock in humans: Clinical evaluation, pathogenesis, and therapeutic approach. In: Shoemaker WC, Ayres S, Grenvik A, Holbrook PR, Thompson WL, eds. *Textbook of Critical Care.* Philadelphia, Pa: WB Saunders; 1989: 1006–1024.

74. Cunnion RE, Parrillo JE. Myocardial dysfunction in sepsis. *Crit Care Clin.* 1989;5:99–118.

75. Parker MM, Shelhamer NH, Natanson C, Alling DW, Parrillo JE. Serial cardiovascular variables in survivors and nonsurvivors of human septic shock: Heart rate as an early predictor of prognosis. *Crit Care Med.* 1987;15:923–929.

76. Calvin JE, Driedger AA, Sibbald WJ. An assessment of myocardial function in human sepsis utilizing ECG gated cardiac scintigraphy. *Chest.* 1981;80:579–586.

77. Parker MM, Shelhamer JH, Bacharach SL, et al. Profound but reversible myocardial depression in septic patients with septic shock. *Ann Intern Med.* 1984;100:483–490.

78. Weisel RD, Vito L, Dennis RC, Valeri CR, Hechtman HB. Myocardial depression during sepsis. *Am J Surg.* 1977;133:512–521.

79. Ognibene FP, Parker MM, Natanson C, Shelhamer JH, Parrillo JE. Depressed left ventricular performance response to volume infusion in patients with sepsis and septic shock. *Chest.* 1988;93:903–910.

80. Jafri SM, Lavine S, Field BE, Bahorozian MT, Carlson RW. Left ventricular diastolic function in sepsis. *Crit Care Med.* 1990;18:709–714.

81. Kimchi A, Ellrodt AG, Berman DS, Riedinger MS, Swan HJC, Murata GH. Right ventricular performance in septic shock: A combined radionuclide and hemodynamic study. *J Am Coll Cardiol.* 1984;4:945–951.

82. Dhaint JF, Lanore JJ, Gournay JM, et al. Right ventricular dysfunction in patients with septic shock. *Intensive Care Med.* 1988;14:488–491.

83. Parker MM, McCarthy KE, Ognibene FP, Parrillo JE. Right ventricular dysfunction and dilatation, similar to left ventricular changes, characterize the cardiac depression of septic shock in humans. *Chest.* 1990;97:126–131.

84. Parker MM, Parrillo JE. Sepsis and myocardial function. In: Reinhart K, Eyrich K, eds. *Sepsis, An Interdisciplinary Challenge.* Berlin, Germany: Springer–Verlag; 1989: 113–124.

85. Parrillo JE, Burch C, Shelhamer JH, Parker MM, Natanson C, Schuette W. A circulating myocardial depressant substance in humans with septic shock. *J Clin Invest.* 1985;76:1539–1553.

86. Newman JH. Sepsis and pulmonary edema. *Clin Chest Med.* 1985;6(3):371–390.

87. Ashbaugh DG, Bigelow DB, Petty TL. Acute respiratory distress in adults. *Lancet.* 1967;2:319.

88. Brighman KL. Specific organ function/dysfunction in sepsis: Pulmonary. In: Sibbald WJ, Spung CL, eds. *Perspective and Sepsis and Septic Shock.* Fullerton, Calif: The Society of Critical Care Medicine; 1986: 147–156.

89. Rinaldo JE, Borovetz H. Deterioration of oxygenation and abnormal lung microvascular permeability during resolution of leukopenia in patients with diffuse lung injury. *Am Rev Respir Dis.* 1985;131:579.

90. Hou S-H, Bushinsky DA, Wish JB, Cohen JJ, Harrington JT. Hospital-acquired renal insufficiency: A prospective study. *Am J Med.* 1983;74:243–248.

91. Knaus WA, Draper EA, Wagner DP, Zimmerman JE. Prognosis in acute organ-system failure. *Ann Surg.* 1985;202:685–693.

92. Menashe PI, Ross SA, Gottleib JE. Acquired renal insufficiency in critically ill patients. *Crit Care Med.* 1988;16:1106–1109.

93. Kreger BE, Craven DE, McCable WR. Gram-negative bacteremia, IV: Re-evaluation of clinical features and treatment in 612 patients. *Am J Med.* 1980;68:344–354.

94. Beaman M, Turney JH, Rodger RS, McGanigle RS, Adu D, Michael J. Changing pattern of acute renal failure. *Q J Med.* 1987;237:15–23.

95. Sprung CL, Peduzzi PN, Shatney CH, et al. The Veterans Administration Systemic Sepsis Cooperative Study Group. Impact of encephalopathy on mortality in the sepsis syndrome. *Crit Care Med.* 1990;18:801–806.

96. Harris RL, Musher DM, Bloom K, et al. Manifestations of sepsis. *Arch Intern Med.* 1987;147:1895–1906.

97. Bolton CF, Young GB. Sepsis and septic shock: Central and peripheral nervous systems. *Crit Care Med.* 1989;17:157–171.

98. Jackson AC, Gilbert JJ, Young GB, Bolton CF. The encephalopathy of sepsis. *Can J Neurol Sci.* 1985;2:303–307.

99. Bowton DL, Bertels NH, Prough DS, Stump DA. Cerebral blood flow is reduced in patients with sepsis syndrome. *Crit Care Med.* 1989;17:399–403.

100. Sacco RL, van Gool R, Mohr JP, Hauser WA. Nontraumatic coma, Glasgow coma score and coma etiology as predictors of 2-week outcome. *Arch Neurol.* 1990;47:1181–1184.

101. Witt NJ, Zochodne DW, Bolton CF, et al. Peripheral nerve function in sepsis and multiple organ failure. *Chest.* 1991;99:176–184.

102. Kinney JM, Duke JH Jr, Long CL. Tissue fuel and weight loss after injury. *J Clin Pathol*. 1970;23(suppl)4:65–68.

103. MacKowiak PA. Microbial synergism in human infections. *N Engl J Med*. 1978;298:21–26.

104. Wilson RF. Prevention and therapy of sepsis in the high-risk surgical patient. In: Reinhart K, Eyrich K, eds. *Sepsis, An Interdisciplinary Challenge*. Berlin, Germany: Springer-Verlag; 1989: 246–283.

105. Meakins JL. Host-defense response to sepsis and septic shock. In: Sibbald WJ, Sprung CL, eds. *Perspectives on Sepsis and Septic Shock*. Fullerton, Calif: Society of Critical Care Medicine; 1986: 113–124.

106. Meakins JL, McLean APH, Kelly R, Bubenik O, Pietsch JB, MacLean LD. Delayed hypersensitivity and neutrophil chemotaxis: Effect of trauma. *J Trauma*. 1982;18:240–247.

107. Alexander JW, Fisher MW. Immunization against *Pseudomonas* infection after thermal injury. *J Infect Dis*. 1974;130:152–158.

108. Kapur MM, Jain P, Gidh M. The effect of trauma on serum C3 activation and its correlation with injury severity score in man. *J Trauma*. 1986;26:464–466.

109. Abraham E. Immunologic mechanisms underlying sepsis in the critically ill surgical patient. *Surg Clin North Am*. 1985;65:991–1003.

110. Wingard DW, Lang R, Humphrey LJ. Effects of anesthesia on immunity. *J Surg Res*. 1967;7:430–432.

111. Scovill WA, Saba TM, Blumenstock FA, Bernard H, Powers SR Jr. Opsonic alpha 2 surface binding glycoprotein therapy during sepsis. *Ann Surg*. 1978;188:521–529.

112. McLoughlin GA, Wu AV, Saporoschetz I, Nimberg R, Mannick JA. Correlation between anergy and a circulating immunosuppressive factor following major surgical trauma. *Ann Surg*. 1979;190:297–304.

113. Dellinger EP, Oreskovich MR, Wertz JM, Lennard ES, Hamaski V. Risk of infection following laparotomy for penetrating abdominal injury. *Arch Surg*. 1984;119:20–27.

114. Meakins JL, Christou NV, Shizgal HM, MacLean LD. Therapeutic approaches to anergy in surgical patients. *Ann Surg*. 1979;190:286–296.

115. Strausbaugh LJ. Hematologic manifestations of bacterial and fungal infections. *Hematol Oncol Clin North Am*. 1987;1:185–206.

116. Emerson WA, Zieve PD, Krevans JR. Hematologic changes in septicemia. *Johns Hopkins Med J*. 1970;126:69–76.

117. Steigbigel RT, Johnson PK, Remington JS. The nitroblue tetrazolium reduction test versus conventional hematology in the diagnosis of bacterial infection. *N Engl J Med*. 1974;290:235–238.

118. Hoeprich PD, O'Grady LF. Manifestations of infectious diseases. In: Hoeprich PD, Jordan MC, eds. *Infectious Diseases: A Modern Treatise of Infectious Processes*. Philadelphia, Pa: JB Lippincott; 1989: 83–94.

119. Bogdonoff DL, Williams ME, Stone DJ. Thrombocytopenia in the critically ill patient. *J Crit Care*. 1990;5:186–205.

120. George JN, Aster RH. Thrombocytopenia due to enhanced platelet destruction by non-immunologic mechanisms. In: Williams WJ, Beutler E, Erslev AJ, Lichtman MA, eds. *Hematology*. New York, NY: McGraw-Hill; 1990: 1351–1370.

121. Kelton JG, Neame PB, Gauldie J, Hirsh J. Elevated platelet-associated IgG in the thrombocytopenia of septicemia. *N Engl J Med*. 1979;300:760–764.

122. Beck EA, Dejana E. Thrombohemorrhagic phenomena associated with infectious diseases. *Semin Hematol*. 1988;25:91–100.

123. Musher DM. Cutaneous and soft-tissue manifestations of sepsis due to Gram-negative enteric bacilli. *Rev Infect Dis*. 1980;2:854–866.

124. Root RK, Jacobs R. Septicemia and septic shock. In: Wilson JD, Braunwald E, Isselbacher KJ, et al, eds. *Harrison's Principles of Internal Medicine*. New York, NY: McGraw Hill; 1991: 502–507.

125. Gramm HJ, Reinhart K, Goecke J, von Buelow J. Symptoms and signs for the early diagnosis of sepsis. In: Reinhart K, Eyrich K, eds. *Sepsis, An Interdisciplinary Challenge*. Berlin, Germany: Springer-Verlag; 1989: 45–57.

126. Krell WS. Pulmonary diagnostic procedures in the critically ill. *Crit Care Clin*. 1988;4:393–407.

127. Young LS. 1990. Gram-negative sepsis. In: Mandell GL, Douglas RG Jr, Bennett JE, eds. *Principles and Practice of Infectious Diseases*. New York, NY: Churchill Livingston; 1990: 611–636.

128. Vender JS. Invasive cardiac monitoring. *Crit Care Clin*. 1988;4:455–477.

129. Goldenheim PD, Kazemi H. Cardiopulmonary monitoring of critically ill patients. *N Engl J Med*. 1984;311:776–780.

130. Amin DK, Shah PK, Swan HJC. The Swan-Ganz catheter: Indications for insertion. *J Crit Illness*. 1986;1:54–61.

131. Amin DK, Shah PK, Swan HJC. The Swan-Ganz catheter: Insertion technique. *J Crit Illness*. 1986;1:38–45.

132. Matthay MA, Chatterjee K. Bedside catheterization of the pulmonary artery: Risks compared with benefits. *Ann Intern Med*. 1988;109:826–834.

133. Connors AF Jr, McCaffree DR, Gray BA. Evaluation of right-heart catheterization in the critically ill patient without acute myocardial infarction. *N Engl J Med*. 1983;308:263–267.

134. Clements FM, de Bruijn NP. Noninvasive cardiac monitoring. *Crit Care Clin*. 1988;4:435–454.

135. Ozier Y, Gueret P, Jardin F, Farcot JC, Bourdarais JP, Margairaz A. Two-dimensional echocardiographic demonstration of acute myocardial depression in septic shock. *Crit Care Med*. 1984;12:596–599.

136. Thomas F, Smith JL, Orme JF Jr, et al. Reversible segmental myocardial dysfunction in septic shock. *Crit Care Med*. 1986;14:587–588.

137. Jardin F, Brun-Ney D, Auvert B, Beauchet A, Bourdarais JP. Sepsis-related cardiogenic shock. *Crit Care Med*. 1990;18:1055–1060.

138. Spinale FG, Smith AC, Crawford FA. Relationship of bioimpedance to thermodilution and echocardiographic measurements of cardiac function. *Crit Care Med*. 1990;18:414–418.

139. Minagi H, Jeffrey RB. Radiologic techniques in the treatment of the critically ill trauma patient. *Crit Care Clin*. 1986;2:821–838.

140. Kronberg FG, Goodwin WJ. Sinusitis in intensive care unit patients. *Laryngoscope*. 1985;95(8): 936–938.

141. Worthen NJ. The use of sonography in the critically ill patient. In: Shoemaker WC, Ayres S, Grenvik A, Holbrook PR, Thompson WL, eds. *Textbook of Critical Care*. Philadelphia, Pa: WB Saunders; 1989: 185–193.

142. Frazee RC, Nagorney DM, Mucha P. Acute acalculus cholecystitis. *Mayo Clin Proc*. 1989;64:163–167.

143. Smith I, Flemming S, Cernaianu A. Mishaps during transport from the intensive care unit. *Crit Care Med*. 1990;18:278–281.

144. Golding RP, Knape P, Strack van Schijndel RJM, de Jong D, Thijs LG. Computed tomography as an adjunct to chest x-rays of intensive care unit patients. *Crit Care Med*. 1988;16(3):211–216.

145. Hoogewoud HM, Rubli E, Terrier F, Hassler H. The role of computerized tomography in fever, septicemia and multiple system organ failure after laparotomy. *Surg Gynecol Obstet.* 1986;162:539–543.

146. Hinsdale JG, Jaffe BM. Re-operation for intraabdominal sepsis: Indications and results in a modern critical care setting. *Ann Surg.* 1984;199:31–36.

147. Hirmer A, Haering R, Peter F. Indication for relaparotomy in postoperative sepsis. In: Schuster HP. Sepsis: Clinical definition and incidence. In: Reinhart K, Eyrich K, eds. *Sepsis, An Interdisciplinary Challenge.* Berlin, Germany: Springer-Verlag; 1989: 284–297.

148. Machiedo, GW, Tikellis J, Suval W, et al. Reoperation for sepsis. *Am Surg.* 1985;51:149–154.

149. Demling RH. Colloid or crystalloid resuscitation in sepsis. In: Sibbald WJ, Sprung CL, eds. *Perspectives on Sepsis and Septic Shock.* Fullerton, Calif: Society of Critical Care Medicine; 1986: 275–300.

150. Rackow EC, Astiz ME, Weil MH. Cellular oxygen metabolism during sepsis and shock: The relationship of oxygen consumption to oxygen delivery. *JAMA.* 1988;259:1989–1993.

151. Rainey TG, English JF. Pharmacology of colloids and crystalloids. In: Chernow B, ed. *The Pharmacologic Approach to the Critically Ill Patient.* Baltimore, Md: Williams & Wilkins; 1988: 219–240.

152. Falk JL, Rackow EC, Weil MH. Colloid and crystalloid fluid resuscitation. In: Shoemaker WC, Ayres S, Grenvik A, Holbrook PR, Thompson WL, eds. *Textbook of Critical Care.* Philadelphia, Pa: WB Saunders; 1989: 1055–1073.

153. Fisher MM. The crystalloid versus colloid controversy. *Clinical Intensive Care.* 1990:52–57.

154. Lucas CE, Ledgerwood AM, Rachwal WJ, et al. Colloid oncotic pressure and body water dynamics in septic and injured patients. *J Trauma.* 1991;31:927–933.

155. Vincent J-L, Armistead CW Jr. Crystalloids versus colloids in septic shock. In: Reinhart K, Eyrich K, eds. *Sepsis, An Interdisciplinary Challenge.* Berlin, Germany: Springer-Verlag; 1989: 231–238.

156. Rackow EC, Falk JL, Fein IA, et al. Fluid resuscitation in circulatory shock: A comparison of the cardiorespiratory effects of albumin, hetastarch, and saline solutions in patients with hypovolemic and septic shock. *Crit Care Med.* 1983;11:839–850.

157. Velanovich V. Crystalloid versus colloid fluid resuscitation: A meta-analysis of mortality. *Surgery.* 1989; 105:65–71.

158. Haupt MT, Rackow EC. Colloid osmotic pressure and fluid resuscitation with hetastarch, albumin, and saline solutions. *Crit Care Med.* 1982;10:159–162.

159. Tullis JL. Albumin: Background and use, I. *JAMA.* 1977;237:355–360.

160. Shoemaker WC, Appel PL, Kram HB, Waxman K, Lee TS. Prospective trial of supranormal valves of survivors as therapeutic goals in high risk surgical patients. *Chest.* 1988;94(6):1176–1186.

161. Fry DE. Multiple system organ failure. *Surg Clin North Am.* 1988;68(10):107–122.

162. Edwards JD, Brown GC, Nightingale P, Slater RM, Faragher EB. Use of survivors' cardiorespiratory values as therapeutic goals in septic shock. *Crit Care Med.* 1989;17(11):1098–1103.

163. Marik PE, Sibbald WJ. Effect of stored-blood transfusion on oxygen delivery in patients with sepsis. *JAMA.* 1993;June 16:3024–3029.

164. Apstein CS, Dennis RC, Briggs L, Vogel WM, Frazer J, Valeri CR. Effect of erythrocyte storage and oxyhemoglobin affinity changes on cardiac function. *Am J Physiol.* 1985;285(Apr, 4 pt 2):H508–H515.

165. Dorinsky PM, Costello JL, Gadek JE. Relationship of oxygen uptake and oxygen delivery in respiratory failure not due to the adult respiratory syndrome. *Chest*. 1988;93(5):1013–1019.

166. Tuchschmidt J, Fried J, Swinney R, Sharna OP. Early hemodynamic correlates of survival in patients with septic shock. *Crit Care Med*. 1989;17(8):719–723.

167. Kariman K, Burns SR. Regulation of tissue oxygen extraction is distributed in adult respiratory distress syndrome. *Am Rev Respir Dis*. 1985;132:109–114.

168. Hotchkiss RS, Karl IE. Reevaluation of the role of cellular hypoxia and the bioenergetics failure in sepsis. *JAMA*. 1992;267:1503–1511.

169. Pasch T, Mahlstedt J, Piche J, Buheitel G, Pscheidl E. Can the outcome after trauma or sepsis be predicted from biochemical or hormonal parameters? *Prog Clin Bio Res*. 1987;236B:85–95.

170. Bakker J, Caffermils M, Leon M, Gris P, Vincent J-L. Blood lactate levels are superior to oxygen-derived variables in predicting outcome in human septic shock. *Chest*. 1991;99(4):956–961.

171. Azimi G, Vincent J-L. Ultimate survival from septic shock. *Resuscitation*. 1986;14(4):245–253.

172. Cady L, Weil MH, Afifi A. Quantitation of severity of critical illness with special reference to blood lactate. *Crit Care Med*. 1973;1:75.

173. Schaer GL, Fink MP, Parrillo JE. Norepinephrine alone versus norepinephrine plus low-dose dopamine: Enhanced renal blood flow with combination pressure therapy. *Crit Care Med*. 1985;13(6):492–496.

174. Desjars P, Pinaud M, Patel G, Tasseau F, Touze M. A reappraisal of norepinephrine therapy in human septic shock. *Crit Care Med*. 1987;15(2):134–137.

175. Meadows D, Edwards JD, Wilkins RG, Nightingale P. Reversal of intractable septic shock with norepinephrine therapy. *Crit Care Med*. 1988;16(7):663–666.

176. Desjars P, Pinaud M, Bugnon D, Tasseau F. Norepinephrine therapy has no deleterious renal effects in human septic shock. *Crit Care Med*. 1989;17(5):426–429.

177. Hesselvik JF, Brodin B. Low-dose norepinephrine in patients with septic shock and oliguria: Effects on afterload, urine flow, and oxygen transport. *Crit Care Med*. 1989;17(2):179–180.

178. Fukuoka T, Nishimura M, Imanaka H, Taenaka N, Yoshiya I, Takezawa J. Effects of norepinephrine on renal function in septic patients with normal and elevated serum lactate levels. *Crit Care Med*. 1989;17(11):1104–1107.

179. Martin C, Eon B, Saux P, Aknin P, Gouin F. Renal effects of norepinephrine used to treat septic shock patients. *Crit Care Med*. 1990;18(3):282–285.

180. Griffel MI, Asiz ME, Rackow EC, Weil MH. Effect of mechanical ventilation on systemic oxygen extraction and lactic acidosis during early septic shock in rats. *Crit Care Med*. 1990;18(1):72–76.

181. Trunkey DD. The treatment of sepsis and other complications in the trauma patient. *Clin Ther*. 1990;12(suppl B):21–32.

182. Simchen E, Sacks T. Infection in war wounds: Experience during the 1973 October war in Israel. *Ann Surg*. 1975;182(6):754–761.

183. Jacob E, Erpelding JM, Murphy KP. A retrospective analysis of open fractures sustained by US military personnel during Operation Just Cause. *Milit Med*. 1992;157(10):552–556.

184. Hardaway RM. Viet Nam wound analysis. *J Trauma*. 1978;18:635–647.

185. Kapusnik JE, Miller RT, Sande MA. Antibacterial therapy in critical care. In: Shoemaker WC, Ayres S, Grenvik A, Holbrook PR, Thompson WL, eds. *Textbook of Critical Care*. Philadelphia, Pa: WB Saunders; 1989: 780–801.

186. Lode H, Kemmerich B. Antimicrobial therapy of septicemia. In: Reinhart K, Eyrich K, eds. *Sepsis, An Interdisciplinary Challenge*. Berlin, Germany: Springer-Verlag; 1989: 780–801.

187. Masur H. Antimicrobials. In: Chernow B, ed. *The Pharmacologic Approach to the Critically Ill Patient*. Baltimore, Md: Williams & Wilkins; 1988: 692–710.

188. Stone HH, Kolb LD, Currie CA. *Candida* sepsis: Pathogenesis and principles of treatment. *Ann Surg*. 1974;179:697–711.

189. Ho M. Nonbacterial infections in the intensive care unit. In: Shoemaker WC, Ayres S, Grenvik A, Holbrook PR, Thompson WL, eds. *Textbook of Critical Care*. Philadelphia, Pa: WB Saunders; 1989: 802–809.

190. Hoyt JW. Pneumonia in the mechanically ventilated patient. Presented at Society of Critical Care Medicine Fellows Symposium; 2 September 1989; Colorado Springs, Colo.

191. Malcolm DS, Zaloga GP. Sepsis and organ failure: Adjunctive pharmacotherapy in sepsis. *Infections in Med*. 1990;June:51–56, July:41–48.

192. Driks MR, Craven DE, Celli BR, et al. Nosocomial pneumonia in intubated patients given sucralfate as compared with antacids or histamine type 2 blockers: The role of gastric colonization. *N Engl J Med*. 1987;317:1376–1382.

193. Garvey BM, McCambley JA, Tuxen DV. Effects of gastric alkalization on bacterial colonization in critically ill patients. *Crit Care Med*. 1989;17:211–216.

194. Kerver AJH, Rommes JH, Mevissen-Verhage EAE, et al. Prevention of colonization and infection in critically ill patients: A prospective randomized study. *Crit Care Med*. 1988;16:1087–1093.

195. Stoutenbeek CP, van Saene HKF. Infection prevention in intensive care by selective decontamination of the digestive tract. *J Crit Care*. 1990;5:137–156.

196. Stoutenbeek CP, van Saene HKF, Miranda DR, Zandstra DF. The effect of selective decontamination of the digestive tract on colonization and infection in multiple trauma patients. *Intensive Care Med*. 1984;10:185–192.

197 McClelland P, Murray AE, Williams PS, et al. Reducing sepsis in severe combined acute renal and respiratory failure by selective decontamination of the digestive tract. *Crit Care Med*. 1990;18:935–939.

198. Cross AS, Sadoff JC, Opal SM, Bhattacharjee AK, Cryz SJ. *The Immunotherapy of Septic Shock: A Process-Oriented Approach*. Washington, DC: Walter Reed Army Institute of Research; 1990: 77–91.

199. Glinz W, Grob PJ, Nydegger UE, et al. Polyvalent immunoglobulins for prophylaxis of bacterial infections in patients following multiple trauma. *Intensive Care Med*. 1985;11:288–294.

200. DiSimone C, Delogu G, Corbetta G. Intravenous immunoglobulins in association with antibiotics: A therapeutic trial in septic intensive care patients. *Crit Care Med*. 1988;16:1–7.

201. Ziegler ED, McCutchan A, Fierer J, et al. Treatment of Gram-negative bacteremia and shock with human antiserum to a mutant *Escherichia coli*. *N Engl J Med*. 1982;307:1225–1230.

202. Calandra T, Glauser MP, Schellekens J, Verhoef J, et al. The Swiss–Dutch J5 Immunoglobulin Study Group. Treatment of Gram-negative septic shock with human IgG antibody to *Escherichia coli* J5: A prospective, double-blind, randomized trial. *J Infect Dis*. 1988;158:312–319.

203. Ziegler EJ, Fisher CJ, Sprung CL, et al. The HA-1A Sepsis Study Group. Treatment of Gram-negative bacteremia and septic shock with HA-1A human monoclonal antibody against endotoxin. *N Engl J Med*. 1991;324:429–436.

204. Kelton JG, Singer J, Rodger C, Gauldie J, Horsewood P, Dent P. The concentration of IgG in the serum is a major determinant of Fc-dependent reticuloendothelial function. *Blood*. 1985;66:490–495.

205. Schumer W. Steroids in the treatment of clinical septic shock. *Ann Surg*. 1976;184:333–341.

206. Bernard GR, Luce JM, Sprung CL, et al. High-dose corticosteroids in patients with the adult respiratory distress syndrome. *N Engl J Med*. 1987;317:1565–1570.

207. Luce JM, Montgomery AB, Marks JD, Turner J, Metz CA, Murray JF. Ineffectiveness of high-dose methylprednisolone in preventing parenchymal lung injury and improving mortality in patients with septic shock. *Am Rev Respir Dis*. 1988;138:62–68.

208. Hooper RG, Kearl RA. Established ARDS treated with a sustained course of adrenocortical steroids. *Chest*. 1990;97:138–143.

209. Sprung CL, Caralis PV, Marcial EH, et al. The effects of high-dose corticosteroids in patients with septic shock: A prospective controlled study. *N Engl J Med*. 1984;311:1137–1143.

210. The Veterans Administration Systemic Sepsis Cooperative Study Group. Effect of high-dose glucocorticoid therapy on mortality in patients with clinical signs of systemic sepsis. *N Engl J Med*. 1987;317:659–665.

211. Bone RC, Fisher CJ, Clemmer TP, Slotman GJ, Metz CA, Balk RA. The Methylprednisolone Severe Sepsis Study Group. A controlled clinical trial of high-dose methylprednisolone in the treatment of severe sepsis and septic shock. *N Engl J Med*. 1987;317:653–658.

212. Peters WP, Johnson MW, Friedman PA, Mitch WE. Pressor effect of naloxone in septic shock. *Lancet*. 1981;1:529–532.

213. Roberts DE, Hall KW, Dobson KE, Light RB. Effects of prolonged naloxone infusion on septic shock. *Lancet*. 1988;2:699–702.

214. Hackshaw KV, Parker GA, Roberts JW. Naloxone in septic shock. *Crit Care Med*. 1990;18:47–51.

215. Alverdy JC, Aoys E, Moss GS. Total parenteral nutrition promotes bacterial translocation from the gut. *Surgery*. 1988;104:185–190.

216. Moore EE. Early postinjury enteral feeding: Attenuated stress response and reduced sepsis. *Contemp Surg*. 1988;32:1–40.

217. Zaloga GP, Chernow B. The multifactorial basis for hypocalcemia during sepsis: Studies of the parathyroid hormone–vitamin D axis. *Ann Intern Med*. 1987;107:36–41.

218. Malcolm DS, Holaday JW, Chernow B, Zaloga GP. Calcium and calcium antagonists in shock and ischemia. In: Chernow B, ed. *The Pharmacologic Approach to the Critically Ill Patient*. Baltimore, Md: Williams & Wilkins; 1988: 889–900.

219. Bosson S, Kuenzig M, Schwartz SI. Verapamil improves cardiac function and increases survival in canine *E. coli* endotoxin shock. *Circ Shock*. 1985;16:307–316.

220. Barton R, Cerra FB. The hypermetabolism multiple organ failure syndrome. *Chest*. 1989;96(5):1153–1160.

221. Pinsky MR. Multiple systems organ failure: Malignant intravascular inflammation. *Crit Care Clin*. 1989;5(2):195–203.

222. Tilney NL, Bailey GL, Morgan AP. Sequential systems failure after rupture of abdominal aortic aneurysms: An unsolved problem in postoperative care. *Ann Surg*. 1973;178:117–122.

223. Fry DE, Pearlstein L, Fulton RL, Polk HC. Multiple system organ failure. *Arch Surg*. 1980;115:136–140.

224. Meakins JL, Wichlund B, Forse A, McLean AP. The surgical intensive care unit: Current concepts in infection. *Surg Clin North Am.* 1980;60(1):117–131.

225. Goris RJ, Boekhorst TP, Nuytinch JK, Gimbrer JS. Multiple organ failure: Generalized autodestructive inflammation? *Arch Surg.* 1985;120:1109–1115.

226. Knaus WA, Wagner DP. Multiple systems organ failure: Epidemiology and prognosis. *Crit Care Clin.* 1989;5(2): 221–232.

227. Richardson JD. Adult respiratory distress syndrome. *Surg Profiles.* 1988;10–15.

228. Bell R, Coalsu J, Smith J. Multiple organ system failure and infection and the adult respiratory distress syndrome. *Ann Intern Med.* 1983;99:293–298.

229. Garrison RN, Fry DE. Enterococcal bacteremial clinical implications and determinants of death. *Ann Surg.* 1982;196:43–47.

230. Keller GA, West MA, Cerra FB, Simmons RL. Multiple systems organ failure: Modulation of hepatic protein synthesis by endotoxin activated Kupffer cells. *Ann Surg.* 1985;201:87–95.

231. Dorinsky PM, Gadek JE. Mechanisms of multiple nonpulmonary organ failure in ARDS. *Chest.* 1989;96(4):885–892.

232. Roussos C, Macklem PT. The respiratory muscles. *N Engl J Med.* 1982;307(13):786–789.

233. Synder JV. Assessment of systemic oxygen transport. In: Snyder JV, Pinsky MR, eds. *Oxygen Transport in the Critically Ill.* St. Louis, Mo: Mosby–Year Book; 1987: 179–196.

234. Kandal G, Aberman A. Mixed venous oxygen saturation: Its role in the assessment of the critically ill patient. *Arch Intern Med.* 1983;143:1400–1402.

235. Shoemaker WC, Appel PL, Kram HB. Tissue oxygen debt as a determinant of lethal and nonlethal postoperative organ failure. *Crit Care Med.* 1988;16(11):1117–1120.

236. Astiz ME, Rackow EC, Kaufman B, Falk JL, Weil MH. Relationship of oxygen delivery and mixed venous oxygenation to lactic acidosis in patients with sepsis and acute myocardial infarction. *Crit Care Med.* 1988;16(7):655–658.

237. Decamp MM, Demling RH. Posttraumatic multiple system failure. *JAMA.* 1988;260(4):530–534.

238. Wilmore DW, Smith RJ, O'Dwyer ST, Jacobs DO, Ziegler TR, Wang X-D. The gut: A central organ after surgical stress. *Surgery.* 1988;104(15):917–923.

239. Border JR. Hypothesis: Sepsis, multiple system organ failure, and the macrophage. *Arch Surg.* 1988;123:285–286.

240. Carrico CJ, Meakins JL, Marshall JC, Fry DE, Maier RV. Multiple-organ-failure syndrome. *Arch Surg.* 1986; 121:196–208.

241. Matuschak GM, Rinaldo JE. Organ interactions in the adult respiratory distress syndrome during sepsis: Role of the liver in host defense. *Chest.* 1988;94(2):400–406.

242. Richardson RS, Norton LW, Soles JE. Gastric blood flow in endotoxin-induced stress ulcer. *Arch Surg.* 1973;106:191–195.

243. DuMoulin GC, Hedley-White J, Paterson DJ. Aspiration of gastric bacteria in antacid-treated patients: A frequent cause of postoperative colonization of the airway. *Lancet.* 1982;1:242–245.

244. Howard RJ. Acute acalculus cholecystitis. *Am J Surg.* 1981;141:194–197.

245. Shoemaker WC, Appel PL, Waxman K, Schwartz S, Chang P. Clinical trial of survivors' cardiorespiratory patterns as therapeutic goals in critically ill postoperative patients. *Crit Care Med.* 1982;10(6):398–403.

246. Parker MM, Shelhamer JH, Natanson C. Serial cardiovascular variables in survivors and nonsurvivors of human septic shock: Heart rate as an early prediction of prognosis. *Crit Care Med.* 1987;15:293.

247. Meguid MM, Campos AC, Hammond WG. Nutritional support in surgical practice. *Am J Surg.* 1990;159 (pt 1):355.

248. Cerra FB, McPherson JP, Konstantimides BS, Konstantimides NN, Teasley KM. Enteral nutrition does not prevent multiple organ failure syndrome (MOFS) after sepsis. *Surgery.* 1988;104(4):727–732.

249. Border J, Hassett J, Labuca J, et al. The gut origin septic states in blunt multiple trauma (ISS 40) in the ICU. *Ann Surg.* 1987;206:427.

250. Peterson VM, Moore EE, Jones TN, et al. Total enteral nutrition versus total parenteral nutrition after major torso injury: Attenuation of hepatic protein reprioritization. *Surgery.* 1988;104:199–207.

251. Kudsk KA, Stone JM, Carpenter G, Sheldon GF. Enteral and parenteral feeding influences mortality after hemoglobin *E. coli* peritonitis in normal rats. *J Trauma.* 1983;23:605–609.

252. Zaloga GP, Knowles R, Black KW, Prielipp R. Total parenteral nutrition increases mortality after hemorrhage. *Crit Care Med.* 1991;19(1):54–59.

Chapter 25

ACUTE RESPIRATORY FAILURE AND VENTILATORY MANAGEMENT

GERALD HARRINGTON, M.D.*; WILLIAM MARX, D.O.†; AND DANIEL P. STOLTZFUS, M.D.‡

*Lieutenant Colonel, Medical Corps, U.S. Army; Department of Surgery, Critical Care Service, Brooke Army Medical Center, San Antonio, Texas 78234-6200

†Lieutenant Colonel, Medical Corps, U.S. Army Reserve; formerly, Director, Surgical Critical Care and Staff, General Surgery Service, Fitzsimons Army Medical Center, Aurora, Colorado 80045-5001; currently, Assistant Professor of Surgery and Critical Care Medicine, Interim Director, Surgical Critical Care, State University of New York Health Science Center of Syracuse, 750 East Adams Street, Syracuse, New York 13210

‡Formerly, Major, Medical Corps, U.S. Army; Staff Anesthesiologist, Staff Intensivist, Anesthesia and Operative Services, Walter Reed Army Medical Center, Washington, D. C. 20307-5001; currently, Assistant Professor of Anesthesiology, University of Florida College of Medicine, Gainesville, Florida 32608-1197; Co-director, Surgical Intensive Care Unit, Veterans Affairs Medical Center, P. O. Box 100254, Gainesville, Florida 32610-0254

INTRODUCTION

Respiratory insufficiency in combat casualties is seen in many different guises depending on the mechanism and the time of appearance (Exhibit 25-1):

- In some casualties, respiratory insufficiency is an immediate and direct consequence of physical trauma to the lungs or the chest wall. An example might be a soldier who is shot through the chest and sustains a massive tension pneumothorax that will cause death within a few minutes unless immediate care is rendered by a medic or a medical officer.
- In other casualties, respiratory insufficiency might develop days after direct trauma to the chest. An example might be a soldier who sustained a gunshot wound of the lung and subsequently develops pneumonia and empyema.
- Unfortunately, some casualties may develop respiratory insufficiency that is, in part, secondary to the therapies given for an injury in some other part of the body. An example might be a soldier who develops pulmonary edema following excessive fluid overload that occurred during the treatment of massive blood loss resulting from a traumatic amputation of a leg.

The most common type of respiratory insufficiency that military anesthesiologists and intensivists (ie, critical care specialists) are likely to see, however, occurs within several days to 1 week following an injury that did not directly involve the lungs or chest wall: the adult respiratory distress syndrome (ARDS). This condition is now recognized as an expression of the systemic inflammatory response syndrome (SIRS) and is related to sepsis.

This chapter is intended to provide practical help to the medical officer who is confronted with casualties whose conditions are of varying degrees of severity, for whom decisions must be made promptly to avoid further morbidity from cerebral hypoxia or

EXHIBIT 25-1

ETIOLOGY OF RESPIRATORY FAILURE IN COMBAT AND CIVILIAN PATIENTS

Pulmonary aspiration

Foreign-body obstruction of the airway

Soft-tissue obstruction of the airway:
- Prolapse of tongue due to unconsciousness
- Prolapse due to facial bone fracture
- Edema and hematoma formation

Pulmonary injury:
- Hemothorax
- Pneumothorax
- Hemopneumothorax
- Lung contusion

Mediastinal emphysema

Rib fractures

Flail chest

Laryngeal fracture (with or without separation)

Tracheobronchial laceration or separation

Acute lung injury secondary to:
- Blast overpressure injury
- Chemical war gas
- Infection
- Hypermetabolism
- Inhalation of combustion products

Hypoventilation secondary to:
- Cervical spinal cord trauma
- Cranial trauma
- Exposure to nerve agent
- Diaphragmatic hernia
- Thoracic wall injury
- Central nervous system depression from drugs or hypoxemia

Adapted with permission from Grande CM, Stene JK, Bernhard WN. Airway management: Considerations in the trauma patient. *Crit Care Clin.* 1990; 6(1):43.

other visceral organ injury. The chapter emphasizes (1) the recognition of respiratory insufficiency and (2) the provision of mechanical ventilation for casualties with respiratory insufficiency at medical treatment facilities from a third-echelon hospital to a medical center in the continental United States.

EPIDEMIOLOGY OF RESPIRATORY FAILURE IN COMBAT CASUALTY CARE

Combat casualties do not commonly present with respiratory insufficiency. Data from the Vietnam War indicate that probably somewhat less than 5% of those killed in action had injuries primarily to the respiratory system exclusive of those who exsanguinated from injuries to the pulmonary vasculature.[1] Respiratory failure at the hospital level may be more common. The total number who die of wounds is about 3% to 4% of hospitalized casualties; it is probably reasonable to assume that all of these casualties—at some time during their hospital stay—would require respiratory support. Data from the Vietnam War indicate that approximately 0.4% of hospitalized casualties died of what would now be called ARDS.[2] Today, many more casualties would probably receive prophylactic respiratory support to prevent respiratory insufficiency, so it is not unreasonable to infer from these data that perhaps 10% of all hospitalized combat casualties are at risk of developing respiratory insufficiency. Furthermore, if nerve agents or enhanced blast munitions were to be used against U.S. military forces in a future hostile action, a much higher percentage of the casualty population will likely need immediate respiratory support. For planning purposes, the Department of Defense's Deployable Medical Systems (DEPMEDS) treatment files predict that in a major, high-intensity war, 17% of hospitalized casualties will require ventilatory support.[3]

Although the civilian experience depends on the type of hospital surveyed, probably no more than several percent of hospitalized patients develop respiratory insufficiency. This assumes that about 5% of patients who are admitted to civilian hospitals are transferred to the intensive care unit (ICU), and that of these, one half require respiratory support for more than 24 hours.[4]

ETIOLOGY OF PULMONARY INSUFFICIENCY

Mechanical Trauma

The battlefield is replete with potential mechanisms for pulmonary injury and the development of respiratory failure. Militarily relevant sources of direct mechanical trauma include penetrating, blunt, and blast injuries to the lungs and the chest wall. In addition, many soldiers with severe penetrating injuries to the brain are not killed outright and require intubation for airway control and mechanical ventilation. The injury to the brain results in destruction of the respiratory centers; therefore, ventilatory drive is absent. During the Vietnam War, this was probably the most common indication for using respiratory support.

Penetrating Injury

Penetrating thoracic injuries may, in turn, cause secondary conditions that result in respiratory insufficiency. Pneumothorax reduces the ability to carry out normal gas exchange. The lack of a negative pressure gradient across the lung parenchyma leads to alveolar collapse and a resulting intrapulmonary shunting of blood. When a sufficient amount of tissue collapses, arterial hypoxemia ensues. *Tension* pneumothorax occurs when air enters the pleural space during inspiration but is unable to escape during exhalation. The progressive accumulation of air produces a shift of the mediastinal structures toward the unaffected side of the thorax. This event worsens gas exchange by compressing the unaffected lung and reduces venous return to the heart, resulting in shock. Hemothorax and hemopneumothorax are found in approximately 50% of casualties with penetrating wounds of the lung.[5] This fact is not surprising, given the close anatomical proximity of bronchioles and arterioles within the lung parenchyma. Small fragments that strike the heart may cause blood to collect within the pericardial space. The increased pressure within the pericardium restricts the ability of the ventricles to accept blood (tamponade). Cardiac output and blood pressure progressively decrease as stroke volume is reduced. If the tamponade is not reversed, cardiovascular collapse and death result.

Blunt Injury

Blunt chest trauma with rib fractures and potential *flail chest* (ie, multiple rib fractures that result in segmental chest wall instability) can occur in a variety of battlefield settings. Underlying pulmonary contusion may be a far more important cause for respiratory failure than the mechanical dysfunction associated with multiple rib fractures.

Blast Injury

Blast injuries from any type of explosion can be categorized as primary, secondary, and tertiary. *Primary* blast injury is due to the direct effect of the pressure wave on the body, and is not common. *Secondary* blast injury occurs when projectiles and debris from the explosion strike the victim. Finally, *tertiary* blast injury, which is the major cause of pure blast injury, occurs when the individual is physically displaced by the bulk flow of gases away from the site of the explosion. The displacement leads to collision with environmental objects and subsequent trauma.[6] A more complete discussion of the medical consequences of blast injury can be found in *The Medical Consequences of Conventional Warfare: Ballistic, Blast, and Burn Injuries*.[7]

The pressure wave from an explosion moves away from the epicenter at supersonic speeds, whether through air or water. As primary blast injury is seen predominantly in the gas-containing organs, the ears, lungs, and gastrointestinal tract are the most readily affected. The ear is the most sensitive, with rupture of the tympanic membrane occurring at pressures above 35 kPa (kilopascals). While injury to the ear causes pain and long-term morbidity, pulmonary damage causes the greatest

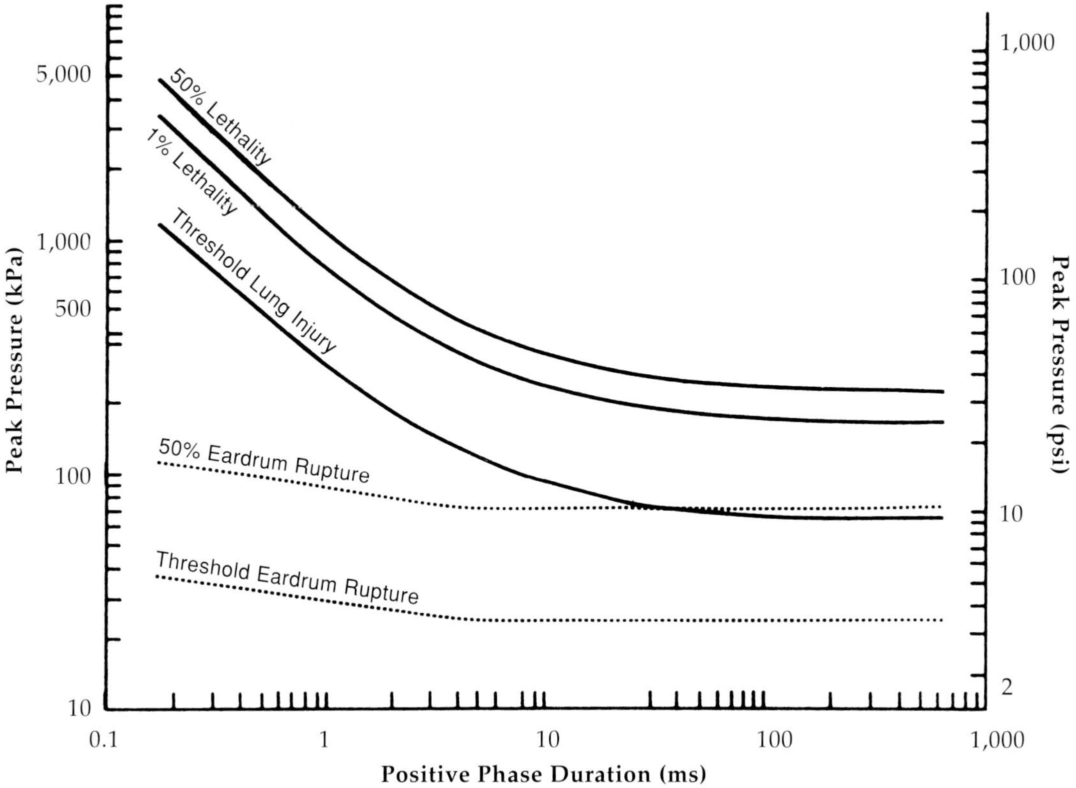

Fig. 25-1. The probabilities of eardrum rupture and death from a pulmonary blast injury. These are shown as functions of both the peak pressure above atmospheric pressure (measured in either kilopascals [kPa] or pounds per square inch [psi]) and the duration of the overpressure (in milliseconds [ms]). For example, a blast wave with a duration of 1 ms that has an overpressure of 5 psi can be expected to cause rupture of the tympanic membranes in a few people. If the overpressure reaches 15 psi, one half of the individuals in the exposed population can be expected to have ruptured tympanic membranes. Much greater pressures are required before pulmonary injury occurs. A blast wave with a duration of 1 msec and a peak overpressure of 50 psi can be expected to cause pulmonary injury in a few people. Doubling that pressure is likely to cause a fatal outcome in about one half of the exposed population. The same lethality is to be expected with a blast wave that lasts 1 s and has a peak overpressure of 12.5 psi. Note that both axes are logarithmic. Adapted from Bowen T, Bellamy RF, eds. *Emergency War Surgery NATO Handbook*. 2nd US rev. Washington, DC: US Department of Defense, Government Printing Office; 1988: 76.

immediate morbidity and mortality (Figure 25-1). Diffuse pulmonary contusions with a marked increase in lung water lead to ventilation–perfusion mismatch and arterial hypoxemia. Disruption of alveoli with the development of alveolar–pulmonary venous communications create the potential for air emboli, which is the most common cause of sudden death in such casualties. The gastrointestinal tract may be disrupted in portions where gas has collected. The colon tends to suffer the most gastrointestinal blast injuries, which are manifested by subserosal and intramural hemorrhage. Gastrointestinal blast injury may result in delayed rupture, days after the traumatic event.[8]

The clinical presentation of each of these injuries depends on the amount of energy transmitted to the various tissues in excess of the tissues' ability to dissipate the delivered forces. Significant pulmonary and gastrointestinal damage is unlikely to have occurred in the absence of tympanic membrane rupture. Arterial air emboli from alveolar–pulmonary venous communications typically present with signs and symptoms of cerebral dysfunction. However, direct trauma to the skull (secondary or tertiary blast injury) is more likely to be the cause of altered neurological function. Evidence of primary blast injury of the lung resembles the diffuse pulmonary contusion seen in blunt chest trauma. Chest pain with tachypnea, use of accessory respiratory muscles, and hemoptysis are common findings. The protean manifestations of *barotrauma* (injury resulting from elevated peak airway pressure) are frequently seen in these patients. Pulmonary contusion, pneumothorax, pneumomediastinum, subcutaneous emphysema, and pulmonary interstitial emphysema can be confirmed with a chest X-ray examination after the patient has been stabilized. Symptoms of blast injury to the lung may be delayed 24 to 48 hours, making differentiation from other forms of acute respiratory failure difficult.

The principles of management are detailed in other textbooks. Briefly summarized, the salient treatment required for improved survival rates of casualties with thoracic injuries is as follows:

- Remove the bloody secretions from the airway.
- Seal open chest wounds.
- Evacuate blood and air from the pleural space.
- Treat hypovolemia.
- Remove blood from the pericardial sac.
- Aggressively treat empyema.

Casualties with blast injuries require additional care. This follows the basic principles of trauma care, with the following caveats directed toward potential complications from the blast:

- Excessive volume resuscitation may complicate the pulmonary contusion present in most of these patients.
- Positive pressure ventilation may increase the severity of barotrauma and increase the possibility of air embolism.
- If oxygenation is inadequate with nasal cannula or mask, continuous positive airway pressure (CPAP) delivered via a tight-fitting mask or endotracheal tube may improve oxygenation without worsening barotrauma.

Thermal Trauma

Although thermal injuries will be encountered on the battlefield, this mode of injury is uncommon in conventional land warfare, occurring in fewer than 10% of all casualties (see Chapter 1, Combat Trauma Overview, Figure 1-4). Thermal injuries are, however, much more common in that subpopulation of soldiers who compose the crew of armored fighting vehicles, and are even more common in sailors and air personnel. In fact, fire and associated smoke inhalation are the most common causes of combat injury on warships.[9] Crewed vehicles—whether ships, tanks, or aircraft—are loaded with munitions and fuel and pose a constant hazard of explosions, fire, and thermal injury secondary to battle damage. Burns to the skin are what we usually think of when thermal injuries are discussed, and in fact, circumferential, full-thickness burns of the thoracic wall may sometimes restrict chest-wall motion to the degree that ventilation is compromised. Escharotomy may be required to improve the restrictive defect. However, the more frequent and more injurious form of thermal injury is damage to the respiratory system caused by inhaling steam and the gaseous and particulate products of combustion such as hydrogen chloride and phosgene from plastic, formaldehyde from wood, and hydrogen cyanide from polyurethane.

Below the level of the vocal cords, thermal injury from heated air is usually prevented by efficient upper-airway cooling. Stridor, hoarseness, and difficulty with phonation all suggest the need to evaluate the upper airway. Injury to the hypopharynx may lead to delayed airway obstruction, making prompt endotracheal intubation a lifesaving maneuver.

These injuries demonstrate a typical acute-lung-injury pattern of increased alveolar-capillary permeability with noncardiac pulmonary edema. Iatrogenic factors may complicate the lung injury: the massive fluid requirements for resuscitation from thermal burns and associated traumatic injuries will invariably worsen pulmonary function. Patients may develop respiratory failure 1 to 2 weeks following thermal injury. When delayed respiratory failure occurs, it is usually caused by infectious complications either within the lung (pneumonia) or at a remote site, giving rise to SIRS, which is the major cause of death.

Inhalation of the toxic products of combustion can induce parenchymal lung damage. The effects may be immediate or delayed for hours. A common, serious pathophysiological effect of inhaling combustion products is carbon monoxide intoxication. The marked affinity of carbon monoxide for hemoglobin (> 200-fold higher than that of oxygen) significantly reduces the oxygen-carrying capacity of blood. A carbon monoxide concentration of 0.1% in ambient air leads to a carboxyhemoglobin concentration of 50%. Carbon monoxide also shifts the oxyhemoglobin dissociation curve to the left, which further reduces oxygen delivery (DO_2) to the tissues. Patients will complain of headache, nausea, and exertional fatigue with moderate carbon monoxide exposure. Damage to the central nervous system (CNS) may occur in up to 30% of affected individuals unless they receive prompt therapy. The classic "cherry red" coloration is not seen with carboxy-hemoglobin concentrations lower than 40%. A far more common manifestation is cyanosis.[10] Lactic acidosis from reduced DO_2 is a common finding with severe intoxication.

The therapy for respiratory injury caused by thermal burn is primarily supportive. Supplemental oxygen and bronchodilators are used to treat hypoxemia and bronchoconstriction. Mechanical ventilation is required for patients with significant acute lung injury. The use of positive end-expiratory pressure (PEEP) increases the functional residual capacity (FRC, the remaining lung volume after passive exhalation) of the lung and allows the fraction of inspired oxygen (FIO_2) to be reduced to nontoxic levels. The U.S. Army Burn Center, Fort Sam Houston, Texas, reports that a mode of ventilation (high-frequency, percussive) that employs repeated cycles of very rapid (several hundred per minute) and small volume (less than the dead-space volume) ventilations may be more efficacious. The mortality rate found in such patients is markedly less (16.4%) than in patients with similar thermal insults who are treated with conventional mechanical ventilation (42.7%). The improved survival may be due to both (*a*) the low airway pressures found in high-frequency percussive ventilation (ie, there is less potential for barotrauma) and (*b*) improved removal of tracheobronchial secretions.[11]

Prophylactic steroids have not proven beneficial for inhalation injury and may increase the risk for subsequent infection. Likewise, antibiotic prophylaxis is no longer used; it may increase the risk for resistant bacterial infection, and has not been shown to reduce morbidity and mortality in clinical trials.[12]

The treatment of carbon monoxide poisoning involves supplying supplemental oxygen to reduce the half-life of carboxyhemoglobin. (With 100% oxygen, the half-life is reduced to 40 min, opposed to 250 min in room air.) Hyperbaric oxygen may be beneficial with severe intoxication; however, this modality is not likely to be available in the combat zone with the possible exception of aboard larger naval vessels.

Chemical Warfare

Almost all chemical war gases cause respiratory insufficiency and manifest a variety of effects that could lead to respiratory failure (see Chapter 30, Anesthesia for Casualties of Chemical Warfare Agents, for a discussion of the respiratory effects of war gases). The four major categories of war gases are nerve, blister, choking, and blood agents. Decontamination procedures are not addressed in this chapter; however, because acute respiratory failure is a common cause of death in affected individuals, medical personnel must ensure that the emergent nature of the situation does not lead to hasty action and inadvertent self-contamination.

Nerve Agents

Nerve agents have the potential to cause vast numbers of casualties. Soldiers must have sufficient personal protective equipment and adequate pharmacological prophylaxis. Military planners must emphasize that medical officers may need to care for mass casualties, all of whom may require mechanical ventilation.

Nerve agents exert their effects by preventing cholinesterase from hydrolyzing acetylcholine (previously released from the nerve terminal). This allows for repetitive stimulation of the postsynaptic receptor, which leads to rapid muscle fatigue. Inhalational or dermal exposures to nerve agents thus present as a cholinergic syndrome, the severity of which depends on the amount of exposure. Respiratory effects of nerve agents include bronchoconstriction and bronchorrhea along with respiratory muscle dysfunction. Organophosphate-induced seizures may further complicate the respiratory embarrassment produced by these agents.

Treatment includes administering both atropine, which blocks the cholinergic receptors, and pralidoxime chloride (2-PAM Cl), which binds to organophosphate and most carbamate nerve agents, releasing the cholinesterase and allowing normal nerve function to resume. Airway control is of paramount importance, as copious secretions may prevent adequate ventilation and oxygenation. If respiratory muscle function is adequate, oral or nasopharyngeal suctioning may be all that is required. However, if respiratory muscle function is poor, endotracheal intubation and mechanical ventilation may be required. Care must be taken to ensure that the lungs are not exposed to the excessively high pressures that result from the intense bronchoconstriction that follows significant nerve agent exposure. Under these circumstances, barotrauma may occur before bronchospasm has subsided. Atropine, inhaled beta agonists such as metaproterenol or terbutaline, and inhalational anesthetics all reverse bronchospasm.[6]

Blister Agents

Blister agents (vesicants), of which the mustards are the best known, are alkylating chemicals that are thought to act by damaging cellular DNA. This leads to cell disruption and death; an intense inflammatory response causes blisters to form. Inhalation of vesicants produces severe tracheitis and bronchitis. Symptoms may not develop for 4 to 6 hours, requiring medical personnel to observe casualties for delayed effects. Bronchopneumonia frequently complicates the recovery of these patients. Progressive, irreversible respiratory insufficiency, developing over months to years after inhalation of mustard, has been described.[13] It appears to be caused by unrelenting fibrosis that leads to stenosis of the entire tracheobronchial tree.

Choking Agents

The war gas that caused the most flagrant example of respiratory insufficiency in World War I was phosgene, a choking agent. Choking agents cause a severe form of respiratory insufficiency and produce significant irritation of the lower respiratory tract. First used in World War I as a toxic agent, phosgene produces distal airway and alveolar inflammation, which eventually causes pulmonary edema. As with blister agents, the effects may be delayed for up to 12 hours; minimal symptomatology may precede the development of fulminant pulmonary edema.

Treatment is entirely supportive. Supplemental oxygen and positive-pressure ventilation may be necessary for severe cases. The effects are self-limiting, but due to the intense inflammatory response elicited, the patient's condition may evolve into ARDS.

Blood Agents

Blood agents such as hydrogen cyanide combine with intracellular cytochrome oxidase and halt cellular respiration. Exposure to large amounts of inhaled hydrogen cyanide causes death within minutes. Exposure to lesser amounts causes vertigo, nausea, vomiting, headache, and tachypnea. Seizures and cardiopulmonary arrest may rapidly ensue if treatment is delayed.

Treatment involves administering amyl nitrate by inhalation or sodium nitrite by vein. Nitrites oxidize the iron moiety of hemoglobin to produce methemoglobin. Methemoglobin scavenges cyanide from the circulating blood, which promotes a concentration gradient for the removal of cyanide from cytochrome oxidase. Intravenous sodium thiosulfate can be administered to provide free sulfur, which will convert cyanide to the far-less-toxic thiocyanate ion. Mechanical ventilation with supplemental oxygen will aid in the resuscitation of apneic casualties; however, expeditious treatment with nitrites is the mainstay of therapy.[6]

Nuclear Warfare

Thermonuclear weapons produce their devastating effects via the release of massive amounts of energy. This energy release produces casualties with three types of injuries: blast, thermal, and radiation. Blast and thermal injuries will be treated in a manner identical to that previously discussed. Neurovascular, gastrointestinal, and hematopoietic syndromes are associated with nuclear radiation injuries. Anesthesiologists and intensivists will encounter the neurovascular and gastrointestinal syndromes only rarely, as these are considered to be uniformly fatal. The hematopoietic syndrome will be the most common radiation injury requiring medical care.

INDIRECT MECHANISMS OF RESPIRATORY INSUFFICIENCY

Respiratory failure in the combat casualty may result from insults other than direct chest trauma. Three of the most frequently encountered etiologies are pulmonary aspiration, hydrostatic pulmonary edema, and permeability pulmonary edema.

Pulmonary Aspiration

Medical personnel should assume that every combat casualty has a full stomach. The combination of a traumatic injury and a full stomach puts soldiers at risk for aspirating blood or regurgitated stomach contents:

> The soldier may have eaten just before being wounded. Even if many hours have passed, pain and anxiety greatly delay gastric emptying. The important interval is not the time since the last meal, but rather the time from the last meal to the time of injury. Regurgitation and aspiration of stomach contents, particularly of volumes greater than 25 mL, with a pH less than 2.5, and in the presence of solid food, place the casualty at high risk for aspiration pneumonitis.[14(p28)]

Aspiration of gastric contents may be asymptomatic or cause several life-threatening syndromes. The underlying common denominator in aspiration is an altered level of consciousness. Many casualties will have head injuries that negate the protective airway reflexes, and many will require general anesthesia or have neurosurgical catastrophes that predispose to aspiration.[15] However, other predisposing conditions (ie, neuromuscular or gastrointestinal disorders) are not common in this population.

Silent aspiration occurs when a small volume of gastric contents is introduced into the trachea. This may occur somewhat frequently in a civilian medical population—elderly and obtunded—who are undergoing elective surgery, receiving therapeutic narcotics, whose level of consciousness is depressed, or while a nasogastric tube is being placed. In a combat situation, silent aspiration is probably less common.

When aspiration occurs, apnea or airway obstruction occur immediately. The acute chemical injury damages the tracheal bronchial tree and alveoli. Pathologic evaluation immediately after aspiration shows bronchiolar epithelial degeneration, pulmonary alveolar edema, and alveolar hemorrhage. Fibrinous exudate, focal atelectasis, and neutrophilic infiltrates occur later. After 24 hours, focal hemorrhage, atelectasis, empyema, fibrin-filled alveoli, and pneumonitis are established.[16] Bacterial pneumonitis can occur within 72 hours, and lung abscesses may occur, usually after days to weeks.

Injury occurs to both Type I and Type II pneumocytes. Type I pneumocytes undergo focal necrosis and the basement membrane is exposed. Fluid fills the alveolar and perivascular spaces. Type II cells are initially edematous, then degenerate. Hyaline membranes form by 48 hours. By 72 hours, alveolar cells regenerate and the inflammatory process abates.

Prevention is the best treatment for aspiration. When prevention fails or is not possible, then making the correct diagnosis, removing large particulate matter, and providing appropriate supportive measures will help improve morbidity and prevent mortality.[17]

Immediate endotracheal intubation is required when apnea occurs. Adequate ventilation should be documented by measuring arterial blood gases or by means of oximetry and capnography, which are discussed later in this chapter.

Airway protection during intubation with cricothyroid pressure should help prevent aspiration. The thumb and middle finger exert pressure lateral to the cricoid cartilage, while the index finger pushes directly down on it. If the technique is properly performed, this technique can prevent regurgitation when intragastric pressures rise to as high as 50 cm H_2O or more. Normal intragastric pressure is usually less than 16 cm H_2O so cricoid pressure should be protective in most instances. As soon as the patient is intubated, the cuff on the endotracheal tube is inflated before manual pressure is released.[18]

Airway obstruction may be due to laryngospasm, edema, mechanical obstruction by foreign material, bronchial inflammation, or bronchospasm. Laryngospasm can be broken with either continuous positive airway pressure or a rapid-acting depolarizing muscle relaxant. If the laryngospasm cannot be broken, surgical control of the airway is mandatory. Nebulized racemic epinephrine may improve airway edema.[15]

Suctioning often clears the airway of foreign debris, but if residual material remains, bronchoscopy will be required. In many instances, aggressive chest physiotherapy will help clear the small airways of particulate matter. This is contraindicated in patients with head trauma or spinal cord injuries, however.

The treatment of aspiration pneumonia should be prophylactic. Elevating the head of the bed to prevent gastroesophageal reflux, neutralizing gastric contents, and prophylactic intubation are of the utmost importance. Once aspiration has occurred, adequate oxygenation is mandatory.[17]

On the battlefield, multiply injured casualties will require intubation. Many will also require urgent or immediate operative intervention. Intubation will prevent further aspiration. Casualties with head injuries will require hyperventilation as well.

Bronchial lavage is no longer believed to be indicated because it may worsen hypoxia. Positive airway pressure should be used for diffuse pneumonitis; however, its use in localized aspiration must be tempered against augmenting ventilation–perfusion mismatch. PEEP may be preferentially distributed to normally compliant units and not improve the FRC in the affected lung region. It must therefore be used with caution.

Appropriate fluid resuscitation should not be tempered by the possibility of lung injury. Fluid overload should be avoided but aggressive resuscitation must not. Cardiovascular stability should be maintained with the proper use of inotropic agents when indicated. In more severe cases, a flow-directed pulmonary artery catheter may be beneficial because it allows optimization of the hemodynamic status of the patient, which should improve survival.

Glucocorticoids have no place in the treatment of aspiration. Glucocorticoids suppress host defense mechanisms and predispose the patient to infection. Prophylactic antibiotics are not used either, as they do not prevent pneumonia and tend to select out resistant organisms, thereby increasing morbidity and mortality.[17]

Hydrostatic Pulmonary Edema

Pulmonary edema is often associated with respiratory failure. The type of pulmonary edema must be determined before the condition can be properly treated. These types are *hydrostatic pulmonary edema,* in which fluid accumulates in the presence of a fairly normal blood–air barrier, and *permeability pulmonary edema,* of which ARDS is the classic manifestation. Hydrostatic pulmonary edema occurs because fluid accumulates in the presence of a fairly normal blood–air barrier. In permeability pulmonary edema, fluid accumulation occurs because the blood–air barrier is abnormal.[19]

Hydrostatic pulmonary edema is usually caused by an increase in the intravascular filtration pressure within the pulmonary microvasculature. The elevated filtration pressure increases the fluid flux into the interstitium. If the capacity of the lymphatic system to reabsorb this fluid is exceeded, then the fluid accumulates in the alveoli. Rarely, fluid may accumulate in two other situations: if plasma oncotic pressure is reduced or if the capacity of the lymphatic system to remove fluid is reduced. The intravascular pressure must rise above 7 to 10 mm Hg for water to flood the interstitial space.

With the increased flux of fluid into the interstitium, the fluid moves down a negative interstitial pressure gradient toward the bronchovascular cuffs. This is where the pulmonary lymphatics begin. If lymphatic uptake is decreased, fluid accumulates around the bronchoalveolar cuff until the interstitial pressure is greater than the airway pressure, at which time fluid enters the alveolus. This is typically seen when the pulmonary artery occlusion pressure (PAOP) exceeds 20 mm Hg.

In the civilian population, the causes of hydrostatic pulmonary edema include cardiac dysfunction, pulmonary venous occlusive disease, neurogenic pulmonary vasoconstriction, pulmonary arterial embolization with air, thrombus, or fat; however, these are rarely seen in young, healthy soldiers. In the combat casualty, the most common causes of hydrostatic pulmonary edema are iatrogenic. Asthma and foreign bodies that cause airway obstruction, and pulmonary lymphatic obstruction may also cause hydrostatic pulmonary edema. Clinically, the classic description is that of respiratory distress with pink, frothy sputum and arterial hypoxemia. In trauma patients, this occurs with massive head injury, chest injury, or large amounts of volume resuscitation.[20]

Patients will occasionally present less dramatically with complaints of mild chest tightness or a pressure sensation, a sensation of being unable to catch the breath, and cough. As the capillary pressure continues to increase, and as the fluid flux becomes more pronounced, the patient will become more symptomatic. The respiratory rate increases and the ventilatory pattern becomes labored. This increases the work of breathing required to achieve adequate lung expansion. Respiratory failure will occur because of muscular exhaustion.

Alveolar flooding is accompanied by arterial hypoxemia. Fluid-filled air spaces prevent the passage of gas into the capillary. These air spaces have low ventilation-to-perfusion ratios (ventilation–perfusion mismatch). As the mismatch increases, the effectiveness of hypoxemic pulmonary vasoconstriction decreases and profound arterial hypoxemia will ensue. Formerly, oxygen was believed to need to diffuse through an abnormally thick layer of water before it reached the red blood cells, but compared to ventilation–perfusion mismatch, this is probably a minor impediment to the exchange of respiratory gases.

The fluid tends to accumulate first in the dependent portions of the lung. Because the pulmonary blood and air flows to the dependent areas are disproportionally small, this fluid accumulation exaggerates the normal propensity for alveoli in the dependent part of the lungs to be underventilated. The pulmonary blood flow is redistributed to less edematous, nondependent alveoli. The FRC decreases with increased critical closing pressure of the alveoli. Other unrelated conditions that decrease FRC (eg, increased intraabdominal pressure, upper abdominal or thoracic incision, and the supine position) can compound the hypoxemia.

The treatment of hydrostatic pulmonary edema must both reverse the changes caused by fluid accumulation and eliminate the underlying disorder that promotes fluid accumulation. The supportive therapy should minimize arterial hypoxemia and decrease the work of breathing. Supplemental oxygen and positive airway pressure are the mainstays of treatment. Administration of supplemental oxygen through nasal prongs or a face mask is useful. However, endotracheal intubation is often required as respiratory failure progresses. If the arterial partial pressure of oxygen (Pa_{O_2}) does not increase after supplemental oxygen therapy is added, then continued hypoxemia is caused by groups of alveoli with low ventilation–perfusion ratios. Positive airway pressure is then delivered as PEEP or CPAP. This will increase the Pa_{O_2} by increasing the FRC of the lungs. (The alveoli are now being ventilated because a higher pressure is being used to force respiratory gas into them.) To decrease the work of breathing, both positive airway pressure and assisted ventilation can be utilized. Positive airway pressure restores lung volume, increases compliance, and increases the cross-sectional area of the airways. It also reduces airway resistance by splinting the airway lumen open. Flow rates will decrease as ventilation becomes less labored, thereby converting a higher-resistance, turbulent flow into a lower-resistant, laminar flow pattern.[21]

Adult Respiratory Distress Syndrome

Lung injury has plagued successful resuscitation of the trauma patient. Lung injury associated with trauma was described in 1932,[22] and ARDS was defined in 1967.[23] For ARDS to occur, the capillary endothelium of the pulmonary vasculature must be injured. This results in dyspnea, hypoxemia, decreased pulmonary compliance, and bilateral pulmonary infiltrates. Pulmonary edema is present but not associated with an increased hydrostatic pressure; it is caused by increased permeability resulting from diffuse alveolar–capillary endothelial injury. ARDS is a common problem affecting previously healthy people. The mortality rate is high: despite vigorous supportive care, it can be greater than 40%.[24]

The syndrome is associated with a wide variety of disease states with multiple underlying etiologies, all demonstrating a single clinical pattern. ARDS can be caused by all types of shock (Exhibit 25-2). A 2.2% incidence of ARDS has been reported

EXHIBIT 25-2

ETIOLOGY OF SHOCK THAT INDUCES THE ADULT RESPIRATORY DISTRESS SYNDROME

- Burns
- Fat emboli
- Lung contusion
- Head trauma
- Near drowning
- Septic states
- Inhalation of toxic gases:
  - Smoke
  - Nitrous oxide
  - Ammonia
  - Chlorine
  - Phosgene
  - Cadmium
- Aspiration of gastric contents
- Drug ingestion
- Pancreatitis
- Multiple transfusions
- Disseminated intravascular coagulation
- Bowel infarction

in casualties with traumatic injuries.[25] The syndrome is more common in casualties with bilateral chest trauma and extensive lung injury than it is in casualties with a localized lung contusion.

Pathophysiology of Alveolar Injury

The normal structural integrity of the alveolus is disrupted in patients with ARDS. Type I pneumocytes cover approximately 95% of the alveolar surface area while Type II pneumocytes cover the remaining 5%. Because of their greater number, Type I pneumocytes are more likely to be injured. Within 24 hours of injury, Type I pneumocytes are destroyed, leaving a denuded basement membrane. Type II pneumocytes, which appear to be more resistant to initial damage, then proliferate and form a continuous layer that covers the previously denuded basement membrane. In addition, the denuded surface may allow aggregates of plasma proteins, cellular debris, fibrin strands, and remnants of surfactant to adhere, which forms the characteristic hyaline membrane. Over the next several days, the alveolar septum thickens, and not only inflammatory cells but also reparative cells proliferate. Hyaline membranes organize, and microatelectasis occurs. The capillary endothelial damage becomes more apparent. Irregularities of the endothelial surface with focal cytoplasmic swelling can be seen, and fibrosis is apparent in the respiratory ducts and bronchioles.[26]

Starling's equation predicts the fluid flux across a semipermeable membrane. It describes the balance between hydrostatic and oncotic pressures acting in opposition across the endothelial barrier. There are two driving forces (the pressure within the capillary, P_c, and the pressure within the interstitium, P_i) and two retaining forces (the colloid osmotic pressure within the capillary, π_c, and the interstitium, π_i). The symbol σ, which is known as the reflection coefficient, represents the impermeability of the membrane to a given substance (ie, if $\sigma = 1$, the membrane is completely impermeable; while if $\sigma = 0$, the membrane is completely permeable). K is a constant representing the filtration coefficient.

Starling's equation states:

$$\text{fluid flux} = K[(P_c - P_i) - \sigma(\pi_c - \pi_i)]$$

Theoretically, the interstitial hydrostatic pressure is slightly negative due to the elastic properties of the lung; therefore, progressively more negative fluid pressures increase the flux into the alveolar space. The small amount of fluid filtered into the interstitial space is readily removed by the extensive pulmonary lymphatic system. Hydrostatic pulmonary edema occurs when the factors favoring fluid flux across the capillary membrane exceed those designed to protect the lungs from developing edema.[19]

The pulmonary edema that characterizes ARDS is caused by alteration of Starling's forces. This alteration is usually due to an abnormally high permeability coefficient; the abnormality is made worse when the capillary hydrostatic pressure increases. The latter abnormality may manifest as elevated pulmonary capillary wedge pressure. Decreased colloid oncotic pressure *can* be caused by severe hypoproteinemia from overhydration with intravenous crystalloid fluid, liver failure, or the nephrotic syndrome; however, it is rarely responsible for lung edema.

Finally, increased interstitial colloid oncotic pressure can occur with increased alveolar capillary membrane permeability (large protein molecules leak out into the interstitium where their oncotic properties attract fluid from the vascular bed). This may be the primary mechanism responsible for the development of pulmonary edema in ARDS. The altered permeability allows the free movement of fluid and protein from the intravascular space, to the interstitial space, to the intraalveolar space. Edema forms at a rate that exceeds the lymphatic system's ability to remove it.

The alteration of the integrity of the alveolar capillaries is believed to result from injuries due to the adverse effects of (*a*) tumor necrosis factor and leukokinin I, which are released from activated macrophages, and (*b*) oxygen free radicals, which are released from neutrophils. Intravascular activation of complement leads to stimulation of neutrophils, sequestration within the capillaries, and subsequent endothelial damage. Patients with ARDS have increased levels of serum C-5A, the activated fifth component of the complement cascade.[26]

Release of C-5A by the alternate pathway causes macrophages and neutrophils to aggregate. The neutrophils release oxygen free radicals; prostaglandins; and granules that contain protease, elastase, coagulase, pepsins and lysozymes. Damage to the basement membrane occurs and increased permeability follows. This allows nonhydrostatic pulmonary edema to form. Arachidonic acid metabolites affect vascular permeability, vascular tone, and airway reactivity, which causes further vasoconstriction and bronchoconstriction.

An additional factor resulting in alteration of the integrity of the alveolar membrane in casualties with massive CNS injury is massive sympathetic discharge, which affects the pulmonary veins. This, in turn, causes profound pulmonary hypertension, which mechanically disrupts the junctions between pulmonary capillary endothelial cells.

Pathophysiology Resulting in Abnormal Gas Exchange

The abnormal gas exchange that occurs in ARDS is due to the increase in extravascular lung water, which tends to close small groups of peripheral alveoli and cause intrapulmonary shunting. This process could be compounded over time by the progressive, extensive fibrosis that occurs in most of these patients. In one study,[27] researchers found that by using multiple, inert-gas elimination techniques in patients with ARDS, some degree of ventilation–perfusion mismatch occurred in 40% of patients. There was no evidence of a diffusion abnormality as it applies to respiratory gas exchange.

ARDS also causes changes in lung mechanics. Both the FRC and pulmonary compliance decrease. Loss of surfactant causes alveolar collapse, leading to further decreases in both FRC and pulmonary compliance. In addition to surfactant abnormalities, flooding of the alveoli decreases alveolar volume and causes further atelectasis. Compliance is further reduced by interstitial and alveolar edema, fibrosis, and the abnormal surfactant.

Clinically, during phase I, the patient will be dyspneic and will demonstrate a respiratory alkalosis with tachycardia and tachypnea (Table 25-1). A latent period, phase II, will occur, lasting from 6 to 48 hours after the injury, during which the patient will appear stable and may appear to be improving. During phase II, the patient will begin to demonstrate an increase in the work of breathing, with hyperventilation and hypocarbia; the lungs become less compliant due to both movement of fluid into the alveoli and loss of surfactant. Decreased alveolar volume and widespread atelectasis are the consequences of these changes (Table 25-2).

Physical examination will demonstrate scattered rales and evidence of the use of the accessory muscles of respiration. The initial chest X-ray examination will be normal, but subsequent radiographs will demonstrate increases in interstitial markings. With continued progression of the disease, the patient will develop acute respiratory failure (phase III). Lung compliance will be markedly decreased due to interstitial and alveolar edema, fibrosis, and abnormal surfactant. Loss of the normal surfactant leads to a decrease in the FRC and thus a further decrease in compliance. Further decreases in the FRC increase the alveolar–arterial oxygen difference and worsen the hypoxia.

The chest radiograph will demonstrate a diffuse interstitial pattern and, in fact, pneumonia is often difficult to rule out. At this time, bronchoalveolar lavage for diagnosis may be indicated to identify the pneumonic process.

The patient may improve at this time. The physical findings will resolve and the chest radiograph will return to normal. More commonly, however, the disease progresses with severe unresponsive hypoxemia, increased intrapulmonary shunting of blood, and metabolic and respiratory acidosis. The radiograph demonstrates honeycombed, patchy, and ill-defined nodular densities.

Treatment

Treatment of the patient with ARDS encompasses measures to (*a*) prevent death from respiratory failure, (*b*) minimize further lung injury, (*c*) provide general support, and (*d*) recognize and treat complications.

The goal of therapy is to provide adequate oxygenation at the lowest possible FIO_2. High inspired oxygen concentrations, as well as high airway pressures, have the potential to significantly exacerbate the acute lung injury.

Initially, the lowest FIO_2 needed to provide an arterial hemoglobin saturation (SaO_2) of 90% or more is used. Continuous pulse oximetry is used to monitor therapy. Decreasing the FIO_2 to 50% is desirable, and to achieve it, end-expiratory pressure is frequently used. PEEP is begun at 5 cm H_2O and increased incrementally with careful attention to cardiac output, pulmonary compliance, and peak inspiratory pressure. The medical officer's clinical judgment may be all that is available to assure optimal oxygenation.

Mechanical ventilation is used to deliver increased FIO_2 and increased tidal volumes. Tidal volumes of 10 to 15 mL/kg should be used initially. Careful attention is required to prevent the increased peak inspiratory pressure from causing barotrauma.

The need for high peak inspiratory pressure may be dictated by decreased compliance of the ARDS lung. However, other causes that may give rise to high peak inspiratory pressure are endotracheal tube displacement, pneumothorax, increased pleu-

TABLE 25-1

CLINICAL FINDINGS IN ADULT RESPIRATORY DISTRESS SYNDROME

Phase	Findings
Phase I: Acute Injury	Normal auscultatory examination Normal chest X-ray examination Tachycardia Tachypnea Respiratory alkalemia on arterial blood gas testing
Phase II: Latent Period (6–48 h)	Minor abnormalities on auscultatory examination Minor abnormalities on chest X-ray examination Tachycardia and tachypnea persist Increased work of breathing Respiratory alkalemia Increased $P_{AO_2} - Pa_{O_2}$
Phase III: Acute Respiratory Failure	High-pitched rales to auscultation Diffuse infiltrates on chest X-ray examination Marked tachypnea and dyspnea Decreased lung compliance Worsening oxygenation and ventilation
Phase IV: Terminal Abnormalities	Severe, unresponsive hypoxemia Increased intrapulmonary shunting Severe metabolic and respiratory acidemia

$P_{AO_2} - Pa_{O_2}$: alveolar-arterial difference in partial pressure of oxygen

TABLE 25-2

PATHOPHYSIOLOGY OF THE ADULT RESPIRATORY DISTRESS SYNDROME

Findings	Mechanisms
Refractory hypoxemia	Increased intrapulmonary shunting Decreased FRC Release of inflammatory mediators
Diffuse infiltrates on chest X-ray examination	Alveolar edema Atelectasis Inflammatory cell infiltrates
Normal PAOP	Endothelial damage results in capillary leakage
Decreased pulmonary compliance	Edema Atelectasis Marked increase in extravascular lung water

FRC: functional residual capacity; PAOP: pulmonary artery occlusion pressure ral effusion, increased lung edema, bronchospasm, mucous plugging, and high flow rates. Adjusting the tidal volume, the level of PEEP, or using paralytic agents to relax the patient's respiratory muscles may be required to decrease barotrauma. The mode of ventilation may be either intermittent, mandatory ventilation (IMV) or assist control (AC), both of which are discussed later in this chapter. Neither mode has been shown to be superior. The mode with which the operator has the most experience should be the mode used.

The use of glucocorticoids in the treatment of ARDS is not resolved. In the past, high-dose glucocorticoids have been advocated, but a prospective randomized trial published in 1987[28] reported that no benefit was seen from the use of glucocorticoids. However, a meta-analysis published in 1995[29] suggests that a subset of patients may benefit from corticosteroids administered during the fibroproliferative phase of the disease process.

Even with aggressive, intensive care, the mortality rate for ARDS remains approximately 50%. Of patients who survive the disease and its complications, most will become clinically asymptomatic. A small percentage, however, will have mild-to-moderate dyspnea on exertion. In the majority, the chest X-ray examination will return to normal, as will their lung volumes. Resting arterial blood gases will tend to be normal but with exercise, approximately half of these patients will have some decrease in their $Pa{O_2}$. Surprisingly, the typical ARDS patient does not die of respiratory insufficiency but of complications of unrelenting sepsis with failure of other organ systems.[30]

Although not presently applicable to combat situations, the use of extracorporeal membrane oxygenation with low-frequency positive pressure ventilation may be of some benefit to patients with ARDS. Although several studies of note have shown no improvement in survival when extracorporeal membrane oxygenation was used for oxygenation, others have used the apparatus with low-frequency positive pressure ventilation to some success. Lung function improved in 73% of patients and 49% survived, compared with the previous mortality rate of 91%.[31] An intra–vena caval blood oxygen–extracorporeal carbon dioxide removal device is presently undergoing clinical trials. Preliminary data indicate that there is no improvement in survival compared with conventional therapy.[32]

DIAGNOSING RESPIRATORY FAILURE

Because the causes of respiratory failure are so varied, astute physicians always search for incipient respiratory failure in their patients. The term *acute respiratory failure* comprises disorders of oxygenation or ventilation or both. Its definition, likewise, has both oxygenation and ventilatory components:

- *hypoxemia*: while breathing room air, the partial pressure of oxygen ($P{O_2}$) is 50 mm Hg or less; and/or
- *ventilatory failure:* the inability to ventilate sufficiently to maintain arterial blood partial pressure of carbon dioxide ($Pa{CO_2}$) less than 50 mm Hg.[21]

Although disorders of oxygenation and ventilation frequently coexist, consideration of each as a separate entity allows for a clearer understanding of the pathophysiological processes that lead to respiratory failure.

Hypoxemia

The signs and symptoms of hypoxemia are the effects of, and the body's response to, insufficient $D{O_2}$ to tissues for metabolic function. Cyanosis is only detectable when the patient's blood contains at least 5 g of deoxygenated hemoglobin per deciliter of blood. Similar findings (ie, signs and symptoms of hypoxemia) are noted when the level of methemoglobin reaches 1.5 g/dL, which may be seen following treatment for cyanide toxicity.[6] Typically, CNS effects are prominent with significant hypoxemia. Confusion, restlessness, and loss of judgment are common manifestations. The lack of available oxygen leads to increased sympathetic tone as the body attempts to compensate for inadequate $D{O_2}$ to the tissues. Lactic acidosis with a compensatory respiratory alkalosis becomes prominent as cells convert to anaerobic metabolism to provide for energy needs.

The major causes of hypoxemia in the trauma patient are a direct result of abnormalities in ventilation–perfusion relationships within alveolar capillary units. The deoxygenated blood that perfuses the alveolar capillaries in areas of hypoventilation within the lung cannot be normally oxygenated. The oxygenation deficit in this circumstance can be corrected by supplemental oxygen. This will increase the relative amount of oxygen within the alveoli in the region of low ventilation.

Although a number of pathophysiological processes produce hypoventilation, atelectasis from direct trauma to the lung parenchyma is the most common. Overly aggressive volume resuscitation with increased lung water is also frequently encountered in the setting of trauma. The second mechanism for the development of arterial hypoxemia, that of right-to-left intrapulmonary shunting of blood, can be thought of as the extreme form of altered ventilation and perfusion. In this instance, pulmonary arterial blood traverses capillaries in regions of complete alveolar collapse or regions that receive no ventilation from airway obstruction. Supplemental oxygen does not correct the oxygenation deficit. Correction is accomplished by inflating these collapsed alveoli, and it is necessary to resort to either continuous positive airway pressure via face mask or endotracheal intubation to improve oxygenation.

In combat medical facilities, supplemental oxygen is delivered from a tank. Oxygen *sieves* (concentrators that can remove and concentrate oxygen from ambient air) will be available in future conflicts to supply supplemental oxygen. In addition to the signs and symptoms of hypoxemia, assessment of the patient's degree of oxygenation requires arterial blood-gas measurement and pulse oximetry. The echelon of combat medical care that will have blood-gas monitoring capabilities is unclear; however, transportable pulse oximetry is available and could be utilized at mobile army surgical hospitals (third echelon), combat support hospitals (third echelon), and possibly even at the clearing station (second echelon).

Ventilatory Failure

Ventilatory failure may result from a number of different pathological processes. The two disorders most commonly associated with respiratory insufficiency leading to ventilatory failure are (1) CNS depression from trauma or drug effect and (2) compromise of the respiratory function of the chest wall. Disorders of the chest wall (eg, flail chest) may occasionally lead to ventilatory failure manifested by hypercarbia. However, associated abnormalities of oxygenation tend to represent the more life-threatening condition. Clinical signs and symptoms of hypercarbia are similar to those noted with hypoxemia, but with these exceptions: cyanosis is absent while oxygenation is maintained, and obtundation is more common than agitation. As it does with failure of oxygenation, optimum determination of the adequacy of ventilation rests on the physician's interpretation of arterial blood-gas determinations. Portable capnography provides a reasonable estimate of arterial carbon dioxide content and may prove useful in situations in which blood gas determinations are not available.[21]

Combined Hypoxemia and Ventilatory Failure in Postoperative Casualties

Postoperative pulmonary complications are among the commonest causes of morbidity and mortality in this patient population. Of all the potential respiratory complications, atelectasis is easily the most common: it may account for up to 90% of postoperative respiratory complications.[33] The degree of involvement may range from a small, insignificant group of airways to complete collapse of an entire lung. Other less common but frequently more life-threatening complications include pneumonia, bronchospasm, pulmonary thromboembolic disease, and respiratory failure. It is possible to define the various abnormalities with a combination of radiographic, laboratory, and clinical features. Chest X-ray examinations, blood-gas measurements, and chest auscultation remain the most valuable techniques to define pulmonary abnormalities and determine the need for more-invasive measures such as bronchoscopy, endotracheal intubation, or pulmonary arteriography.[34]

Upper abdominal and thoracic surgery carry the greatest risk for postoperative pulmonary dysfunction. Splinting to ease pain reduces the patient's ability to cough and breathe deeply, both of which predispose to distal airway plugging and collapse. The splinting results in a reduced vital capacity that leads to hypoventilation, while the airway plugging causes atelectasis and hypoxemia. Another important factor, a direct result of general anesthesia, is depression of mucociliary transport. Abnormal ciliary action and production of mucus are both worsened by lengthening anesthesia time. Cigarette smoking potentiates this abnormality.

Surgical procedures also predispose to premature closure of the distal airways. Supine positioning, increased abdominal girth and breathing at reduced lung volumes are nonpulmonary factors that contribute to premature airway closure. Interstitial edema, airway obstruction from secretions and bronchoconstriction, and loss of surfactant are pulmonary factors that tend to promote airway closure and atelectasis.[34]

A routine program of respiratory therapy before, during, and after surgery can reduce the number of postoperative respiratory complications and improve patient outcome when they do arise. The first few hours after the operation are the most critical for preventing respiratory complications. Alveolar collapse, with the resulting loss of FRC, may be prevented or reversed by deep breathing. Maneuvers that utilize forced exhalation (eg, blow bottles) do not effectively prevent airway collapse and may, in fact, promote this problem if an ineffective inspiration precedes the forced exhalation. Deep-breathing exercises, with inspiration to total lung capacity, are easily the most effective, cost-efficient means to prevent and reverse atelectasis (and hence, most pulmonary complications). Incentive spirometers allow patients to participate in their therapy and free the respiratory therapist to perform other duties. Most studies have found that intermittent positive-pressure breathing is, at best, equal to, and in most cases, inferior to incentive spirometry as a prophylactic measure to prevent postoperative pulmonary complications.[33]

The likelihood that a patient will develop postoperative respiratory complications is directly related to the type of surgical procedure and the duration of surgery and anesthesia; the patient's smoking history, preexisting pulmonary disease, obesity, and overall physical condition; and other factors.[35] For the most part, soldiers are in excellent physical condition and do not demonstrate significant preexisting lung disease.

MANAGING RESPIRATORY FAILURE

Although exsanguination is the most common cause of early death among combat casualties, medical officers must not forget that the first step to be taken in the management of any trauma victim is to assure a patent airway.[36] Respiratory failure must be recognized and treated promptly. Upper airway obstruction may not be obvious on initial assessment in the field, and may recur anytime during the medical-evacuation process. All military medical personnel should be trained in simple maneuvers to relieve upper airway obstruction. Should a hypovolemic trauma casualty require endotracheal intubation and positive-pressure mechanical ventilation, it is especially important that cardiovascular resuscitation be continued, to mitigate against the possible adverse effects of the positive pressure.

Supportive Care

Respiratory care begins with the use of supplemental oxygen. The most common methods to employ this drug are nasal cannulae and face masks. The FIO_2 actually achieved with a nasal cannula is dependent upon the patient's inspiratory flow rate and respiratory rate. A variety of masks are available for oxygen therapy. Higher percentages of FIO_2 may be obtained by use of the partial rebreathing mask or the nonrebreathing mask. The latter is the type most frequently applied to patients following general anesthesia, and is available in deployable medical facilities, including field echelons. The use of such a mask, which utilizes *three* unidirectional valves, ensures that carbon dioxide will not be rebreathed.

The next most common form of respiratory care used for patients is incentive spirometry. The success of this therapy in expanding the patient's FRC depends on both achieving adequate inspiratory volume and sustaining maximum inspiratory effort. Although preoperative teaching is often done in the setting of elective surgery, this obviously will not be possible in the combat casualty setting.

Intratracheal suctioning is important in maintaining the patency of the proximal airway and in preventing secretions from obstructing the alveoli. This is particularly true in the casualty with a penetrating chest wound, where the potential exists for bleeding into the airway. The casualty can drown in his own blood. Intratracheal suctioning is not entirely benign: it can be associated with complications such as trauma to the tracheal mucosa with resultant hemorrhage, hypoxia, and the vasovagal response leading to bradycardia and hypotension.

Endotracheal Intubation

Although most patients who require endotracheal intubation will also require mechanical ventilatory support, there are clinical situations in which intubation should proceed independent of the criteria defining respiratory failure. Intubation is required to provide airway protection and to prevent aspiration in a patient who is semicomatose. The treatment of upper-airway obstruction following direct maxillofacial trauma and the prevention of complete airway obstruction following thermal burn injuries are two other clinical examples. A full discussion of the methods of endotracheal intubation is found in Chapter 3, Airway Management.

Prolonged endotracheal intubation brings with it many possible complications. The posterior arytenoid cartilages are the most common sites for laryngeal damage, which is caused by the anterior bend imposed on the endotracheal tube at this point. Although the definition of prolonged translaryngeal intubation and the timing of tracheostomy are not yet answered in the medical literature, most clinicians consider 14 to 21 days to be a safe period before performing a tracheostomy.[37]

The complications of an elective tracheostomy are generally greater than those of translaryngeal intubation, although the overall incidence of complications is still low (3%). Early stomal bleeding is common; bleeding after 48 hours is more worrisome because it may indicate a catastrophic complication: a fistula between the trachea and the innominate artery. Tracheal–innominate artery fistulae occur infrequently but have a high mortality.

An increased incidence of bacteremia and nosocomial pneumonia are other problems associated with tracheostomy. Studies[38] have shown that up to 87% of patients with tracheostomies experience chronic aspiration. For example, tracheal stenosis is a common, clinically significant complication. The reported incidence varies, but exceeds that seen in patients with endotracheal tubes.[37] The most common site for tracheal stenosis is the stoma itself. A 75% reduction in the diameter of the trachea may occur before symptoms are manifested. The patient who is developing tracheal stenosis—who experiences stridor at rest—probably has a tracheal diameter less than 5 mm.

PHYSIOLOGICAL EFFECTS OF MECHANICAL VENTILATION

Once an endotracheal tube is used for ventilation, the patient's natural mechanism for the warming and humidification of inspired air are bypassed. Immediately following intubation and the institution of mechanical ventilation, patients may experience physical and psychological discomfort, which results in coughing and agitation. Most patients—especially those who are awakening, alert, or mildly obtunded—attempt to "fight" the ventilator.[39] Nearly constant medical supervision is required, and restraints may be necessary to avoid self-extubation.

Pulmonary Effects

Positive pressure applied during inspiration results in an alteration of the normal ventilation–perfusion matching. During spontaneous ventilation, most pulmonary blood flow and ventilation occurs in the dependent parts of the lungs. This relationship is changed during mechanical ventilation such that the greatest ventilation now occurs in the superior aspects of the lung. This is most likely the result of changes in the diaphragmatic shape and motion following positive airway pressure. The result is an increase in the physiological dead space following the institution of mechanical ventilation.

The use of positive-pressure ventilation may also create changes in the lung mechanics. Reductions in the FRC and pulmonary compliance may result in an increase in the work of breathing, and increased minute ventilation requirement.

The application of expiratory distending pressure results in an improvement of gas exchange and pulmonary compliance secondary to an increase in lung volumes. The mechanism of the increase in FRC is not clearly known but probably is the result of one or more of the following:

- an increase in the transpulmonary pressure;
- "recruitment" of atelectatic alveoli, resulting in their reexpansion; or simply
- the maintenance of alveolar patency, which was achieved during inspiration.

It is unlikely that the application of PEEP can open atelectatic alveoli that were not reexpanded during positive-pressure ventilation. Expiratory distending pressure also causes a decrease in the closing volume below the FRC, which mitigates against airway collapse during exhalation.

Conversely, an increase in lung volume may be detrimental if the FRC exceeds the normal volume. Excessive increases in FRC reduce pulmonary compliance and increase the pulmonary vascular resistance and dead space. Contrary to earlier beliefs, applying expiratory distending pressure actually *increases* total lung water, although oxygenation usually improves.

Cardiovascular Effects

The effects of expiratory distending pressure can be divided into (*a*) the effects on pulmonary vascular resistance and (*b*) the effect on cardiac output. The pulmonary vascular resistance is lowest when the FRC is normal. If the FRC is returned to normal by the recruitment of atelectatic alveoli, and venous admixture is decreased, hypoxic pulmonary vasoconstriction will be reduced. In contrast, if the alveolar pressure is increased beyond normal (thoracic overinflation), pulmonary capillary pressure will rise, resulting in an increase in the pulmonary vascular resistance.

The varying effect of expiratory distending pressure in different patients depends on thoracic compliance, which governs the transmission of pressure to the pleural space and great vessels. When the pulmonary compliance is low (eg, in a patient with ARDS), a minimal amount of expiratory distending pressure is transmitted to the pleural space. Thus, these patients frequently tolerate high levels of PEEP relatively well. If, however, the thoracic compliance decreases from abdominal distention or postoperative atelectasis, much of the expiratory distending pressure will be transmitted to the pleural space. This results in a potentially significant decrease in both venous return and cardiac output. The treatment is to increase the peripheral venous pressure, usually by volume administration. The extent to which this complication occurs may also be minimized by permitting spontaneous breaths through the use of IMV. Negative-pressure, spontaneous breaths serve to minimize the effect of expiratory distending pressure by augmenting venous return.

The effect of expiratory distending pressure on ventricular afterload differs between ventricles. An increase in right ventricular afterload is not predictable and depends upon the amount of increase in the pulmonary vascular resistance. At higher levels of PEEP (> 15–20 cm H_2O), right ventricular dilation occurs resulting in a shift of the intraventricular septum and possibly contributing to a decreased left ventricular stroke volume and cardiac output.[40] In this setting, the PAOP or pulmonary capillary wedge pressure (PCWP) may not reflect the true left ventricular end diastolic volume. As a result of an increased pleural pressure, the left ventricle may be compressed (ie, assisted). A failing left ventricle performs better when the afterload has been reduced.

Renal Effects

High levels of expiratory distending pressure have been associated with decreased urinary output. Animal studies comparing continuous, positive airway pressure to spontaneous breathing (ie, IMV) with PEEP failed to implicate reduced cardiac output as the etiologic factor.[41] Two possible explanations are (1) an increase in venous pressure, resulting in a decreased glomerular filtration rate and (2) an alteration of the distribution of intrarenal blood flow.

COMPLICATIONS FROM MECHANICAL VENTILATORY SUPPORT

A variety of complications may occur during mechanical ventilation. Two of the most important are cardiovascular depression and barotrauma. First, positive-pressure ventilation necessarily increases intrathoracic pressure. The increased intrathoracic pressure reduces venous return to the heart, and, therefore, right ventricular preload. This has two effects: (1) the reduction in preload results in a decrease in cardiac output; and (2), right-ventricular afterload increases, probably as a result of direct compression of the pulmonary vasculature. These two detrimental effects act in concert to reduce cardiac output, and both effects tend to be magnified by hypovolemia and PEEP.[21]

The second major complication of positive-pressure ventilation is barotrauma. The spectrum of barotrauma extends from pulmonary interstitial emphysema through pneumomediastinum, pneumothorax, and subcutaneous emphysema.[42] Current theories on barotrauma relate the initial event as alveolar rupture with dissection of air along the vascular sheath to the mediastinum. Once air enters the mediastinum, it may track along the fascial planes into the pleural space, subcutaneous tissue, or retroperitoneum.[43] It is the development of pneumothorax, and in particular, of tension pneumothorax, that represents the greatest threat to the patient. Peak airway pressure is believed to be the primary factor related to the development of barotrauma. No barotrauma was found in one series of patients whose peak airway pressure could be maintained at less than 50 cm H_2O.[42] Although experts debate the maximal pressure that can be tolerated without barotrauma, the practice of minimizing peak airway pressure to forestall the development of barotrauma is standard for managing patients with respiratory failure.

The finding of pulmonary interstitial emphysema on chest X-ray examination should alert the clinician to the real possibility that the patient may soon develop a pneumothorax. Because pneumothorax may present abruptly, the diagnosis should be made on the basis of clinical examination. The combination of respiratory distress, hypotension, hyperresonance, diminished breath sounds, and tachycardia should lead the clinician to evacuate the presumed pneumothorax with a large-bore needle placed in the second or third intercostal space in the midclavicular line on the affected side. Following immediate decompression by needle drainage, a tube thoracostomy should be performed, with the tube connected to a Heimlich valve or a water seal to preclude reaccumulation of air in the pleural space.

ETHICAL DILEMMAS IN USING LIMITED LIFE-SUSTAINING THERAPY

"Battlefield military medicine has a threefold mission: to save lives, to alleviate suffering, and to return soldiers to duty."[15(p192)] The question exists as to whether mechanical ventilation is a useful component of the medical officer's armamentarium for the treatment of combat casualties. In other words, is it likely that the casualty who requires mechanical ventilation will be returned to the battlefield? Probably not, with these two exceptions: when perioperative ventilation is used for residual anesthetic effects, and when mechanical ventilation is used to support casualties of chemical war gases. However, the mission of battlefield medicine is also to save lives, and the use of mechanical ventilation to accomplish this goal is without dispute.

When the number of mechanical ventilators is limited, medical officers will be required to decide which patients will receive them. This decision may be based on several considerations. Probably the most important, and least-biased, factors are (*a*) the expected reversibility of the inciting injury and (*b*) the predicted patient outcome. For example, the casualty who develops ARDS will most likely require at least 2 to 3 weeks of mechanical ventilatory support. In addition, the mortality rate exceeds 40%.[24] If this patient receives a ventilator, several others with an expected quick recovery may either sustain neurological injury or death if no respirator is available for respiratory support. A second example is the patient who develops multiple organ failure. If three or more organ systems have failed for at least 3 days in the ICU, the mortality exceeds 95% to 97%.[44]

Another factor that must be considered when a limited number of mechanical ventilators is available is the medical officer's experience and skill in managing critically ill patients *nonmechanically*.

MECHANICAL VENTILATION AND COMBAT CASUALTIES

The medical officer working in the combat casualty environment must (*a*) understand the types of pulmonary injuries that may occur and (*b*) be able to evaluate the need for mechanical ventilatory support. The decision to use a mechanical device to assist ventilation is primarily based on the patient's inability to sustain sufficient gas exchange. The most common reason for requiring positive-pressure ventilation is refractory hypoxemia. Historically, this use of positive-pressure ventilation dates back to 1938 for the treatment of pulmonary edema.[45]

Military anesthesiologists and critical care specialists must understand the design of mechanical ventilators, be able to choose the proper mode of ventilation, and be able to select the appropriate initial ventilatory settings. These required settings include tidal volume, rate, peak gas flow, inspiratory-to-expiratory ratio, and the fractional concentration of oxygen. A further challenge to medical officers is the lack of sophisticated monitoring for casualties who are mechanically ventilated. Thus, a good understanding of pulmonary physiology and astute clinical-assessment skills are required to determine if the patient is appropriately ventilated and oxygenated.

In contrast to the Vietnam War, where the capability for mechanical ventilation was very limited, in future conflicts, state-of-the-art ventilators may be available to save the lives of casualties who would otherwise die. During the months following the 2 August 1990 invasion of Kuwait by the Iraqi army, the Department of Defense purchased many types of mechanical ventilators, which were sent to the Saudi Arabian theatre. An unexpected problem arose, however: although many different kinds of ventilators were available, most of them were unfamiliar to young physicians new to the military.

Additional problems relating to the provision of mechanical ventilation in the field were the need for oxygen, oxygen blenders, PEEP valves, and spirometers. The principal problem on the battlefield is the availability of compressed oxygen. During the Vietnam War, oxygen was provided principally in cylinders, with replenishment by liquid oxygen. In future conflicts, there are no plans for pipeline oxygen supply in the land hospitals; however, there should be an increased availability of liquid oxygen. Use of oxygen sieves may become commonplace. The logistics of continual provision of filled oxygen tanks is significant.

Indications for Mechanical Ventilation

A combat casualty's need for mechanical ventilatory support generally falls under one of three categories: impaired oxygenation, inadequate ventilation (eg, the central ventilatory drive or the functional integrity of the thoracic cage is impaired), or an excessive amount and/or inefficiency of respiratory work. A number of clinical problems are associated with more than one of these deficiencies (Exhibit 25-3).

Several of these indications are self-explanatory; however, a few merit specific comments. Oxygen itself may be toxic to the pulmonary system when administered in a high quantity. If a peripheral oxygen saturation above 90% cannot be obtained within a reasonable amount of time (< 12 h) by the use of a face mask–nonrebreathing apparatus (FIO_2 > .80), then endotracheal intubation and mechanical ventilation should be instituted. Improved oxygenation may be achieved by manipulation of the FIO_2, mean airway pressure, or the pattern of ventilation.

Although patients in cardiovascular collapse or shock may not meet the arterial blood-gas criteria for respiratory failure, supportive care for these patients includes using mechanical ventilation to reduce work demands placed on a patient with inadequate cardiac output. Data from animal studies support this approach, as mortality was reduced in the group of animals in shock that were supported with mechanical ventilation.[39]

EXHIBIT 25-3

INDICATIONS FOR MECHANICAL VENTILATION

Impaired Oxygenation

- Direct thoracic trauma with resulting pneumothorax
- Hemothorax or pulmonary contusion
- Hypovolemia and shock
- Pulmonary edema
- Progressive atelectasis
- Pneumonia or aspiration pneumonitis
- Adult respiratory distress syndrome

Impaired Ventilation

- Postoperative state with residual anesthesia
- Head injury
- Chemical warfare injury
- Quadriplegia from spinal cord trauma
- Diaphragmatic injury
- Fractured ribs or flail chest

Excessive Respiratory Work

- Multiple trauma
- Compensation for severe metabolic acidemia
- Severe bronchospasm
- Sepsis or multiple organ dysfunction

Functional Design of Mechanical Ventilators

The type of ventilator is designated by its mechanism of cycling (ie, the event that terminates inspiration). There are three principal types of cycling: pressure, volume, and time. Both volume and time allow for a constant level of tidal volume. The tidal volume varies during use of pressure-cycled ventilators whenever pulmonary compliance or airway resistance change. An important component of the ventilator's design is its driving power (ie, what empowers positive pressure); either compressed gas (usually oxygen) or electrical power may be used. Most modern ventilators, and all that are designed for use in ICUs, are electrically powered, have an internal battery for back-up power, and are often controlled by a microprocessor. For medical officers, this advantage is significant: it reduces the amount of compressed oxygen that must be supplied to support field hospitals.

Simplistic, mechanical ventilators have only a few components: a gas-controller device, blender, humidifier, PEEP generator, and the circuit tubing. The gas-controller device provides flow either on demand, based on input from a sensor, or by continuous flow.

The limitations of specific ventilators are discussed later in this chapter.

Pressure Cycled

In pressure-cycled ventilators, inspiration ends when a preset pressure is reached in the proximal airway, as sensed by a manometer placed within the ventilator circuit. The Bennett PR-2 is an example of this type of ventilator, and is available in military warehouses. It is one of the first kinds of ventilators sent to Saudi Arabia in 1990. However, a pressure-cycled ventilator is used mainly in the patient who is comatose, quadriplegic, or postoperative from general anesthesia; or who has a large leak around the endotracheal tube and an anesthesiologist or clinician who is experienced in reintubation is unavailable. Many limitations discourage the use of the PR-2.

Volume Cycled

In volume-cycled ventilators, the inspiratory phase ends when a preset volume is delivered to the patient. This is the most common type of cycle mechanism on modern ventilators and on all machines classified as "ICU ventilators." Ventilators of this type that were sent to the Persian Gulf War to support U.S. and coalition forces include the Bear 33, Lifecare PLV-100 and PLV-102, Bennett MA-1, and the Puritan-Bennett Companion. A safety feature of an appropriately set peak airway pressure prevents excessive pressure in the airway if either pulmonary compliance or airway resistance change suddenly. When this "pop-off" pressure is reached, the remainder of the tidal volume vents out of the circuit and remains undelivered to the patient. Volume cycling also has some limitations, including the need for a good seal around the endotracheal tube, and an inspiratory time that is unresponsive to the patients' own respiratory pattern.

Time Cycled

In time-cycled ventilators, the inspiratory phase ends when the selected time is reached. Ventilators of this type include the Servo 900C (Siemens-Elema, Solna, Sweden); the Evita (Dragerwerk, Bonn, Germany); and the Univent-750 (Impact Instrumentation, West Caldwell, N.J.). The Univent-750 was designed as a transport ventilator and large quantities were sent to the Persian Gulf during Operation Desert Storm. Similar to the volume-cycled ventilator, the time-cycled ventilator delivers a relatively constant tidal volume. Tidal volume is determined by either (*a*) the inspiratory time and the peak inspiratory flow rate or (*b*) the minute ventilation and the respiratory rate. For example, if the inspiratory time is 1 second, and the peak flow rate is 60 L/minute, then the set tidal volume will be 1,000 mL. The Evita, also a time-cycled ventilator, is an extremely flexible and capable ICU ventilator and was supplied in large quantity to receiving hospitals in the U.S. Army Seventh Medical Command, in Germany.

Flow Cycled

Pressure-support ventilation is generally viewed as a mode of ventilation and may be performed on either volume-cycled or time-cycled machines. Nevertheless, the mechanism for termination of inspiration (cycling) is unique in that flow to the patient stops when the patient's intrinsic inspiratory flow falls below a certain percentage of the initial effort.

This topic is discussed more fully below.

Modes of Positive-Pressure Ventilation

There is no uniformly accepted terminology for the different ventilatory modes. The application of positive airway pressure can be divided according to the timing during inspiration or exhalation, or during both phases. When comparing the following modes of ventilation, one general concept should be remembered: positive intrathoracic pressure may contribute to decreased venous return and, therefore, to inadequate cardiac output. The degree to which this complication becomes clinically significant depends on the duration and level of positive airway pressure, whether any spontaneous (negative-pressure) breaths occur, and the patient's preceding intravascular volume and cardiac status.

Inspiratory Positive Pressure

Controlled Mechanical Ventilation. In the controlled mechanical ventilation (CMV) mode, the ventilator initiates positive-pressure inspiratory cycles independent of the patient's spontaneous efforts. This method is indicated when the patient is apneic secondary to heavy sedation, paralysis, or coma; or when neuromuscular pathology, including quadriplegia, has occurred. A problem arises when the patient tries to breathe spontaneously: the patient may compete with the ventilator. The result will be a patient who is at best uncomfortable, and at worst subject to pulmonary overinflation and barotrauma. All inspiratory cycles are positive pressure, thus decreased venous return and decreased cardiac output are common. If the patient does not initiate spontaneous efforts, then the entire work of breathing is provided by the ventilator. This allows the patient to rest, but also may lead to atrophy of the diaphragm and intercostal muscles.

Assist-Control Ventilation. Again, all inspiratory cycles are positive pressure with the AC mode of ventilation. Any breaths taken above the rate set by the physician must be triggered by a spontaneous effort. Competition between the patient and the ventilator is therefore avoided, which reduces the potential for barotrauma. The primary advantages of AC ventilation are that (1) respiratory muscles rest when the peak flow is high enough to decrease the patient's work of breathing and (2) the patient determines the P_{CO_2} and the pH. Unfortunately, respiratory alkalosis is frequently observed in critically ill patients. When AC ventilation is used, the medical officer must remember that the set respiratory rate is only a back-up if the patient's spontaneous rate falls below that frequency. The actual frequency of full tidal-volume breaths will be determined by the patient's spontaneous rate or the set, mechanical rate—whichever is the greater number.

Intermittent, Mandatory Ventilation. The IMV mode allows unlimited, negative-pressure, spontaneous breaths between the delivered mechanical breaths. As a result, this mode can be used across a spectrum of minimal to complete ventilatory support, offering flexibility to the physician whose patient load requires a large number of ventilators or who is attempting to wean a patient from the ventilator. IMV is indicated primarily during weaning. However, when the respiratory rate and tidal volume are set high enough to provide most of the patient's minute ventilation requirement, the patient can rest, and the work of breathing can be reduced. The use of IMV has several advantages (Exhibit 25-4).

Synchronized, Intermittent, Mandatory Ventilation. The synchronized, intermittent, mandatory ventilation (SIMV) mode was designed to improve patient comfort and to prevent the stacking of breaths (ie, repeated inhalations without full exhalation) that may lead to barotrauma. As with IMV, the set rate is the minimum number of positive-pressure breaths that the patient will receive regardless of his intrinsic central respiratory drive. However, in SIMV, the patient's spontaneous breathing and the ventilator are coordinated by means of a circuit manometer, which detects the onset of a spontaneous breath. Within a "window" during which the ventilator should cycle (eg, every 6 s when the set rate is 10 breaths per minute), if the patient makes a spontaneous effort, the mechanical breath will be triggered and superimposed at the beginning of the patient's respiratory cycle, rather than randomly throughout. This timing should help avoid barotrauma by synchronizing the ventilator-delivered breath with the inspiratory effort of the patient. The only significant disadvantage of the IMV or SIMV ventilatory mode is the potential increase in work of breathing imposed by the demand valve incorporated into the ventilator.

EXHIBIT 25-4

ADVANTAGES OF INTERMITTENT, MANDATORY VENTILATION

Distribution of ventilation is more normal

Physiological dead space is reduced

Detrimental effects on the cardiovascular system are minimized

Some degree of respiratory muscle tone is maintained

Respiratory alkalemia is minimized

Pressure Support Ventilation. The pressure support (PS) mode of ventilation is triggered by the negative flow created by a patient's spontaneous breath. The initial use of this mode was the intermittent, positive-pressure breathing (IPPB) device. The level of pressure support set by the physician provides for positive airway pressure for the duration of spontaneous inspiration. Depending on the type of ventilator employed, the pressure returns to the end-expiratory pressure level when the inspiratory flow drops below a preset absolute rate or percentage of the initial inspiratory flow rate. This pressure augmentation results in reduced work of breathing, which compensates for the increased resistance from the endotracheal tube, ventilator circuit, and mechanical demand valve (which may be difficult to trigger). The total respiratory rate, tidal volume, and length of inspiration remain under the patient's control; the result is markedly increased patient comfort. Pressure support is usually used in conjunction with SIMV, which provides back-up ventilation in the event that patient-initiated efforts become inadequate (eg, excessive sedation, metabolic encephalopathy).

The disadvantages of pressure-support ventilation are that (1) the inspiratory cycle uses positive pressure and (2) the delivered tidal volume varies when changes in either airway resistance or pulmonary compliance occur.

The initial assist-pressure setting can be estimated at approximately one half the peak airway pressure. An in-line expiratory spirometer should be used to measure spontaneous breaths (5–7 mL/kg exhaled tidal volume is a reasonable goal). None of the ventilators that were sent to the Persian Gulf War in 1990 had this capability.

Inverse-Ratio Ventilation. As a patient's respiratory gas exchange becomes progressively inadequate, increasing the inspiratory-to-expiratory ratio to greater than 1 may lead to significant improvement (by elevating the mean airway pressure). The most likely mechanism for this improvement is an increase in lung volume resulting from the recruitment of atelectatic alveoli through the generation of intrinsic end expiratory pressure or so-called "auto-PEEP." Inverse-ratio ventilation may be accomplished in the pressure or volume control ventilatory modes. The pressure control variety is achieved by maintaining the set pressure limit for a fixed period of time. The volume control mode of IRV results when the inspiratory flow rate is reduced to the point whereby inspiratory time exceeds expiratory time.[39] Because this pattern of ventilation is nonphysiological, sedation is usually required for the patient.

High-Frequency Ventilation. High-frequency ventilation can be provided in three modes: high-frequency, positive-pressure ventilation; high-frequency jet ventilation; and high-frequency oscillation. The advantages of high-frequency ventilation are that the mean and peak airway pressures decrease, resulting in minimized risks of barotrauma and cardiovascular impairment. The Food and Drug Administration approves the use of high-frequency ventilation in adults for only one condition: bronchopleural fistula. The results of high-frequency ventilation in patients with ARDS have been very disappointing, but there may be some use for it in treating inhalation injury.[11]

Expiratory Positive Pressure

The application of positive pressure during exhalation, whether it occurs in the spontaneous or the mechanically ventilated patient, is called expiratory distending pressure (EDP). The two principal methods of delivery are (1) CPAP, which uses positive airway pressure throughout the spontaneous ventilatory cycle, and (2) PEEP, which uses positive pressure during the exhalation fraction of the cycle.

Expiratory distending pressure can be applied via either a flow resistor or a threshold device placed in the expiratory limb of the ventilatory circuit. The result is that expiration is retarded, prohibiting full exhalation, which, in effect, maintains alveolar distension. The flow resistor accomplishes this by changing the size of the orifice for gas flow, whereas the threshold device allows no expiratory flow until the pressure exceeds the set valve pressure. The threshold device is preferred because it can accommodate a sudden increase in expiratory pressure (eg, during coughing) without allowing a build-up of pressure in the ventilator circuit.

Continuous, Positive Airway Pressure

Large, patient-initiated decreases in airway pressure are associated with increased work of breathing. CPAP may reduce the work of breathing by giving an inspiratory assist, which leads to an almost passive inspiratory cycle. Continuous, positive airway pressure delivered via a face mask may have a limited role in the treatment of combat casualties because of the frequent occurrence of obtundation, which increases the risk for pulmonary aspiration of gastric contents. With proper patient selection, however, continuous, positive airway pressure has certain advantages: (1) the maintenance of the patient's ability to cough, (2) the maintenance of the patient's ability to warm and humidify the inspiratory gases, and (3) the avoidance of complications associated with endotracheal intubation. The primary disadvantage is gastric distension (and the concomitant increased risk of aspiration), which can be minimized by the placement of a nasogastric sump.

Clinical Use of Positive End-Expiratory Pressure

The use of PEEP merits specific attention not only because this technique is popular but also because the misconceptions regarding its use are numerous. The only valid reason for using PEEP is to increase lung volume—specifically, the FRC. The FRC is composed of the residual volume and the expiratory reserve volume. This lung capacity provides for a reservoir of oxygen-filled alveoli and permits gas exchange between inspirations. The FRC is frequently decreased following trauma or surgery (Table 25-3).

In most patients, the length of the expiratory cycle far exceeds the inspiratory. If alveoli are permitted to close during the expiratory time, then intrapulmonary shunting, resulting in hypoxemia, may occur. This premise was used to defend the "super" PEEP that was used during the 1970s, when PEEP levels greater than 20 cm H_2O were titrated until the shunt fraction was decreased to the lowest possible level.[46] No prospective study has demonstrated improved patient outcome with the use of these high levels of PEEP, leading most clinicians to use PEEP in restricted amounts (eg, < 15 cm H_2O).[47]

TABLE 25-3

CAUSES OF DECREASED FUNCTIONAL RESIDUAL CAPACITY

Cause	Effect
Residual anesthetic	Shifts the CO_2 response curve or alters central respiratory control, resulting in shallow tidal volume breathing
Abdominal distension	Compresses the diaphragm and the lower pulmonary segments
Splinting of chest-wall movements secondary to thoracic pain	Pain prevents deep breathing, which results in collapsed alveoli
Excessive airway secretions or obstruction	Work of breathing increases as the airway is blocked

INITIATING MECHANICAL VENTILATION

The initial settings that are selected for mechanical support depend on the indication for which the patient requires ventilatory support. Exhibit 25-5 is a brief guide to setting the ventilator.

Tidal Volume and Respiratory Rate

The recommended initial settings for nonrespiratory failure–ventilatory support are a tidal volume of 10 to 15 mL/kg and a respiratory rate of 7 to 10 breaths per minute, resulting in a minute ventilation of 70 to 150 mL/kg/min. The patient who is comatose or who remains under the influence of sedatives will generally be normocarbic at 80 mL/kg/min. Higher rates should be used for the initial setting when

- hypocapnic therapy is needed to treat increased intracranial pressure,
- a severe metabolic acidosis needs immediate compensation,
- a large amount of sodium bicarbonate has been administered,
- a thermal burn has created hypermetabolism, or
- pulmonary vascular occlusion has caused an increase in physiological dead space.

The selection of respiratory rate in the AC mode only determines the minimum amount of ventilation that will be ensured if the patient loses his respiratory drive. Thus, the selected setting should provide for approximately 70% to 80% of the minute ventilation required for the patient to maintain normocarbia. To obtain the maximal benefit from SIMV, once the patient is stable, the respiratory rate should be set at the minimum amount necessary to prevent respiratory acidosis.

Calculation of the tidal volume should be set on the patient's *actual* weight if the weight above the estimated lean amount is the result of obesity. Increased weight gain following fluid resuscitation does not necessitate increasing the tidal volume. Not all the set tidal volume will be delivered to the patient's alveoli because of dead space (anatomical and artificial) and volume loss (from the compliance of the ventilator circuit tubing). When the patient reaches a peak airway pressure of 40 to 60 cm H_2O during ventilation, the average amount of volume lost is 3 to 4 mL/cm H_2O pressure.[12]

Fraction of Inspired Oxygen

Many of the ventilators sent to the Persian Gulf in support of Operation Desert Storm in 1990 required an additional, external oxygen blender to provide oxygen in a relatively safe range (> room air [.21] and < 1.0). All FIO_2 settings—even on a sophisticated ICU ventilator—should be confirmed by an oxygen analyzer that is placed within the inspiratory limb of the patient's breathing circuit. The initial setting for FIO_2 will depend on whether pulmonary injury has occurred. In a postoperative patient who has sustained only an extremity or lower-abdominal wound, a slight increase in the FIO_2 to .40 will usually suffice. If significant pulmonary injury has occurred, then an initial FIO_2 of 1.0 should be selected. All attempts should be made to use the lowest concentration of oxygen that provides at least 90% oxygen saturation

EXHIBIT 25-5

MODES AND SETTINGS OF POSITIVE PRESSURE VENTILATION

Volume-Cycled Ventilators

Apnea	*Spontaneous Ventilation*
Control Mode	*Assist-Control/Synchronized, Intermittent, Mandatory Ventilation*
1. TV: 10–15 mL/kg	1. TV: 10–15 mL/kg
2. Not applicable	2. Sensitivity: –2 to –2.5 cm H_2O
3. Respiratory rate: 8–12 breaths per min	3. Respiratory rate: AC: set default rate to 6–8 breaths per min in case of apnea; SIMV: to rest the patient, ensure that 80% of breaths are mechanically provided
4. Not applicable	4. PF: 3.5–4.0 • minute ventilation

5. Expiratory time should exceed inspiratory time by 2:1
6. Keep PAP < 30–40 cm H_2O
7. Add PEEP in 2- to 4-cm H_2O increments if hypoxemia persists on FIO_2 > 50%
8. Set PL at 15–20 cm H_2O above PAP during a normal breath or < 80 cm H_2O

Pressure-Cycled Ventilators

1. TV: starting at 20 cm H_2O, increase peak pressure until tidal volume is adequate by clinical examination or arterial blood gas criteria
2. Respiratory rate: provides for a minimum amount if patient becomes apneic. Set to provide 70%–80% of minute ventilation
3. FIO_2: an in-line O_2 analyzer is strongly recommended
4. Patient interaction: the spontaneously breathing patient may not tolerate this type of ventilator, necessitating either weaning or changing to a different mode of ventilation

Time-Cycled Ventilators

1. TV: set the inspiratory time and PF to provide the calculated tidal volume
2. Respiratory rate: ensures a minimal amount of ventilation
3. As the PF determines the TV, it is necessary to check the inspiratory-to-expiratory time ratio with each rate change

AC: assist-control ventilation; FIO_2: fraction of inspired oxygen; PAP: peak airway pressure; PEEP: positive end-expiratory pressure; PF: peak flow; PL: pressure limit; SIMV: synchronized,intermittent, mandatory ventilation; TV: tidal volume

of the arterial hemoglobin. High oxygen concentrations are toxic to the lungs and may result in numerous complications. These include a deterioration in ventilation–perfusion matching, absorption atelectasis, decreased mucociliary clearance, and ARDS.[48] Decreasing the FIO_2, utilizing a pulse oximeter as a monitor, may be safely done in increments of 5% to 10% every 5 minutes.

Inspiratory Flow Rate

The peak inspiratory flow rate is particularly important. If it is set too high, ventilation is maldistributed throughout the lungs. If set too low, the expiratory time may be shortened, creating a problem for patients with obstructive airway disease. In all cases, the peak inspiratory flow rate must exceed the patient's intrinsic demand if further respiratory work by the patient is to be avoided. A setting that is 3.5- to 4-fold greater than the patient's minute volume requirement is usually adequate. When increasing the peak flow rate, the physician will generally observe a rise in the peak airway pressure. Occasionally, the peak airway pressure will decrease, signifying that intrinsic (or auto-) PEEP is occurring. This will resolve with lengthening of the expiratory time.

Additional Settings

The remainder of the mechanical ventilator settings are often overlooked by medical officers but will be set by a respiratory therapist. These include the inspiratory-to-expiratory ratio, the selection of an inspiratory waveform (square, ramp, sine), and a variety of alarms. The most important alarm, which is accompanied by a release mechanism, is the peak airway pressure. Initially, this should be set for approximately 15 to 20 cm H_2O higher than the peak pressure measured during unlabored, mechanical breathing. These additional settings are important for the intensivist when a patient is particularly difficult to ventilate.

Stabilizing the Patient in Acute Respiratory Failure

The approach to initiating mechanical support in the patient in acute respiratory failure differs from the previous discussion. The initial settings recommended above are merely a guideline for initiating mechanical support. As a result of either hypermetabolism or increased dead-space ventilation, a combat casualty's minute ventilation requirement may be as high as 25 to 30 L/min. Respiratory muscle fatigue appears to be a common component of acute respiratory failure regardless of the etiology.[49] The initial goal is to ensure a good quality of rest and recovery. Using a constant tidal volume of 10 to 15 mL/kg, the respiratory rate should be increased until the patient is comfortable and rested. When these high levels of mechanical support are required, bedside supervision by an intensivist is necessary to avoid (*a*) excessive elevation of airway pressure and (*b*) air-trapping, which results from an inadequate expiratory time. Although the AC mode may allow the greatest decrease in the patient's work of breathing, a very tachypneic or anxious patient may cause excessive triggering and stacking of ventilations. Occasionally, the patient may need to be sedated and paralyzed so that hemodynamic compromise can be minimized and the elimination of carbon dioxide can be improved.

Patients who do not respond initially to treatment for sepsis or shock should be considered for early intubation and mechanical ventilatory support. Considerable oxygen can be consumed by the diaphragm alone (as much as 30%–40% of the body's total amount) in the state of shock or acute respiratory failure.[50]

Following a period of stabilization, a progressive amount of work should be assumed by the patient to prevent atrophy and promote conditioning.[51]

MONITORING THE EFFECTIVENESS OF VENTILATION AND OXYGENATION

Monitors used in patients with acute respiratory failure may be characterized as invasive or noninvasive, and intermittent or continuous. A monitor may either follow only the progression of disease or give concomitant information regarding the effect of therapy.

Oxygen Concentration

The F_{IO_2} delivered to the patient is one of the most important and easiest parameters to measure. Once the F_{IO_2} is known, other indices—all of which serve as markers for the severity of pulmonary dysfunction—can be calculated:

- the difference between the partial pressure of oxygen within the alveoli and that present within the arterial blood ($P_{AO_2} - Pa_{O_2}$); normal is 5 to 10 mm Hg;
- the ratio of arterial to alveolar partial pressure of oxygen (Pa_{O_2}/P_{AO_2}); normal is 0.75; and
- the ratio of arterial partial pressure of oxygen to the fraction of inspired oxygen (Pa_{O_2}/F_{IO_2}); normal is 250 mm Hg.

Pulse Oximetry

The pulse oximeter is a continuous monitor that detects the percentage of total hemoglobin saturated with oxygen. This is achieved by using a photoelectric tube to measure the amount of light transmitted at two different wavelengths. Only the arterial component of the blood in the tissue is analyzed. This is done by simultaneously measuring pulsatile flow and subtracting the background absorption, which is the nonpulsatile venous and capillary blood. Because of a different stereochemistry of hemoglobin molecules, saturated and un-

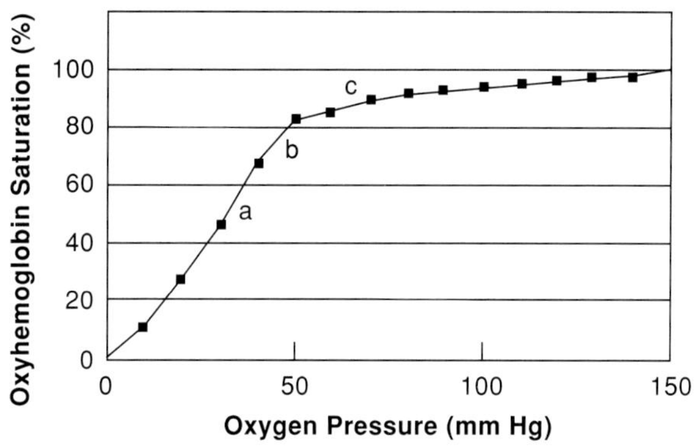

Fig. 25-2. The sigmoid shape of the oxyhemoglobin dissociation curve, with its nonlinear relation between the partial pressure of oxygen dissolved in blood and the percentage of oxygen saturation of hemoglobin, must be borne in mind when interpreting blood gas data. The shape and position of the curve can be estimated in terms of these three points, which fix the relation between partial pressure and saturation: (**a**) the oxygen pressure at which hemoglobin is 50% saturated (P_{50}), (**b**) the oxygen pressure of mixed venous blood, which is normally 75% saturated ($S_{mv}O_2$), and (**c**) the partial pressure at which hemoglobin is 90% saturated.

saturated hemoglobin display unique absorption spectrums. To use this information clinically, the physician must know the three key points on the oxyhemoglobin dissociation curve (Figure 25-2):

a. the P_{50}, the Po_2 at which 50% of the hemoglobin molecules are saturated, which normally occurs at 27 mm Hg;
b. the mixed venous saturation ($S_{mv}O_2$) (75%), corresponding to a Po_2 of 35 to 40 mm Hg; and
c. the "knee" of the curve at 90% saturation of hemoglobin molecules, at a Po_2 of approximately 60 mm Hg.

This technology has several limitations: pulse oximetry (*a*) does not compute carboxyhemoglobin or methemoglobin as desaturated hemoglobin, (*b*) is inaccurate in instances of severe anemia ($\leq$ 7 g/dL), and (*c*) does not measure venous oxygen saturation because venous blood is only slightly pulsatile. The latter situation may occur when large amounts of PEEP are applied. One important point is that the patient's Po_2 may decrease from 400 to 100 mm Hg, representing a significant change in pulmonary function, yet the pulse oximeter saturation display does not change.

The Persian Gulf War was the first conflict in which pulse oximeters were widely available for patient monitoring. Oximeters were present at all anesthetizing locations, within the ICUs, and in the emergency departments.

Gas-Exchange Indices

Partial Pressure of Arterial Oxygen

Factors other than the gas-exchange capability and efficiency of the lung may affect the Pao_2. Two clinical situations that exemplify this point are (1) shock, during which the venous Po_2 is markedly reduced, and (2) a state of increased Vo_2. The desaturating effect of venous hypoxemia is exacerbated in the presence of lung pathology, contributing to intrapulmonary shunting. Hence, when hypoxemia (low Po_2) occurs, it is not a correct assumption that the patient's clinical problem is one of strictly pulmonary pathology. Conversely, if the Po_2 is completely normal for a given Fio_2, the lungs are assumed to be functioning normally. The Po_2, when measured by an arterial blood-gas determination, is the accepted standard for measuring oxygenation.

Arterial blood gases as a monitor of oxygenation have the limitation of reflecting the clinical state at only one moment. Furthermore, the Pao_2 measures only the oxygen dissolved in the blood, which is only a small fraction of the total amount of oxygen delivered to the tissues. Most of the arterial oxygen content is that portion of oxygen bound to hemoglobin. However, the Pao_2 is the major determinant of the position on the oxygen–hemoglobin dissociation curve and thus determines the arterial hemoglobin oxygen saturation.

Alveolar–Arterial Oxygen Tension Difference

The difference between the partial pressure of oxygen in the alveoli and in the arteries (PAO_2 – Pao_2) is a specific indicator of pulmonary pathology, but this index has a significant practical limitation: the clinician must know the Fio_2. Multiple determinations of the calculated value for PAO_2 – Pao_2 are accurate predictors of pulmonary injury *only* when the Fio_2 has remained constant. PAO_2 – Pao_2 is calculated using the following equation:

$$PAO_2 - Pao_2 = Fio_2\,(P_B - P_{H_2O}) - Pco_2/R.Q.$$

where P_B represents barometric pressure (760 mm Hg at sea level); P_{H_2O} represents partial pressure of fully saturated water vapor (47 mm Hg); and *R.Q.* represents the respiratory quotient, assumed to be 0.8 with a normal diet. The normal value for PAO_2 –

Pa_{O_2} is less than 10 mm Hg for a healthy, young adult.

The Ratio of Arterial to Alveolar Oxygen Tension

The arterial-to-alveolar oxygen tension ratio (Pa_{O_2}/PA_{O_2}) remains more stable with alteration in the FI_{O_2}, and this calculation can be employed to predict the expected Pa_{O_2} when the FI_{O_2} is altered. The normal value is 0.75.

The Ratio of Arterial Oxygen to Inspired Oxygen

The arterial-to-inspired oxygen ratio (Pa_{O_2}/FI_{O_2}) is the simplest index to calculate, as it does not require use of the alveolar gas equation. The normal value is greater than 250 mm Hg.

Right-to-Left Shunting

Right-to-left intrapulmonary shunting of blood leads most of the hypoxemia seen with severe respiratory failure. The shunt equation applicable to severe respiratory failure is

$$Qs/Qt = Cc_{O_2} - Ca_{O_2}/Cc_{O_2} - Cv_{O_2}$$

where *Qs* represents the flow to the shunt, *Qt* represents the total pulmonary blood flow, and Cc_{O_2} represents the oxygen content of pulmonary capillary blood, which equals (1.34 mL O_2/g Hb) • (Hb g/dL) • (% S_{O_2}). The pulmonary capillary blood is assumed to be fully saturated (S_{O_2} = 100%). Ca_{O_2} represents the arterial oxygen content and Cv_{O_2} represents the pulmonary venous oxygen content whose hemoglobin oxygen saturations can be directly measured. This equation discounts the small contribution of dissolved oxygen in computing the various oxygen contents.

If FI_{O_2} = 1.0, then the following simplified shunt equation may be used:

$$Qs/Qt = P(A - a)_{O_2}/20$$

Monitoring Mechanical Ventilation

The importance of bedside patient observation cannot be overemphasized. Much information is gained by attentively watching the patient's spontaneous ventilatory efforts and use and coordination of the thoracoabdominal muscles of inspiration. In addition to the more-specific pulmonary pathologies, tachypnea is an early sign of shock or sepsis.

Airway Pressures

The peak and plateau airway pressures are monitored in all patients in respiratory failure who are supported by mechanical ventilation. From these measurements the dynamic and static compliance may be calculated as follows:

$$Cd = \text{change in volume}/(PAP - PEEP)$$

$$Cs = \text{change in volume}/(PLP - PEEP)$$

where *Cd* represents dynamic compliance, *Cs* represents static compliance, *change in volume* represents ventilator tidal volume, *PAP* represents peak airway pressure, *PEEP* represents positive end-expiratory pressure, and *PLP* represents plateau pressure. Actual tidal volume should be corrected by subtraction of the volume lost for circuit expansion (3–4 mL/cm H_2O peak airway pressure).

A single, discrete value cannot be given be given for the dynamic compliance, which is flow dependent. Static compliance has the range 75 to 125 mL/cm H_2O. The normal values are position dependent, and, for supine measurements, the normal value should be reduced approximately 30%.

The measurement of dynamic compliance is affected by the airway resistance, the compliance of the pulmonary parenchyma, and the compliance of the chest wall. The difference in peak and plateau pressures (normal = < 10 cm H_2O) indicates the difference between these two compliances and is independent of airway resistance.[52] If this difference is large, then therapeutic intervention should be directed toward minimizing or eliminating the contributing factors (Exhibit 25-6). Bronchospasm is a common cause of increased airway resistance during mechanical ventilation. Stan-

EXHIBIT 25-6

FACTORS CONTRIBUTING TO INCREASED AIRWAY RESISTANCE

Airway secretions

Kinked endotracheal tube

Narrow internal diameter of the endotracheal tube

Condensed water in the ventilator tubing

Bronchospasm

dard medical therapy includes inhaled beta agonists, inhaled anticholinergic agents, theophylline, and steroids.

If both the peak and plateau airway pressures are elevated and there is minimal difference between the dynamic and static compliances, then the compliance of either the pulmonary parenchyma or the chest wall has been reduced. Most commonly, this is the result of pulmonary injury (Exhibit 25-7). All medical officers caring for patients on mechanical ventilation must remember that the peak airway pressure is not infrequently elevated as a result of the selection of ventilatory settings (peak inspiratory flow, tidal volume, and respiratory rate), an example of iatrogenic noncompliance.

Capnography

Whenever possible, end-tidal carbon dioxide ($ETCO_2$) monitoring (capnography) should be used in every patient on mechanical ventilation. The initial widespread clinical use of capnography was to confirm the correct placement of an endotracheal tube. If direct visualization and placement of an endotracheal tube between the vocal cords is not achieved, capnography is the only other absolute confirmation of correct placement. A malpositioned endotracheal tube is a greater problem in a critically ill patient in the ICU than in an anesthetized, paralyzed patient in the operating room. Patients in the ICU are obviously intubated for longer periods of time, are more mobile, more interactive, often more agitated, and are not continuously observed at the bedside, compared to patients in the operating room. Self-extubation is a recognized complication in all ICUs, with an estimated occurrence of 11% to 13%.[53] In addition, because of patient movement and respiratory therapies, disconnections in the airway circuitry (ventilator tubing, humidifier, nebulizer) occur frequently. Capnography provides immediate detection of airway obstruction, extubation, or ventilator disconnection. The presence of a regularly occurring exhaled carbon dioxide waveform confirms the continued presence of an intratracheal tube. The use of pulse oximetry is not a replacement for monitoring these events, as pulmonary oxygen reserve may allow sufficient gas exchange for several minutes.

An idealized normal capnogram is shown in Figure 25-3. In contrast to pulse oximetry, monitoring of exhaled carbon dioxide can provide more information than just the $ETCO_2$ (recorded in mm Hg or % CO_2). From the shape of the waveform, we can infer several observations such as the adequacy of alveolar emptying and the magnitude of pulmonary dead space. A well-defined plateau tells us that alveolar emptying is adequate and pulmonary dead space is minimal; therefore, $ETCO_2$ closely matches $PaCO_2$.

The difference between $PaCO_2$ and $ETCO_2$ is normally 4 to 7 mm Hg for most monitors currently available. An increase in this gradient in a patient on mechanical ventilation suggests the further development of physiological dead space. Exhibit 25-8 lists frequent clinical causes of increased dead space ventilation.

EXHIBIT 25-7

CLINICAL CAUSES OF REDUCED PULMONARY COMPLIANCE

- Pulmonary edema
- Pneumonia
- Atelectasis
- Pulmonary fibrosis
- Pneumothorax or hemothorax
- Pulmonary aspiration
- Chemical pneumonitis

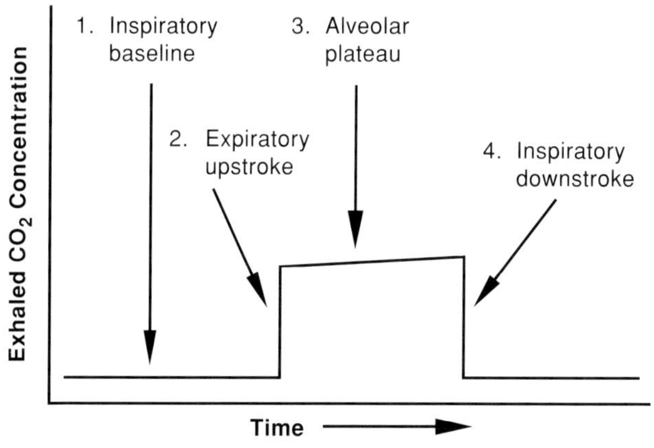

Fig. 25-3. Idealized capnogram waveform, with time plotted on the x axis and exhaled carbon dioxide concentration on the y axis. The numbered segments indicate the four phases of the ventilatory cycle. Adapted with permission from Benumof JL. *Anesthesia for Thoracic Surgery.* 2nd ed. Philadelphia, Pa: WB Saunders; 1995: 244.

Analysis of the carbon dioxide waveform also provides information regarding bronchospasm (the slope of the ascending segment) and the competency of the ventilator expiratory valve (baseline rebreathing of CO_2 > 2–4 mm Hg). One study[54] indicated that a rise or reappearance of exhaled carbon dioxide is one of the first indicators of the return of spontaneous circulation following a cardiopulmonary arrest. Additional studies have demonstrated that $ETco_2$ monitoring may be a good indicator of both the adequacy of pulmonary blood flow and cardiac output, and also a good prognostic indicator of the success of cardiopulmonary resuscitation.[55]

Exhaled Volume Monitoring (Spirometry)

It is crucial that exhaled tidal or minute volume be monitored while mechanical ventilation is used. Several of the ventilators that were sent to the Persian Gulf War—including the Univent 750, Bear 33, Lifecare PLV-100 and Lifecare PLV-102—did not have built-in exhaled volume monitoring. Monitoring of exhaled volume is particularly important when using either a pressure-cycled or a time-cycled mechanical ventilator. The use of these ventilators does not ensure the maintenance of a constant minute ventilation and a stable Pco_2 level. Even during the use of volume-cycled ventilation, measurement of exhaled volume serves as an additional monitor warning of a disconnection, a malfunctioning inspiratory or expiratory valve, an endotracheal or tracheostomy cuff leak, or a marked change in the pulmonary compliance (eg, pneumothorax).

EXHIBIT 25-8

FACTORS CONTRIBUTING TO INCREASED DEAD SPACE

Pulmonary
- Bronchospasm
- Chronic obstructive pulmonary disease
- Excessive positive end-expiratory pressure

Circulatory
- Hypovolemia
- Hypotension
- Reduced cardiac output
- Pulmonary embolism (thrombus, air, fat)

Clinical Examination of the Patient–Ventilator Unit

The clinical examination of the patient receiving mechanical ventilation (ie, the patient–ventilator *unit*) is the most important "monitor" of all. The first observation to make is determining whether the patient is ventilating spontaneously. If the patient demonstrates a lack of ventilatory effort, it usually reflects one or more of the criteria discussed in Exhibit 25-9. If the patient is making spontaneous ventilatory efforts, then ensure that the ventilator is not in the CMV mode, as this setting does not allow for ventilation beyond that designated by the set rate.

It is equally important to evaluate how well the mechanical support is meeting the patient's ventilatory requirements. If purpose of mechanical ventilation is to better meet the patient's ventilation and oxygenation needs, then allowing the patient to perform an excessive amount of the work of breathing defeats the purpose of mechanical support. The amount of minute ventilation required to maintain normocarbia can provide useful information as to the amount of dead space ventilation and the overall metabolic state in the setting of trauma and serious infection.

The level of peak airway pressure is a major risk factor for the development of barotrauma. For this reason, should the airway pressures be increased or noted to be rising, it is prudent to evaluate the patient for reversible causes of airway pressure elevation.

Lastly, should the patient demonstrate agitation while receiving mechanical ventilation, one should always first assume that the problem rests not with the patient, but rather with the ventilator itself or the manner in which it is being employed. By fully evaluating the ventilator and assuring that there are no malfunctions or inappropriate ventilatory settings, the clinician can avoid a potential catastrophe.

Oxygen Delivery

The gas exchange capability of the lung, as assessed by the Pao_2, $AaDo_2$, or other indices, is only one of the components that determines Do_2 to tissues. The two other major components are the level of hemoglobin and the cardiac output. (The comments in this chapter are limited to respiratory insufficiency; the reader can find a more detailed discussion in Chapter 24, The Syndromes of Systemic Inflammatory Response and Multiple Organ Dysfunction.) However, a number of studies[56–59] give credence to the importance of the calculation of both Do_2 and Vo_2 by use of a pulmonary artery

EXHIBIT 25-9

CRITERIA FOR OPTIMAL VENTILATOR USE

1. **Is the patient ventilating spontaneously?**

   If *NO*, then

   a. The settings (TV, rate) for mechanical support exceed the patient's requirement.

   b. The patient's apneic threshold has been altered (eg, narcotics, benzodiazepines).

   c. pH compensation is needed for a severe metabolic alkalosis.

   d. The patient does not have an intact central ventilatory drive (eg, due to a closed head injury or coma).

   e. The patient's thoracic or diaphragmatic muscular function is inadequate (eg, due to nerve agents, extreme fatigue, malnutrition).

   If *YES*, then

   a. Change from control mode to either AC or SIMV, and

   b. Evaluate how hard the patient is working while maintaining this spontaneous ventilation (eg, respiratory rate, diaphoresis, pulse, mental status).

2. **What is the minute ventilation requirement?**

   a. The requirement will vary frequently in the same patient based on the physical demands and the therapies being performed.

   b. The daily trend in mechanical ventilation provides information as to overall patient status in sepsis and trauma.

3. **Is the peak airway pressure too high (ie, progressively increasing or > 50 cm H_2O)?**

   If *YES*, then

   a. Evaluate dynamic (TV/PAP – PEEP) and static (TV/plateau – PEEP) compliances.

   b. Evaluate whether bronchospasm or secretions are causing increased airway resistance.

4. **Is the patient fighting the ventilator?**

   If *YES*, then evaluate for the following:

   a. Secretions and the need for suctioning,

   b. Bronchospasm, and

   c. Stacking of breaths or "auto-PEEP" because of too short an expiratory time or too high a sensitivity setting.

REMEMBER: the patient is "fighting" for his life. *Do not sedate and paralyze the patient* until you are confident that the ventilator is not malfunctioning and that the settings chosen are appropriate for the patient's needs.

TV: tidal volume; AC: assist control; SIMV: synchronized, intermittent, mandatory ventilation; PAP: peak airway pressure; PEEP: positive end-expiratory pressure

catheter. Several clinical states including sepsis and ARDS are characterized by what appears to be a pathological oxygen-supply dependency. Systemic oxygen need may reach levels as high as 21 mL/kg/min.[60] (Arterial and mixed-venous oxygen contents and the cardiac index must be measured simultaneously to allow these calculations.)

The usefulness of augmenting cardiac output has been difficult to demonstrate in several clinical trials. In both the surgical setting and the setting of myocardial infarction,[61] pushing cardiac output with inotropic drugs has not been associated with improved outcome. These studies are difficult to perform, since critically ill patients are sometimes hard to match—but meta-analysis and further clinical trials will elucidate the true effects of artifically increasing oxygen delivery. At this time, the question remains only partially answered and is the source of considerable controversy among practitioners across the country.[62,63]

Chest Radiography

Daily chest X-ray examinations are an accepted ICU monitor for patients in respiratory failure. Several studies have validated the importance of daily chest X-ray examinations in critically ill unstable or mechanically ventilated patients: approximately 14% to 15% of chest X-ray examinations demonstrate unexpected findings that lead to a change in management.[64,65]

Most chest X-ray examinations taken of critically ill patients are made by a portable device at the bedside. These films are taken from an anterior-posterior rather than the standard posteroanterior orientation. This is important for several reasons. The distance from the X-ray beam to the intrathoracic structures is not constant, and objects that are far from the film (cardiac silhouette) are magnified. Critically ill patients, particularly those in respiratory failure, are often tachypneic, and obtaining an end-inspiratory chest film is difficult because they cannot hold their breath. It should be remembered that a chest X-ray examination cannot properly evaluate upper-airway obstruction; however, careful attention not infrequently reveals tracheal abnormalities. One example of this is tracheal or left main bronchus deviation when a traumatic aortic dissection occurs. The information that can be obtained from a chest X-ray examination depends on the respiratory status of the casualty: whether the patient's ventilations are spontaneous or mechanically assisted.

Spontaneously Ventilating Patients. Chest radiography is used to evaluate the patient for pulmonary parenchymal injury. The presence of a radiological density may represent collapse of alveoli (eg, atelectasis); or alveolar consolidation from water (pulmonary edema), blood (aspiration or bronchoalveolar hemorrhage); or infected secretions (pneumonia). These fluids are indistinguishable radiologically, and clinical examination or other diagnostic tests must be conducted to discern the actual cause. The chest X-ray examination may also detect pathology in the pleural space (eg, pneumothorax, hemothorax, or effusion). Frequently, chest X-ray examinations done in this patient population are performed in the supine position, and a pneumothorax may be missed. One helpful radiological sign is the "deep sulcus sign," a clear costophrenic angle that often extends well below the normal location for the diaphragm.

Additionally, radiological assessment of the heart, great vessels, and pulmonary vasculature offers information pertinent to the patient's intravascular volume status, the presence of congestive heart failure, or the possible occurrence of a pulmonary embolism. The latter should be suspected when a pleura-based, wedge-shaped infiltrate (Hampton's hump) or regional oligemia (Westermark's sign) are seen on a chest roentgenogram.

Mechanically Ventilated Patients. Patients who require mechanical ventilation may benefit from additional radiographic monitoring for potential complications. A daily chest X-ray examination is a good method to use for confirming a safe location for an endotracheal tube. Although other monitors (such as capnography) exist to confirm intratracheal placement, a chest X-ray examination will reveal the exact location of the cuff and the tip of the endotracheal tube. To prevent either intubation of the right main bronchus or accidental extubation, the optimal distance from the carina to the tip of the endotracheal tube is 3 to 7 cm. The carina is used as a reference point because the relationship of the endotracheal tube tip to the clavicle changes, depending on the angle at which the film was exposed. Tracheostomy tubes are much more secure, and less frequent radiological monitoring is required.

Mechanical ventilation may be associated with barotrauma. This is more common when peak airway pressures exceeding 40 to 50 cm H_2O have been employed. Barotrauma may take several forms including pneumothorax, pneumomediastinum, pneumoperitoneum; or subcutaneous emphysema of the chest wall, neck, or even the eyes. Patients in respiratory failure who require high levels of ventilatory support, particularly once evidence of barotrauma is present, need frequent, routine chest X-ray examinations, as well as an additional one whenever a clinical deterioration in either hemodynamic or respiratory status occurs. A small pneumothorax in a patient being supported with positive-pressure ventilation may at any time become a tension pneumothorax with the accompanying hemodynamic compromise.

Hemodynamic Monitoring

Although arterial, central venous, and pulmonary artery–catheter monitoring are important in monitoring the critically ill patient, a full discussion of hemodynamic monitoring is beyond the scope of this chapter. Further information may be found in Chapter 5, Physiological Monitoring.

WEANING FROM MECHANICAL VENTILATION

Weaning the patient from mechanical ventilation refers to shifting to partial ventilatory support while observing the patient's response to the increased work of breathing associated with spontaneous ventilation. Weaning is frequently unnecessary in patients who are mechanically supported for a brief period of time following surgery or another medical illness and who have not suffered from malnutrition. These patients should not have developed respiratory muscle fatigue.

Discontinuation of mechanical ventilation should be considered only if the underlying cause of the respiratory failure (eg, treated pneumonia, resolved sepsis, arousal from coma) has been reversed. Discontinuation is likely to prove possible only if the following preconditions have been met:

- the central respiratory drive is intact, ensuring normocarbia;
- muscular strength is adequate to maintain a clear airway and provide for full spontaneous breathing;
- the patient is hemodynamically stable (ie, shock is resolved, intravascular volume restored); and
- carbon dioxide production is not elevated.

Medical officers, however, must consider not only the casualty's condition but also the need for aeromedical evacuation to a higher echelon of care. The U.S. Air Force is reluctant to evacuate casualties on ventilators and, in fact, refused to do so during the Persian Gulf War. (See Chapter 27, Military Medical Evacuation, for a more complete discussion of this subject.)

Many criteria have been published to evaluate a patient's ability to be successfully weaned from mechanical ventilatory support (Exhibit 25-10). Some of these criteria are subjective and thus require good clinical acumen as to the physiological capability of the patient. Even objective criteria that can be measured and quantified have been questioned, as there are patients who do successfully wean from mechanical support despite their not meeting the weaning criteria.[66,67] In addition, certain of the quantitative measurements are frequently not performed properly and thus may give false information. Nevertheless, combining criteria into a decision tree (Figure 25-4) is usually helpful in deciding if and when to wean. Application of the decision tree presupposes that the patient is not sedated to the point where the ventilatory drive is blunted.

Several of these indicators (negative inspiratory force, minute ventilation, and maximum voluntary ventilation) were evaluated in one study.[68] If the minute ventilation was less than 10 L, then the maximum voluntary ventilation was 2-fold greater than the minute volume, and the negative inspiratory force was greater than –30 cm H_2O. All patients were successfully extubated in this study. These parameters are probably of greater use in short-term ventilator use than they are in prolonged, when the clinical judgment of the physician is as valid as the measured criteria.

Patients who required prolonged (> 30 d) mechanical ventilation have been shown to have a hospital mortality identical to patients who required only short-term mechanical ventilation.[69] Thus, these patients deserve a well-conceived plan for the goal of successful extubation and separation from mechanical ventilatory support.

EXHIBIT 25-10

CRITERIA FOR WEANING FROM VENTILATORS

Respiratory or Metabolic Demand or Both

Respiratory rate < 25

Minute ventilation < 10 L/min

Dead space ventilation < 30%–40% of total ventilation

Oxygenation

Pa_{O_2} > 60 mm Hg on F_{IO_2} < 50%

PEEP < 5 cm H_2O

Intrapulmonary shunt < 30%

Adequate hemoglobin concentration (7–10 g/dL)

Respiratory Muscle Strength

Tidal volume > 5 mL/kg

Vital capacity > 10 mL/kg

Negative inspiratory force > –30 cm H_2O

Maximal voluntary ventilation > 2-fold the resting minute ventilation

Pa_{O_2}: partial pressure of arterial oxygen; PEEP: positive end-expiratory pressure

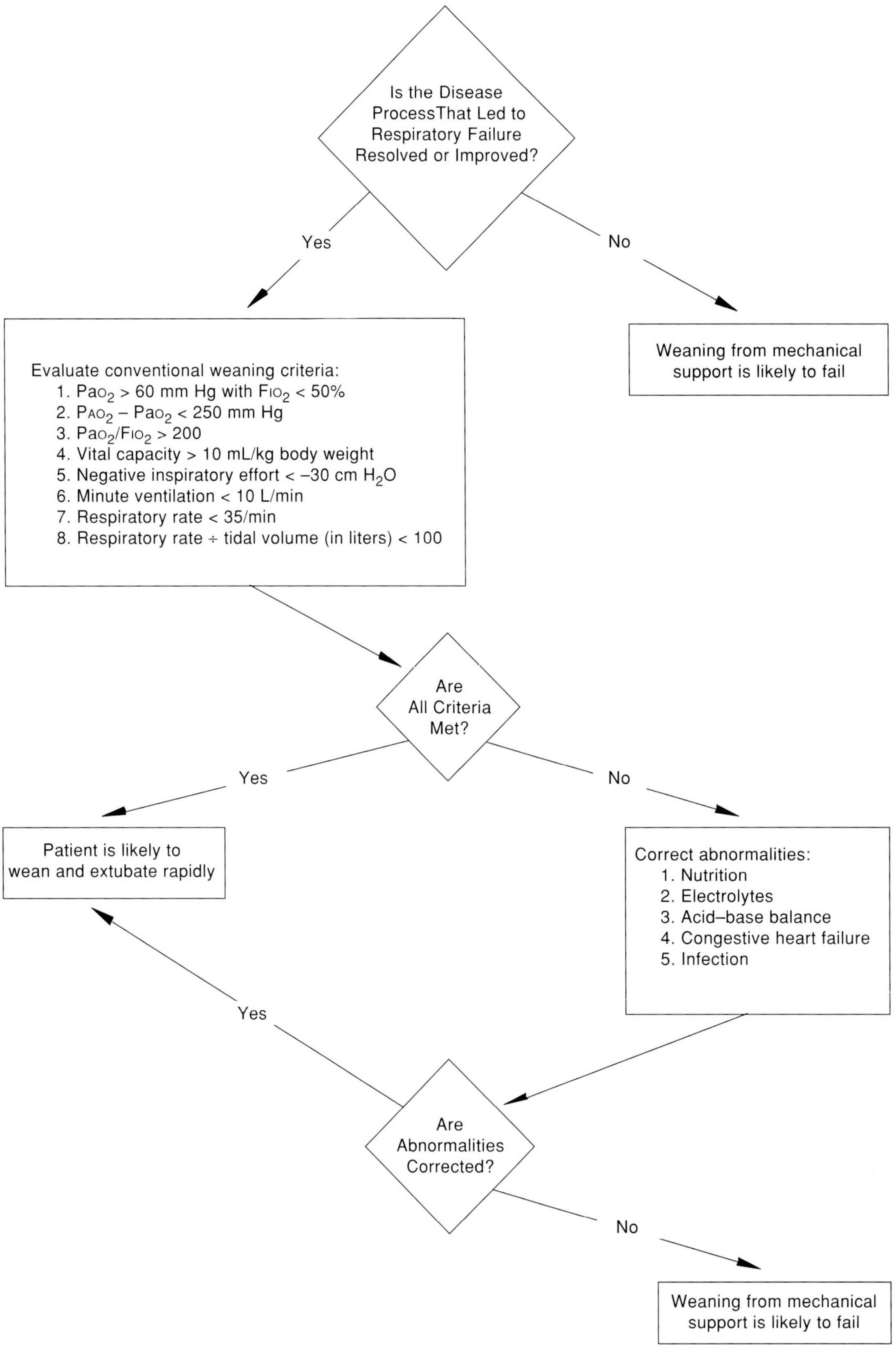

Fig. 25-4. Decision tree for weaning from mechanical ventilation.

The first step in weaning a patient who has been dependent on mechanical ventilatory support is to optimize the patient's general status (Exhibit 25-11). This may seem obvious, but it is not fully appreciated and is frequently overlooked completely—especially when too much attention is directed toward purely respiratory indices. Even if the patient demonstrates no respiratory distress, it is unwise to wean a patient who appears to be in any form of shock. By definition, the term "shock" means that the supply of blood and nutrients (oxygen and glucose) to organs or tissues has not met the demand. If such a patient were required to sustain full spontaneous ventilation, the increase in oxygen demand could worsen the balance between systemic oxygen delivery and systemic oxygen need. For example, in sepsis, oxygen utilization by the diaphragm can be very high and, in fact, can constitute nearly 30% to 40% of the body's total V_{O_2}.[50]

Several clinical conditions may lead to an elevated production of carbon dioxide, necessitating a higher minute ventilation to maintain normocarbia. Patients who are febrile, agitated, in pain, or who have suffered traumatic injuries, thermal burns, or seizures produce increased carbon dioxide. Excessive carbon dioxide production may also arise iatrogenically as a result of excessive carbohydrate administration. (For a more complete discussion, see Chapter 23, Metabolic Derangements and Nutritional Support.)

It is often impossible to determine the exact cause of a patient's failure to wean, but recent discussion has focused on respiratory muscle fatigue and disuse atrophy as two important causes. It may be clinically impossible to distinguish between these two causes. Respiratory muscle fatigue has been suspected clinically for some time and electromyographic evidence supports this concern.[70] The clinician must remain alert to mechanical factors that exacerbate rather than aid respiratory muscle fatigue. Most intensivists know that increased airway resistance results from using a small endotracheal tube ($\leq$ 7.0 mm internal diameter). A tracheostomy, by increasing the diameter and shortening the length of the airway, may reduce the resistance. Occasional patients may wean best by simply proceeding to extubation, totally eliminating the resistance of the artificial airway. (This is becoming less necessary as advanced mechanical ventilators with multiple ventilatory modes are developed.)

The three principal weaning modalities are (1) a progressive reduction of mechanical support through the use of IMV, (2) T-piece trials, whereby the patient is disconnected from the ventilator and attached to a T-piece for progressively longer intervals, and (3) pressure-support weaning. The literature does not support the superiority of any one method.[67]

T-piece trials should be initiated in 5-minute intervals, with the physician or nurse at the bedside to evaluate any significant changes in the patient's respiratory rate, pulse, or subjective complaints of excessive work. T-piece trials use intermittent periods of vigorous breathing intended to increase the patient's respiratory endurance. Rest periods are

EXHIBIT 25-11

FACTORS THAT MAY PREVENT DISCONTINUATION OF MECHANICAL VENTILATION

The patient must not be malnourished. Diaphragmatic muscle loss is nearly linearly related to the degree of malnutrition.[1,2]

Significant acid–base and electrolyte abnormalities must be corrected, including metabolic alkalosis that demands hypoventilation to normalize the serum pH.

Hypophosphatemia may also contribute to respiratory muscular weakness.

Left-ventricular failure leading to reduced pulmonary compliance may be an occult cause of persistent failure to wean from mechanical support.

Airway secretions may be a significant problem to the patient after extubation, during which time small-airway obstruction leads to atelectasis and bronchospasm.

Sources: (1) Bell RM, Bynoe RP. Nutrition and respiration. *Prob Crit Care.* 1987;1(3):413–434. (2) Lewis MI, Belman MJ. Nutrition and the respiratory muscles. *Clin Chest Med.* 1988;9(2):337–348.

important to the success of this method. The definition of quality respiratory rest (ie, the respiratory muscles are resting) has been clouded by recent studies showing significant amounts of respiratory work with AC ventilation. In addition, the optimal rest time between periods of T-piece work has not been answered in the literature. Our practice has been to allow for a minimum of one hour between exercise periods and rest the patient with full ventilatory support overnight.

SIMV is another ventilatory strategy commonly used in weaning. Quite simply, the number of mechanical breaths per minute provided to the patient are gradually reduced over several days to weeks. As the number of mechanical breaths is reduced, the patient must assume a greater amount of the work of breathing. The potential disadvantage of this strategy is the increase in work of breathing due to the resistance inherent in the inspiratory demand valves used in modern mechanical ventilators.[71] This work may be sufficient to cause the weaning attempt to fail in some patients (eg, those patients with severe obstructive lung disease or significant respiratory muscle atrophy).

Another relatively new strategy for weaning has been the use of pressure support ventilation, either in conjunction with or in place of SIMV. Pressure support ventilation permits the mechanical flow of fresh gas after the patient initiates a breath. Because the patient retains control of the total respiratory rate and the depth and duration of assisted breaths, they are generally more comfortable while receiving mechanical ventilatory support. This mode offsets the increased work of breathing inherent in the ventilator circuit due to resistance to gas flow in the circuit. Most authorities do not recommend reducing the SIMV rate below four breaths per minute unless pressure support ventilation is utilized concomitantly.

Several general comments should be made regarding medical plans for ventilatory weaning:

- Adequate rest periods are essential to prevent respiratory muscle fatigue.
- The physician must constantly assess the patient's progress during weaning.
- Arterial blood gas measurements are no substitute for clinical judgment.
- Hypercarbia is a late finding of inadequate respiratory muscle strength.
- The patient must be observed for tachypnea, paradoxical respiratory movements, use of accessory muscles of inspiration, and diaphoresis.

VENTILATORS AVAILABLE FOR COMBAT CASUALTY CARE

A large number of mechanical ventilators are in the inventories of the medical departments of the U.S. armed forces. The following section discusses the Puritan-Bennett PR-2 (manufactured by the Bennett Medical Equipment, Los Angeles, Calif.), which is pressure cycled; the Bear 33 (manufactured by Bear Medical Systems, Riverside, Calif.) and the Lifecare PLV-100 and PLV-102 (manufactured by Lifecare Corporation, Lafayette, Colo.), which are volume cycled; the Bennett MA-1 (manufactured by Bennett Medical Equipment, Los Angeles, Calif.), which is also volume cycled; and the Impact Uni-Vent Model 750 M (manufactured by Impact Instrumentation, West Caldwell, N.J.), which is time cycled.

These ventilators are available for use with deployed medical units.

Puritan-Bennett PR-2

The Puritan-Bennett PR-2 is basically a converted intermittent, positive-pressure breathing machine and requires a source of compressed gas to function. The PR-2 is unique among the ventilators under discussion here because it is pressure cycled. The patient's tidal volume cannot be directly set, but is a result of the pressure limit and the inspiratory time. The limitations of the PR-2 in providing mechanical ventilatory support to combat casualties are as follows:

- If the patient's compliance decreases or airway resistance increases (a change in the patient's position, secretions in the airway, bronchospasm, or patient agitation), the same settings of airway pressure will result in a decreased tidal volume and hypoventilation. Thus, we strongly advise that (*a*) exhaled tidal volume be monitored and (*b*) an alarm be attached.
- The patient may continue to spontaneously breathe; however, competition may occur as there is no mechanism to provide synchronization with the patient's efforts. This may result in high airway pressures and barotrauma.

- There is inaccurate control of F_{IO_2} from breath to breath when oxygen enrichment is used. The higher the patient's minute ventilation, the lower the F_{IO_2}.
- When the respiratory rate increases and the pressure is kept constant, inspiration may end prematurely because the constant flow rate results in higher peak airway pressures closing the inspiratory valve.
- To provide PEEP, an external valve must be attached to the exhalation limb.
- These ventilators have limited peak flow capabilities and may not be able to provide for the traumatized casualty whose minute ventilation demands are excessive.

Bear 33 and Lifecare PLV-100 and PLV-102

The Bear 33 and the Lifecare PLV-100 and PLV-102 ventilators are all portable, electrically powered, microprocessor controlled, and volume cycled. They do not require a separate source of compressed gas unless oxygen enrichment is used. All these ventilators can function in AC and SIMV modes, with some limitations. All have an internal battery and may be connected to an external battery as well. The limitations of these ventilators are as follows:

- "Apnea, breathing-circuit disconnections, leaks, exhalation-valve failures and occlusions may remain undetected...."[72(p107)] Thus, it is recommended that an exhaled volume monitor be used with these ventilators. There is no built-in capability for monitoring exhaled volume.
- The provision for enriched oxygen supply is passive and, except in the PLV-102, requires an externally attached H-valve mechanism. Three problems may be encountered:
  1. the potential misassembly of the H-valve, which may lead to obstruction during patient inspiration;
  2. the inaccuracy of the inspired oxygen concentration, which mandates the use of an oxygen analyzer (the F_{IO_2} will be ± 10% if the patient has a *stable* minute ventilation pattern, and greater if the patient is unstable);
  3. the automatic increase in tidal volume, which occurs with increased oxygen flow (in the Bear 33 and PLV-100), may cause increased airway pressure and barotrauma.
- "Substantial increases in work of breathing varied with each ventilator so that the work of breathing approached that of a patient with high airway resistance: Bear 33, 41%; Lifecare PLV-100 and PLV-102, 88%...."[72(p107)] While supported on these ventilators, the patient may appear dyspneic, and weaning by IMV is likely to be unsuccessful unless an external H-valve attachment is assembled.
- If a microprocessor failure occurs, the Bear 33 will not return to the previously set parameters, but will revert to "apnea settings" of a tidal volume of 500 mL and a respiratory rate of 16 breaths per minute.
- Lead–acid batteries are used in all these ventilators. The life of this type of battery will be shortened if it is allowed to remain discharged. If fully functioning and charged, the internal battery life is expected to be 1 to 3 hours.
- To provide PEEP therapy, an external valve needs to be attached on the exhalation limb.

Bennett MA-1

The Bennett MA-1 has been used for many years in ICUs. This ventilator is electronically powered and volume cycled (termination of inspiration). Its limitations are as follows:

- There is no built-in monitoring of exhaled volume.
- An externally attached H-valve apparatus must be used to allow IMV to be used. Hence, IMV is not synchronized and mechanical breaths may "stack" on top of spontaneous breaths.
- To provide PEEP, an external valve must be attached to the exhalation limb.

Impact Uni-Vent Model 750 M

The Impact Uni-Vent Model 750 is the newest ventilator to be accepted for military use. The Impact is a portable, electrically controlled, time-cycled, pressure-limited mechanical ventilator. It is microprocessor-controlled and is capable of control, AC, or SIMV ventilatory modes. It has an internal battery with a fully charged time capability of 9 hours. This mechanical ventilator does require a source of compressed gas to provide patient flow, except during spontaneous breaths in the SIMV mode. The limitations are as follows:

- There is no built-in capability for exhaled volume monitoring.
- To institute PEEP therapy, an external PEEP valve needs to be attached and several control settings must be adjusted to allow monitoring of the amount of PEEP within the patient's circuit.
- The work of breathing is not well studied for this ventilator. An optional demand valve (connected to a source of compressed gas) is available, which provides an inspiratory flow of 60 L/min and is reported to provide a small pressure assist (support) of 2 to 3 cm H_2O.
- If the optional demand valve is not used, room air will be entrained through the antiasphyxiation port during the patient's spontaneous breaths. This will decrease the fractional concentration of oxygen provided to the patient.
- There is no measurement of the size of spontaneous breaths taken during SIMV.
- The digital display of peak inspiratory pressure is hard to quantitate in the most common range of pressures (10–50 cm H_2O).

Many of the mechanical ventilators projected for use in the combat casualty setting are different from those used in most peacetime hospitals. For this reason, it would be prudent for medical personnel who may be called on to care for patients with these ventilators to familiarize themselves with their operating capabilities.

SUMMARY

Respiratory failure of a magnitude that requires mechanical ventilation can be expected to occur in 10% to 15% of hospitalized casualties. The most likely causes are ARDS, severe brain injury, and severe torso injury during the postoperative phase. The diagnosis of respiratory failure depends on the observation of hypoxemia ($PaO_2 \leq 50$ mm Hg while breathing room air) and ventilatory failure ($PaCO_2 >$ 50 mm Hg). Although these findings indicate the presence of severe pathophysiology, respiratory support with supplemental oxygen, incentive spirometry, and intratracheal suctioning may decrease the need for intubation and mechanical ventilation.

Mechanical ventilation has several beneficial effects, including eliminating the work of breathing for the casualty, maximizing the concentration of inspired oxygen, and ventilating collapsed and poorly ventilated alveoli. The latter changes cause a decrease in the amount of intrapulmonary shunting and an increase in the functional residual capacity of the lung. However, high airway pressure during expiration—especially in the presence of hypovolemia—may lead to decreased venous return to the heart, a fall in cardiac output, and a decrease in oxygen delivery. Barotrauma leading to tension pneumothorax is a potentially fatal complication of mechanical ventilation but is unlikely to occur if peak airway pressure is maintained below 50 cm H_2O.

Military anesthesiologists and intensivists must understand the design of deployable mechanical ventilators, be able to choose the proper mode of ventilation, and be able to select the appropriate initial ventilatory settings. These required settings include tidal volume, rate, peak gas flow, inspiratory-to-expiratory ratio, and the fractional concentration of oxygen. In addition, anesthesiologists and intensivists must be familiar with the logistics of oxygen supply.

Mechanical ventilators use three types of cycling: pressure, volume, and time. Both volume- and time-cycled ventilators allow for a constant level of tidal volume, which makes them more effective than pressure-cycled ventilators whenever pulmonary compliance or airway resistance is elevated. The initial settings that are selected for mechanical support depend on the indication for which the patient requires ventilatory support. Plausible initial settings are tidal volume, 10 to 15 mL/kg; respiratory rate, 7 to 10 breaths per minute; and inspired oxygen concentration, 40%. Both the respiratory rate and the oxygen concentration may have to be increased, and flow rates and end expiratory pressures adjusted, if pulmonary injury is present. A variety of parameters may be measured to judge the effectiveness of ventilation and oxygenation (eg, systemic DO_2 and the magnitude of the arterial-venous shunt), but useful information is also obtained from the subjective appearance of the casualty. In addition, in deployable hospitals, from the practical standpoint, an assessment as to the effectiveness of ventilation will depend on measurement of PaO_2 and $PaCO_2$ measured with a blood gas analyzer, SaO_2 measured with a pulse oximeter, a chest radiogram, and the airway flow and pressure measurements from the controls and sensors of the mechanical ventilator. The goal is to maximize oxygenation while minimizing airway pressures and inspired oxygen concentration.

Discontinuation of mechanical ventilation should be considered only if the underlying cause of the respiratory failure has been reversed. Multiple criteria have been advanced to guide the weaning process once the decision has been made to discontinue mechanical support. Among them are (*a*) PaO_2 greater than 60 mm Hg when FIO_2 is less than 0.5, (*b*) the ability to produce a spontaneous vital capacity greater than 10 mL/kg, and (*c*) the ability to generate a negative inspiratory effort greater than 30 cm H_2O. None of these criteria are absolute. Premature discontinuation of mechanical ventilation and extubation to make possible rapid evacuation—especially when it is by air—is to be avoided in combat casualties.

REFERENCES

1. Bellamy RF. Colonel, Medical Corps, US Army. Personal communication, July 1994. The single most useful database describing combat wounds and the circumstances of wounding is the Wound Data and Munitions Effectiveness Team (WDMET) study prepared by the US Army Materiel Command during the Vietnam War. These data are stored at the National Naval Medical Center, Bethesda, Maryland. Access is controlled by the Uniformed Services University of the Health Sciences, Bethesda, Maryland 20814-4799; telephone (301) 295-6262. Three summary volumes contain extensive abstracts of the statistical data and can be obtained from Defense Documentation Center, Cameron Station, Alexandria, Virginia 22304-6145; telephone (703) 545-6700 and (703) 274-7633.

2. Arnold K, Cutting RT. Causes of death in United States military personnel hospitalized in Vietnam. *Milit Med.* 1978;143:161–164.

3. Wright S. US Army Medical Department Center and School, Fort Sam Houston, Tex. Personal communication, 29 July 1993.

4. Whatmore D. Lieutenant Colonel, Medical Corps, US Army. Personal communication, August 1994.

5. McNamara J, Messersmith J. Thoracic injuries in combat casualties in Vietnam. *Ann Thor Surg.* 1970;10(4): 389–401.

6. Bowen TE, Bellamy RF, eds. *Emergency War Surgery NATO Handbook.* 2nd rev US ed. Washington, DC: Department of Defense, Government Printing Office; 1988.

7. Bellamy RF, Zajtchuk R, eds. *Medical Consequences of Conventional Warfare.* In: Zajtchuk R, Jenkins DP, Bellamy RF, eds. *Textbook of Military Medicine.* Washington, DC: US Department of the Army, Office of The Surgeon General, and Borden Institute; 1991.

8. Huller T, Bazini Y. Blast injuries of the chest and abdomen. *Arch Surg.* 1970;100:24–30.

9. Blood CG. Analyses of battle casualties by weapon type aboard US Navy warships. *Milit Med.* 1992;157(3):124–130.

10. Fein A, Leff A, Hopewell P. Pathophysiology and management of the complications resulting from fire and the inhaled products of combustion. *Crit Care Med.* 1980;8(2):94–98.

11. Rue LW, Cioffi WG, Mason AD, McManus WF, Pruitt BA. Improved survival of burned patients with inhalation injury. *Arch Surg.* 1993;128:772–780.

12. Levine B, Petroff P, Slade C, Pruitt B. Prospective trials of dexamethasone and aerosolized gentamicin in the treatment of inhalation injury in the burned patient. *J Trauma.* 1978;18(2):188–193.

13. Freitag L, Firusian N, Stamatis G, Greschuchria D. The role of bronchoscopy in pulmonary complications due to mustard gas inhalation. *Chest.* 1991;100:1436–1441.

14. Bellamy RF, ed. *Combat Casualty Care Guidelines: Operation Desert Storm.* Washington, DC: US Department of the Army, Office of The Surgeon General, and Borden Institute; 1991: 28.

15. Dolev E. Wartime trauma: Lessons and perspectives. *Internat Anes Clin*. 1987;25(1):191–202.

16. Teabeaut J. Aspiration of gastric contents: An experimental study. *Am J Pathol*. 1951;28:51.

17. Patterson A. *Pulmonary Aspiration Syndromes in Respiratory Failure*. Chicago, Ill: Yearbook Medical Publishers; 1986.

18. Fanning G. The efficacy of cricoid pressure in preventing regurgitation of gastric contents. *Anesthesia*. 1970;32(6):553–555.

19. Allen S, Drake R, Williams J, Laine G, Gabel J. Recent advances in pulmonary edema. *Crit Care Med*. 1987;15(10):963–970.

20. Grande CM, Stene JK, Bernhard WN, Barton CR. Trauma anesthesia and critical care: the concept and rationale for a new subspecialty. *Crit Care Clin*. 1990;6(1):1–11.

21. Tobin MJ, Yang K. Weaning from mechanical ventilation. *Crit Care Clin*. 1990;6(3):725–747.

22. Moon VH, Kennedy PJ. Pathology of shock. *Arch Path*. 1932;14:360–371.

23. Ashbaugh D, Bigelow D, Petty T, Levine B. Acute respiratory distress in adults. *Lancet*. 1967;2(7511):319–323.

24. Milberg JA, Davis DR, Steinberg KP, Hudson LD. Improved survival of patients with acute respiratory distress syndrome (ARDS): 1983–1993. *JAMA*. 1995;273(4):306–309.

25. Olcott C, Barber R, Blaisdell F. Diagnosis and treatment of respiratory failure after civilian trauma. *Am J Surg*. 1971;122:260–268.

26. Hammerschmidt D, Weaver L. Association of complement activation in elevated plasma C5A with ARDS: Pathophysiological relevance and possible prognostic value. *Lancet*. 1980;1:947–949.

27. Sutter PM, Schlobohm RM. Determination of functional residual capacity during mechanical ventilation. *Anesthesiology*. 1974;41:605–607.

28. Bernard GR, Luce JM, Sprung CL. High dose corticosteriods in patients with the Adult Respiratory Distress Syndrome. *N Engl J Med*. 1987;317(25):1565–1570.

29. Kollef MH, Schuster DP. The acute respiratory distress syndrome. *N Engl J Med*. 1995;332(1):27–35.

30. Montgomery AB, Stager MA, Carrico J. Cause of mortality in patients with the adult respiratory distress syndrome. *Am Rev Respir Dis*. 1985;132(5):485–489.

31. Zapol WM, Snider MT, Hill JD. Extracorporeal membrane oxygenation in severe acute pulmonary failure: A randomized prospective study. *JAMA*. 1979;242(20):2193–2196.

32. Abrams JH, Gilmour IJ, Kriett JM, et al. Low frequency positive pressure ventilation with extracorporeal carbon dioxide removal. *Crit Care Med*. 1990;18(2):218–220.

33. Van de Water J, Watring W, Linton L. Prevention of postoperative pulmonary complications. *Surg Gynecol Obstet*. 1978;135:129.

34. Latimer RG, Dickman M, Day WC, Gunn ML, Schmidt CD. Ventilatory patterns and pulmonary complications after upper abdominal surgery determined by preoperative and postoperative computerized spirometry and blood gas analysis. *Am J Surg*. 1971;122(5):622–632.

35. Ward RJ, Danzier F, Bonica JJ, Allen GD, Bowes J. An evaluation of postoperative respiratory maneuvers. *Surg Gynecol Obstet*. 1966;123:51–54.

36. Committee on Trauma, American College of Surgeons. *Advanced Trauma Life Support Program for Physicians: Instructor Manual*. 5th ed. Chicago, Ill: American College of Surgeons; 1993.

37. Berlauk JF. Prolonged endotracheal intubation *vs* tracheostomy. *Crit Care Med*. 1986;14(8):742–745.

38. Nash M. Swallowing problems in the tracheotomized patient. *Otolaryngol Clin North Am*. 1988;21(4):701–709.

39. Marini J, Wheeler A. Mechanical ventilation. In: *Critical Care Medicine—The Essentials*. Baltimore, Md: Williams & Wilkins; 1989: 65.

40. Biondi JW, Shulman DS, Soufer R, et al. The effect of incremental positive end-expiratory pressure on right ventricular hemodynamics and ejection fraction. *Anesth Analg*. 1988;67(2):144–151.

41. Shelhamer JH, Natanson C, Parrillo JE. Positive end-expiratory pressure and adults. *JAMA*. 1984;251(20): 2692–2695.

42. Petersen GW, Baier H. Incidence of pulmonary barotrauma in a medical ICU. *Crit Care Med*. 1983;11(2):67–69.

43. Haake R, Schlictig R, Ulstad D, Henschen R. Barotrauma, pathophysiology, risk factors and prevention. *Chest*. 1987;91(4):608–613.

44. Knaus WA, Wagner DP. Multiple systems organ failure: Epidemiology and prognosis. *Crit Care Clin*. 1989;5(2): 221–232.

45. Barach A, Martin J, Eckman M. Positive pressure respiration and its application to treatment of acute pulmonary edema. *Ann Int Med*. 1938;12:754.

46. Gallagher TJ, Civetta JM, Kirby RR. Terminology update: Optimal PEEP. *Crit Care Med*. 1978;6(5):323–326.

47. Petty TL. The use, abuse, and mystique of positive end-expiratory pressure. *Am Rev Respir Dis*. 1988;138(2): 475–478.

48. Lodato R. Oxygen toxicity. *Crit Care Clin*. 1990;6(3):749–765.

49. Tobin M, Lodato R. Respiratory monitoring in the ICU. *Pulmonary and Critical Care Update*. 1988;3(22):1.

50. Roussos C, Macklem P. The respiratory muscles. *N Engl J Med*. 1982;307(13):786–797.

51. MacIntyre NR. Respiratory function during pressure support ventilator. *Chest*. 1986;89(5):677–683.

52. Hubmayr RD, Gay PC, Tayyab MM. Respiratory system mechanics in ventilated patients: Techniques and indications. *Mayo Clin Proc*. 1987;62(5):358–368.

53. Coppolo DP, May JJ. Self-extubations: A 12-month experience. *Chest*. 1990;99(5):1319–1320.

54. Garnett AR, Ornato JP, Gonzales ER, Johnson EB. End-tidal carbon dioxide monitoring during cardiopulmonary resuscitation. *JAMA*. 1987;257(4):512–515.

55. Sanders AB, Kern KB, Otto CW, Milander MM, Eury GA. End-tidal carbon dioxide monitoring during cardiopulmonary resuscitation: A prognostic indication for survival. *JAMA*. 1989;2629100:1347–1351.

56. Shoemaker WC, Appel PL, Kram HB, Waxman K, Lee TS. Prospective trial of supranormal values of survivors as therapeutic goals in high-risk surgical patients. *Chest*. 1988;94(6):1176–1186.

57. Wolf Y, Cotev S, Perel A, Manny J. Dependence of oxygen consumption on cardiac output in sepsis. *Crit Care Med*. 1987;15(3):198–203.

58. Cain SM. Supply dependence of oxygen uptake in ARDS: Myth or reality? *Am J Med Sci.* 1984;288(3):119–124.

59. Gutierrez G, Pohil RJ. Oxygen consumption is linearly related to O_2 supply in critically ill patients. *J Crit Care.* 1986;1(1):45.

60. Mohsenifar Z, Goldback P, Tashkin D, Campisi D. Relationship between O_2 delivery and O_2 consumption in the Adult Respiratory Distress Syndrome. *Chest.* 1983;84(3):267–271.

61. Yu M, Takanishi D, Myers SA, et al. Frequency of mortality and myocardial infarction during maximizing oxygen delivery: A prospective, randomized trial. *Crit Care Med.* 1995;23(6):1025–1032.

62. Knox JB. Oxygen consumption–oxygen delivery dependency in adult respiratory distress syndrome. *New Horizons.* 1993;1(3):381–387.

63. Demling RH. Adult respiratory distress syndrome: Current concepts. *New Horizons.* 1993;1(3):388–401.

64. Brunel W, Coleman D, Schwartz D, Peper E, Cohen N. Assessment of routine chest roentgenograms and the physical examination to confirm endotracheal tube position. *Chest.* 1989;96(5):1043–1045.

65. Strain DJ, Kinasluity GT, Vereen LE, George RB. Value of routine daily chest X-rays in the medical intensive care unit. *Crit Care Med.* 1985;13(7):534–536.

66. Sporn PH, Morganroth ML. Discontinuation of mechanical ventilation. *Clin Chest Med.* 1988;9(1):113–126.

67. Morganroth M, Grum C. Weaning from mechanical ventilation. *J Intern Care Med.* 1988;3(2):109.

68. Sahn SA, Lakshninarayan S. Bedside criteria for the discontinuation of mechanical ventilation. *Chest.* 1973;63(6):1002–1005.

69. Morganroth ML, Morganroth JL, Nett LM, Perry TL. Criteria for weaning for prolonged mechanical ventilation. *Arch Intern Med.* 1984;144(5):1012–1016.

70. Cohen C, Zagelbaum G, Gross D, Roussos C, Macklem P. Clinical manifestations of inspiratory muscle fatigue. *Am J Med.* 1982;73(3):308–316.

71. Hughes C, Poparich J. Overcoming common problems with mechanical ventilation valve systems. *J Crit Illness.* 1988;1:13.

72. ECRI. Portable volume ventilators. *Health Devices.* 1988;17(4):107–131. Special issue.

Chapter 26

ACUTE RENAL FAILURE

JACK MOORE, Jr., M.D.*

*Colonel, Medical Corps, U.S. Army, (ret); formerly, Chief, Nephrology Service, Walter Reed Army Medical Center, Washington, D. C.; Nephrology Consultant to The Surgeon General; and Associate Professor of Medicine, Uniformed Services University of the Health Sciences, 4301 Jones Bridge Road, Bethesda, Maryland 20814-4799; currently, Associate Professor of Medicine, Division of Renal Diseases and Hypertension, Department of Medicine, The George Washington University Medical Center and School of Medicine, Washington, D. C. 20037

INTRODUCTION

Acute renal failure (ARF) is a disorder manifested by a sudden decline in renal function and is characteristically accompanied by (*a*) changes in the concentrations of electrolytes and nitrogenous waste products in the blood and (*b*) a reduction in urinary output. While ARF has diverse etiologies, most patients sustain injury from renal ischemia, nephrotoxins, or both. ARF usually occurs in the setting of serious injury or illness, and as such, substantially affects morbidity and mortality.

The morbidity and mortality of ARF depend on several factors including the etiology and clinical features of the disease as well as the patient's underlying condition. The mortality of ischemic, oliguric ARF, usually occurring in patients who have sustained trauma or patients with medical or surgical illnesses with shock, exceeds 50%, and may be higher depending on the patient population under study. Conversely, ARF accompanied by substantial urinary output (ie, nonoliguric ARF, in which nephrotoxins play an important role in the pathogenesis[1]) is usually associated with a lower mortality.[2] Finally, covariables such as age and associated extrarenal organ involvement adversely affect outcome.

These patients do not die of renal failure per se, but the presence of renal failure substantially increases the mortality. The availability of dialysis to control fluid and electrolyte imbalances and nitrogenous waste retention has prolonged the duration of illness, with patients surviving 4 to 6 weeks instead of several days. Nonetheless, many eventually succumb to overwhelming infections (approximately 70%) or pulmonary complications (approximately 30%). The impact of multiple organ failure on survival with ARF is such that when ARF develops without concomitant extrarenal organ failure, as is often seen in obstetrical and radiocontrast injury, the mortality is usually lower than 10%.[3]

Although we have the capability to provide dialysis to the combat casualty, it has become axiomatic that dialysis and modern critical care medicine have not exerted an important effect on the mortality associated with ARF. The reasons for this are not clear; they may relate to an increase in the mean age of the population that sustains ARF or to increased comorbidity in this population. Nonetheless, our current efforts are directed toward preventing ARF, providing better nutrition, and developing more effective drugs to treat infection. Because there is little reason to believe that improvements in dialysis will affect outcome in the majority of patients, we have sought to expand our understanding of the pathophysiology of ARF, with the ultimate goal of preventing renal injury.

It is not the purpose of this chapter to exhaustively review the literature on either experimental or clinical ARF. Such purpose, given the thousands of papers that have been written on this subject, would be unrewarding. The principles outlined herein are designed to assist medical officers, including nephrologists, in the prevention, diagnosis, and management of ARF in combat casualties.

MILITARY HISTORY

World War II

ARF has been recognized as a serious problem for military physicians since 1941, when E. G. Bywaters and D. Beall[4] published their classic description of rhabdomyolysis and myoglobin-induced ARF in four patients who sustained crush injuries in the bombings of London, England, during World War II. Since then, our understanding of the pathophysiology of ARF has increased, and our treatment options have expanded substantially. However, posttraumatic ARF continues to be associated with a persistently high mortality,[5] and is a complex medical problem for those who plan the delivery of military healthcare during wartime.

The salient features of the incidence, treatment, and outcomes of combat casualty–associated ARF in U.S. military forces in modern armed conflicts have been reviewed in detail[6] and are summarized here to emphasize the lessons learned.

During the World War II era, blood chemistry analyzers were primitive and not widely available; thus, ARF was usually recognized by the presence of oliguria, hypertension, and pulmonary edema, and only occasionally by azotemia—making it likely that only severe ARF was recognized. Nonoliguric ARF was undoubtedly under-diagnosed. Using data that had been collected and analyzed during 1944 and 1945, but not published until 1952, the Board for the Study of the Severely Wounded[7] included records of patients who were oliguric during shock and died within 24 hours of injury. Inclusion of these patients probably led to over-emphasis of the role of parenchymal ARF in their mortality. The cited mortality of ARF—90%—is therefore problematic, although that figure became accepted as the standard mortality of ARF in its untreated state. A more accurate interpretation of the data would place the mortality between 70% and 80%. ARF's severity may well have been increased by the medical realities of the war: evacuation times exceeded several hours, and shock was treated with plasma because supplies of blood and crystalloid fluids like saline were limited. Accordingly, some of the lessons learned from the study of ARF during the World War II era may not be applicable currently: more effective therapy of shock in subsequent conflicts radically changed the apparent incidence and clinical characteristics of ARF.

Korean War

Nonetheless, recognition of the impact of ARF in World War II led to anticipation of the problem of posttraumatic ARF in troops engaged in the Korean War. At that time, early forms of hemodialysis had been developed and were utilized at a center for kidney treatment established at Wonju, Korea, in 1951. The incidence of ARF during the Korean War was approximately 1 per 200 seriously wounded. The decrease in the mean duration of shock and more-rapid evacuation of wounded, in conjunction with successful use of hemodialysis in the combat zone, resulted in substantial reductions in the observed mortality due to ARF: down to 53% to 60%. In this conflict, ARF was the subject of careful clinical observation, which indicated that the mortality was often due to shock and multiple organ failure.[8,9] Concomitantly, although the overall mortality of patients with ARF remained quite high, two tenets of the treatment of established ARF were developed:

1. Attempts were made to provide nutritional support utilizing high-caloric, low-volume fluid regimens developed for use in oliguric patients.
2. Hemodialysis was utilized in an effort to attenuate the effects of uremia.

Vietnam War

Many of the lessons learned in Korea were used to advantage during the Vietnam War. The 629th Medical Renal Detachment was formed at Brooke General Hospital in 1965 and was attached to the Third Field Hospital in Saigon in 1966. Other renal units were placed at Clark Air Force Base in the Philippines and on two U.S. Navy hospital ships. These renal intensive care units had the capability of delivering complete care to casualties with ARF. Nephrologists prescribed and supervised dialysis, which was performed by nurses and corpsmen trained in dialysis. These personnel comprised "K" teams, which gained a substantial body of experience in the management of ARF and the numerous medical problems with which it was associated.

During the Vietnam War, two factors contributed to the decrease in the incidence of ARF to approximately 1 per 600 seriously wounded:

1. Rapid volume resuscitation of casualties, instituted near the geographical site of injury, was widely practiced in Vietnam and reduced the duration of shock.
2. The use of helicopters substantially reduced evacuation times.

Nonetheless, the 55% to 65% mortality of ARF was nearly identical to that seen in the Korean War, despite the facts that hemodialysis was utilized extensively for more severe forms of ARF and peritoneal dialysis was utilized in milder forms of ARF (eg, hemoglobinuria associated with malaria).

During the Vietnam War, medical officers reported several landmark studies of casualties with ARF. In 1974, W. J. Stone and J. H. Knepshield[10] described their experience with 62 casualties with ARF who received care in the renal unit of the 629th Medical Detachment in Saigon, and noted a 69% mortality despite the liberal use of dialysis. Sepsis, respiratory failure, bleeding, and hyperkalemia were the causes of death; the two former causes accounted for 89% of the total mortality. In 1972, R. E. Lordon and J. R. Burton[11] described their experience with 67 casualties with ARF treated at Clark Air Force Base. Although frequent dialysis was utilized, the mortality was 63%. These investigators also emphasized the role of infection in ARF, which accounted for 72% of the deaths. In 1975, J. D. Conger[12] conducted a prospective trial of "prophylactic" dialysis compared with dialysis for more conventional indications in 18 patients treated for ARF aboard the USS *Sanctuary*. This study purported to examine the role of prophylactic dialysis; however, it is more accurately characterized as a study of intensive dialysis. Although differences in mortality between patients who received intensive prophylactic dialysis compared with those dialyzed for conventional indications failed to reach statistical significance, the former group suffered fewer complications. The collective experience with the management of ARF in the Vietnam War served to validate the role of hemodialysis in the management of posttraumatic ARF. Because hemodialysis was simultaneously being widely applied in the civilian treatment of ARF, due in part to the pioneering efforts of R. C. Swann and J. P. Merrill[13] in Boston in 1953, it became an accepted treatment modality for most patients with ARF. Selected features of the experience with ARF in conflict are presented in Figures 26-1 and 26-2.

A new expression of ARF, in which renal dysfunction developed over several days, became evident in both the Vietnam War and the civilian sector during the period 1965 through 1974.[14,15] ARF was noted to develop in critically ill patients with multiple organ failure and was attributed to multiple etiologies, including sepsis and exposure to nephrotoxic drugs. Although some patients required only conservative management, others required dialytic support. At present, the concept of ARF developing without overt shock has reached its fullest expression in the patient with multiple organ failure.[16] Patients with ARF in association with multiple organ failure now represent a large fraction of patients with ARF seen in peacetime, and providing support to them represents a major mechanism for regular and reserve medical officers' maintaining their "go-to-war" skills.

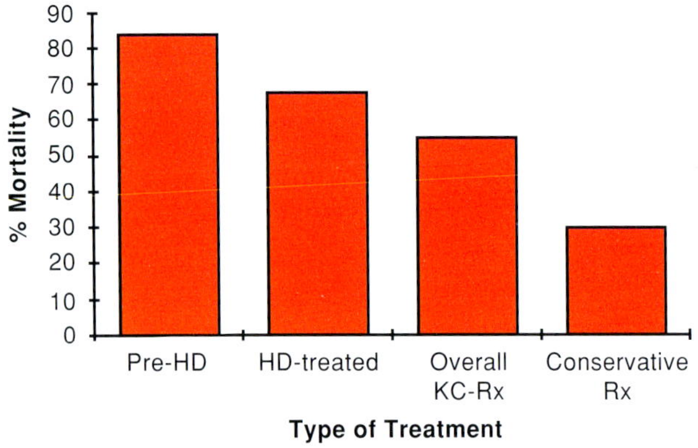

Fig. 26-1. Mortality of casualties from acute renal failure during the Vietnam War. Pre-HD refers to patients who were treated before hemodialysis was available. KC refers to patients who were treated in the specialized Kidney Center in the 3rd Field Hospital in Saigon. Data source: Butkus DE. Post-traumatic acute renal failure in combat casualties: A historical review. *Milit Med.* 1984;149:117–124.

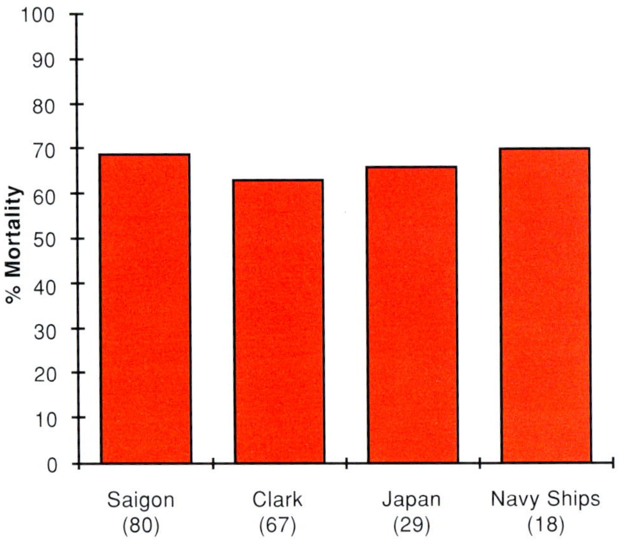

Fig. 26-2. Mortality of casualties from acute renal failure in the Vietnam War, stratified as to the location of their dialysis treatment. The numbers in parentheses represent the number of patients treated in each location. Adapted with permission from Butkus DE. Post-traumatic acute renal failure in combat casualties: A historical review. *Milit Med.* 1984;149:121. *Military Medicine,* Official Journal of the Association of Military Surgeons of the United States (AMSUS).

Military and Civilian Experience Since Vietnam

The experience gained from the wartime treatment of ARF, augmented by knowledge gained from the care and study of patients with ARF since the mid-1970s, has engendered several principles that guide our planning for the care of combat casualties:

1. ARF is a substantial problem in casualties with serious injuries and is often heralded by oliguria due to shock.
2. Identification of patients at high risk for ARF is possible, although there is surprisingly little objective evidence that such identification has been clinically effective.
3. ARF may develop at any time during the treatment and management of the seriously wounded, and even after initial stabilization may result from injury induced by anesthesia, hemolysis, sepsis, or drug toxicity.
4. Given the widespread application of dialysis, casualties rarely die of ARF but instead die of the infections and sequelae of multiple organ failure that accompany severe injuries.

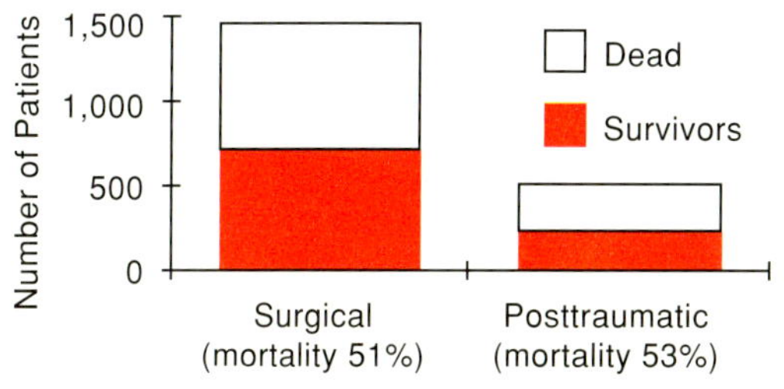

Fig. 26-3. Mortality of acute renal failure between 1970 and 1979 in surgical and trauma patients. Data source: Finn WF. Recovery from acute renal failure. In: Brenner BM, Lazarus M. *Acute Renal Failure*. Philadelphia, Pa: WB Saunders; 1983: 755.

A comprehensive review of the mortality of different forms of ARF, factored for the era in which it occurred, has been provided by W. F. Finn,[17] part of whose data are summarized in Figure 26-3.

Deployable Medical Systems

To provide healthcare for casualties of future conflicts, the Department of Defense has revised doctrine to include the concept of Deployable Medical Systems (DEPMEDS).[18] Military and civilian medical experts, many with experience in conflict, drew up a list of disorders likely to be encountered in combat. Projected incidence data and treatment protocols were defined for each of these patient conditions (this subject is discussed more fully in Chapter 6, Deployable Hospitals). More than 20% of identified patient conditions would be expected to be accompanied by the development of ARF in at least a cohort who sustain the illness or injury. In general, it is estimated that 5% of casualties who sustain either moderately severe, multiple, fragment injuries to the thorax or abdomen; isolated extremity injuries with muscle damage; or severe malaria will potentially require dialytic support at the fourth echelon. Ten percent of casualties who sustain either severe injuries to the thorax or abdominal cavities, alone or in combination, or major crush injuries, particularly of the lower extremities, are expected to require dialysis. Obviously, such figures could vary depending on the location of the conflict, its intensity, the types of weapons systems utilized, and the triage and evacuation policies of the theater commander. For example, given equal rates and severity of injury, there would likely be more ARF in a conflict in an arid environment, in which water supplies are limited and personnel are dehydrated, than in a more temperate climate.

Under the DEPMEDS doctrine, all equipment and consumable supplies required to perform hemodialysis are in a self-contained module. Only electrical generators are not included in the module. The cohort of personnel required to provide dialysis are delineated, and include a nephrologist, a dialysis-trained nurse, and corpsmen trained in dialysis. This team is similar to the "K" teams of Korea and Vietnam.

Civilian Disasters

Although much of the contingency planning for the delivery of care to patients with ARF in future conflicts is based on experience gained in prior conflicts, these concepts have been validated recently in a peacetime situation analogous to combat. The earthquake in 1988 in Armenia produced more than 600 patients with ARF secondary to crush injury. An international team of medical personnel, in conjunction with support from the dialysis industry, was rapidly mobilized to provide personnel and supplies for over 400 patients, at times administering 150 dialysis treatments per day. The magnitude of the disaster required that more than 80,000 lb of dialysis supplies be shipped from the United States. Intrinsic resources in Armenia and in Moscow were utilized for at least one third of the patients.[19] Because much more ARF could have been encountered if more casualties had survived, the magnitude of the problem of ARF in this setting underscores the need for the capability to rapidly mobilize large quantities of consumable supplies, sophisticated medical equipment, and appropriately trained personnel. It is this expeditious deployability of healthcare—eliminating the need to preposition personnel, supplies, and equipment—that is the basic tenet of DEPMEDS.

PATHOGENESIS OF ACUTE RENAL FAILURE

Classic Mechanisms of Renal Failure

The pathogenesis of ARF has been the subject of considerable experimental study, clinical observation, and review.[20–30] Information obtained from nearly all experimental models of ARF indicates that both renal blood flow and the glomerular filtration rate decline early after the initial insult. This early period, lasting from hours to days, is termed the *initiation* phase. Gradually, renal blood flow returns toward normal, while the glomerular filtration rate remains depressed. This period, which may last from days to weeks, is called the *maintenance* phase. In general, when ARF persists for longer than 3 months, end-stage renal disease is assumed.

Four mechanisms have been proposed to explain the pathophysiology of ARF (Exhibit 26-1). These mechanisms—renal vasoconstriction, reduction in glomerular filtration, tubular obstruction, and back leak of filtrate—have been identified and delineated using models in which the renal artery is either clamped or infused with norepinephrine, or in which hemorrhage of sufficient severity is produced to result in sustained systemic hypotension. This latter model is of particular interest as it closely mimics the clinical setting of posttraumatic ARF, and because the kidney is exposed to the multiplicity of hormonal and neurogenic alterations that accompany shock. A similar model involves the injection of glycerol into a large muscle of an animal, which results in muscle necrosis and vascular pooling in the involved extremity, and is closely analogous to crush injury.

The classic mechanisms of ARF can be divided into (*a*) those that exert primarily vascular effects and (*b*) those that exert tubular effects. The vascular mechanisms include reductions in both renal blood flow and the intrinsic filtration capability of the glomeruli. The tubular mechanisms include tubular obstruction by casts and back leak of filtrate. Undoubtedly, all four mechanisms participate in the injury seen in existent models of ARF. The contribution of each, however, is likely to differ depending on the model used. Thus, reduced renal blood flow is the prominent feature of ARF induced by hemorrhagic hypotension, while intratubular obstruction by casts is more prominent in ARF induced by glycerol. Models most useful for the study of clinical ARF combine features of all suspected mechanisms.

EXHIBIT 26-1

CLASSIC MECHANISMS OF ACUTE RENAL FAILURE

Vascular Mechanisms
- Renal vasoconstriction
  - Reduced blood flow
  - Increased resistance
- Reduced glomerular filtration
  - Endothelial morphology
  - Reduced glomerular area

Tubular Mechanisms
- Luminal obstruction
  - Cellular debris
  - Casts
- Back leak of filtrate
  - Inulin
  - Other markers

Vascular Mechanisms

An early decrease in renal blood flow and an increase in renal vascular resistance are consistent findings in virtually all types of experimental ARF. The reduction in renal blood flow results in integrated hormonal, neural, and intrinsic renal responses, all of which are designed to restore the extracellular fluid, renal blood flow, and renal function. ARF is the result when these mechanisms fail.

Reduced Extracellular Fluid Volume. Sensor mechanisms for detection of decreased extracellular fluid include baroreceptors located throughout the body. These receptors are sensitive to mechanical stretch and transmural pressure. Intrathoracic volume receptors exist in both the atria and the pulmonary capillaries. Activation of these receptors results in increased traffic both in sympathetic fibers and in cranial nerves IX and X, the latter to centers in the hypothalamus and medulla. Arterial volume sensors in the carotid sinus have been postulated to provide stimuli for the kidney to retain sodium and water, although the mechanisms of their actions have not been completely defined. Finally, baroreceptors located in the juxtaglomerular apparatus of the kidney are exquisitely sensitive to reductions in renal perfusion pressure. Their activation initiates the release of renin and the subsequent formation of the vasoconstrictor angiotensin II, and release of the sodium-retaining hormone aldosterone. Effector mechanisms react to reduced renal blood flow and induce vasoconstriction and sodium and water retention, both of which are designed to restore the extracellular fluid. These mechanisms include catecholamines, angiotensin II, arginine vasopressin, aldosterone, vasoconstrictor prostaglandins, and intrinsic renal tubular events, which participate in an integrated response.

Decreased Glomerular Filtration. The second vascular mechanism that occurs is decreased filtration capability of the glomeruli. Filtration is a function of the intrinsic permeability characteristics of the glomerular capillary membrane, the surface area available for filtration, and the net pressure for filtration (defined by Starling forces) across the glomerular capillaries. The aggregate capability for filtration is expressed by the term K_f, and is reduced pari passu the reduction in renal blood flow, as the latter is a major determinant of glomerular filtration rate. Such reduction may be due either to a direct effect of ischemia on the basement membrane of the capillary or to reduction in the surface area of the capillary, perhaps mediated by angiotensin II.

Tubular Mechanisms

Obstruction. Obstructing casts originate from cellular debris, principally sloughed epithelial cell fragments and brush border membranes, which coalesces with Tamm-Horsfall mucoprotein of uroepithelial origin. The resultant obstruction of the tubular lumen raises intratubular pressure in excess of glomerular filtration pressure, so that glomerular filtration ceases.

Back Leak. The second tubular mechanism is back leak of filtrate, in which a marker of glomerular filtration rate, usually inulin, can be shown to traverse the damaged tubular epithelium from the tubular lumen into the renal circulation. Such movement of solute could be due either to disruptions in intercellular bridges or, most likely, to impairment in the ability of epithelial cells to restrict the transcellular movement of normally excluded solutes.

The Nature of Cellular Injury

If the four events detailed above were sufficient explanations for the mechanisms of ARF seen after ischemic or nephrotoxic injury, we could infer that maneuvers successful in ameliorating one or more factors might exert a beneficial effect on the incidence or severity of renal injury. Unfortunately, the results of such strategies have been largely inconsistent and only variably successful. The lack of success could result from an inability to distinguish precisely between the initiation phase of ARF, when damage could putatively be reversed, and the maintenance phase, when injury is established. Alternatively, the factors believed to be operative in the classic explanation of the pathophysiology of ARF may be epiphenomena.

Since the early 1980s, our understanding of the pathogenesis of ARF has been amplified substantially by investigation into the cellular basis of ischemic and toxic renal injury.[31] Research utilizing kidney, heart, and liver tissue has formed a base for additional studies with renal tubular epithelia, mesangial and endothelial cells, as well as subcellular constituents. These studies have provided information that has vastly improved our understanding of the mechanisms by which ischemic and nephrotoxic injury occur. Our current research seeks to formulate unifying hypotheses of renal injury, with the understanding that whole-organ injury is predicated on, and best understood in the context of, injury to its constituent cells.

Ischemia initiates a cascade of events that result in cell death. Changes in cellular metabolism, alterations in cation adenosine triphosphatases (ATPases), activation of phospholipases, generation of toxic free radicals, and changes in the intrinsic nature of the renal epithelial membrane itself[32] have been studied in a variety of models of ARF. While the nature of the cellular response to injury varies somewhat depending on the model, these responses are sufficiently homogenous that inferences about possible therapeutic maneuvers can be made.

Two of the central events in the cell's response to ischemia are (*a*) the simultaneous reduction in the availability of adenosine 5′-triphosphate (ATP) and other high-energy phosphate compounds and (*b*) an increase in the formation of adenine nucleotide degradation products.[33] Without an adequate supply of ATP to maintain normal function, the cell's ability to maintain its metabolic integrity is severely compromised. Thus, diminished activity of the sodium-potassium ATPase results in the accumulation of intracellular sodium and swelling of the cell. Similarly, inhibition of the calcium ATPase results in cytosolic and mitochondrial calcium overload, with impairment of the functional integrity of the electron transport chain.[34,35] These findings have led to the use of stimulators of sodium-potassium ATPase such as thyroid hormone, which has been found to be beneficial in a number of different models of ARF.[36] Similarly, some investigators[37] have demonstrated a beneficial effect of calcium channel blocking agents such as verapamil.

The results of ischemia are (*a*) the metabolism of ATP to hypoxanthine and (*b*) loss of nucleosides from the cell.[30] This latter event inhibits the regeneration of ATP and cell recovery. During reperfusion, the enzyme xanthine oxidase, which is formed during periods of ischemia from xanthine dehydrogenase, converts hypoxanthine to xanthine, with the concomitant generation of toxic free radicals through iron-requiring reactions known as the

Haber-Weiss and Fenton reactions.[38–40] Inhibition of xanthine oxidase by allopurinol prevents the irreversible degradation of hypoxanthine, so that when ischemia resolves, purine salvage pathways can utilize adenine nucleotides for resynthesis into ATP.[41]

Activation of phospholipase A_2 results in peroxidation of lipids in the cell membrane, a phenomenon that can be measured by the accumulation of malondialdehyde. Phospholipase A_2 is activated by excessive concentrations of calcium, which may result from diminished activity of calcium ATPase. Moreover, with reperfusion, enzymatic changes occur that result in the formation of large quantities of hydrogen peroxide and the hydroxyl ion.[39,40] These moieties are extremely toxic to cell contents. In the laboratory, the use of free radical scavengers such as superoxide dismutase and dimethyl thiourea has shown some promise in abrogating renal injuries caused by oxygen-derived free radicals.[42]

Taken collectively, the voluminous literature that has appeared since the early 1980s on the cellular basis of ARF demonstrates how much our understanding of this condition has expanded. As we will see later, however, the therapeutic maneuvers that follow from this understanding have not yet reached the stage of widespread clinical application.

CLINICAL ASPECTS OF ACUTE RENAL FAILURE

No single definition of ARF is accepted by all clinicians, although many accept the diagnosis if the serum creatinine concentration increases by 50% above its baseline. The blood urea nitrogen (BUN) concentration is affected by diet, hydration, and medications; therefore, it is not, by itself, a particularly valid marker of renal function. Acute renal dysfunction commonly is detected by alterations in volume of urine, particularly acute *oliguria,* which is defined as urinary output less than 400 mL/d, or approximately 20 mL/h. Acute *anuria* is defined as urinary output less than 50 to 100 mL/d, but this is an uncommon manifestation of ARF. *Polyuria* in the context of acute renal dysfunction should be reserved to describe urinary output of several liters of urine daily. Individuals who excrete urine in these amounts are often found to have partial urinary tract obstruction. The term *nonoliguric* characterizes the substantial portion of patients who have significant ARF, yet maintain urinary output of 1 to 2 L/d.

Distinguishing Between Acute Oliguria and Acute Renal Failure

Operationally, the differences between acute oliguria and ARF are substantial (Exhibit 26-2). The former term implies that there may be a reversible aspect of the renal dysfunction (ie, prerenal or postrenal injury), while the latter connotes injury that may require days to weeks to resolve.

Prerenal azotemia is renal dysfunction that results from any absolute or relative deficiency of blood or extracellular fluid. The consequent reduction in renal blood flow results in activation of the effector mechanisms that already have been mentioned. Urinary flow and sodium excretion decrease because the physiological response to perceived volume depletion is to conserve salt and water avidly.

Postrenal azotemia, which is generally caused by obstruction of the urinary tract, elicits physiological responses that are similar to those seen in prerenal azotemia. The causes of obstructive injury deserve emphasis, as they may not be seen frequently by nonsurgical physicians. First, obstruction of the ureters above the level of the bladder

EXHIBIT 26-2

DIFFERENTIAL DIAGNOSIS OF OLIGURIA

Prerenal Azotemia
- Absolute blood loss
- Absolute or relative loss of extracellular fluid
- Heart failure
- Liver failure
- Nephrotic syndrome

Postrenal Azotemia
- Intravesicular obstruction
- Retroperitoneal hemorrhage
- Ureteral injury with single kidney

Intrinsic Acute Renal Failure
- Renal ischemia
- Nephrotoxins
- Acute glomerulonephritis
- Acute tubulointerstitial nephritis

may result from pelvic trauma or surgery, in which the ureters can be obstructed by blood or by inadvertent ligation. Rarely, obstruction may be the first sign of a leaking aorta or vena cava. In this situation, blood causes a desmoplastic response resulting in encasement of the ureters. Obviously, supravesicular obstruction will only induce substantial renal failure should both ureters be involved, or if the patient has only one kidney, a condition that occurs in 1 in 900 to 1,000 individuals. Second, individuals who are susceptible to renal calculi may experience episodes of nephrolithiasis if climatic conditions are unfavorable (eg, dehydration in the desert). However, renal calculus disease will cause oliguria or ARF or both if the stones are bilateral, or if the stones form in a patient who has a single kidney. And third, because it is virtually routine to place an indwelling bladder catheter in seriously injured casualties, many cases of oliguria due to postrenal causes should be detected and definitively treated early, before substantial reduction in renal function occurs. The most common cause of urinary tract obstruction is an indwelling bladder catheter that has become occluded or dislodged; therefore, the integrity of the drainage system should be verified at the first sign of diminishing urinary output.

Intrinsic ARF has a variety of causes. Moreover, any prerenal or postrenal condition can result in established ARF if uncorrected for sufficient time. The period that must elapse before reversible injury becomes irreversible is variable. Thus, relatively trivial insults result in renal injury in some patients, while substantial insults can be tolerated by others before renal dysfunction is irreversible. Such differences may result from the kidneys' autoregulatory ability. In the otherwise healthy human, the lower limit of mean arterial pressure for autoregulation is approximately 60 to 70 mm Hg. This corresponds to systolic blood pressures of 80 to 90 mm Hg. The time that renal blood flow can be maintained under more severe hypotensive conditions is unknown.

Other factors besides those related to volume depletion—including hypercapnia and hypoxemia, frequent concomitants of acute respiratory failure—can also result in decreased renal blood flow.[43] Cross-clamping of the aorta results in the same response even if a surgically induced alternate pathway for perfusion, around the aortic cross-clamp, is provided to the kidneys.[44] Agents that disrupt the balance between systemic and intrarenal vasoconstrictor and vasodilatory hormones, which participate in the maintenance of renal blood flow, are associated with marked reductions in renal blood flow. These agents, including the nonsteroidal antiinflammatory agents and angiotensin-converting enzyme inhibitors, are particularly injurious when the extracellular fluid volume is subnormal, and renal blood flow is predicated on the balance between vasoconstrictor and vasodilator hormones.[45] Finally, it is intuitive that renal injury might be more likely or more severe with a combination of injurious factors than with a single factor. Given the dependence of the kidneys on renal blood flow for oxygen delivery, any situation in which oxygen is reduced would make the kidneys more susceptible to either ischemic or nephrotoxic insult.

Renal ischemia accounts for ARF in most patients, although nephrotoxic injury has become increasingly important in peacetime medical practice.[1] Patients who sustain nephrotoxic injury often have sepsis, and the coexistent hemodynamic changes associated with sepsis often result in renal ischemia and undoubtedly enhance the injurious effects of nephrotoxic substances, drugs, or diagnostic agents.

The military physician's task is to distinguish between oliguria that results from correctable causes (ie, prerenal or postrenal failure) and established ARF. Although the spectrum of causes of ARF in a peacetime environment is quite broad, relatively few disorders cause ARF on the battlefield; and many of the rarer causes of ARF in peacetime practice, such as acute glomerulonephritis, are not likely to be encountered at all by medical officers dealing with combat-associated ARF. Finally, the distinction between ischemic and nephrotoxic causes is often artificial because a substantial portion of patients have elements of both types of injury.

Diagnostic Assessment

Collectively, the history, physical examination, biochemical analyses of serum and urine, urinalysis, and judicious use of renal imaging studies almost always provide the information needed by the clinician to determine whether there is a readily reversible cause of acute renal dysfunction or the patient has established ARF. Medical treatment facilities in the combat zone will have limited laboratory capability, but rearward facilities, particularly fixed general hospitals, may have a wide range of sophisticated diagnostic equipment. At times, the volume status of the patient is difficult to assess, and measurement of central venous pressure or pulmonary capillary wedge pressure is necessary.

However, hemodynamic monitoring, while providing valuable information, can be time-consuming to institute, and may delay fluid resuscitation and prolong renal ischemia.

Patient History

The medical officer's review of available records, including flow sheets, nurses' notes, and medications, is essential, particularly in patients who develop ARF during hospitalization. Recent hypotension, either profound or subtle but sufficient to cause decreased renal perfusion, may have occurred, and daily weights and accurately measured urinary outputs may be of substantial value.

The patient's history of drug therapy is also important, as many drugs, particularly antibiotics and nonsteroidal antiinflammatory agents, can cause nephrotoxic injury either alone or in concert with decreased renal perfusion. Aminoglycoside antibiotics are associated with nephrotoxicity in approximately 10% of patients. Risk factors for toxicity include heart failure, liver disease, and other states associated with decreased renal perfusion.[46] The most powerful predictor of toxicity is the duration of therapy. Renal toxicity is seldom seen with fewer than 5 to 7 days of therapy; the incidence increases substantially if therapy exceeds 10 days.

Many patients with ARF have few symptoms and signs other than those related to the causative disorder. Symptoms are related to the rapidity of onset and severity of dysfunction and the patient's underlying condition, and may include nausea, vomiting, or altered mental status. A diffuse bleeding diathesis, with gastrointestinal, nasotracheal, and puncture-site hemorrhage, may occur with severe azotemia. Typically, however, azotemia is largely asymptomatic unless the BUN and creatinine exceed 100 to 120 mg/dL and 6 to 8 mg/dL, respectively; or if azotemia develops extremely rapidly (eg, over 24–48 h). Acidemia can be asymptomatic; however, if severe, it may result in hypotension from depression of myocardial performance or reduction in peripheral resistance. Hyperkalemia may result in cardiac arrhythmias and skeletal muscle weakness. The latter may be extremely difficult to detect in the critically ill patient. All the features described above can be caused by factors other than azotemia.

Some patients develop symptoms of volume overload rapidly, which may reflect aggressive fluid therapy. Fluid therapy is frequently continued in oliguric patients for several hours, until the significance of diminishing urinary output is finally appreciated. Although oliguria is the most common manifestation, nonoliguric ARF is frequently seen with nephrotoxic injury. As has been mentioned, polyuria is characteristic of urinary tract obstruction, and anuria is typical of vascular catastrophes or complete urinary tract obstruction.

Physical Examination

The physical examination is useful in helping to determine whether the patient is volume depleted or volume overloaded, or the urinary tract is obstructed. Crucial elements include assessments of skin turgor and edema, and the cardiac, pulmonary, and genitourinary examinations. Accurate weights or fluid flow sheets or both, blood pressure assessment for orthostatic hypotension, and proof of a properly draining urinary tract are essential.

Biochemical Analyses of Blood and Urine

The concentrations of BUN and creatinine increase steadily during the course of ARF because production remains relatively constant while excretion is profoundly decreased. Daily increments of BUN and creatinine usually average at least 20 to 30 mg/dL and 1.3 to 1.5 mg/dL, respectively. More-rapid incremental changes in the BUN may reflect excessive catabolism or gastrointestinal hemorrhage, while excessive increments in the serum creatinine may reflect muscle necrosis from rhabdomyolysis. Although the measurement of renal function using the serum creatinine concentration is not as accurate as calculating clearances from timed urine collections, it is sufficiently accurate for diagnosing posttraumatic renal dysfunction and for initiating rational therapy.

Other abnormalities commonly encountered include metabolic acidosis, which results from retention of endogenously produced acid. The serum bicarbonate concentration averages 17 to 18 mmol/L in uncomplicated cases. Hyperkalemia may result from limited excretion and acidemia. Potassium concentrations usually range from 5.0 to 6.5 mmol/L. Hyperphosphatemia occurs because phosphate excretion is negligible. In the absence of major tissue destruction, phosphate concentrations rarely exceed 8 mg/dL. However, such levels, in conjunction with the inhibition of the effect of vitamin D and the resistance to the actions of parathyroid hormone that occur in ARF,[47] result in hypocalcemia. In the absence of obvious blood loss, the hematocrit should fall over 5 to 7 days to a level of 0.23 to 0.27, and may reflect volume overload, covert blood loss, and bone marrow suppression.

Urinalysis

Biochemical and microscopical analyses of the urine are extremely important in treating patients with ARF, as the tests may provide evidence of prerenal or postrenal azotemia, or may support the diagnosis of established ARF. The patient with prerenal azotemia should have concentrated urine with high urine-to-plasma ratios of urea, creatinine, and osmolality, and a low urinary sodium concentration. Similar values are found in patients with acute urinary obstruction. The patient with established ARF usually loses the ability both to concentrate the urine and to conserve urinary sodium, with low urine-to-plasma ratios of solute and high urinary sodium concentrations. Similar values are found in patients with ARF from chronic obstruction of the urinary tract. Indices of renal function such as the fractional excretion of sodium and the renal failure index are manipulations of these basic data, all of which should be interpreted cautiously if the patient has received diuretics in the 12 to 18 hours prior to their determination.[48] Nonetheless, biochemical analyses of urine can accurately distinguish between prerenal or postrenal failure and established ARF in nearly 90% of cases.

The information gleaned from the microscopical examination of the urine is so critical that the physician should examine it personally. The urine sediment is typically relatively unremarkable in prerenal and postrenal azotemia, although it may contain hyaline and granular casts. Hematuria may be present if a catheter is in place. Conversely, the sediment in ARF contains many granular casts, and, most importantly, renal tubular epithelial cells and other cellular debris, which give rise to a very "dirty" sediment. Experienced observers can distinguish between prerenal or postrenal failure and established ARF on the basis of the sediment in approximately 85% to 90% of cases.

Radiographic Studies

Imaging of the kidneys in patients with ARF should be limited to those studies that demonstrate whether there are two kidneys, calculi, and urinary tract obstruction. Although a technically well-done renal ultrasound examination is the imaging test of choice, ultrasound is not now available in the combat zone, and such capability may be limited even further to the rear. Thus, plain radiographs of the abdomen should be obtained, and may suffice to determine the number of kidneys and to demonstrate radiopaque calculi. Because the renal shadows are often obscured by bowel gas, computed axial tomography, which is available at fourth-echelon hospitals, is far superior and should be performed if the question of urinary obstruction cannot be resolved. Such scans should always be performed without radiocontrast agents to avoid further injury from these agents. Nuclear medicine scans have virtually no role in the evaluation of the patient with suspected ARF. In patients with true anuria, selective angiography of the renal vessels may be required to evaluate whether a vascular catastrophe has occurred.

PREVENTION OF ACUTE RENAL FAILURE

There has been a resurgence of interest in preventing ARF in patients known to be at high risk since, despite aggressive therapy, established ARF remains associated with substantial mortality. Moreover, advances in the understanding of the abnormalities of cell biology that occur in ARF have suggested avenues for new therapeutic regimens. Finally, we have developed sufficient expertise to be able to predict with some accuracy who is at risk for the development of ARF. Prospective identification of high-risk patients should allow for proactive intervention to prevent the occurrence of ARF. This assumes that preventing ARF may be more rewarding than improving the quality of care of patients with established ARF.

Identification of High-Risk Patients

A number of investigators have conducted studies of patients with ARF and have identified clinical scenarios in which patients are likely to be at high risk for ARF. These studies have also shown that ARF is almost always multifactorial (ie, it seldom results from a single insult).

In 1983, S. H. Hou and her colleagues[49] prospectively studied more than 2,000 consecutive hospital admissions and found 129 episodes of ARF in 109 patients, for an incidence of 4.9%. She further delineated those factors that appeared to be causal in the development of ARF. Decreased renal perfusion accounted for 54 (42%) of the episodes. Among the causes of decreased renal perfusion were volume depletion in 41%, cardiac dysfunction in 30%, and sepsis in 19%. ARF developed postoperatively in 23 patients (18%); however, only 12 of the patients had documented hypotension. ARF in association with cardiac and vascular surgery had incidence rates of 15% and 8%, respectively. Administration of radiocontrast agents was associated with ARF in 16 (12%) of the episodes, although such injury was only rarely seen in patients who had normal serum creatinine concentrations at the time the contrast medium was administered. Aminoglycoside administration accounted for 9 (7%) of the episodes, while miscellaneous causes, such as the hepatorenal syndrome or unknown causes, were implicated in 27 (21%) of the episodes. Of particular interest was the investigators' inference that 55% of all episodes were partly iatrogenic.

A similar analysis had been performed in 1982 by H. H. Rasmussen and L. S. Ibels,[50] who studied 143 patients with hospital-acquired ARF for the purpose of identifying risk factors and the nature of the acute insults with which ARF was associated. The presence of hypertension, preexistent renal disease, and diabetes were the most prominent risk factors associated with the development of ARF. Sepsis, administration of nephrotoxins such as aminoglycoside antibiotics or radiocontrast agents, myoglobinuria from rhabdomyolysis, and volume depletion were the most common acute insults resulting in ARF. The investigators noted that 48% of the patients had more than one risk factor, and 62% had more than one acute insult. More importantly, analysis of the entire dataset demonstrated that the number of acute insults was additive as a determinant of both the incidence and severity of ARF.

In research published in 1990, F. Jochimsen and colleagues[51] extended and expanded these observations in a prospective analysis of 261 patients who had ARF and were in an intensive care unit. Two groups of patients, 95 with ARF severe enough to require dialytic support, and 166 patients whose ARF did not require dialysis, were studied. Bleeding, volume depletion, sepsis, administration of antibiotics, cirrhosis, and diabetes were identified as the risk factors associated with more-severe ARF. Patients with multiple risk factors were far more likely to develop ARF than patients with a single risk factor.

These studies, in conjunction with the clinical experience of most nephrologists, reinforce the concept that patients without preexisting comorbidity appear to be relatively resistant to the development of ARF and may be able to withstand a single insult without developing ARF. For example, uncomplicated gastrointestinal hemorrhage in otherwise healthy patients rarely results in ARF.[52] Likewise, uncomplicated myocardial infarction is also infrequently associated with ARF.[53]

In victims of trauma, the nature of the injury in large part determines whether the patient will be at risk for the development of ARF. Thus, patients who sustain only isolated limb or head injuries rarely develop multiple organ failure and ARF. Conversely, injuries to the abdomen, with or without other injuries, are accompanied by the development of ARF in a substantial number of patients.

In the conflict setting, casualties who develop oliguria can be categorized into three groups. The first consists of patients in whom relative or absolute hypotension has been present for varying times before medical care is instituted. These patients are frequently in shock. Resuscitative efforts may be successful in restoring urinary output and renal function. In such patients, the incidence and severity of renal dysfunction, manifested by oliguria and prerenal azotemia, are functions of (*a*) how long the renal insult has been present and (*b*) how efficacious are the efforts to restore effective circulatory function. These patients are at high risk for subsequent renal injury, and every effort must be made to prevent further ischemic or nephrotoxic injury.

The second group includes casualties who have sustained severe and prolonged insults, for whom resuscitative efforts have not been successful, and in whom ARF has become established. The duration or intensity of shock may have resulted in additional ischemic injury to the brain, heart, gastrointestinal tract, or liver. These patients may often require surgery, and the presence of multiple organ failure predicts substantial morbidity and mortality. Many of these patients will require prolonged and aggressive nutritional and dialytic support.

The third group of casualties consists of those who develop ARF while under medical care, during or after initial evaluation, stabilization, evacuation, and treatment. These patients may not be oliguric; thus, ARF may be detected by biochemical analysis of their blood. Hypotension may have been part of their presenting picture, and sepsis may have been associated with renal ischemia. Often these patients have undergone or will undergo surgery, or require the administration of nephrotoxic drugs or diagnostic agents. Renal injury may have to be tolerated as part of the cost of effective treatment for the casualty's condition. A small fraction of this group develop ARF because the urinary tract may have been, or has become, obstructed.

While therapeutic efforts may differ somewhat among these three groups, the basic principles of the initial assessment of the patient with ARF are applicable to all. Moreover, the information gained from risk-factor identification and analysis, coupled with an enhanced understanding of the pathophysiology of ARF, has provided opportunities for proactive intervention to protect renal function. Before examining methods of renal protection in detail, we must first discuss volume expansion and the pharmacological agents that are used in such management strategies.

Volume Expansion

The beneficial effects of volume expansion have been known for years. Although the mechanism or mechanisms by which volume expansion abrogates renal injury are not completely defined, at least four mechanisms are thought to be operative. First, volume expansion exerts a salutary effect on renal hemodynamics by inhibiting intrarenal renin release, with a reduction in the concentration of the vasoconstrictor angiotensin II. Second, it decreases the activity of the catecholamine-mediated renal nerves by direct intranephronal mechanisms; consequently renal blood flow is maintained. Third, volume expansion results in a decrease in the activity of the intrathoracic baroreceptors that play a central role in the control of renal blood flow. Diminution in their activity results in both decreased traffic in the renal nerves and minimal renal vasoconstriction. The importance of these baroreceptors is illustrated by their role in hypotension with cardiac failure. This situation, in which the atrial baroreceptors are distended and less active than when they are collapsed, results in a lesser decrease in renal blood flow than does equivalent hypotension from absolute volume depletion. And fourth, some data suggest that saline may exert a beneficial effect by inducing a solute diuresis, an effect that may be independent of the renin-angiotensin axis.[54]

There is evidence that volume expansion can reduce the incidence or severity of clinical ARF. The reduction in the rate of ARF per seriously injured casualty from the Korean War to the Vietnam War has been mentioned previously, and is undoubtedly due in large part to rapid and aggressive volume resuscitation of casualties prior to their transport to definitive medical care. Other evidence comes from studies of rhabdomyolytic-induced ARF. In 1979, F. Eneas, P. Y. Schoenfeld, and M. H. Humphreys[55] reported a salutary effect of bicarbonate diuresis in patients with rhabdomyolysis. In other forms of ARF (eg, those induced by cis-platinum and amphotericin), volume expansion with hypertonic saline or mannitol clearly results in attenuation of renal injury.[56] However, studies utilizing mannitol must be interpreted cautiously regarding the effects of volume expansion, because the contribution of mannitol may be as a volume expander, osmotic diuretic, or both.

In summary, volume expansion, usually done with normal saline but occasionally with isotonic fluids containing alkali or other base precursors, is generally accepted as beneficial in the prevention of ARF. This is particularly true if hypovolemia is present, because interpretation of the numerous studies examining the role of volume expansion in the prevention or attenuation of ARF suggests that volume expansion may prevent incipient ARF in many situations of prerenal failure. A trial of volume expansion can be both diagnostic and therapeutic, in the sense that it can reduce the contribution that renal ischemia makes to the pathogenesis of ARF. Moreover, a large body of clinical experience supports the concept that the volume-expanded state confers protection against renal injury. This concept has implications for fluid and nutritional support of troops deployed to arid regions, in whom subclinical volume depletion of several liters may occur rapidly unless adequate salt and water are provided. In such situations, maintenance of an adequate extracellular volume may be the most important mechanism by which ARF can be prevented.

Pharmacological Interventions

A number of agents have been evaluated in experimental and clinical studies for their ability to abrogate or attenuate the untoward effects of ischemia or nephrotoxins.[57] Many of these have been used in the management and, at times putatively, in the prophylaxis of ARF (Table 26-1). Most studies with loop and osmotic diuretics and vasodilators have been conducted in either laboratory or clinical ARF after the renal injury has been induced. Newer agents—including dopamine, adenine nucleotides, calcium channel–blocking agents, atrial natriuretic factor, and thyroid hormone—and agents that (*a*) interfere with the generation of or (*b*) scavenge toxic free radicals have received much attention recently. This discussion concentrates on agents that are presently in unrestricted clinical use, and provides a brief overview of the rationale for the use of the remaining agents.

TABLE 26-1

AGENTS USED IN THE PREVENTION OF ISCHEMIC ACUTE RENAL FAILURE

Agent	Status
Furosemide	In use
Mannitol	In use
Dopamine (low-dose)	In use
Thyroid hormone	Clinical trials
Adenine nucleotides	Causes hypotension
Xanthine oxidase inhibitor	Transplant trials
Free-radical scavengers	Clinical trials
Calcium channel blockers	Clinical trials
Prostaglandins	Causes hypotension
Atrial natriuretic factor	Used with dopamine

Loop and Osmotic Diuretics

The use of loop diuretics (ie, a class of diuretic agents that act by inhibiting reabsorption of sodium and chloride in Henle's loop) in both laboratory and clinical ARF is based on three theoretical constructs. First, furosemide is a renal vasodilator that might contribute to the restoration or maintenance of renal blood flow in the presence of renal ischemia. Second, loop diuretics also increase tubular flow rate, potentially abrogating the effects of intratubular obstruction. Third, because the vast majority of renal oxygen consumption is utilized to reabsorb sodium, inhibiting sodium reabsorption by the renal tubules should reduce renal oxygen consumption and renal work.

Furosemide has been shown in controlled clinical trials to promote urinary output in patients with ARF.[58,59] These trials contained small numbers of patients, so their conclusions may be flawed. Nonetheless, many patients' urinary output increased, although neither the severity, duration, nor outcome of ARF was affected. A more problematic issue is the role of furosemide in "converting" oliguric to nonoliguric ARF. A substantial proportion of oliguric patients increase their urinary output when given furosemide. Whether this is due to abrogation or attenuation of the severity of ARF, or is simply a marker of those patients with reversible, or intrinsically mild, ARF, is not known. No studies have been conducted sufficiently early in the course of incipient ARF to demonstrate whether furosemide exerted a beneficial effect on renal function.[60]

The osmotic diuretic mannitol has long been considered a renal protective agent, largely based on studies such as those performed in 1961 by K. G. Barry and colleagues,[61] who utilized mannitol infusions prior to aortic cross-clamping in the operating room and demonstrated preservation of renal blood flow. Mannitol is a renal vasodilator and increases tubular flow rate. In contrast to loop diuretics, mannitol expands the extracellular fluid volume, which may account for its beneficial effect in some situations. It has also been shown experimentally to prevent endothelial swelling associated with ischemia.[62] However, there has never been convincing evidence that it exerts a beneficial effect on overall mortality if administered after ARF is established, and no controlled prospective studies utilizing mannitol early in oliguria (ie, in the initiation phase of ARF) have been conducted. Nonetheless, substantial uncontrolled clinical experience suggests that mannitol prevents ARF both in vascular surgery procedures and in rhabdomyolysis.

Vasoactive Agents

A number of vasoactive agents have been utilized in various models of ARF and have been used in a limited fashion in clinical ARF. These agents have been used to promote renal vasodilation with the goal of minimizing the adverse effects of renal vasoconstriction. Acetylcholine, vasodilatory prostaglandins, antibodies to renin, and dopamine have all been utilized. Although many laboratory studies have shown that these agents can restore renal blood flow toward normal values, only dopamine has been widely utilized in clinical ARF because the other agents have unacceptable hemodynamic toxicity.

Both experimental and clinical studies suggest a beneficial role of dopamine in ARF, although in clinical studies, proof of its efficacy is largely anecdotal. In 1979, A. Lindner and colleagues[63] studied the effects of dopamine with and without furosemide in a canine model of nephrotoxic ARF. Treatment with both agents resulted in improvement in both renal blood flow and urinary flow rate, and attenuated the fall in glomerular filtration rate compared with values in control animals or those animals who received either dopamine or furosemide alone. In contrast, in 1988, L. J. Pass and colleagues[64] studied the effects of dopamine with and without mannitol in dogs undergoing thoracic aortic cross-clamping. No beneficial effect on any measure of renal function was noted in any group.

Regarding its use in clinical ARF, low-dose (ie, renal dose) dopamine, 1 to 3 μg/kg/min, has been administered in situations characterized by oliguria and incipient decreased renal function. In many circumstances, dopamine is associated with a modest increase in systemic arterial pressure while urinary output increases. Whether the increase results from the effect on systemic arterial pressure or from intrarenal vasodilation cannot be discerned from clinical studies. In 1982, R. F. Davis and colleagues[65] studied (without control subjects) the effects of low-dose dopamine in 15 adults with oliguria after cardiac surgery. Dopamine infusion was associated with (*a*) improved creatinine and osmolar clearances, (*b*) improved urinary flow rate and sodium excretion, and (*c*) reduced plasma renin activity, when compared with such values in the patients prior to administration of dopamine. Moreover, in a prospective trial of patients undergoing liver transplantation, prophylactic dopamine was associated with less ARF. In 1987, R. J. Polson and colleagues[66] studied 34 patients who underwent 36 liver transplants. Nineteen patients (21 operations) received low-dose dopamine prophylactically, while 15 patients did not. The incidence of renal dysfunction was 9.5% in the dopamine group, compared with 67% in the control group. Overt ARF was not seen in the dopamine group but was seen in 27% of the control group. Dopamine is widely used in intensive care units in patients with oliguria or other early signs of renal dysfunction. Although (*a*) the effects of low-dose dopamine on renal function; (*b*) the incidence or severity, or both, of ARF; (*c*) the need for dialysis; and (*d*) mortality have not been studied in a rigorous fashion, dopamine has been associated with improvement in urinary output in the majority of patients, with minimal toxicity. However, it should not be used in any patient whose extracellular fluid volume is not adequate.

Experimental Drugs

A number of additional agents have shown promise in experimental ARF. However, there is limited clinical experience with these agents, in some cases because of their toxicity and in others because of their relatively recent availability. Adenine nucleotides, generally in the form of adenosine triphosphate combined with magnesium chloride (ATP-$MgCl_2$), have been used extensively, and are of interest because of their ability to attenuate the severity of renal injury even when given after the insult.[67] Their mechanism of action may be twofold: first, they result in a marked increase in renal blood flow; and second, they provide the precursors necessary for injured cells to resynthesize ATP, levels of which are markedly depressed after an ischemic insult.[68] Unfortunately, ATP-$MgCl_2$ causes profound hypotension in humans, which severely limits its usefulness.

Other agents, such as calcium channel–blocking agents and atrial natriuretic factor, have shown promise in experimental ARF. Although a substantial literature on the role of calcium channel–blocking agents in ARF is available, it remains unclear whether any beneficial effect is due to hemodynamic effects or effects on intracellular redistribution of calcium.[69] These agents are currently undergoing clinical trials.

The administration of thyroid hormone abrogates or attenuates renal injury in a variety of models of ARF.[36] It appears to operate by increasing either the activity or the amount of the tubular cells' sodium-potassium ATPase. Thyroid hormone is of interest for two reasons. First, it appears to be relatively nontoxic and has few hemodynamic effects. Second, it appears to be effective even after renal injury occurs. Clinical studies with this drug are ongoing.

Finally, free radical scavengers (eg, superoxide dismutase) and inhibitors of reactions that generate free radicals (eg, allopurinol and deferoxamine) have been subjects of intense investigation. As yet, however, controlled clinical studies in patients with ARF are not available. Allopurinol inhibits xanthine oxidase, which contributes to the generation of toxic free radicals during reperfusion via the Haber-Weiss reaction. Superoxide dismutase has been demonstrated to be effective in preventing ischemic damage in kidneys procured for organ transplantation.[70] Of interest is the fact that deferoxamine, an iron-chelating agent, substantially reduces the severity of ARF in glycerol models. Because iron participates in the Haber-Weiss reaction, chelation of iron may reduce toxic free-radical formation. Deferoxamine has been shown to minimize the untoward effects of such radicals on renal function.[71]

Thus, many of the recent investigations into the prevention of ARF have utilized agents that might be beneficial, based on observations of the cellular nature of injury induced by renal ischemia. Investigators have focused more on the response of individual cells or their constituents to injury than on the whole organ's response to injury. The use of these agents may become widespread if efficacy can be demonstrated in clinical trials. Some of these experimental drugs are promising because of their ability to exert beneficial effects even when administered after renal injury. It is likely that efficacy will be linked to cytoprotective effects rather than to effects on renal hemodynamics. A new generation of agents that may protect or restore renal function after injury is exciting but unlikely to be available for a few years for use in combat casualties with ARF.

PROTECTION FOR PATIENTS IN INCIPIENT RENAL FAILURE

Patients with incipient or established ARF may receive pharmacological therapy from our current armamentarium for a number of different goals. One goal is to promote urinary flow, with or without an improvement in glomerular filtration itself. A second goal is to prevent the occurrence, or lessen the severity, of ARF. Based on these goals, the following protocol, for patients with acute oliguria and for those at high risk for renal dysfunction, has been developed.

Pharmacological Therapy of Acute Oliguria

As early as possible after oliguria ensues, the extracellular fluid must be determined to be adequate—either clinically or by clinical impression validated by the results of invasive hemodynamic monitoring. If the extracellular fluid is not adequate, then normal saline, in 500-mL increments, should be administered intravenously until either the central venous pressure or the pulmonary capillary wedge pressure is higher than 15 mm Hg. Then graded doses of 1, 5, and 10 mg/kg of furosemide are administered—at hourly intervals—to clearly normovolemic patients. Furosemide will often restore urinary output. If there is no response to the 5-mg/kg dose, then 5 mg of metolazone, a proximally acting diuretic, should be given 30 minutes before the 10-mg/kg furosemide dose is administered. If there is no response to this final furosemide-metolazone challenge, then the patient should be considered to be resistant to diuretics. Resumption of urinary output at any dose of diuretic, however, obviates further doses. Low-dose dopamine (1–3 µg/kg/min), which often promotes urinary flow even without affecting systemic arterial pressure, is infused throughout the diuretic challenge. In patients in whom oliguria is associated with rhabdomyolysis, or who have undergone vascular surgical procedures with aortic cross-clamping, or who have undergone cardiac bypass, a mannitol-bicarbonate solution (100 g of 20% mannitol in 5% dextrose in water to which 3 ampules of sodium bicarbonate have been added) can be used to assist in restoring urinary output. Mannitol may serve as a volume expander in these situations. However, accurate assessment of the patient's volume status is critical if mannitol is to be administered, as it may precipitate pulmonary edema in the borderline hypervolemic patient. Mannitol should not be used in patients with serum sodium concentrations lower than 125 mmol/L: life-threatening hyponatremia may ensue as mannitol causes water to move from the cells into the extracellular fluid. Neither furosemide nor dopamine is likely to be effective, and the former may be harmful if the patient is volume depleted; thus, the extracellular fluid must be adequate.

Concomitant with the measures described above, an indwelling bladder catheter should be placed, or the existent catheter should be flushed. A renal ultrasound examination should be obtained emergently. Ultrasound equipment will not be available in field medical treatment facilities, but integrity of the bladder catheter should be ensured in all patients.

Prevention of Acute Renal Failure in High-Risk Patients

The same protocol can be used in patients at high risk for developing oliguria or established ARF or both. Many of these patients will need to undergo surgery imminently, and some will have undergone surgery recently. One standard practice is to obtain baseline measures of renal function (ie, a current BUN and creatinine concentration) and a urinalysis. An expanded extracellular fluid should be maintained in these patients, either as determined on clinical grounds or, preferably, with some form of hemodynamic monitoring. For patients who will undergo vascular procedures, a portion of administered fluids should include mannitol 1 g/kg, given as a 20% solution. Maintenance of an expanded extracellular fluid is probably the most powerful protection against renal ischemia associated with alterations in systemic arterial pressure from the adverse hemodynamic effects of anesthesia and blood loss during surgery.

In oliguric patients and in those at high risk for renal injury, potentially nephrotoxic drugs should be used judiciously. Loading doses of drugs are not altered, but the use of known nephrotoxins should be modified by either prolonging the dosing interval or giving reduced doses at regular intervals. Renal function should be assessed by measuring the serum creatinine at least daily. Since measurement of drug levels will not be available in battlefield medical treatment facilities, some nephrotoxic injury is likely. Other drugs, particularly nonsteroidal antiinflammatory agents that are useful as analgesics, should be used with caution; alternative analgesics are available.

To illustrate these principles, medical officers should consider the following discussion, which describes a situation that occurs frequently in combat and is likely to lead to ARF. Rhabdomyolytic-induced ARF, a classic example of posttraumatic ARF,[72] commonly occurs after a missile or crush injury of an extremity (as a result of a compartment syndrome) or with heat stroke. Even though there are a number of nontraumatic causes of rhabdomyolysis (Exhibit 26-3),[73] this discussion is confined to the traumatic causes, as they are likely to be encountered in battle injuries.

Muscle necrosis results from direct trauma or from the impairment of the blood supply. Muscle cells depend on oxygen delivery to maintain their cellular integrity. As ischemic injury occurs, muscle cells swell and eventually lyse. The release of intracellular contents causes predictable alterations in blood chemical values, and, with sufficient severity, leads to ARF or death. Muscle contains myoglobin, a respiratory protein that contains a globin chain and a heme moiety. The latter contains iron and is the delivery system for oxygen for the muscle cells. Myoglobin is carried in the circulation loosely bound to an α_2 globulin up to a concentration of approximately 23 mg/dL; if this concentration is exceeded, myoglobin circulates freely. As the molecular weight of myoglobin is 17,000 daltons, it is readily filtered by the glomeruli. In normal individuals, myoglobin is excreted if urinary flow rates and pH are optimal. One gram of muscle contains 4 mg of myoglobin.

However, there are situations that preclude the uneventful excretion of myoglobin. These situations include volume depletion and acidic urine. If sufficient quantities of myoglobin reach the kidney in the presence of these conditions, ARF is likely to occur. Volume depletion contributes to the toxicity of myoglobin via four mechanisms:

1. Renal blood flow is reduced, and the kidneys are subject to ischemic injury, with the consequences that have been discussed previously.
2. The relatively low urinary flow rates associated with volume depletion serve to increase the concentration of myoglobin in the tubules. Myoglobin precipitates with low-molecular-weight proteins in tubular fluid, which obstructs the tubular lumen, preventing flow.
3. In acidic urine, myoglobin dissociates into two moieties: globin and ferrihemate. This latter substance is extremely toxic to renal tubular cells.[74]
4. When ferrihemate is transported into cells, iron is released. When reperfusion occurs, the iron is a source of toxic free radicals through the Haber-Weiss and Fenton reactions.

ARF induced by rhabdomyolysis is one of the most severe forms of ARF. A substantial portion of patients who sustain muscle injury sufficient to induce ARF die of shock or hyperkalemia. The latter results from the release of intracellular potassium, the concentration of which in muscle is approximately 140 mmol/L. Other intracellular products released include organic acids; purine precursors such as uric acid; creatine, which is ultimately dehydrated into creatinine; other muscle enzymes; and proteins, which serve as procoagulants on their release.

EXHIBIT 26-3

CAUSES OF RHABDOMYOLYSIS

Trauma

Electrolyte Disorders

- Hypokalemia
- Hypophosphatemia

Myopathies From Enzyme Deficiencies*

- Phosphorylase deficiency (McCardle's disease, ie, type 5 glycogenosis)
- Phosphofructokinase deficiency (Tarui's disease)
- Carnitine palmityl transferase deficiency

Myopathies From Toxins*

- Alcohol-induced myopathies
- Carbon monoxide–induced myopathies

Idiopathic Paroxysmal Myoglobinuria*

*Not discussed in this chapter

Patients with rhabdomyolytic ARF present with overt trauma; oliguria or anuria; hypotension; and severe biochemical abnormalities, including hyperkalemia, metabolic acidemia, hyperphosphatemia, hypocalcemia, hyperuricemia; and elevations of enzymes principally found in muscle, particularly creatine kinase. Renal failure develops quickly as a consequence of both renal ischemia (from shock) and the nephrotoxicity of myoglobin. The profound depression of glomerular filtration, in conjunction with an excessive catabolic rate and the release of creatine from damaged muscle, results in a creatinine concentration that is disproportionately elevated compared with the BUN concentration. Moreover, the rate of production of creatinine continues to be excessive as long as damaged muscle is present; thus, the daily increment in the serum creatinine concentration may exceed 4 to 6 mg/dL.

The prevention of rhabdomyolytic-induced ARF follows logically from an understanding of its pathogenesis. First, volume depletion must be corrected rapidly and the extracellular fluid should be expanded. Casualties who sustain crush or other injury of an extremity are often in shock, and may lose liters of extracellular fluid into the injured extremity. In situations where muscle groups are enclosed by nondistensible fascial planes, such swelling may contribute to further muscle necrosis. Nonetheless, volume depletion and shock must be treated aggressively in an effort to correct renal ischemia. Renal blood flow must be restored before attempts to augment urinary flow can be made.

Tubular flow can be enhanced by expansion of the extracellular fluid with mannitol. In addition to its effects on renal blood flow owing to its ability to expand the extracellular fluid, mannitol is also an osmotic diuretic and will increase bulk fluid flow through the tubules. This effect serves to enhance the excretion of myoglobin and to restore tubular patency. Alkalinization of the urine is also crucial. Because myoglobin dissociates into its toxic components in an acidic milieu, prevention of further dissociation is facilitated by infusing isotonic sodium bicarbonate at rapid rates. This fluid, in addition to serving as a urinary alkalinizing agent, is also an effective volume expander. Low-dose dopamine infusion, even in the presence of normal blood pressure, should be started.

The aggressive character of this form of ARF usually necessitates early and vigorous hemodialysis if renal resuscitation is unsuccessful.[75] These casualties are extremely catabolic, and hemodialysis should be applied early, before the plasma concentrations of potassium or nitrogenous waste result in cardiac death or uremia, respectively. Additionally, surgical expertise is required to determine the extent of surgical debridement necessary, and whether and when fasciotomies should be performed. Because limb salvage is secondary to preservation of life, fasciotomies should be utilized liberally—certainly if there is any question about the vascular integrity of a limb.

CONSERVATIVE TREATMENT OF ESTABLISHED ACUTE RENAL FAILURE

Despite protective and resuscitative efforts, however, many patients will not respond to the maneuvers outlined above, and are assumed to have established ARF. We must then determine clinically whether conservative or dialytic therapy is indicated. Part of such determination includes an assessment of the optimal timing and type of dialysis, should it be required. Because the fundamental assumption in the treatment of ARF is that injured kidneys can recover, the major goal of therapy is to support the patient until this occurs. An ancillary goal is to provide an optimum milieu for both nutritional support and prevention or treatment of infection (infection being by far the major cause of death in ARF). To these ends, the assistance of experts in nutritional care and infectious diseases is critical in the management of these patients. Two management strategies can be used for patients with established ARF: conservative management and management with some form of dialysis. Many of the principles of conservative management of course also apply to patients who require dialysis.

Some patients with ARF, particularly those who remain nonoliguric and in whom catabolism is not excessive, can be managed without dialysis. Conservative management requires meticulous attention to nutritional support, fluid and diuretic therapy, and acid–base and electrolyte balance, the use of drugs, and general medical care.

Nutritional Support

The subject of nutritional support in ARF was reviewed in 1994.[76] One of the seminal studies that supported the use of nutritional support in ARF was conducted in 1967 by H. A. Lee, P. Sharpstone, and A. C. Ames.[77] These investigators studied 45 patients with ARF who were treated with casein hydrolysate and lipid, and noted diminished weight loss and more prompt recovery of renal function. Then in 1973, R. M. Abel and colleagues[78] prospectively studied 53 patients with ARF. These investigators utilized a combination of hypertonic dextrose and essential amino acids, compared with glucose alone, in cohorts of 28 and 25 patients, respectively. Of the patients receiving the protein-glucose solution, 75% recovered from ARF, compared with 44% of the patients receiving glucose alone ($P < .02$). Of the patients who required dialysis, 65% of those given amino acids and glucose survived, while only 18% of those given glucose alone survived.

In 1975, S. M. Baek, G. G. Makabali, and C. W. Bryan-Brown[79] studied 129 patients with postoperative ARF and noted a reduction in mortality from 70% in patients given glucose alone to 46% in patients treated with amino acids. The improvement in mortality was particularly impressive in patients who had sepsis.

However, the results of a number of other studies of nutritional support of patients with ARF have not been consistently positive, and the optimal nutritional regimen has not yet been defined. Moreover, no studies have been conducted in prospectively defined groups in which disease etiology and severity have been stratified. Nonetheless, many investigators believe that nutritional support of patients with ARF is beneficial, and it is often provided to patients.

A large body of clinical experience suggests that most fluid administered to patients with ARF should be nutritionally supportive, because these patients have limited ability to excrete fluids. All fluids should be administered only as they meet a specific need of the patient, and "maintenance fluids" should be carefully prescribed. Nutritional support should be initiated within the first 48 hours after the injury in most patients with posttraumatic ARF, because nutritional support clearly attenuates the hypercatabolism that many of them exhibit.

Fluids used to provide nutritional support (the "renal-failure" fluids) consist of hypertonic glucose and amino acid solutions, and should be supplemented by lipid emulsions to provide additional calories. Energy requirements are best calculated on the basis of basal metabolic requirements, with additional requirements predicated on a *stress factor* related to the type and severity of the underlying illness. Energy requirements (*ER*) in kilocalories per day can be expressed in the formula

$$ER = \text{basal requirements} \bullet \text{stress factor}$$

A factor of 1.25 accounts for the increased energy requirements of ill patients who are not paralyzed. The stress factor is 1.30 to 1.50 for patients who have sustained multiple trauma or who have infection.[80] Basal metabolic requirements and stress factors are discussed in detail in Chapter 23, Metabolic Derangements and Nutritional Support.

In general, a minimum of 30 to 50 kcal/kg/d is required by most critically ill patients. Carbohydrate should account for 60% to 70% of the calories, while most of the remainder should be provided as fat. Excessive carbohydrate administration will cause carbon dioxide accumulation and respiratory distress; thus, judicious use of lipid emulsions is critical.[81] Fluid regimens should provide as many calories in as small a volume as possible; thus, 50% to 70% dextrose is often required. Lipid can be administered through a peripheral vein, as the solutions are not hypertonic.

Because of azotemia, the quantities of protein must be limited to 0.8 to 1.0 g/kg/d unless the patient is on dialysis. Amino acids are lost across the dialysis membrane at a rate of 10 to 15 g per treatment, and must be replaced in addition to the basal requirement of amino acids.[82] Protein should be of high biological value and contain mostly essential amino acids, including branched-chain amino acids. Solutions containing casein hydrolysates or amino acid preparations in which nonessential amino acids predominate may result in excessive azotemia without attenuation of catabolism.

Enteral alimentation is preferable to parenteral alimentation if the patient's condition permits. Small-diameter polyethylene feeding tubes are placed through the patient's nose for instillation of solutions of either essential amino acids or a mixture of essential and nonessential amino acids. Not only is enteral feeding associated with fewer complications, but some evidence also suggests that feeding facilitates the maintenance of the integrity of the bowel mucosa, which may prevent endotoxemia and gut-associated sepsis, both of which can induce multiple organ failure.[83] Moreover, the presence of nutrients in the bowel will maintain the enzymes necessary for enteral nutrition and permit a smooth transition to enteral feedings when the patient's condition permits. However, enteral solutions will often cause diarrhea if administered in too large quantities or at too rapid a rate. The use of infusion pumps, which facilitate constant instillation of solution, greatly reduces this complication.

However, many patients with posttraumatic ARF will have undergone abdominal surgery, and enteral feedings will not be possible. Moreover, the magnitude of nutritional support required by hypercatabolic patients often precludes the use of enteral feedings. Should total parenteral nutrition (TPN) be required, access to the central circulation is obtained through the subclavian or the internal or external jugular veins. The catheter site should be inspected and redressed daily, using strict aseptic techniques, and the catheter used exclusively for TPN. If these guidelines are followed, catheter-related infection is uncommon.

The composition of enteral or parenteral fluid can be varied according to the needs of the patient. Sodium can be added or deleted depending on the volume status and the serum sodium concentration. Often, sodium is administered as the acetate salt; the eventual metabolism of acetate to bicarbonate tends to abrogate the acidemic effects of TPN solutions. Potassium supplementation is seldom required initially, but is generally required after several days of TPN when the rate of catabolism has slowed and anabolism has begun. The serum phosphate concentration is high initially but can fall to dangerously low levels after several days of therapy, and may require addition of phosphate to the TPN as either the potassium or sodium salt.

The success of nutritional support in patients with ARF depends on

- avoidance of infection in patients treated with TPN,
- attenuation of catabolism,
- establishment of relatively normal biochemical values in plasma, and
- maintenance of stable extracellular fluid.

A standard monitoring scheme should be followed, so that electrolyte disturbances can be anticipated and corrected before they become severe. The serum glucose should be monitored several times daily, and hyperglycemia should be treated with insulin. Although patients with renal dysfunction have prolonged serum half-life of insulin, they also exhibit insulin resistance. In general, insulin administration is required in virtually all patients treated with TPN. Once daily insulin requirements have become stable, the requisite amount of insulin can be administered in the TPN solution by constant infusion. Surveillance of glucose levels should be continued, however, as sudden hyperglycemia is often the first sign of an incipient infection.

Fluid and Diuretic Therapy

Fluid intake should be limited to the measured urinary output, with additional fluid given for measured gastrointestinal losses and estimated insensible losses. As has been emphasized previously, much of the administered fluid should be nutritionally supportive; the remainder is often required for medication administration. As a general rule, all medications should be administered in as concentrated a form as possible. Most nonoliguric patients excrete no more than 1 to 1.5 L of urine per day. This loss, coupled with gastrointestinal and insensible losses, may be sufficient to allow required fluids in the form of nutrition and medications to be administered. Because most patients excrete urine that is hypotonic to plasma, with urinary sodium concentrations of 60 to 90 mmol/L, fluid that is equivalent in electrolyte composition should be administered. Replacement of urinary fluid and electrolyte losses in this fashion will tend to minimize water excess or deficit and avoid hyponatremia or hypernatremia, respectively. The serum sodium concentration should be monitored frequently as a guide to the patient's water balance, and should kept in the range of 130 to 150 mmol/L.

Ideally, the patient treated conservatively will lose no more than 0.5 to 1.0 kg of body weight per day. However, some nonoliguric patients will not excrete sufficient urine to allow for effective nutritional support, particularly if large quantities of other fluids (eg, antibiotics) must be administered, and they will gain weight. In such patients, urinary output can be augmented, if necessary, with low-dose dopamine infusions and intermittent doses of loop diuretics. There appear to be few adverse effects of low-dose dopamine infusions. However, excessive use of loop diuretics may result in metabolic alkalemia, deafness, and potassium depletion, the latter of which results in impairment of glucose homeostasis and proper muscle function. Osmotic diuretics such as mannitol should be avoided in most patients with established ARF, as they can induce hyponatremia if a diuresis does not result, hypernatremia if excessive free-water diuresis is induced, or pulmonary edema if urinary output declines. Thiazide diuretics are not effective in ARF, and potassium-sparing diuretics are contraindicated.

Management of Acid–Base Disturbances

The major acid–base disturbances that occur in patients with ARF are metabolic alkalosis and metabolic acidosis. The more immediate threat is from metabolic acidosis, which results from both excessive generation of acid and the inability to excrete acids. Metabolic alkalosis usually results from inadequate replacement of nasogastric fluid losses, particularly in nonoliguric patients, in whom chloride, and to a certain extent, potassium, loss represents the primary pathophysiological mechanism.

Metabolic Acidosis

Metabolic acidosis is manifested by a depressed serum bicarbonate concentration and, usually in posttraumatic ARF, an anion gap. The concentration of lactic acid is often elevated in these patients, as are concentrations of other organic acids (such as from phosphate and sulfate salts) when renal failure is severe. In uncomplicated cases of ARF, the serum bicarbonate concentration will average 16 to 18 mmol/L, and the serum pH will average 7.34 to 7.37. This degree of acidemia is not associated with untoward effects. In fact, the rightward shift of the oxyhemoglobin curve will result in more effective oxygen delivery to tissue. If acidosis is more severe, cardiovascular complications such as arrhythmias and hypotension may ensue.

The treatment of metabolic acidosis is relatively simple,[84] although recent questions have been raised regarding the efficacy of bicarbonate administration in correcting the hemodynamic abnormalities in critically ill patients.[85] Nonetheless, nonoliguric patients can receive sufficient alkali, usually in the form of sodium bicarbonate, to correct their base deficit and ongoing losses. In patients who are not excessively catabolic, such ongoing losses should amount to approximately 1 mmol HCO_3/kg/d. In certain patients, the alkali requirement can be met with oral preparations. Sodium bicarbonate tablets, however, result in excessive eructation. A combination of citric acid and sodium citrate (Sholl's solution), which contains 1 mmol HCO_3 equivalent per milliliter, can be used. In severe cases, hemodialysis can be used to remove extracellular fluid volume so that sodium bicarbonate can be administered in large quantities. The concentration of bicarbonate or equivalent base in the dialysate can be manipulated to meet the needs of the patient.

Metabolic Alkalosis

Metabolic alkalosis is characterized by an elevated serum bicarbonate concentration and a depressed serum chloride concentration. The actual pH of the blood depends on whether (*a*) the alkalosis is an isolated acid–base disturbance or (*b*) there are other disturbances. Substantial alkalosis has a number of untoward effects, including

- hypokalemia, which can result in muscle weakness and cardiac arrhythmias;
- respiratory muscle weakness, which may retard successful weaning from the ventilator;
- compensatory respiratory acidosis, because the response to pure metabolic alkalosis is to retain carbon dioxide, and patients on assisted ventilation may become acidotic in an attempt to return the alkaline pH toward more normal values;
- arterial hypoxemia, which is the result of the alveolar hypoventilation required to produce hypercarbia; and
- impaired oxygen delivery to tissues, because the oxyhemoglobin dissociation curve is shifted to the left, for any given partial pressure of oxygen; therefore, less oxygen is delivered to tissue.

Metabolic alkalosis is largely preventable, particularly if intravascular volume (sodium chloride) and potassium depletion are avoided. Excessive diuretic-induced volume and electrolyte losses should be replaced. Moreover, because nasogastric suction removes volume, potassium, and acid from the body, inhibition of gastrointestinal acid secretion by histamine-receptor blocking agents will reduce net proton loss from the body. In this regard, ranitidine is preferable to cimetidine, since alterations in mental status are seen more frequently with the latter.

The treatment of established metabolic alkalosis includes correction of both intravascular volume deficits and potassium depletion. Potassium deficits can be substantial, on the order of several hundred millimoles. In the rare situation in which volume and potassium repletion do not correct alkalosis, carbonic anhydrase inhibitors can be used to promote urinary bicarbonate loss. However, in the vast majority of patients with ARF, these drugs will be ineffective. In oliguric patients, the volume space for correction of volume deficits may not exist. Thus, dilute hydrochloric acid can be infused into a central vein in nonoliguric patients or into the venous return of a dialyzer in patients on dialysis.[86] With this therapy, the difference between the measured and the desired serum chloride concentration is multiplied by the product of the body weight (in kilograms) and 0.27 (the volume of distribution of chloride). The amount of chloride, in milliequivalents, is administered as an equal amount of 1.0 N hydrochloric acid diluted in dextrose and water. Finally, hemodialysis utilizing especially prepared dialysate solutions can remove excessive bicarbonate and replace potassium and sodium chloride losses.

Management of Electrolyte Imbalances

Hyperkalemia

Hyperkalemia is potentially the most dangerous of all metabolic complications of ARF, as lethal cardiac dysrhythmias can result with little warning. Hyperkalemia results from a number of different mechanisms, including the following:

- Transcellular shifts of potassium for hydrogen occur during metabolic acidemia, when the body attempts to buffer protons intracellularly. Although it has been classically taught that for each 0.1 change in the pH, there is a reciprocal 0.6 mEq change in the serum potassium concentration, some researchers[87] now think that this does not occur when the metabolic acidosis is due to organic (ie, lactic) acid accumulation. Rather, transcellular shifts occur only when hydrogen is accompanied by an anion such as chloride, which is restricted from transcellular movement.
- Excessive production of potassium also occurs when there is breakdown of tissue in conjunction with inability to excrete potassium. Tissue destruction is common in rhabdomyolysis, but may also be seen with ischemia of the gastrointestinal tract and after vascular surgery, in which tissue viability may be in question.
- Interference with potassium excretion by drugs may also occur. Nonsteroidal agents and β-adrenergic blocking agents may interfere with and impair renal excretion of potassium.
- Finally, renal dysfunction itself severely limits the ability to excrete potassium. Although fecal potassium excretion often increases by as much as 35% in patients with chronic renal failure, this adaptive mechanism is unusual in ARF, and is probably why patients with ARF do not tolerate the levels of hyperkalemia that are tolerated by patients with chronic renal failure.

The causes of hyperkalemia in ARF include minimal urinary excretion (fecal excretion is possible, but takes days) and release of potassium ions from injured tissue. In addition, hyperkalemia is aggravated by metabolic and respiratory acidemia and insulin resistance; and is worsened by the presence of drugs with potassium effects (eg, nonsteroidal antiinflammatory drugs, extravascular influsion drugs).

Determining the mechanism of hyperkalemia may assist the physician in choosing the most appropriate therapy, because hyperkalemia can be controlled with exchange resins, glucose and insulin, and bicarbonate. The most important therapy, however, is that which antagonizes the effect of hyperkalemia on cardiac muscle. Thus, the initial diagnostic maneuver after hyperkalemia is first noted is to obtain an electrocardiogram. If there are any abnormalities, calcium chloride should be administered immediately. Then, more definitive steps can be taken to resolve the problem.

Phosphate Abnormalities

Hyperphosphatemia is the most common abnormality of divalent ion metabolism in ARF and can usually be controlled by the frequent oral administration of aluminum-containing antacids, either aluminum hydroxide or aluminum carbonate. These agents are administered as suspensions, 30 to 60 mL every 3 to 4 hours, until the serum phosphate concentration approaches normal values, after which they can be administered less frequently. Although such agents bind phosphorus most effectively in the stomach (ie, when given with food), they are effective even in the absence of enteral nutrients, in which situation they interrupt the enteric recirculation of phosphorus. Aluminum toxicity should not be considered a problem in patients with ARF, as it is in those with chronic renal disease. Aluminum-containing antacids are often ineffective until they have been administered for several days. Even then, they may not control the serum phosphate concentration, in which case sucralfate can be administered four to six times daily in doses of 1.0 g. Finally, hyperphosphatemia almost always responds to the provision of adequate nutrition, particularly if appropriate concentrations of branched-chain amino acids and effective nonnitrogen-to-nitrogen caloric ratios are met. Presumably, effective nutritional support retards catabolism and promotes anabolism, so that phosphorus is transported into cells.

Hypophosphatemia has a number of untoward effects, the most common of which are (*a*) impaired muscle function and (*b*) reduced extraction of oxygen from hemoglobin.[88] The most frequent adverse clinical effect is diffuse muscle dysfunction, which may involve both skeletal and cardiac muscle. Skeletal muscle dysfunction may severely retard efforts to wean the patient from the ventilator. More-severe hypophosphatemia can result in rhabdomyolysis. The second-most-frequent effect is a shift in the oxyhemoglobin dissociation curve, so that less oxygen is delivered at a given partial pressure. Other effects of hypophosphatemia on the hematopoietic system include (*a*) hemolytic anemia due to red blood cell ATP depletion and the inability to maintain membrane fluidity and (*b*) white blood cell dysfunction.

Hypophosphatemia in ARF is commonly a consequence of overaggressive therapy of hyperphosphatemia, and it occasionally occurs in patients who have received TPN. The serum phosphorus can be expected to fall 0.3 mg/dL/d in patients who are receiving TPN. Thus, patients who have baseline normal phosphate concentrations can be expected to develop significant hypophosphatemia in 5 to 10 days. When hypophosphatemia develops, phosphorus should be added to the TPN solution. Symptomatic hypophosphatemia is common when the serum phosphate concentration is below 1.8 mg/dL. In such situations, replenishment of phosphate stores should be considered. Phosphate repletion can be accomplished by a number of different maneuvers.[88]

Calcium Abnormalities

Hypocalcemia results not only from hyperphosphatemia but also from resistance to the actions of vitamin D and parathyroid hormone. Unless the patient is symptomatic, has signs such as Chvostek's sign, or has electrocardiographic changes associated with hypocalcemia, the more judicious initial treatment is to lower the elevated serum *phosphate* concentration toward normal. As the serum phosphate concentration becomes more normal, the serum calcium concentration will begin to rise. If necessary, elemental calcium can be administered as enteral or parenteral nutritional supplements. Should clinical symptoms or electrocardiographic changes consistent with hypocalcemia become evident, calcium should be administered intravenously. There are a number of preparations, including the chloride, lactate, or gluceptate salts, that can be utilized.

APPROACHES TO DIALYSIS

Conservative therapy of ARF requires meticulous management, and attention to the routine details of patient care requires considerable effort. However, the severity of renal dysfunction, with its resultant catabolism and metabolic perturbations, may eventually require dialysis support. Thus, when or if conservative management is inappropriate or unsuccessful, dialysis is indicated. Three approaches to blood-purification therapy can be utilized to attenuate the effects of nitrogenous waste retention, electrolyte imbalance, and circulatory overload: conventional hemodialysis, peritoneal dialysis, and hemofiltration.[89]

Conventional Hemodialysis

Hemodialysis has traditionally been the therapy of choice for posttraumatic, hypercatabolic ARF, and has been designated as the mainstay of renal replacement therapy in the DEPMEDS doctrine. Removal of urea nitrogen, creatinine, other retained waste products, potassium, sodium, and water is efficient, as metabolic homeostasis can usually be achieved and then maintained with a 3- to 4-hour treatment conducted three to five times weekly. Modern artificial kidneys achieve BUN and creatinine clearances in excess of 175 mL/min and have ultrafiltration rates of 4 to 5 milliliters per millimeter of transmembrane pressure per hour. With typical operating parameters, BUN and creatinine concentrations can be reduced by 30% to 40%, and 2 to 3 L of extracellular fluid can easily be removed during a 4-hour treatment. Many modern dialysis membranes are made of cuprophane, a substance that may occasionally induce hypoxemia in the initial period of the dialysis treatment by activating components of the complement cascade, resulting in stasis of leukocytes in the pulmonary circulation. Although alternative materials for dialysis membranes are available, they are associated with excessive clotting in the artificial kidney. Fortunately, the hypoxemia associated with cuprophane membranes is transient. The cuprophane membrane is configured in either parallel-plate or hollow-fiber geometry. Although parallel-plate membranes are easier to use, they are associated with slightly higher rates of clotting than are the hollow-fiber type. Polyethylene tubing to conduct blood flow to and from the artificial kidney is required and must be compatible with both the artificial kidney and the dialysis machine.

Hemodialysis operates through a combination of diffusive and convective transport. Solute removal by diffusion depends on the size of the solute molecules; the thickness and surface area of the artificial membrane; and the rates of blood and dialysate flow, which are countercurrent to each other. Solute removal by convection depends on the rate of fluid (ie, solvent) transport across the membrane. Fluid removal depends on a pressure gradient across the membrane, which is generated by a combination of the patient's blood pressure and resistance to blood flow through the angioaccess, and pressure applied from the dialysate side of the membrane. This cumulative pressure, known as the *transmembrane* pressure, can be varied by the operator to enhance or retard fluid removal.

Circulatory Access

Obtaining access to the circulation for hemodialysis is often quite difficult in critically ill patients. Hemodialysis requires a blood flow of at least 200 to 250 mL/min, which is generated through the use of a blood pump intrinsic to the dialysis machine. Angioaccess is typically achieved with double-lumen dialysis catheters, which are placed percutaneously in the subclavian, internal jugular, or femoral vein. The first location is preferable, since an occlusive bandage can easily be applied to prevent contamination. These catheters should be dressed only by dialysis personnel, and are routinely left in place for several weeks. Catheter-related infection is extremely rare if the catheters are used only for dialysis. Percutaneous access for conventional hemodialysis is preferable to arteriovenous shunts: the latter must be placed surgically and are often complicated by infection and bleeding. Recently, double-lumen catheters that have a synthetic polyester cuff have been used with some success. These catheters are surgically placed in the subclavian vein, where their properties are equivalent to those of conventional percutaneous catheters. However, for rapid access to the circulation for dialysis, we prefer the percutaneous approach.

Although some patients with ARF tolerate hemodialysis without problems, hemodynamic instability and hypotension are relatively common for at least three reasons:

1. The blood pump generates blood flow that is independent of the patient's blood pressure.
2. The efficiency of solute removal with hemodialysis induces osmolar shifts, which are thought to induce hypotension.
3. The use of acetate as a base replacement in the dialysate can result in peripheral vasodilation and impaired myocardial contractility, particularly in patients with liver dysfunction who cannot rapidly metabolize acetate to bicarbonate (this has been abrogated by the virtual universal use of bicarbonate dialysate in critically ill patients).

Anticoagulation of the blood with heparin is generally required, although there are several alternatives to conventional anticoagulation if bleeding is a risk.[90] There is substantial experience utilizing the technique of heparin-free dialysis, in which the artificial kidney is flushed with saline several times each hour. Unfortunately, this not only dramatically reduces the efficiency of the dialysis procedure, it also limits the amount of fluid that can be removed in a standard treatment period. The judicious use of low doses of heparin is associated with acceptable patency of the extracorporeal circuit without untoward bleeding. In general, we should administer 15 units of heparin per kilogram of body weight as a loading dose, then 750 to 1,000 units per hour as a constant infusion. Either dose is easily alterable, depending on the level of anticoagulation, which is measured by the activated clotting time using a portable monitor and disposable tubes coated with platelet activating factor. The desired end point of the test is between 160 and 180 seconds, and this method allows for rapid and repetitive assessment of the effects of heparin administration. Such techniques as regional anticoagulation with heparin or citrate, with protamine or calcium rescue respectively, or anticoagulation with prostacyclin, largely have been abandoned. Prostacyclin produces severe hypotension, which makes maintenance of the extracorporeal circuit impossible.

Sorbent-Based Dialysis Delivery System

The large water requirements of conventional hemodialysis can be avoided by the use of sorbent-based dialysis delivery systems.[91] These systems regenerate spent dialysate, and require approximately 6 L of water, as opposed to the nearly 250 L of water required by conventional hemodialysis. Bicarbonate, calcium, potassium, and other desired solutes can be added to the dialysate as needed. Waste products that diffuse from the blood into the dialysate are adsorbed onto different layers of a sorbent cartridge, resulting in the maintenance of the desired type of dialysate (Figure 26-4).

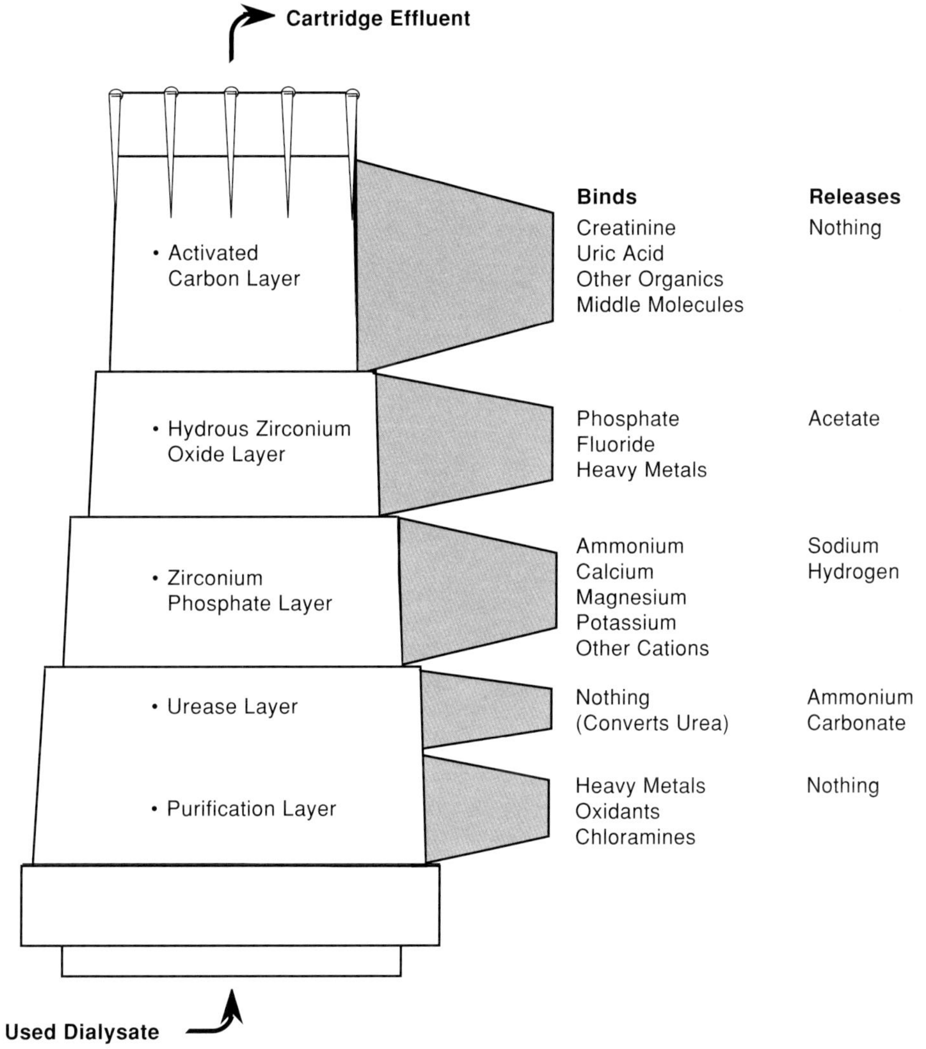

Fig. 26-4. The single-use sorbent cartridge is commercially available in a number of different sizes. It consists of several components, which, from the bottom of the cartridge up, include scavenger (ie, purification), urease, zirconium phosphate, hydrated zirconium oxide, and activated carbon layers. The scavenger layer consists of activated carbon and zirconium oxide. This layer removes trace metals such as copper and oxidizing agents such as chloramine, which would otherwise inactivate the second layer. The second layer consists of urease. This catalyzes the reaction of urea into ammonia and carbamic acid, which in aqueous solution form ammonium in equilibrium with ammonia, and bicarbonate. The third layer consists of zirconium phosphate, which serves as a cation exchanger. Thus, the ammonium ions that result from the urease layer, in addition to calcium, magnesium, and potassium, are exchanged for sodium and hydrogen ions in a ratio of 8:1 by the zirconium. The fourth layer, of zirconium oxide, serves as an anion exchanger, in which phosphate is exchanged for acetate. The final layer consists of activated carbon, which adsorbs creatinine, uric acid, and other organic compounds. The use of this sorbent-based system allows dialysis to be conducted using potable water, rather than water that would otherwise have to be treated with filters, deionizers, and reverse osmosis membranes. Reprinted with permission from Organon Teknika Corp. *Sorbent Dialysis Primer*. Durham, NC: Organon Teknika Corp; 1988: 3.

The major drawback of the sorbent-based system is that the sorbent cartridge has a finite capacity. That is, the ability of the cartridge to remove urea is limited by the ability of the zirconium-phosphate layer to exchange ammonium, which is derived from the urease-based catalysis of urea, for sodium and hydrogen. When this layer is saturated, additional ammonia cannot be processed and can diffuse into the patient. The capacity of the cartridge to handle urea depends on its size. High-capacity cartridges can remove 28 g of urea nitrogen (ie, 60 g or 1,000 mmol of urea). Detection of ammonia is facilitated by the use of ammonia test strips. When hypercatabolic patients are dialyzed and excessive urea must be removed, either the dialysate must be monitored for ammonia or, more commonly, the cartridge can simply be replaced with a fresh cartridge halfway through the treatment.

Equipment and Support

The machinery and other technical requirements for hemodialysis are substantial. Modern machines are equipped with numerous safety features and monitoring devices. Because many are based on solid-state circuitry, a surge-free electrical current is required. Electrical generators or fixed-facility power plants must be capable of providing 110- to 120-V, 50-Hz power to support machines that are manufactured in the United States. These machines are sufficiently complex that several weeks are required to train operators. Relatively sophisticated medical maintenance support and spare-part backup, primarily in the form of spare circuit boards, are required, as user-based maintenance capabilities are minimal. Supply modules have been configured that contain all the material necessary to conduct dialysis. The machines contained in a DEPMEDS module (deployed at the third echelon) are slightly larger than a large suitcase, and weigh approximately 50 lb.

Hemodialysis is conducted by dialysis technicians, who are corpsmen who have special training in dialysis, and who are supervised by nurses who have undergone similar specialized training. A 6-month course for dialysis technicians is conducted at Walter Reed Army Medical Center (WRAMC) in Washington, D. C., and a course has recently been started for registered nurses who wish to become dialysis nurses. Technicians and nurses alike then receive personnel skill identifiers that facilitate their assignment to facilities where dialysis will be provided. The standards of practice required to care for the typical patient with ARF are that one technician provide treatment to a single patient. Moreover, a registered nurse with experience in dialysis should be present in any location where patients are being dialyzed. Dialysis personnel are also trained in assisting nephrologists in the placement and subsequent care of catheters for dialysis. Because a typical dialysis treatment requires nearly 1 hour of preparation, 4 hours for the actual treatment, and nearly 1 hour to prepare for the next patient, hemodialysis is a labor-intensive process.

Peritoneal Dialysis

Peritoneal dialysis was used during the Vietnam War for milder forms of ARF. This form of dialysis, in which the peritoneal membrane serves as the dialyzing membrane, is inherently much less efficient than hemodialysis. Access to the peritoneal cavity is achieved via either the percutaneous placement of a stiff peritoneal catheter or, preferably, the placement of a softer, curled catheter through a small incision using local anesthesia and direct visualization of the peritoneal cavity. As with hemodialysis, solutes are removed by a combination of diffusion and convection. Ultrafiltration is caused by the movement of water from the blood into the peritoneal cavity in response to the placement of hypertonic dextrose (1.5%, 2.5%, or 4.25%) into the peritoneal cavity. Solute and fluid removal rates are substantially slower than those achieved with hemodialysis, with BUN and creatinine clearances approximating 15 and 5 mL/min under optimum conditions.

Peritoneal dialysis has some advantages over other forms of dialysis:

- Anticoagulation is not required; thus, patients who are at high risk of bleeding, or in whom bleeding might be catastrophic, can receive therapy.
- There is very little hemodynamic stress, and patients with hypotension who cannot be hemodialyzed can undergo peritoneal dialysis successfully.

However, for military medicine, the disadvantages outweigh the advantages:

- The casualty must have an intact peritoneal cavity. Only rarely can patients successfully undergo acute peritoneal dialysis after abdominal surgery.
- Peritoneal dialysis also requires large quantities of dextrose-containing fluid; delivery, storage, and maintenance of sterility of this fluid represent logistical challenges.

Although peritoneal dialysis has been used in patients with posttraumatic ARF,[92,93] the disadvantages make it of limited use in posttraumatic renal failure, and there is no provision for this form of therapy in our current DEPMEDS planning.

Hemofiltration

Hemofiltration is the newest form of therapy available and has shown promise in the management of critically ill patients.[94,95] This approach to dialysis utilizes a polysulfone membrane configured in a hollow-fiber geometry. Both hydraulic conductivity and solute passage are substantially greater than they are with hemodialysis. Solute removal occurs through convection, in which transport of the solute depends on the solute's being swept along by the moving stream of solvent (ie, solvent drag) and not on the size of the solute molecule. As long as the size of the solute does not exceed the size of the pore in the membrane, the solute will be cleared with its solvent. However, the concentration of solute in the blood will not change.

The porosity of the hemofilter membrane is such that large volumes of fluid can be removed. Ultrafiltration rates of 50 to 60 mL/min are theoretically achievable; in practice, removal of more than 1 L/h is commonplace. However, because the concentration of undesired substances in the blood does not change, other maneuvers must be utilized to effect a substantial reduction of nitrogenous waste concentration. One such method is to replace fluid removed by the hemofilter concurrently, usually in a postfilter mode, with appropriate quantities of sterile, pyrogen-free, isotonic, electrolyte-balanced fluid. This method is true hemofiltration, and is effective in controlling concentrations of nitrogenous waste products in the blood.

Continuous Arteriovenous Hemofiltration

No blood pump is required in continuous arteriovenous hemofiltration (CAVH), as the patient's systemic arterial pressure determines the rate of blood flow through the extracorporeal circuit. Other determinants of the efficacy of this system include the type of cannulae used for angioaccess and the length of tubing utilized for ultrafiltrate collection. CAVH requires that a large artery and vein be cannulated or that an external arteriovenous shunt be surgically placed. The term CAVH should be reserved for the use of a hemofilter and postfilter replacement fluid therapy (ie, hemodilution), in which the goal of therapy is control of nitrogenous waste and circulatory overload in the oliguric or anuric patient with ARF. The enormous quantities of intravenous-quality fluid required to achieve reductions in concentrations of nitrogenous waste make this form of therapy logistically problematic in a wartime setting.

Slow, Continuous Ultrafiltration

Slow, continuous ultrafiltration (SCUF) is identical to CAVH except that no replacement fluid is administered. Instead, the hydraulic conductivity of the hemofilter is utilized, along with the patient's own blood pressure, to remove an isotonic ultrafiltrate of plasma. This is very effective therapy for volume overload. Concentrations of substances in the blood do not change, and waste removal is limited to the amount of ultrafiltrate removed. Thus this therapy is not effective by itself for azotemia. Conversely, it can be utilized effectively for both acidemia and hyperkalemia, since excessive fluid can be removed, allowing space for bicarbonate, glucose, and insulin. However, because neither acid nor potassium is actually removed from the body in substantial quantities by this procedure, SCUF is probably best considered as a temporizing measure to be utilized until the patient can be treated with hemodialysis.

Continuous Arteriovenous Hemodiafiltration

The newest form of therapy available is a hybrid of CAVH and SCUF, called continuous arteriovenous hemodiafiltration (CAVH-D).[96,97] In this technique, SCUF is performed with the simultaneous infusion of an electrolytically balanced solution countercurrent to the blood path in the hemofilter apparatus. Such fluid can be pumped with an intravenous fluid–control device, at a rate of 1 L/h; peritoneal dialysate is often used as the fluid. Although the system is relatively inefficient, the mixture of convective- and diffusion-based transport does remove unwanted solutes from the body. Bicarbonate or base-precursors, usually acetate or lactate, diffuse from dialysate into blood, and when metabolized by the liver to bicarbonate, result in the attenuation of acidemia. However, since dialysate flows are approximately 1 L/h, the quantities of fluid required are similar to those required by true CAVH.

There are several advantages of SCUF, with or without hemodiafiltration, over hemodialysis in critically ill patients[98,99]:

1. Because no blood pumps or dialysis machines are required, the machinery and personnel requirements for SCUF are sub-

stantially less than for hemodialysis. The cognitive and technical requirements that are necessary to be able to supervise or perform SCUF or its variants are readily taught by nephrologists to registered nurses with critical care training, and to internists or intensivists or both.[100] Many of the graduate medical education programs in the military provide this form of training to appropriate resident physicians.
2. Compared with hemodialysis, there is very little hemodynamic instability or hypotension attributable to the extracorporeal procedure itself. The reasons for this are not clear but probably relate to the fact that SCUF does not produce changes in plasma osmolality as does hemodialysis.
3. The membrane material in hemofilters appears to be more biocompatible than hemodialysis membranes; thus, allergic reactions and sequestration of leukocytes are uncommon.
4. Critically ill patients with ARF have enormous nutrient requirements; it is not uncommon for such patients to need 3 to 5 L of parenteral nutrition daily. Removal of these substantial volumes of fluid with conventional hemodialysis is often hindered by refractory hypotension; thus, optimal nutritional support cannot be provided.
5. The use of SCUF does not preclude intermittent hemodialysis. In fact, many patients with ARF who require dialytic support may need virtually continuous volume control, with only intermittent solute removal. Thus, in my experience at WRAMC (1980–1985) with 101 patients dialyzed for ARF, volume overload was by far the most frequent cause for intervention, while azotemia, hyperkalemia, and acidemia were indicated far less frequently.[101] Many patients with oliguric ARF can be treated successfully with SCUF and only intermittent hemodialysis.

DIALYTIC MANAGEMENT OF ACUTE RENAL FAILURE

The decision to provide dialytic therapy to a critically ill casualty is one that should not be made lightly, and should be made by a nephrologist in consultation with the primary physician after the risks and expected benefits are weighed. At the very least, the decision to provide dialysis involves commitment of substantial personnel, supply, and time. Dialysis should never be offered to casualties who have been triaged as expectant. As a general rule, dialysis should be provided as far rearward in the theater as possible, and should be considered a support measure to allow the casualty to be evacuated as soon as possible to a site of definitive medical care. Given the nature of the injuries and illnesses that are associated with ARF, even with the most favorable circumstances and outcomes, survivors of ARF are virtually never fit to return to any form of duty for 3 to 6 months.

The goals of dialysis are

- to maintain relatively normal electrolyte concentrations;
- to maintain predialysis BUN concentration of 80 to 90 mg/dL and creatinine concentration of 6 to 8 mg/dL;
- to maintain an extracellular fluid volume that permits required fluid administration and acceptable oxygenation-ventilation parameters; and
- to eliminate or prevent manifestations of uremia.

Indications for Dialysis

In modern nephrologic practice, there are no absolute indications for or contraindications to dialysis, so that virtually any casualty who is not in the expectant triage category may be considered a candidate for dialysis, even those for whom dialysis would have been considered contraindicated in earlier years. The expanded applicability of dialysis is undoubtedly a result of both a better appreciation of the physiological events that accompany dialysis and more advanced physiological monitoring systems. I have successfully dialyzed patients with both closed and open head injuries, patients actively bleeding from gastrointestinal or pulmonary sources, and patients with virtually refractory hypotension. However, these patients require intensive resources that are exceedingly scarce in field hospitals, and the decision to utilize them must be made in the context of the whole theater's need for dialysis support.

The usual indications for dialysis include intractable volume overload, refractory metabolic acidemia, uncorrectable hyperkalemia, and substantial azotemia, usually defined as concentrations of BUN and creatinine greater than 110 to 120 mg/dL and 7

EXHIBIT 26-4

INDICATIONS FOR DIALYSIS OF PATIENTS WITH ACUTE RENAL FAILURE

Intractable metabolic acidemia

Intractable volume overload

Intractable hyperkalemia (dialysis is the definitive therapy)

Uremic pericarditis

Uremic encephalopathy

Dialyzable toxin ingestion

Gastrointestinal hemorrhage after localization

Bleeding diathesis prior to surgery

to 9 mg/dL, respectively (Exhibit 26-4). These levels of azotemia may prompt many nephrologists to institute dialysis even without uremia. Moreover, overt uremia (manifested by pericarditis, altered mental status, or bleeding diathesis) signifies that dialysis should be instituted as soon as possible. Finally, hypercatabolic ARF, in which the daily incremental changes in BUN or creatinine or both exceed 40 mg/dL and 3 mg/dL, respectively, may occur frequently in wartime and generally requires dialysis.

Volume Overload

Intractable volume overload in the oliguric patient is the most common indication for dialytic support, and is manifested by progressive weight gain, substantial edema, and, more importantly, by accumulation of fluid in the lungs with progressive hypoxemia. Accumulation of ascitic fluid may further compromise respiratory function. If possible, a diagnosis of intravascular volume overload made on clinical grounds should be corroborated by central venous pressure or hemodynamic monitoring. Although many patients will exhibit salt and water accumulation secondary to adult respiratory distress syndrome, hypoalbuminemia, or myocardial dysfunction, fluid accumulation in these latter circumstances is exceedingly more difficult to remove with an extracorporeal circuit than is true intravascular volume overload. Injudicious use of SCUF or hemodialysis may result in profound hypotension and retard recovery from ARF.

In patients for whom volume removal is intended, blood pressure can be sustained by a number of different maneuvers:

- Many patients are already receiving vasoactive drugs when dialytic support must be provided. Maintenance of a successful extracorporeal circuit may require that these agents be continued, often in higher doses. Dopamine can be used in doses of up to 10 µg/kg/min; higher doses are not usually effective.
- If myocardial performance is depressed as manifested by low cardiac output, then dobutamine, in doses of 1 to 10 µg/kg/min, is the preferred agent. In my experience, there is no added efficacy for the two drugs together compared with their use alone. Levophed, administered as an infusion of 4 µg/min, may be required for severe hypotension, as may be combinations of isoproterenol, epinephrine, or calcium.
- Correction of metabolic acidemia by infusion of sodium bicarbonate may restore response to pressor agents. Salt-poor albumin (25%) will often reverse hypotension on dialysis by mobilizing edema into the vascular space.[102]
- Similarly, packed red blood cells can be administered through the venous line of the dialysis circuit, particularly if the hematocrit is lower than 0.30. There is little to be gained by raising the hematocrit past this point. Higher hematocrit values (*a*) are associated with an increased incidence of membrane clotting and (*b*) reduce the efficiency of the dialysis procedure by increasing plasma oncotic pressure, which tends to retard fluid removal from the blood across the dialysis membrane. However, in general, if the systolic blood pressure cannot be maintained above 100 mm Hg, dialysis will not be possible. Even with SCUF circuits, a mean arterial pressure of at least 60 mm Hg is required.

Metabolic Acidemia

Refractory metabolic acidemia responds to dialysis because organic acids such as lactic acid are readily removed by the dialysis membrane. In addition, the dialysate contains either a base precursor, such as acetate, or a base such as bicarbonate, which diffuses into the patient's blood owing to a favorable concentration gradient. The usual bicarbonate concentration in such situations can range from 25 to 35 mmol/L. Finally, even with SCUF alone, the removal of extracellular fluid will provide space for sodium bicarbonate to be infused into the patient.

Hyperkalemia

Uncorrectable hyperkalemia also favorably responds to dialysis. The removal of potassium is extremely rapid, and overt cardiac toxicity can often be attenuated within the first hour of dialysis. The concentration of potassium in the dialysate should be prescribed for the individual patient. Extremely low potassium dialysate concentrations, such as 0 or 1 mmol/L, should be used only with extreme caution, because rapid shifts of potassium from the blood to the dialysate may be associated with cardiac arrhythmias. It is often more prudent to begin with a 3- to 4-mmol potassium bath and to lower the concentration periodically during the treatment. Although SCUF removes only limited amounts of potassium from the body, removal of extracellular fluid will provide space for the administration of calcium, glucose and insulin, or bicarbonate as necessary.

Uremia

Azotemia is a sign: elevated concentrations of nitrogenous waste products in the blood. Uremia, however, is a syndrome. Thus, patients can be azotemic but not uremic. The detection of severe uremia in critically ill patients can be exceedingly difficult. Classically, uremia is described as a constellation of abnormalities thought to be due to retention of toxins that have not been precisely defined. Elevated concentrations of BUN and creatinine, while considered markers of toxin retention, may not be toxic themselves, as there is not a linear relation between their concentration and the severity of symptoms. Pericarditis, nervous system abnormalities, and bleeding are the typical major clinical features of severe uremia. In general, the medical officer should not attribute any of these disorders to uremia unless the BUN and creatinine concentrations exceed 100 to 120 mg/dL and 6 to 9 mg/dL, respectively. Critically ill patients with ARF will often have coexistent liver, cardiac, hematological, or central nervous system dysfunction from either their primary illness or the effects of drugs or anesthetics. The contribution that renal failure makes in such generalized physiological dysfunction is often hard to determine.

Uremic Pericarditis. Uremic pericarditis may only be manifested by a three-component friction rub, which can be evanescent and extremely difficult to detect in a patient maintained on a ventilator. The electrocardiographic changes that accompany uremic pericarditis are sufficiently nonspecific as to be unhelpful. In the absence of chest pain, this complication of ARF can be extremely difficult to detect, although it may occur in as many as 15% of patients. Although an echocardiogram can readily detect a pericardial effusion, many patients have pericarditis without effusion. Moreover, echocardiograms will not be available in the combat theater. Thus, increasing size of the cardiac silhouette on chest radiograph or progressive hypotension, particularly if the patient is on dialysis, may be the only clues to the presence of uremic pericarditis. The treatment for pericarditis in this setting is the institution or intensification of hemodialysis.[103] Generally, patients will respond quickly to the former. The development of pericarditis in a patient already receiving dialysis for ARF is of concern, and should lead to a search for pericardial infection.

Neurological Abnormalities. The neurological abnormalities seen in ARF are quite diverse and include abnormalities of both central and peripheral nervous system function. Alterations in mental status range from minor abnormalities in sophisticated cortical function to profound coma. The latter is virtually never seen in patients with ARF unless there is a contributing cause besides renal failure. Neuromuscular irritability, manifested by hyperreflexia and clonus, can be seen with severe azotemia. Neurological abnormalities respond only variably to dialysis, because they are seldom caused by renal failure alone. Furthermore, peripheral neuropathies and clonus may be masked by the neuromuscular paralytic agents that are often used in ventilated patients.

Bleeding Disorders. Bleeding disorders occur frequently in patients with ARF. It is been my practice to attempt to determine the precise cause of bleeding rather than to attribute it a priori to uremia. These patients may bleed from any of the disorders that cause bleeding in critically ill patients without ARF. For example, gastrointestinal hemorrhage may be due to stress ulcers or ischemic areas of bowel. There may be deficiencies or inhibitors of coagulation factors. Because dialysis generally requires anticoagulation, it is appropriate to eliminate those causes of bleeding that are not due to renal failure before instituting dialysis. Moreover, if hemodialysis is not available or if the patient must undergo surgery before it can be arranged, nondialytic measures can be attempted. One of the most effective is the infusion of desmopressin acetate, a vasopressin derivative, which is administered at a dose of 0.3 µg/kg in 50 mL of 5% dextrose in water 4 to 6 hours prior to surgery or other intervention. This therapy is more effective than the infusion of fresh frozen plasma and can be repeated several times in a 2- to 3-day period.[104]

It has been known for years that uremia is associated with inhibition of platelet function, so that despite adequate numbers, platelets do not function properly.[105] Bleeding due to uremia is usually diffuse and is manifested by oozing from the gastrointestinal tract as well as from venipuncture sites. Bleeding may also involve serous surfaces such as the pleural and pericardial membranes. Uremic bleeding generally improves with the institution of hemodialysis, although it seldom responds to just one treatment. When hemodialysis is instituted for bleeding, the activated clotting time should be followed carefully, as these patients may require little heparin. Moreover, hypotension during dialysis should be avoided, as it is difficult to determine quickly at the bedside whether it is due to fluid removal or bleeding into the pericardial sac with acute pericardial tamponade, and the hemodialysis treatment may have to be aborted.

Hypercatabolism

Hypercatabolic ARF is the most dramatic form of ARF likely to be encountered after trauma, and is manifested by the rapid development of severe azotemia and concomitant fluid and electrolyte and acid–base disturbances.[106] Rhabdomyolytic-induced ARF commonly results in this syndrome. Casualties with multiple injuries will also occasionally exhibit this picture. Early recognition of the hypercatabolic nature of a patient's ARF is important, as dialytic support, in conjunction with nutrition, is vital if the patient is to have an opportunity to recover. Dialysis is generally begun earlier in this form of ARF than in other forms, as intensive, often daily dialysis is usually required to control metabolic abnormalities. Peritoneal dialysis is ineffective, and SCUF and CAVH are best considered temporizing measures until conventional hemodialysis can be instituted.

Complications of Dialysis

Although the decision to dialyze is made by the nephrologist after the risks and benefits of such therapy are considered, the actual treatment itself is conducted by either a dialysis technician or a nurse. Hemodialysis is associated with a number of potential complications that mandate that it be conducted by trained personnel (Exhibit 26-5).[107] The most common complication is hypotension, which may be seen at any time from the initiation of the treatment until its conclusion. Its management has been previously discussed. Maneuvers to be utilized by dialysis personnel in response to hypotension are outlined by the nephrologist at the onset of each treatment. All agents administered during hemodialysis should be infused into the blood lines distal to the artificial kidney so as to prevent rapid clearance of the drug or clotting of the membrane. Over the first hour of dialysis, the blood flow should gradually be increased from 100 to 125 mL/min to 200 to 250 mL/min. Acutely ill patients may not tolerate higher blood flows; such flows are unnecessary, as very effective dialysis is achieved with blood flows of 250 mL/min.

Other complications are related more to the technical aspects of hemodialysis.[108] These include hemolysis from (*a*) trace metal contamination of the water used for dialysate or (*b*) excessive dialysate temperature. With either situation, the blood in the blood lines becomes a translucent, cranberry red. The procedure must be stopped instantly and the entire extracorporeal circuit discarded. Abnormalities in the electrolyte composition of the dialysate

EXHIBIT 26-5

ACUTE COMPLICATIONS OF HEMODIALYSIS

Hypotension

Disequilibrium syndrome

Hemorrhage

Arrhythmias

Pulmonary dysfunction

Technical errors: dialysate composition, water/air embolism, kidney rupture may result in progressive hyponatremia or hypernatremia: either situation will result in progressive deterioration in the patient's mental status. If a sorbent-based system is used, the dialysis technician should be instructed to conduct dialysis with dialysate composed of bicarbonate as the base, with a sodium concentration of 128 to 130 mmol/L. The dialysate sodium concentration will rise as dialysis proceeds, since the reaction of urea with the zirconium phosphate layer of the sorbent cartridge will liberate sodium into the bath. Dialysate electrolyte composition is monitored on-line with a conductivity meter, however, and malfunction is uncommon. Occasionally, an artificial kidney will have a defective seal and will rupture during the treatment. The blood pump must be stopped instantly and the lines clamped to prevent the patient's exsanguination. Finally, air may enter the circuit from a defective blood line or if the technician uses an "air rinse" to clear the lines at the conclusion of the treatment. Air will be trapped in the patient's right atrium and ventricle, and may result in cardiac collapse. The treatment involves placing the patient on the left side so that the air rises to the top of the cardiac chamber. Small quantities will gradually be reabsorbed, but larger quantities may have to be aspirated by a percutaneously placed intracardiac catheter.

Practical Aspects of Dialysis

Monitoring of the patient during the dialysis procedure is extremely important and is the responsibility of dialysis personnel. Vital signs should be recorded every 15 minutes. Bed scales will not be available in the theater; therefore, the blood pressure and pulse are useful indicators of the patient's ability to tolerate removal of extracellular fluid. Often, overt hypotension will be preceded by an increase in the pulse rate, and should be avoided to prevent ischemia from damaging other organs and further injuring the kidneys. In general, critically ill patients should undergo hemodialysis while on a cardiac monitor, and should receive supplemental oxygen to attenuate the almost universal fall in oxygen tension seen with the treatment. No other treatments, including wound care, should be performed during hemodialysis.

Conversely, SCUF or CAVH-D are prescribed and initiated by nephrologists and dialysis personnel but are conducted by intensive care unit personnel. The nephrologist and dialysis personnel should obtain angioaccess, set the operating parameters of the system, and ensure that the system is operating correctly. Operating parameters to be established include

- the level of anticoagulation that is desired,
- the dosage of heparin that is required to maintain this level,
- limits of ultrafiltration rates that are acceptable, and
- the types and frequency of monitoring techniques that are to be used.

Intensive care personnel should ensure that nurse providers receive in-service training from dialysis personnel, who should remain available for consultation and assistance. However, one of the principal reasons for choosing SCUF or CAVH-D over hemodialysis is that there are relatively few dialysis-trained personnel in the theater. Widespread availability of SCUF and CAVH-D permit dialytic therapy of ARF to be made available to more casualties than could be managed by dialysis personnel alone.

SCUF and CAVH-D are remarkably free of complications, given the severity of illness in the patients to whom these therapies have been applied.[109] Hypotension due to either procedure is uncommon, since the patient's mean arterial pressure is the driving force for ultrafiltration. Should hypotension occur, ultrafiltration will slow down or stop entirely. However, a diminution in the ultrafiltration rate is also a signal that the filter may be clogging with blood clots. If filtration begins to slow, nursing personnel should check both the activated clotting time, to ensure that it is within the prescribed range, and the patient's blood pressure. The only other significant complication of either treatment is bleeding from the catheter sites. This is extremely common in the first few hours after their placement, but will generally respond to a pressure dressing applied for a few hours.

The desired ultrafiltration rate is established by the needs of the patient. In general, most patients will require several hundred milliliters of fluid removal per hour to permit nutrition and antibiotic administration, in addition to removal of the excessive salt and water that have accumulated during the days prior to initiation of the procedure. Fluid removal across a hemofilter is governed by the same Starling forces that govern fluid removal across a capillary. Thus, the forces tending to result in fluid removal include the mean arterial pressure, which is dependent on the blood flow, and the pressure exerted by the column of fluid in the collection tube. Blood flows in a typical patient may range from 60 to 100 mL/min, depending on the type of angioaccess and the size of the cannulated artery. The pressure exerted by the column of fluid in the collection tube depends on the length of the tube. Excessive ultrafiltration can be slowed by shortening this tube. The principal force that retards fluid removal is the oncotic pressure of the blood, which is predicated on the hematocrit and the protein concentration in the blood. Hematocrits greater than 0.30 and plasma protein concentrations greater than 6 to 7 mg/dL are associated with low ultrafiltration rates. The net ultrafiltration rate is a balance between these forces. A convenient method of determining whether ultrafiltration is too excessive is to check the hematocrit at both the arterial and the venous sides of the hemofilter. The arteriovenous difference should not exceed 10% to 15%.

If CAVH-D is being performed, we should remember that a liter of dialysate will be collected each hour, in addition to the volume of ultrafiltrate. Total ultrafiltrate should be measured each hour; this is greatly facilitated by placing a large-capacity collection bag on a small scale so that weight changes can be monitored, rather than volume changes manually measured, each period.

Because SCUF results in an isotonic ultrafiltrate of plasma, the biochemical composition of plasma can be checked simply by sampling the ultrafiltrate periodically. This minimizes the need for peripheral venipunctures in fully anticoagulated patients. However, because CAVH-D results in some diffusive transport, this method is not valid in patients undergoing this form of therapy.

Timing and Frequency of Dialysis

Hemodialysis is an intermittent procedure that requires 3 to 4 hours. It may be required daily in some patients, while two to three treatments per week may suffice in others. With the four goals of dialysis in mind—to maintain relatively normal electrolyte concentrations; predialysis BUN concentration of 80 to 90 mg/dL and creatinine concentration of 6 to 8 mg/dL; extracellular fluid volume that permits required fluid administration and acceptable oxygenation–ventilation parameters; and to eliminate or prevent manifestations of uremia—the decision to dialyze is made anew each day. This decision is made far easier when the patient's biochemical values, weight, and accurate flow sheets are available for the nephrologist on a timely basis. Because dialysis is as scarce a resource as is, for example, the operating room, close coordination between intensivists, surgeons, and nephrologists will permit the patient to receive optimum care.

PROGNOSIS AND OUTCOME OF ACUTE RENAL FAILURE

The mortality of ARF has remained relatively constant since the introduction of dialysis during the Korean War. This fact can be interpreted in different ways:

- Regarding posttraumatic ARF, it is possible that we now provide dialysis to patients who, because of better resuscitation procedures than in the past, might previously have died of shock without ever developing the need for dialysis.
- Regarding patients who develop ARF in the context of nephrotoxic injury or surgery, it is possible that these patients are older and have more associated comorbidity than patients previously offered dialysis.
- Alternatively, dialysis may not contribute to the overall management of patients with ARF, and may represent an expensive, albeit ineffective, technology.

Most nephrologists feel that dialysis does add substantially to the care of patients with ARF, and that our inability to effectively treat infections and the complications of nonrenal organ failure are the principal reasons why the mortality of ARF has remained so high. To provide insight into better ways to treat patients with ARF, I will review some of the extensive experience that has been gained over 4 decades of treatment of ARF. Several studies examined are probably of more historical than practical interest, as they reflect experience of the decades of the 1960s through the 1980s. General improvements in medical intensive care since the mid-1980s have made analysis of older experiences very problematic in terms of applying their conclusions to current patient populations. Recent studies, which incorporate techniques and practices still in use, may provide more useful information.

In 1960, P. E. Teschan and his colleagues[110] reported their experience with prophylactic hemodialysis in the treatment of 15 patients with ARF at the Institute of Surgical Research at Brooke Army Medical Center, San Antonio, Texas. Teschan postulated that the uremic syndrome represented a generalized toxic state in which harmful, albeit dialyzable, substances resulted in cumulative injury of many tissues, leading to sepsis and other complications that would result in death. He reasoned that prophylactic dialysis would remove these toxins and prevent both uremia and its lethal sequelae. He dialyzed patients when their BUN concentrations approached 120 mg/dL, and reported a marked attenuation of uremia, as manifested by improved mental status, appetite, and reduced bleeding. Moreover, he noted an improvement in the resistance to infection and a reduction in the severity of infection.

Teschan's results extended those of R. C. Swann and J. P. Merrill,[13] who in 1953 reported their extensive experience with dialysis of patients with ARF in Boston, Massachusetts. These two reports, in conjunction with reports of the results of dialysis being performed in U.S. military hospitals in Korea, led to the widespread application of dialysis for the treatment of ARF. However, the reports of subsequent experience failed to demonstrate a convincing effect of dialysis on the overall mortality of ARF.

In 1973, A. C. Kennedy and colleagues[111] analyzed their experience with 251 patients with ARF treated between 1959 and 1970, including 133 patients (53.8%) with ARF in the surgical setting. Of this group, 32 (24%) sustained ARF from multiple injuries, while the remainder developed ARF after surgical procedures, generally of the abdomen. The mortality in the trauma group was 50%, while the overall mortality in the group was 58%. One hundred twenty-four of the patients underwent dialysis, including all but one of the patients who sustained multiple trauma. The investigators determined that nearly two thirds of the deaths, particularly in the group sustaining trauma, were due to the effects of the trauma itself. Complications including pneumonia, gastrointestinal hemorrhage, cardiac failure, and sepsis played a role in at least 30% of the deaths. Moreover, when analyzed separately, the investigators believed that sepsis was directly responsible for 40% of all deaths.

In 1972, R. B. Stott and his colleagues[112] reported their experience from 1969 to 1971 with 109 patients with established ARF. While the overall mortality of the group was 57%, the investigators stratified their patients into two ARF groups: medical and surgical-traumatic. The latter group, consisting of 55 patients, experienced a 65% mortality. In patients who had proven sepsis, the mortality was 72%; patients in whom sepsis was not suspected had a mortality of 47%.

In 1978, McMurray and colleagues[113] reported their experience with 276 patients with ARF from 1967 to 1975, of whom 240 required dialysis. There were 117 surgical patients and 49 trauma patients, in whom the mortality was 44% and 35%, respectively. These investigators stratified their patients for complications, and found that survivors experienced a mean of 2.2 complications, while nonsurvivors experienced a mean of 3.8 complications ($P < .001$). In contrast to many studies, these investigators were also able to demonstrate an adverse impact of age: older patients fared significantly worse than younger patients. The impact of advancing age has long been considered a powerful predictor variable, although this has not been demonstrated in all studies.

G. S. Routh and colleagues[114] conducted an analysis of 114 patients who were dialyzed for ARF between 1969 and 1978. In their study, published in 1980, the patients were divided into two groups: 58 patients, primarily with multiple organ failure, who were treated in an intensive care unit, and 56 less severely ill patients, who were treated in a renal intensive care unit. The mortality in the former group was 64%; in the latter group, 37%. These investigators also demonstrated the adverse impact of comorbidity and documented that sepsis was the most common cause of death. Of interest is the fact that ARF itself was believed to be the cause of death in only two patients.

In 1972, D. Kleinknecht and colleagues[115] provided a convincing argument for the aggressive use of dialysis in ARF with a study that compared outcomes in two groups of patients treated with different degrees of dialytic support. These investigators analyzed 500 patients with ARF seen between 1966 and 1970. The patients were divided into two groups of 279 and 221 patients. Patients in Group I, who would serve as historical controls, were dialyzed only when their BUN concentration exceeded 350 mg/dL; patients in Group II underwent early and frequent dialysis to maintain BUN concentrations less than 200 mg/dL, and, for the most part, they received nutritional support. Dialysis exerted a salutary effect on two important parameters: (1) the frequency of gastrointestinal hemorrhage was reduced from 26% in Group I to 18% in Group II ($P < .20$), as was the mortality from such hemorrhage (55% vs 27%, $P < .01$). And (2), although the frequency of sepsis was not altered, the mortality from sepsis decreased from 24% in Group I to 12% in Group II ($P < .02$).

The results of J. D. Conger's[12] experience with intensive hemodialysis in the Vietnam War, published in 1975, were discussed earlier in this chapter; in conjunction with the experience of the investigators cited above, Conger's results were partly responsible for providing an intellectual basis for a change in the way patients with ARF were routinely managed after the early 1970s. From then on it would be usual for patients with substantial ARF to receive dialytic and nutritional support prior to the onset of overt uremia and severe biochemical abnormalities. Notwithstanding the lack of properly designed, prospective, controlled studies comparing patients treated with and without dialysis, studies published during the 1980s on the outcome of ARF reflect this aggressive approach to dialysis, and have largely concentrated on identifying risk factors that affect prognosis. Thus, several studies were published in the 1980s on the outcome of ARF. These studies are important because they reflect the practices that will likely be employed in treating future combat-casualty-associated ARF. These practices include the aggressive use of dialysis, combined with intensive nutritional support, general intensive care management, and powerful antibiotics. The current approach of most nephrologists is based on the concepts of Teschan[110] and Champion[106] and incorporates an aggressive, multidisciplinary approach to patients with posttraumatic ARF.

J. Lien and V. Chan[116] conducted a retrospective analysis of 84 patients with ARF treated by hemodialysis between 1980 and 1984. In their study, published in 1985, the overall mortality was 63.7%. These investigators identified several risk factors that were different between survivors and nonsurvivors, including malnutrition, jaundice, hypotension, the need for assisted ventilation, heart failure, and sepsis.

In 1988, J. W. Lohr, M. J. McFarlane, and J. J. Grantham[117] reported on 126 patients who received dialysis for ARF between 1979 and 1985. Dialysis was routinely employed for BUN and creatinine concentrations greater than 100 and 10 mg/dL, respectively. The overall mortality was 75%, and was dependent on five variables that adversely affected survival: hypotension, assisted ventilation, congestive heart failure, proven or suspected sepsis, and gastrointestinal dysfunction. Moreover, these investigators quantified these covariables and demonstrated an inverse relation between survival and the number of covariables. If no factors were present, the survival was 62%, while if four or more factors were present, the survival was only 2.7%.

Also in 1989, F. Liano, F. A. Garcia-Martin, and A. Gallego[118] published the results of a prospective analysis of their experience with ARF (1979–1985), during which period they studied a cohort of 228 patients, of whom 87 were treated with hemodialysis. These investigators found that coma, hypotension, and the requirement for assisted ventilation adversely affected survival, which was only 44%. None of the patients died of ARF directly.

Finally, in 1986, D. M. Gillum and colleagues,[119] one of whom was J. D. Conger, extended Conger's previous observations on the use of dialysis in ARF by conducting a prospective, controlled study of intensive dialysis in ARF. Thirty-four patients with ARF were matched for etiology and a number of clinical characteristics, including nutrition and other support, and were divided into two groups: the first group received intensive dialysis to maintain BUN and creatinine concentrations less than 60 and 5 mg/dL, respectively; the second group was more routinely dialyzed and maintained BUN and creatinine concentrations less than 100 and 9 mg/dL, respectively. There were no significant differences in complication rates or in mortality, which was 59% in the intensive group and 47% in the nonintensive group. This study has been criticized for its small sample size, however, by proponents of dialysis. Interestingly, some investigators[120] questioned whether hemodialysis, because of its hemodynamic stress, delays the recovery from acute renal failure.

The experience at WRAMC has been similar. We analyzed our experience with 101 patients dialyzed for ARF at WRAMC during the period 1980 through 1985 and published the results in 1985.[101] The overall mortality was 64%, and infection was directly responsible for nearly half the deaths. Our experience since then has corroborated that previous experience. Patients rarely die of pericarditis, gastrointestinal hemorrhage, or other features of uremia itself. They die of infection. The lungs and intra-abdominal viscera are the presumed sites of the majority of these infections, based on the types of organisms recovered from blood cultures. We rarely see lethal infections from the urinary tract or indwelling catheters. Instead, the principal organisms are Gram-negative organisms, which are resistant to many antibiotics, and fungi. These infections are notoriously difficult to treat and are often unresponsive to all forms of antibiotics and antifungal agents. Although there are exceptions, in general, patients who develop ARF and require dialysis either recover in the first 10 to 14 days after the renal failure ensues, or they only rarely recover.[121]

The studies described above have been conducted with the goal of identifying factors that affect prognosis, and have largely been based on cohorts in which dialysis was provided. Despite differences in study design, patient populations, and treatment protocols, the findings are consistent.[122] Risk factors, which appear as covariables in statistical analyses, can be identified that exert a predictable effect on outcome, and the more risk factors that are present, the worse the outcome. Dialysis has not measurably reduced the substantial mortality associated with ARF.

The whole problem of the mortality of ARF and the impact of dialysis on its outcome has been reviewed.[2,123,124] Not surprisingly, the vast majority of the available literature implicates the devastating effects of multiple organ failure and infection on mortality. Little evidence exists to suggest that improvements in the quality or quantity of dialysis would have any impact on outcome. J. S. Cameron[123] summarized the data from a number of different studies, in which the effects of organ failure and sepsis were analyzed for their contribution to mortality. In the aggregate, these data suggest that an identifiable cohort of patients who develop ARF may be doomed despite our best efforts. Predictive functions utilizing clinical variables can predict outcome correctly in 70% to 80% of patients.[49,125] Nonetheless, no predictive equation predicts outcome infallibly, and the datasets on which such equations are based have included patients with substantial comorbidity and advanced age compared with the young, previously healthy soldiers who will develop ARF in wartime. It is possible that casualties in future conflicts who develop ARF will provide the best evidence for the salutary effects of aggressive dialytic and general intensive care support.

SUMMARY

Casualties with ARF are both a medical and a logistical problem for military medical personnel. The condition was first recognized during World War II and has been associated with a persistently high mortality in subsequent conflicts, despite improvements in the evacuation and treatment of casualties with ARF in the theater.

ARF usually results from either ischemic or nephrotoxic injury; commonly, both forms of injury exist in a given casualty. Multiple theories have been advanced regarding the pathophysiology of ARF. None are completely satisfactory, and knowledge of cellular and molecular biology has increased our understanding of this disorder. Both renal ischemia and nephrotoxic injury result in structural and functional abnormalities of the renal epithelium that subserve clinical injury. A number of promising therapeutic maneuvers, many based on a more in-depth understanding of the disorder, are presently in clinical trials and may soon be available for use.

The approach to the patient with suspected ARF involves ensuring adequacy of the volume of the extracellular fluid, patency of the urinary tract, and elimination of all factors that could potentially damage the kidneys. The determination as to whether oliguria results from prerenal, postrenal, or intrinsic renal causes is critical. The diagnosis of ARF can usually be made from the history, physical examination, microscopical and chemical analyses of the urine, and simple radiographic tests. Patients with oliguria should be challenged with graded doses of diuretics, after the extracellular fluid volume has been restored, to promote urinary flow. Patients who do not have oliguria are easier to manage in terms of fluid balance, nutrition, and dialysis requirements. Nutritional support is an important aspect of the care of the patient with ARF, who requires a relatively large amount of energy delivered in a small volume of fluid.

The therapeutic options available for casualties with established ARF include conservative management and dialysis. A number of different types of dialysis care are available, including conventional hemodialysis and peritoneal dialysis. With newer, more biocompatible membranes, hemofiltration, ultrafiltration, or a combination of these treatments can be used. The indications for hemodialysis include intractable metabolic and circulatory volume abnormalities. Absolute contraindications include refractory hypotension and having been triaged as expectant. Despite the widespread availability of dialysis, the mortality of combat- and trauma-associated ARF remains high. The most common cause of death is infection, usually associated with multiple organ failure.

The casualty with ARF is a formidable medical and logistical challenge. Despite advancements in our knowledge of renal disease, the mortality of ARF remains high. We can expect improvement in the outcome of this disorder when we have better ways to prevent and treat infection and multiple organ failure.

REFERENCES

1. Anderson RJ, Linas SL, Berns AS, et al. Nonoliguric acute renal failure. *N Engl J Med*. 1977;296:1134–1138.

2. Diamond JR, Yoburn DC. Nonoliguric acute renal failure. *Arch Intern Med*. 1982;142:1882–1884.

3. Corwin HL, Bonventre JV. Factors influencing survival in acute renal failure. *Semin Dialysis*. 1989;2:220–225.

4. Bywaters EG, Beall D. Crush injuries with impairment of renal function. *Br Med J*. 1941;1:427–432.

5. Butkus DE. Persistent high mortality in acute renal failure: Are we asking the right questions? *Arch Intern Medicine*. 1983;143:209–212.

6. Butkus DE. Post-traumatic acute renal failure in combat casualties: A historical review. *Milit Med*. 1984;149:117–124.

7. Beecher HK, ed. The Board for the Study of the Severely Wounded, North African–Mediterranean Theater of Operations. *The Physiologic Effects of Wounds*. In: *Surgery in World War II*. Washington, DC: US Department of the Army Medical Department, Office of The Surgeon General; 1952.

8. Teschan PE, Post RS, Smith LH, et al. Post-traumatic renal insufficiency in military casualties, I: Clinical characteristics. *Am J Med*. 1955;18:172–186.

9. Teschan PE, Post RS, Smith LH, et al. Post-traumatic renal insufficiency in military casualties, II: Management, use of an artificial kidney, prognosis. *Am J Med*. 1955;18:187–198.

10. Stone WJ, Knepshield JH. Post-traumatic acute renal insufficiency in Vietnam. *Clin Neph*. 1974;2:186–190.

11. Lordon RE, Burton JR. Post-traumatic renal failure in military personnel in Southeast Asia. *Am J Med*. 1972;53:137–147.

12. Conger JD. A controlled evaluation of prophylactic dialysis in post-traumatic acute renal failure. *J Trauma*. 1975;15:1056–1063.

13. Swann RC, Merrill JP. The clinical course of acute renal failure. *Medicine*. 1953;32:215–292.

14. Fischer RP, Polk HC. Changing etiologic patterns of renal insufficiency in surgical patients. *Surg Gynecol Obstet*. 1975;140:85–86.

15. Shin B, Mackenzie CF, Cowely RA. Changing patterns of posttraumatic acute renal failure. *The American Surgeon*. 1979;3:182–189.

16. Decamp ME, Demling RH. Posttraumatic multisystem organ failure. *JAMA*. 1988;260:530–534.

17. Finn WF. Recovery from acute renal failure. In: Brenner BM, Lazarus M. *Acute Renal Failure*. Philadelphia, Pa: WB Saunders; 1983: 753–771.

18. Scotti MJ, chairman. Defense Medical Standardization Board. *DEPMEDS Policies/Guidelines: Treatment Briefs*. Fort Detrick, Frederick, Md: 1990.

19. Collins AJ. Kidney dialysis treatment for victims of the Armenian earthquake. *N Engl J Med*. 1989;320:1292–1292.

20. Harrington JT, Cohen JJ. Current concepts: Acute oliguria. *N Engl J Med*. 1975;292:89–91.

21. Levinsky NG. Pathophysiology of acute renal failure. *N Engl J Med*. 1977;296:1453–1458.

22. Stein JH, Lifschitz MD, Barnes LD. Current concepts on the pathophysiology of acute renal failure. *Am J Physiol*. 1978;234:F171–181.

23. Schrier RW. Acute renal failure. *Kidney Int*. 1979;15:205–216.

24. Oken DE. On the differential diagnosis of acute renal failure. *Am J Med*. 1981;71:916–920.

25. Oken DE. Hemodynamic basis for human acute renal failure (vasomotor nephropathy). *Am J Med*. 1984;76:702–710.

26. Wilkes BM, Mailloux LU. Acute renal failure: Pathogenesis and prevention. *Am J Med*. 1986;80:1129–1136.

27. Myers BD, Moran SM. Hemodynamically mediated acute renal failure. *N Engl J Med*. 1986;314:97–105.

28. Anderson RJ, Schrier RW. Acute tubular necrosis. In: Schrier RW, Gottschalk, CW, eds. *Diseases of the Kidney*. 4th ed. Boston, Mass: Little, Brown; 1988: 1413–1446.

29. Badr KF, Ichikawa I. Prerenal failure: A deleterious shift from renal compensation to decompensation. *N Engl J Med*. 1988;319:623–629.

30. Kon V, Yared A, Ichikawa I. Role of renal sympathetic nerves in mediating hypoperfusion of renal cortical microcirculation in experimental congestive heart failure and acute extracellular fluid volume depletion. *J Clin Invest*. 1985;76:1913–1920.

31. Weinberg JM. The cellular basis of nephrotoxicity. In: Schrier RW, Gottschalk, CW, eds. *Diseases of the Kidney*. 4th ed. Boston, Mass: Little, Brown; 1988: 1137–1196.

32. Molitoris BA, Falk SA, Dahl RH. Ischemia-induced loss of epithelial polarity: Role of the tight junction. *J Clin Invest*. 1989;84:1334–1339.

33. Cunarro JA, Schultz SE, Johnson WA, Weiner MW. Effects of ischemia on metabolite concentrations in dog renal cortex. *Renal Physiol*. 1982;5:143–155.

34. Cheung JY, Bonventre JV, Malis CD, Leaf A. Calcium and ischemic injury. *N Engl J Med*. 1986;314:1670–1675.

35. Burke TJ, Arnold PE, Gordon JA, Bulger RE, Dobyan DC, Schrier RW. Protective effect of intrarenal calcium membrane blockers before or after renal ischemia. *J Clin Invest*. 1984;74:1830–1841.

36. Siegel NJ, Gaudio KM, Cooper K, et al. Accelerating recovery from acute renal failure: Exogenous metabolic augmentation. *Mol Physiol*. 1985;8:593–598.

37. Schrier RW, Arnold PE, Van Putten VJ, Burke TJ. Cellular calcium in ischemic acute renal failure: Role of calcium entry blockers. *Kidney Int*. 1987;32:313–321.

38. Weisfeldt ML. Reperfusion and reperfusion injury. *Clin Res*. 1987;35:13–20.

39. Southorn PA, Powis G. Free radicals in medicine, I: Chemical nature and biologic reactions. *Mayo Clin Proc*. 1988;63:381–389.

40. Southorn PA, Powis G. Free radicals in medicine, II: Involvement in human disease. *Mayo Clin Proc*. 1988;63:390–408.

41. Cunningham SK, Keaveny TV, Fitzgerald P. Effect of allopurinol on tissue ATP, ADP and AMP concentrations in renal ischemia. *Br J Surg*. 1974;61:562–565.

42. Paller MS, Hoidal JR, Ferris TF. Oxygen free radicals in ischemic acute renal failure in the rat. *J Clin Invest*. 1984;74:1156–1164.

43. Kraman S, Khan F, Patel S. Renal failure in the respiratory care unit. *Crit Care Med*. 1979;7:263–268.

44. Meyers BD, Miller DC, Mehigan JT. Nature of the renal injury following total renal ischemia in man. *J Clin Invest*. 1984;73:329–341.

45. Lifshiftz MD. Renal effects of non-steroidal anti-inflammatory agents. *Lab Clin Med.* 1983;102:313–318.

46. Moore RD, Smith CR, Lipsky JJ, Mellits ED, Lietman PS. Risk factors for nephrotoxicity in patients treated with aminoglycosides. *Ann Intern Med.* 1984;100:352–357.

47. Llach F, Felsenfeld AJ, Haussler MR. The pathophysiology of altered calcium metabolism in rhabdomyolysis-induced acute renal failure. *N Engl J Med.* 1981;305:117–123.

48. Miller TR, Anderson RJ, Linas SL, et al. Urinary diagnostic indices in acute renal failure: A prospective study. *Ann Intern Med.* 1978;89:45–50.

49. Hou SH, Bushinsky DA, Wish JB, Cohen JJ, Harrington JT. Hospital-acquired renal insufficiency: A prospective study. *Am J Med.* 1983;74:243–248.

50. Rasmussen HH, Ibels LS. Acute renal failure: Multivariate analysis of causes and risk factors. *Am J Med.* 1982;73:211–218.

51. Jochimsen F, Schafer J, Maurer A, Distler A. Impairment of renal function in medical intensive care: Predictability of acute renal failure. *Crit Care Med.* 1990;18:480–485.

52. Kim V, Kark AE, Rudick J. Factors influencing mortality in surgical treatment for massive gastroduodenal hemorrhage. *Am J Gastro.* 1974;62:24–30.

53. Krug H, Raszeja-Wnic B, Wochowiak A. Intravascular coagulation in acute renal failure after myocardial infarction. *Ann Intern Med.* 1974;81:494–498.

54. DiBona GF. Hemodynamic support: Volume management and pharmacological cardiovascular support. *Semin Nephrol.* 1994;14:33–40.

55. Eneas F, Schoenfeld PY, Humphreys MH. The effect of infusion of mannitol–sodium bicarbonate on the clinical course of myoglobinuria. *Arch Int Med.* 1979;139:801–804.

56. Hayes DM, Cvitkovic E, Golbey RB. High dose cis-platinum diammine dichloride: Amelioration of renal toxicity by mannitol diuresis. *Cancer.* 1977;39:1372–1377.

57. Fischereder M, Trick W, Nath KA. Therapeutic strategies in the prevention of acute renal failure. *Semin Neph.* 1994;14:41–52.

58. Brown CB, Ogg CS, Cameron JS. High dose frusemide in acute renal failure: A controlled trial. *Clin Neph.* 1981;15:90–96.

59. Kleinknecht D, Ganeval D, Gonzalez-Duque LA, Fermanian J. Furosemide in acute oliguric renal failure: A controlled trial. *Nephron.* 1976;17:51–58.

60. Nierenberg DW. Furosemide and ethacrynic acid in acute tubular necrosis. *Western J Med.* 1980;133:163–170.

61. Barry KG, Cohen A, Knochel JP, et al. Mannitol infusion, II: The prevention of acute functional renal failure during resection of an aneurysm of the abdominal aorta. *N Engl J Med.* 1961;264:967–971.

62. Flores J, DiBona DR, Beck CH, Leaf A. The role of cell swelling in ischemic renal damage and the protective effect of hypertonic solute. *J Clin Invest.* 1972;51:118–126.

63. Lindner A, Cutler RE, Goodman WG. Synergism of dopamine plus furosemide in preventing acute renal failure in the dog. *Kidney Int.* 1979;16:158–166.

64. Pass LJ, Eberhart RC, Brown JC, Rohn GN, Estrera AS. The effect of mannitol and dopamine on the renal response to thoracic aortic cross-clamping. *J Thorac Cardiovasc Surg.* 1988;95:608–612.

65. Davis RF, Lappas DG, Kirklin JK, Buckley MJ, Lowenstein E. Acute oliguria after cardiopulmonary bypass: Renal functional improvement with low-dose dopamine infusion. *Crit Care Med.* 1982;10:852–856.

66. Polson RJ, Park GR, Lindop MJ, Farman JV, Calne RY, WIlliams R. The prevention of renal impairment in patients undergoing orthotopic liver grafting by infusion of low dose dopamine. *Anesthesia.* 1987;42:15–19.

67. Siegel NJ, Glazier WB, Chaudry IH, et al. Enhanced recovery from acute renal failure by the postischemic infusion of adenine nucleotides and magnesium chloride in rats. *Kidney Int.* 1980;17:338–349.

68. Stromski ME, Cooper K, Thulin G, et al. Postischemic ATP-$MgCl_2$ provides precursors for resynthesis of cellular ATP in rats. *Am J Physiol.* 1986;250:F834–837.

69. Schrier RW, Burke TJ. Calcium-channel blockers in experimental and human acute renal failure. *Adv Nephrol.* 1988;17:287–300.

70. Schneeberger H, Illner WD, Abendroth D, et al. First experience with superoxide dismutase in kidney transplantation—Results of a double-blind randomized study. *Trans Proc.* 1989;21:1245–1246.

71. Paller MS Hedlund BE. Role of iron in postischemic renal injury in the rat. *Kidney Int.* 1988;34:474–480.

72. Knochel JP. Rhabdomyolysis and myoglobinuria. *Semin Neph.* 1981;1:75–86.

73. Grossman RA, Hamilton RW, Morse BM. Non-traumatic rhabdomyolysis and acute renal failure. *N Engl J Med.* 1974;291:807–811.

74. Braun SR, Weiss FR, Keller AI, Preuss HG. Evaluation of the renal toxicity of heme proteins and their derivatives: A role in the genesis of acute tubular necrosis. *J Exp Med.* 1970;131:443–460.

75. Silva H, Pomeroy J, Rae AI, Rosen SM, Shaldon S. Daily hemodialysis in "hypercatabolic" acute renal failure. *Br Med J.* 1964;2:407–410.

76. Seidner DL, Matarese LE, Steiger E. Nutritional care of the critically ill patient with renal failure. *Semin Neph.* 1994;14:53–63.

77. Lee HA, Sharpstone P, Ames AC. Parenteral nutrition in renal failure. *Postgrad Med.* 1967;43:81–87.

78. Abel RM, Beck CH, Abbot WM, Ryan JA, Barnett GO, Fischer JE. Improved survival from acute renal failure after treatment with intravenous essential L-amino acids and glucose. *N Engl J Med.* 1973;288:965–969.

79. Baek SM, Makabali GG, Bryan-Brown CW. The influence of parenteral nutrition on the course of acute renal failure. *Surg Gynecol Obstet.* 1975;141:405–411.

80. Wesson DE, Mitch WE, Wilmore DW. Nutritional considerations in the treatment of acute renal failure. In: Brenner BM, Lazarus M. *Acute Renal Failure.* Philadelphia, Pa: WB Saunders; 1983: 618–642.

81. Askanazi J, Nordenstrom MD, Rosenbaum SH, et al. Nutrition for the patient with respiratory failure: Glucose vs fat. *Anesthesiology.* 1981;54:373–377.

82. Rosen H, Meroney WH, Levenson SM. Plasma amino acids in patients with renal failure: Effect of extracorporeal hemodialysis. *Clin Sci.* 1958;17:653–666.

83. Cerra FB, Shronts EP, Kostantinides NN. Enteral feeding in sepsis: A prospective randomized, double-blind trial. *Surgery.* 1985;98:632–639.

84. Hood VL, Tannen RL. Lactic acidosis. *The Kidney* (National Kidney Foundation). 1989;22(1):1–6.

85. Cooper DJ, Walley KR, Wiggs BR, Russell JA. Bicarbonate does not improve hemodynamics in critically ill patients who have lactic acidosis. *Ann Intern Med.* 1990;112:492–498.

86. Shavelle HS, Parke R. Postoperative metabolic alkalosis and acute renal failure: Rationale for the use of hydrochloric acid. *Surgery*. 1975;78(4):439–445.

87. Adrogue HJ, Madias NE. Changes in plasma potassium concentration during acute acid–base disturbances. *Am J Med*. 1981;71:456–467.

88. Rubin MF, Narins RG. Hypophosphatemia: Pathophysiological and practical aspects of its therapy. *Semin Nephrol*. 1990;10:536–545.

89. Twardowski SJ. Blood purification in acute renal failure. *Ann Intern Med*. 1984;100:447–449. Editorial.

90. Lohr JW, Schwab SJ. Minimizing hemorrhagic complications in dialysis patients. *J Am Soc Nephrol*. 1991;2:961–975.

91. Shapiro WB. The current status of sorbent hemodialysis. *Semin Dialysis*. 1990;3:40–45.

92. Firmat J, Zucchini A. Peritoneal dialysis in acute renal failure. *Contrib Nephrol*. 1979;17:33–38.

93. Tzamaloukas AH, Garella S, Chazan JA. Peritoneal dialysis for acute renal failure after major abdominal surgery. *Arch Surg*. 1973;106:639–643.

94. Kaplan AA, Longnecker RE, Folkert VW. Continuous arteriovenous hemofiltration: A report of six months' experience. *Ann Intern Med*. 1984;100:358–367.

95. Synhaivsky A, Kurtz SB, Wochos DN, Schniepp BJ, Johnson WJ. Acute renal failure treated by slow continuous ultrafiltration. *Mayo Clin Proc*. 1983;58:729–733.

96. Ronco C, Brendolan A, Bragantini L, et al. Arteriovenous hemodiafiltration associated with continuous arteriovenous hemofiltration: A combined therapy for acute renal failure in the hypercatabolic patient. *Blood Purif*. 1987;5:33–40.

97. Pattison ME, Lee SM, Ogden DA. Continuous arteriovenous hemodiafiltration: An aggressive approach to the management of acute renal failure. *Am J Kid Dis*. 1988;11(1):43–47.

98. Dicarlo JV, Dudley TE, Sherbotie JR, Kaplan BS, Costinaro AT. Continuous arteriovenous hemofiltration/dialysis improves pulmonary gas exchange in children with multiple organ system failure. *Crit Care Med*. 1990;18:822–826.

99. Voerman HJ, Strack van Schijndel RJ, Thijs LG. Continuous arterial-venous hemodiafiltration in critically ill patients. *Crit Care Med*. 1990;18:911–914.

100. Carson JL. Clinical competence in continuous arteriovenous hemofiltration. *Ann Intern Med*. 1988;108:900–902.

101. Bennett R, Hodder R, Gouge S, Moore J. Acute renal failure: Impact of etiology and treatment on outcome. *Kidney Int*. 1985;27;133A.

102. Jardin F, Prost JF, Ozier Y, Margairaz A. Hemodialysis in septic patients: Improvement in tolerance of fluid removal with concentrated albumin as the priming fluid. *Crit Care Med*. 1982;10:650–652.

103. Renfrew R, Buselmeier TJ, Kjellstrand CM. Pericarditis and renal failure. *Ann Rev Med*. 1980;31:345–360.

104. Mannucci PM, Remuzzi G, Pusineri F, et al. Deamino-8-D-arginine vasopressin shortens the bleeding time in uremia. *N Engl J Med*. 1983;308: 8–12.

105. Minno GD, Martinez J, McKean M, De La Rosa J, Burke JF, Murphy S. Platelet dysfunction in uremia. *Am J Med*. 1985;79:552–559.

106. Champion H, Long W, Smith H, et al. Indications of early hemodialysis in multiple trauma. *Lancet*. 1974;1: 1125–1127.

107. Carson JL. Clinical competence in acute hemodialysis. *Ann Intern Med*. 1988;108:632–634.

108. Bregman H, Daugirdas JT, Ing TS. Complications during hemodialysis. In: Daugirdas JT, Ing TS, eds. *Handbook of Dialysis*. Boston, Mass: Little, Brown; 1994: 149–168.

109. Golper TA. Continuous arteriovenous hemofiltration in acute renal failure. *Am J Kid Dis*. 1985;6:373–386.

110. Teschan PE, Baxter CR, O'Brien TF, Freyhof JN, Hall WH. Prophylactic hemodialysis in the treatment of acute renal failure. *Ann Intern Med*. 1960;53:992–1016.

111. Kennedy AC, Burton JA, Luke RG, et al. Factors affecting the prognosis in acute renal failure. *Quart J Med*. 1973;165:73–86.

112. Stott RB, Cameron JS, Ogg CS, Bewick M. Why the persistently high mortality in acute renal failure? *Lancet*. 1972;2:75–79.

113. McMurray SD, Luft FC, Maxwell DR, et al. Prevailing patterns and predictor variables in patients with acute tubular necrosis. *Arch Intern Med*. 1978;138:950–955.

114. Routh GS, Briggs JD, Mone JG, Ledingham IM. Survival from acute renal failure with and without multiple organ dysfunction. *Quart J Med*. 1980;56:244–247.

115. Kleinknecht D, Jungers P, Chanard J, Barbanel C, Ganeval D. Uremic and non-uremic complications in acute renal failure: Evaluation of early and frequent dialysis on prognosis. *Kidney Int*. 1972;1:190–196.

116. Lien J, Chan V. Risk factors influencing survival in acute renal failure treated by hemodialysis. *Arch Intern Med*. 1985;145:2067–2069.

117. Lohr JW, McFarlane MJ, Grantham JJ. A clinical index to predict survival in acute renal failure patients requiring dialysis. *Am J Kid Dis*. 1988;11(3):254–259.

118. Liano F, Garcia-Martin FA, Gallego A. Easy and early prognosis an acute tubular necrosis: A forward analysis of 228 cases. *Nephron*. 1989;51:307–313.

119. Gillum DM, Dixon BS, Yanover MJ, et al. The role of intensive dialysis in acute renal failure. *Clin Neph*. 1986;5:249–255.

120. Conger JD. Does hemodialysis delay recovery from acute renal failure? *Semin Dialysis*. 1990;3:146–148.

121. Spurney RF, Fulkerson WJ, Schwab SJ. Acute renal failure in critically ill patients: Prognosis for recovery of kidney function after prolonged dialysis support. *Crit Care Med*. 1991;19:8–11.

122. Halstenberg WK, Goormastic M, Paganini EP. Utility of risk models for renal failure and critically ill patients. *Semin Nephrol*. 1994;14:23–32.

123. Cameron JS. Acute renal failure—The continuing challenge. *Quart J Med*. 1986;228:337–343.

124. Smithies MN, Cameron JS. Can we predict outcome in acute renal failure? *Nephron*. 1989;51:297–300.

125. Rasmussen HH, Pitt EA, Ibels LS, McNeil DR. Prediction of outcome in acute renal failure by discriminant analysis of clinical variables. *Arch Intern Med*. 1985;145:2105–2018.

Chapter 27

MILITARY MEDICAL EVACUATION

COLIN A. B. McLAREN, QHP, MB, ChB, FC ANAES*; LOUIS M.GUZZI, M.D.†; AND RONALD F. BELLAMY, M.D.‡

*Formerly, Air Commodore, Consultant Adviser Anaesthetics, The Royal Air Force (ret); Central Medical Establishment, Kelvin House, Cleveland Street, London, W1P 5FB, England; Currently, Consultant Anaesthetist, 12 Broadacres, Broad Town, Wootton Bassett, Wiltshire, SN4 7RP, England

†Major, Medical Corps, U.S. Army; Chief, Combat Trauma Research, Walter Reed Army Institute of Research, Washington, D. C. 20307-5100

‡Colonel, Medical Corps, U.S. Army; Managing Editor and Officer in Charge, Textbook of Military Medicine, Borden Institute, Walter Reed Army Medical Center, Washington, D. C. 20307-5001

INTRODUCTION

Unless an army is prepared to deploy its major medical assets, including its hospitals, into the middle of a battlefield, it must be capable of carrying out that "undeniable but unavoidable evil of evacuation of the sick and wounded,"[1] in the words of Nikolai I. Pirogov, one of the founders of 19th century military surgery. Pirogov's use of the word "evil" may seem extreme, but harmful effects can arise during evacuation, especially when it is viewed simply as transportation.

That military medical evacuation is more than transportation is clear from its official definition. According to U.S. Army Field Manual (FM) 8-10-6, *Medical Evacuation in a Theater of Operations*, military medical evacuation includes[2(p4-1)]:

- collecting the wounded,
- performing triage,
- providing an evacuation mode or transportation,
- providing medical care en route, and
- anticipating complications and being ready to perform emergency medical interventions.

Evacuation is not an end in itself but, at a minimum, is a tool that makes possible more effective treatment. At the same time, by allowing the deployment of the most logistically demanding, immobile, and vulnerable medical assets far to the rear, evacuation simplifies the commander's combat service support mission. Ideally, treatment is ongoing during evacuation.

Implicit in the official definition of medical evacuation is the fact that the act of evacuating casualties covers a wide spectrum of contingencies that range from

- manual evacuation (by two-man carry) of the casualty to a sheltered site 100 m distant, to
- ground ambulance evacuation to a battalion aid station several kilometers distant, to
- helicopter evacuation to a mobile army surgical hospital (MASH) 30 km distant, to
- *intra*theater (ie, tactical) aeromedical evacuation by fixed-wing aircraft to a communication zone hospital 300 km distant, to
- *inter*theater (ie, strategic) aeromedical evacuation by long-range transport to a hospital in the zone of the interior 10,000 km distant.

Not surprisingly, the indications for evacuation, the medical diagnoses of the evacuees, and the differing technical characteristics of the means of evacuation interact to produce a variety of potential medical treatment problems. However, certain basic medical truths predicated on human anatomy and physiology remain constant and cannot be ignored without dire consequences for the casualty. The potential medical "evil" of evacuation, especially that which may arise from the physiological threat of aeromedical evacuation, is the primary subject of this chapter.

HISTORY

Most ancient armies had medical staffs to look after their sick and wounded, but it would seem that their chief responsibility was to attend to the well-being of officers and princes.[3] The problems of removing the sick and wounded from the battlefield were probably not viewed as one of the functions of the medical staff but rather as a logistical problem that needed to be solved: the dead and dying on the battlefield interfered with the fighting. Such considerations no doubt motivated the first well-documented instance of evacuation, namely, when Scipio temporarily broke off his ultimately successful attack on Hannibal in the climactic battle of the Second Punic War at Zama in 202 BC:

> The space between the two corps which still remained on the field was by now covered with blood, corpses, and wounded men, and the physical obstacle created by the enemy's rout presented a difficult problem to the Roman general. Everything combined to make it hard for him to advance without losing formation: the ground slippery with gore, the corpses lying in blood-drenched heaps, and the spaces between encumbered with arms that had been thrown away at random. However, Scipio first arranged for his wounded to be carried to the rear....[4(p477)]

It is unclear when the rationale for evacuation was first looked on as medical rather than as the logistical process of "clearing the battlefield." Certainly by the Napoleonic era, some military surgeons recognized that early evacuation from the battlefield even before the fighting had ended was a necessary prerequisite for effective treatment. Foremost among them was Dominique-Jean Larrey, who was surgeon to Napoleon's Imperial Guard.

Larrey's recognition of the need to improve evacuation preceded any of Napoleon's battles, and he presented his conclusions regarding evacuation at a conference held on 17 November 1789. This conference was convened in Paris by the National Convention of the Revolution to study Larrey's report describing the medical treatment of French troops fighting in the battles of Limbourg and Speyer.[5] At this time, the treatment, or lack of it, depended on the result of the battle: success meant that the casualty would receive some sort of treatment, albeit 48 hours after wounding, whereas defeat meant no care and almost certain death.

Larrey pursued his ideas despite his initial lack of success. He developed the use of horse-drawn vehicles to evacuate the sick and wounded from the battlefield via the *ambulance volante* (ie, flying ambulance), which was first used in 1797 on the battlefield of Konigstein, in the Taunus mountains of the Rhineland Palatinate. Although Larrey's flying ambulances were available in only a tiny part of Napoleon's army, their ability to provide rapid and humane evacuation was widely recognized. James McGrigor, Wellington's outstanding chief medical officer in the Peninsular campaign, in attempting to justify the acquisition of similar vehicles, wrote the following classic description of evacuation gone wrong:

> The suffering of the sick and wounded was very great.... They suffered so much by the transport [ie, slow, clumsy ox-carts—*RFB*], the weather, and the privation...that...many of the wounded and those ill of dysentery arrived in so bad a state as only to survive a few days....[6(p121)]

Other modes of transportation were adopted for the evacuation of casualties during the 19th century. Florence Nightingale was instrumental in organizing hospital ships to evacuate the sick and wounded during the Crimean War. (The first reports of the use of ships for the transfer of the wounded had occurred during the Eighth Crusade, when galleys were used to move them to Damietta.[3]) At the same time, the rapid growth of railways as the principal mode of transportation offered an alternative. Given the appalling state of the roads in any battle area and the congestion of vehicles traveling to the battle area (causing delays with the ambulances traveling in the opposite direction), and the ever-increasing size and complexity of the rail networks, it is not surprising that several countries investigated the possibility of using the railway systems to permit rapid evacuation of large numbers of sick and wounded in warmth, light, and relative comfort, where they could continue receiving medical and nursing care.

The first examples of medical evacuation by rail occurred in 1859, during the Italian War, when large numbers of French casualties were moved via railway. The seriously wounded were transported in baggage cars, the less seriously wounded in passenger cars.[3] During the American Civil War, many attempts were made to organize a satisfactory evacuation service using railway trains. After many experiments, the Union Army developed a well-organized ambulance train service, which, as well as carrying the sick and wounded, had facilities to maintain treatment and provide catering during the journey. In some of the campaigns, the distance from the front line to the base hospitals was several hundred miles. In 1864, the Army of the Cumberland River made use of three trains per day to transfer the sick and wounded back to Louisville, Kentucky. The Confederate forces were not so lucky: only irregular service was available, with none of the amenities available to the Union forces.[3]

Owing to the leadership of Jonathan Letterman, the chief medical officer of the Army of the Potomac, by the end of the American Civil War military medical evacuation was seen as a systematic process to be carried out by a dedicated corps of specialists under the command and control of the medical department. Letterman's influence was such that he was able to get the U.S. Congress to enact a law codifying the organization and function of ambulance corps and ambulance trains.[7] Many of the subsequent developments in military medical evacuation revolved around the technical characteristics of the evacuation vehicles, but the correctness of Letterman's doctrinal and organizational innovations is still considered beyond dispute.

By the second half of the 20th century, aircraft had become the preferred evacuation vehicle in western armies, but use and acceptance came slowly. The first aircraft did not fly until 1903; however, the future use of rapid air transport of the sick and wounded had already been conceived by imaginative minds:

- Jules Verne, in his book *Robert le Conquerant*, published in 1854, described the use of an airship to rescue injured and shipwrecked seamen.[8]
- War historians have described the use of hot-air balloons to evacuate the sick and wounded during the siege of Paris during the Franco–Prussian War (1870–1871); unfortunately, however, this romantic description cannot be supported by fact.[9]
- In the last decade of the 19th century, the Dutch Surgeon General de Mooy described and illustrated his concepts of air evacuation (Figure 27-1).

Only 7 years after the Wright brothers' first flight, two U.S. Army officers had developed an airplane for the transport of casualties but the venture did not receive War Department backing. A second attempt to obtain U.S. Army funding for the construction of an airplane to transport the severely wounded was made during a conference in Baltimore, Maryland, only to be followed by an editorial in the following day's *Baltimore Sun* (23 October 1912) that stated: "Surely the hazard of being severely wounded was sufficient without the additional hazard of transportation by airplane."[10] A similar fate followed the first demonstration flight in the United Kingdom, which took place in 1913 and lasted exactly 45 seconds. The surrogate patient's shouts of fear as he slid gently across the wing toward the pusher propeller caused a rapid landing and a complete lack of interest by the army general staff who were present.[11]

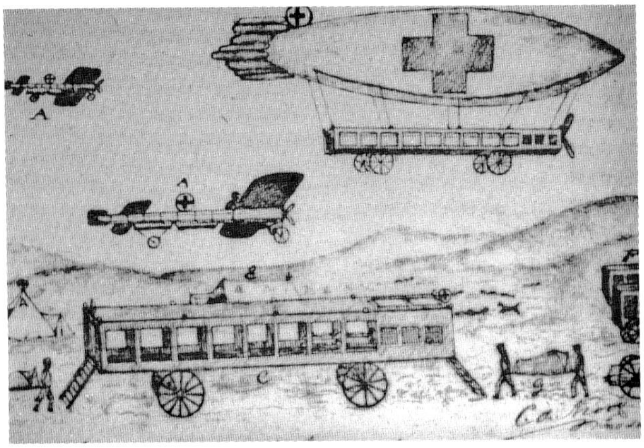

Fig. 27-1. Aeromedical evacuation as envisioned by Dutch Surgeon General de Mooy during the late 19th century. Photograph: Reprinted from Vincent A. Le transport des blesses par avion. *Rev Int Croix Rouge*. 1924;6:720–723.

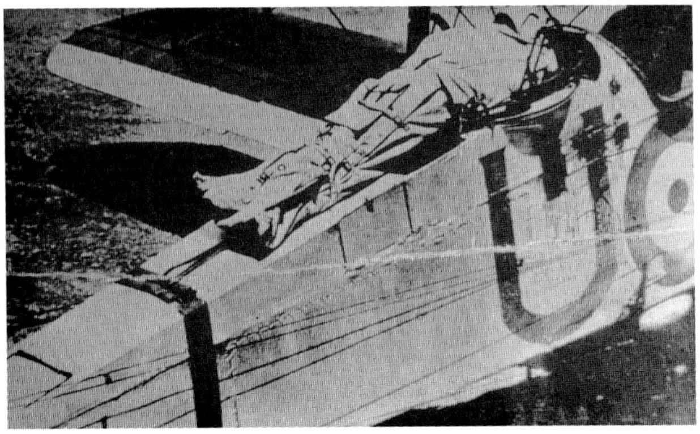

Fig. 27-2. Rarely, aircraft were used to evacuate casualties during World War I. Reprinted from Andrews DR. Helicopter ambulances in critical care. *J R Army Med Corps*. 1994:140:22.

Aircraft were used to evacuate casualties during World War I (Figure 27-2), but the first use of an airplane specifically modified for casualty evacuation appears to have occurred in 1920 during a British expedition to what is now Somalia.[12] The mass transportation of sick and wounded by air first occurred during the Spanish Civil War (1936) and was carried out by the newly formed German Luftwaffe. The Condor Squadrons, flying unheated and unpressurized Junkers JU 52s, transported sick and wounded back to Germany in a few hours rather than the days that would have been required for road, rail, and sea transport.[13] The resulting improvement in the morale of the sick and wounded were exactly the same as Larrey had described 140 years earlier.[14] The full development of German aeromedical evacuation occurred during the early years of World War II and especially during the Russo–German campaign, where the great distances made evacuation by air especially desirable (Figure 27-3).

During the fall of 1942, far-sighted U.S. military medical authorities, in recognition of the value of aeromedical evacuation, established three patient categories that would justify trans-Atlantic evacuation to the continental United States (CONUS): (1) emergency cases for whom essential treatment was not locally available, (2) casualties whose air evacuation the chief surgeon deemed a military necessity, and (3) casualties who required prolonged hospital and convalescent care. Nevertheless, by the end of 1943, only 116 patients had been evacuated by air from the European Theater of Operations. By the last year of the European war, from 2,000 to 4,000 casualties per month were being evacuated to CONUS by air. This number, although large, needs to

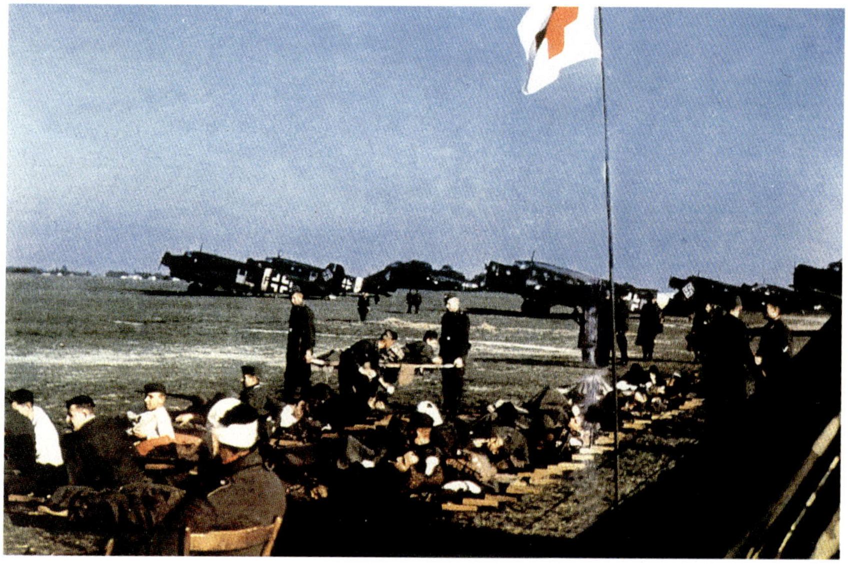

Fig. 27-3. A German aeromedical staging base in the southern portion of the eastern front during 1943. The JU 52s shown here could carry up to 12 litter casualties; their short takeoff and landing capability were impressive (the minimum runway length was about 400 m). The relatively idyllic circumstance shown here was exceptional. More representative of German aeromedical evacuation was the situation at Stalingrad during the great battle in 1942–1943, in which 25,000 German casualties were evacuated under appalling weather conditions and in the face of overwhelming Soviet military strength. Reprinted with permission from Carell P. *Der Russlandkrieg: Fotografiert von Soldaten* [in German]. Frankfurt, Germany: Verlag Ullstein GmbH; 1967: 320–321.

be put in perspective; casualties returned by air constituted only about 10% of the total number of evacuees from Europe. The great majority were sent home by ship.[15]

Because of its success in World War II and rapid developments in aviation technology, aeromedical evacuation from the hospital level soon came to dominate all other forms of military medical evacuation. The Secretary of Defense directed in September 1949 that all evacuation of sick and wounded, both in peace and in war, shall be accomplished by air whenever aircraft are available and proper medical treatment can be provided to the patient en route.[16] The rationale for this policy, which remains in effect, is stated in Table 27-1.

The various modes of transportation that are used in military medical evacuation should not be thought of as mutually exclusive. In fact, more than one type of evacuation vehicle is commonly needed. The complexity and interrelation of evacuation assets was nowhere more obvious than in the European Theater of Operations at the end of World War II, in which evacuation was carried out every using almost every type of land, sea, and air vehicle (Figure 27-4). Although the U.S. Army's experience since World War II has emphasized evacuation by air at all echelons, the number of casualties generated in a high-intensity war and the conditions present in such a war may allow only for ground evacuation. For example, medical planning for a war between North Atlantic Treaty Organization (NATO) and Warsaw Pact countries envisioned the extensive use of hospital trains in addition to tactical medical evacuation flights from the corps communication zone. Military anesthesia providers need to maintain a broad perspective when thinking about medical evacuation if for no other reason than to ensure that the system is resilient.

Although air transportation has become the dominant mode of evacuation, its utility is based on a frequently unrecognized assumption; namely, that a forward air base would always be available for use as an evacuation and holding center. The British experience in the Falklands War in 1982 showed that this is not always true. No forward air base was available initially, which made it impossible to fly treated casualties out of the combat zone. This would have been difficult even if an airfield had been available because the distance between the Falkland Islands and the nearest British air base, on Ascension Island, is 4,000 miles (6,400 km). The solution to the problem was to evacuate casualties by helicopter to a hospital ship, which then sailed to neutral territory (Uruguay), from where the casualties were evacuated by air.[17]

TABLE 27-1

ADVANTAGES OF AEROMEDICAL MEDICAL EVACUATION

Advantage	Rationale
Speed	The "Golden Hour" of resuscitation can be better utilized by rapid and safe air transport of the casualty. The value of rapid evacuation to a Level-1 trauma center has been well-demonstrated in civilian medicine.
Range	Transport of casualties over long distances in a relatively short period of time allows fewer tertiary centers to support several units.
Trafficability	Rotor-wing aircraft can pick up patients in relatively inaccessible areas and transport them quickly and safely. The minimal landing requirements provide this feature.
Flexibility	A casualty can be airlifted quickly to that medical installation where appropriate specialized care may be available, thereby bypassing unnecessary delays.
Comfort and Morale	Because of the speed and comfort of flight, the soldier knows that if injured, he can be transported to the appropriate medical treatment facility quickly and in stable condition.
Economy of Resources	Because one large hospital is able to accommodate several battle areas, fewer facilities need to be set up.

The hospital ship was obtained by converting the cruise liner SS *Uganda*, the conversion being carried out in only 4 days. The vessel, which was equipped with a helicopter landing pad, full hospital facilities, and an intensive care unit, was only 15 minutes' flying time from the land battles. International Red Cross regulations required that once on board the hospital ship, all casualties had to be evacuated from the war zone. Their repatriation required the good offices of the Uruguayan authorities, who permitted their transfer by sea (in small survey vessels), over 1,500 km from the Falkland Islands to Montevideo, for onward air transportation to the United Kingdom. Five hundred eighty casualties were evacuated by this route.[17] The experience of the SS *Uganda* constitutes one of the few recent instances in which a hospital ship has been used as a evacuation vehicle in addition to functioning as a hospital. Much more common is the use of hospital ships as deployable hospitals.

The British experience in the Falkland Islands has led to a reevaluation of the role of hospital ships in any future conflict, resulting in the U.S. Navy's converting two supertankers into the hospital ships *Comfort* and *Mercy*, two 1,000-bed hospitals with full facilities. However, few countries can afford the luxury of maintaining permanent, fully equipped hospital ships. A less expensive system has been developed, whereby hospital facilities such as wards, operating theaters, radiographic units, laboratories, and intensive care facilities have been modularized, based on the International Standards Organization's (ISO's) standard container. The number of units can be varied as required and rapidly installed in any suitable ship.

The ships must have unobstructed deck space, such as is usually found on fleet auxiliaries, tank-landing ships, or roll on–roll off merchant ferries. The great advantage of the modular system is that the vessel can carry out its ordinary task until it is required for medical duties. The benefits offered by the Rapid Deployment Hospital Ship program are low cost, a dual role for the ship, extremely rapid conversion into the war role, a controlled hospital environment, and the possibility that any of the modules can be transferred to land, if required. This excellent, low-cost facility was used when a British Naval Auxiliary vessel was converted into a 100-bed facility in a short time and sailed to the Persian Gulf during the hostilities there (1990–1991).

In describing the evolution of military medical evacuation in the 20th century, evacuation from forward hospitals to hospitals in the communication zone or CONUS has been emphasized almost exclusively. However, regardless of how successfully this link in the evacuation chain functions, it remains totally dependent on the casualty's first having been evacuated from the battlefield. Even

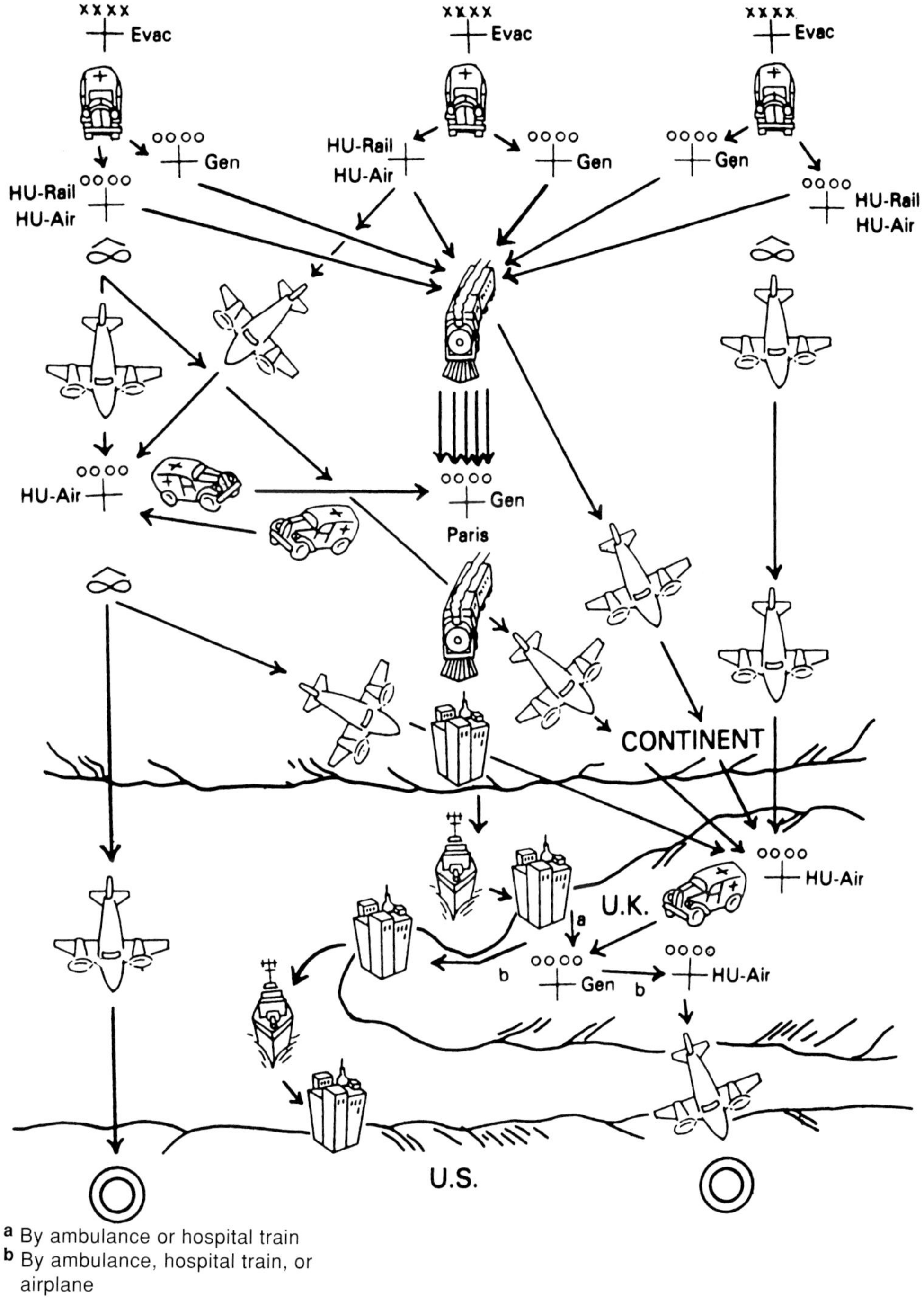

Fig. 27-4. This cartoon shows how evacuation was carried out in and from the European Theater of Operations in World War II. The built-in redundancy allowed for maintenance of the casualty flow even if the activity of one form of evacuation was impaired (eg, when aeromedical evacuation was hindered by bad weather). It is important to recognize that evacuation in and from the theater of operations depends totally on the casualty's arriving at this echelon after successful evacuation from the unit, division, and corps levels. The symbols indicate army-level, general, and evacuation hospitals. HU: holding units. Reprinted from Cosmas GA, Cowdrey AE. *Medical Service in the European Theater of Operations*. Washington DC: Center of Military History, US Army; 1992: 335.

with the field ambulances of Larrey and Letterman, the casualty would first have to be taken to a collection point from where he could be removed from the battlefield. Extracting casualties from the battlefield, frequently while under enemy fire—the most difficult, arduous, and dangerous segment of the evacuation chain—remained the province of medics, litter bearers, and nonmedical soldiers, who all depended on human muscle power to move the casualty. The advent of mechanized warfare in World War II made possible an alternative approach, namely, the use of equipment: first, armored fighting vehicles; and second, small, fixed-wing aircraft and helicopters. The latter had a revolutionary effect on evacuation because it made possible the speedy transportation of casualties directly from the scene of wounding on the battlefield to a surgical hospital.

Helicopter evacuation from the battlefield first occurred in 1944 in Burma, but first assumed prominence in the Korean War, during which approximately 17,700 casualties were evacuated from the battlefield to hospitals.[18] Although more than 300,000 casualties were evacuated from Korea to Japan during the Korean War, the true value of air evacuation was in the timely pick-up and transport of the soldier from the point of wounding to the point where he was seen by a medical officer. It was widely recognized by medical authorities, both military and civilian, that timely evacuation, together with the use of whole blood and antibiotics, were the three factors responsible for the low mortality during the Korean War.

During the Vietnam War, between 850,000 and 900,000 allied military personnel and Vietnamese civilians underwent aeromedical evacuation. At least 90% of all hospitalized U.S. Army battle casualties were evacuated by helicopter at one time or other during their treatment.[18] There can be no doubt that the helicopter, by making unnecessary many long and difficult litter carries as well as uncomfortable trips in ground ambulances, made life much more tolerable for both casualties and medics (Figure 27-5).

Nevertheless, helicopter evacuation of casualties directly from the battlefield was not without drawbacks. For example, when compared with fixed-wing aircraft, helicopters have limited operational ranges. On an extensive battlefield such as characterized the Persian Gulf War, direct helicopter evacuation from the site of injury to the hospital level is usually impractical. In addition, darkness and weather conditions at times interfere with aeromedical evacuation. More importantly, helicopter evacuation from the battlefield can be very dangerous. It has been estimated that one third of all air ambulance pilots in the Vietnam War sustained either battle or nonbattle injuries, and medical evacuation helicopters sustained more than three times more battle damage than helicopters used in combat and combat support missions.[18] Although regulations initially precluded making casualty pick-ups from landing zones that were subject to enemy fire, this became commonplace in both the Korean and Vietnam wars. The heroism of helicopter crews made possible the evacuation of casualties that in many instances, in retrospect, seems impossible.

Even so, helicopter evacuation from the high-intensity battlefield is probably suicidal. In fact, U.S. Army regulations do not foresee casualty extraction by helicopter occurring forward of the battalion aid station when enemy air-defense artillery capabilities are substantial; thus, the need for evacuation vehicles capable of functioning far forward

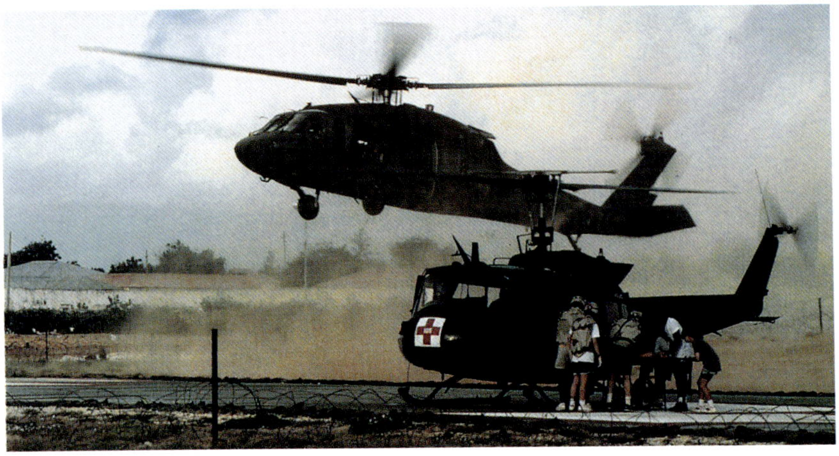

Fig. 27-5. A scene from the Somalia peacekeeping operation. A casualty is being removed from a UH-1 medical evacuation helicopter while a UH-60 hovers in the background. The latter is now the US Army's primary air ambulance, replacing the former, which has served with distinction since its introduction in 1959. The UH-60 has greater range and speed, and superior aivonics compared with the UH-1 but, suprisingly, can carry no more casualties. Photograph: Public Affairs, Office of The Surgeon General, US Army.

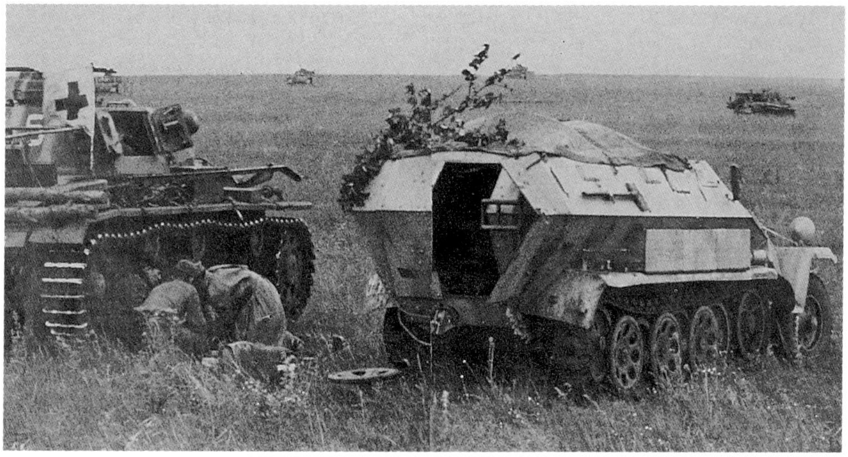

Fig. 27-6. Evacuation during an armored battle fought in central Russia during summer, 1943. The armored unit's medical officer rode into battle in the tank shown on the left and was accompanied by an armored personnel carrier, which was used to evacuate the casualty. First aid and preparation of the casualty for evacuation took place in the open. Although the casualty was protected from small-arms fire and fragments from shells during evacuation, the small internal volume of the armored personnel carrier precluded effective ongoing care. Futhermore, the separation of the physician and the casualty during evacuation no doubt resulted in increased mortality and morbidity. Reprinted with permission from Pielkalkiewicz J. *Unternehmen Zitadelle* [in German]. Bergisch Gladbach, Germany: Gustaf Lübbe Verlag GmbH; 1983.

under enemy fire.[2(p4-12)] The precedent for the use of armored fighting vehicles for this purpose dates from early in World War II, when German armored formations used half-track vehicles for casualty evacuation (Figure 27-6). More recently, many other armies have used armored personnel carriers for evacuating casualties under enemy fire. The Israelis have even used their main battle tank—the Merkava—for this purpose. The Merkava's engine is in the front, which leaves a space in the rear—accessed by an armored door—that can be used for carrying several casualties.

LOGISTICAL AND OPERATIONAL ASPECTS

The schematic diagram that is part of the front matter of this book shows the organization for evacuation as it existed in the U.S. Army at the time of publication. For purposes of this chapter, the system used to evacuate sick and wounded soldiers will be studied in three segments: (1) the unit (ie, the medical platoon) and the division level, (ie, the medical company or medical battalion, which usually have no surgical capabilities); (2) the corps level and the communication zone, which contain the deployable hospitals; and (3) the domestic system, which is operated by the U.S. Air Force.

Unit and Division Levels

Evacuation at the unit level can be by ground or by air. The type of vehicle used depends on the warfighting scenario. In a high-intensity war, it is likely that 90% of casualty evacuation will be by ground, with the remaining 10% by air (—RFB, personal observation, 1994). In a low-intensity war, most evacuation can be expected to be by air. Evacuation at the unit level is regulated by the battalion surgeon or the medical company commander; at the division level, by the division medical operations center.[2(p4-2)]

Ground Evacuation

As previously indicated, aerial transport may not be feasible because of enemy action. Furthermore, bad weather, darkness, and distance may preclude aeromedical evacuation. Ground ambulances may be used at these times. These ambulances, which are *organic* (ie, intrinsic; included in the Table of Organization and Equipment) to the U.S. Army Medical Department units that are responsible for transporting the sick and wounded, have the basic supplies and are staffed with ambulance personnel qualified in basic emergency medical care and treatment procedures. An ambulance crew consists of a driver and an additional soldier, both of whom are medical aidmen. Current ground ambulances include the following vehicles[2(pp10-1–10-16)]:

- M1010 truck ambulance, $1\frac{1}{4}$ ton 4 x 4. This truck is designed to transport the sick and wounded and is the standard field ambulance of medical units at the division and higher-level units where suitable roads exist. The patient compartment is separated from the remainder of the vehicle and has a heater and a surgical light. The capacity is 4 litter patients, or 8 to 10 ambulatory patients, or a combination of litter and ambulatory patients (eg, 2 litter and 5 ambulatory patients).
- High-mobility, multipurpose, wheeled vehicle (HMMWV, M996 and M997) truck ambulance, 4 x 4, armored tactical vehicles. The HMMWV is designed to be used cross-country and over all types of terrain. Depending on the configuration, the vehicle can carry 2 to 4 litter patients, or 6 to 8 ambulatory casualties, or a mixture of litter and ambulatory casualties. These vehicles can be modified for operation in a nuclear, biological, or chemical warfare environment.
- M113 carrier, personnel, full-tracked, armored. The M113 can carry up to 10 ambulatory or 4 litter patients.

The M792 (Gamma Goat), M170, and M718 evacuation vehicles are being phased out of the U.S. Army's inventory. Any military vehicle may be adapted for carrying patients as the situation allows, but safety and stability during transport are important priorities that need to be satisfied by any putative ambulance.

Air Evacuation

An assigned mission of the U.S. Army is to provide air transportation for the sick and wounded within the combat zone. The major objective of air transportation is the expedient delivery of the casualty to the care level necessary for survival. The flexibility and rapid deployment of air services make this an optimal method of delivery. Air transport involves the use of either fixed- or rotor-wing aircraft.

Organization of U.S. Army Air Evacuation

A soldier injured in a forward area may initially receive first aid from an aidman. Then the soldier may be transported by ground to the battalion aid station, where the injury is reassessed; if evacuation is necessary, it is the U.S. Army's responsibility to provide appropriate ground or air evacuation. The latter is usually provided by the medical air ambulance company. The medical company's air ambulance is normally assigned to the corps medical brigade and is attached to the medical evacuation battalion for command and control.[2(p3-7)]

The capabilities of the medical air ambulance company include

- aeromedical evacuation of critically wounded or other patients;
- extrication and then air evacuation of personnel from crashed aircraft;
- emergency aid at air-crash sites, in-flight medical treatment, and surveillance of patients en route to treatment facilities;
- expeditious delivery of medical personnel and material to meet emergency treatment requirements within a combat zone; and
- in-flight emergency medical care.

The core of the air ambulance company is its air ambulance platoon. Military physicians need to be aware of the composition and skill level of this platoon. Each consists of a platoon leader, two section leaders, nine evacuation pilots, one platoon sergeant, six air ambulance aidmen, six crew chiefs, and one voice-radio operator. Each platoon is authorized six UH-60A helicopters. Each helicopter has an assigned crew consisting of a crew chief, two pilots, and an air ambulance aidman. All are proficient in emergency medical treatment. Although each air ambulance has a capacity for six litter patients or nine ambulatory patients (the UH-1), or four litter and seven ambulatory patients (the UH-60A), the combat load for each is three litter and four ambulatory patients.[2(p10-27)]

The situation may occur when nonmedical aircraft such as the U.S. Army's CH-47 Chinook will be used for evacuation at the division level. This helicopter can carry up to 24 litter patients.

Only approved and tested equipment may be taken aboard aircraft, and each type of aircraft has its own list of approved equipment. Medical personnel should consult with the crew chief or senior medic of the particular aeromedical evacuation ambulance to ascertain what equipment is presently available and approved.

Air Ambulance Operations

Air ambulances are used as far forward as possible and as the numbers of combat casualties allow. Ambulances should be used only if the landing zone is both free of hostile fire and secure. If it is not, the pilot must be notified. The base of operations must be located and operated so that it can respond as quickly as possible when there are casualties on the battlefield. In the absence of clear guidelines as to the casualty's destination, the pilot is the final authority.

All medical officers of deployable units should know how to arrange aeromedical evacuation. FM 8-10-6 should be consulted for a detailed description of the official procedure; a brief overview follows. Requests for air ambulance evacuation must contain concise, accurate, and reliable information so that appropriate equipment can be provided and flights planned. The commander of the air ambulance team supporting the division decides whether to accept the mission, based on meteorological conditions or the availability of aircraft. All U.S. Army aeromedical evacuation requests should provide information in the sequence provided in FM 8-10-6 (Exhibit 27-1).

EXHIBIT 27-1

SEQUENCE OF INFORMATION REQUIRED IN U.S. ARMY AEROMEDICAL EVACUATION REQUESTS

LINE 1:	Location of pick-up site
LINE 2:	Radio frequency, call sign and suffix
LINE 3:	Number of patients by precedence, as described in FM 8-10-6 (p7-1)
LINE 4:	Special equipment required (eg, ventilator)
LINE 5:	Number of patients and type of injury
LINE 6:	Security of pick-up site
LINE 7:	Method of marking pick-up site
LINE 8:	Patient nationality and status
LINE 9:	Nuclear, biological, and chemical contamination

Adapted from Department of the Army. Field Manual 8-10-6. *Medical Evacuation in a Theater of Operations.* Washington DC: Headquarters, DA; 31 October 1991: pp 7-3–7-5.

Assignment of Medical Evacuation Priority

FM 8-10-6 specifies the following categories of precedence and the criteria used for their assignment:

> Priority I—URGENT is assigned to emergency cases that should be evacuated as soon as possible and within a maximum of 2 hours to save life, limb, or eyesight; to prevent complications of serious illness; or to avoid permanent disability.
> Priority IA—URGENT-SURG is assigned to patients who must receive surgical intervention far forward to save life and stabilize for further evacuation.
> Priority II—PRIORITY is assigned to sick and wounded personnel requiring prompt medical care. This precedence is used when (*a*) the individual should be evacuated within 4 hours or his medical condition could deteriorate to such a degree that he will become an URGENT precedence, or (*b*) requirements for special treatment are not available locally, or (*c*) will suffer unnecessary pain or disability.
> Priority III—ROUTINE is assigned to sick and wounded personnel requiring evacuation but whose condition is not expected to deteriorate significantly. The sick and wounded in this category should be evacuated within 24 hours.
> Priority IV—CONVENIENCE is assigned to patients for whom aeromedical evacuation is a matter of medical convenience rather than necessity.[2(p7-1)]

Civilian Approaches to the Assignment of Evacuation Priority

The assignment of evacuation priorities according to FM 8-10-6 is, by its very nature, subjective. In an effort to bring objectivity to the determination of the need for helicopter evacuation to a trauma center, civilian emergency medical systems have adopted the use of triage scoring systems. The civilian approach needs to be understood by military anesthesiologists because a modification may be applicable to military medical evacuation:

- The Trauma Score (Exhibit 27-2) is a composite that includes measures of the status of the cardiovascular, respiratory, and central nervous systems. (It incorporates the

EXHIBIT 27-2

TRAUMA SCORE USED IN CIVILIAN EVACUATION

Trauma Score Component	Value	Points	Score
A. Respiratory Rate			
Number of respirations in 15 s, multiplied by 4	10–24	4	
	25–35	3	
	> 35	2	
	< 10	1	
	0	0	
			A. ______
B. Respiratory Effort			
Normal	Normal	1	
Shallow—markedly decreased chest movement or air exchange	Shallow	0	
Retractive—use of accessory muscles or intercostal retraction	Retractive	0	
			B. ______
C. Systolic Blood Pressure			
Systolic cuff pressure, either arm, auscultate or palpate	> 90	4	
	70–90	3	
	50–69	2	
	< 50	1	
No carotid pulse	0	0	
			C. ______
D. Capillary Refill			
Normal—forehead, lip mucosa, or nail-bed color refills in 2 s	Normal	2	
Delayed—more than 2 s of capillary refill	Delayed	1	
None—no capillary refill	None	0	
			D. ______

E. Glasgow Coma Scale (GCS)	Value	Total Glascow Coma Scale Points	Score	
1. Eye Opening				
Spontaneous	4	14–15	5	
To voice	3	11–13	4	
To pain	2	8–10	3	
None	1	5–7	2	E. ______
2. Verbal Response				
Oriented	5			
Confused	4			
Inappropriate words	3			
Incomprehensible words	2			
None	1			
3. Motor Response				
Obeys commands	6			
Purposeful movement (pain)	5			
Withdraw (pain)	4			
Flexion (pain)	3			
Extension (pain)	2			
None	1			

Total GCS points (1 + 2 + 3) ______

Trauma Score ______
(Total points A + B + C + D + E)

Reprinted with permission from Champion HR, Sacco WJ, Carnazzo AJ, et al. Trauma score. *Crit Care Med.* 1981;9:672.

Glasgow coma scale as its central nervous system component.) The best feature of the Trauma Score is that it measures the physiological state at the scene of the injury. Patients who require prompt diagnosis and definitive care at a Level 1 trauma center are those with a score of 12 or less.[19]

- The CRAMS scale was developed by S. P. Gormican in 1982 and modified by T. P. Clemmer in 1985 (Exhibit 27-3).[20] It is a simple and easy scale to remember, with the letters of the acronym representing *c*irculation, *r*espiration, *a*bdomen, *m*otor, and *s*peech.

EXHIBIT 27-3

MODIFIED CRAMS SCALE USED IN CIVILIAN MEDICAL EVACUATION

Circulation
- 2: Normal capillary refill and blood pressure > 100 mm Hg systolic
- 1: Delayed capillary refill or blood pressure 85–99 mm Hg systolic
- 0: No capillary refill or blood pressure < 85 mm Hg systolic

Respiration
- 2: Normal
- 1: Abnormal (labored, shallow, or rate > 35)
- 0: Absent

Abdomen
- 2: Abdomen and thorax not tender
- 1: Abdomen and thorax tender
- 0: Abdomen rigid, thorax flail, or deep penetrating injury to either chest or abdomen

Motor
- 2: Normal (obeys commands)
- 1: Responds only to pain, no posturing
- 0: Postures or no response

Speech
- 2: Normal (oriented)
- 1: Confused or inappropriate
- 0: Unintelligible or no sounds

____ **Total CRAMS Score**

Reprinted with permission from Clemmer TP, Orme JF Jr, Thomas F, et al. Prospective evaluation of the CRAMS scale for triaging major trauma. *J Trauma*. 1985;25:189.

Recommended equipment for civilian helicopter evacuation is shown in Exhibit 27-4. A simplified triage flow sheet (Figure 27-7) and a recommendation for helicopter transport at all times (Exhibit 27-5)[21] are also included to allow some familiarity with civilian decision making. Additional recommendations have been set forth for the transport of the critically ill patient and have been reviewed and approved by The Association of Air Medical Service.[22]

Corps and Communications Zones: Zone of the Interior

Much of the medical evacuation that occurs at the corps level and above will involve the U.S. Air Force. However, the corps level medical evacuation battalion has as one of its missions the task of evacuating casualties from the division to the corps level, and does this by using the army's ground or air assets.

Evacuation from the division is regulated by the division Medical Operations Center and the medical group Medical Regulations Officer.[2(p4-2)] Evacuation from the corps level to the communication zone and higher is the mission of the Military Airlift Command of the U.S. Air Force. Medical regulating at this level proceeds from the patient administrator of a given hospital to the medical group and medical brigade Medical Regulating Office to the theater-level Joint Medical Regulating Office. Medical regulating for evacuation from the communications zone to the zone of the interior is carried out by the Armed Services Medical Regulating Office.

It is important that military anesthesiologists recognize that when the casualty initially enters the U.S. Air Force's medical evacuation system, he will be at a Mobile Aeromedical Staging Facility (MASF). The function of this unit is to collect casualties, not to provide treatment. Physicians are not assigned to a MASF and casualties should not be sent there unless they are in stable condition. Furthermore, the MASF does not have a holding capability; patients are not to remain there longer than 6 hours.[2(p6-9)]

Tactical Evacuation System

The tactical evacuation system provides for the airlift of patients within the corps level and from the corps level to the communication zone. Most of these casualties will have had initial surgery and should be in stable condition. U.S. Air Force guidance indicates that mission duration will not exceed

EXHIBIT 27-4

RECOMMENDED CIVILIAN HELICOPTER CHECK LIST

In Side Wall Blue Pouches:
- 1 pair wrist restraints
- 1 roll 2-in. cloth tape
- 2 oral airways (small, medium)
- 1 30-mL syringe
- 1 10-mL syringe
- 2 pairs eyeglasses
- Masks and gloves

In Front Wall Pockets:
- 2 survival kits
- 2 life vests
- Doppler flow probe and acoustic coupler
- 2 lithium-powered batteries
- Obesity blood-pressure cuff
- Large adult blood-pressure cuff
- Passenger guide

On Side Wall:
- Suction cannister with suction tubing and yankeur
- 2 oxygen regulators
- Personal mask resuscitation bag, with mask

In Clam Shell:
- 2 head rolls
- Cervical collars (small, medium, large)
- 1 spider strap
- Pediatric immobilizer with pump

In Airway Seat:
- Large survival kit
- 1 life vest

In Side Seat Drawer:
- 4 D-cell batteries
- 2 reflective vests
- 1 syringe pump
- 1 syringe pump charger
- 2 spare stretcher brackets
- 1 flashlight
- 1 L normal saline
- 500 mL Tridil*
- Charcoal and ipecac syrup†
- Foam ear plugs
- Charger for PROPAC‡ monitor and pulse oximeter

Between Bench and Side Seat:
- Military antishock trousers bag

In Side Rear Pouch:
- 1 trauma dressing
- 1 sterile drape
- 2 reflective vests
- 1 camp light

Under Bench Seat:
- Linen
- Pneumatic shock garments, adult and pediatric, with pump
- Clipboard with flight charts

Under Side Seat:
- Elastic bracket for lithium-powered battery

On Wall Next to Side Seat:
- Backup stretcher
- KED extraction splint§
- Scoop stretcher
- Blue interhospital patient-attendant bag
- Red scene bag

Behind Side Seat:
- 3 oxygen tanks

With Stretcher:
- Oxygen tank and regulator
- PROPAQ monitor with cables and cuff

Also Aboard Helicopter:
- 1 spare headset
- 2 fire extinguishers
- Portable, free-standing suction unit¶
- Suction kits and 1 yankeur
- Charger for lithium-powered battery

---

*Nitroglycerin in 1,2,3-propanetriol trinitrate, manufactured by Du Pont Multi-Source Products, Garden City, NY
†Syrup of Ipecac, manufactured by Roxane Laboratories, Inc, Columbus, Oh
‡Manufactured by Protocol Systems, Inc, Beaverton, Ore
§Kendrick Extraction Device, manufactured by Medix Choice, Santee, Calif
¶Portable: Continuous and Programmable Intermittent Suction System, Model 326/326M, manufactured by Impact Instrumentation, Inc, West Caldwell, NJ

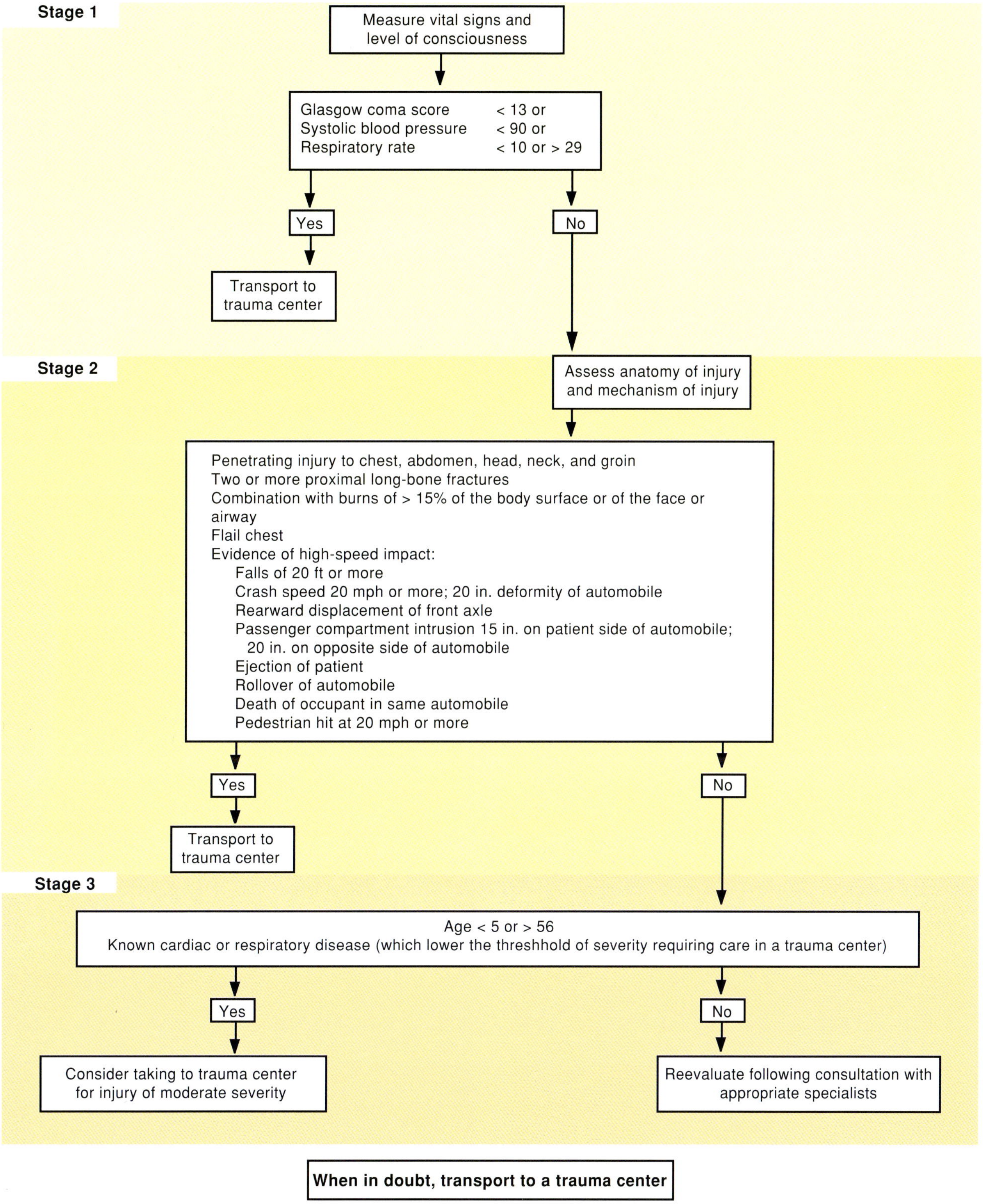

Fig. 27-7. Civilian triage decision scheme. In stage 1, if easily determined clinical indices such as the Glasgow coma score, systolic blood pressure, and respiratory rate are abnormal, the patient should be flown directly to a trauma center. Stage 2 is implemented in patients in whom these indices are not grossly abnormal. The anatomical location of the injury and its mechanism are used as discriminators. In stage 3, extremes of age and the known presence of cardiopulmonary disease are used as further triage discriminators. Adapted with permission from Champion HR. Helicopter triage. *Emerg Care Q*. 1986;2:13–21.

EXHIBIT 27-5

SIMPLIFIED CIVILIAN EVACUATION POLICY

A helicopter should be used for patient transport under any of the following conditions:

Urban and suburban environments

Transport time to the trauma center > 15 min by ambulance

Ambulance transport impeded by access to or egress from the accident scene

Presence of multiple casualties

Rural environment

Time to local hospital via ambulance > time to trauma center via helicopter

Wilderness rescue

Reprinted with permission from Champion HR. Helicopter triage. *Emerg Care Quart*. 1986;2:20.

4 hours. The most commonly used aircraft is the C-130 Hercules (Figure 27-8).[2(p10-45)] The C-130 is a long-range, high-wing, four turboprop–engine aircraft. The fuselage is divided into the cargo compartment and the flight deck. It can be fully pressurized, heated, and air conditioned. The C-130 can maintain a sea-level cabin pressure at an altitude up to 19,000 ft and an 8,000-ft cabin pressure at an altitude of 35,000 ft. It can land and take off on runways as short as 600 m, a capability that allows for rapid transportation of personnel and equipment to and from the battlefield. The C-130 can readily be configured for aeromedical evacuation by using seat and litter provisions stowed in the cargo compartment, but military anesthesia providers should not expect to find extensive resources available for treatment. Depending on inherent equipment and the model of the aircraft, it can hold a maximum of 74 litter patients, 92 ambulatory patients, or various combinations (Figure 27-9).

Strategic Evacuation System

The mission of the strategic evacuation system is to provide controlled evacuation of stable patients to medical treatment facilities that are located outside the theater of operations—frequently in CONUS. U.S. Air Force guidance on mission duration

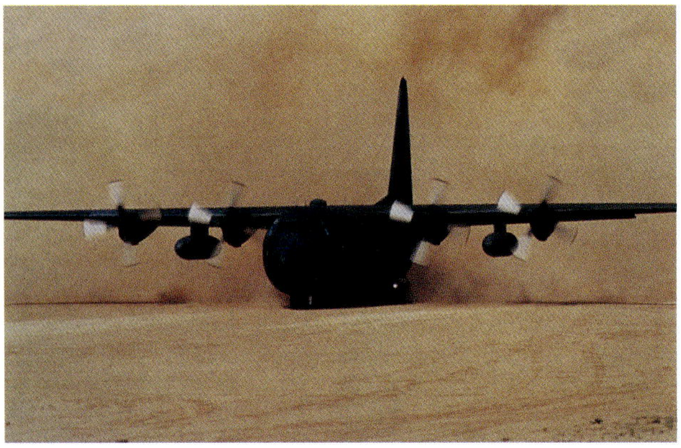

Fig. 27-8. A C-130 Hercules taking off somewhere in the Kuwaiti Theater of Operations during the Persian Gulf War. The original design of the C-130 dates from 1951. The rugged construction of these aircraft allows them to use unprepared runways, as are found forward on the battlefield. Photograph: Defense Audio-Visual Agency, Still Media Depository, Washington, DC.

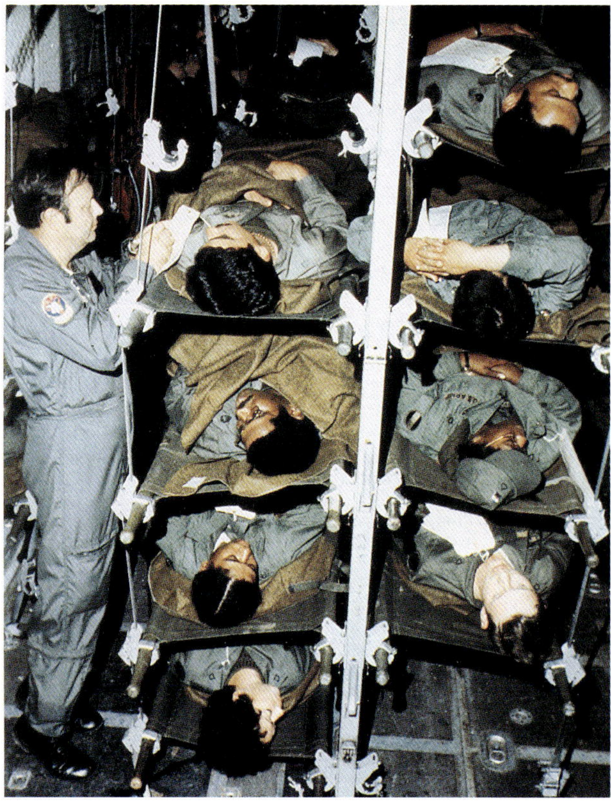

Fig. 27-9. This photograph, taken during an exercise in 1980, shows the extremely tight space available for individual casualties. The space and the sparse medical equipment provided markedly limit the provision of in-flight medical care. Photograph: Defense Audio-Visual Agency, Still Media Depository,Washington, DC.

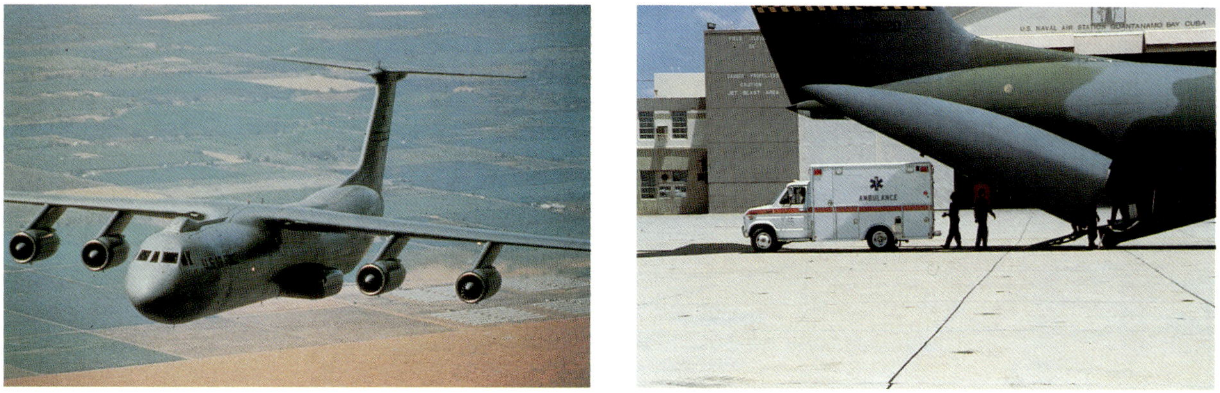

Fig. 27-10. The C-141 Starlifter (**a**) and its loading ramp (**b**). This aircraft was the mainstay of the US Air Force's strategic aeromedical evacuation system during both the Vietnam and the Persian Gulf wars. Photographs: Courtesy of Lieutenant Colonel Charles Beading, MD, Medical Corps, US Air Force, Flight Surgeon, Uniformed Services University of the Health Sciences, Bethesda, Md.

is 7 to 14 hours. The aircraft currently used is the C-141 Starlifter (Figure 27-10).[2(p10-46)] The C-141 is a long-range, high-speed, high-altitude aircraft designed for the airlift of combat support equipment, troops, or aeromedical evacuation patients. It is powered by four jet engines, cruises at 550 mph at an altitude of 30,000 ft, and has a range of 5,250 miles. When used for aeromedical airlift, a self-contained comfort pallet can be placed in the forward section of the cargo compartment. Conditions aboard a typical strategic aeromedical evacuation flight during the Persian Gulf War era are shown in Figure

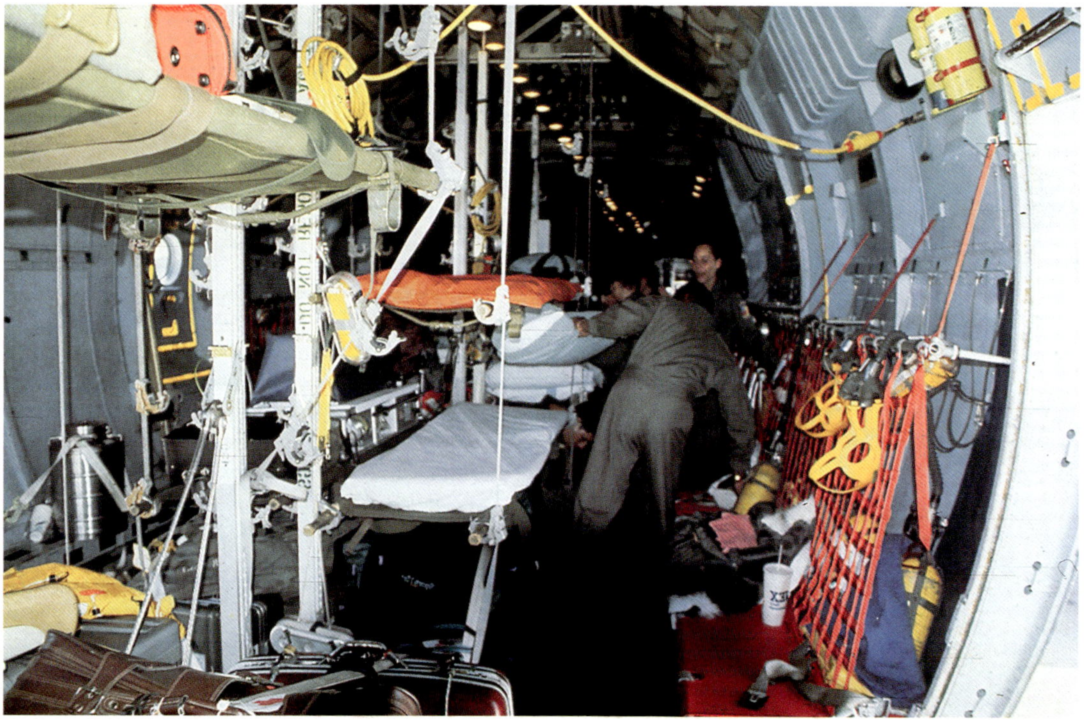

Fig. 27-11. In-flight conditions for casualties aboard a C-141 during a strategic aeromedical evacuation. Access to patients and the availability of medical equipment are superior to that on the C-130. Photograph: Courtesy of Lieutenant Colonel Charles Beading, MD, Medical Corps, US Air Force, Flight Surgeon, Uniformed Services University of the Health Sciences, Bethesda, Md.

a

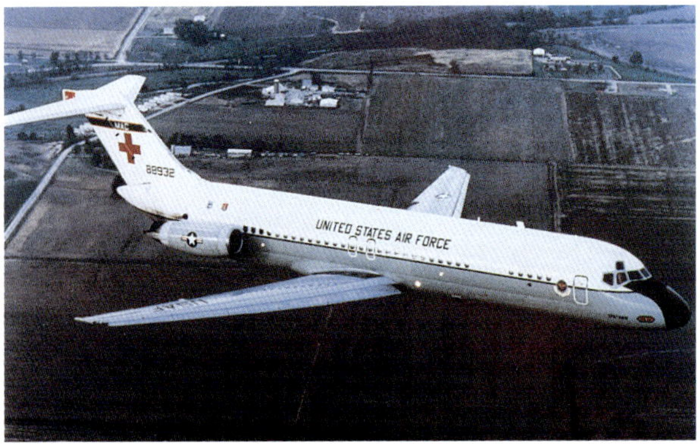

b

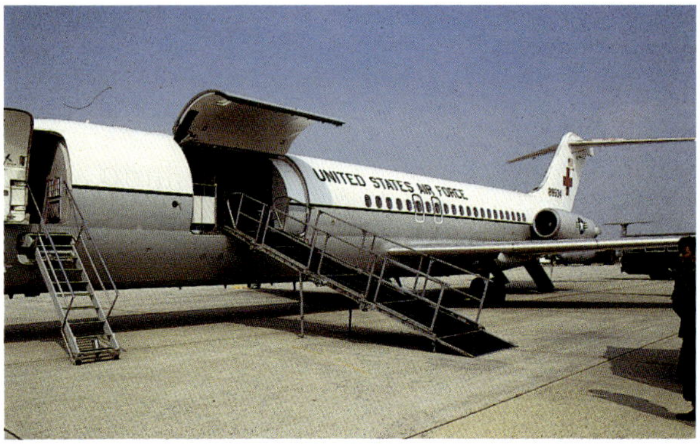

Fig. 27-12. The C-9 Nightingale (**a**), a modified version of the commercial DC-9 and the only US Air Force aircraft especially designed for aeromedical evacuation. (**b**) The loading ramp. Photographs: Courtesy of Lieutenant Colonel Charles Beading, MD, Medical Corps, US Air Force, Flight Surgeon, Uniformed Services University of the Health Sciences, Bethesda, Md.

27-11. Maximum capacity of the aircraft is 103 litters or 147 ambulatory patients, or various combinations of litter and ambulatory patients. The conditions are much better than in the C-130. Patients are not overcrowded, hot meals are provided, and the cabin temperature is better controlled than in tactical aircraft. Oxygen and electrical outlets permit the use of complex medical equipment en route. However, dehydration may occur because the flights are long and the ambient humidity is low (5%–30%). There has been recurrent interest in configuring and outfitting a small number of C-141s as flying intensive care wards.

Domestic Aeromedical Evacuation System

The U.S. Air Force's daily system of flights within CONUS has flight crews and aircraft dedicated to aeromedical evacuation of military casualties. The aircraft currently used is the C-9 Nightingale, which is a modified version of the commercial DC-9.[2(p10-45)] The T-tailed aircraft is powered by twin, aft-mounted jet engines and cruises at 500 mph. Its range exceeds 2,300 miles. The C-9 is the only U.S. Air Force aircraft specifically designed for aeromedical evacuation. An integral folding ramp enables efficient enplaning and deplaning of litter patients (Figure 27-12). The C-9 can hold a maximum of 40 litter patients, 40 ambulatory patients, or a variety of combinations of litter and ambulatory patients (Figure 27-13). The environment on board is comparable to first-class accommodations on a commercial airline. Most specialized equipment available on a hospital ward can be provided on a C-9, including isolation and humidity control.

Although the domestic system is in operation daily, it is during emergencies, when military casualties of accidents and disasters require evacuation to specialized hospitals within CONUS, that its function is most clearly illustrated, as in the following incident.

The air force's domestic aeromedical evacuation system was activated in March 1994 after two army training planes (a four-engine turboprop C-130 Hercules transport plane and a single-engine F-16D) crashed and burned while attempting to land at Pope Air Force Base, North Carolina. Twenty-three paratroopers died and 83 others sustained burns or other injuries in the accident. The severely burned survivors were aeromedically evacuated to the burn center at Brooke Army Medical Center, Fort Sam Houston, San Antonio, Texas.[23]

> While the injured were being triaged and treated at Womack Army Medical Center, Fort Bragg, North Carolina; [civilian hospitals in Fayetteville and Chapel Hill]; and Portsmouth [Virginia] Naval Hospital; the Aeromedical Evacuation Coordination Center (57th Aeromedical Evacuation Squadron) at Scott Air Force Base (AFB), Illinois...was dispatching two C-9As and medical crew members to Fayetteville.
> In the meantime, the Air Education and Training Command (Randolph AFB, San Antonio [Texas]) provided a twin-jet T-43 A...to fly a burn team from Brooke Army Medical Center to Pope AFB.
>
> . . . .
>
> [T]he first C9-A departed Pope AFB the following morning for Kelly AFB, San Antonio, with 11 patients on litters, nine of whom were on ventilators. All had second- and third-degree burns covering from 30% to 80% of their bodies.... The second C-9A made the flight about 5 hours later with nine

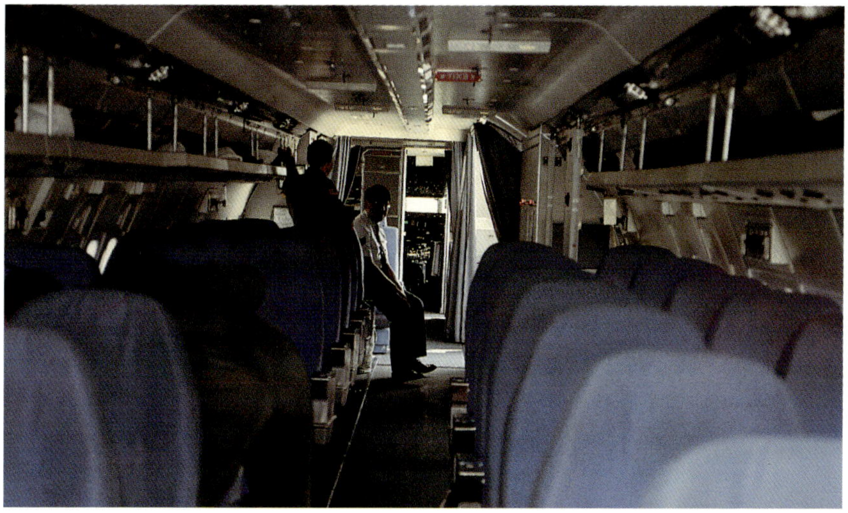

a

b

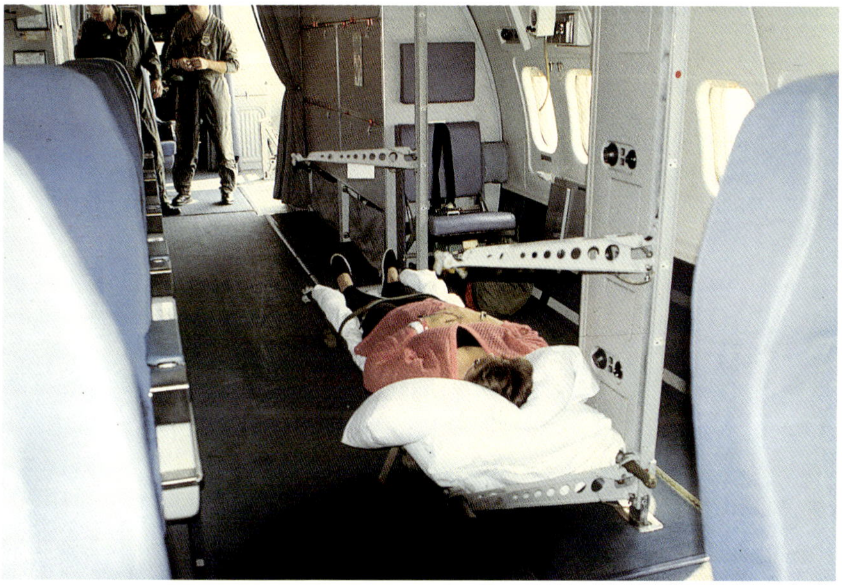

Fig. 27-13. (**a, b,** and **c**) Patient conditions aboard the C-9 Nightingale. Photographs: Courtesy of Lieutenant Colonel Charles Beading, MD, Medical Corps, US Air Force, Flight Surgeon, Uniformed Services University of the Health Sciences, Bethesda, Md.

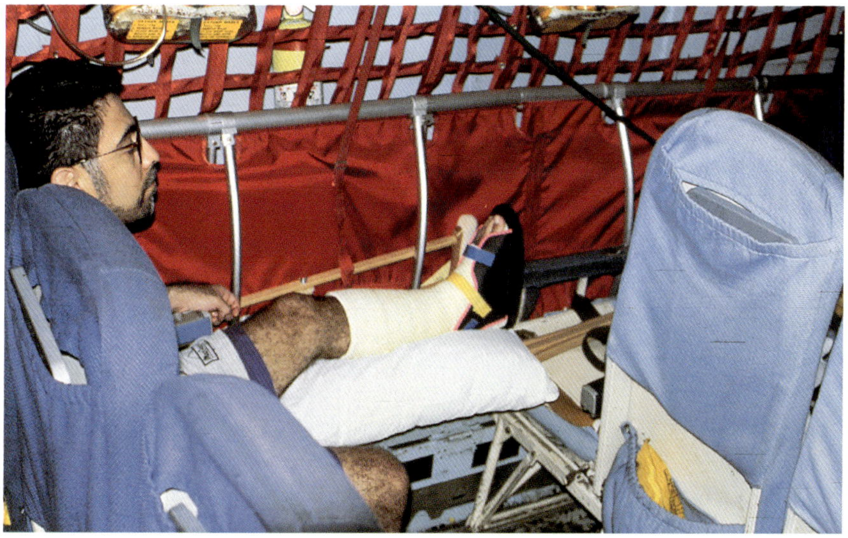

c

EXHIBIT 27-6

U.S. AIR FORCE CLASSIFICATION OF PATIENTS SCHEDULED FOR AEROMEDICAL EVACUATION

Class 1. Neuropsychiatric Patients

1A. Severe psychiatric litter patients requiring the use of restraining apparatus, sedation, and close supervision at all times.

1B. Psychiatric litter patients of intermediate severity requiring tranquilizing medication or sedation, not normally requiring the use of restraining apparatus, but who react badly to air travel or who may commit acts likely to endanger themselves, others, and/or the safety of the aircraft. Restraining apparatus should be available for use.

1C. Psychiatric walking patients of moderate severity who are cooperative and who have proved reliable under observation.

Class 2. Litter Patients (Other Than Psychiatric)

2A. Immobile litter patients unable to move about of their own volition under any circumstances.

2B. Mobile litter patients able to move about of their own volition in an emergency.

Class 3. Walking Patients (Other than Psychiatric)

3A. Nonpsychiatric and nonsubstance abuse patients who require medical treatment, assistance, or observation en route.

3B. Recovered patients who are returning to their units and require no medical attention en route.

3C. Ambulatory drug or alcohol substance-abuse patients.

Class 4. Infant Category

4A. Infants under 3 years of age, occupying a seat or in a bassinet or car seat secured in an ambulatory seat.

4B. Recovered infants under 3 years of age, occupying a seat or in a bassinet or car seat secured in an ambulatory seat.

4C. Infants in an incubator.

4D. Infants younger than 3 years of age on a litter.

4E. Outpatients under 3 years of age on a litter for comfort.

Class 5. Outpatient Category

5A. Ambulatory outpatients, non psychiatric and non substance abuse, who are traveling for an outpatient visit and do not require a litter or medical assistance in flight.

5B. Ambulatory drug- or substance-abuse outpatients going for treatment.

5C. Psychiatric outpatients going for treatment.

5D. Outpatients on a litter for comfort or safety.

5E. Returning outpatients on a litter for comfort or safety.

5F. Other returning outpatients.

Class 6. Attendant Category.

6A. Medical attendants, either physician, nurse, or technician, who are assigned to give specialized medical treatment or nursing care to a particular patient.

6B. Nonmedical attendants, either relatives or friends, who may assist with the patient's care and who may also require support.

Sources: (1) Department of the Army. Field Manual 8-10-6. *Medical Evacuation in a Theater of Operations.* Washington DC: Headquarters, DA; 31 October 1991: p F-1. (2) Department of the Air Force. *Physicians' Roles and Responsibilities in Aeromedical Evacuation.* Washington, DC: Secretary of the USAF; 1995: in press. Air Force Joint Manual 41-306.

patients on litters, five of whom were on ventilators. Two patients already had undergone leg amputations.

. . . .

[T]he flights were cleared to fly directly to San Antonio and thus were able to do so in less than 2 hours.[23(p1225)]

Military anesthesiologists need to be aware that to overcome shortfalls of strategic evacuation capability during a major war, the air force, in conjunction with a number of airlines and the U.S. Department of Transportation, has expanded the existing Civilian Reserve Air Force program to provide aircraft dedicated to aeromedical evacuation. The primary aircraft to be provided to support aeromedical airlift is the B-767. Once activated, each B-767 would be reconfigured from its civilian passenger configuration to an aeromedical configuration in about 18 hours.

Because casualties who enter the U.S. Air Force medical evacuation system during wartime should be medically stable, the prioritizing of precedence for picking up and moving casualties is more commonly applicable to emergency situations such as peacetime disasters[24]:

- URGENT: pick up immediately
- PRIORITY: pick up within 24 hours
- ROUTINE: pick up within 72 hours

The air force places considerable importance on the classification of patients to be evacuated (Exhibit 27-6).[2(pF-1)] The great majority of combat casualties will be placed into Classes 2A and 2B.

MEDICAL IMPLICATIONS OF BIOPHYSICAL EFFECTS OF AEROMEDICAL EVACUATION

Many potential problems are associated with aeromedical evacuation, but most of the unique threats are specific to long-range flight at high altitude and are a consequence of human adaptations to life at sea level. The modern jet must fly at the highest possible levels (9,000–12,000 m) for reasons of speed, fuel economy, and comfort. At 12,000 m the barometric pressure is only 140 mm Hg. At this level, the partial pressure of oxygen is approximately 30 mm Hg, which cannot sustain human life. Jet aircraft can operate at such altitudes only because the pressurized cabin was developed, which maintains ambient cabin altitude at a barometric pressure equivalent to that found between 1,500 and 2,600 m. Despite all the problems of living in a strange environment, "aeromedical transport of patients presents no problems so long as one remembers that man is adapted for life at sea level."[25(p237)]

Barometric Pressure

Barometric pressure falls as a function of height above the surface of Earth (Figure 27-14). This fact explains not only the etiology of hypoxia at altitude

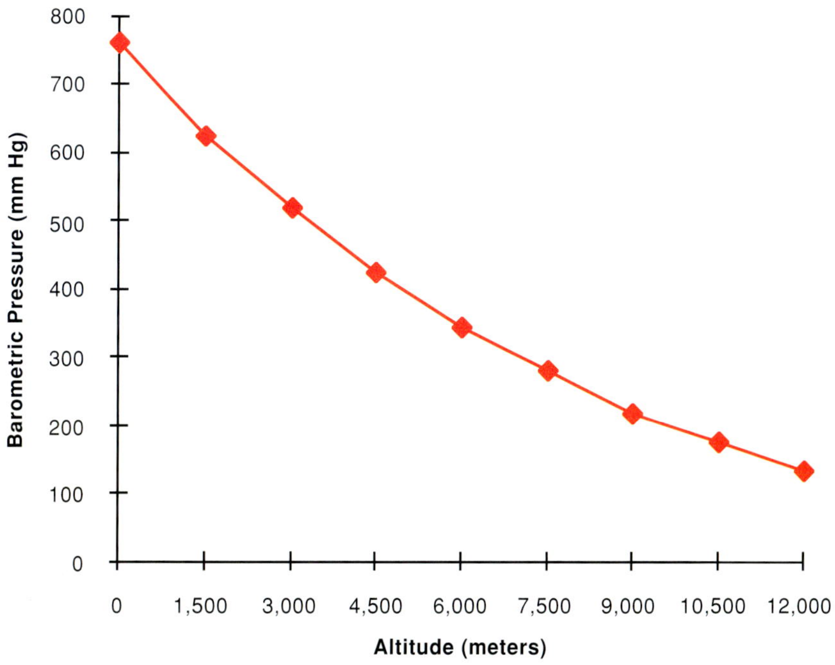

Fig. 27-14. Barometric pressure as a function of altitude.

but also why gas trapped within body cavities, as well as gas used to fill medical devices, can constitute a significant hazard to casualties undergoing aeromedical evacuation. The effect of falling barometric pressure is understandable in terms of the gas laws of Boyle and Dalton. Boyle's law states that at a constant temperature, the volume of a gas is inversely proportional to the pressure to which it is subjected. As altitude increases in an unpressurized aircraft and as barometric pressure decreases, gas in a closed or semiclosed space expands. All common drug vials, albumin infusions, and medical containers act like closed spaces when taken to altitude.

Patients with pneumothorax, bowel obstruction, and other conditions in which gas is trapped in a closed space are at risk. The most serious problem occurs in casualties who have an untreated pneumothorax. In properly treated casualties, a chest tube attached to a one-way valve will have been inserted and left in place until the air leak has sealed. However, if undetected prior to evacuation, the volume of trapped gas will increase as the ambient pressure falls, producing a degree of cardiorespiratory embarrassment that may require urgent decompression. Therefore, in cases of suspected pneumothorax, it is essential to obtain a chest radiograph prior to evacuation. It is much easier for the physician and safer for the patient to delay the evacuation, or, if evacuation must take place, to insert the chest tube, before departure. The alternative is being presented with the need to perform an arduous and dangerous act during the flight.

Expansion of gas in the intestinal tract can also give rise to problems. Although only small volumes are involved, there is a theoretical risk that the expansion of the gas could produce damage to anastomotic suture lines following intestinal surgery or dehiscence of the abdominal incision. One of the earlier tenets of air evacuation was to defer moving recently operated patients for at least 14 days although, based on Israeli experience with aeromedical evacuation starting with the Yom Kippur War and continuing through the Lebanon War of 1982, recent abdominal surgery is no longer considered a contraindication if the gastrointestinal tract is kept decompressed with a nasogastric tube.[26]

In a group of patients with paralytic ileus who were treated with hyperbaric oxygen, studies have shown that high concentrations of oxygen can reduce abdominal distension. It is possible to move casualties who have had recent operations if the patients receive 100% oxygen (via mask or endotracheal tube) during the flight.[27]

Of paramount importance is the status of the endotracheal tube or tracheostomy cuff balloon, which will expand at increasing altitude. This expansion can preclude patient ventilation and cause pressure necrosis of the tracheal wall. Although the volume of air used to inflate the cuff of an endotracheal tube used for ventilatory support is small, the changes in volume can produce complications even when using the modern, low-pressure, high-volume cuffed endotracheal tube. It is essential that the cuff be inflated with either saline or water to overcome this further complication of a change in ambient pressure.

During long-range medical evacuation, many casualties will be receiving intravenous fluids, the daily requirements of which have been carefully calculated. The fall in ambient pressure in the aircraft cabin can cause an appreciable acceleration of the rate of infusion because the volume of air in the intravenous infusion set will increase with increasing altitude. A drip chamber with a total volume of 9 mL that contains 2 mL of fluid at sea level will be completely empty at 2,000 m. It is therefore essential to monitor the drip rate, if infusion pumps are not in use. Care must be taken to ensure that adequate replacement fluid volumes are available (it is very difficult to obtain extra supplies while flying at 10,000 m). A final precaution to be observed is that all infusion fluid should be carried in flexible plastic containers, *not* in glass bottles, which could explode during the flight.

The problems associated with expansion of gas in closed spaces is found in air-pressure splints including pneumatic antishock garments (PASGs) and even certain types of stretchers. As ambient pressure decreases, the transmural pressure across the wall of the PASG will increase, causing it to inflate and thereby compress the casualty's incarcerated extremities and lower trunk. This effect is especially noticeable above 1,000 m. If the trousers are inflated while in flight, the opposite effect occurs during descent of the aircraft: the PASG becomes flaccid and therefore less effective than expected. Careful attention must be paid to changes in altitude to avoid mishaps en route. Experiments in a decompression chamber confirmed the theoretical consideration that there will be considerable increase in the volume of air in the splint as ambient pressure falls: measurements indicate a change in volume of almost 50% for every 1,000 ft, or about 16% per 100 m in altitude (—*CABMcL*, personal observation). In other words, the contained volume doubles for every 610 m increase in altitude. This finding is of importance in helicopter transfers, where air splints are used frequently.

The vacuum stretcher consists of a mattress containing a vast number of polystyrene beads. In its softened state, it is molded around the casualty, giving support and a degree of comfort. As the air is extracted from the mattress, the beads expand so that the mattress makes a total-body splint. However, as the ambient pressure falls, support decreases, requiring the further evacuation of air to maintain the support. During the descent, the support pressure increases and it is essential to maintain close control of the mattress's rigidity.

Oxygenation

While changes in air pressure are critical, given their potential for causing complications, of even greater importance is the need to deliver an adequate amount of oxygen not only to the patient but to the flight crew as well. The degree of hypoxia depends on the partial pressure of oxygen (PO_2) in the atmosphere. The PO_2 decreases in direct proportion to the decrease in pressure because the concentration of atmospheric oxygen remains about 21%. Therefore, at sea level, with barometric pressure approximately 760 mm Hg, the PO_2 in dry air is 169 mm Hg (21% of 760 mm Hg). At 3,000 m, where the barometric pressure is about 500 mm Hg, the partial pressure is 105 mm Hg (21% of 500 mm Hg). At the summit of Mount Everest (8,848 m or 29,028 ft, which is slightly below the normal cruising altitude of modern jet transports), the measured barometric pressure is 253 mm Hg and the estimated PO_2 is 53 mm Hg. Owing to the presence of water vapor in the lung and depending on the respiratory rate, the partial pressure of alveolar oxygen (PAO_2) will be lower to a variable extent. The measured PAO_2 on the summit of Mount Everest is 35 mm Hg, from which an arterial PO_2 (PaO_2) of only 28 mm Hg can be calculated.[28]

A simple consideration of the effect of barometric pressure on PO_2 explains why signs of hypoxia become increasingly obvious in even healthy persons as they fly higher than 3,000 m without supplemental oxygen. As PO_2 falls, the amount of oxygen transported by hemoglobin also falls, but the reduction is not a linear function of PaO_2 because the shape of the oxyhemoglobin dissociation curve is sigmoidal (see Figure 25-2 in Chapter 25, Acute Respiratory Failure and Ventilatory Management). At sea level, the PAO_2 is 100 mm Hg, which results in an arterial oxygen saturation of 95%. As a person goes to higher altitude, the PO_2 in the surrounding air decreases, resulting in a decrease in the amount of transported oxygen. The PO_2 in blood in the lungs and arteries decreases to the point that at 3,000 m, the PaO_2 is about 60 mm Hg and the hemoglobin in the arteries is only about 87% saturated (Figure 27-15). Because of the sigmoid shape of the oxyhemoglobin dissociation curve, a further increase in altitude results in a precipitous fall in oxygen saturation, such that at an altitude corresponding to the summit of Mount Everest, the estimated arterial oxygen saturation is only about 50%—substantially below the normal oxygen saturation of venous blood at sea level.

The importance of understanding the physics and physiology of hypoxia and oxygen delivery stems from the fact that battlefield casualties may have impaired pulmonary compliance, hypovolemia, anemia secondary to acute blood loss, acidosis, and also be hypothermic—factors that impair oxygen pickup in the lungs and oxygen delivery at the cellular level. Studies carried out early in the Vietnam War heightened concern about arterial desaturation occurring during high-altitude aeromedical evacuation. It was not unusual to find casualties being prepared for aeromedical evacuation with an arterial PO_2 of 50 mm Hg or less, breathing room air with a PO_2 of 150 mm Hg. Because the PO_2 is about 118 mm Hg in the cabin of a C-141 pressurized to about 2,400 m, a real potential existed for fatally low arterial oxygen saturations to develop.[29]

Accordingly, supplemental oxygen is needed by many casualties during aeromedical evacuation. The amount necessary to maintain a PaO_2 at 100 mm Hg is shown in the upper curve in Figure 27-15. In some cases, the fraction of inspired oxygen (FIO_2) needed is so high that elective intubation with positive pressure ventilation may be necessary to prevent significant desaturation at altitudes higher than 2,000 m.[30] However, because of the logistical and manpower constraints associated with the aeromedical evacuation of casualties who need mechanical ventilation, such casualties should be evacuated only in very unusual circumstances.

Almost all the oxygen transported by blood is carried by the hemoglobin in red blood cells; at sea level, only 0.2 mL of oxygen per 100 mL of blood is being carried in direct solution in the plasma. Therefore, the casualty's hemoglobin concentration and blood volume become important determinants of oxygen transport. Severely anemic or hypovolemic casualties are at risk during aeromedical evacuation even if their arterial oxygen saturation exceeds 90%. Hemoglobin levels should be measured prior to transfer in casualties who had sustained acute blood loss; the lowest acceptable level is approximately

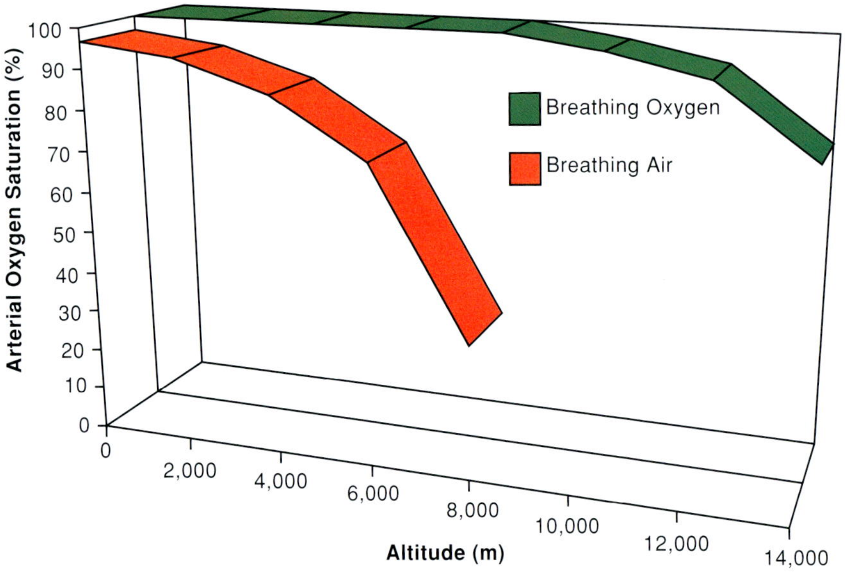

Fig. 27-15. Maintenance of arterial PO_2 with supplemental oxygen.

7.5 g of hemoglobin per deciliter of blood. A level of 10 g/dL will have already set into motion the several physiological compensatory mechanisms and so the casualty will be able to tolerate air transport.[31]

Blood volume cannot be so easily checked but is an equally important determinant of oxygen transport. A study carried out on casualties waiting to be evacuated from Vietnam found that 13 of 43 were hypovolemic, and an additional 8 were hypervolemic. Hematocrit values were not useful indicators of volume status, although anemic casualties were usually hypovolemic. Hypovolemia was especially common in casualties who were evacuated within 2 to 3 days of being wounded.[29]

Gravitational and Accelerative Forces

While not commonly thought of as causing patient problems, the effects of gravitational forces (*g*) can be quite detrimental during aeromedical evacuation. An individual sitting in a seat has a force equal to his weight, which is pressing against the seat. The intensity of this force, equal to the pull of gravity at the surface of Earth, is said to be 1*g*. The factors influencing gravitational forces are weight and its distribution; gravitational pull; and acceleration, which is caused by the movement of the vehicle. The most important effect of acceleration is on the circulatory system because blood, being mobile, can be translocated from one part of the body to another. Other tissues can also be displaced and distorted by accelerative forces, but they usually remain functional.

Both positive and negative gravitational forces affect casualties on medical evacuation flights. At accelerations greater than 4*g*, the systemic arterial pressure at the level of the heart falls to approximately 40 mm Hg. Therefore, a decrease in cardiac output may occur, which is secondary to venous pooling of blood in the lower extremities. Because of this complication, patients with compromised cardiac function should be positioned with the head toward the rear of the aircraft.[32]

The contrary process is also possible, because negative gravitational forces can cause a tremendous increase in arterial pressure that, when transmitted to the head, can cause blood pressure to rise as high as 400 mm Hg. This extreme pressure increase may cause a paradoxical effect via the baroreceptor reflex, with slowing and even stopping of the heart. The cerebrospinal fluid in the cranial vault may act as a buffer to the expansion of the intravascular blood volume. However, some small vessels on the surface may rupture and subarachnoid hemorrhages have developed in animals exposed to negative gravitational forces. For these reasons, a casualty with a head injury or increased intracranial pressure should be positioned with his head toward the front of the aircraft.[33]

Thermal Stress

Battlefield casualties may have been exposed to the elements for extended periods. Extremes of heat and cold can both cause medical problems. The vascular system's compensatory vasoconstriction and vasodilation associated with thermal regulation may cause significant fluid shifts and thereby make more difficult the assessment of the adequacy of volume restoration. The volume-depleted hypothermic patient, whose hemodynamics may be fairly normal while the vascular bed is contracted, becomes hypotensive as the vascular bed dilates in response to warmth.

The temperature at Earth's surface is approximately 20°C; the temperature at 10,000 ft is 0°C. While most rotor-wing flights are at a lower altitude than 10,000 ft, the thermal losses to radiation, evaporation, conduction, and convection may be significant and underestimated. Attempts to provide at least a physiologically normal temperature will decrease oxygen consumption and improve the medical officer's ability to assess the patient.

Noise and Vibration

Rotor-wing aircraft and ground ambulances create a significant amount of noise and vibration that are difficult to moderate. These factors may affect electrocardiographic monitoring, noninvasive blood pressure monitoring, pulse oximetry, and the auscultatory efforts of the monitoring team. Because of these limitations, the medical officer must be able to perform some form of adaptive monitoring procedure. These include palpating and assessing radial, brachial, and femoral pulses, and correlating them to mean arterial pressure; observing respiratory excursion and patterns of breathing for any acute changes in status; and intervening appropriately. The simplicity and reliability of mechanical monitors will commonly be lost during transport. The noise levels, especially in tracked vehicles and at aircraft takeoff and landing, are a potent source of stress. Taking clinical measurements on unconscious patients may cause sharp rises in pulse, blood pressure, and respiration rate if protective earplugs are not used. The noise levels, especially when associated with vibrational frequencies above 10 Hz, are more detrimental to patient care than are the physiological effects of the vibration.

The speed of transit can also affect the low-frequency vibrations to which casualties can be subjected. In a study of four different types of ground ambulances, marked increases in two low-frequency areas (at 4–8 Hz and 16–28 Hz) occurred when the ambulances traveled between 30 and 45 mph. The tests were repeated in ambulances fitted with a "floating" stretcher. The results confirmed that the vibrations can be damped down in the specific frequency areas, but the cost of fitting this type of stretcher would be prohibitive.[32]

Fatigue and Sleep Lag

The evacuation of patients over many thousands of miles, through several time zones and different ambient temperatures, gives rise to general fatigue, due largely to disturbances of the circadian rhythms (ie, jet lag).[34] In addition, even in a fit person, the long flight at reduced barometric pressure, with the resulting lowered oxygen tensions, gives rise to serious fatigue problems. The level of degradation of performance is difficult to quantify, but experimental work in a decompression chamber showed a marked reduction in the appreciation and performance of tests when initially attempted, although once learned, there were no problems with retention of the newly acquired skills.[35] A general level of fatigue is demonstrated by patients during long-distance transfer flights, especially when overnight stops are necessary. The marked improvement as a result of direct flights was first noted in the German sick and wounded who were being evacuated during the Spanish Civil War: even though the aircraft were unpressurized and unheated, nonstop flights were considered better for the patients.[25]

Workers in New Zealand have a possible treatment for jet lag. The pineal gland (ie, the "third" eye) secretes melatonin, which is considered to be one of the principal factors in setting the biological clock. Preliminary findings indicate that when research subjects take formulations of melatonin, compared with a placebo, the effects of jet lag are markedly reduced.[36]

MEDICAL DETERMINANTS OF SAFE EVACUATION

Specific medical factors, such as abdominal and eye injuries, may increase the risk of medical evacuation. Clearly, other factors (eg, enemy action and mechanical problems associated with the design and operation of the aircraft) may adversely affect the evacuee, but they will not be discussed here.

In-Flight Medical Problems of Long-Range Aeromedical Evacuation

Only limited historical data have been gathered on the medical aspects of aeromedical evacuation. The most useful data are from the Vietnam War;

although long-range casualty evacuation occurred during both Operation Just Cause in Panama (1989) and the Persian Gulf War (1990–1991), the number of American casualties was too small to draw meaningful conclusions, although much interesting anecdotal information was collected.

The Vietnam War

The low frequency of death observed during aeromedical evacuation (< 1 per 20,000 casualties evacuated) during the Vietnam War does not necessarily mean that nonlethal medical problems were similarly infrequent. In lieu of data from a more recent war, the U.S. Air Force medical evacuation experience in the early years of the Vietnam War, in which casualties were evacuated through an aeromedical staging facility in the Philippine Islands prior to being evacuated to Japan, is of interest. Of some 20,000 casualties already in the evacuation chain, many (68 of 128 in one check) were found to have developed signs and symptoms indicative of the possible development of potentially serious complications. Complications were especially common in three categories of casualties[29(p276)]:

1. Vascular injuries. Of 347 casualties who had vascular reconstruction, 187 were found during aeromedical evacuation to have developed signs and symptoms suggestive of a complication (ie, a cool, pulseless extremity; excessive pain in the limb; excessive drainage; fever). No fewer than 57 of the 187 (approximately 30%) required an extremity amputation.
2. Chest injuries. Of 629 casualties who had chest trauma, 137 were found to have a pneumothorax or a hemothorax. One third of this group, 46 casualties, presented with respiratory distress, and 16 of 17 in whom arterial blood-gas measurements were made had a PaO_2 less than 80 mm Hg while breathing room air. It seems likely that these casualties had pathologically low arterial oxygen saturation during evacuation. Thirty-one casualties of the group of 137 had a nonfunctioning chest tube in place. Heimlich valves had been used in some patients and in several this was defective, allowing air to remain in the pleural space.
3. Abdominal injuries. Of 626 casualties with abdominal trauma, 117 had signs and symptoms during the evacuation that indicated the need for reoperation. Among the more common indications were dehiscence, evidence of peritonitis, intestinal obstruction, stress ulcer hemorrhage, hemorrhage from an abdominal wound, and wound sepsis.

It should be understood that (*a*) these complications were apparent after 6-hour evacuation flights, (*b*) many of the complications had probably existed prior to evacuation but had not been diagnosed, and (*c*) these casualties probably were evacuated prematurely. The Vietnam aeromedical evacuation experience strongly suggests that the medical problems that do develop are much more likely to be associated with the original injury than with abnormal environment in the evacuation.

Operation Just Cause and the Persian Gulf War

The distinguishing military medical characteristics of Operation Just Cause in Panama was the paucity of third-echelon medical assets deployed with the combat units. Although a surgical team was present to perform emergency lifesaving surgery on the critically wounded, initial surgery was performed on most casualties in military hospitals in San Antonio, Texas. After receiving first aid at the unit level and MASF, these casualties, together with those who had already been operated on, were evacuated in C-141s, which soon became aerial emergency and intensive care wards. Not surprisingly, "In-flight care for these fresh combat casualties was a challenge for the usual crew of two flight nurses and three aeromedical evacuation technicians."[37(p943)]

In contrast to Operation Just Cause, the Persian Gulf War was characterized by a long buildup period during which extensive third-echelon medical assets were deployed. Even so, the anticipated casualty rates were so high that the need to evacuate fresh, unstable casualties was thought to be highly likely. As a result of the Panama experience and breaking with the tradition existing since World War II, medical commanders decided to assign physicians to at least some tactical and strategic air evacuation flights so as to optimize the success of lifesaving, in-flight, medical interventions.[37] Fortunately, actual U.S. and Allied casualties were only a tiny fraction of those anticipated, and the need for lifesaving interventions was correspondingly small.

The experiences in both of these wars suggest that injury-related complications, rather than the adverse physiological conditions of the evacuation environment, will be the major source of problems.

Furthermore, it seems likely that the proportion of evacuated casualties who develop injury-related complications during evacuation will be inversely related to the interval between wounding and evacuation (ie, the more quickly the casualty is evacuated after wounding, the more likely it is that a complication will develop). Therefore, both during mass casualty situations and when the theater evacuation policy is very short (eg, during a short but intense conflict), military anesthesia providers should be especially alert to the possibility of in-flight medical problems.

Civilian Experience

A relevant civilian experience also supports the view that medical problems during evacuation are more likely to be due to the original injury than due to evacuation per se. After resuscitative surgery (usually a laparotomy) was carried out in a rural hospital, patients were transferred to a regional trauma center within 48 hours of injury. No deaths occurred during evacuation, but 8 of the 19 patients studied developed tachycardia or became hypotensive; 7 of the 8 unstable patients subsequently died. Transport time averaged 2.4 hours. All but 3 of the patients had blunt trauma as the mechanism of their injuries. A physician and a nurse accompanied all patients, all received intravenous fluids, and all but 2 were mechanically ventilated.[38]

Patient Conditions Leading to Medical Instability

The major constraints placed on battlefield evacuation from and to the first and second echelons of care arise not so much from the conditions of the casualties but from enemy action and the availability of the means of evacuation. Evacuation from higher echelons may, however, be constrained by the aeromedical evacuation policy of the U.S. Air Force, which is based on the realization that some patients' medical conditions predispose to in-flight complications. The air force does not recognize any absolute contraindication to aeromedical evacuation, but a variety of conditions either constitute relative contraindications to evacuation or require that arrangements be made for specialized treatment if evacuation is to proceed.[2(pE-3),31]

When they enter the U.S. Air Force medical evacuation system, casualties should be stable enough to tolerate a 1- to 24-hour trip with a high probability that complications will not occur. The necessary degree of stabilization depends on the operational situation: tactical missions are typically shorter than strategic missions. Therefore, less-stable patients might tolerate tactical evacuation, but strategic evacuation might be highly detrimental.

Abdominal Injuries

Patients with abdominal injuries should be carefully evaluated by a general surgeon prior to flight. Use of nasogastric or rectal tubes or both should be considered to avoid both the distention frequently encountered with a nonfunctioning bowel and the gas-volume changes associated with varying barometric pressure. Extra colostomy bags should accompany the patient. Drainage is more profuse at altitude because of gas expansion. It is essential that military surgeons close all abdominal incisions with retention sutures to minimize in-flight dehiscence due to expansion of intraabdominal gas.

Cardiovascular Disease

Patients with severe cardiovascular disease usually have reduced tolerance to hypoxia, but they generally do well during flight if provided supplemental oxygen. With appropriate preparation monitoring, patients with recent myocardial infarctions can usually be moved by airlift. Unstable patients requiring in-flight cardiac monitoring will be moved with a medical attendant, and the referring medical treatment facility must provide an air force–approved monitor. Patients who have had a myocardial infarction should not be evacuated for at least 10 days, and should have been free of pain for 5 days. If monitored, such patients must be accompanied by a physician.

Thoracic Injuries

Chest tubes should be left in place in casualties with thoracic injuries. However, each chest tube will require a Heimlich valve and an underwater chest drainage system approved for air evacuation use. Ideally, patients with recently removed chest tubes should not be airlifted until the following conditions are met:

- at least 24 hours have elapsed since the chest tube was removed;
- normal expiratory and lordotic chest radiographs have been taken at least 24 hours after removal of the chest tube (just prior to airlift, if possible), with an interpretation in the patient's medical record; and

- an occlusive dressing has been placed at the site where the chest tube was removed.

Eye Injuries

Penetrating eye wounds or surgery or both can sometimes introduce air into the globe of the eye, making it susceptible to the effects of oxygen deficiency and, especially, decreased barometric pressure. Presence of gas in the posterior chamber comes as close to constituting an absolute contraindication to high-altitude aeromedical evacuation as there is likely to be. A delay in evacuation, or an altitude restriction, is recommended for such patients.

Hematological Considerations

Ideally, patients should have a preflight hemoglobin concentration of 10 g/dL or a hematocrit of 0.30. Severely traumatized patients may have readings below those levels, and supplemental oxygen may be required. Hemoglobin concentration can be as low as 8.5 g/dL if the patient's condition is chronic, stable, and not due to bleeding.

Infectious Disease

Patients in the infectious stage of a serious communicable disease need to be segregated from the other evacuees.

Maxillofacial Injuries

Due to the increased potential for nausea and vomiting, patients with wired, immobilized upper and lower jaws must have a quick-release mechanism applied or have easy access to wire cutters in their possession. Premedication with an antiemetic should be considered.

Neurological Injuries

The decreased Po_2 at altitude can cause increased intracranial pressure in casualties with head injuries. Low-flow oxygen and an altitude restriction should be considered for flight. Noise, vibration, and thermal stresses can precipitate seizures, and adequate antiseizure medication levels should be established before flight. Valsalva's maneuver should be avoided by patients at risk from increased intracranial pressure. Therefore, administrating a preflight decongestant and inserting a polyethylene tube into the patient's middle ears should be considered, especially if the patient is comatose. Patients who have had a craniotomy should not be evacuated for at least 48 hours after surgery, and should be awake and alert. The subtle changes in neurological status that are usually discovered during routine neurological checks are very difficult to detect during flight; patients requiring close observation are poor candidates for aeromedical evacuation. Stable, comatose patients can be transported. Decreased humidity at altitude dictates that patients with a loss of corneal blink reflex be provided with bilateral eye patches and eye ointment or liquid tears. Intraventricular monitoring cannot be accomplished during flight.

Orthopedic Injuries

Ideally, casts on recent fractures should be at least 48 hours old. All casts should be bivalved unless that would jeopardize the stability of the fracture. Free-swinging weights for traction are unacceptable for flight. Cervical traction is available via a Collins traction device; however, a medical officer must be present when the device is applied. Patients using crutches should travel by litter because of the safety factors involved in moving about on unstable aircraft. Crutches should accompany the patient and be stowed aboard the aircraft.

Thermal Injuries

In general, casualties with thermal injuries should not be evacuated during the period of fluid sequestration (ie, the first 48 h). Thermal injuries should be covered with occlusive dressings. Escharotomies are required for full-thickness circumferential burns. Extra burn dressings for in-flight reinforcement should be provided. Limited infusion pumps and poor in-flight refrigeration capabilities preclude the use of total parenteral nutrition. Infusions of 10% dextrose in water with necessary electrolytes should be ordered as a short-term substitute. Phosphorous injuries should be covered with saline-soaked dressings. Large vesicles and bullae should be protected during the evacuation with large, bulky dressings.

Vascular Injuries

Vascular repairs should be clearly recorded on Patient Evacuation Form DD 602 or 1380. Casts that are less than 48 hours old should be bivalved and windowed over the injured area in case excessive swelling occurs during flight.

Psychiatric Illness

Severely ill psychiatric patients (Classification 1A) require a litter, leather wrist and ankle restraints, and sedation. Patients whose psychiatric illnesses are of intermediate severity (Classification 1B) require a litter and sedation, and restraints must be available. All psychiatric patients on litters must be searched, and all sharp objects such as razor blades and pocket knives must be removed as part of the antihijacking procedure. A secondary search must be accomplished just before enplaning.

Drug and Alcohol Abuse

Soldiers who are being treated for drug and alcohol abuse should undergo 3 to 5 days of detoxification before they are airlifted. An aeromedical evacuation mission is not equipped to deal with acute withdrawal symptoms.

Preparation for Evacuation

Initial Assessment

The Advanced Trauma Life Support (ATLS) course of the American College of Surgeons is taught to military physicians as part of the Combat Casualty Care Course.[39] Prior to evacuation, the initial assessment of the casualty's condition is based on the ATLS ABCs (*a*irway, *b*reathing, and *c*irculation) and the extent and location of injury, especially when the time available for battlefield medical implementation of ATLS is short and injuries may have been missed.

The "Golden Hour" concept, which arises from the civilian trauma experience, suggests that if a trauma patient with a survivable injury who is in clinical shock does not receive the definitive care necessary to reverse the process within the first hour after entering the shock state, the long-term survivability drops below 10%. This is independent of the quality of care after that 60-minute period.[30] In the context of combat casualty care, providing care within the Golden Hour is important, because about 90% of the total combat mortality occurs within the first hour after wounding (see Chapter 1, Combat Trauma Overview, for a more complete discussion). In Vietnam, transport took 35 minutes after the patient was loaded.[40] The Germans[41] and Swiss[42] can transport at least 90% of their population in 15 minutes or less, but of course conditions for civilian aeromedical evacuation in these countries are more favorable than they were in Vietnam: there is no need to pick up casualties from a dense jungle or from a landing zone exposed to enemy small-arms fire.

The chaos of the battlefield or aid station may preclude an organized approach to each casualty. However, the rules of assessment, resuscitation, and stabilization must be followed in an orderly manner. This provides as safe a mechanism as possible for the transport of the trauma patient.

Supplies and Equipment Required From the Originating Medical Treatment Facility

The MASF does not have any equipment that can be given in replacement: all equipment and supplies that each casualty will need during the entire evacuation process must be supplied by the originating medical treatment facility (MTF) and accompany the casualty to the aeromedical staging facility. U.S. Army anesthesiologists should be aware of the following U.S. Air Force requirements for supplies and equipment[31]:

- Patient medications. Patients transported intratheater should be given a 3-day supply of medications and supplies; intertheater patients should be given a 5-day supply.
- Intravenous fluids. The referring MTF should provide a 3-day supply of intravenous fluids and infusion equipment, including all necessary supplies for antibiotic administration, if required.
- Special medical equipment. Special equipment includes cardiac monitors, ventilators, Stryker frames, continuous-suction units, pulse oximeters, oxygen analyzers, and restraints.

As a rule, dressings will be reinforced but not changed during flight due to the relatively unclean in-flight environment. Serious complications such as bleeding, increased pain, or swelling may require wound inspection. Routine dressings will be provided by the air evacuation crew; however, unique dressings or dressings for patients with excessively draining wounds should be provided by the originating MTF.

Physician's Orders

Although the recommendation has been made that flight surgeons augment the basic air evacuation crew on selected tactical and strategic evacuation missions,[37] the absence of physicians on most U.S. Air Force aeromedical evacuation missions emphasizes the absolute criticality that clear and concise orders, covering the entire patient transfer, be written on the Patient Evacuation Tag, DD Form 602. The referring physician is legally responsible for all medical care until the patient reaches the destination facility.

Stretchers and Securing the Casualty in the Aircraft

The first principle of aeromedical evacuation is that the casualty must be securely fastened to the evacuation platform. If a casualty has an extremity fracture, the fracture must be immobilized for both safe and humane transportation. This is especially necessary when bumpy ground evacuation is expected.

At this time, there are at least 30 different types of stretchers available for use by NATO forces, constructed from various materials, but still based on the Swiss designs of 1912 and 1922. This multiplicity of stretchers can lead to problems in locating the stretcher in the different types of transport. With the wealth of new materials available at the end of the 20th century, it seems remarkable that a suitable stretcher has not been developed that is compatible with the road, rail, sea, and air requirements. In a mass casualty situation, the loading of stretcher patients is important: more seriously ill casualties must be positioned to ensure all-around access for the medical and nursing team. Also, adequate facilities must be available at the departure airhead to enable rapid loading of the casualties. It is also necessary to have the ground facilities to maintain full medical care for at least 24 hours, should there be a delay in the evacuating flights.

The differing aircraft likely to be used have loading doors at varying heights above ground. Some, like the C-130 Hercules and the C-141 Starlifter, can of course be loaded directly, but when commercial jets such as the VC-10, Lockheed 1001, and Boeing 737, 747, and 767 are used in medical evacuation, special loading ramps are necessary.

In all forms of transportation, but especially by air, it is essential to ensure that the patients are securely strapped to their stretchers,. These, in turn, are located on the fixed stretcher supports to minimize the acceleration and deceleration forces that are generated during ground transportation and takeoff and landing of fixed-wing aircraft.

Stretchers are traditionally placed longitudinally, with the casualty traveling head first, whatever form of transport is being employed. Many have suggested that the ideal siting of stretchers would be transverse: across the aircraft cabin. This siting would lessen the fore-and-aft movements of body fluids during the acceleration and deceleration phases of travel.

Stryker frames are generally indicated for paraplegia, quadriplegia, cervical fractures, severe burns, and those patients requiring total assistance. Patients with cervical injuries and wearing halo traction may be transported on a regular litter or, if stabilized, they may be transported as ambulatory patients. All components of the Stryker frame must be sent with the casualty from the originating MTF to allow continuity of patient care and turning of patients throughout transfer. Stretcher frames and the stretcher harness must be stressed to at least 6*g* to give a wide margin of safety should it be necessary to abandon the takeoff in a fixed-wing aircraft.

Catheters

Intravenous Infusions. The military anesthesiologist must be extremely attentive to the establishment, securing, and maintenance of intravenous lines. These lines are important for the continued resuscitation of the casualty as well as for the administration of needed pain medication and other drugs. The establishment of large, easily accessible, secure lines should be uppermost in the anesthesiologist's mind, as these lines may provide the only means of drug delivery.

Patients who require intravenous fluids on the ground will also require them during the flight, owing to the excessively dry cabin environment. Catheter function should be assessed prior to transport to ensure that the catheter is securely in place. Patients requiring antibiotics without fluid replacements should be switched to a heparin lock with heparin flushes provided. A 3-day supply of intravenous fluid should accompany each patient who requires intravenous fluids.

Urinary Catheters. Indwelling urinary catheters and drainage bags in use before transport should be left in place during evacuation, or inserted before the flight if urinary retention is a problem. The internal balloon should be filled with sterile, normal saline or water instead of air to avoid gas expansion during the flight.

Nasogastric Tubes. Nasogastric tube insertion is recommended for patients with abdominal wounds, abscesses or obstructions, paraplegia or quadriplegia, or the potential for paralytic ileus. Limited suction capabilities are available aboard the aircraft; however, the distal end of the tube may be left to drain by gravity into a glove or bag.

Respiratory Support

The utmost concern in the mind of every anesthesiologist is the adequacy of the patient's airway and therefore of the patient's ventilation. The need to establish a definitive airway rapidly is foremost in ATLS instruction. Several aspects of the maintenance of a patent airway during aeromedical evacuation deserve special mention.

Airway Management. Endotracheal tubes should be used if the patient requires assisted ventilation and should be inserted before aeromedical evacuation begins. Balloon cuffs should be filled with normal saline instead of air, as gas expansion at altitude may cause tracheal damage.

Airway Stability. Several questions must be answered while the casualty is being prepared for evacuation. Is the patient breathing spontaneously? Will the patient's airway need attention? What is the potential that the patient's airway will be compromised? The significance of the airway in air ambulance transport revolves around the ability to control ventilation and the need for personnel (nurses, medics, respiratory technicians) and equipment to aid that ventilation. Coexisting injuries may compromise the airway, such as cervical instability and severe facial trauma including LeFort fractures. The military anesthesiologist must remember that airway problems are especially common in casualties with burn injuries.

Tracheostomies. Tracheotomy tubes should be changed before flight and an extra tube should be sent with the patient.

Ventilators. Ventilator-dependent patients will be accompanied by a respiratory therapist or other appropriate medical attendant from the referring MTF. The apneic patient requires full ventilatory support from a respirator that will provide automatic control. There are many such machines available, but in the context of military aeromedical evacuation, it is likely that compactness and durability will be preferred to sophistication (ie, a multitude of dials and controls, such as those seen in intensive care units). A further constraint is the mode of operation. All but the simplest ventilators require a compressor to provide the gas that drives the ventilator. Transportation ventilators must be lightweight, rugged, durable, and simple to operate. Manual ventilation may be all that is available on a helicopter flight.

Humidifiers. Because the ambient cabin humidity during long-distance aeromedical evacuation is usually between 5% and 20%, marked insensible water loss and drying of the respiratory tract should be expected. This consideration applies to all patients but especially to those in whom the normal humidifying function of the nose is prevented, such as casualties with a tracheostomy or an endotracheal tube. It will therefore be necessary to provide adequate humidification to avoid the problems of ventilating with dry gases.

There are many humidifiers, as there are ventilators, but the simplest, and therefore the most appropriate, device is the small condenser humidifier, which can be plugged into the ventilating circuit. A lightweight item, it works by passing the fresh gases through the condenser foil on which the water vapor in the expired air condenses. The water is then available to humidify the inspired oxygen. A bonus, of course, is the degree of heat conservation achieved during the respiratory cycle. The efficiency of the "Swedish nose" (the Humid-Vent Heat-Moisture Exchanger, manufactured by Gibeck Respiration Co., Uplands, Väsby, Sweden) is such that a relative humidity of approximately 50% can be maintained during the transfer.[43]

Oxygen. There are many simple devices available to deliver oxygen, ranging from nasal cannulae and the simple mask, which deliver variable concentrations and flows of oxygen, to fixed-dilution Venturi masks, which are capable of delivering 24% to 50% oxygen. It is difficult to tap into the main aircraft oxygen supplies, so the source of oxygen for patients must be cylinders; however, when required in large numbers, oxygen cylinders produce a severe weight penalty. A further problem is the availability of adequate numbers of the appropriate cylinder sizes. It is therefore necessary to consider alternative sources of oxygen for in-flight use.

Liquid oxygen, despite being considered in some quarters to be dangerous cargo on aircraft, offers an excellent alternative means, as can be seen from the volumes of gaseous oxygen available from one 30-L flask of liquid oxygen: one such flask is equivalent to 18 large cylinders of compressed gas, with the obvious weight savings. The problem of fitting a heat exchanger to avoid freezing of the delivery outlet can be overcome without much difficulty. The pressure-swing absorber system (ie, the oxygen concentrator) must also be considered as a source of additional oxygen. The concentrator works by forcing dried ambient air, at a low pressure, through fractionating columns of zeolite crystals. As air passes through the zeolite, all other constituents of air are removed except oxygen and argon. At the delivery end of the unit, a mixture of up to 95% oxygen and 5% argon is obtained, at a rate of 4 L/min. Of course, this is not the standard required for medical oxygen, but is a perfectly satisfactory oxygen supply. There have been no reports of the effects of ventilating with a mixture of oxygen and argon. The oxygen concentrator requires a power source to drive the compressor and produce a continuous supply of oxygen, but little maintenance. If the flow through the columns is increased, a higher volume of oxygen is produced, but the percentage of oxygen falls in direct relation to the increased flow through the columns.

Fracture Stabilization

The problems that increasing and decreasing gravitational forces exert on fractures during aircraft acceleration and deceleration have already been discussed. It is during the transport of patients with severe fractures that the problems assume great importance.

Most patients transported by air or ground ambulance will be immobilized on stretchers or gurneys. The ability to maintain in-line traction for cervical injuries as well as continued support for long-bone fractures is essential. The goal is to prevent the conversion of stable injuries to unstable injuries. It is necessary in all cases of spinal fracture, especially the cervical spine, with or without paralysis, to ensure that the degree of traction on the spine is maintained accurately. Although modern jets will be flying above the weather, there is still the problem of clear-air turbulence. When this happens, the gravitational forces exerted as the aircraft is bounced about can increase 4- to 5-fold, so that a traction weight of 10 lb will immediately increase to 40 or 50 lb, with the obvious deleterious effects on the patient, even though such forces occur for extremely short periods of time.

The Stryker frame or its derivatives used for transferring patients with spinal fractures did not address the problems of (*a*) rapid increases in forces exerted and (*b*) difficulty in moving the frame and patient.[44] The Povey turning frame addresses many of the problems experienced with the Stryker frame.[45] It weighs only 70 lb and can easily be moved. The traction weights are maintained horizontally, eliminating the high vertical-acceleration forces. The weights can also be maintained during any necessary nursing procedure. The Povey frame takes up much less space on the aircraft, and the amount of whip during turbulent conditions is much reduced.

The whole frame can be turned through 360° while head and neck traction are maintained. This is important for the nursing care of patients with fracture and paralysis. In the quadriplegic patient, it is essential to maintain full nursing care to the skin, which, deprived of sensory input, can rapidly become broken and develop serious infection at the damaged area.

Historically, motion sickness does not appear to have been a significant problem in transporting physiologically stable casualties. In all cases of spinal injury it is essential to ensure that a nasogastric tube is passed prior to takeoff, as one of the immediate and fatal complications of such injuries is acute dilation of the stomach, leading to massive emesis. The presence of the tube will permit continuous aspiration of the stomach, thus avoiding the complication.

Casualty Assessment and Monitoring

Ideally, the same monitoring equipment found in an intensive care unit in a fourth-echelon hospital (or a Level-1 trauma hospital) would be available throughout the evacuation chain. Obviously, however, logistical realities constrain equipment availability. Inspection of the patient is probably still the best monitor available. As with the ventilators, it is necessary that all items used must be rugged, lightweight, and compatible with the aircraft type. The power supplies in aircraft vary so, as the degree of sophistication of the electronic monitors used increases, it is necessary to know the type of airplane to be used.

All monitoring equipment generates a degree of electromagnetic interference, which can interfere with navigational or communication equipment of the aircraft. It is therefore necessary for all monitors to be tested for such interference. Standards have been formulated, but at this time very few of the items tested have received a seal of approval on first testing.[46]

It would seem logical to employ battery-operated monitoring equipment in an attempt to avoid electromagnetic induction. There are, however, problems with the type of battery available during air transport. The sight of an acid-filled battery being carried aboard—even the nonspill type—will raise concerns about safety. The duration of battery life is also an important consideration as the battery chargers available for use give rise to an induction field, which precludes their used in flight. Several monitoring packages are now being produced that will, it is hoped, satisfy the safety requirements.

SUMMARY

The requirement to evacuate the sick and wounded is of much greater importance in military medicine than it is in civilian medical practice. This fact is a consequence of one of the distinguishing characteristics of military medicine: the provision of care by echelons. The nature of evacuation and the conditions under which it is carried out differ according to the echelons. At one extreme is the army's evacuation from the battlefield of gravely wounded, unstable combat casualties by ground ambulance or rotor-wing aircraft. At the other extreme is the air force's intertheater (strategic) evacuation of stable combat casualties by long-range jet transport. The medical complications of evacuation arise primarily from the basic injury, but aspects of the somewhat unphysiological environment of high-altitude, long-range aeromedical evacuation may contribute to morbidity and even mortality. Foremost among these are (*a*) decreased barometric pressure, which can cause expansion of abnormal collections of gas trapped within the body; and (*b*) decreased PO_2, which may give rise to arterial desaturation and defective oxygen transport. It is imperative that military anesthesiologists understand how to order and to carry out evacuation from the battlefield and from the levels of care in which they ordinarily practice. Recognizing the capabilities and limitations of the evacuation assets serving each level of care is especially important.

REFERENCES

1. Pirogov NI. *Nacala Obcsej Voenno-Polevoj Chirurigii.* (*Origins of Military Field Surgery.*) St. Petersburg, Russia: 1857. In German: *Grundziige der Allgemeinen Kriegscherurgie*. Leipzig, Germany: 1864. No English translation is available.
2. Department of the Army. *Medical Evacuation in a Theater of Operations*. Washington DC: Headquarters, DA; 31 October 1991. Field Manual 8-10-6.
3. Ransom JE. Care of the sick and wounded in early wars. *CIBA Symposium*. 1947;8:541–542.
4. Polybius; Scott-Kilvert I, trans. *The Rise of the Roman Empire*. London, England: Penguin Books; 1979: 477.
5. Uzac M, Suffrin-Herbert M. *Neuvieme Question*. Paris, France: Premier Congress International de l'Aviation Sanitaire; 1929.
6. Blanco RL. *Wellington's Surgeon General: Sir James McGrigor*. Durham, NC: Duke University Press; 1974: 121.
7. Letterman J. *Medical Recollections of the Army of the Potomac*. New York, NY: D Appleton and Company; 1866: 171.
8. Meneces ANT. The transport of casualties by air. *J Roy Army Med Corps*. 1951;96:1–12.
9. Lam DM. To pop a balloon: Aeromedical evacuation in the 1879 siege of Paris. *Aviat Space Environ Med*. 1988;59:998–991.
10. William AW The flying ambulance. *Milit Surg*. 1943;92:443–446.
11. McLaren CAB. Aeromedical evacuation. *Aviat Med Q*. 1987;1:41–49.
12. Scholl MD, Geshekter CL. The Zed Expedition: The world's first air ambulance? *J R Soc Med*. 1989;82:679.
13. Kowalzig H. Long distance transportation of the wounded at high altitudes. *Deut Militarzt*. 1940;5:10–14.
14. Schmidt F. Transport of the wounded by plane. *Deut Militarzt*. 1940;5:7–10.

15. Cosmas GA, Cowdrey AE. *Medical Service in the European Theater of Operations*. Washington, DC: Center of Military History, US Army; 1992: 106.

16. Futrell RF. Development of aeromedical evacuation in the USAF: 1909–1960. USAF Historical Division, Air University. 1960: 507. Cited in: Mabry EW, Munson RA, Richardson LA. The wartime need for aeromedical evacuation physicians: The U.S. Air Force experience during Operation Desert Storm. *Aviation, Space, and Environmental Medicine*. 1993;Oct:941–946.

17. Marsh AR. A short but distant war. *J R Soc Med*. 1983;76:972–982.

18. Dorland P, Nanney J. *Dust Off: Army Aeromedical Evacuation in Vietnam*. Washington, DC: Center of Military History, US Army; 1984: 9.

19. Champion HR, Sacco WJ, Carnazzo AJ, Copes W, Foulty W. Trauma score. *Crit Care Med*. 1981;9:673–676.

20. Clemmer TP, Orme JF, Thomas F, Brooks KA. Prospective evaluation of the CRAMS scale for triaging major trauma. *J Trauma*. 1985;25:188–191.

21. Champion HR. Helicopter triage. *Emerg Care Q*. 1986;2:13–21.

22. Association of Air Medical Services. Position paper on the appropriate use of emergency air medical services. *J Air Med Transport*. Sept 1990;29–33.

23. Medical News and Perspectives. *JAMA*. 1994;271(16):1225–1228.

24. US Departments of the Army and the Air Force. *Worldwide Aeromedical Evacuation*. Washington, DC: HQ DA, DAF; 1979. Air Force Regulation 164-5, Army Regulation 40-535.

25. Parson CJ, Bobechko. Aeromedical transport: Its hidden problems. *Can Med Assoc J*. 1982;126: 237–243.

26. Dolev E. Early evacuation of patients from the battlefield after laparotomy: Experience in Vietnam, Israel and the Falklands. *Milit Med*. 1987;152: 57–59.

27. Loder RE. Use of hyperbaric oxygen in paralytic ileus. *Br Med J*. 1977;1(6074):1448–1449.

28. West JB. *Everest: The Testing Place*. New York, NY: McGraw-Hill Book Company; 1985.

29. Whelan TJ, Burkhalter WE, Gomez A. Management of war wounds. *Curr Probl Surg*. 1967;Sept:339.

30. Stene JL, Grande CM. *Trauma Anesthesia*. Baltimore, Md: Williams & Wilkins; 1991: Chap 15.

31. Department of the Air Force. *Physicians' Roles and Responsibilities in Aeromedical Evacuation*. Washington, DC: Secretary of the USAF; 1995: in press. Air Force Joint Manual 41-306.

32. Snook R, Pacifico R. Ambulance ride: Fixed or floating stretcher. *Br Med J*. 1976;2:405–407.

33. Hippke E. Transport of the sick and wounded. *Milit Surg*. 1940;86:439–440.

34. Siegel PV. Time zone effects. *Science*. 1969;164:1249–1255.

35. Denison DM, Ledwith F, Poulton EC. Complex reaction times at simulated cabin altitudes of 5,000 feet and 8,000 feet. *Aerospace Med*. 1966;37:1010–1013.

36. Petrie K, Conaglen JV, Thompson C, Chamberlain K. Effect of melatonin on jet lag after long haul flights. *Br Med J*. 1989;298:745–747.

37. Mabry EW, Munson RA, Richardson LA. The wartime need for aeromedical evacuation physicians: The US Air Force experience during Operation Desert Storm. *Aviation, Space, and Environmental Medicine*. 1993;Oct:941–946.

38. SR Sharar, GK Luna, Rice CL, Valenzuela TD, Copass MK. Air transport following surgical stabilization: An extension of regionalized trauma care. *J Trauma*. 1988;28:794–797.

39. Committee on Trauma, American College of Surgeons. *Advanced Trauma Life Support Program for Physicians: Instructor Manual*. 5th ed. Chicago, Ill: American College of Surgeons; 1993.

40. Neel S. Army aeromedical evacuation procedures in Vietnam. *JAMA*. 1968;204:99–103.

41. Burghart H. Helicopter rescue for traffic accidents: The West German experience. *Emerg Med Serv*. 1986;June:72–74.

42. Brismar B, Dahlgren BE, Larsson J. Ambulance utilization in Sweden: Analysis of emergency ambulance missions in urban and rural areas. *Ann Emerg Med*. 1984;13:1037–1039.

43. Mapleson WW. Assessment of the condenser humidifier. *Br Med J*. 1963;1:300–305.

44. Stryker H. A device for turning the frame patient. *JAMA*. 1939;113:1731–1732.

45. Povey RW. New turning-frame. *Br Med J*. 1968;2:114.

46. Nish WW, Walsh FW, Land P, Swedenburg M. Effect of electromagnetic interference by neonatal transport equipment on aircraft operation. *Aviat Space Environ Med*. 1989;60:599–600.

Chapter 28

SYSTEMIC HYPOTHERMIA

T. CAMERON MACCAUGHELTY, M.D.*; BRIAN G. MCALARY, M.D.†; AND MICHAEL MOON, M.D.‡

*Formerly, Lieutenant Colonel, Medical Corps, U.S. Army Reserve; Group Surgeon, 11th Special Forces Group (Airborne), U.S. Army First Special Forces; Commanding Officer, 306th U.S. Army Reserve Field Hospital; currently, Chief of Anesthesiology, Illinois Valley Community Hospital, 925 West Street, Peru, Illinois 61354

†Formerly, Commander, Medical Corps, U.S. Navy; Director of Medical Corps Programs, Health Sciences Education and Training Command, National Naval Medical Center, Bethesda, Maryland; and Chairman, Department of Anesthesiology, National Naval Medical Center, Bethesda, Maryland 20889-5600; currently, Lecturer and Consultant in Anesthesia and Critical Care, 9260 Broken Timber Way, Columbia, Maryland 20145

‡Colonel, Medical Corps, U.S. Army; Staff Anesthesiologist, Madigan Army Medical Center, Fort Lewis, Washington 94831-5000

INTRODUCTION

Military operations in cold environments have the potential to create vast problems for military medical services. Everything is more difficult to do. Evacuation of casualties is impeded. Infectious diseases are much more common. And cold by itself becomes an agent of injury, as was pointed out in 390 BC by the Greek essayist and general, Xenophon, in his *Anabasis*, a description of a 4th-century BC military expedition through Asia Minor.[1] But perhaps the most spectacular manifestation of cold as a source of attrition in the warfare of the ancient world was that of Hannibal, who may have lost as many as 50% of his men, many from hypothermic injury, while crossing the Alps in 218 BC.[2]

The spectrum of cold injury extends from (*a*) transient injury to the most superficial layers of the skin, through (*b*) full-thickness necrosis of varying amounts of the soft tissue of the hands and feet, to (*c*) fatal systemic hypothermia. By far the most common medical treatment problems caused by military operations in cold environments in past wars have been those associated with damage to superficial tissues in the extremities. Such local cold injury is known by a variety of names: immersion foot, trench foot, and frostbite are the best known. During World War I, cold-induced casualties included 38,000 Italian, 80,000 French, and 115,000 British troops. World War II produced 90,000 cold-induced U.S. casualties and 100,000 German.[3] Similar observations are applicable to more recent wars. During the Korean War, cold weather contributed to at least 10% of U.S. casualties,[3] and during the Falklands War in 1982, hypothermia and local cold injuries were quite common.[3–5]

Systemic hypothermia is less well known but is certain to be a much greater therapeutic challenge for military trauma anesthesiologists than is local cold injury. Strangely enough, not a single official history of the U.S. Army Medical Department in World War II mentions this condition, including *Cold Injury, Ground Type*, the volume that is dedicated to cold injury.[6] It is inconceivable that the condition did not occur. Systemic hypothermia was known to contribute to wartime death by drowning. In fact, the Nazi hypothermia "experiments," the scientific validity of which has recently been debunked, were allegedly prompted in part by the high mortality rate among downed German pilots and U-boat crews.[3,7]

It is reasonable to assume that the contribution of systemic hypothermia to combat mortality was obscured by more-dramatic conditions such as battlefield trauma and disease. Soldiers found frozen to death on the battlefield and whose demise was attributed to "exhaustion" or "exposure" were, no doubt, victims of systemic hypothermia. Certainly, the nearly 10% of George Washington's troops who were reported to perish during the cold winter of 1777 and 1778 died of systemic hypothermia.[3,4] Because such casualties die on the battlefield, the importance of systemic hypothermia would not have been recognized at the hospital level. With more rapid means of evacuation from the battlefield, however, it is likely that cases of systemic hypothermia will be seen more frequently in future wars.

Soldiers fighting on a wintry battlefield are not the only candidates for systemic hypothermia. The battle casualty with substantial blood loss who undergoes a lengthy laparotomy or thoracotomy, and who receives inadequately warmed intravenous fluids in a suboptimally climate-controlled field hospital, is obviously at risk for developing intraoperative hypothermia—with its attendant potential for hemodynamic and coagulation abnormalities. The military anesthesia provider's experience with systemic hypothermia is much more likely to be based on casualties who become hypothermic in the operating room than on casualties whose hypothermia was caused by environmental exposure. Ironically, hypothermia was recognized as a problem for the U.S. Army Medical Department during the Persian Gulf War—a war fought in the desert—but not in World War II or Korea:

> Hypothermia was a frequent and significant clinical problem for combat hospitals. Preoperative and intraoperative hypothermia consumed vast amounts of additional oxygen, personnel, and [intensive care unit] resources. DEPMEDS [the Department of Defense's Deployable Medical Systems] provides for warming blankets for the operating room beds, but lacks other methods for active rewarming.[8(p10-37)]

The infrequent observation of intraoperative hypothermia in past wars may reflect the simple fact that no device for measuring intraoperative core temperature has yet been fielded. PROPAQ monitors (manufactured by Protocol Systems, Beaverton,

Ore.), which are fielded, have a thermistor port, but the thermistor itself is not part of the DEPMEDS equipment. DEPMEDS does, however, field a thermometer that reads as low as 21°C, which will permit diagnoses of hypothermia to be made more commonly in the future.

NORMAL THERMOREGULATION

Man, like other mammals and birds, is a homeothermic animal and thus strives to maintain body temperature within a narrow range despite changes in environmental temperature. There is a normal diurnal variation in temperature in healthy individuals, with the nadir typically occurring between the hours of 0200 and 0400. Oral temperatures of 36.1°C (97°F) are common on morning arising and increase gradually during the day to reach a peak of 37.2°C (99°F) or slightly higher between the hours of 1800 and 2200.[9] This normal pattern is not reversed in individuals who work a night shift.

Temperature Measurement

Most scientific literature uses the term *core temperature* as a basis of reference. The precise definition of core temperature and the most appropriate site or sites for its measurement have, nonetheless, been elusive. Despite the inconsistency of rectal temperature and its lack of intrinsic thermal significance, most clinical knowledge of body temperature depended for years on this site of measurement.[10] Tympanic membrane temperature closely approximates the temperature of the blood supplying the hypothalamus, site of the temperature regulation control center.[11] The tympanic membrane, situated at the base of the middle cerebral fossa and separated from the internal carotid artery by a thin layer of bone, would seem the ideal, easily accessible location for measuring core temperature.[10,12]

With the thermistor tip placed in the mid esophagus, investigators from Yale University determined no significant difference between esophageal and pulmonary artery temperatures during either steady-state conditions or hypothermia and rewarming in patients undergoing cardiac surgery.[13] Positioning the esophageal probe where they heard the loudest heart sounds, anesthesiologists at the Arizona Health Sciences Center showed that esophageal temperature and tympanic membrane temperature have a correlation coefficient greater than 0.75.[14] Furthermore, these investigators demonstrated similar correlation for nasopharyngeal and bladder temperatures. Although conceding that tympanic membrane temperature (measured in this study with a Model 6000 monitor manufactured by Mon-a-therm, Inc., St. Louis, Mo.) best approximates the true value for core temperature, they recommend using esophageal, nasopharyngeal, and bladder temperatures because of possible trauma to the tympanic membrane.[14,15] Whichever site is chosen, a device capable of recording low temperatures must be used so that unsuspected hypothermia will not be missed.[16]

Neural Temperature Control

The hypothalamus contains the negative-feedback integrative centers that initiate adaptive responses to perceived changes in temperature. The central temperature control center responds to a variety of stimuli including endocrine influences (eg, the thermogenic effect of progesterone), exercise, sweating, flushing, and mental stress. Peripheral nerve endings innervating the skin, many areas in the body core, and nervous elements in the spinal cord and brain stem are known to be sensitive to temperature changes.[17,18] Preoptic anterior hypothalamic nuclei monitor core temperature. The hypothalamus responds to the rate of firing of thermosensitive neurons, which is partially dependent on the rate of change of the stimulus. Thus, it is possible to abolish shivering by slightly increasing skin temperature at the onset of shivering, thereby allowing core cooling to continue.[19] For example, when deep divers are warmed with flowing hot water, they may continue to become hypothermic although their perception is that they are warm. Radiant heat from a fireplace may produce the sensation of warmth, prevent vasoconstriction, and thereby hasten the development of hypothermia in an otherwise cold room.[19] This fact may explain the observation of Napoleon's chief surgeon, Baron Dominique Larrey, who, noting the effects of the Russian winter on the troops of the Grande Armèe, found that victims of the cold who were placed closest to the campfire usually died.[3,20,21]

Heat Production

At the basal metabolic rate, heat is produced at 40 to 60 kcal per square meter of body surface area per hour.[3,22] The ultimate source of heat production is from the action of adenosine triphosphatase (ATPase) on adenosine 5′-triphosphate (ATP) in the sodium pump of all biologically active cell membranes.[9] The core organs (brain, liver, spleen, heart, and kidneys) contribute almost 60% of basal heat production,[19] despite constituting only about 10% of body weight. Nonshivering thermogenesis is enhanced by an increase in catecholamines, thyroxine, and adrenocorticoids. Basal heat production can be markedly increased by muscle activity and shivering.

Preshivering enhancement of muscular tone increases heat production by up to 100%.[22] Visible shivering can increase heat production (and oxygen consumption) by 500%.[23,24] Because of fatigue and glycogen depletion, this degree of heat production from shivering is limited to a few hours.[22] Thermoregulatory shivering demonstrates a waxing and waning pattern (4–8 Hz) and differs distinctly from generalized postanesthetic tremor.[25] Unfortunately, activity and shivering are uneconomical ways to increase heat production because they are often accompanied by increased skin and muscular blood flow, which further increases heat loss (Figure 28-1).[19,23]

Heat Loss

Humans are essentially warm-weather, subtropical animals that do not physiologically tolerate or adapt well to cold environments.[4,26,27] Unclothed, we probably could not survive at temperatures much below 21°C (71°F).[22] Human adaptation is primarily behavioral and intellectual: constructing shelters and acquiring clothes and artificial heat. Thermally, the body can be envisioned as a core, consisting of the vital organs and a shell, the inner layer of which comprises the skeletal muscle mass, and the superficial layer of which includes superficial muscle, subcutaneous fat, and skin.[19,21,27,28] Ninety-five percent or more of daily heat production must be lost to the environment.[22] This loss occurs through the shell and the respiratory tract by radiation, conduction, convection, and evaporation.

Radiation

Radiation (the transfer of heat between objects by electromagnetic waves) normally accounts for 55% to 70% of heat loss. The amount of heat loss depends on the temperature gradient between the body surface and the environment, and the amount of exposed body surface area. The uncovered head can be an important source of radiant heat loss. Due to poor vasoconstriction of the face and scalp, at 4°C (39°F), one half the total basal metabolic heat production can be lost from an exposed head.[19,29]

Conduction and Convection

Conduction refers to the transfer of thermal energy through direct contact. Normally, only 2% to 3% of heat loss occurs via conduction to other objects; however, the loss dramatically increases (up to 5-fold) during contact with cold ground or snow. Water's thermal conductivity is some 30-fold greater than that of air, and immersion causes extremely rapid heat loss. Approximately 1,500 passengers on the *Titanic* died in 0°C water in less than 2 hours.[30] Insulation (both clothing and subcutaneous fat) can prolong survival times.[30–32]

After heat is moved from the body's core to the shell by conduction, it can be dissipated by air movement over the skin—a process called *convection*. Heat loss by convection is quite variable and depends on wind velocity (with the cooling effect varying approximately as the square root of the wind velocity)[29] and the degree of insulation provided by clothing. Wet garments, rather than trapping air next to the skin and retarding convective heat loss, become effective conductive heat transmitters.

Evaporation

Evaporation is the conversion of a liquid to its gaseous phase. The conversion of 1 g of water from a liquid to a gas requires 0.58 kcal.[22,28,29] In humans, heat loss by evaporation from the skin and respiratory tract generally accounts for 20% of total heat loss, but this can be increased remarkably by sweating.[22,29] Relative humidity and ambient temperature markedly affect the degree of heat loss by evaporation, with the greatest loss occurring in dry, cold environments.[3]

Heat Conservation

By means of a remarkable ability to decrease or increase blood flow, primarily through cutaneous arteriovenous shunts[33] in the extremities, the human body regulates delivery of heat to its surface. Cutaneous blood flow can decrease from its normal 300 to 500 mL/min to 30 mL/min and can increase to more than 3 L/min with maximum vasodilation.[22,27,34] Capillary flow, as well as arteriovenous shunt flow, decreases with higher degrees of vasoconstriction.[35]

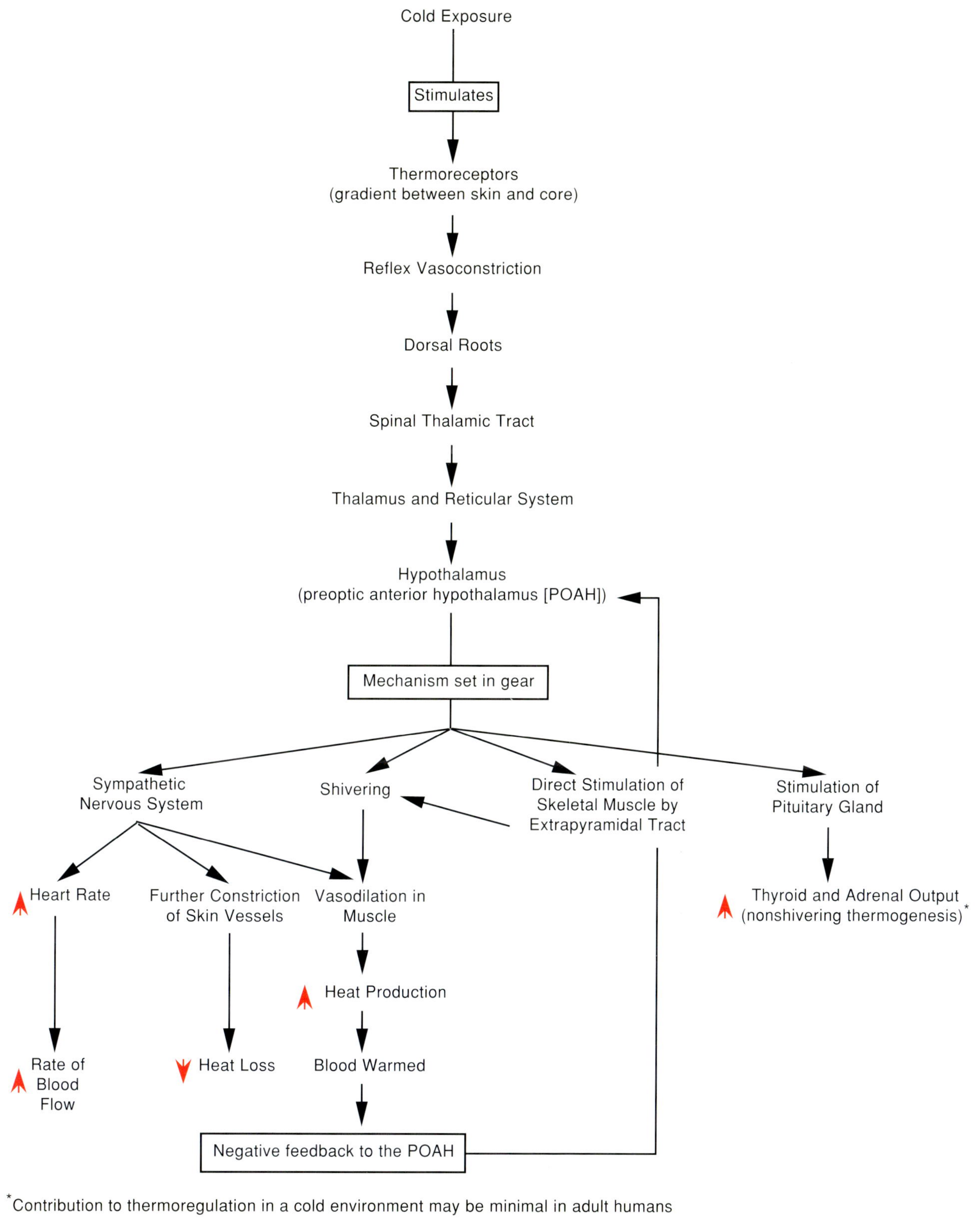

Fig. 28-1. The stepwise and integrated physiological response to cold in the normal human.
Adapted with permission from Reuler JB. Hypothermia: Pathophysiology, clinical settings, and management. *Ann Intern Med*. 1978;89:520.

DEFINITION AND CLASSIFICATION OF HYPOTHERMIA

In humans, hypothermia is defined as a core temperature less than 35°C (95°F).[3,19,22,28,29] In addition to the hypothermia that is deliberately induced in certain surgical patients, there are two broad categories of pathological hypothermia:

1. *primary* (accidental), in which an otherwise healthy person is exposed to a cold environment and the thermoregulatory system's compensation is inadequate[36]; and
2. *secondary*, in which another illness or condition predisposes the individual to accidental hypothermia.[3,22,29,36]

Further subdivisions into *acute* and *chronic* (which afflicts particularly the elderly who live in insufficiently heated winter houses) and *immersion* and *nonimmersion* have been made.[3,36] Another supplemental subclassification distinguishes *very rapid* (usually immersion) hypothermia, in which the cold stress quickly exceeds the body's ability to produce heat and maintain core temperature, and *intermediate* (exhaustion) hypothermia, in which the individual's heat production is able to maintain core temperature against a cold stress only as long as sufficient energy sources are available.[19] In very rapid hypothermia, heat production is unimpaired and the person will have little difficulty rewarming on removal from cold stress. In intermediate hypothermia, heat production is markedly impaired when exhaustion ensues, and "even a relatively mild degree of cold exposure may be sufficient to cause continued cooling."[19(p102)] (This subject is also discussed in Chapter 23, Metabolic Derangements and Nutritional Support.) Primary hypothermia is the concern of this chapter, although military anesthesia providers should bear in mind that they are most likely to encounter casualties with secondary hypothermia: injured soldiers in a cold operating room tent.

A number of diverse clinical conditions lead to impaired thermoregulation, and can generally be classified as central, peripheral, metabolic, pharmacological or toxicological, and dermatological (Exhibit 28-1). Of these, the most significant are probably

- spinal cord transection, which, by interrupting the spinothalamic tract, breaks the afferent thermoregulatory loop;
- trauma associated with hypotension and hypovolemia, which results in generalized vasoconstriction and decreased metabolic heat production;
- general anesthetics, which shift the threshold for vasoconstriction and shivering to a lower temperature range; and
- acute ethanol ingestion, which causes generalized vasodilation and thereby increases heat loss.

CLINICAL AND LABORATORY MANIFESTATIONS

Hypothermia per se is not lethal to tissue: cellular death occurs only with denaturation when ice crystals are formed. "What does occur as cells are gradually cooled is a progressive decrease in functional performance that ultimately kills the organism."[37(p620)] Hypothermia is known to affect most organ systems, the metabolism, and the blood and its chemistry (Table 28-1), but the effects of hypothermia depend on the degree of cooling. Three stages of hypothermia are commonly recognized: mild (> 32°C), moderate (32°C–26°C), and severe (< 26°C). Much of the material that follows is summarized in Table 28-2.

Organ-System Effects

Central Nervous System Effects

An initial deterioration in mental status may progress to dysarthria, incoordination, withdrawal, irritability, apathy, disorientation, confusion, and finally to lethargy, intermittent stupor, and frank coma. Visual evoked potentials decrease[38] and the latency period of somatosensory evoked potentials is prolonged[39] by hypothermia. Although cerebrovascular autoregulation is reportedly preserved to 25°C,[3] hypothermia produces a predominance of slower-frequency waves on the electroencephalogram, which eventually becomes electrical silence at 19°C to 20°C.[3,19] Hyporeflexia progresses to areflexia and is accompanied by an increase in rigidity.[19]

Cardiac Effects

In hypothermia, the usual cause of death is progressive deterioration in cardiopulmonary function. Following an initial increase in heart rate and blood pressure, hypothermia causes a progressive bradycardia and myocardial depression, eventu-

EXHIBIT 28-1

CLINICAL CONDITIONS POSSIBLY RESPONSIBLE FOR IMPAIRED THERMOREGULATION

Central Nervous System Conditions (Affecting Hypothalamic Function)
- Cranial trauma (especially basilar fractures)
- Chronic subdural hematomas, and intracerebral hemorrhages
- Central nervous system infection
- Cerebrovascular accidents
- CNS infiltrative lesions including neoplasms, systemic lupus erythematosus, and sarcoidosis
- Spontaneous periodic hypothermia
- Shapiro's syndrome (dysgenesis of the corpus callosum)
- Wernicke's encephalopathy

Peripheral Conditions
- Neoplasms, especially Hodgkin's disease and other lymphomas[1,2]
- Peripheral neuropathies
- Spinal cord transection*
- Trauma associated with hypotension and hypovolemia*
- Carcinomatosis
- Pancreatitis
- Miliary tuberculosis
- Myocardial dysfunction with decreased cardiac output

Metabolic Conditions
- Hypothyroidism (myxedema)
- Hypoglycemia
- Hypopituitarism
- Hypoadrenalism
- Ketoacidosis
- Anorexia nervosa
- Marasmus and kwashiorkor

Pharmacological/Toxicological Conditions
- General anesthetics*
- Major conduction anesthetics,(ie, subarachnoid block and epidural)
- Ethanol ingestion, acute and chronic*
- Barbiturates
- Phenothiazines
- Benzodiazepines
- Cyclic antidepressants
- Lithium
- Carbon monoxide
- Clonidine
- Narcotics

Dermatological Conditions
- Burns
- Epidermolysis bullosum
- Exfoliative dermatitis

*Most important

(1) Buccini RV. Hypothermia in Hodgkin's disease. *N Engl J Med*. 1985;312:244. (2) Chang M, Gill T. Hypothermia, neurologic dysfunction, and sudden death in a man with carcinoma. *South Med J*. 1981;74:1509.

TABLE 28-1

PHYSIOLOGICAL DERANGEMENTS ASSOCIATED WITH PROLONGED HYPOTHERMIA

System	Effects
Central Nervous	Incoordination Disorientation Confusion
Cardiac	Decreased heart rate, mean arterial pressure, cardiac output Conduction slows, T waves are inverted, QT interval increases ST elevation occurs between 32°C–33°C (J wave) Atrial and ventricular fibrillation occur < 30°C
Respiratory	Respiratory rate increases early on Anatomical and physiological dead spaces increase (at 25°C)
Renal	Cold diuresis occurs late in the course of the injury, leading to volume depletion, oliguria, and azotemia
Hematological	Hemoconcentration occurs, with increased hematocrit and hemoglobin levels Disseminated intravascular coagulation can occur from peripheral microvasculature failure
Metabolic	Hyperglycemia and mild ketosis Lactic acidosis
Gastrointestinal	Decreased intestinal motility (at < 34°C) Hemorrhagic pancreatitis is seen occasionally in fatal cases

Notes:

- The metabolism of all drugs is decreased in hypothermia, as is the liver's ability to detoxify drugs. This should be considered when administering medications to hypothermic patients.
- In the absence of other overriding medical considerations (eg, severe trauma), no one is dead until *warm* and dead.

Source: Bellamy RF, ed. *Combat Casualty Care Guidelines: Operation Desert Storm*. Washington, DC: Office of The Surgeon General, Walter Reed Army Medical Center, and Borden Institute; 1991: 154.

ally terminating in asystole or ventricular fibrillation. Some controversy exists over whether asystole or ventricular fibrillation is the more common terminal rhythm.[3,21,40] Rather clearly, the conduction system is sensitive to cold, and both PR and QT intervals are characteristically prolonged.[3] Ventricular irritability develops near 29°C, and there are reports of ventricular fibrillation in hypothermic patients induced by mechanical stimulation secondary to placement of pulmonary artery catheters, esophageal probes, and endotracheal tubes.[19,37,41]

The J wave (also known as the Osborne wave) is said to be present in up to 90% of hypothermic patients (Figure 28-2).[37] This positive–negative deflection immediately follows the QRS complex—probably caused by delayed depolarization of the left ventricle—and is occasionally observed in patients with subarachnoid hemorrhage, left ventricular ischemia, and in some healthy young adults.

Respiratory Effects

After an initial increase in respiratory rate following sudden exposure to cold, respiratory rate, tidal volume, minute ventilation, and the respiratory response to carbon dioxide all progressively decrease.[22,42,43] Despite a decrease in carbon dioxide production, minute ventilation becomes inadequate to remove carbon dioxide below approximately 32°C.[3,22] The cough reflex and ciliary motility are depressed, resulting in an impaired ability to deal with frequently encountered bronchorrhea and pulmonary edema.[3,19,22] Autopsy findings often include not only pulmonary edema but also parenchymal hemorrhages.[22,44]

TABLE 28-2

CHARACTERISTICS OF THE THREE STAGES OF HYPOTHERMIA

Stage	Core Body Temperature (°C)	Core Body Temperature (°F)	Characteristics
Mild	37.6	99.6 ± 1	Normal rectal temperature
(> 32°C)	37	98.6 ± 1	Normal oral temperature
	36	96.8	Increase in metabolic rate
	35	95.0	Urinary temperature 34.8°C; maximum shivering thermogenesis
	34	93.2	Amnesia; dysarthria, and poor judgment develop; normal blood pressure; maximum respiratory stimulation
	33	91.4	Ataxia and apathy develop
Moderate	32	89.6	Stupor; 25% decrease in oxygen consumption
(26°C–32°C)	31	87.8	Extinquished shivering thermogenesis
	30	86	Atrial fibrillation and other arrhythmias develop; poikilothermia; pulse and cardiac output 67% of normal; insulin ineffective
	29	85.2	Progressive decrease in level of consciousness, pulse, and respiration; pupils dilated
	28	82.4	Decreased ventricular fibrillation threshold; 50% decrease in oxygen consumption and pulse
	27	80.6	Loss of reflexes and voluntary motion
Severe	26	78.8	Major acid–base disturbances; no reflexes or response to pain
(<26°C)	25	77	Cerebral blood flow 33% of normal; cardiac output 45% of normal; pulmonary edema may develop
	24	75.2	Significant hypotension
	23	73.4	No corneal or oculocephalic reflexes
	22	71.6	Maximum risk of ventricular fibrillation; 75% decrease in oxygen consumption
	20	68	Lowest resumption of cardiac electromechanical activity; pulse 20% of normal
	19	66.2	Flat EEG
	18	64.4	Asystole
	16	60.8	Lowest adult accidental hypothermia survival
	15.2	59.2	Lowest infant accidental hypothermia survival
	10	50	92% decrease in oxygen consumption
	9	48.2	Lowest therapeutic hypothermia survival

Reprinted with permission from Danzl DF. Accidential hypothermia. In: Rosen et al, eds. *Emergency Medicine: Concepts and Clinical Practice.* 3rd ed. St. Louis, Mo: Mosby-Year Book; 1992.

Vascular, Renal, and Gastrointestinal Effects

Vascular and Renal Effects. The remarkable ability of the body to constrict blood vessels in the extremities produces an initial, relative, central hypervolemia, which is interpreted as a volume overload leading to suppression of the antidiuretic hormone and the well-known cold diuresis. As

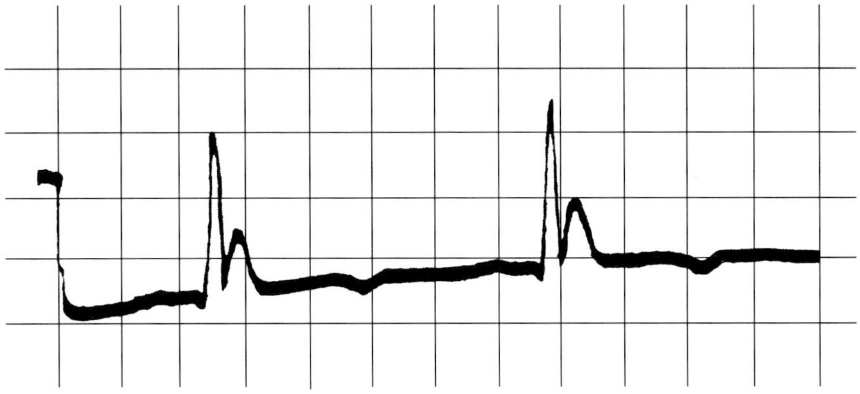

Fig. 28-2. This electrocardiograph shows typical J waves (also called Osborne waves), which follow the QRS complex that develops at temperatures below 32°C.

renal tubular dysfunction progresses, little of the glomerular filtrate is reabsorbed, and this, combined with shifts of fluid from the intravascular space, produces hypovolemia.

Gastrointestinal Effects. Gastrointestinal hemorrhage and pancreatitis are common autopsy findings.[21,45] Gastrointestinal motility decreases concomitant with the decline in metabolic rate. Functional hepatic impairment occurs with little if any structural damage,[37] altering the rate of clearance and metabolism of many drugs.

Metabolic and Hematological Effects

Metabolic Effects. Following an initial increase in metabolic rate up to 6-fold greater than the basal rate[3,22–24,46] at 35°C, hypothermia slows all metabolic processes, with the metabolic rate decreasing to 50% of normal at core temperatures of 28°C to 30°C.[28,42] A reduction in metabolism and oxygen consumption of 7% per degree Celsius decrease in temperature is widely reported.[16,42]

Hematological Effects. As a consequence of hemoconcentration and a reported[40,47] 2% increase in viscosity per degree Celsius decrease in temperature, hematocrit usually increases along with significant "sludging" and interference with tissue perfusion.[3,21,36] Platelet and leukocyte counts are frequently depressed because of splenic and hepatic sequestration.[28,42] Platelet sequestration occurring in the portal bed is largely reversible on rewarming.[48,49]

Blood Chemistry Abnormalities

Electrolytes and Serum Glucose

Preexisting clinical conditions can result in transcellular membrane shifts of electrolytes and produce significant alterations. Unfortunately, there are no predictable changes in serum sodium, chloride, potassium, magnesium, calcium, or phosphate[3,22]; therefore, frequent laboratory determinations are necessary during resuscitation from hypothermia. Cold- and catecholamine-induced glycogenolysis and decreased insulin secretion[37] cause an initial hyperglycemia that proceeds to hypoglycemia with glycogen depletion.[3] Note that insulin is ineffective below 30°C.[3] Therefore, persistent hyperglycemia during rewarming can indicate diabetic ketoacidosis, pancreatitis, or both.

Dissolved Gases and the Acid–Base Balance

The solubility of gases in liquids increases at colder temperatures; therefore, the partial pressures of both oxygen and carbon dioxide (Po_2 and Pco_2) decrease in the hypothermic patient. The partial pressure of arterial oxygen (Pao_2) declines 7.2% per degree Celsius decrease, and the partial pressure of arterial carbon dioxide ($Paco_2$) declines 4.4% per degree Celsius decrease.[50] Because blood samples are warmed to 37°C before determination of Po_2 and Pco_2, temperature correction of both of these laboratory values was formerly advocated. Such temperature correction of Po_2 is useful clinically. A Pao_2 of 60 mm Hg at 27°C corresponds to a Pao_2 of 130 at 37°C.[3] The lower Pao_2 at 27°C represents not oxyhemoglobin desaturation but simply a lower partial pressure of oxygen due to its increased liquid solubility at the lower temperature.

The situation with appropriate evaluation of pH and $Paco_2$ is somewhat more complicated but has now essentially been resolved in favor of *not* correcting for temperature when measuring pH and Pco_2.[3,51,52] The word *correcting* is to be understood in the following sense: commercially available pH meters automatically warm a blood sample to 37°C, the temperature at which the pH is actually measured. There are two options for reporting the results of this measurement: (1) to report the results at 37°C or (2) to "correct" them to the original temperature of the sample. Because pH normally increases as temperature falls, the uncorrected pH measured at 37°C will be lower than the pH corrected to the hypothermic casualty's actual body temperature.

Studies of cold-blooded (ie, ectothermic) vertebrates show that their blood pH increases and their P_{CO_2} decreases as their body temperatures cool.[51–53] Some of the decrease in P_{CO_2} results from the increased solubility of carbon dioxide at the lower blood temperature, but there is also decreased carbon dioxide production incident to the decreased metabolic rate. In these animals, total body carbon dioxide content[3,51] does not change with decreasing temperature because ventilation decreases less than does metabolism. As body temperature falls, the pH of the blood of these animals increases in such as way as to remain slightly alkalotic. By way of contrast, in some small hibernating mammals, pH does not change as temperature falls. These animals hypoventilate and their total body carbon dioxide increases. Thus, their blood becomes progressively acidotic.

There are two basic approaches to managing pH alterations during hypothermia, both of which resemble the natural physiological responses described above. In the technique called *alpha-stat pH management*, chemical neutrality is maintained by allowing pH to increase as temperature falls. Conversely, in the approach known as *pH-stat management*, pH is maintained constant at 7.4 regardless of the temperature.[51,52]

Alpha-stat pH management employs uncorrected blood gases, whereas pH-stat management utilizes corrected gases and strives to maintain a constant pH of 7.4 regardless of the temperature. The former term derives from the alpha imidazole ring on the histidine moiety of various body proteins.[51,52] The neutral pH of water (ie, that pH at which $[H^+] = [OH^-]$ is 6.8 at 37°C),[53] and the normal 0.6 pH units of alkalinity of human blood may well be important for enzymatic function.[3,51–5] In addition,

> [m]any essential enzymes (such as lactic dehydrogenase, sodium-potassium-adenosine triphosphatase, and cytochrome C reductase) have been found to be temperature sensitive and to exhibit optimum activity when pH is increased during hypothermia.[51(p1643)]

The key factor is probably chemical neutrality rather than a specific hydrogen ion concentration.

Several studies done in endotherms, including humans, have demonstrated improved cardiac performance and electrical stability when the pH under hypothermic cardiopulmonary bypass was deliberately determined by noncorrected laboratory values.[55,56] For example, the pH determined at 37°C might be found to be 7.4, which would correspond to a pH of 7.7 when measured at 28°C. Similarly, increased cerebral blood flow was also seen when the *noncorrected* values for P_{CO_2} and pH were used and the animals were allowed to remain hypocarbic and alkalotic.[57] In a 1986 study[58] of 181 cardiopulmonary bypass patients, 40% of those managed with the pH-corrected technique developed spontaneous ventricular fibrillation, whereas only 20% of those managed with the noncorrected technique did so.

Other authorities have also concluded that pH correction can be deleterious in the patient with hypothermia:

> Potentially deleterious effects of this alkalosis on other organ systems have yet to be identified. However, it is clear that maintaining the corrected pH at 7.4 and P_{CO_2} at 40 mm Hg during hypothermia depresses cerebral and coronary blood flow and cardiac output, and increases the incidence of lactic acidosis and ventricular fibrillation. A correction of pH and P_{CO_2} in hypothermia is unnecessary and potentially deleterious.[3(p46)]

In other words, attempting to maintain an actual pH of 7.4 in a hypothermic casualty will have a deleterious effect because the corresponding uncorrected pH is profoundly acidotic.

CLINICAL PREVENTION AND TREATMENT

In cold environments, body temperature can be maintained by increasing body heat production, decreasing body heat loss, and supplying external heat sources. However, hospital operating rooms are kept cool and patients undergoing surgery are not warmly clothed, so the most practical and efficient methods to decrease heat loss (ie, clothing and shelter—our primary adaptations to cold) are contravened. This is especially true in field hospitals that are deployed in tents. The fact that casualties are not kept warm during surgery led directly to the development of the medical unit, self contained, transportable (MUST) and DEPMEDS hospitals, which allowed temperature-controlled interiors.

All anesthetized patients become hypothermic in rooms cooler than 20°C unless preventive measures are used.[59,60] Ambient temperatures must be 24°C to 26°C to prevent a decrease in esophageal temperature.[60] Radiation and convection account for approximately 80% of heat loss, and most of this occurs during the first hour of anesthesia.[42,60] Methods of heat conservation *must* be a priority of the operating room staff and *must* begin before the casualty is brought into the operating room. In addition to increasing the ambient temperature, the operating room staff must also ensure that the casualty—particularly his head—is covered as much as possible,[19] and must minimize evaporative heat loss from open surgical wounds, especially those of the trunk.

All the methods described below, except cardiopulmonary bypass, increase temperature rather slowly, in the range of 0.5°C to 1.5°C per hour.[3,61] There is no proof that rapid rewarming improves survival rates.[3]

Supplemental Warming Devices

Warm blankets provide some conductive heat transfer as well as decrease radiant and convective heat loss.[42] Although not available in DEPMEDS-equipped hospitals, the "space blanket," a reflective blanket using aluminized Tyvek (manufactured by King-Seeley Thermos Co., Winchester, Mass.) is particularly useful when 60% or more of the body surface area can be covered.[62] In 1980, researchers conducted a study of patients undergoing major vascular procedures with an average operating room time of 6 hours. Before they were draped for surgery, the patients were placed in operating rooms that were cold (14°C–18°C) or warm (23°C–26°C). The latter group also received intravenous fluids and blood that were warmed to 37.5°C and were placed on a heating blanket at 37.8°C. The researchers were able to confirm greater heat loss prior to draping in the cold-room group, but were unable to demonstrate a difference in outcome. The key factor seemed to be the ability of the patients to compensate for internal heat loss that had occurred over an extended period of time. Because many procedures do not last 6 hours, and because the patients in this (and other) studies initially lose more heat in cold operating rooms,[60] operating rooms need to be warmed.[42]

Placing blankets that contain warm, circulating fluid between the operating-table mattress and the patient does *not* prevent intraoperative hypothermia when used alone.[63,64] This finding is not surprising because (*a*) there is little well-perfused tissue in contact with the blanket and (*b*) the thermal conductivity of the usual operating-table mattress is rather low. (However, these blankets have caused burns.[42]) Warmed, humidified, inspired gases used in conjunction with a warming blanket, however, produce a synergistic effect and better temperature preservation than when either is used alone.[64]

The efficacy of warmed, humidified gases as a method of conserving heat is easily understood when it is appreciated that a patient breathing dry gases at *room* temperature can consume 25 kcal/h (about one third of the basal heat production) in warming that air to *body* temperature.[42,65] Several studies have demonstrated the efficacy of passive heat and moisture exchangers in significantly reducing the rate of fall of core temperature,[65–67] especially when lower fresh-gas flows are used. In addition to preventing the expenditure of approximately 25 kcal/h to warm and humidify dry room-temperature gases,[3,42,65] heated (45°C), humidified gases delivered at 20 L/min provide about 30 kcal/h heat exchange to a patient with a core temperature of 28°C (Table 28-3).[61]

In awake hypothermic volunteers, one group of researchers[68] demonstrated an increase in the rate of core rewarming of 0.3°C/h for each 10 L/min increase in ventilation of moist air with an inspiratory temperature of 44°C. Clearly, lesser rates of heat transfer occur if the gases are cooler and if the patient's core temperature is higher.[61] Other groups of researchers[61,69] performed their calculations using 45°C as an accepted maximum airway temperature, and still others[70] used inspired gases at 42°C to 47°C at the Y connector of the anesthesia tubing.

In one notable study,[71] however, researchers studied dogs that had been mechanically ventilated for 6 hours. The group monitored temperatures at the internal end of the endotracheal tube and demonstrated an acute airway injury consisting of

> diffuse mucosal degeneration with focal necrosis, shedding and sloughing of the pseudostratified columnar epithelium, and an acute inflammatory response in the submucosal tissue [when] average tracheal temperature exceeded 40°C.[71(pA490)]

These investigators did not control the peak temperature, however, and report peaks of 46°C "when the average tracheal temperature was

TABLE 28-3

ESTIMATED HEAT GAIN FROM ENDOGENOUS AND EXOGENOUS SOURCES

Heat Source	Calories Provided at Core Temperature 28°C*
Normal metabolic rate	70 kcal/h
Maximum shivering	350 kcal/h
Heated (45°C) humidified O_2 at 20 L/min	30 kcal/h
Heated (45°C) intravenous fluid (1 L)	17 kcal
Heated (45°C) peritoneal dialysis fluid (1 L);	17 kcal
flow rate 5 L/h over 1h	85 kcal/h
Heated (42°C) cardiopulmonary bypass perfusate (1 L);	17 kcal
flow rate 28 L/h	476 kcal/h
Trunk immersion in 45°C water:	
Vasoconstriction	600 kcal/h
Vasodilation	2,400 kcal/h

*A 70-kg human requires a gain of 60 kcal of heat to increase body temperature 1°C
Reprinted with permission from Bangs C, Hamlet MD. Hypothermia and cold injuries. In: Auerbach BS, Geehr EC, eds. *Management of Wilderness and Environmental Emergencies*. St. Louis, MO: Mosby-Year Book; 1983: 38. Original data source: Myers RAM, Britten JS, Cowley RA. Hypothermia: Quantitative aspects of therapy. *Journal of the American College of Emergency Physicians*. 1979:8(12):523–527.

42°C."[71(pA490)] In addition to retarding heat loss and providing heat gain, heated and humidified gases stimulate pulmonary cilia and retard cold-induced bronchorrhea.[3,72]

Blood and Fluid Warmers

Approximately 15 kcal (20% of basal heat production) are required to warm 1 L of 20°C intravenous fluid to 30°C.[42,61] Because general anesthesia ablates shivering and produces increased blood flow to the skin, rendering the normally homeothermic human a poikilotherm (ie, an ectotherm)[17,36,73] and therefore unable to increase caloric production, a patient's temperature will decrease more rapidly when challenged with cold intravenous fluids. The rapid administration of cold (4°C) blood products represents a considerable thermal challenge, one that is capable of reducing temperature approximately 0.5°C for every liter transfused over a 15-minute interval.[42] In addition to long-available heating systems (eg, the Dupaco Hemokinititherm Fluid Warmer, manufactured by Dupaco, Oceanside, Calif., which uses a countercurrent multiplier system of tubing immersed in a container of warmed water), the Level 1 Fluid Warmer (manufactured by Life Systems, Inc., Southfield, Mich.), is now available and can warm fluid and cold blood to 35°C at flows up to 500 mL/min.[74] Additionally, glucose-free intravenous fluids in flexible plastic containers can be preheated in a microwave oven.[3,75,76] (Preliminary testing of the warming characteristics of each oven should be done, and the fluid should be thoroughly mixed before it is administered.[3]) Packed red blood cells can be mixed with warm, calcium-free, isotonic crystalloid,[77] or can be prewarmed in a standard operating room fluid-warming cabinet,[78] provided moderate temperature ranges and proper temperature control are maintained.

Treatment in the Postanesthesia Care Unit

The methods of treatment previously discussed should be continued for casualties in the postanesthesia care unit who have subnormal temperatures. To prevent or diminish postanesthesia shivering and its consequent increase in oxygen consumption, high-risk casualties with temperatures lower than 35°C should be kept intubated, sedated, and paralyzed until they are rewarmed. The rewarming rate is the same when using either radiant heat lamps or heated blankets changed every 30 minutes,[79] and both methods are more effective than only one application of a warmed blanket.[80] Radiant heat and other methods of skin-surface warming also prevent or inhibit shivering.[19,37,81] A new device, the Bair Hugger (manufactured by Augustine Medical, Inc., Eden Prairie, Minn.), provides a microenvironment of warmed air through slits in a disposable blanket made of paper and plastic. In a postoperative patient lacking thermoregulatory responses, the Bair Hugger effectively transferred sufficient heat to increase the mean body temperature approximately 1.5°C/h,[82] and should be similarly effective during anesthesia. Spinal and epidural anesthetics may extend the risk of hypothermia longer into the recovery period than does general anesthesia, by virtue of the prolonged sympathectomy and associated vasodilation[83] combined with their interruption of afferent fiber activity from peripheral thermoreceptors.[36] But military trauma anesthesiologists must remember that an awake, nonshivering, postoperative patient is not necessarily a normothermic one, and rewarming may well still be required.

Nonhypothermic Shivering

Although the precise mechanism of nonhypothermic shivering remains unclear, even nonhypothermic postanesthetic tremor exacts a high metabolic cost[25] and must be curtailed in patients who are less able to tolerate the increased oxygen consumption. Meperidine, but not morphine or fentanyl, often stops postanesthetic shivering.[84–86] This may be because residual anesthetic inhibits descending cortical control, which, in turn, results in reflex hyperactivity.[25] A dose of 12.5 mg to 25 mg, administered intravenously, is effective in 67% to 73% of patients, and 50 mg is successful in 89%.[84]

Core Rewarming Techniques

The first report of core rewarming appeared in 1957 in *Time* magazine: 78 L of warm saline was used as a mediastinal irrigation via thoracotomy.[87] Intragastric and intracolonic warm irrigation have also been used. Cardiopulmonary bypass is the most rapidly effective means of active body core rewarming[3,21,61] and can, moreover, sustain viability until adequate myocardial function resumes. Although less effective, hemodialysis is also an effective modality. Heated peritoneal dialysis is the most efficacious technique of core rewarming, second only to cardiopulmonary bypass and hemodialysis.[3,61,72,88] This is a relatively simple procedure to perform by either a "mini-laparotomy" or the percutaneous approach, using isotonic dialysate at 40°C to 50°C.[3,88–90] Peritoneal dialysis with 45°C dialysate at 5 L/h will provide 85 kcal/h, which should increase core temperature about 1°C/h (see Table 28-3).[61]

Surface Rewarming Techniques

Although it has been calculated to yield up to 2,400 kcal of heat transfer per hour,[61] active external rewarming by immersing the casualty's trunk in 45°C water may be dangerous, especially if active core-rewarming methods are not simultaneously used.[3,30,37,40,91] Reflex vasodilation from external heat application can cause *rewarming shock* as circulating vascular volume in an already hypovolemic core is diverted to the peripheral circulation.[30,37,40,92] This is a much greater problem in patients with chronic exposure hypothermia[30,61] than in patients with sudden immersion hypothermia, who have not yet developed hypovolemia. In addition, cardiopulmonary resuscitation is impossible with a patient immersed in a water bath.

An effective field device for surface rewarming that relies on a charcoal-fueled heating element to provide energy was developed by the Norwegian military and is available for use in the U.S. Army: the Heatpac Personal Heater (manufactured by Alcatel Innova A/S, P.O. Box 60, Økern, 0508 Oslo 5, Norway; and distributed by Norsk Enterprises Inc., Alexandria, Va.). The Heatpac is a 23-cm x 12-cm x 6-cm package weighing 500 g with a combustion time of 6 to 20 hours and heat output of 40 to 250 W. The proprietary charcoal fuel pack weighs 120 to 160 g. The heat energy from charcoal combustion is distributed via a 1.5-V, D-cell–driven electric fan and a series of gas ducts. Carbon monoxide pollutants are scavenged by a catalyst. The unit has been field-tested by the U.S. armed forces and found to be a practical adjunct in the treatment of hypothermic casualties. The Heatpac has been adapted successfully to the U.S. casualty evacuation bag (National Stock Number [NSN] 6530-01-109-9030). Test documentation may be requested from Norsk Enterprises Inc. or the U.S. Army Medical Bioengineering Research and Development, Fort Detrick, Frederick, Maryland 21701-5010. Heatpac is available in the inventories of the North Atlantic Treaty Organization countries and the U.S. Army:

- the charcoal heater bag is NSN 6530-01-255-0835,
- the heating unit alone is NSN 6530-01-254-6492, and
- the charcoal element is NSN 6530-01-254-4130.

CARDIOPULMONARY RESUSCITATION

The presence of such severe prognostic signs as rigor mortis; livor mortis; and fixed, dilated pupils are not reliable criteria for withholding cardiopulmonary resuscitation (CPR) in casualties with hypothermia.[3,93] Considerable controversy still exists, however, regarding the initiation, maintenance, and techniques of CPR in the pulseless, apneic, severely hypothermic (< 30°C) person.[3,37,94,95] The recommendation to search for a pulse for 1 full minute has been made.[94] The clinical aphorism that a patient is not dead until he is *warm* and dead continues to apply.

CPR requires protocol modification with progressive degrees of hypothermia. This fact is explicitly recognized in the most recent recommendations for the treatment of systemic hypothermia made by the American Heart Association (Figure 28-3)[96]; (note that the American Heart Association's temperature criteria for the severity of hypothermia are different from those given in Table 28-2). Patients are divided into two categories by this protocol: those with both pulse and breathing present and those with pulse or breathing or both absent. Those with spontaneous cardiac and respiratory activity are further stratified by core temperature. Above 34°C, passive rewarming (which in the field means placing the casualty in a warm environment, or covering with blankets or a warm sleeping bag) is all that should be necessary. Patients with core temperatures between 30°C and 34°C may benefit, in addition to passive rewarming, from active external rewarming using the Heatpac Personal Heater. Those whose core temperature is below 30°C and who have a supraventricular rhythm and stable vital signs should undergo active internal rewarming. In the field, this means intravenous infusion of warm (43°C) fluids; breathing warm (42°C–46°C), humidified oxygen; and, possibly, peritoneal lavage with warm (43°C), potassium-free fluid.

Active internal rewarming using extracorporeal bypass incorporating a heat exchanger is an extremely effective modality but is not available in DEPMEDS-equipped hospitals. A procedure similar to hemodialysis was originally proposed, with blood being taken from the femoral artery, passed through a heat exchanger, and then transfused into the femoral vein. Nowadays, however, femoral vein–to–femoral artery bypass with a pump is used because the amount of blood that can be warmed is greatly increased. If the casualty is being ventilated and has effective cardiac action, an oxygenator is not absolutely necessary but is included in the circuit because of the propensity of such patients to develop ventricular fibrillation—even when treated prophylactically with antifibrillatory bretylium tosylate and while avoiding fibrillary stimuli (eg, chest compression and placement of intracardiac catheters).

The vulnerability of hypothermic patients to ventricular fibrillation is an important issue. In fact, some authorities[97,98] recommend that CPR be avoided in the severely hypothermic patient until asystole or ventricular fibrillation can be electrocardiographically demonstrated. As myocardial tissue cools, the function of the conduction system degrades and dispersion of relative refractory periods occurs. These phenomena may contribute to the propensity for malignant dysrhythmias that is seen with severe hypothermia. A continuum of effects is seen:

- The higher pacing centers are progressively inactivated, starting with the sinus node.
- Prolongation of intervals and changes in T-wave morphology is noted.
- The terminal deflection of the QRS, the J-wave, is classically seen. (Although Osborne, their discoverer, asserted that J-waves were the result of injury, this is now believed to be unlikely.[98])
- At 32°C, atrial dysrhythmias are expected.
- As the core temperature approaches 28°C, ventricular fibrillation may occur with minimal stimulation.

Unfortunately, these dysrhythmias are refractory to the standard dosages of antidysrhythmics, as well as to electrical defibrillation, below 28°C to 30°C.[99] This phenomenon included ventricular fibrillation that is unresponsive to lidocaine and procainamide. Bretylium tosylate has been credited with effective chemical defibrillation,[100] following earlier reports wherein bretylium's prophylactic role, as opposed to its therapeutic one, was experimentally appreciated.[101]

Airway security is an important goal in the severely hypothermic patient who is at increased risk for aspiration. However, endotracheal intubation itself can cause iatrogenic dysrythmogenic problems. The key is gentle manipulation of the airway at the time of intubation.[102] The goal of minimizing stimulation during intubation is emphasized.[103] Nasotracheal intubation is advocated by some.[104,105]

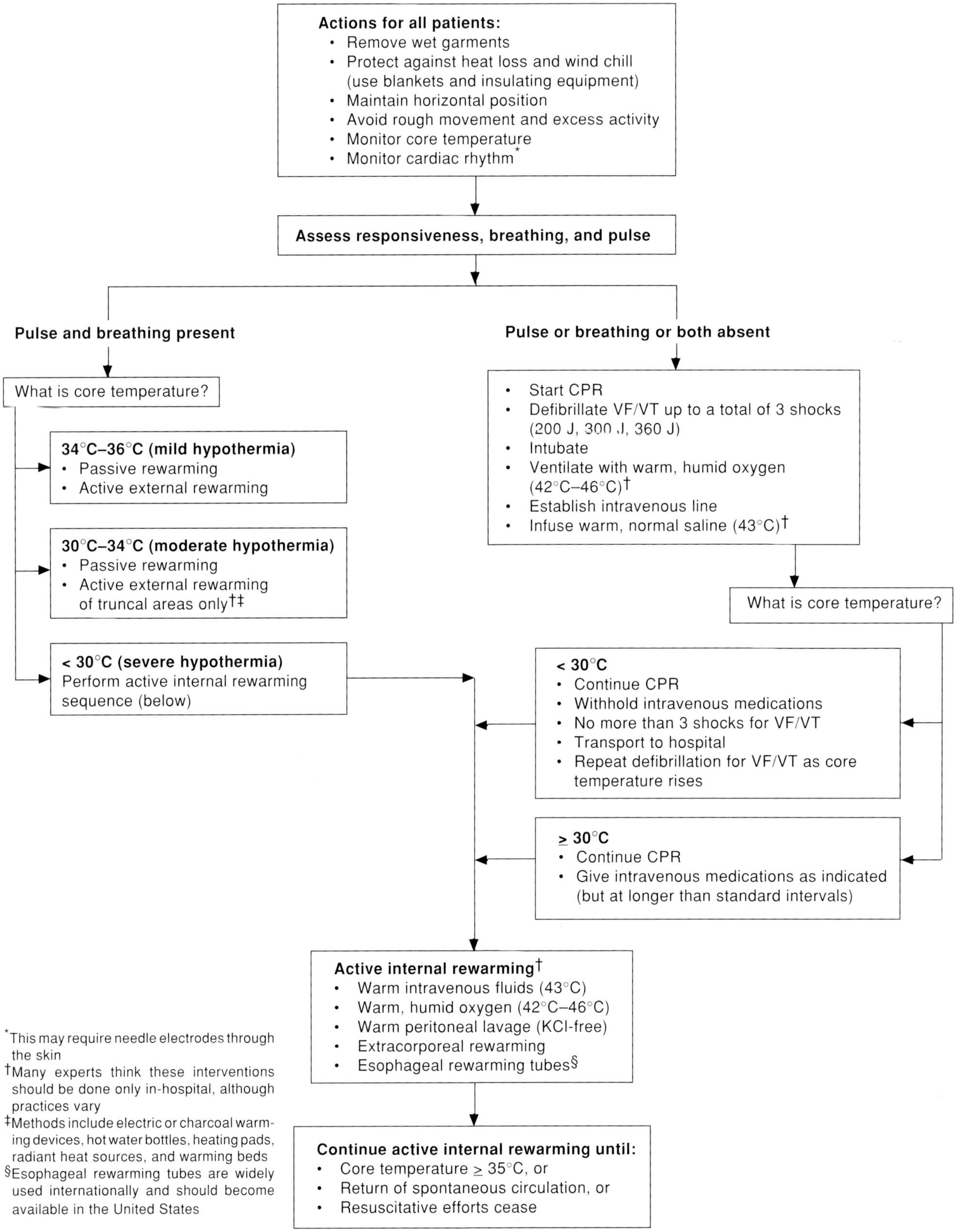

Fig. 28-3. Algorithm for the treatment of hypothermia. CPR: cardiopulmonary resuscitation; VF: ventricular fibrillation; VT: ventricular tachycardia. Reprinted with permission from Emergency Cardiac Care Committee and Subcommittees, American Heart Association. Guidelines for cardiopulmonary resuscitation and emergency cardiac care. *JAMA*. 1992;268:2245.

It should be borne in mind, as previously mentioned, that avoiding respiratory alkalosis is important. Accordingly, low ventilatory rates (eg, 5 breaths per min) are indicated in the severely hypothermic patient.

The American Heart Association recommendations for managing the pulseless, apneic, hypothermic patient are to begin CPR and to attempt defibrillation if ventricular fibrillation is diagnosed. The latter intervention is unlikely to be successful if the core temperature is below 30°C. Rapid rewarming using a femoral-to-femoral bypass should begin as soon as possible. An oxygenator is required when the heart is arrested. Blood is taken from the femoral vein, passed through an oxygenator and heat exchanger, and then pumped back into the femoral artery. Although in the past, access to the femoral vessels required their surgical exposure, there has been increasing success using percutaneous techniques, which greatly simplifies this intervention.[106] Bypass rewarming is continued until the patient is hemodynamically stable or cardioversion at 28°C to 30°C is successful. Given the lack of cardiopulmonary bypass capability in the combat zone, the only therapeutic option for hypothermic casualties who are both apneic and in cardiac arrest is to perform a thoracotomy, through which open-chest cardiac massage and warmed saline pericardial irrigation can be carried out.

Closed-chest cardiac massage in severely hypothermic patients has not been exhaustively studied, but it has proven to be effective. Recommendations to alter the absolute or relative rates of ventilation and closed chest massage are based on clinical experience and animal experimentation. CPR rates of massage and ventilation that are one-half normal are indicated in severe hypothermia. Both the reduced metabolic demand of hypothermic patients and the desirability of avoiding potentially deleterious alkalosis underlie the rationale. One group of researchers investigated changes in regional blood flow that were the result of hypothermia-induced cardiac arrest in pigs. Initially, the hypothermic pigs had lower perfusion indices than their normothermic counterparts, probably due to decreases in chest-wall compliance. Hypothermia reduced the cardiac output 50%; cerebral blood flow, 55%; and myocardial blood flow, 31% vis à vis arrested normothermic pigs. Interestingly, within 20 minutes of cardiac arrest and initiation of CPR, the normothermic group suffered continued decline in these parameters so that there was no significant difference between the two groups.[107]

The controversial issue of blood-gas interpretation remains unresolved. Nevertheless, treatment of profound acidosis using the alpha-stat method has been demonstrated clinically[108] in a severely hypothermic patient. This approach challenges the recommendation of some authorities[22] to defer bicarbonate treatment until the patient's temperature has reached 32°C to 35°C.

The determination of death is complicated by not only the unreliability of pupillary signs but also the invalidity of electrocardiography and electroencephalography, the standard assessment tools.[109] A definitive end point of resuscitation is irreversibility of arrest in a patient whose core temperature is 35°C or higher.

OTHER CONCERNS OF SPECIAL INTEREST

In addition to the matters previously discussed and their application to anesthesiologists both inside and outside the operating room, hypothermia has some other effects of particular concern to military trauma anesthesiologists and critical care specialists:

- Minimal alveolar concentrations of halothane and isoflurane decrease with temperature in a manner similar to the decrease in oxygen consumption (ie, a 5% decrease compared to a 7% decrease in oxygen consumption per degree Celsius decrease in temperature).[16,42,110]
- Although data do not exist for all drugs used by anesthesiologists, the functional hepatic impairment caused by hypothermia increases the half-life of free morphine from 3.7 minutes at 37°C to 98 minutes at 25°C.[37] We can logically deduce that other narcotics, barbiturates, and benzodiazepines would be similarly affected by hypothermia.
- The effect of neuromuscular blocking drugs is enhanced and generally prolonged by hypothermia.[111–114]
- In addition to its other effects on pulmonary function, hypothermia both significantly increases pulmonary vascular resistance and inhibits hypoxic pulmonary vasoconstriction.[115]

SUMMARY

Environmental cold has the potential to cause two significant problems for the military anesthesia provider practicing combat casualty care: local cold injury, of which frostbite is the best known, and systemic hypothermia. The morbidity resulting from the former may cause significant attrition, but the condition is unlikely to be fatal. The importance of the latter as a source of combat mortality seems to be underrated, possibly because death in such casualties is usually ascribed to more obvious physical trauma or disease. It may also be that the lack of a means to accurately measure core temperature in the field means that there is no way to diagnose systemic hypothermia.

Normal thermoregulation depends on a sequence of events that starts with the activation of peripheral thermoreceptors, the integration of the afferent signals in the preoptic nucleus of the hypothalamus, and the activation of efferent pathways that cause vasoconstriction in the skin and the fibrillary contraction of skeletal muscles known as shivering. The latter mechanism increases the production of heat, while the former decreases heat loss. The mechanisms responsible for thermoregulation in the otherwise healthy combat casualty are likely to be impaired by the casualty's trauma—the decreased heat production associated with shock and the increased heat loss from large, open wounds or surgical incisions—and by the general anesthesia, which, although it makes possible the needed resuscitative surgery, may also prevent peripheral vasoconstriction and shivering. To make matters worse, the casualty may arrive from the field already hypothermic, and the ambient temperature within the typical combat zone operating room, especially if the facility has deployed in tents, is likely to be either too cold or too hot.

It is essential that military anesthesia providers assure that there is no further cooling of the hypothermic casualty in the operating room. Although the mildly hypothermic combat casualty (core temperature > 34°C) may initially require only passive external rewarming, conditions may develop during a long operation that will magnify the heat loss. External active rewarming, and such active internal rewarming modalitics as intravenous infusion of fluids heated to 43°C and even peritoneal lavage with warm saline, should be undertaken prophylactically. Casualties whose core temperatures are below 30°C will certainly need active internal rewarming, as they are at grave risk of developing ventricular fibrillation. If available, active internal rewarming using a pump oxygenator and femoral-to-femoral bypass should be instituted. Hypothermic combat casualties who have sustained cardiac arrest are unlikely to be salvageable. Closed-chest massage should be started while active rewarming proceeds. Defibrillation may be possible but is unlikely to be successful until core temperature reaches 30°C to 32°C. In lieu of cardiopulmonary bypass, open-chest cardiac massage with lavage of the heart and mediastinum with warm saline may be all that can be done.

REFERENCES

1. Xenophon; Warner R, trans. Marching through the snow. In: *The Persian Expedition*. London, England: Penguin Books; 1972: Book 4: 196–201.

2. Polybius; Scott-Kilvert I, trans. The second Punic War. In: *The Rise of the Roman Empire*. London, England: Penguin Books; 1979: Book 3: 211, 229.

3. Danzl DF, Pozos RS, Hamlet MP. Accidental hypothermia. In: Auerbach PS, Geehr EC, eds. *Management of Wilderness and Environmental Emergencies*. St. Louis, Mo: CV Mosby; 1989: 35–76.

4. Francis TJR. Non-freezing cold injury: A historical review. *J Roy Nav Med Serv*. 1984;70:134–139.

5. Andrews RP. Cold injury complicating trauma in the subfreezing environment. *Milit Med*. 1987;152:42–44.

6. Whayne TF, DeBakey ME. *Cold Injury, Ground Type*. In: Coates JB Jr, ed. *Medical Department, US Army in World War II*. Washington, DC: US Department of the Army, Office of The Surgeon General; 1958.

7. Berger RL. Nazi science—The Dachau hypothermia experiments. *New Engl J Med*. 1990;322:1435–1440.

8. US Army Office of The Surgeon General, Professional Services Directorate. *Operation Desert Storm: Professional Afteraction Review*. Phoenix, Ariz: US Department of the Army, Office of The Surgeon General; June–July 1991.

9. Petersdorf RG. Hypothermia and hyperthermia. In: Wilson JD, Braunwald E, Isselbacher KJ, et al, eds. *Harrison's Principles of Internal Medicine*. New York, NY: McGraw-Hill; 1991: 2194–2200.

10. Benzinger M. Tympanic thermometry in surgery and anesthesia. *JAMA*. 1969;209:1207–1211.

11. Benzinger TH, Taylor GW. Cranial measurements of internal temperature in man. In: Hardy JD, ed. *Temperature: Its Measurement and Control in Science and Industry*. New York, NY: Reinhold; 1963: 111–120. Out of print.

12. Severinghaus JW. Temperature gradients during hypothermia. *Ann NY Acad Sci*. 1962;80:515–521.

13. Weintraub A, Hines, R, Carp D. Temperature monitoring during cardiac surgery: Does site make a difference? *Anesthesiology*. 1986;65A:A529.

14. Cork RC, Vaughan RW, Humphrey LS. Precision and accuracy of intraoperative temperature monitoring. *Anesth Analg*. 1983;62:211–214.

15. Wallace CT, Marks WE, Adkins WY, Mahaffey JE. Perforation of the tympanic membrane, a complication of tympanic thermometry during anesthesia. *Anesthesiology*. 1974;41:290–291.

16. Conroy JM, Fuhrman TM, Alpert CC, Wallace CT, Baker JD. The big chill: Intraoperative diagnosis and treatment of unsuspected preoperative hypothermia. *South Med J*. 1988;81:397–399.

17. Hammel HT. Anesthetics and body temperature regulation. *Anesthesiology*. 1988;68:833–835.

18. Simon E. Temperature regulation: The spinal cord as a site of extrahypothalamic thermoregulatory functions. *Rev Physiol Biochem Pharmacol*. 1974;71:1–76.

19. Lloyd EL. Hypothermia and cold. *Sci Prog*. 1989;73:101–116.

20. Brantigan CO, Patton B. Clinical hypothermia, accidental hypothermia and frostbite. In: Goldsmith HS, ed. *Lewis Practice of Surgery*. New York, NY: Harper and Row; 1978. Out of print.

21. Moss J. Accidental severe hypothermia. *Surg Gynecol Obstet*. 1986;162:501–503.

22. Bangs C, Hamlet MP. Hypothermia and cold injuries. In: Auerbach PS, Geehr EC, eds. *Management of Wilderness and Environmental Emergencies*. New York, NY: Macmillan; 1983: 27–63.

23. Horvath SM, Spurr GB, Hutt BK, Hamilton LH. Metabolic cost of shivering. *J Appl Physiol*. 1956;8:595–602.

24. Iampietro PF, Vaughan JA, Goldman RF, Kreider MB, Masucci F, Bass DE. Heat production from shivering. *J Appl Physiol*. 1960;15:632–634.

25. Sessler DI, Israel D, Pozos RS, Pozos M, Rubinstein EH. Spontaneous post-anesthetic tremor does not resemble thermoregulatory shivering. *Anesthesiology*. 1988;68:843–850.

26. Post PW, Daniels F, Binford RT. Cold injury and the evolution of "white" skin. *Hum Biol*. 1975;47:65–80.

27. Purdue GF, Hunt JL. Cold injury: A collective review. *J Burn Care Rehabil*. 1986;7:331–342.

28. Reuler JB. Hypothermia: Pathophysiology, clinical settings, and management. *Ann Intern Med*. 1978;89:519–527.

29. Edlich RF, Chang DE, Birk KA, Morgan RF, Tafel JA. Cold injuries. *Compr Ther*. 1989;15:13–21.

30. Martin TG. Near-drowning and cold water immersion. *Ann Emerg Med*. 1984;13:263–273.

31. McCallum AL, McLellan BA, Reid SR, Courtade W. Two cases of accidental immersion hypothermia with different outcomes under identical conditions. *Aviat Space Environ Med.* 1989;60:162–165.

32. Hayward MG, Keatings WR. Roles of subcutaneous fat and thermoregulatory reflexes in determining ability to stabilize body temperature in water. *J Physiol.* 1981;320:229–251.

33. Sessler DS, Olofsson CI, Rubinstein EH, Beebe JJ. The thermoregulatory threshold in humans during halothane anesthesia. *Anesthesiology.* 1988;68:836–842.

34. Rowell LR. The cutaneous circulation. In: Ruch TC, Patton HD, eds. *Physiology and Biophysics.* Vol 2, 20th ed. Philadelphia, Pa: WB Saunders; 1973: 185–193.

35. Coffman JD, Cohen AS. Total and nutritional blood flow in the finger. *Clin Sci.* 1972;42:243–250.

36. Mitchell D, Laburn HP. Pathophysiology of temperature regulation. *Physiologist.* 1985;28:507–517.

37. Ferguson J, Epstein F, van de Leuv J. Accidental hypothermia. *Emerg Med Clin North Am.* 1983;1:619–637.

38. Russ W, Kling D, Loesevitz A. Effect of hypothermia on visual evoked potentials in humans. *Anesthesiology.* 1984;61:207–210.

39. Sebel PS, Bruijn H, Neville WK. Effect of hypothermia on median nerve somatosensory evoked potentials. *Anesthesiology.* 1986;65:A154.

40. Harnett RM, Pruitt JR, Sias FR. A review of the literature concerning resuscitation from hypothermia, I: The problem and general approaches. *Aviat Space Environ Med.* 1983;54:425–434.

41. Coniam SW. Accidental hypothermia. *Anesthesiology.* 1979;34:250–252.

42. Lilly RB Jr. Inadvertent hypothermia: A real problem. In: *American Society of Anesthesiologists Refresher Courses.* Vol 15. Philadelphia, Pa: JB Lippincott; 1987: Chap 8.

43. Cooper KE, Sheilage M, Riben P. Respiratory and other responses in subjects immersed in cold water. *J Appl Physiol.* 1976;4:903–910.

44. Hirvonen J. Necropsy findings in fatal hypothermia cases. *Forensic Science.* 1976;8:155–164.

45. Paton BC. Accidental hypothermia. *Pharmacol Ther.* 1983;22:331–377.

46. Bay J, Nunn JF, Prys-Roberts C. Factors influencing arterial Po_2 during recovery from anesthesia. *Br J Anaesth.* 1968;40:398–406.

47. Kanter GS. Hypothermic hemoconcentration. *Am J Physiol.* 1968;214:856–859.

48. Patt A, McCroskey BL, Moore EE. Hypothermia induced coagulopathies in trauma. *Surg Clin North Am.* 1988;68:775–785.

49. Thomas R, Hessel EA, Harker LA, Sands MP, Dillard DH. Platelet function during and after deep surface hypothermia. *J Surg Res.* 1981;31:314–318.

50. Kelman GR. Nunn JF. Nomograms for correction of blood Po_2, Pco_2, pH, and base excess for time and temperature. *J Appl Physiol.* 1966;21:1484–1490.

51. Swain JA. Hypothermia and blood pH. *Arch Int Med.* 1988;148:1643–1646.

52. Tinker JH. *Cardiopulmonary Bypass: Current Concepts and Controversies.* Philadelphia, Pa: WB Saunders; 1989.

53. Rahn H, Reeves RB, Howell BJ. Hydrogen ion regulation, temperature, and evolution. *Am J Respir.* 1975;112:165–172.

54. Somero GN, White FN. Enzymatic consequences under alphastat regulation. In: Rahn H, Prakash O, eds. *Acid–Base Regulation and Body Temperature.* Hingham, Mass: Martinus Nijhoff; 1985: Chap 4.

55. Becker H, Vinten-Johansen J, Buckberg GD. Myocardial damage caused by keeping pH 7.40 during systemic deep hypothermia. *J Thorac Cardiovasc Surg.* 1981;82:810–820.

56. Swain JA, White FN, Peters RM. The effect of pH on the hypothermic ventricular fibrillation threshold. *J Thorac Cardiovasc Surg.* 1984;87:445–451.

57. Kopf GS, Mirvis DM, Myers RE. Central nervous system tolerance to cardiac arrest during profound hypothermia. *J Surg Res.* 1975;18:29–34.

58. Kroncke GM, Nichols RD, Mendenhall JT. Ectothermic philosophy of acid–base balance to prevent fibrillation during hypothermia. *Arch Surg.* 1986;121:303–304.

59. Vole RJ. Postoperative accidental hypothermia. *Anesthesiology.* 1969;24:449.

60. Morris RH. Operating room temperature and the anesthetized, paralyzed patient. *Arch Surg.* 1971;102:95–97.

61. Myers RAM, Britten JS, Cowley RA. Hypothermia: Quantitative aspects of therapy. *Journal of the American College of Emergency Physicians.* 1979;8:523–527.

62. Bourke DL, Wurm H, Rosenberg M, Russell J. Intraoperative heat conservation using a reflective blanket. *Anesthesiology.* 1984;60:151–154.

63. Morris, RH, Kumar A. The effect of warming blankets on maintenance of body temperature of the anesthetized, paralyzed adult patient. *Anesthesiology.* 1972;36:408–411.

64. Tollofsrud SG, Gundersen Y, Anderson R. Perioperative hypothermia. *Acta Anaesthesiol (Scand).* 1984;28:511–515.

65. Haslam KR, Nielsen CH. Do passive heat and moisture exchangers keep the patient warm? *Anesthesiology.* 1986;64:379–381.

66. Weeks D. Evaluation of a disposable humidifier for use during anesthesia. *Anesthesiology.* 1981;54:337–340.

67. Chalon F, Markham FP, Ali MM, Ramanathan S, Turndorf H. The Pall Ultipor breathing filter—An efficient heat and moisture exchanger. *Anesth Analg.* 1984;63:566–570.

68. Morrison JB, Conn ML, Hayward JS. Thermal increment provided by inhalation rewarming from hypothermia. *J Appl Physiol.* 1979;46:1061–1065.

69. Hayward JS, Steinman AM. Accidental hypothermia: An experimental study of inhalation rewarming. *Aviat Space Environ Med.* 1975;46:1236–1240.

70. Pflug AE, Aasheim GM, Foster C, Martin RW. Prevention of post anesthesia shivering. *Can Anaesth Soc J.* 1978;25:43–49.

71. Sims NM, Geoffrian BS, Welch JP, Jung W, Burke JF. Respiratory tract burns caused by heated humidification of anesthetic gases. *Anesthesiology.* 1986;65:A490.

72. Harnett RM, Pruitt JR, Sias FR. A review of the literature concerning resuscitation from hypothermia, II: Selected rewarming protocols. *Aviat Space Environ Med.* 1983;54.487–495.

73. Roe CF. Temperature regulation and energy metabolism in surgical patients. *Prog Surg.* 1973;12:96–127.

74. Browne DA, De Boeck, Morgan M. An evaluation of the Level 1 blood warmer series. *Anesthesia*. 1990;45:960–963.

75. Anshus JS, Endahl GL, Mottley JL. Microwave heating of intravenous fluids. *Am J Emerg Med*. 1985;3:316–319.

76. Werwath DL, Schwab CW, Scholten JR. Microwave ovens: A safe new method of warming crystalloids. *Am Surg*. 1984;50:656–659.

77. Judkins D, Iserson KV. Rapid admixture blood warming. *J Emerg Nurs*. 1991;17(3)146–150.

78. Boyan CP. Cold or warmed blood for massive transfusions. *Ann Surg*. 1964;160:282–286.

79. Vaughn MS, Vaughn RW, Cork RC. Radiation versus conduction for post op rewarming of adults. *Anesthesiology*. 1980;53:S195.

80. Murphy MT, Lipton JM, Giesecke AH. Post-anesthetic shivering: Effect of localized radiant heat versus warmed blanket treatment. *Anesthesiology*. 1986;65:A306.

81. Kalant H, Le AD. Effects of ethanol on thermoregulation. *Pharmacol Ther*. 1984;23:313–364.

82. Sessler DI, Moayeri A. Skin-surface warming: Heat flux and central temperature. *Anesthesiology*. 1990;73:218–224.

83. Vaughn MS, Vaughn RW, Cork RC. Postoperative hypothermia in adults: Relationship of age, anesthesia, and shivering to rewarming. *Anesth Analg*. 1981;60:746–751.

84. Claybon LE, Hirsh RA. Meperidine arrests postanesthesia shivering. *Anesthesiology*. 1980;53:S180.

85. Pauca AL, Savage RT, Simpson S, Roy RC. Effect of pethidine, fentanyl, and morphine on post-operative shivering in man. *Acta Anaesthesiol Scand*. 1984;28:138–143.

86. Burks LC, Aisner J, Fortner CL, Wiernik PH. Meperidine for the treatment of shaking chills and fever. *Arch Intern Med*. 1980;140:483–484.

87. Coughlin F. Heart warming procedure. *N Engl J Med*. 1973;290:326.

88. Reuler JB, Parker RA. Peritoneal dialysis in the management of hypothermia. *JAMA*. 1978;240:2289–2290.

89. Lash RF, Burdete JA, Ozdil T. Accidental profound hypothermia and barbiturate intoxication—Report of rapid "core" rewarming by peritoneal dialysis. *JAMA*. 1967;201:269–270.

90. Pickering BG, Bristow GK, Craig DB. Case history number 97: Core rewarming by peritoneal irrigation in accidental hypothermia with cardiac arrest. *Anesth Analg*. 1977;56:574–577.

91. Miller JW, Danzl DF, Thomas DM. Urban accidental hypothermia: 135 cases. *Ann Emerg Med*. 1980;9:456–461.

92. Ponning PE, Skulberg A, Abyholin F. Accidental hypothermia: Review of the literature. *Acta Anaesthesiol Scand*. 1986;30:601–613.

93. Standards and guidelines for cardiopulmonary resuscitation (CPR) and emergency cardiac care (ECC). *JAMA*. 1986;255:2905–2984.

94. Steinman AM. Cardiopulmonary resuscitation and hypothermia. *Circulation*. 1986;74:(4)29–32.

95. Ornato JP. Special resuscitation situations: Near drowning, traumatic injury, electric shock, and hypothermia. *Circulation*. 1986;74:(4)23–36.

96. American Heart Association. Emergency Cardiac Care Committee and Subcommittees. American Heart Association guidelines for cardiopulmonary resuscitation and emergency cardiac care. *JAMA*. 1992;268:2171–2259.

97. Zell SC, Kurtz KJ. Severe exposure hypothermia: A resuscitation protocol. *Ann Emerg Med.* 1985;14:339–345.

98. Solomon A, Barish R, Browne B, Tso E. The electrocardiographic features of hypothermia. *J Emerg Med.* 1989;7:169–173.

99. Dronen S, Nowak RM, Tomlanovich MC. Bretylium tosylate and hypothermic ventricular fibrillation. *Ann Emerg Med.* 1980;9:335.

100. Danzl DF, Sowers BF, Vicario SJ, Thomas DM, Miller JW. Chemical ventricular defibrillation in severe accidental hypothermia. *Ann Emerg Med.* 1982;11(12):698–699.

101. Buckley JJ, Bosch OK, Bacaner MB. Prevention of ventricular fibrillation during hypothermia with bretylium tosylate. *Anesth Analg.* 1971;50:587–593.

102. Miller JW, Danzl DF, Thomas DM. Hypothermia treatment. *Ann Emerg Med.* 1981;10:396–397. Authors' reply.

103. Miller JW. Hypothermia. In: Kravis TC, Warner CG, eds. *Emergency Medicine: A Comprehensive Review.* 2nd ed. Rockville, Md: Aspen Publishers; 1987: Chap 45: 639–656.

104. Miller JW, Danzl DF, Thomas DM. Urban accidental hypothermia: 135 cases. *Ann Emerg Med.* 1980;9:456–461.

105. Danzl DF, Thomas DM. Nasotracheal intubations in the emergency department. *Crit Care Med.* 1980;8:677–682

106. Laub GW, Banaszak D, Kupferschmid J, Magovern GW, Young JC. Percutaneous cardiopulmonary bypass for the treatment of hypothermic circulatory collapse. *Ann Thor Surg.* 1989;47:608–611.

107. Maningas PA, DeGuzman LR, Hollenbach SJ, Volk KA, Bellamy RF. Regional blood flow during hypothermic arrest. *Ann Emerg Med.* 1986;15:390–396.

108. Cohen DJ, Cline JR, Lepinski SM, Brown M, Ireland K. Resuscitation of the hypothermic patient. *Am J Emerg Med.* 1988;6:475–478.

109. Gregory RT, Patton JF. Treatment after exposure to cold. *Lancet.* 1972;1:377.

110. Vitez TS, White PF, Eger EI. Effects of hypothermia on halothane MAC and isoflurane MAC in the rat. *Anesthesiology.* 1974;41:80–81.

111. Miller RD, Rodericks LL. Pancuronium-induced neuromuscular blockade and its antagonism by neostigmine at 29, 37, and 41°C. *Anesthesiology.* 1977;46:333–335.

112. Flynn PJ, Hughes R, Walton B. Use of atracurium in cardiac surgery involving cardiopulmonary bypass with induced hypothermia. *Br J Anaesth.* 1984;56:967–972.

113. Buzello W, Schluermann D, Schindler M, Spillner G. Hypothermic cardiopulmonary bypass and neuromuscular blockade by pancuronium and vecuronium. *Anesthesiology.* 1985;62:201–204.

114. Heier T, Caldwell JE, Sessler DI, Miller RD. Mild intraoperative hypothermia increases duration of action and recovery time of vecuronium. *Anesth Analg.* 1990;70:S153.

115. Benumof JL, Wahrenbrock EA. Dependency of hypoxic pulmonary vasoconstriction on temperature. *J Appl Physiol.* 1977;42:56–58.

Chapter 29

MALIGNANT HYPERTHERMIA

STEVEN M. KARAN, M.D.*; AND SHEILA M. MULDOON, M.D.†

*Major, Medical Corps, U.S. Army; Assistant Professor of Anesthesiology, Uniformed Services University of the Health Sciences
†Chairman, Department of Anesthesiology, Uniformed Services University of the Health Sciences, 4301 Jones Bridge Road, Bethesda, Maryland 20814-4799

INTRODUCTION

Despite screening efforts to remove them from combat roles, soldiers who are susceptible to malignant hyperthermia will be deployed to the battlefield. A soldier may be unknowingly susceptible, or may have a first-degree relative who has been diagnosed since the soldier arrived in the combat theater. Rarely, the soldier may have concealed his or her susceptibility.

The diagnosis and treatment of malignant hyperthermia in the combat environment differs from that during peacetime. Peacetime care relies on heightened awareness, capnographic monitoring, and a readily available supply of dantrolene (the specific agent for the prevention and treatment of malignant hyperthermia). This combination has reduced fatal outcomes to 2% to 3%.[1–4] The management of malignant hyperthermia in combat must rely on diagnosis and treatment in light of the available resources. Therefore, to approach this level of success on the battlefield, heightened awareness and increased vigilance, rather than the availability of advanced monitors, must be emphasized. Although all efforts will be made to provide the most advanced equipment available, this equipment may not always perform optimally in a hostile environment.

CLINICAL SYNDROME

Fulminant Malignant Hyperthermia

Malignant hyperthermia is a pharmacogenetic disorder of skeletal muscle metabolism that is expressed as a broad clinical spectrum. The term malignant hyperthermia is most commonly used to refer to a fulminant presentation that begins at the time of an anesthetic induction, but the spectrum also encompasses episodes that develop later in the anesthetic course and progress less rapidly.

Masseter muscle rigidity, which occasionally progresses to fulminant malignant hyperthermia, and less well-defined or documented entities (ie, stress or exercise-induced hyperthermic responses) are also included in the spectrum. When the susceptible patient is anesthetized with triggering agents, the fulminant episode presents as tachypnea and tachycardia that can rapidly progress to arrhythmias, muscle rigidity, and high fever. Rhabdomyolysis can lead to myoglobinuria, acute renal failure, and disseminated intravascular coagulation. Death results from arrhythmias, inability to ventilate, cardiovascular collapse, or brain damage.

A fulminant malignant hyperthermia episode can occur at induction, hours into a stable anesthetic, in the recovery room, or on the ward. The rate of progression varies from minutes to hours, and appears to be independent of the time of onset. The clinical signs reflect the body's inability to respond to an extraordinary increase in metabolic demand. When the demand can no longer be sustained, organ-system failure occurs and accelerates the syndrome. The ability to recognize the clinical syndrome is complicated by (*a*) its rare occurrence, (*b*) the lack of a noninvasive screening test, and (*c*) the well-known fact that 50% of patients with fulminant episodes will have had at least one previous, uneventful exposure to triggering agents. Although contracture testing with halothane and caffeine has been useful in predicting malignant hyperthermia susceptibility in humans, this test is unacceptable for general screening due to (*a*) the complexity of the testing conditions and (*b*) its invasiveness (the testing requires a skeletal muscle biopsy). For the same reasons, contracture testing has no place in the management of an acute episode of malignant hyperthermia. In addition, like all other diagnostic tests, it is not 100% sensitive or specific. A detailed discussion of halothane and caffeine contracture testing follows later in this chapter.

Potent inhalational anesthetics and succinylcholine can initiate the malignant hyperthermia syndrome in susceptible individuals. Factors that may influence the onset include

- the patient's genetic predisposition,
- stress,
- trauma,
- the potency and dosage of the triggering agent, or
- the presence of nondepolarizing neuromuscular blocking agents or other nontriggering anesthetics in the anesthetic technique.

Although the exact site (or sites) for the initiation of the syndrome is still unknown, data on human subjects and swine document that aerobic and anaerobic metabolism in skeletal muscle increase very early in the clinical syndrome.[5] Elevations in carbon dioxide and lactic acid production in the muscle cause both a decrease in venous pH and an increase in venous carbon dioxide content.[6] The sympathetic nervous system responds to this hypermetabolic state with a massive release of catecholamines, which increases minute ventilation and cardiac output. Tachycardia and blood pressure elevations appear early. Tachypnea is also an early sign in patients who are allowed to ventilate spontaneously; however, this sign is often masked in controlled ventilation with muscle relaxation (the current clinical practice). In this setting, elevation of the end-tidal carbon dioxide is the earliest clinically detectable sign of the syndrome.

Once metabolic demand exceeds the body's ability to compensate, core temperature begins to rise because the body is no longer able to dissipate the heat generated from the skeletal muscle. Temperature can increase more than 1°C every 15 minutes; however, this rate will vary depending on conditions such as the ambient temperature, site and size of the surgical incision, and measures of heat preservation employed for the patient.

In a review of cases published in 1970, (prior to the discovery of dantrolene therapy) muscle rigidity was found in 70% of the patients.[7] The progression of muscle rigidity usually parallels the progression of the clinical syndrome and can interfere with perfusion and with ventilation. Less frequently, severe rigidity can occur immediately after the administration of succinylcholine, and has been associated with profound fasciculations. Alterations in skeletal muscle membrane permeability lead to elevations in serum potassium, sodium, calcium, phosphate, myoglobin, and creatine kinase (CK, formerly called creatine phosphokinase [CPK]).[8]

Ventricular arrhythmias result from hypoxia, hyperkalemia, severe acidosis, or increased catecholamine release. Although patients can appear cyanotic, mottled, or their blood can appear dark in the surgical field, arterial blood-gas analysis rarely identifies gross hypoxia. Peripheral vasoconstriction and decreasing cardiac function probably account for regional hypoperfusion, which compounds the metabolic disorder. Without prompt treatment, death is inevitable if the syndrome has progressed to this point. Even after treatment, the patient is at risk for recrudescence of the syndrome for up to 24 hours.[9]

Masseter Muscle Rigidity

Trismus, masseter muscle spasm, and masseter muscle rigidity all describe rigidity of the jaw muscles after the administration of succinylcholine. This transient phenomenon occurs despite flaccid paralysis of the extremities. Tachycardia, ventricular arrhythmias, and elevations in end-tidal carbon dioxide are common. Discontinuing the triggering agents usually permits an uneventful recovery; however, progression to the fulminant episode can begin immediately. More commonly, progression to the fulminant episode develops 20 to 30 minutes after the resolution of masseter muscle rigidity. Therefore, monitoring for the syndrome should continue during this period. Serum creatine kinase levels, which peak 8 to 12 hours after induction, will be elevated (5,000–10,000 international units) and can be markedly elevated especially if a second dose of succinylcholine was administered. Patients should be monitored postoperatively for the resolution of rhabdomyolysis and myoglobinuria to decrease the risk of renal complications.

The incidence of masseter muscle rigidity progressing to the fulminant episode is unknown, and until this question is answered, induction techniques that are closely associated with the development of masseter muscle rigidity should be limited. The incidence of masseter muscle rigidity following an intravenous induction is greatly reduced compared to that seen with inhalational induction.[10] Therefore, the use of intravenous succinylcholine following induction with a potent inhalational agent should be avoided.[11] If an inhalational induction is required, intubation can be accomplished with a short-acting, nondepolarizing muscle relaxant or by deepening the level of anesthesia. In situations when rapid airway control is mandatory, no other muscle relaxant can match succinylcholine's combination of rapid onset and short duration of action. The onset time of nondepolarizing muscle relaxants can be decreased by doubling or tripling the recommended dose for intubation, but this markedly prolongs the duration of action. Before nondepolarizing muscle relaxants are administered in this fashion, four factors must be considered:

1. the plan of action if ventilation is not improved following adequate muscle relaxation,
2. the resources available for mechanical ventilation in the postoperative period,
3. the number of soldiers requiring surgical procedures, and
4. the length of the anticipated surgical procedure.

Although masseter muscle rigidity was originally described as an early sign of malignant hyperthermia, the validity of this idea and the operating room management of this condition are being reevaluated.[12–14] The following facts have become accepted:

1. Although masseter muscle rigidity can follow both intravenous and inhalational inductions, it is far more likely in the latter (1:4,000 vs 1:100).[10,15,16]
2. Most of the data concerning masseter muscle rigidity is in the pediatric population, presumably because inductions with inhalational anesthetics are more frequent in children.
3. In vitro halothane and caffeine contracture testing (discussed later in this chapter) is positive for malignant hyperthermia after clinical masseter muscle rigidity in approximately 50% of pediatric patients and 25% of adult patients.[17–19]
4. Succinylcholine transiently increases the basal tension of masseter muscles, possibly by a mechanism similar to its action on extraocular muscles. The relationship between this modest increase in tension and masseter muscle rigidity or malignant hyperthermia is unknown.[20,21]

Why the incidence of masseter muscle rigidity is more common after an inhalational induction remains elusive. Because inductions with inhalational anesthetics are rare in adults, it is unknown if the incidence in this population is the same as in children, or if age is a factor. Reporting slight increases in masseter tension as actual instances of masseter muscle rigidity may account for some of the disparity; however, data from one hospital center that examined 42,000 children showed a 10-fold increase in masseter muscle rigidity following induction with inhalational anesthetics (1:370) versus induction with intravenous agents (1:3,879).[10] When the incidence of masseter muscle rigidity following induction with inhalational anesthetics is applied to halothane and caffeine contracture data, the incidence of masseter muscle rigidity continues to be markedly higher than the currently accepted incidence of malignant hyperthermia (1:370 • 50% = 1:740). Once the role that inhalational agents or endogenous catecholamines play in sensitizing the masseter muscles is determined, we may have a better understanding of the physiology of this phenomenon. Until then, patients with marked increases in jaw tension (ie, the anesthesia provider is unable to open the patient's mouth) should be identified and treated as susceptible to malignant hyperthermia.

Stress-Induced Malignant Hyperthermia

In susceptible swine breeds, the malignant hyperthermia syndrome can be triggered by environmental stresses that include heat, exercise, fear, and excitement. These stresses have occasionally been implicated in humans, but convincing and complete data are hard to obtain.[22–25] Malignant hyperthermia triggered by combat stress has not been reported. Patients who are identified as susceptible to malignant hyperthermia—either by clinical episode or by contracture testing—but who have no history of an adverse reaction to stress are not likely to experience an adverse reaction to stress in the future. Activity need not be limited in this group, although patients must avoid the triggering anesthetics. If a susceptible patient has experienced a reaction to stress, that stress and similar stresses should be avoided or approached with caution.

BATTLEFIELD RESOURCES

Combat anesthesia depends on both the battlefield environment and the supply of anesthetic equipment on the battlefield. Sophisticated techniques can be performed even under austere conditions with a basic minimum of equipment (Exhibit 29-1).[26] As new advances in anesthetic management occur, the specific equipment will change; however, the principle of optimizing care with limited resources will not change. To achieve the goals of early diagnosis and treatment of malignant hyperthermia, the monitors that are available at each level will be evaluated. Achieving this goal will reduce the morbidity and mortality of malignant hyperthermia patients and therefore will reduce the amount of resources devoted to their postoperative care. Clinical suspicion is the cornerstone for detecting malignant hyperthermia in any environment. This section will also include a discussion of the role of the clean anesthesia machine, the malignant hyperthermia cart, and laboratory testing.

Levels of Equipment Availability

The signs of malignant hyperthermia can present in almost any order or combination. However, the

EXHIBIT 29-1

LEVELS OF EQUIPMENT AVAILABILITY

Equipment Level 1
- Ohio 885A Field Anesthesia Machine
- Ohmeda Universal Vaporizer Portable Anesthesia System
- Pulse oximeter
- Basic blood pressure monitoring equipment
- Blood-warming and -delivery system
- Oxygen source
- Fundamental airway and ventilation equipment including suction
- Intravenous fluid administration equipment
- Intravenous and inhalation drugs

Equipment Level 2
- All equipment included in equipment level 1, plus:
- Temperature-monitoring device
- Automatic pneumatic blood pressure device
- Electric or compressed gas-driven ventilator
- Blood autotransfusion equipment

Equipment Level 3
- All equipment included in equipment levels 1 and 2, plus:
- Capnograph
- Invasive blood pressure monitor
- Electrocardiograph

Adapted from Condon BC, Temo JM, Crowl FD, et al. Anesthesia guidelines. In: Bellamy RF, ed. *Combat Casualty Care Guidelines: Operation Desert Storm*. Washington, DC: US Department of the Army, Office of The Surgeon General, and Borden Institute; 1991: 24.

progression of the syndrome usually follows a general pattern (Table 29-1). Because the scope and availability of laboratory facilities will vary, laboratory signs will be discussed later in this section. When only the first level of equipment is available, early diagnosis involves the recognition that nonspecific signs (ie, an elevated heart rate and blood pressure) are out of proportion to the expected condition. If the patient is breathing spontaneously (mechanical ventilators are not included at this level), tachypnea will probably be the earliest sign. Rhythm irregularities can be detected by the pulse oximeter and confirmed with a finger on the pulse. Skeletal muscle rigidity may be detected by

- masseter muscle spasm at the time of intubation,
- increasing difficulty with ventilation, or
- the surgeon's complaint of inadequate muscle relaxation.

Late signs will include an elevated temperature detected by touch or by warm carbon dioxide–absorption canisters, the exhaustion of carbon dioxide canisters (indicating increased carbon dioxide production), or dark blood on the surgical field (indicating a relative hypoxia).

Additional equipment at the second level of availability includes automated blood pressure- and temperature-monitoring devices. Due to high levels of ambient battlefield noise (like those experienced during Operation Desert Storm), the automated blood pressure device may be the only reliable, noninvasive means for monitoring blood pressure. Although the temperature monitor provides objective data, its usefulness in diagnosing malignant hyperthermia is limited: elevated temperature is a *late* sign.

Additions at the third level of equipment availability include capnographic and electrocardiographic monitoring. The capnograph identifies one of the earliest signs of the syndrome and is easily applied to any anesthetic procedure. This combination makes it an ideal monitor for the detection of malignant hyperthermia. Changes in venous blood-gas analysis, serum lactate, oxygen consumption, and cardiac output also occur very early in the syndrome; but these changes cannot be detected, continuously monitored, or easily applied to the battlefield with current monitoring technology. Although pulse oximetry can alert the clinician to ongoing arrhythmias, electrocardiographic monitoring is needed for identifying and treating complex arrhythmias. Electrocardiography can also be useful in detecting changes in serum potassium levels.

The Clean Anesthesia Machine

A *clean* anesthesia machine is one that either (*a*) has never been used to administer a potent inhalational agent or (*b*) has been made safe for use with malignant hyperthermia–susceptible patients. This item may be taken for granted in most operating suites in the continental United States, but it is not included in the equipment provided at any of the three levels of equipment availability. Three steps are required to create a clean anesthesia machine from one that has already been exposed to potent

TABLE 29-1

DETECTING CLINICAL SIGNS OF MALIGNANT HYPERTHERMIA AT EACH LEVEL OF EQUIPMENT AVAILABILITY

Signs of Malignant Hyperthermia in Common Order of Progression (top = early; bottom = late)	Equipment Level 1	Equipment Level 2*	Equipment Level 3†
Increased CO_2 production and/or minute ventilation	Tachypnea Hot or expired CO_2 canister		Capnograph
Increased O_2 consumption	Dark blood on surgical field		
Increased cardiac output			
Increased pulse	Stethescope Palpation Pulse oximeter		ECG
Increased blood pressure	Manual cuff	Automated cuff	Invasive monitoring
Arrhythmias	Palpation Pulse oximeter		ECG
Rigidity	Touch Ventilation difficulties		
Temperature elevation	Touch Hot CO_2 canisters	Temperature monitor	

*Includes means available in Level 1
†Includes means available in Levels 1 and 2

inhalational anesthetics. First, because the rubber parts of anesthesia machines will retain potent inhalational anesthetics, the fresh gas hose, ventilator bellows, and circuit (if nondisposable) must be replaced with new or disposable parts. Second, the machine must be flushed with a high fresh gas flow (10 L/min) for 10 minutes. Finally, the vaporizers should be removed or drained to prevent any possibility that they will be turned on during the perioperative period. A nonrebreathing system (eg, the Mapleson or Jackson-Rees anesthesia breathing circuits) can also serve as a clean anesthesia machine when attached to an oxygen source with adequate fresh gas flow.

The Malignant Hyperthermia Cart

The rationale for a malignant hyperthermia cart is to have the supplies required for treatment of malignant hyperthermia assembled and ready so the response time for treatment of an episode can be decreased (Table 29-2). Supplies and medications available for anesthetists are found in two medical material sets (MMSs, which are discussed in Chapter 6, Deployable Hospitals): MMS D301, Operating Room, and MMS D306, Pharmacy. Recommendations are under study to create a separate MMS for anesthesia equipment and medications. Currently, MMS D301 contains six vials of dantrolene (20 mg per vial), lidocaine, calcium chloride, epinephrine, and sodium bicarbonate. Because the average adult requires 160 to 200 mg of dantrolene at the beginning of treatment, coordination with the pharmacy will be necessary to ensure the smooth and rapid administration of the initial dose. An additional 30 vials of dantrolene are contained in MMS D306, along with procainamide, dextrose 50%, insulin, mannitol, furosemide, and sterile water. The current supply of sterile water is contained in 5-mL vials (60 mL of sterile water is required to dissolve each vial of dantrolene). Therefore, another recommendation has been made to include two 500-mL

TABLE 29-2

SUPPLIES FOR MALIGNANT HYPERTHERMIA CART

Supply	Quantity	Purpose
Dantrolene	At least 36 vials	——
Sterile water for injection	3 L	Reconstitution of dantrolene
50-mL syringes and large-gauge needles	12	Draw up dantrolene
Lidocaine	5 ampules	Bolus and continuous infusion
Procainamide	5 ampules	Bolus and continuous infusion
Dextrose 50%	4 ampules	Treatment of hypokalemia
Mannitol 25%	100 g (8 ampules)	Renal protection
Furosemide	200 mg	Renal protection
Sodium bicarbonate	50 meq (10 ampules)	Treatment of metabolic acidosis
Epinephrine	1 mg (4 ampules)	Treatment of hypotension
Calcium chloride 10%	4 ampules	Treatment of hyperkalemia
Normal saline (refrigerated)	6 L	For injection and irrigation

Also included on the cart: crushed ice or ice maker, irrigating Foley catheter, rectal tube, cooling blanket, central venous access kits, pulmonary artery catheter, new fresh gas hose, carbon dioxide–absorption canisters, anesthesia breathing circuit, ventilator bellows, blood-collection tubes, lab slips, labels

bags of sterile water to MMS D301 and four 500-mL bags of sterile water to MMS D306 for more-rapid mixing of dantrolene.

Laboratory Testing

Laboratory tests that aid in making the diagnosis include

- arterial and venous blood-gas analyses;
- serum potassium, glucose, sodium, and calcium;
- prothrombin and partial thromboplastin times;
- serum creatine kinase; and
- serum and urinary myoglobin.

Laboratory support will be crucial in confirming the diagnosis of malignant hyperthermia and in managing advanced cases. Severe metabolic and electrolyte disturbances require frequent laboratory analyses in both the initial treatment and the recovery phases. The most valuable tests of the initial treatment phase are the arterial blood-gas analyses and serum potassium levels, while serum creatine kinase and myoglobin levels are useful in preventing renal damage in the recovery phase.

BATTLEFIELD MANAGEMENT

Early recognition of the syndrome, discontinuation of the triggering agent or agents, rapid administration of dantrolene, and prompt initiation of supportive care are the four cornerstones of successful management. It is unlikely that the coordination of this complex process will progress smoothly unless a plan has already been discussed and implemented. Although the Malignant Hyperthermia Hotline [(800) 644-9737] is theoretically available for assistance in the management of suspected cases, communication linkage to this resource from the battlefield is doubtful. The management of the patient with a fulminant episode, masseter muscle rigidity, and a history of malignant hyperthermia needs to be considered in light of these constraints.

A Fulminant Episode

Treatment of a fulminant malignant hyperthermia episode requires that two distinct approaches be initiated simultaneously: (1) preparation and administration of dantrolene sodium, and (2) initiation and maintenance of supportive care. Assistance from other medical personnel is essential if these tasks are to be completed rap-

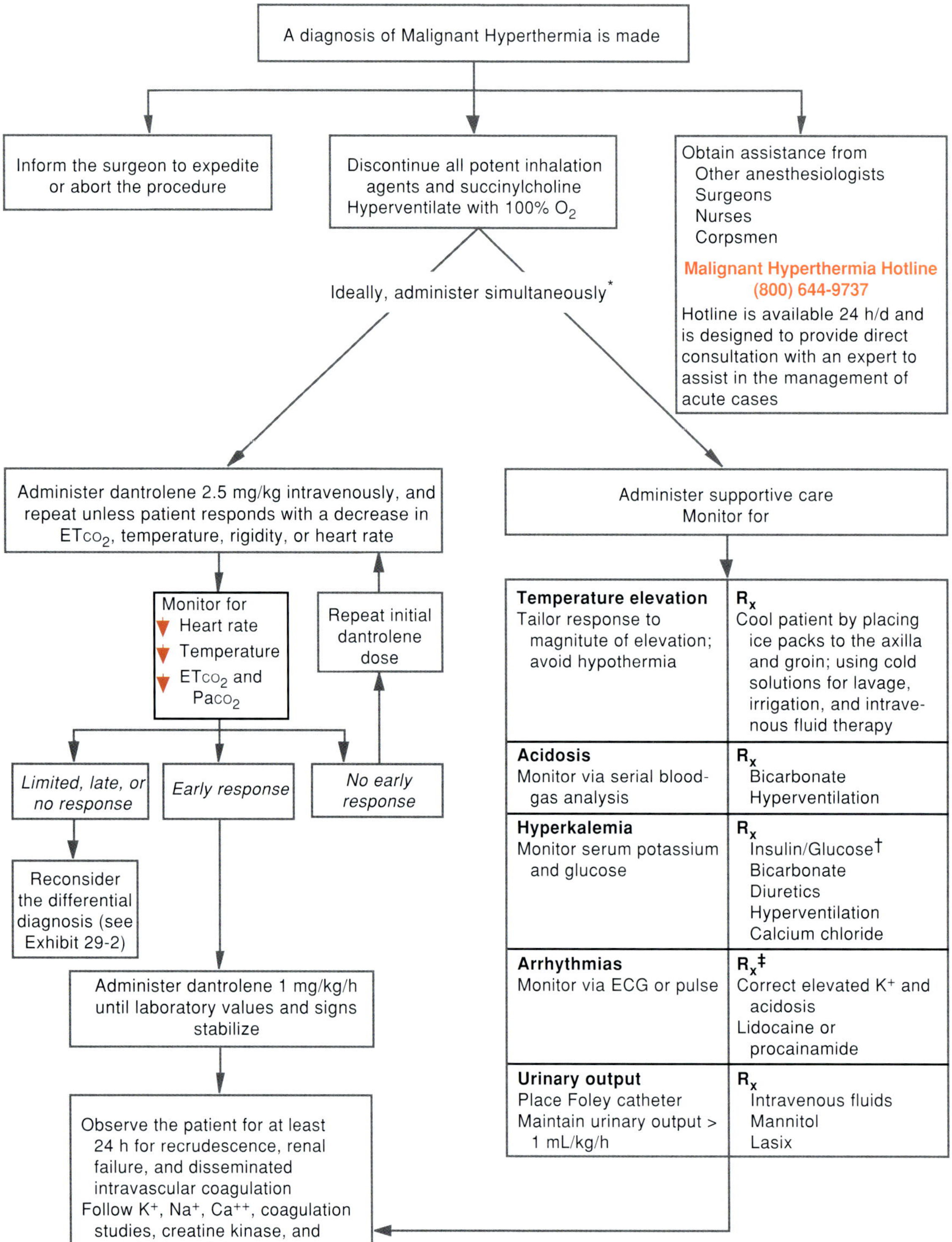

*When resources are limited, administer dantrolene first; otherwise, administer simultaneously with supportive care

†10 units regular insulin in 1,000 mL 10% dextrose in water

‡If arrhythmias persist or are life threatening, continue to correct hyperkalemia and acidosis, and administer lidocaine 1 to 2 mg/kg or procainamide 2–3 mg/kg intravenously as needed. Avoid calcium channel–blocking agents

Fig 29-1. Management of a patient with fulminant malignant hyperthermia. The Malignant Hyperthermia Hotline should be contacted as soon as possible after the working diagnosis is made.

idly and with the recommended priority (Figure 29-1). If another anesthesia provider is unavailable, an operating room nurse or technician or a surgeon can assist.

Potent inhalational agents and succinylcholine infusions must be stopped and the patient hyperventilated with 100% oxygen at high rates of flow. These two actions will limit the patient's exposure to the triggering agents and enhance the elimination of the inhaled agents. Switching to a clean anesthesia machine will further enhance the elimination of inhaled agents; however, this task is usually difficult, time-consuming, and unnecessary. In less severe cases, or in brief exposures, these two actions may be adequate to stop the syndrome. In severe cases, even vigorous manual ventilation cannot return carbon dioxide levels to normal. Even if the syndrome is halted with supportive care alone, the administration of dantrolene is still recommended because resources for observation in an intensive care unit may be extremely limited.

Dantrolene Therapy

Intravenous administration of dantrolene (2.5 mg/kg) is recommended, as dantrolene not only reverses the episode but also decreases the postoperative complications. Myocardial depression or severe rigidity can lead to inadequate muscle perfusion and therefore limit the delivery of the drug to its site of action.[27] If the patient does not respond to the first bolus, additional doses should be administered until decreased carbon dioxide, temperature, rigidity, and heart rate have been achieved. Once the acute episode is controlled, dantrolene should be continued at 1 to 2 mg/kg/h for a minimum of 2 hours, or until the clinical and laboratory signs have returned to baseline (with the exception of creatine kinase and myoglobin).

Dantrolene is supplied in a lyophilized form and has a shelf life of 3 years. It is reconstituted with sterile water (50 mL for each 20-mg vial) due to its high osmotic content. Dantrolene is almost insoluble in water, but the manufacturer's addition of mannitol (3 g) and sodium hydroxide to each vial has rendered the drug soluble and therefore preparation time has been reduced to 2 to 3 minutes. The pH of the reconstituted solution is 9.5; therefore, dantrolene should be administered in a large vein to decrease the risks of thrombophlebitis and tissue necrosis from extravasation.

Dantrolene is the most effective treatment for both arrhythmias and elevated temperatures because it reverses the abnormal metabolic state. Arrhythmias result from the combination of hypoxia, acidosis, hyperkalemia, hypercarbia, and elevated endogenous catecholamines. Lidocaine (1–2 mg/kg) or procainamide (2–3 mg/kg) should be administered as needed for persistent or life-threatening arrhythmias. If control of heart rate is necessary, short-acting β-adrenergic blocking agents should be used instead of calcium channel–blocking agents. (Hyperkalemic cardiovascular collapse has been reported with the combination of dantrolene and calcium channel–blocking agents.[28,29])

Recrudescence

After an adequate clinical response, tachycardia may return as the patient emerges from the anesthetic. A titration of narcotics or benzodiazepines is useful in this situation. Recrudescence of the syndrome is managed with the same urgency as the original episode. Recrudescence has occurred up to 24 to 30 hours later; therefore, continued monitoring in the postoperative period is advocated.[9] If the patient fails to respond or only partially responds to appropriate therapy, then treatment of malignant hyperthermia should continue but other diagnoses should be considered (Exhibit 29-2). Pheochromocytoma and thyroid storm mimic malignant hyperthermia and can be confused with malignant hyperthermia crises.

EXHIBIT 29-2

DIFFERENTIAL DIAGNOSIS OF MALIGNANT HYPERTHERMIA

Hypoxia
Hypercarbia
Sepsis
Light anesthesia
Thyroid storm
Pheochromocytoma
Drug reaction
Cocaine toxicity
Intracranial trauma
Neuroleptic malignant syndrome
Hypoxic encephalitis
Factitious malignant hyperthermia
Iatrogenic hyperthermia

Therapeutic Cooling

Lowering the patient's temperature reduces oxygen consumption and prevents brain injury. Core cooling, which is more effective than surface cooling, is accomplished by using refrigerated solutions for gastric and rectal lavage, wound irrigation, and intravenous infusion. Surface cooling is more effective when ice packs are placed in the groin and axilla. Drastic cooling of the room or placing the patient in an ice bath may actually be counterproductive, as they will induce shivering and vasoconstriction. Once the patient's temperature is controlled, continued monitoring is necessary to detect hypothermia or recrudescence of the syndrome.

Acid–Base Disturbances

Serial measurements of arterial blood gases are essential for assessing and correcting the metabolic and respiratory acidoses as well as in evaluating the effectiveness of therapy. Overaggressive bicarbonate therapy risks severe alkalosis and requires additional ventilation to eliminate the excess carbon dioxide produced. During rapid ventilation, a stable plateau phase may be impossible to obtain on the capnogram. Therefore, blood-gas analysis is necessary to validate the accuracy and trend of the capnograph. Finally, arterial blood-gas analyses can be used to determine oxygen consumption if cardiac output and mixed venous oxygen are known.

Hyperkalemia

The most life-threatening serum abnormality is hyperkalemia. It results from leakage out of damaged muscle cells and from acidosis when a hydrogen ion is exchanged for a potassium ion. This abnormality should be corrected with glucose, insulin, and bicarbonate therapy. Hypokalemia can follow the initial hyperkalemia; therefore, frequent measurements of serum potassium and glucose are required. Currently, calcium therapy is reserved for life-threatening arrhythmias or inotropic support, as it may increase intracellular calcium levels through calcium-induced calcium release. Hypocalcemia, which is common and detected on the electroencephalogram as a prolongation of the QT interval, is refractory to calcium therapy. Changes in phosphate, sodium, and chloride may also occur and usually correct with control of the syndrome.

Late Complications

Late complications include renal failure, disseminated intravascular coagulation, and neurological deficits. Reversal of these complications is difficult and frequently not possible; therefore, early diagnosis and treatment are essential to limit or prevent damage. Renal protection is achieved by maintaining urinary output at 1 to 2 mL/kg/h and should continue until urinary myoglobin has cleared and creatine kinase levels have peaked. Central venous pressure monitoring can be helpful in guiding this therapy. Creatine kinase and urinary myoglobin elevations usually peak 12 to 24 hours after the event, and should be followed every 8 hours until they approach baseline. They reflect the destruction of skeletal muscle and leakage of enzymes from intact skeletal muscle cells, possibly due to increased intracellular osmotic pressure.[30] Continued elevation of these parameters can indicate a partially treated case or recrudescence of the syndrome. Disseminated intravascular coagulation results from hemolysis, released tissue thromboplastin, and hypoperfused tissue. Serial laboratory evaluation of prothrombin time, partial thromboplastin time, fibrinogen, and fibrin split products will help to identify this complication before clinical signs appear. Treatment of disseminated intravascular coagulation in malignant hyperthermia is managed as it is from any other source. Neurological complications include delayed awakening (possibly due to cerebral edema) and permanent neurological deficit secondary to hypoxia or hypotension.

Masseter Muscle Rigidity

When an anesthetized patient is found to have masseter muscle rigidity, the anesthesia provider has three treatment options:

1. Cancel the operation.
2. Continue the operation but convert to a nontriggering anesthesia technique.
3. Continue the operation as planned.

The differential diagnosis of a "stiff jaw" must also be considered and ruled out (Exhibit 29-3). The status of the patient, the estimated length of the surgery, the resources available to initiate and sustain treatment of a fulminant episode, and the anesthesia provider's own familiarity with the treatment of malignant hyperthermia must all be considered. The conservative approach, option 1, is to stop the anesthetic, observe for signs of ma-

EXHIBIT 29-3

DIFFERENTIAL DIAGNOSIS OF MASSETER MUSCLE RIGIDITY

Inadequate skeletal muscle relaxation
Temporomandibular joint disease
Myotonia congenita
Abnormal physiological response to succinylcholine

lignant hyperthermia and renal dysfunction, identify the patient as susceptible to malignant hyperthermia, and return to the operating room another day with a nontriggering anesthetic.[1,3] This approach is supported by the facts that (*a*) morbidity and mortality continue to be associated with malignant hyperthermia and (*b*) the anesthesia provider cannot predict the severity or progression of the syndrome once masseter muscle rigidity is identified. Discontinuing the anesthetic is the safest approach in the face of limited resources, but will not be possible when the surgery is life or limb saving. When surgery must be performed, convert to a nontriggering technique, administer dantrolene 2.5 mg/kg, maintain adequate urinary output, and proceed with the surgery with heightened vigilance.

In options 2 and 3, surgery is permitted to proceed even when it is not emergent. Clinical malignant hyperthermia only infrequently follows masseter muscle rigidity; therefore, the argument can be made that the operation can continue as long as the anesthesia provider is equipped to monitor for malignant hyperthermia and to treat it if the syndrome occurs. Supporters of option 2 believe that masseter muscle rigidity is part of the spectrum of malignant hyperthermia; therefore, they convert to a nontriggering technique to prevent further exposure.[2] The patient is (*a*) identified as susceptible to malignant hyperthermia and (*b*) administered only nontriggering anesthetics for future surgeries. Supporters of option 3 do not believe that masseter muscle rigidity is part of the spectrum of malignant hyperthermia.[10,14] Following this reasoning, triggering agents are continued.

All three options have limited support in the literature, but more information is needed to determine the true relationship of masseter muscle rigidity and malignant hyperthermia. Until this question is answered adequately, the conservative options, 1 and 2, appear better suited for the treatment of masseter muscle rigidity.

A History of Malignant Hyperthermia

Soldiers who are susceptible to malignant hyperthermia are not eligible for combat duty. Despite this policy, however, the situation will undoubtedly arise in which a wounded soldier reports with a questionable or even a documented history of malignant hyperthermia. In combat, there will be no practical means to document a questionable history; therefore, the management of such a casualty will not differ from that of a soldier with a documented history. Whenever possible, the casualty should be evacuated to a combat support hospital, where equipment and personnel are less limited. If evacuation is not possible, a safe anesthetic can be administered with additional preparation. The anesthetic technique will depend on both the casualty's condition and the proposed procedure, and may involve monitored care, regional anesthesia, or a nontriggering general anesthetic technique. Whichever technique is chosen, the anesthetic machine must be prepared, dantrolene must be on hand, and extra personnel should be alerted in anticipation of any signs of malignant hyperthermia. The rubber parts of the field machine will retain potent inhalational anesthetics and therefore must be replaced with new or disposable parts, and flushed clear with a high fresh gas flow.[31] The vaporizer should be drained or removed.

When time is limited, an alternative to the field anesthesia machine is a clean Mapleson system with an oxygen source. If possible, use either the operating room with the best ventilation system or the one in which the lowest level of potent inhalational agents was used that day. If the operating rooms are designed to accommodate two separate anesthetizing locations in the same room, arrangements should be made so that a triggering anesthetic is not being administered at the second location. End-tidal carbon dioxide monitoring should be used whenever possible. Because nitrous oxide will probably not be available, nontriggering techniques that do not rely on this agent must be employed. Intravenous techniques include infusions of pentothal, ketamine, narcotics, or propofol; titrated combinations of benzodiazepines; ketamine and narcotics; or neuroleptic anesthesia. An extended observation period (4–6 h) is required, and the recovery personnel must be educated in the signs of malignant hyperthermia. Although most Malignant Hyperthermia Hotline consultants no longer believe that pretreatment with dantrolene (2.4 mg/kg, administered intravenously) is required, the decision to pretreat with dantrolene is left to the individual anesthesia provider and circumstance. While preoperative administration of dantrolene will provide a measure of reassurance to the clinician in an emergent situation or when the certainty of a clean environment is questionable, it may deplete a limited supply of the drug or cause postoperative weakness in the patient. Oral dantrolene premedication has no place in this setting. If dantrolene is administered, a Foley catheter is required because the mannitol in the intravenous formulation has a diuretic effect.

EPIDEMIOLOGICAL AND GENETIC FACTORS

Incidence

The prevalence of the malignant hyperthermia gene and the incidence of the syndrome remain unknown in the general population. Determinations of prevalence and incidence are complicated by the following factors:

- The human genetic defect or defects responsible for the malignant hyperthermia syndrome remain elusive.
- The presentation of the clinical syndrome is variable.
- Greater awareness of the disease has resulted in treatment of suspicious episodes before true diagnosis-confirming signs develop.
- A simple and accurate screening test is lacking.

In light of these difficulties, the incidence of malignant hyperthermia is estimated to be in the range of 1:4,200 to 1:250,000 anesthetics, depending on the patient population and criteria used in the analysis.[7,32,33] It is impossible to predict (*a*) whether an episode of malignant hyperthermia will occur in the operating room during the next armed conflict or (*b*) if an individual soldier is susceptible to malignant hyperthermia. No acute episodes of malignant hyperthermia were reported during Operation Desert Storm. However, seven soldiers were identified as susceptible (via their family histories) and removed from the combat area for further evaluation. Susceptible soldiers probably will be deployed during future conflicts, but their number is likely to be small.

Although at this time it is impossible to influence the incidence of malignant hyperthermia in the military, proper planning and vigilance will limit the morbidity and mortality of this disease. Fatal outcomes continue to decline. Since 1970, mortality has fallen from 70% to 2% to 3%; this decline is a direct result of both widespread education of anesthetists concerning malignant hyperthermia and the availability of dantrolene therapy.[4,7]

Genetics

An autosomal dominant pattern of inheritance was suggested in the first reported case of malignant hyperthermia.[34] Features of this mode of inheritance are that it (*a*) appears in every generation, (*b*) is transmitted to approximately one half the offspring of affected family members, (*c*) does not appear in the offspring of unaffected family members, and (*d*) is not influenced by the gender of the affected family member for transmission. However, as more families were investigated, the autosomal dominant pattern was not always evident. In 1982, the families of 93 malignant hyperthermia–susceptible patients were reviewed to determine their mode of inheritance.[35] Only 52% of the families were identified as clearly or possibly autosomal dominant (Table 29-3). The concept of multiple gene defects as an explanation for the apparent heterogeneity of the syndrome has several supporters.[35–37] The inheritance of malignant hyperthermia will remain incompletely understood until the genetic defect or defects that give rise to malignant hyperthermia are identified.

TABLE 29-3

INHERITANCE PATTERN OF 93 FAMILIES WITH MALIGNANT HYPERTHERMIA

Genetic Pattern	Present in Families (%)
Clearly autosomal dominant	38
Possibly autosomal dominant	14
Associated with dominant myopathies	3
Isolated	17
Questionable recessive (isolated)	21
Insufficient information	7

Adapted with permission from McPherson EW, Taylor CA. The genetics of malignant hyperthermia: Evidence for heterogeneity. *Am J Med Genetics*. 1982;11:277.

PATHOPHYSIOLOGY

The clinical presentation of malignant hyperthermia is the result of abnormal calcium regulation in skeletal muscle following exposure to triggering anesthetic agents. Original theories postulating a central nervous system origin for malignant hyperthermia could not explain why the syndrome was initiated in a caudal animal preparation or following total spinal blockade.[5,38] The sympathetic nervous system was ruled out as the initiating site for malignant hyperthermia when researchers studying swine found that metabolic changes preceded increases in sympathetic tone and temperature.[39] Data from the same study also showed that uncoupling of oxidative phosphorylation could not explain the heat production during a malignant hyperthermia episode. A distinctive myopathic defect is unlikely in malignant hyperthermia. Skeletal muscle from susceptible individuals usually exhibits no characteristic histological defect; however, variable nonspecific changes are seen. Conclusive evidence supporting skeletal muscle as the functional site of the defect has been found in both the swine model and in human data.[40,41] These data include

1. the observation that during a fulminant episode, a patient experienced total-body rigidity, with the exception of the one extremity that was protected by a tourniquet;
2. the development of in vitro contractures to halothane in biopsied muscle samples from susceptible patients; and
3. elevated levels of creatine kinase and myoglobinemia following fulminant episodes.

The Excitation–Contraction Coupling Pathway

A brief review of the excitation–contraction coupling pathway will provide a framework to understand the current theories in the pathogenesis of malignant hyperthermia (Figure 29-2). Although normal excitation–contraction coupling is not completely understood, skeletal muscle contractions start with an action potential at the neuromuscular junction that rapidly spreads over the sarcolemma and into the transverse tubule (T) system (invagination of the sarcolemma).[42] This electrical signal results in the rapid release of calcium from the terminal cisternae of the sarcoplasmic reticulum. It is yet to be discovered how the signal traverses from the T system to the sarcoplasmic reticulum, but a calcium-release channel that forms a bridge between the two structures has been identified.[43] This channel is now known as the ryanodine receptor. Ryanodine, an alkaloid insecticide, binds to the channel with high affinity and specificity and causes skeletal muscle contraction. During normal skeletal muscle contraction and relaxation, the calcium-release channel will close shortly after activation. The myoplasmic calcium concentration reaches a plateau and therefore facilitates relaxation by allowing calcium uptake to exceed calcium release. Skeletal muscle relaxation is accomplished by the return of calcium to the sarcoplasmic reticulum. Calcium uptake into the sarcoplasmic reticulum is an active process performed by a calcium pump, the major portion of which is a 100-Kd (kilodalton) protein.

Early investigations noted that skeletal muscle from susceptible individuals developed contractures at lower caffeine concentrations than normal muscle.[44] This focused investigators' attention on the sarcoplasmic reticulum, because caffeine produces contractures in skeletal muscle at that site.[45] However, biochemical studies failed to reveal either the specific defect in sarcoplasmic reticulum or a site where anesthetic agents would increase the release of calcium. Because calcium regulation is the primary function of the sarcoplasmic reticulum in skeletal muscle, calcium regulation in the excitation–contraction coupling pathway was also investigated.

The identification of dantrolene's pharmacological site of action supported this approach, because its site of action is thought to be somewhere between the transverse tubule and the sarcoplasmic reticulum.[27] Direct evidence of defective intracellular calcium regulation was provided by two separate methods of measuring myoplasmic calcium concentrations. In one study[46] utilizing fura-2 (an intracellular calcium-selective dye), elevations in myoplasmic calcium were found to correlate with the force of in vitro contracture in susceptible swine muscle induced by halothane or caffeine. In the other study,[47] calcium-selective microelectrodes detected myoplasmic calcium concentrations that increased when the malignant hyperthermia syndrome was triggered in swine, and reversed following the administration of dantrolene. Prolonged elevation of myoplasmic calcium (*a*) produces muscle contracture and a sustained contraction and (*b*) appears to be the source of the metabolic disturbances during a malignant hyperthermia episode.

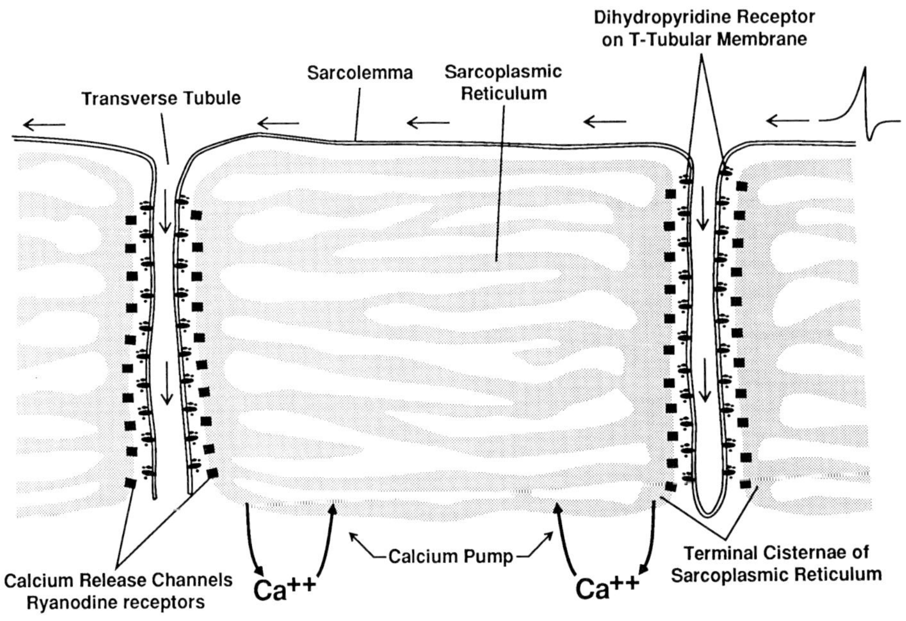

Fig. 29-2. This skeletal muscle transverse tubule–sarcoplasmic reticulum system illustrates the cellular components involved in excitation-contraction coupling. An action potential begins at the top right corner of the figure and traverses the sarcolemma and transverse tubules, as the arrows depict. This electrical activity is transformed into the release of calcium from the terminal cisternae of the sarcoplasmic reticulum. Although the exact mechanism is unclear, the dihydropyridine receptor on the T-tubular membrane and the nearby calcium-release channels and ryanodine receptors on the terminal cisternae appear to have major roles. During normal excitation–contracting coupling, calcium is released from the terminal cisternae through the open calcium-release channels. This increases the myoplasmic calcium concentration and initiates contraction. Closure of the calcium-release channels and uptake of the myoplasmic calcium by the calcium pumps have the net effect of decreasing the myoplasmic calcium concentration, thus limiting contraction. In malignant hyperthermia, calcium hemostasis is abnormal, as evidenced by elevated myoplasmic calcium concentrations. The elevated myoplasmic calcium concentrations may be the result of an abnormality of the dihydropyrimidine receptor, ryanodine receptor, or some modulator of these receptors. Adapted with permission from Muldoon SM, Karan SM. Hyperthermia and hypothermia. In: Rogers MC, Tinker JH, Covino BG, Longnecker DE, eds. *Principles and Practice of Anesthesiology*. St Louis, Mo: Mosby–Year Book; 1993: 2504.

Either alone or in combination, exaggerated calcium release or depressed calcium uptake can produce an elevation of the myoplasmic calcium concentration.

Because calcium uptake appears to be unaffected in susceptible muscle, recent investigation is focused on identifying defects in calcium release or regulation. This approach is supported by the facts that (1) dantrolene has no effect on calcium uptake in the sarcoplasmic reticulum and (2) dantrolene also reduces calcium release in the sarcoplasmic reticulum.[28] A mechanism for abnormal calcium release was first described in 1981, when a researcher postulated that calcium-induced calcium release was responsible for the abnormal contractures induced by caffeine or halothane in biopsied skeletal muscle from malignant hyperthermia–susceptible patients.[48] (The term calcium-induced calcium release describes the observation that skeletal muscle sarcoplasmic reticulum will release calcium when calcium is applied to its cytoplasmic surface.) Calcium-induced calcium release is activated by calcium, halothane, and caffeine, and is inhibited by high magnesium, calmodulin, tetracaine, and ruthenium red[49,50]; it is also associated with the sarcoplasmic reticulum terminal cisternae, site of the ryanodine receptor, and may be activated or inhibited by ryanodine.[51] Abnormal calcium-induced calcium release has also been reported in the swine model. While one researcher[52] reports that susceptible swine have a lower calcium threshold to initiate calcium-induced calcium release, others[53] report that susceptible swine have a higher rate of calcium-induced calcium release. To date, biochemical evidence of a ryanodine receptor abnormality exists only in swine.[54] Other investigators suggest that the calcium-release channel is normal but the structures that modulate its function are abnormal.[55,56] Alternative theories to a defect in the ryanodine receptor include the dihydropyridine receptor,[55] hormone-sensitive lipase,[56] phospholipase A_2,[57] and inositol 1,4,5,-triphosphate phosphatase[58] deficiency. In light of the broad spectrum of clinical presentation of malignant hyperthermia, more than one defect will probably be identified with the malignant hyperthermia syndrome. Advances in genetic analysis may provide some answers for this complex disease.

Defect Linked to Chromosome 19

The first major genetic breakthrough was the linkage of a possible malignant hyperthermia defect to chromosome 19q12-13.2 by two independent laboratories (Figure 29-3).[59,60] Linkage is said to occur when two distinct genes on the same chromosome tend to be inherited together. The likelihood of linkage is increased as the distance between the genes is decreased. The *lod* score (logarithm of the odds) quantifies the likelihood of linkage. Linkage is considered proven when the lod score is 3 (1,000:1 in favor of linkage) and ruled out when the lod score is –2. With the knowledge that porcine malignant hyperthermia is genetically linked to the glucose phosphate isomerase (GPI) locus, a team of researchers examined three extended Irish families who expressed malignant hyperthermia susceptibility as an autosomal dominant trait for linkage to the human GPI locus.[59] Human GPI was previously mapped to chromosome 19q12-13.2, an area with several well-defined polymorphic loci from which lod scores could be determined. The lod score for linkage between malignant hyperthermia susceptibility and the genetic marker CYP2A was 5.65. The researchers concluded that in both humans and swine, malignant hyperthermia is probably due to mutations in homologous genes, and that the malignant hyperthermia defect in humans is probably located in the CYP2A area. Other research supports this conclusion by demonstrating a linkage (lod score 4.20) between the ryanodine receptor gene and malignant hyperthermia susceptibility in nine families with ryanodine gene polymorphisms (two or more expressions of the same gene).[60] Eleven families in the study did not exhibit polymorphism of the gene; this suggests another genetic site for the malignant hyperthermia defect.

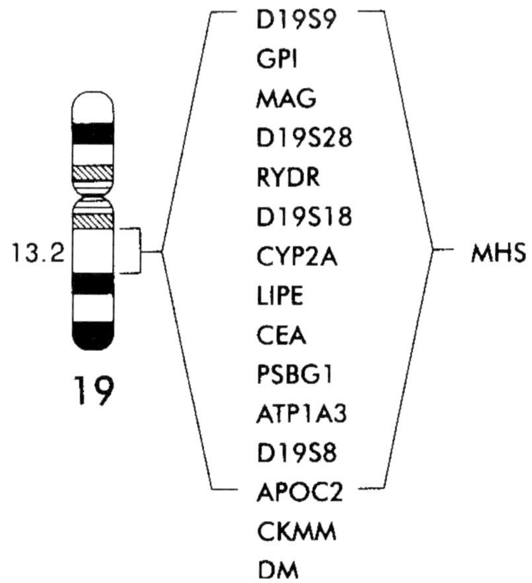

MHS: malignant hyperthermia susceptibility
GPI: glucose phosphate isomerase
MAG: myelin-associated glycoprotein
RYDR: ryanodine receptor
CYP2A: cytochrome P450, subfamily 11A
LIPE: hormone-sensitive lipase
CEA: carcino-embryonic antigen
PSBG1: pregnancy-specific B-1-glycoprotein 1
ATP1A3: ATPase; Na^+, K^+, a3 polypeptide
APOC2: apolipoprotein C-11
CKMM: creatine kinase, skeletal muscle
DM: dystrophia myotonica

Fig. 29-3. Regional localization of gene and DNA-segment markers on chromosome 19. This type of genetic map only gives information as to the sequence of markers on a gene, but gives no information as to the size of the marker or the distance between markers. Using *lod* scores (logarithm of the odds), researchers have linked malignant hyperthermia susceptibility to chromosome 19 between markers D19S9 and APOC2. Genes located within this region are considered to be candidates for the elusive, defective "gene" for malignant hyperthermia. Markers identified with a D and followed by a sequence of numbers and letters have not yet been identified as part of a known gene sequence. Adapted with permission from Levitt RC, McKusick VA, Fletcher JE, Rosenberg H. *Nature*. 1990;345:298. Letter. © Macmillan Magazines Ltd.

Single-Point Mutation of Ryanodine-Receptor Gene

The second breakthrough in the genetics of malignant hyperthermia was reported in 1991. This research identified a single-point mutation of the porcine ryanodine-receptor gene, which results in the substitution of a cysteine for an arginine at position 615 in the ryanodine receptor of susceptible swine.[61] The mutation was present in five of six breeds and was present at the same frequency as porcine stress syndrome for that breed. In the sixth breed, Hampshire, porcine stress syndrome has not been reported.

Using this information, another team of researchers examined 35 families whose members are susceptible to malignant hyperthermia for the corresponding human ryanodine gene mutation.[62] In one family, three members were identified as heterozygous for the substitution. Genetic identification of susceptibility was consistent with the results of prior halothane and caffeine contracture testing. This family was originally identified when the proband exhibited masseter muscle spasm after the administration of succinylcholine. Although the study identifies a common defect in porcine and human malignant hyperthermia, it also indirectly indicates genetic heterogeneity in human malignant hyperthermia.

The most convincing data supporting genetic heterogeneity in human malignant hyperthermia were provided in 1991.[37] In three susceptible families, linkage measurements were calculated for the ryanodine receptor gene, CYP2A, and several other markers in the area of 19q12-13.2. Malignant hyperthermia susceptibility did not cosegregate with any of the previously identified markers or genes. Although linkage for the human lipase gene was not calculated in this report, it can also be eliminated as a candidate gene in these families, because the human lipase gene is flanked on both sides by markers that were tested for linkage. Even though the data do not identify a new site for the malignant hyperthermia defect in these families, they support the evidence for at least one additional genetic locus for the syndrome.

Advances in the pathophysiology of malignant hyperthermia will continue to rely on the application of genetic analysis to families whose susceptibility has been delineated through halothane and caffeine contracture testing. Likewise, animal models will continue to be invaluable in the search for other causes of malignant hyperthermia. If porcine malignant hyperthermia proves to be a homogeneous defect, the model may only apply to a small percentage of humans susceptible to the syndrome. Perhaps other models (canine, equine, goat) will provide new clues to explain the clinical syndrome of human malignant hyperthermia.

EVALUATION OF SUSCEPTIBILITY

No simple screening test or minimally invasive diagnostic test exists to identify patients susceptible to malignant hyperthermia. Although physical examination can identify loosely associated abnormalities that are common in the general population, the syndrome lacks a distinct physical sign to identify susceptible patients. Numerous tests have tried to identify susceptible patients. These include serum creatine kinase, serum cholinesterase levels, chemiluminescence, human leukocyte antigen, platelet nucleotide depletion test, erythrocyte fragility, and the calcium uptake test in muscle. While some of these tests may be useful under restricted conditions, they have not been successful when applied to a larger population of patients. The only tests that reliably identify patients who have exhibited the clinical syndrome are the halothane and caffeine contracture tests.[63] However, these tests require not only a skeletal muscle biopsy, they also require the biopsy to be performed at a malignant hyperthermia diagnostic center because the muscle must remain viable throughout the testing period (tests must be completed within 5 h of the biopsy) and cannot be preserved or frozen. Only 12 medical centers in North America provide diagnostic contracture testing. Tests that show some promise for the future include genetic analysis[64] and phosphorus nuclear magnetic resonance spectroscopy.[64,65] Although further development of these tests is necessary, they provide hope for a simpler and more accurate diagnostic test in the future.

Physical findings that have been associated with malignant hyperthermia include increased muscle bulk, hyperextensible joints, strabismus, and scoliosis. Rare diseases such as Duchenne and Becker type muscular dystrophies, myotonia congenita, central core disease, King-Denborough syndrome, Schwartz-Jampal syndrome and osteogenesis imperfecta have been linked to malignant hyperthermia, but these are highly unlikely to be seen on the battlefield. A history of muscle cramps

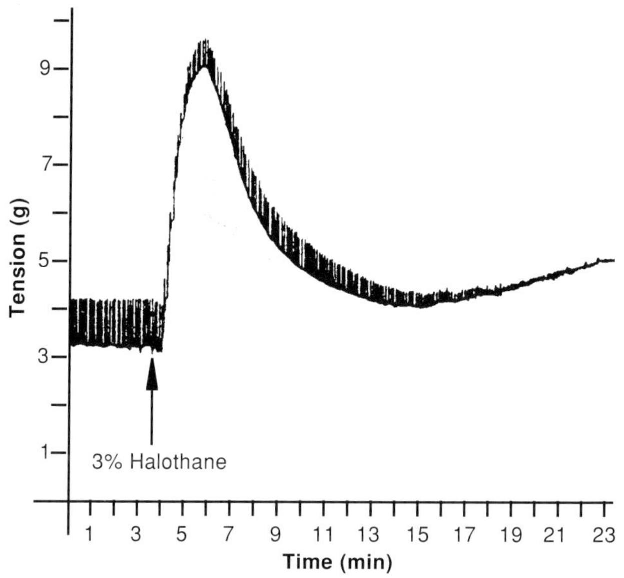

Fig. 29-4. This tracing illustrates an abnormal contracture response of human skeletal muscle to 3% halothane. A strip of muscle (2–3 cm, 100–200 mg) is tied with silk thread at both ends. One end is attached to a hook in the tissue bath, while the other is attached to a strain-gauge transducer. The muscle strip is submerged in Krebs solution and oxygenated via a sintered disk with a mixture of 95% oxygen and 5% carbon dioxide. Transmural electrical stimulation is applied to the muscle strip via platinum electrodes. The muscle is electrically stimulated for a minimum of 15 minutes, or until a stable baseline tension is obtained. A twitch height of greater than 0.5 g tension to the electrical stimulation is considered viable for testing. Halothane is delivered to the tissue bath by adding it to the mixture of oxygen and carbon dioxide. A response is considered positive when baseline tension increases by greater than 0.7 g within 10 minutes of exposure to 3% halothane. A normal skeletal muscle response to halothane is an increase in twitch tension height without an increase in baseline tension. Reprinted with permission from Muldoon SM, Karan SM. Hyperthermia and hypothermia. In: Rogers MC, Tinker JH, Covino BG, Longnecker DE, eds. *Principles and Practice of Anesthesiology*. St Louis, Mo: Mosby–Year Book; 1993: 2508.

or heat intolerance has no predictive value for the occurrence of malignant hyperthermia.

The halothane and caffeine contracture tests are the most widely accepted diagnostic tests for the identification or conformation of malignant hyperthermia susceptibility; however, due to the constraints already discussed, these tests will not be available on (or near) the battlefield. The response of skeletal muscle to halothane is the most specific test for malignant hyperthermia, but it is the least sensitive (Figure 29-4). Caffeine will produce a contracture in any skeletal muscle, but this response will occur at a lower dosage in susceptible individuals. Besides requiring a biopsy from the vastus lateralis muscle (3 cm • 1 cm), these contracture tests have other drawbacks:

- They require a significant amount of technical expertise to perform.
- They are performed at only 12 sites in North America.
- A diagnostic gray zone exists when the muscle responds to halothane or caffeine but not strongly enough to meet the positive requirements. By applying a wide spectrum of susceptibility, these patients are usually identified as positive at the lower end of the spectrum.
- At this time, false-positive results cannot be identified because these patients will not be exposed to triggering agents.
- Although no false-negative results have been reported, few reports exist of patients with negative contracture results and subsequent exposure to triggering agents.[66]

Any soldier who exhibits the clinical syndrome does not need contracture testing prior to future anesthetics, (eg, if further surgery were necessary before the soldier could be discharged from the military). Contracture testing is most useful in confirming suspicious episodes and in helping to identify susceptible family members. Soldiers who have not exhibited the clinical syndrome, but have been informed they may be susceptible, should be evaluated with contracture testing as soon as possible. Malignant hyperthermia diagnostic evaluations can be arranged for armed forces personnel or their dependents by contacting the following address or commercial telephone number:

Uniformed Services University of the Health Sciences
Department of Anesthesiology
Director, Malignant Hyperthermia Diagnostic Center
4301 Jones Bridge Road
Bethesda, Maryland 20814-4799
Telephone: (301) 295-3140

SUMMARY

Malignant hyperthermia is a rare pharmacogenetic disease that can be expressed on exposure to triggering anesthetic agents. No simple, widely applied test exists to screen for susceptible individuals. The hypermetabolic syndrome is identified by increases in carbon dioxide production, lactic acid production, muscle rigidity, and sympathetic tone. Temperature elevation is a late sign. Treatment consists of prompt recognition of the clinical syndrome, removal of the triggering agents, rapid administration of dantrolene, and supportive care. Successful management of malignant hyperthermia is possible, even in austere conditions, when treatment plans are formulated in advance and are tailored to the resources available.

REFERENCES

1. Muldoon SM, Karan SM. Hyperthermia and hypothermia. In: *Principles and Practice of Anesthesiology*. Rogers M, Tinker J, Covino B, Longnecker D, eds. St Louis, Mo: Mosby–Year Book; 1993: 2499–2520.

2. Gronert GA, Schulman SR, Mott J. Malignant hyperthermia. In: Miller R, ed. *Anesthesia*. New York, NY: Churchill, Livingstone; 1990: 935–956.

3. Rosenberg H, Seitman D. Pharmacogenetics. In: Barash PG, Cullen BF, Stoelting RK, eds. *Clinical Anesthesia*. Philadelphia, Pa: JB Lippincott; 1989: 459–472.

4. Ellis FR, Halsall PJ, Christian AS. Clinical presentation of suspected malignant hyperthermia during anaesthesia in 402 probands. *Anaesthesia*. 1990;45:838–841.

5. Gronert GA, Ahern CP, Milde JH. Treatment of porcine malignant hyperthermia: Lactate gradient from muscle to blood. *Can Anaesth Soc J*. 1986;33:729–736.

6. Gronert GA, Theye RA. Halothane-induced porcine malignant hyperthermia: Metabolic and hemodynamic changes. *Anesthesiology*. 1976;44:36–43.

7. Britt BA, Kalow W. Malignant hyperthermia: A statistical review. *Can Anaesth Soc J*. 1970;17:293–315.

8. Harrison GG. Porcine malignant hyperthermia. In: Britt BA, ed. *Int Anesthesiol Clin: Malignant Hyperthermia*. 1978:17:25–61.

9. Mathieu A, Bogosian AJ, Ryan JF. Recrudescence after survival of an initial episode of malignant hyperthermia. *Anesthesiology*. 1979;51:454–455.

10. Littleford JA, Patel LR, Bose D. Masseter muscle spasm in children: Implications of continuing the triggering anesthetic. *Anesth Analg*. 1991;72:151–160.

11. Delphin E, Jackson D, Rothstein P. Use of succinylcholine during elective pediatric anesthesia should be reevaluated. *Anesth Analg*. 1987;66:1190–1192.

12. Rosenberg H, Shutack JG. Masseter muscle spasm in children. *Anesth Analg*. 1991;73:361–362. Letter.

13. Patel LR, Littleford JA. Masseter muscle spasm in children. *Anesth Analg*. 1991;73:362–363. Reply to letter.

14. van der Spek AF. Triggering agents continued after masseter spasm: There is proof in this pudding! *Anesth Analg*. 1991;73:364–365.

15. Carroll JB. Increased incidence of masseter spasm in children with strabismus anesthetized with halothane and succinylcholine. *Anesthesiology*. 1987;67:559–561.

16. Schwartz L, Rockoff MA, Koka BV. Masseter spasm with anesthesia: Incidence and implications. *Anesthesiology*. 1984;61:772–775.

17. Ellis FR, Hallsall PJ. Suxamethonium spasm: A differential diagnostic conundrum. *Br J Anaesth*. 1984;56:381–384.

18. Rosenberg H, Fletcher JE. Masseter muscle rigidity and malignant hyperthermia susceptibility. *Anesth Analg*. 1986;65:161–164.

19. Allen GC, Rosenberg H. Malignant hyperthermia susceptibility in adult patients with masseter muscle rigidity. *Can J Anaesth*. 1990;37:31–35.

20. van der Spek AF, Fang WB, Ashton-Miller JA. The effects of succinylcholine in mouth opening. *Anesthesiology*. 1987;67:459–465.

21. van der Spek AF, Fang WB, Ashton-Miller JA. Increased masticatory muscle stiffness during limb muscle flaccidity associated with succinylcholine administration. *Anesthesiology*. 1988;69:11–16.

22. Britt BA. Combined anesthetic- and stress-induced malignant hyperthermia in two offspring of malignant hyperthermic–susceptible parents. *Anesth Analg*. 1988;67:393–399.

23. Gronert GA, Thompson RL, Onofrio BM. Human malignant hyperthermia: Awake episodes and correction by dantrolene. *Anesth Analg*. 1980;59:377–378.

24. Grinberg R, Edelist G, Gordon A. Postoperative malignant hyperthermia episodes in patients who received "safe" anaesthetics. *Can Anaesth Soc J*. 1983;30:273–276.

25. Wingard DW. Malignant hyperthermia—acute stress syndrome of man? In: Henschel EO, ed. *Malignant Hyperthermia: Current Concepts*. East Norwalk, Conn: Appleton-Century-Crofts; 1977: Chap 6: 79–95.

26. Condon BC, Temo JM, Crowl FD, et al. Anesthesia guidelines. In: Bellamy RF, ed. *Combat Casualty Care Guidelines: Operation Desert Storm*. Washington, DC: US Department of the Army, Office of The Surgeon General, and Borden Institute; 1991: 21–40.

27. Harrison GG. Dantrolene—dynamics and kinetics. *Br J Anaesth*. 1988;60:279–286.

28. Rubin AS, Zablocki AD. Hyperkalemia, verapamil, and dantrolene. *Anesthesiology*. 1987;66:246–249.

29. Saltzman LS, Kates RA, Corke BC. Hyperkalemia and cardiovascular collapse after verapamil and dantrolene administration in swine. *Anesth Analg*. 1984;63:473–478.

30. Wasserman K, Hansen JE, Sue DY. Facilitation of oxygen consumption by lactic acidosis during exercise. *NIPS*. 1991;6:29–34.

31. Beebe JJ, Sessler DI. Preparation of anesthesia machines for patients susceptible to malignant hyperthermia. *Anesthesiology*. 1988;69:395–400.

32. Ording H. Incidence of malignant hyperthermia in Denmark. *Anesth Analg*. 1985;64:700–704.

33. Ellis FR, Halsall PJ. Malignant hyperpyrexia. *Br J Hosp Med*. 1980;24:318–327.

34. Denborough MA, Lovell RH. Anesthesia deaths in a family. *Lancet*. 1960;2:45.

35. McPherson EW, Taylor CA. The genetics of malignant hyperthermia: evidence for heterogeneity. *Am J Med Genet*. 1982;11:273–285.

36. Nelson TE, Flewellen EH, Gloyna DF. Spectrum of susceptibility to malignant hyperthermia—diagnostic dilemma. *Anesth Analg*. 1983;62:545–552.

37. Levitt RC, Nouri N, Jedlicka AE. Evidence for genetic heterogeneity in malignant hyperthermia susceptibility. *Genomics*. 1991;11:543–547.

38. Gronert GA, Milde JH, Theye RA. Role of sympathetic activity in porcine malignant hyperthermia. *Anesthesiology*. 1977;47:411–415.

39. Berman MC, Harrison HH, Bull AB. Changes underlining halothane-induced malignant hyperpyrexia in Landrace pigs. *Nature*. 1970;225:653–655.

40. Ellis FR, Harriman DG, Keaney NP. Halothane-induced muscle contracture as a cause of hyperpyrexia. *Br J Anaesth*. 1971;43:721–722.

41. Satnick JH. Hyperthermia under anesthesia with regional muscle flaccidity. *Anesthesiology*. 1969;30:472–474.

42. Endo M. Calcium release from the sarcoplasmic reticulum. *Physiol Rev*. 1977;57:71–108.

43. Lai FA, Meissner G. The muscle ryanodine receptor and its intrinsic Ca^{2+} channel activity. *J Bioenerg Biomembr*. 1989;21:227–246.

44. Kalow W, Britt BA, Terreau ME. Metabolic error of muscle metabolism after recovery from malignant hyperthermia. *Lancet*. 1970;2:895–898.

45. Weber A. The mechanism of action of caffeine on sarcoplasmic reticulum. *J Gen Physiol*. 1968;52:760–772.

46. Iaizzo PA, Klein W, Lehmann-Horne F. Fura-2 detected myoplasmic calcium and its correlation with contracture force in skeletal muscle from normal and malignant hyperthermia susceptible pigs. *Pflugers Arch*. 1988;411:648–653.

47. Lopez JR, Alamo L, Jones DE. Ca^{2+} in muscles of malignant hyperthermia susceptible pigs determined in vivo with Ca^{2+} selective microelectrodes. *Muscle Nerve*. 1986;9:85–86.

48. Endo M. Mechanism of calcium-induced calcium release in the SR membrane. In: Ohnishi ST, Endo M, eds. *The Mechanism of Gated Calcium Transport Across Biological Membranes*. New York, NY: Academia Press; 1981: 257–264.

49. Ohnishi ST. Calcium-induced calcium release from fragmented sarcoplasmic reticulum. *J Biochem*. 1979;86:1147–1150.

50. Nelson TE. Effect of calmodulin on calcium pulse-induced calcium release from fragmented skeletal sarcoplasmic reticulum. *Fed Proc*. 1984;43:498.

51. Meissner G. Ryanodine activation and inhibition of the Ca^{2+} release channel of sarcoplasmic reticulum. *J Biol Chem*. 1986;261:6300–6306.

52. Nelson TE, Sweo T. Ca^{2+} uptake and Ca^{2+} release by skeletal muscle sarcoplasmic reticulum: Differing sensitivity to inhalational anesthetics. *Anesthesiology*. 1988;69:571–577.

53. Ohta T, Endo M. Ca-induced Ca-release in malignant hyperthermia susceptible pig skeletal muscle. *Am J Physiol*. 1989;256:C358–367.

54. Mickelson JR, Gallant EM, Litterer LA. Abnormal sarcoplasmic reticulum receptor in malignant hyperthermia. *J Biol Chem*. 1988;263:9310–9315.

55. Ervasti JM, Mickelson JM, Louis CF. Transverse tubule calcium regulation in malignant hyperthermia. *Arch Biochem Biophys*. 1989;269:497–506.

56. Levitt RC, McKusick VA, Fletcher JE. Gene candidate. *Nature*. 1990;345:297–298. Letter.

57. Cheah KS, Cheah AM. Skeletal muscle mitochondrial phospholipase A_2 and the interaction of mitochondria and sarcoplasmic reticulum in porcine malignant hyperthermia. *Biochim Biophysica Acta*. 1981;638:40–49.

58. Foster PS, Gesini E, Claudianos C. Inositol 1,4,5,-triphosphate phosphatase deficiency and malignant hyperpyrexia in swine. *Lancet*. 1989;2:124–127.

59. McCarthy TV, Healy JM, Heffron JJ. Localization of the malignant hyperthermia susceptibility locus to human chromosome 19q12-13.2. *Nature*. 1990;343:562–564.

60. MacLennan DH, Duff C, Zorzato F. Ryanodine receptor gene is a candidate for predisposition to malignant hyperthermia. *Nature*. 1990;343:559–561.

61. Fujii J, Otsu K, Zorzato F. Identification of a mutation in porcine ryanodine receptor associated with malignant hyperthermia. *Science*. 1991;253:448–451.

62. Gillard EF, Otsu K, Fujii J. A substitution of cysteine for arginine 614 in the ryanodine receptor is potentially causative of human malignant hyperthermia. *Genomics*. 1991;11:751–755.

63. Larch MG, and the North American Malignant Hyperthermia Group. Standardization of the caffeine halothane muscle contracture test. *Anesth Analg*. 1989;69:511–515.

64. Olgin J, Rosenberg H, Allen G. A blinded comparison of noninvasive, in vivo phosphorus nuclear magnetic resonance spectroscopy and the in vitro halothane/caffeine contracture test in the evaluation of malignant hyperthermia susceptibility. *Anesth Analg*. 1991;72:36–47.

65. Olgin J, Zohar A, Rosenberg H. Non-invasive evaluations of malignant hyperthermia susceptibility with phosphorous nuclear magnetic resonance spectroscopy. *Anesthesiology*. 1988;68:507–513.

66. Allen GC, Rosenberg H, Fletcher JE. Safety of general anesthesia in patients previously tested negative for malignant hyperthermia susceptibility. *Anesthesiology*. 1990;72:619–622.

Chapter 30

ANESTHESIA FOR CASUALTIES OF CHEMICAL WARFARE AGENTS

DAVID J. BAKER, M. PHIL., D.M., FFARCS*; AND J. M. RUSTICK, M.D.†

*Department of Clinical Neurological Sciences, University of Southampton, United Kingdom
†Director of Military Medical Research, Public Safety Group, 12608-B Lakeridge Drive, Woodbridge, Virginia 22192

INTRODUCTION

Chemical agents (ie, substances intended for use in military operations to kill, seriously injure, or otherwise incapacitate through pathophysiological effects[1,2]) were first used on a wide scale in modern times during World War I. Although in recent years the demise of the Warsaw Pact has markedly lessened the threat of a major war fought with unconventional weapons, the same cannot be said for what may happen in the Third World. In fact, there is evidence that chemical agents have been used in at least seven military actions since 1965 (Exhibit 30-1). While the list of chemical warfare agents most likely to proliferate is not especially long (Exhibit 30-2), there is nothing to say that a country seeking to develop a surreptitious chemical warfare capability may not use a nontraditional agent as a weapon. Even traditional agents may be used in a nontraditional manner. An excellent example of this is Iraq's use of the *mixture* of GB (sarin) and GF (this agent does not have a common name), which together pose a threat via both the respiratory and the transdermal routes of exposure. As treaties banning the use of chemical warfare agents become more numerous, the more likely we are to encounter the unexpected.

The trauma anesthesia provider is usually concerned with the management of casualties injured by physical forces such as blunt and penetrating injury and blast.[3] The American College of Surgeons' standard Advanced Trauma Life Support (ATLS) teaching[4] is geared to rapid assessment and management of such casualties of conventional warfare. The concept of injury from chemical agents, however, extends the notion of trauma into a new and often more difficult area, where the injury may not always be immediately obvious and may also still be developing during the period of initial assessment. Since the risk of injury from chemical agents in warfare has not diminished in recent years, the military anesthesia provider must always be prepared for the possibility that casualties might suffer from chemical as well as from physical trauma. To a certain extent, the existence of thermal injury in warfare, an injury so very different from the much more common ballistic trauma that has historically dominated warfare, serves to remind us of the need to be prepared to treat unusual injuries. The absence of chemical casualties in World War II and subsequent actions where North Atlantic Treaty

EXHIBIT 30-1

ALLEGED USES OF CHEMICAL WARFARE AGENTS IN THIRD-WORLD COUNTRIES BEFORE THE PERSIAN GULF WAR

Egypt in South Yemen in 1963–1968

Vietnam in Laos, 1975–1978

Ethiopia against Eritrean and Somalia-backed rebels, 1976– ?

Vietnam in Cambodia, 1978– ?

China and Vietnam, 1979

Iraq against Iran, 1984–1988

Iraq against the Kurds, 1988

EXHIBIT 30-2

CHEMICAL AGENTS MOST LIKELY TO BE PROLIFERATED

Nerve Agents
- GA: Tabun
- GB: Sarin
- GF: (no common name)
- GB/GF Mixture

Vesicant Agents
- HD: Sulfur mustard

Choking Agents
- CG: Phosgene

Blood Agents
- AC: Hydrogen cyanide

Incapacitating Agents
- BZ: (no common name)

Vomiting and Riot Control Agents
- DM: Adamsite
- CS: Tear gas

Organization forces were involved has perhaps induced a false sense of security. However, there have been other wars in which chemical weapons have been used with devastating effect.[5–7] Fears during the Persian Gulf War (1990–1991) highlighted real problems posed by the threat of chemical weapons and enforced new thinking about management of chemical casualties. This was particularly true for anesthesia, and at the time of writing there is again an increased awareness among military medical officers of the potential problems.[8]

The nature of chemical weapons and the formal management of chemical casualties are discussed in *Medical Aspects of Chemical and Biological Warfare*, a volume of the *Textbook of Military Medicine* series, and will not be further discussed here except to mention that the two main chemical threats are

- nerve agents, which kill by causing respiratory paralysis due to their irreversible inhibition of acetylcholinesterase, with consequent accumulation of acetylcholine in nicotinic and muscarinic receptors, and
- vesicants, of which the sulfur mustards are best known, and which incapacitate by causing second-degree chemical burns of the skin.

This chapter covers some of the particular problems posed to military anesthesia providers by the management of the chemical injury itself and by surgical anesthesia for trauma casualties who may also have been exposed to chemical agents. With the ever-increasing number of agents now regarded as potential threats, the approach will be to look at the injury primarily from a pathophysiological standpoint rather than from that of agent specificity.

In general, the involvement of the military anesthesia provider will focus on three broad categories of casualties:

1. those with potentially fatal exposure to a chemical agent, who need immediate, lifesaving airway management but who will not require a general anesthetic;
2. those with combined ballistic and chemical agent injuries, who will require anesthesia for the management of the conventional injury; and
3. those who have received pyridostigmine prophylaxis against chemical agents, and who will also require anesthesia for the management of a conventional injury.

Chemical injury may affect almost all the systems of the body but particularly the respiratory and nervous systems. Military anesthesia providers may be directly concerned with these in all stages of management of the wounded, including resuscitation, preoperative stabilization, perioperative and postoperative care, intensive care, and recovery. Chemical injury can affect all these stages, creating clinical problems in their own right and complicating conventional management of injuries that require surgery. Anesthesiologists, as a result of their training, are well placed to grasp the clinical problems arising from chemical injury. The pharmacology and toxicology of the agents will be familiar, as will the nature of the neuromuscular paralysis and respiratory complications such as pulmonary edema and respiratory distress syndrome, which are the life-threatening aspects of chemical injury.

Conventional teaching of chemical warfare injury has often tended to view the subject in isolation. No doubt based on the initial use of poison gas in 1915, the use of chemical arms is often viewed as a special event that will create mass casualties from only one cause. This ignores the subsequent use of poison gas in World War I, wherein the gas was usually disseminated from shells fired in conjunction with conventional high-explosive shells. Thus, casualties with combined ballistic and chemical injuries occurred. Exactly how common such casualties were in World War I is not known. However, of the 546 American soldiers who died following exposure to gas in the period March to November 1918, 6% also had ballistic injuries.[9] Given the tactical doctrine of chemical agent powers such as the former Soviet Union, which took an integrated approach to the use of chemical weapons (seeing them as part of the ordinary armamentarium available to field commanders, as opposed to being special "weapons of mass destruction"), combined ballistic and chemical casualties should be expected whenever chemical weapons are used.[10] During the Iran–Iraq War, when chemical agents were used the most extensively since World War I (Exhibit 30-3), chemical weapons were also used in a localized, tactical way, particularly as part of defensive infantry actions. The consequence of these developments is that wounding by chemical agents should not be viewed in isolation. It may now be appropriate to think of wounding in three main classes:

1. conventional traumatic wounding, where the tissues are disrupted by externally impressed forces;

EXHIBIT 30-3

IRANIAN EXPERIENCE WITH CHEMICAL WARFARE AGENTS

During the Iran-Iraq War, modern medicine was applied to the treatment of injuries caused by sulfur mustard, tabun, Lewisite, and the biological agent mycotoxin.[1,2] Although data are limited, there are a number of lessons that we should note. The most unexpected was the surprisingly low mortality: fewer than 1% of the estimated 27,000 Iranian chemical casualties.[3]

Troops with organophosphate exposure fell into four categories. Those with the greatest exposure died in the field. The number appears to have been very small even though most of the Iraqi attacks were made against unprotected Iranian troops. Those most severely injured who reached medical aid were unconscious and unresponsive, and often in respiratory arrest. The seriously intoxicated had symptoms of dizziness, disorientation, anxiety, salivation, and respiratory difficulty. Those with relatively mild symptoms were often physically difficult to manage because of their disorientation. By far the largest number of casualties required no treatment other than decontamination.

Treatment of mustard exposure during the Iran-Iraq War reflects the experience gained in the management of burn wounds during the 80 years since World War I. Treatment begins with early and thorough decontamination. Early in the course of injury, blistering may not be present. Still, removal of contaminated clothing is important to limit the casualty's contact time with the agent. Shaving of the affected areas followed by washing mechanically removes and dilutes the agent. Aspiration of blisters, removal of necrotic tissue, and treatment of the skin lesions with silver sulfadiazine cream forms the basis for treatment of skin injury. Respiratory exposure to mustard creates its own set of problems. Depending on the degree of injury, the treatment must be adjusted to the degree of injury. Humidified air or oxygen helps to prevent airway obstruction. Bronchodilators, mucolytics, and expectorants are useful. In cases of serious injury, mechanical ventilation with positive end-expiratory pressure and acid–base balance control are used to support the casualty until the injuries resolve. Injury to the eyes is treated with irrigation and sodium sulymid. Pain is treated with systemic medications. Because of weight loss, often in excess of 10 kg, nutritional support is instituted to help reduce the significant mortality associated with negative nitrogen balance. Once the patient reaches a setting for definitive care, therapy is divided into two parts: a general supportive treatment for sepsis and dehydration, and treatment to eliminate toxins from the body.[1]

Significant observations from the Iran-Iraq War include the following:

- Decontamination, using soap and water and shaving body hair, was done early. This protected medical personnel and simplified further treatment.
- Comatose casualties of nerve agents who did not have cardiovascular problems were treated with large doses of atropine, 50 to 200 mg administered intravenously. Most casualties received 2 mg every 8 hours. Comatose casualties with significant cardiovascular deterioration (such as bradycardia after 2 mg of intravenous atropine) were most often found not to survive.
- Mustard, although it dates from World War I, continues to be an important chemical agent. It is a vesicant but also has effects on multiple organ systems.

(1) Colardyn F, de Keyser H, Ringoir S, de Bersaques J. Clinical observation and therapy of injuries with vesicants. *Journal de Toxicologie Clinique et Experimentale*. 1986;6(4):237–246. (2) Kadivar H, Adams SC. Treatment of chemical and biological warfare injuries: Insights derived from the 1984 Iraqi attack on Majnoon Island. *Milit Med*. 1991;156:171–177. (3) Hammick M. All stick and no carrot. *International Defense Review*. 1991;(Dec):1323–1327.

2. toxic wounding, where the body systems are poisoned; and
3. environmental wounding, where the body is damaged by excesses of heat and cold.

Casualties may occur from any combination of all three categories.

In a mixed chemical and conventional environment, the number of casualties with combined (both conventional penetrating and chemical) wounds could be considerable. Not only will these numbers cause potential problems for military anesthesia providers, but other aspects of combat casualty care will also be affected. One study[11] used the U.S. Marine Surgical Data Base from the Vietnam War to calculate a figure of potential protective mask failures secondary to conventional wounds of the head and neck (including the trachea, oral cavity, etc). These researchers predicted that 34% of casualties presenting at a hospital would have wounds that interfered with proper sealing of fielded gas masks. Since this study makes no attempt to consider wounds that would disrupt other components of mission-oriented protective posture (MOPP) gear, 34% may indeed be a conservative estimate.

ASPECTS OF TOXIC AGENTS OF IMPORTANCE IN MILITARY ANESTHESIA

Recent changes in thinking about the status and definition of toxic warfare agents are of particular importance to military anesthesia providers. Conventionally, riot control agents, herbicides, smoke, and flame are excluded from the definition of chemical agents, although their clinical effects (ie, they kill, seriously injure, or otherwise injure via their pathophysiological effects) bring them within the classical definition of chemical agents. *Biological* agents, on the other hand, are defined as living organisms, the use of which is intended to kill or incapacitate man in warfare.[2] Under the 1972 Biological Warfare Convention, toxins, which originally could only be produced by living organisms, were included with the biological agents, despite the fact that they are, in fact, chemical substances with unusually high molecular weights.

Although we could argue that all agents designed to incapacitate or kill are, by definition, biological, since the target is man and not his machines, the traditional view of chemical and biological agents has persisted. Clinically, however, the separation of chemical and biological weapons has now become increasingly difficult: new technologies have expanded the number of potential agents in both classes—particularly in the toxins, which lie midway between the two. Developments in biotechnology mean that the synthesis of toxins is now feasible, and that their use as sophisticated chemical agents is more likely.[12]

The Spectrum of Toxic Hazards in Warfare

Medically, it is now desirable to integrate traditional definitions of chemical and biological agents into a unified concept known as the chemical–biological warfare spectrum of toxic agents. This is shown diagonally in Exhibit 30-4, where the agents are arranged in order of ascending molecular weight, with conventional chemical agents on the left and the self-reproducing agents such as bacteria and viruses on the right. Toxins and other agents of biological origin occupy the middle.

The spectral, rather than the agent-specific, view is important clinically because pathophysiological mechanisms that should be considered in medical management are common to agents from different parts of the spectrum. Neuromuscular paralysis and pulmonary edema are two examples. Failure of the neuromuscular junction, for example, can be caused by two agents as chemically different as a nerve agent and botulinum toxin. The clinical result, however, is the same, and in severe cases the primary lifesaving measure is artificial ventilation. Similarly, there are many agents of which the end result is pulmonary edema. The spectral concept is a reminder to military anesthesia providers that

EXHIBIT 30-4

THE SPECTRUM OF CHEMICAL–BIOLOGICAL WARFARE AGENTS

Low Molecular Weight →		**High Molecular Weight**
Nerve agents	Neuropeptides	Bacteria
Pulmonary irritants	Toxins	Viruses
Vesicants		Rickettsiae
Cyanogens		

Adapted with permission from Baker DJ. Chemical and biologic warfare. Part 2. In: Baker DJ. Extreme environmental conditions. In: Grande CM, ed. *Textbook of Trauma Anesthesia and Critical Care*. St. Louis, Mo: Mosby–Year Book; 1993: Chap 108: 1331.

medical management must respond to system dysfunction, not simply to etiology.

Characteristics of Toxic Agents

The characteristics of toxic agents may be divided into the operational and the pathophysiological. The operational aspects are not discussed in this chapter. The pathophysiological aspects of toxic agents are of particular importance to military physicians, however, and include (*a*) toxicity, (*b*) latency of onset, and (*c*) transmissibility.

Toxicity

Toxic agents can kill or incapacitate. The biological effects of potential agents may be estimated from animal studies and data from accidental exposure, but there may be considerable difference from one species to another. The clinical importance of toxicological data is to give some idea of the substances' hazards to man. There are a number of ways of expressing toxicity of agents (Table 30-1); the following are the most common:

- Ct is the product of the concentration of an airborne agent multiplied by the time it was inhaled, given a standard rate of respiration. The Ct product applies to the middle range of exposure but is inaccurate at very high or very low levels. The units of Ct are mg • min/m^3. The relationship of Ct to absorbed dose is a function of the rate of respiration or the total exposed skin area. This should always be specified when quoting Ct values, and is conventionally accepted as 10 to 15 L/min.
- LCt_{50} and ICt_{50} are the Ct values for a specified route of absorption that will kill (lethal, L) or incapacitate (I) 50% of the exposed population.
- LD_{50} and ID_{50} are the doses for a specified route of absorption that will kill (L) or incapacitate (I) 50% of the exposed population.

Latency

Latency of action is a clinically important property of toxic agents. All agents have a latent period, ranging from a few seconds in the case of cyanide to several hours in the case of some vesicants. Biological agents such as *Brucella* can have a latent period as long as 3 weeks. A patient presenting with few symptoms after exposure may develop more, and more dramatic, symptoms later. Because of this, detecting the use of a toxic agent by the immediate effects on those who have been exposed may not always be possible. Specific latency may be modified by physical factors such as ambient temperature and the amount of exertion after exposure. Latency often decreases as absorbed dose increases.

TABLE 30-1

RELATIVE TOXICITIES OF SOME IMPORTANT BIOLOGICAL AND CHEMICAL WARFARE AGENTS*

Agent	LCt_{50} (mg•min/m^3)	LD_{50}
Botulinum toxin†		0.15 µg/kg
Soman	40–60	0.025 mg/kg, IV
Sarin	70–100	0.01 mg/kg, IV
Tabun	150	0.08 mg/kg, IV
Cyanide	2,000–5,000	1.0 mg‡
Sulfur mustard	1,500	100.0 mg/kg

* Values are based on experimental and extrapolated data from accidential exposure. Toxicities are expressed as LCt_{50}, the median lethal exposure delivered by inhaling a concentration C for a time t in minutes; and LD_{50}, the conventional median lethal dose.
†Estimated respiratory value for man
‡Respiratory value
Adapted with permission from Baker DJ. Chemical and biologic warfare. Part 2. In: Baker DJ. Extreme environmental conditions. In: Grande CM, ed. *Textbook of Trauma Anesthesia and Critical Care*. St. Louis, Mo: Mosby-Year Book; 1993: Chap 108: 1332.

Transmissibility

Toxic agents may affect not only the casualty but also the casualty's medical attendants. In the case of biological agents, the risk of transmission by infection is widely recognized. For chemical agents, the risks are of contact and inhalational transmission to medical personnel if the casualty is not properly decontaminated. Transmissibility is an important characteristic that distinguishes toxic from conventional weapons. *All* casualties of toxic agents must *always* be regarded as risks to their attendants, who may not themselves have been involved in the original attack. This point has considerable significance for the operating theater team involved with the management of such casualties.

PROTECTION, DETECTION, AND DECONTAMINATION

Protection against chemical warfare agents and their detection and decontamination are considered in detail elsewhere,[1] but it is essential that military anesthesia providers be familiar with these concepts, as they affect field anesthetic practice in many ways.

It is the policy of the U.S. military not to perform surgery in a contaminated environment. The casualty should be adequately decontaminated before being taken into the preoperative area or operating room. Clothing should be removed, and the skin and hair decontaminated with hypochlorite. A casualty should not enter the "clean" operating room or the collective protective ensemble (CPE) until decontamination is accomplished; once this is done, the danger from contamination is nil.

Although the desired aim of field anesthesia is to work either on decontaminated casualties or in some form of CPE, it may be necessary in extreme circumstances for hospital-based anesthesia providers to work in an individual protective ensemble (IPE, which is the British equivalent of MOPP gear), particularly in the early stages of resuscitation and triage. Since individual protection involves isolating the operator from the contaminated environment by means of a protective suit and respirator, it follows that many of the normal tactile skills available to the anesthesia provider will be lost or severely impaired, particularly since the casualty may also be similarly isolated. In full MOPP gear, even assessing for something so simple as the casualty's color will be difficult. Simple pulse measurement may not be possible, although radial pulses are palpable through an Mk 4 suit (ie, a kind of IPE) when inner gloves are left out of the operator's ensemble (—*DJB*, personal observation, 1990).

It is clear that only the simplest lifesaving measures are available to the military anesthesia provider in full MOPP gear, although these must include definitive securing of the airway. If necessary, it may be necessary to break the casualty's own IPE to gain access since the danger of airway obstruction outweighs the consequences of further contamination—particularly where there is no direct hazard from a liquid agent. Nevertheless, a surgeon who operates on a contaminated casualty risks spreading contamination into the casualty, a very bad practice indeed.

Although CPE offers greater freedom to work on casualties contaminated with toxic agents, anesthesia providers should be aware of the limitations of collective protection and the importance of careful decontamination, and check the casualty's contamination monitoring before entering the CPE. Experience from the 1991 Persian Gulf War emphasizes the cramped conditions of anesthesia providers working in CPE.[8] The transit period for any patient through the airlock system is particularly dangerous since it may not be physically possible for a paramedical or anesthetic attendant to be present.

Toxic agents may be delivered as vapor, liquid, or a particulate or liquid aerosol. The possibility that chemical agents can be absorbed onto a carrier dust that will deliver point concentrations of agent directly to the alveoli is an ominous new development. For the anesthesia provider dealing with a potentially contaminated patient, the risks are from direct contact with liquid agent on the patient's clothing, from the vapor the liquid emits, and from reaerosolization of powders.

The simplest method of detecting liquid agents uses special detector papers (although the range of agents detected is limited at this time). The most useful technique for vapor analysis available for use in the operating room is the chemical agent monitor (CAM), which detects nerve and vesicant chemical warfare agents and is used to identify the presence of chemical agent vapors in decontamination operations. This device uses ion-cluster acceleration as the basis for analysis. This technique is similar in principle to mass spectrometry but depends on forming hydrated ion clusters with the toxic agent rather than on accelerating small ions. In CAM, the vapor is sucked into a sampling port, where a radioisotope is used to ionize the toxic agent to form the ion clusters. These are then accelerated down a high-voltage drift tube and the collected current characteristics are analyzed at one end. In its original form, CAM could be preset to detect either mustard or nerve agent. A modification allows detection of several other agents, all of which can be detected using the drift-tube technique. CAM may be used preoperatively to check the decontamination of patients. One problem that may arise is the slow clearance time of the instrument when background levels of agent are high. Individual chemical agent detectors (ICAD), worn by individual medical personnel, may provide the earliest warning while contaminated patients are being handled. The ICAD will identify nerve, blister, blood, and choking agents and will warn by audio and visual alarms.

The possibility that chemical agents are absorbed onto dusts, or that toxins are delivered as solid aerosols, should be considered with the greatest care. The presence of dust on a patient should be treated with suspicion, particularly since there is no simple toxin-detection device available and these agents are likely to be delivered in solid aerosol form.

If liquid agent is on a casualty, careful decontamination is required. There are two main methods, wet and dry. Wet decontamination involves the use of oxidizing solutions containing hypochlorite, which effectively oxidizes liquid agents such as mustard and nerve agents. Thickened nerve agents such as thickened GD may have a consistency similar to that of glue and require scraping off before decontamination can proceed further. Dry decontamination (which is not currently used by U.S. forces) uses fuller's earth, an absorbent clay, to remove liquid agent. It should be understood that absorption and removal of the chemical agent does not decrease the agent's toxicity, so care must be taken with the discarded material. Fuller's earth is available in puffer bottles and impregnated pads that may be applied directly to the contamination. The proper sequence of decontamination consists of first removing clothing, then decontaminating the skin. Following decontamination, it is essential that the patient be monitored carefully to allow further medical intervention. An important point is that in serious toxic injury, the normal ATLS processes should be dynamically integrated with the decontamination processes. Proper assessment and definitive airway management will be difficult until decontamination has been achieved.

SITES OF INJURY BY TOXIC AGENTS

In traumatic injury, the mechanism of injury may be known and often will be a useful predictor of the damage.[13] Similarly, the knowledge that a toxic injury has been caused by a particular agent (eg, an organophosphate) will alert the anesthesia provider to a specific pattern of damage. Knowledge of the nature of the toxic agent is more important than knowledge of the nature of a traumatic force; however, although information may be available at primary casualty assessment, it cannot be guaranteed. Casualties with immediately life-threatening conditions such as apnea or cardiac arrest should receive immediate treatment before decontamination. Decontamination typically takes 10 to 15 minutes, but death from respiratory failure due to exposure to nerve agents can occur within 5 minutes of exposure. In fact, respiratory support must begin before the casualty is brought to the hospital—or to the battalion aid station, for that matter. The casualty will not wait until he arrives at the medical facility to stop breathing. Nevertheless, excluding life-threatening emergencies due to exposure to chemical agents, it is helpful to classify toxic injury in terms of the damage that may be caused by a range of different agents at key anatomical sites rather than simply as a pattern of injury from a specific agent.

The Skin and Viscera

The skin may be affected by vesicants and toxins. Many agents acting on the skin exhibit considerable latency. Although damage to the skin may be classed as incapacitating rather than life-threatening, the agents concerned, if inhaled, may have additional serious effects on the respiratory tract. Therefore, during assessment, skin lesions should be regarded as a warning of possible accompanying respiratory damage. Sulfur mustard was the vesicant most widely used in World War I. Much clinical experience was gained at the time, but since then, there have been only isolated case reports in which the effectiveness of modern medical therapy can be assessed (see Exhibit 30-1).[14]

The viscera may be affected by vesicants if ingested, and by nerve agents following local or systemic poisoning. Ingestion of nerve agents will produce particularly marked intestinal actions, which are probably of central nervous system origin rather than due to local cholinergic action.

The Central and Peripheral Nervous Systems and the Eyes

The central nervous system is affected by a wide range of agents including nerve agents and toxic neuropeptides. Central nervous system symptoms following nerve agent intoxication will be accompanied by peripheral nervous system symptoms in both the voluntary and autonomic systems. Symptoms caused by neurotoxins, however, may be varied, ranging from modification of thought processes and mild delusions to frank coma. A careful assessment of the casualty's level of consciousness is therefore of great importance in the assessment of any toxic casualty. Again, the latency periods will be variable and observation over a lengthy period may be required. At the level of the brainstem, the central nervous system is affected by nerve agents that produce central respiratory failure, and also by cyanogen agents.

Paralysis caused by nerve agents is accompanied by other signs of poisoning (eg, miosis, excessive secretions), and the differential diagnosis from other types of paralysis such as that caused by neurotoxins is not difficult. Paralysis is accompanied by apnea, so an unventilated patient with paralysis is unlikely to be seen at the hospital level. Paralysis from nerve agents lasts 2 to 3 hours at most and should not be confused with the more prolonged paralysis caused by other agents such as botulinum toxin.

The peripheral motor and autonomic nerves are the sites of action of nerve agents and neurotoxins. Neuromuscular paralysis will therefore require differential diagnosis among several possible causes both prejunctional and postjunctional. This may be facilitated by the use of nerve stimulation techniques, which are discussed later in this chapter.

Vesicant agents cause damage to the eye and loss of vision by blepharospasm and corneal ulceration. Nerve agents may produce a variable loss of visual acuity due to miosis and central nervous system effects on the visual pathway. Loss of accommodation follows spasm of the ciliary muscle.

The Respiratory Tract

Toxic agents may seriously affect all stages of respiration (Table 30-2). In toxic injury, the respiratory tract is particularly vulnerable and its management must take a high priority. Careful clinical examination is of vital importance. While examinations such as radiography and blood gas analyses may be available, simple clinical examination will reveal much of value and must be undertaken as soon as the patient is decontaminated and out of MOPP gear. Five important points to remember are the following:

1. The presence of burns on the skin may indicate similar lesions within the respiratory tract.
2. The casualty's color and the nature of the respirations may point to impending respiratory failure.
3. The presence of paradoxical respiratory movements may indicate upper respiratory blockage of large and small airways.
4. The presence of rales at the bases of the lungs will indicate the development of pulmonary edema.
5. The presence of pathological amounts of secretions in the airway in a casualty who is likely to have been exposed to a nerve agent is strong evidence that too little atropine has been given.

Certain toxins as well as inhaled vesicants have particularly short latency periods, but the latency of onset of symptoms in the chest after toxic injury may be very variable. Any casualty with a suspected respiratory injury should be admitted to a hospital for a mandatory 24-hour observation, during which the respiratory tract should regularly be assessed for the development of signs.

MANAGEMENT OF ANESTHESIA AFTER TOXIC INJURY

The management of toxic casualties is an unfamiliar task for most anesthesiologists, but the specialty should be involved at the earliest stages of planning of facilities to deal with the problem. Besides formulating plans to deal with mass or limited casualties, planning must include flexibility for the effects of unexpected chemical casualties on the operation of a forward surgical facility. Although intelligence may give good warning of a toxic attack, the information cannot be guaranteed, particularly in rapid-response operations. All ordinary anesthetic and surgical procedures are hampered by the chemical environment, either from the results of an attack or simply from the threat of

TABLE 30-2

EFFECTS OF TOXIC AGENTS ON RESPIRATION

Respiratory Component	Effect	Toxic Agent
Central Nervous System	Depression of respiratory drive and convulsions leading to apnea	Nerve agents, cyanide, neuropeptides
Peripheral Nervous System	Neuromuscular paralysis of respiratory muscles	Nerve agents, neurotoxins
Nasopharynx	May become blocked by excess secretions	Lung-damaging agents, nerve agents
	Prodromal rhinitis and rhinorrhea	Vesicants
	Sneezing	Early symptom of mustard
Larynx	Irritation, laryngeal spasm	Upper-respiratory irritant lung-damaging agents
		Riot-control agents, particularly CS and CR (tear gas)
		Nerve agents (theoretical)
Large Airways	Blocked by secretions	Variety of agents
	Blocked by inhaled vomitus	Nerve agents
	Sloughing of walls of trachea and main bronchi, produces "pseudodiphtheritic" membrane, serious cause of large airway obstruction, leading to bronchopheumonia and death	Mustard agents
Small Airways	Blocked by secretions	
	Cholinergic innervation affected; bronchospasm (relieved by atropine)	Nerve agents
	Chemical bronchiolitis, followed by serious bronchospasm	Mustard agents
Alveoli	Toxic pulmonary edema	Variety of agents, especially lung-damaging agents (latency 6–24 h)
		Vesicant agents, particularly if inhaled at high ambient temperatures[1]

[1]Willems JL. Clinical management of mustard gas casualties. *Annales Medicinae Militaris Belgicae.* 1989;3(suppl)1–61:47, 51.

it, enforcing the use of IPE-MOPP. The planning stage should therefore ensure that the possibility of toxic attack is understood, that equipment is designed to be simple and straightforward in use, and that medical and paramedical personnel are adequately trained.

When reviewed, experience in the Persian Gulf War showed that a number of personnel discontinued the use of pyridostigmine without medical advice.[15] Had there been actual exposure to nerve agents, these troops and their missions would have been at risk. Anesthesiologists, particularly those in forward areas, are among the most suitable medical personnel to educate the troops to the necessity of using such pretreatment as pyridostigmine and to allay fears with regard to potential side effects.

U.S. military doctrine does not have anesthesiologists or surgeons checking decontamination procedures. By doctrine, noncommissioned officers do decontamination and watch casualties during that procedure. The following are potential areas of responsibility in the management of casualties from toxic attack:

- managing casualty reception, including checking of decontamination procedures, particularly for casualties in severe respiratory and neuromuscular distress;
- preoperatively assessing the whole patient, who may be suffering from both traumatic and toxic injury;
- assessing the likely impact of prophylactic measures (eg, pyridostigmine bromide), toxic agents, and therapeutic measures on the subsequent action of anesthetic drugs and agents;
- providing advice to surgeons on the morbidity factors associated with the toxic injury in otherwise uncomplicated surgery;
- managing casualties perioperatively;
- managing postoperative complications, which may be toxic, anesthetic, or surgical, or any combination; and
- managing patients who require postoperative intensive care.

The importance of decontamination has been emphasized previously. However, although decontamination is vital for the safety of casualties and medical personnel alike, it must not be allowed to interrupt the continuous process of resuscitation and assessment during triage. Decontamination and monitoring must at all times be dynamic and integrated with primary and continuing medical care. Initially, the casualty arriving at a surgical facility may have to be managed by medical attendants wearing MOPP gear, but the aim should be to get the casualty into CPE as soon as possible to facilitate examination and initial treatment.

Types of Casualties

The following types of casualties may be anticipated following actions where chemical weapons have been employed:

- traumatic casualties, uncontaminated with chemical agents;
- traumatic casualties, contaminated;
- toxic casualties;
- iatrogenic toxic casualties, produced as a result of the side effects of antidotes to toxic agents;
- combined traumatic and toxic casualties;
- thermal stress casualties (these will usually be suffering from heat stress as a result of wearing MOPP gear, but hypothermia may also occur); and
- psychological casualties (combat stress reaction may be common in toxic warfare).

Triage of Casualties

Triage of casualties with conventional traumatic wounds is considered in detail in Chapter 1, Combat Trauma Overview. It is important, however, to apply a system of triage to casualties affected solely by chemical agents. The following is the authors' suggestion (with the U.S. Army's triage designations in parentheses):

- T1 (Priority I and Priority IA): the casualty requires immediate lifesaving treatment. This will almost certainly involve securing the airway, starting intermittent positive-pressure ventilation (IPPV), and continuing pharmacological measures such as atropine, oximes, and benzodiazepines for nerve agent poisoning. Agents causing this type of immediately life-threatening injury will be nerve agents, lung-damaging agents (ie, phosgene), cyanides, and toxins.
- T2 (Priority II): some delay in management is possible. Respiration may be compromised by direct airway problems and by developing neuromuscular paralysis but not to the extent that immediate intervention is indicated. Placing the casualty in this triage category may be influenced by military intelligence about the toxic agent used. If considerable latency of action is likely (eg, with vesicants and some lung-damaging agents), close observation of the casualty is indicated to look for signs of developing vesication in the airway, and pulmonary edema.
- T3 (Priority III): minimal effects from the toxic agent. The casualty may be returned to duty after a period of observation.
- T4 (Priority IV): expectant treatment category. Casualties will usually be placed in this category because facilities available for their medical care are limited (eg, long-term IPPV) in relation to the facilities needed for a larger number of less-seriously injured casualties. Unlike traumatic wounds, there are few toxic injuries in which

the acute phase cannot be managed in the field given sufficient intensive care resources. However, some chemical injuries (eg, extensive vesicant burns) will require long-term hospitalization, which will not be practical in a field hospital.

Casualty-Management Phases

The anesthesiologist who assesses casualties with toxic injuries for surgery must be aware of the preceding medical management, which should have been documented on the casualty card accompanying the patient. The nature of the agent used, the likely exposure time, pretreatment, and early therapy are of importance. The following five phases may be identified:

1. Preattack. Casualties may have been taking pyridostigmine bromide, the drug currently contained in the nerve agent pretreatment sets (which are discussed later in this chapter) if a nerve agent attack was thought to be imminent. The state of MOPP at the time of attack is important.
2. Self-aid. Casualties may have administered autoinjectable atropine, oximes, and benzodiazepine before or after a nerve agent attack. The possibility exists that the injection may have been given without subsequent chemical agent attack. Atropine intoxication is a theoretical possibility at this stage, causing the casualty to be confused and compounding his heat stress, although the amount of atropine in three MARK I autoinjectors is unlikely to cause significant confusion in the average 70-kg soldier.
3. Buddy-aid. The chemically injured casualty may receive further autoject medication from a comrade, but U.S. military doctrine has no provision or method for a buddy to provide airway management or IPPV in a masked casualty.
4. Initial medical care (battalion aid station), including initial triage decontamination and ventilatory assistance.
5. Hospital level, including decontamination and monitoring with continued integrated medical support. A full ATLS primary survey should be possible at this stage to establish airway, breathing, and circulation, and to determine disability and exposure. The full ATLS primary survey can be carried out only in a decontaminated casualty.

During the first four phases, the casualty may be relatively isolated from the medical attendants both by IPE and by the use of casualty bags during transport. Even simple maneuvers such as measuring pulse and respiration may be difficult. At the third echelon, noninvasive monitoring should be possible and may include pulse oximetry and capnography. Simple observations of color and mode of respiration, together with auscultation of the lungs, will provide much valuable information at this time. The anesthesia provider may be actively involved with T1 (Priority I and Priority IA) casualties at the third echelon in securing the airway and assessing neuromuscular deficit. The use of an endotracheal tube with early IPPV and positive end-expiratory pressure (PEEP) may be highly desirable, and a laryngeal mask or esophageal occlusion device may be helpful.[16] (Techniques for securing the airway are discussed in Chapter 3, Airway Management.) It is important with toxic casualties to remember the omnipresent risk of vomiting and aspiration. Pharyngeal and bronchial secretions are a major feature of intoxication by several agents, particularly nerve agents, and although efficient suction for clearance is vital, the presence of excessive secretions indicates the need for more atropine. In fact, one of the end points for atropine administration is minimal secretions.

Preoperative Assessment and Examination

The military anesthesia provider preoperatively assessing any casualty must bear in mind the overall classification of casualties stated above. In particular, the possibility of contamination of a patient who has not yet sustained toxic injury must be considered. In a casualty with combined injuries, the anesthesia provider must remember that the casualty may have received pyridostigmine pretreatment, antimuscarinics such as atropine and oximes after agent exposure, and opiates after wounding. All of these will interact with the conduct of general anesthesia.

Toxic agents may radically alter the normal pattern of anesthesia. It is therefore vital that any preoperative assessment should attempt to gain as much information as possible about the circumstances and timing of toxic wounding, together with any information that might be available about the nature of the agents used. Examination should concentrate on the key respiratory and nervous system sites that will interfere with subsequent general anesthesia. The possibility of latency of onset of signs and symptoms is particularly important, as these may lead to onset of pulmonary edema or other respiratory pathology during the anesthetic course.

The usual preoperative investigations will be required, but these may usefully be supplemented by some assessment of the level of acetylcholinesterase, which is depressed by nerve and mustard agents. In the field hospital, direct estimation of acetylcholinesterase will be difficult, but whether abnormal serum butyrylcholine esterase (also called plasma cholinesterase) is present can be determined using the dibucaine test, which is familiar to anesthesiologists investigating prolonged, pathological action of succinylcholine in a patient.[17] Butyrylcholine esterase will be depressed by nerve agents to an extent similar to acetylcholinesterase when exposure has been severe and the levels of both enzymes are close to zero. Wherever possible, X-ray examinations of the chest should be performed—particularly after exposure to lung-damaging agents, which carry a high risk of causing pulmonary edema. Radiographic evidence of alveolar membrane damage may lag behind the development of pulmonary edema but may be apparent on auscultation of the chest.

Only limited time may be available for preoperative examination, but care should be taken to determine the casualty's color and the rate and depth of respiration. Diminished air entry to the lungs may indicate the presence of secretions, which are a major problem with nerve agents and indicate the need for further administration of atropine. Bronchospasm and bronchiolitis may be signs of inhaled vesicant agent vapor as well as conventional lung-damaging agents, particularly at high ambient temperatures. Unfortunately, the findings of bronchospasm and bronchiolitis within 3 to 4 hours of mustard exposure indicate severe lung damage, and the casualty should be classified in the expectant category.

Cardiovascular assessment should follow the ATLS procedure, but it is important to note that the normal relationship between pulse and blood pressure in a casualty with traumatic injuries combined with nerve agent poisoning may be totally unreliable, due primarily to administered atropine. In casualties with nerve agent injuries who have been inadequately treated, the normal relationship between pulse and blood pressure may also be absent owing to the widespread action of the organophosphate at vagal and sympathetic ganglionic sites alike. The alimentary system is unstable following nerve agent poisoning, and the risk of vomiting is high. Simple examination of the extremities will reveal possible fasciculations and weakness following nerve agent exposure. If train-of-four testing is possible at this stage, a characteristic depolarization block with no fade is most likely to be found.[18]

Anesthetic Induction, Maintenance, and Recovery

Toxic injury may have serious effects on induction of emergency general anesthesia. Shock and toxic airway injury can both produce ventilation–perfusion inequality, giving rise to less-effective preoxygenation. Therefore, as far as possible, the toxic injury should be stabilized before the start of surgical anesthesia. The responses to the inducing agent will require careful titration; normal doses of intravenous induction agents may not apply. With many toxic injuries, both the risk of vomiting and the need for controlled induction with cricoid compression are increased. If assistance is not available, induction should be performed in the lateral position. The action of succinylcholine will be considerably prolonged if used after nerve agent exposure. This effect will also be noted after pyridostigmine pretreatment, owing to the anti–butyrylcholine esterase action of the carbamate anticholinesterase.[19]

The respiratory uptake of anesthetic vapors and alveolar ventilation will be affected by degrees of shunt and pulmonary edema during balanced anesthesia. Careful titration of the balance is required.

The characteristics of nondepolarizing muscle relaxants may be particularly affected in patients poisoned with nerve agents. Since organophosphates cause an increase of acetylcholine at the cholinergic junctions, including the neuromuscular junction, the normal pharmacological actions of nondepolarizing blocking agents will be antagonized. For a severely poisoned casualty, the degree of acetylcholinesterase inhibition will be greater than 70%.[20] There is little or no clinical experience regarding the actions of muscle relaxants under these conditions, but the buildup of acetylcholine at the postjunctional folds will antagonize the action of nondepolarizing blocking agents, leading to higher-than-expected doses. A casualty who has suffered severe nerve agent poisoning requiring IPPV may have a sufficient depolarization block from the acetylcholine increase to permit surgery, in which case the use of nondepolarizing blocking agents may be unnecessary. Clinical experience in this area is very scarce. There is, however, a theoretical advantage in using nondepolarizing agents in this situation, since the occupancy of the receptor sites by the drug may protect the endplate from long-term postoperative damage.

In field surgery, where the operating load may be heavy, predictability of recovery is very important and is the principal advantage of using balanced anesthesia in this situation. The many possible interactions of toxic agents with the techniques of balanced anesthesia, in which multiple drugs are administered, are likely to disturb this predictability and lead to postoperative complications. The normal physiological indicators of balanced anesthesia, such as pulse rate and blood pressure, may be compromised by the effects of toxic agents. The reversal of nondepolarizing blocking agents may be particularly affected, and recurrent paralysis may occur following nerve agent poisoning. Generally, the likelihood of continuing postoperative intensive care will be greater when conventional and toxic injuries are combined. Given the potential problems for balanced general anesthesia arising from the effects of toxic agents, there may be considerable advantages in using regional blocks for general surgery in this situation. Spinal and epidural anesthesia may be highly unpredictable from a cardiovascular point of view, where the autonomic nervous system is affected by nerve agents.

TOXIC AGENT COMPLICATIONS OF MILITARY ANESTHESIA

The postoperative complications may be significant in patients whose field surgery is complicated by chemical injury. The most important complications from toxic injury of concern to the anesthesia provider are to the respiratory and nervous systems.

Respiratory Complications

Respiratory complications take the form of damage to the airways and alveoli. Vesicant agent exposure causes slow-healing ulceration of the upper respiratory tract and large airways. If sloughing of the pseudodiphtheritic membrane occurs, there will be blockage of bronchi with subsequent collapse.[21] Bronchopneumonia is a common sequel to these events and was a primary cause of death from mustard poisoning during World War I. Bronchoscopic intervention may be required in such cases. Cases of mustard inhalation reported from the Iran–Iraq War have shown that mustard will affect the terminal airways, in some cases causing a chemical bronchiolitis. This can give rise to severe bronchospasm, which may present difficulties in weaning from a ventilator (—*DJB*, personal observation, 1988). In some casualties, intractable bronchostenosis developed after several years.[22]

Pulmonary edema occurs with vesicants only after extremely high exposure or as a terminal event days after exposure. After an extremely high exposure, patchy pulmonary edema may occur within hours of exposure and is also a preterminal event. It is unlikely that a surgical procedure would be undertaken under either of these circumstances. The value of early IPPV with PEEP and high-dose steroid therapy is controversial. Development of the adult respiratory distress syndrome is possible, and early recognition of the syndrome is important. The problem of doing so is compounded by the fact that such cases will often be managed in clinically unsophisticated facilities, where blood gas analysis and other routine intensive care investigations may not always be available.

For postoperative casualties with toxic injuries, some form of simple intensive care facility is necessary for the respiratory care of the more severely affected. The equipment required may be simple but should be capable of ventilating casualties who have significant adverse changes in pulmonary compliance. Evacuation of ventilator-dependent patients may be desirable in certain circumstances.

Neurological Complications

The therapy of nerve agent poisoning emphasizes the early use of antimuscarinic drugs and oximes to regenerate acetylcholinesterase, in conjunction with pyridostigmine pretreatment.[1,23] This regime should be effective in most cases, but severely poisoned casualties will require ventilatory support. If nerve agent intoxication was sufficient to remove all remaining acetylcholinesterase after pyridostigmine pretreatment (about 60% of the original store), a period of time will be required for the carbamylated enzyme to be released at the neuromuscular junction. Total ventilatory support may be required during this period. If pretreatment has been effective, this should last only a matter of hours. The nature of the neuromuscular block during this period will be a classical depolarization with a nondecremental response to train-of-four stimuli at 2 Hz. However, military anesthesia providers must recognize that long-term ventilatory support, indicative of long-term paralysis, is uncommon. With no pretreatment, individual case reports indicate that paralysis and the need for ventilatory support do not persist for more than 2 to 3 hours.[24]

The experience with nerve agents is in contrast to what is seen with organophosphate *pesticide* poisoning,[25] in which the initial block, during the cholinergic phase, may disappear within a few hours. After about 18 hours, however, the block recurs, this time having the characteristics of nondepolarizing block with a decremental response to train-of-four stimulation monitoring. This recurrent paralysis has been termed the *intermediate* syndrome, and is the phase of neurotoxicity when nerve conduction itself is affected, giving rise to sensory and motor dysfunction. The final phase may be mediated by direct neurotoxic actions of organophosphate pesticides rather than through acetylcholinesterase. The neuromuscular block of the intermediate syndrome may be persistent, lasting in some instances as long as several weeks. It may be analogous to the much-debated concept of dual block seen after multiple doses of succinylcholine.[26] If the intermediate syndrome occurs, improvement may be seen in neuromuscular transmission following administration of neostigmine.[25] There is supporting evidence, from studies using single-fiber electromyography following low-dose sarin exposure in volunteers, that subclinical, nondepolarizing neuromuscular failure occurs even at modest levels of acetylcholinesterase inhibition 3 days after exposure.[27] It is important for military anesthesia providers to know that the intermediate syndrome has *not* been seen in thousands of experimental animals and in the limited number of humans inadvertently exposed to *nerve* agents. Furthermore, recently published experiences with organophosphate pesticide poisoning suggest that the delayed respiratory insufficiency is due to pulmonary complications such as secondary pneumonia rather than to respiratory muscle insufficiency per se.[28]

The use of diazepam may prevent neurological complications from seizure activity as well as decrease spasm from excessive acetylcholinesterase stimulation.

Nondepolarizing Neuromuscular Blocking Agents in Organophosphate Poisoning

Although the intermediate syndrome has not been described in experimental animals or in humans after nerve agent exposure, it should be kept in mind that the experience with humans is quite limited. It is possible that the intermediate syndrome may become apparent given large numbers of nerve gas casualties. If so, theoretical and experimental considerations suggest the following therapeutic approach. Nerve agents cause a prolonged depolarization at the neuromuscular junction, which may lead to secondary changes in the acetylcholine receptors. One therapeutic possibility to avoid the intermediate syndrome is to block the receptor sites with long-acting, nondepolarizing blocking agents such as curare or pancuronium. Competitive denial of access of acetylcholine to the receptors may alter the processes leading to the development of the intermediate syndrome. With the present state of knowledge regarding the long-term block following exposure to nerve agents, this approach can only be regarded as conjecture. However, the anesthesia provider will feel confident in the use of the nondepolarizing drugs in long-term ventilation in the intensive care unit and will have available a therapeutic tool in an area that has little else to offer at present. Further research on the long-term block is needed before any definitive advice can be given.

PYRIDOSTIGMINE PRETREATMENT AND GENERAL ANESTHESIA

Pretreatment with carbamate anticholinesterases is now an established technique whenever there is a risk of exposure to nerve agents. The drug used at the present time is pyridostigmine bromide, 30 mg given every 8 hours. The first large-scale use of pyridostigmine under field conditions occurred during the Persian Gulf War,[15] based on efficiency studies in animals.[29] The complete rationale and use of pyridostigmine pretreatment is described in U.S. Army Field Manual 8-285, *Treatment of Chemical Agent Casualties and Conventional Military Chemical Injuries*.[1] This use of pyridostigmine may have important consequences of which military anesthesia providers must be aware.

Pharmacology

Pyridostigmine bromide is a dimethyl carbamate compound containing a quaternary amine site. It does not, therefore, readily penetrate the blood–brain barrier. In usual doses, its actions are peripheral, and only high doses might cross the barrier and have central nervous system actions. Like other carbamates such as neostigmine and physostigmine, pyridostigmine is an anticholinesterase compound. Therefore, it has the same action as the organophosphates, but unlike the latter it forms a reversible complex with acetylcholinesterase. Pyridostigmine has no significant plasma-protein binding, indicating that there should be no drug interactions involving competition for binding sites. Seventy percent to 90% of the absorbed dose is excreted unchanged in the urine. At the normal pretreatment dose of 30 mg every 8 hours, the anticholinesterase level returns to within 10% of normal 12 hours after the last dose.[30]

Mild and reversible symptoms associated with taking the prescribed prophylactic dose have been well described (Table 30-3).[15] Another study[8] found that more than 10% of 200 uninjured personnel who were taking pyridostigmine pretreatment reported significant side effects including abdominal cramps, increased volume and frequency of stools, flatulence, increased salivation, sweating, headache, and various eye signs including difficulty in focusing and dimness of vision. Isolated reports of more-serious problems such as hypertension were also reported.[8] In addition, two women with body weights of 45 to 50 kg experienced increased salivation, severe abdominal cramps, nausea, diaphoresis, and muscular twitching—all signs of pyridostigmine overdose. Symptoms were found to usually begin within hours of taking the first tablet and were often decreased if the pyridostigmine was taken with a meal.

TABLE 30-3

EFFECTS OF PYRIDOSTIGMINE PRETREATMENT*

Effect	Range of Incidence (%)
Gastrointestinal symptoms	≥ 50
Urinary urgency and frequency	5–30
Headaches, rhinorrhea, diaphoresis, tingling of extremities	< 5
Need for medical visit	1
Discontinuation on medical advice	< 0.1

*Based on reports from medical personnel providing care to 41,650 soldiers (6.5% women) who took pyridostigmine bromide orally, 30 mg every 8 h for 1–7 d. Drug administration resulted in 483 clinic visits, and use of the drug was discontinued in 28 soldiers.

Reprinted from Keeler JR, Hurst CG, Dunn MA. Pyridostigmine used as a nerve agent preteatment under wartime conditions. *JAMA*. 1991;266(5):694.

Protective Action Against Organophosphates

At the pretreatment dosage schedule, pyridostigmine combines with part of the acetylcholinesterase enzyme store to produce a carbamylated complex, which is resistant to subsequent attack by an organophosphate. If a person taking this regime is exposed to nerve agent in a potentially lethal dose, the remaining free acetylcholinesterase will bind irreversibly to the organophosphate, causing a buildup of acetylcholine. However, the carbamylated portion of the enzyme spontaneously breaks down, regenerating free enzyme and effectively providing an autotransfusion of enzyme at the postjunctional membrane. This process does not require the presence of oxime; oxime has no effect on the carbamate–enzyme bond. This new free enzyme is not attacked by nerve agent, because the latter is rapidly broken down in plasma after exposure. There is a considerable safety margin in normal acetylcholinesterase levels present at the neuromuscular junction, and the amount of enzyme released from the pyridostigmine complex is sufficient to restore neuromuscular transmission. The restoration of enzyme in conjunction with the usual resuscitative measures offers a therapeutic solution to the potentially lethal poisoning by nerve agent.

Interactions Between Pyridostigmine and Drugs Used in General Anesthesia

U.S. Army Lieutenant Colonel Jill R. Keeler has reviewed the possible interactions of pyridostigmine pretreatment on the subsequent management of general anesthesia, based on the known pharmacological activity at cholinergic synapses, and her papers should be consulted for a thorough review of the subject.[19,31] There is very little clinical information on which to draw to confirm these possibilities. The degree of interaction will be related to the amount of acetylcholinesterase inhibition. At the usual pyridostigmine pretreatment dosage, this is usually 40%. Military anesthesia providers should allow for changes in the normal pharmacokinetic profile produced by delayed gastric emptying caused by factors such as traumatic wounding. In this situation, the degree of enzyme inhibition may be less predictable. The possible effects may best be considered in terms of the anesthetic process.

Premedication

In field anesthesia, formal premedication may be comparatively rare. Opioids will often have been administered for pain following wounding. Antimuscarinic drugs are usually given as part of the induction. The cholinergic agonist activity of pyridostigmine would be expected to antagonize the action of such agents as atropine and hyoscine. In most Priority I, IA, and II casualties with either traumatic or toxic wounding or both, the notion of conventional premedication is largely academic; however, the anesthesia provider should be aware of the potential problem and be prepared to administer larger-than-usual doses of atropine.

Induction Agents

Sodium thiopental can provoke asthma in susceptible subjects. Pyridostigmine, through its muscarinic activity, may aggravate this situation but clinical evidence is not available. Thiopental is not considered by some to be an induction agent of choice in a hypotensive battle casualty, particularly when time for preoperative stabilization may be limited. The drug causes a fall in cardiac index, stroke volume, and blood pressure. In theory, pyridostigmine may cause a fall in cardiac output due to its vagal action and subsequent bradycardia. There is, therefore, a risk of synergism between the two drugs, and thiopental may best be avoided. Arylcyclohexamines such as ketamine have an established place in field surgery because they provide good cardiovascular support. Heart rate, contractility, cardiac output, and blood pressure are all maintained owing to sympathetic activity. These will tend to antagonize the muscarinic actions of pyridostigmine. Both pyridostigmine and ketamine increase oral secretions. This may increase the risk of laryngospasm following sensitization of the larynx by ketamine.

Neuromuscular Blocking Agents

Balanced anesthesia involving the use of relaxants with endotracheal intubation and IPPV is highly desirable in field surgery because (*a*) delayed gastric emptying associated with stress during combat means that patients presenting for operation must be assumed to have full stomachs, and (*b*) in a situation where casualties may be numerous and the operative flow heavy, predictable anesthesia and recovery are essential. To achieve success when relaxants are in use, the effects of pretreatment on their characteristics should be considered. As an anticholinesterase, pyridostigmine can affect neuromuscular blockade in three ways: by directly affecting depolarization block, by antagonizing nondepolarizing block, and by effects on repeated stimuli used to assess the degree of nondepolarization block.

Action of Pretreatment on Depolarization Block

Depolarization-blocking drugs such as succinylcholine and decamethonium are structurally related to acetylcholine and work effectively as agonists. In normal neuromuscular transmission, acetylcholine reacts with receptors at the postjunctional folds to produce a depolarization, which induces a muscle action potential in the fiber controlled by the junction. The depolarization is usually short-lived owing to the rapid hydrolysis catalyzed by acetylcholinesterase. Unlike acetylcholine, depolarizing blocking agents are not affected by acetylcholinesterase, and the depolarization they produce lasts for a longer period than acetylcholine lasts. It might be expected that pyridostigmine and the standard depolarization blocking agents would be synergistic in their actions, but the degree of significance of the interaction at the targeted pyridostigmine-induced acetylcholinesterase inhibition level of 30% to 40% has yet to be determined. Apart from considerations of synergism, a more important effect of pyridostigmine is on butyrylcholine esterase. This enzyme is found at many sites in the body, including the plasma, where it is responsible for the normal hydrolysis of succinylcholine. The genetic homozygotic and heterozygotic possibilities controlling the enzyme give rise to the well-recognized syndrome of succinylcholine apnea. Pyridostigmine may cause an unpredictable extension in the duration of action of succinylcholine.

Action of Pyridostigmine on Nondepolarizing Agents

Carbamate anticholinesterases such as neostigmine and pyridostigmine are used routinely to reverse the action of nondepolarizing blocking drugs. They do this by inhibiting the catalytic breakdown of acetylcholine at the postjunctional folds. The concept of giving the reversal drug before the relaxant, however, is far less familiar and may be expected to produce changes in the rate of onset and the minimum level of paralysis produced. Experimental studies[32] have indicated that pyridostigmine does not significantly alter the characteristics of neuromuscular block in adductor pollicis in the isolated human forearm, and therefore the clinical significance may be minimal. Since more central muscles, such as the diaphragm, may have a higher safety margin of neuromuscular transmission, the results on adductor pollicis are a good indicator that pretreatment is unlikely to produce significant clinical effects on the subsequent use of nondepolarizing blocking agents. In practical terms, careful titration of the dose of blocking agents will be necessary to ensure ideal clinical conditions. Electrophysiological studies following pyridostigmine pretreatment have shown little change in jitter, indicating no significant neuromuscular effect of the pretreatment schedule itself.[27]

Effect of Pretreatment on Neuromuscular Monitoring

Train-of-four stimulation monitoring is widely used to assess the degree of recovery of neuromuscular block. Pyridostigmine has a prejunctional, as well as a postjunctional, action. The prejunctional neuromuscular site is thought to be the determinant of fade through a positive feedback mechanism.[33] Therefore, alterations of the conventional fade–block relationship[18] may be possible, and predictions of neuromuscular block may be inaccurate. Experimental evidence in the isolated forearm indicates that the hysteresis relationship between T1 and T4 (of the train-of-four) during onset and recovery of relaxation (differential fade) is unaltered by pyridostigmine.[31]

Inhalational Anesthetics

The anticholinesterase activity of pyridostigmine may give rise to bronchospasm in patients with asthmatic tendency. Inhalational anesthetics such as isoflurane, enflurane, and halothane have a bronchodilator effect, which might antagonize any sensitization of the bronchi by pyridostigmine. In addition, the inhalational agents potentiate the actions of nondepolarizing neuromuscular blocking drugs. This may be an advantage in pyridostigmine-pretreated patients in removing the need for increased dosage of relaxant drugs.

Military Clinical Experience

During the 1991 Persian Gulf War, the number of casualties sustained by the alliance forces was relatively low. Some of these were taking pyridostigmine in anticipation of nerve agent attack. In three casualties with gunshot wounds who were taking pyridostigmine pretreatment and who also required surgery, a technique of total intravenous anesthesia using ketamine, midazolam, and vecuronium was used. Atropine premedication was required because of significant salivation. There was no obvious extension of the action of suxamethonium bromide used for intubation, but there were indications that a larger-than-usual dose of vecuronium was required. It is not clear whether this was due to the total intravenous anesthesia technique or to the pyridostigmine pretreatment. The casualties were all operated on at least 7 hours after taking the last dose of pyridostigmine, and by this stage only about 10% of the acetylcholinesterase could be expected to be complexed. Although these findings are anecdotal, they are a useful indicator for general anesthesia following pyridostigmine pretreatment. The observations on the side effects, in particular, are at variance with previous studies, although it should be noted that the battlefield observations were uncontrolled.

SUMMARY

In the past, military anesthetic policy and experience have largely been involved with conventional physical trauma rather than chemical injury. The continuing risk of casualties from chemical warfare agents enforces a wider view, encompassing casualties who may be suffering from physical, toxic, or environmental trauma, or from any combination. Chemical agent injury may affect all body systems, and military anesthesia providers may be involved in its management either directly or as part of the perioperative management of coincident physical trauma. Chemical casualties should be expected at any time during conflict and not just in unique circumstances, and chemical weapons should now be considered as tactical weapons rather than necessarily as weapons of mass destruction. Preparations for chemical agent casualties should, therefore, be made in all military actions, particularly those involving rapid-response forces in unusual areas.

The concept of chemical weapons has now been extended to cover agents previously described as toxins or biological agents. A spectrum of toxic agents exists, in which agents that differ considerably in their physical nature may have common pathophysiological pathways of clinical damage.

The chemical–biological warfare spectrum reminds military anesthesia providers of the need to respond to the dysfunction of systems rather than solely to the specific management of individual toxic agents. All agents in the spectrum possess three main characteristics: toxicity, latency of action, and transmissibility. The serious consequence of transmissibility is that toxic agents, unlike other weapons, pose a continuing danger to medical attendants down the evacuation line.

Military anesthesia providers must be totally familiar with current teaching about protection, detection, and decontamination of toxic agents. The use of CAM and ICAD will facilitate all practices. IPE-MOPP gear may be required for anesthesia providers working at early stages of casualty management. These protective ensembles will enforce isolation from the casualty and make difficult the contact necessary for simple monitoring and airway management. When the casualty's life is threatened, it may be necessary to remove his respirator to gain access to the airway, since the dangers from the existing respiratory failure may outweigh the risks from further inhalation of the agent. Collective protection offers greater freedom for casualty assessment, resuscitation, and anesthesia, but conditions may be cramped.

Much as the knowledge of the type of trauma sustained may be a useful predictor of the nature of physical injury, so knowledge of the toxic agent may also predict the extent of toxic injury. This is particularly true in the case of long-latency agents, where the symptoms and signs may not yet have fully developed. In some instances, specific knowledge of the agent used may not be available, and treatment should be based on the casualty's presenting signs and symptoms. Toxic agents may affect the skin, viscera, blood, mitochondria, central and peripheral nervous systems, and the respiratory system. In the last category, agents may affect the respiratory center, respiratory muscles, nasopharynx, larynx, large and small airways, and the alveoli. Careful clinical assessment of all systems is vital. Signs present in one system may provide valuable clues about developing pathology in others.

The responsibilities of the anesthesia provider in the management of toxic injury start with planning in the preattack phase. Specific responsibilities include being knowledgeable about the hospital's plans for casualty reception, including decontamination and resuscitation of chemical casualties. Military anesthesia providers will be intimately involved in preoperative assessment of prophylactic measures, toxic agent effects, and therapeutic measures on the subsequent course of anesthesia. They may be asked to advise surgeons on toxic morbidity factors; the perioperative management of casualties with combined conventional and chemical injuries; and the management of toxic, anesthetic, and surgical postoperative complications, including intensive care.

A system of triage must be created for casualties who have been exposed to toxic agents, and conventional triage systems should be modified to take account of toxic factors. Careful preoperative assessment is required, since toxic factors may radically alter the normal patterns of anesthesia. The respiratory and neuromuscular systems are particularly important. Induction and maintenance of, and recovery from, general anesthesia may all be affected by toxic injury and its therapy. A casualty's responses to neuromuscular blocking drugs may particularly be altered after nerve agent exposure. The action of succinylcholine may be prolonged and the nondepolarizers antagonized. Nerve agent paralysis itself may permit surgical intervention but is likely to be unreliable. Given the problems posed to general anesthesia, careful consideration must be given to the use of regional anesthetic techniques; spinal and epidural anesthesia may, however, provoke unstable cardiovascular responses after nerve agent attack.

Postoperative complications may be significant. Serious and frequently fatal damage to the large and small airways can result from the inhalation of droplets or vapor of vesicant agent. Pulmonary edema is a consequence of several toxic agents, including conventional lung-damaging agents (eg, phosgene) and vesicants (eg, mustard gas). Neurological complications may follow nerve agent poisoning. Evidence from organophosphate pesticide poisoning, but not so far with nerve agents, indicates a relapse of neuromuscular paralysis 24 hours after exposure and following apparent recovery with atropine and oxime treatment (the intermediate syndrome). The recurring paralysis is nondepolarizing in nature. There may also be a later stage of peripheral neuropathy. Toxic complications will increase the likelihood of postoperative intensive care.

Pretreatment with pyridostigmine as a prophylaxis against nerve agent poisoning has several implications for military anesthetic practice. Inhibition of butyrylcholine esterase may cause the action of succinylcholine to be prolonged. Although experimental studies have not indicated significant antagonism of the action of nondepolarizing relaxants, clinical experience in this area is scarce. Reports of casualties who had taken pyridostigmine, and who subsequently received total intravenous anesthesia for surgery following traumatic, not toxic agent, injuries, indicate that the amount of vecuronium required may possibly be increased. At present, it may be said that pyridostigmine pretreatment adds to the uncertainty of clinical anesthesia for incidental operative intervention.

There has been very little recent experience of anesthesia after toxic injury in warfare, and the subject still remains one of speculation. Good planning and familiarity with standard procedures will reduce the undoubted difficulties likely to be encountered in the anesthetic interface with casualties of toxic weapons.

Acknowledgment

The authors thank Frederick R. Sidell, M.D., Chief, Chemical Casualty Care Office, and Director, Medical Management of Chemical Casualties Course, U.S. Army Medical Research Institute of Chemical Defense, Aberdeen Proving Ground, Maryland, for his expert scientific and doctrinal review of this chapter in its developmental stages.

REFERENCES

1. US Departments of the Army, the Navy, and the Air Force. *Treatment of Chemical Agent Casualties and Conventional Military Chemical Injuries*. Washington, DC: HQ DA, DN, DAF; 28 February 1990. Army Field Manual 8-285, Navy Medical Pamphlet 504, Air Force Manual 160-11.

2. Command of the Defence Council. *Medical Manual of Chemical Defence Against Chemical Agents*. London, England: Ministry of Defense, Her Majesty's Stationery Office; 1987: JSP 312, ¶ 1010.

3. Bellamy RF, Zajtchuk R, eds. *Conventional Warfare: Ballistic, Blast, and Burn Injuries*. Part 1, vol 5. In: Zajtchuk R, Jenkins DP, Bellamy RF, eds. *Textbook of Military Medicine*. Washington, DC: US Department of the Army, Office of The Surgeon General, and Borden Institute; 1991: Chaps 5, 9.

4. Committee on Trauma, American College of Surgeons. *Advanced Trauma Life Support Program for Physicians: Instructor Manual*. 5th ed. Chicago, Ill: American College of Surgeons; 1993.

5. United Nations. Report of the specialists appointed by the Secretary-General to investigate allegations by the Islamic Republic of Iran concerning the use of chemical weapons. New York, NY: UN; 26 March 1984. UN Document S/16433.

6. United Nations. Report of the mission dispatched by the Secretary-General to investigate allegations of the use of chemical weapons in the conflict between Iran and Iraq. New York, NY: UN; 12 March 1986. UN Document S/17911.

7. United Nations. Report of the mission dispatched by the Secretary-General to investigate allegations of the use of chemical weapons in the conflict between the Islamic Republic of Iran and Iraq. New York, NY: UN; 8 May 1987. UN Document S/18852.

8. Restall J. Consultant Advisor in Anaesthetics, Royal Army Medical Corps, United Kingdom. Personal communication, 1992.

9. Gilchrist HL. Statistical consideration of gas casualties. In: Weed FW. *Medical Aspects of Gas Warfare*. Vol 14. In: Ireland MW. *The Medical Department of the United States Army in the World War*. Washington, DC: Government Printing Office; 1926: Chap 8: 275–277.

10. Hemsley J. *The Soviet Biochemical Threat to NATO*. London, England: Royal United Services Institute/Macmillan; 1987.

11. Colardyn F, de Keyser H, Ringoir S, de Bersaques J. Clinical observation and therapy of injuries with vesicants. *Journal de Toxicologie Clinique et Experimentale*. 1986;6(4):237–246.

12. Geissler E, Lohs KH. The changing status of toxin weapons. In: Geissler E, ed. *Biological and Toxin Weapons Today*. Stockholm, Sweden: SIPRI; 1986: Chap 3.

13. Grande CM. Mechanisms and patterns of injury: The key to anticipation. *Crit Care Clin*. 1990;6:25–36.

14. Ruhl CM, Park SJ, Danisa O, et al. A serious skin sulfur mustard burn from an artillery shell. *J Emerg Med*. 1994;12:159–166.

15. Keeler JR, Hurst CG, Dunn MA. Pyridostigmine used as a nerve agent pretreatment under wartime conditions. *JAMA*. 1991;266(5):693–695.

16. Grob D, Harvey AM. Effects in man of the anticholinesterase compound sarin (isopropyl methyl phosphonofluoridate). *J Clin Invest*. 1958;37:350–368.

17. Kalow W, Ganest K. A method for the detection of atypical forms of human serum cholinesterase: Determination of dibucaine numbers. *Can J Biochem*. 1957;35:339.

18. Ali HH, Savarese JJ. Monitoring of neuromuscular function. *Anesthesiology*. 1976;45:216–249.

19. Keeler JR. Drug interaction of combined use of nerve agent pretreatment with anesthetics, analgesics and other battlefield medications. Aberdeen Proving Ground, Md; 1988. US Army Medical Research Institute for Chemical Defense TR-88-08.

20. Grob D, Harvey JC. Effects in man of the anticholinesterase compound sarin (isopropyl methyl phosphonofluoridate). *J Clin Invest*. 1958;37:350–368.

21. Willems JL. Clinical management of mustard gas casualties. *Annales Medicinae Militaris Belgicae*. 1989;3(suppl)1–61:47, 51.

22. Freitag L, Firusian N, Stamatis G, Greschuchna D. The role of bronchoscopy in pulmonary complications due to mustard gas inhalation. *Chest*. 1991;100:1436–1441.

23. Gall D. The use of therapeutic mixtures in the treatment of cholinesterase inhibition. *Fund Appl Toxicol*. 1981;1: 214–216.

24. Sidell F. Chief, Chemical Casualty Care Office, and Director, Medical Management of Chemical Casualties Course, US Army Medical Research Institute of Chemical Defense. Aberdeen Proving Ground, Md. Personal communication, August 1994.

25. Senanayake N, Karralliede L. Neurotoxic effects of organophosphorus insecticides: An intermediate syndrome. *N Engl J Med*. 1987;316:761–763.

26. Churchill-Davidson HR, Christie TH, Wise RP. Dual neuromuscular block in man. *Anesthesiology*. 1960;21:144.

27. Baker DJ. *The Clinical Neurophysiology of Organophosphate Poisoning*. Southampton, United Kingdom: University of Southampton; 1986: Chap 8. Thesis.

28. Tsao TC-Y, Juang Y-C, Lan R-S, Shieh W-B, Lee C-H. Respiratory failure of acute organophosphate and carbamate poisoning. *Chest*. 1990;98(3):631–636.

29. Kluwe WM, Chinn JC, Feder P, Olson C, Joiner R. Efficacy of pyridostigmine pretreatment against acute soman intoxication in a primate model. Proceedings of the Sixth Medical Chemical Defense Bioscience Review. Aug 1987;227–234. AD B121516.

30. Moylan-Jones RJ. The pharmacokinetics of pyridostigmine in humans, II: Multiple dose studies. Chemical Defence Establishment, Porton Down, UK; 1979. CDE Technical Paper 258.

31. Keeler JR. Interactions between nerve agent pretreatment and drugs commonly used in combat anesthesia. *Milit Med*. 1990;155(2):527–533.

32. Turner GA, Williams JD, Baker DJ. Effects of pretreatment with pyridostigmine on subsequent activity of alcuronium in non-anaesthetized subjects. *Br J Anaesth*. 1990;16:365–369.

33. Bowman WC. Prejunctional and postjunctional cholinoceptors at the neuromuscular junction. *Anesth Analg*. 1980;59:935–942.

Chapter 31

A BRIEF HISTORY OF MILITARY ANESTHESIA

MARY ELLEN CONDON-RALL, Ph.D.*

*Military Studies Branch, Center of Military History, Department of the U.S. Army, Washington, D. C. 20005-3402

INTRODUCTION

For 150 years, the medical departments of the U.S. military have provided state-of-the-art anesthesia within the limitations imposed by the battlefield. From the Mexican War (1846–1848), when the first anesthetic was administered during military surgery, to the Persian Gulf War (1990–1991), military medicine has adapted civilian advances in anesthesiology for use in wartime. Those advances included new drugs, new techniques, new machines, and an expanded role for the anesthesia provider. In turn, the civilian practice of anesthesiology has benefited from lessons learned on the battlefield.

For most of this period, civilian anesthetists counseled the military about what to bring and what to leave at home during deployment. Complex and cumbersome machines, logistical priorities, and the need for simplicity at the front complicated the provision of modern anesthesia in war. By the Vietnam War, however, the military had its own anesthesia specialists and was no longer dependent on civilian medicine for advice. In the 1960s, the field of military anesthesia produced intensive care specialists and a decade later, practitioners of critical care. Critical care medicine led to a natural alliance of military and civilian anesthesiology in the treatment of trauma.

This chapter is intended to be a brief survey, not a comprehensive study, of the events surrounding the history of military anesthesia.

EARLY ANALGESICS

Man has tried to conquer pain since the beginning of recorded history. Primitive peoples sought pain relievers in herbs, roots, seeds, flowers, opium, mandrake, hemlock, the mulberry tree, and even the garden lettuce, among other remedies. A sea sponge saturated with the juices of soporific plants became the major analgesic of the Middle Ages, although drugged wine, "not enough drug to be poisonous," but sufficient to put one to sleep, was considered the safest anesthetic. By the middle of the 17th century, whiskey, gin, and rum had replaced most drugs, considered unsafe since there was no way to standardize dosage, although occasionally physicians used opium. The search for a successful anesthetic continued, but, "in practice, the reduction of pain depended upon the speed of the surgeon."[1(p44)]

The fear of pain kept patients from committing themselves to the surgeon's knife. Many preferred to risk death than to undergo the terrible agony of an operation while fully conscious. Once strapped to the table, some screamed and struggled, begging the surgeon to be quick; some "fell into a trance-like state," which made the operation easier but did not bode well for their recovery; some cursed or prayed; some endured bravely and quietly; others wept and fainted (Figure 31-1). All suffered "severe nervous

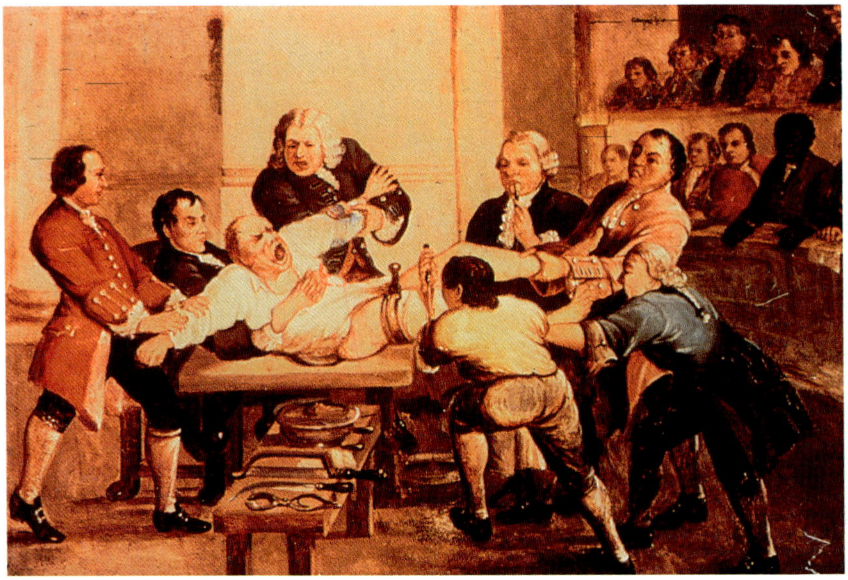

Fig. 31-1. Surgery and anesthesia before ether (ca 1800). Photograph: Courtesy of William Clayton Petty, MD, Captain, Medical Corps, US Navy, Bethesda, Md.

shock" and afterward a "long period of depression,"[2(pp505–506)] which interfered with healing and delayed convalescence. Only recently have scientists discovered that severe pain actually produces chemical imbalances in the brain that can cause depression and death. The 19th-century British surgeon Sir Benjamin Richardson wrote:

> I have heard many express that if they had known beforehand what the suffering was, and the effects subsequently endured, they would rather have faced death than such a fearful struggle for continued existence.[2(pp505–506)]

The presence of pain also interfered with the development of surgery as a science. Because of the patient's fear of pain, and the surgeon's unwillingness to operate except in traumatic amputations or as a last resort, when all else had failed, operations were few in number. They also were few in kind, because of the necessity of devising operations that could be done quickly. In the 18th century, these were chiefly confined to the surface of the body, including excision of tumors, amputation of limbs, various plastic operations, cataract removal, lithotomy, and herniotomy. With pain such a barrier to good surgery and the saving of life, it is not surprising that men through the centuries have sought ways to alleviate it.[2]

THE EVOLUTION OF ANESTHESIA

The search for a successful anesthetic received great impetus with the discovery of gases and their effects on respiration. In 1772, the Englishman Joseph Priestley discovered nitrous oxide gas (Figure 31-2). Twenty-eight years later, Humphry Davy determined that nitrous oxide destroyed physical pain and suggested the anesthetic possibilities of the agent (Figure 31-3). In 1818, Michael Faraday noted the soporific effects of sulfuric ether after breathing the gas himself and anesthetizing a cat. His achievement received little attention. In 1824, Henry Hill Hickman, another Englishman, successfully anesthetized animals with carbon dioxide, introducing the principle of anesthesia by inhalation. His published results became the first separate publication on anesthesia. In their day, Davy's, Faraday's, and Hickman's discoveries received slight notice.[1,3]

Hypnosis as a method of pain relief received impetus from the work of Franz Anton Mesmer (1734–1815) of Vienna, which advocated "animal magnetism" as a cure for body ailments. Although contemporary physicians and scientists thought of him as a quack, Mesmer had followers in Britain, the United States, and India who claimed to have performed operations under mesmerism. Apostles of somnambulism, a development of mesmerism, became convinced of its ability to relieve pain during surgical procedures. Also, James Braid of Manchester believed that hypnotism could either moderate the pain or produce a state whereby the patient was unaware of the pain. Although other practitioners of surgery failed to produce painless operations with this method, their attempts helped to establish a mind-set for the possibility and acceptance of surgery without pain.[1,3]

Pain continued to dominate surgery and interfere with its advancement as a science. Then the discovery of ether anesthetic changed everything.

The Discovery

The search for painless surgery has many precursors, but four names will always be linked with its discovery, each vying for the honor of being the discoverer of anesthesia and each with his own partisans. Crawford W. Long (Figure 31-4), a Georgia physician, in 1842 excised two tumors from a patient under ether but delayed publication of the event and lost the worldwide recognition he might have received.

Horace Wells, a dentist from Hartford, Connecticut, used nitrous oxide (laughing gas) in his practice in 1844 but was unable to stage a successful public demonstration of the gas in surgery in Boston, Massachusetts. Although ridiculed after his failure, he continued to use nitrous oxide on his own patients. William T. G. Morton, a Boston dentist, used ether to extract a patient's abscessed tooth (Figure 31-5). Morton had witnessed Wells's experiments with nitrous oxide and had followed the suggestion of Charles Thomas Jackson, a chemist, to use pure ether instead of laughing gas.

On 16 October 1846, a little more than a fortnight after the painless tooth extraction, Morton successfully demonstrated ether anesthesia in a surgical operation at Massachusetts General Hospital. This staging of the first successful demonstration of ether anesthesia resulted in a gradual acceptance and graded application of this method for painless surgery. Jackson claimed the triumph for himself because of his suggestion to use ether instead of nitrous oxide.

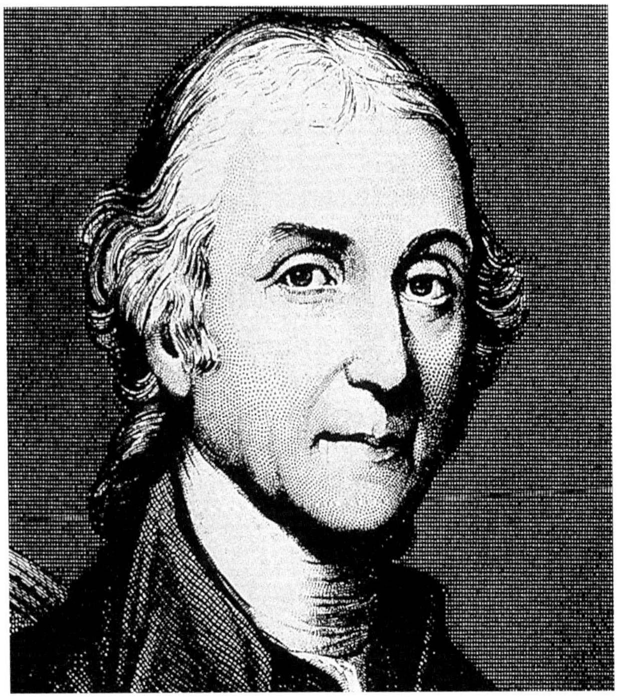

Fig. 31-2. Joseph Priestley (1733–1804) is the man most responsible for introducing modern chemical and physical studies of gases. A politically controversial, nonconformist minister, he produced and described nitrous oxide in 1772. Photograph: Reprinted with permission from Thomas KB. *The Development of Anaesthetic Apparatus*. Oxford, England: Association of Anaesthetists of Great Britain and Ireland, Blackwell Scientific Publications; 1975: 106.

a

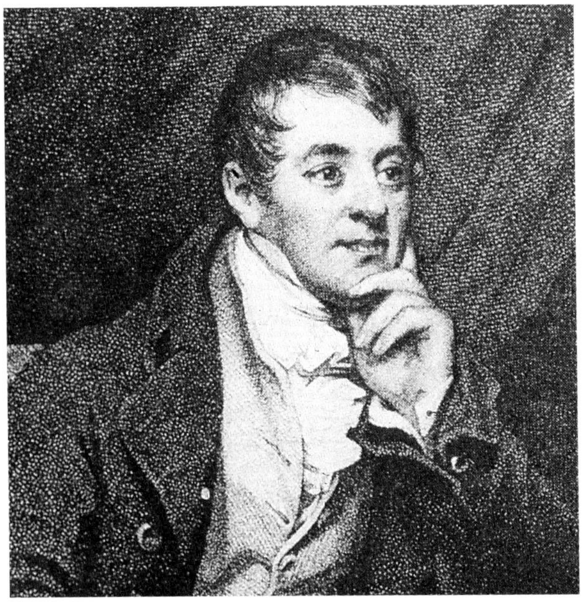

b

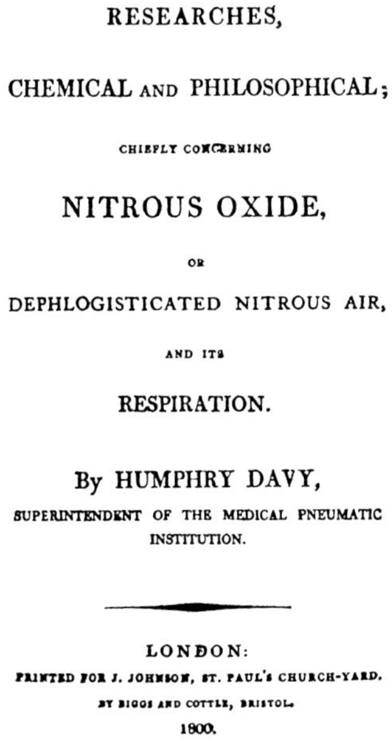

RESEARCHES,

CHEMICAL AND PHILOSOPHICAL;

CHIEFLY CONCERNING

NITROUS OXIDE,

OR

DEPHLOGISTICATED NITROUS AIR,

AND ITS

RESPIRATION.

By HUMPHRY DAVY,

SUPERINTENDENT OF THE MEDICAL PNEUMATIC INSTITUTION.

LONDON:

PRINTED FOR J. JOHNSON, ST. PAUL'S CHURCH-YARD,

BY BIGGS AND COTTLE, BRISTOL.

1800.

Fig. 31-3. (**a**) Sir Humphry Davy (1778–1829) was the first to describe the analgesic properties of nitrous oxide. This steel engraving was made from a portrait by Thomas Phillips, which was painted in 1826 when Davy was President of the Royal Society. (**b**) In 1800, at the age of 22, Davy published his first major contribution in what became a magnificently productive career. Photograph (a): Reprinted with permission from Nuland SB. *The Origins of Anesthesia*. Birmingham, Alabama: The Classics of Medicine Library, Gryphon Editions, Ltd; 1983: 190. Photograph (b): Reprinted with permission from the American Society of Anesthesiologists, Park Ridge, Ill.

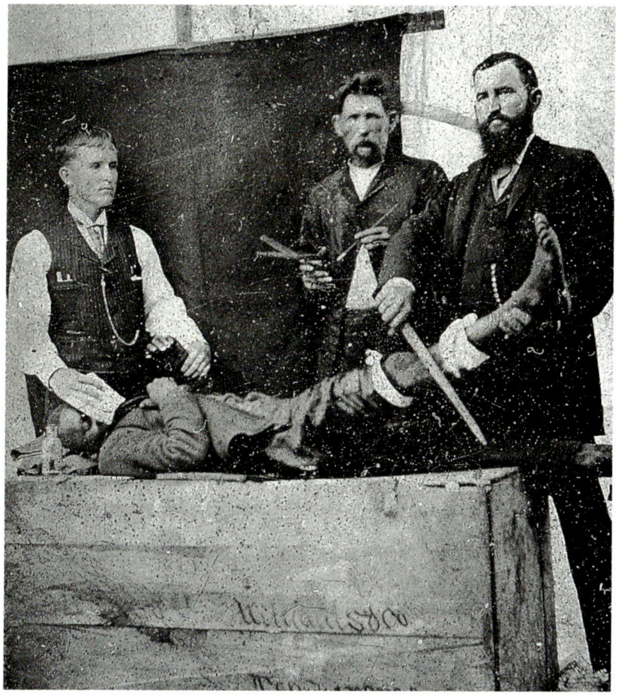

Fig. 31-4. Crawford Williamson Long administered ether for a surgical procedure 4 years before the public demonstration of ether anesthesia by William T. G. Morton. This photograph, one of the few known of Long (1815–1878), from Jefferson, Georgia, was probably taken between 1854 and 1861. It depicts a staged demonstration of an amputation under ether anesthesia. Long is believed to represent the "surgeon"; his brother, the "anesthetist," holds an ether-impregnated cloth over the mouth and nose of the "patient." Photograph: Reprinted with permission from Special Collections, Briscoe Library of The University of Texas Health Science Center, San Antonio, Tex.

a

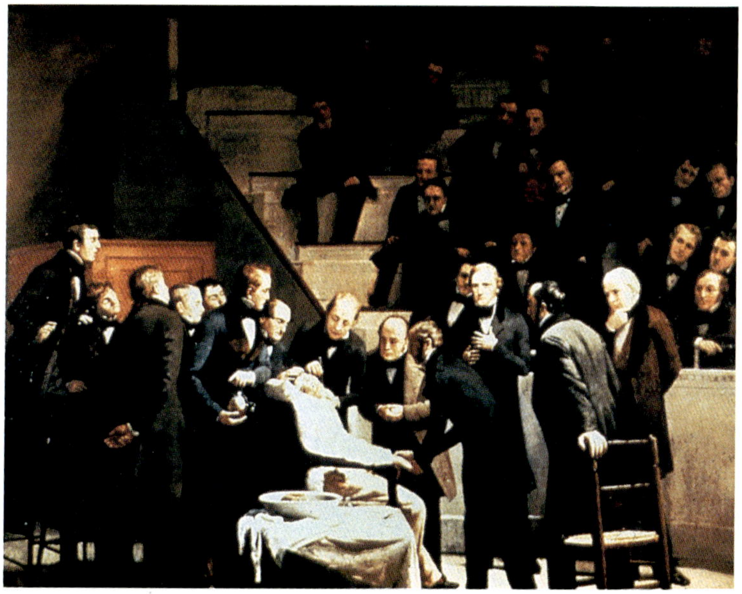

b

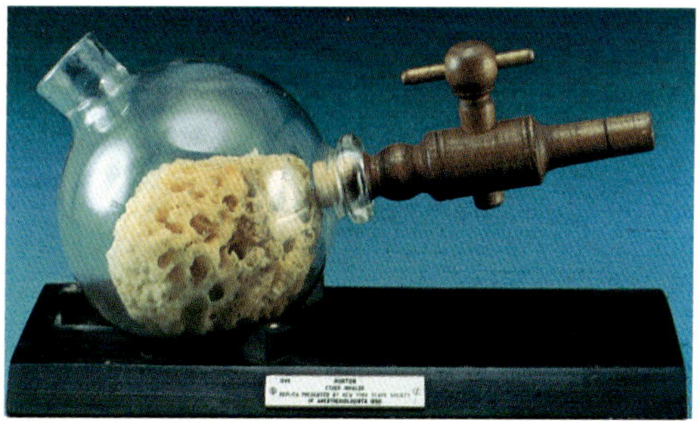

Fig. 31-5. (**a**) This famous painting by artist Robert Hinckley (1853–1941), "The First Operation With Ether," shows William Thomas Green Morton (1819–1868) first publicly administering sulfuric ether to a surgical patient on 16 October 1846 in the Massachusetts General Hospital surgical amphitheater. (**b**) Morton's ether inhaler (1846). This is a replica of the apparatus used in the first successful public demonstration of ether anesthesia. Photograph (a): Reprinted from John Knowles, MD, and Henry R. Viets, MD, Boston, Mass. In: *JAMA*. 1965;194(2):cover. Photograph (b): Reprinted with permission from the Charles King Collection of Historic Anaesthetic Apparatus (Colour Slide Collection), Association of Anaesthetists of Great Britain and Ireland, London, England.

Like so many other discoveries, ether anesthesia was the culmination of many hours of research and discovery, and to many belong the credit. Regardless of who gets the honor, ether anesthesia remains one of the most important discoveries in the history of medicine and an essential element in the development of the art of surgery.[1,4]

Improvements in ether administration began appearing from the time of its discovery. The original method of dropping ether on cloths and inhaling it from them gave way to ether administration by means of an inhaler apparatus, which produced more uniformly successful results. The first ether inhaler, designed by William Morton and used by him from the first, consisted of a glass globe containing an air hole, a glass tube, and a mouthpiece with valves that permitted the patient to inhale a mixture of ether and air into his lungs and exhale the breathed vapor into the room.

By the spring of 1847, nasal inhalation—breathing ether through the nose—was in use. A simple sea sponge shaped to fit the face and then saturated with ether replaced Morton's cumbersome glass vessel. Meanwhile, Morton patented his invention and tried unsuccessfully to sell it to the U.S. government for use on the Mexican front.[1,5]

The Mexican War

Military anesthesia received its baptism of fire during the Mexican War (1846–1848), when a U.S. Army contract physician directed the use of diethyl ether to an accidentally injured teamster in General Winfield Scott's command. In the spring of 1847, using an ether-dispensing apparatus that he had brought with him to Veracruz, Edward H. Barton, surgeon of the Third Dragoons, Cavalry Brigade, Twiggs' Division, successfully anesthetized the patient before the amputation of both legs. An eyewitness to the surgery proclaimed:

> The unfortunate man was soon rendered completely insensible to all pain, and indeed, to everything else, and the limb was removed without the quiver of a muscle.[6(p30)]

The first military use of anesthesia was a resounding success.

Despite this triumph, a number of surgeons remained skeptical of the new discovery, complaining of its dangerous side effects. U.S. Army surgeon John B. Porter attributed severe hemorrhage during an amputation in summer, 1847,

> to the pernicious influence of the ether. [He remarked that] anesthetics poison the blood and depress the nervous system, and, in consequence, hemorrhage is more apt to occur, and union by adhesion is prevented.[7(p18)]

He considered anesthetic agents to be unnecessary and even injurious in the treatment of gunshot wounds and, at the end of the war, decided never to use them again. Future anesthesiologists would know that ether evaporates more quickly at warmer temperatures; that soldiers in pain, shock (ie, hypovolemia), and hemorrhage respond differently to the anesthetic; and that a low cardiac output increases sensitivity to the depressant action of anesthetics.[7–9]

Porter also believed painless surgery to be an unnecessary interference in the soldier's development of healthy, masculine endurance, a view held by military surgeons on both sides of the Atlantic. "Heroic manly fortitude, heightened by the 'excitement' of battle, rendered soldiers insensitive to the pain of 'almost any operation,'"[10(p150)] declared British military surgeon Rutherford Alcock. At this time, most military surgeons scoffed at surgical anesthesia as a product "of misguided effeminate sentimentalism."[10(p146)] In 1847, this viewpoint, plus fear of the unfamiliar, prejudice, and staunch opposition to change, blinded army surgeons to the value of ether. As a result, they used anesthesia sparingly during the Mexican War and forfeited an opportunity to contribute significantly to the growth of the new science.[1,10]

In 1849, however, the almost universal acceptance of ether anesthesia prompted the U.S. Army to order an allowance of 2 lb of sulfuric ether for every 100 men, officially sanctioning the drug's use. The army added chloroform, discovered in 1847, to its list of regular drugs for the purpose of testing its advantages in surgical operations. Although occasional sudden convulsions and deaths were attributed to chloroform, the drug had certain advantages over ether: small doses of chloroform would put the patient to sleep quickly and peacefully; and the drug was neither flammable, a matter of considerable concern during the days of operations by candlelight, nor odorous like ether. Therefore, chloroform was more pleasant to take.

The administration was made easier by Englishman John Snow's development of a chloroform inhaler (Figure 31-6). This device, composed entirely of metal, a conductor of heat, and placed in contact with water to regulate temperature, enabled the anesthetist to control the strength of the

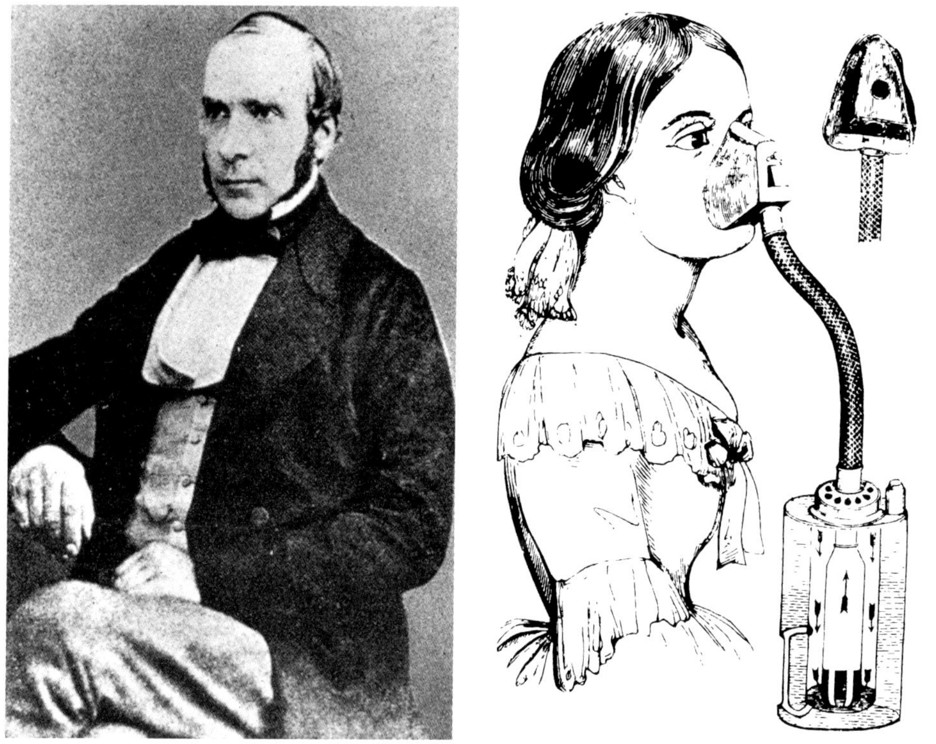

Fig. 31-6. (**a**) The Englishman John Snow (1813–1858) was the first physician to specialize in anesthesia. (**b**) He produced this chloroform inhaler in February 1848. Snow devoted his life to making the art of anesthesiology a science; he also made lasting contributions to epidemiology. Photographs: Reprinted with permission from Shephard DAE. History of anaesthesia: John Snow and research. *Can J Anaesth.* 1989;36(2):224, 230.

vaporized air. Chloroform became the drug of choice for British surgeons. U.S. surgeons used chloroform for eye surgery but preferred ether for other operations, considering its odor the only significant drawback. Military surgeons used both anesthetics.[7,11,12]

During the War in the Crimea (1853–1856), the British army used chloroform almost exclusively, and the French employed the agent often. George H. B. Macleod, a British surgeon, became convinced of chloroform's attributes as a result of his experiences during the war. The Crimean War

> has shown that chloroform, both directly and indirectly saves life; that it abates a vast amount of suffering; that its use is as plainly indicated in gunshot as in other wounds; that if administered with equal care, it matters not whether the operation about to be performed be necessitated by a gunshot wound, or by any of the accidents which occur in civil life.[13(p126)]

Although sulfuric ether and chloroform became the two most popular anesthetics before the American Civil War, civilian physicians tried other agents. Surgeons at the Massachusetts General Hospital preferred chloric ether, which is chloroform dissolved in alcohol in assorted ratios, to regular chloroform or ether. Other products cited in the literature of the time included morphine, cocaine, ethylene, amylene, and a method called "the vapor of Benzid." Some very conservative surgeons used none of the anesthetic agents then on the market, relying instead on the old standbys of alcohol and opium. One surgeon declared: "[I]f my patients will have an anesthetic agent [I] will give them as much good whiskey as they will drink."[7(p19)] Some surgeons believed that opium prevented inflammation by lowering irritability.[7]

Between the Mexican War and the American Civil War, most surgeons practiced anesthesia conservatively and selectively, using it only some of the time and only on people meeting certain criteria. The Massachusetts General Hospital performed one of three "potentially painful" operations without anesthesia in 1847 and 1848.[10(p190)] The patient's age, gender, condition, and the type of operation to be performed influenced the surgeon's decision about whether to anesthetize. Children received anesthesia more than anyone else. Women received anesthesia in 69% of minor operations, and men in 50%.[10(p191)] Surgeons made the judgment that men did not need anesthesia as much as women and children.

Both military and civilian surgeons performed surgical anesthesia for amputations more than for any other type of operation, considering it more humane. Many mid–19th-century surgeons believed that surgical anesthesia killed about 5% more patients than operations without anesthetics.[10(p220)] Contemporary statistics retrieved later proved this conclusion incorrect: infection from industrial injuries probably caused deaths that were originally attributed to the anesthetic in operations on seriously injured persons. Still, in the 19th century, surgeons practiced selective anesthetization. They wished "to balance life saving and painkilling, the need to reconcile a universal science with human variability."[10(p238)]

The American Civil War

Mid–19th-century attitudes about anesthetics influenced who received anesthesia early in the American Civil War (1861–1865). Soldiers were at the mercy of military surgeons, who, as in the Mexican War, had almost total control over anesthetic policy.[10] By late 1862, however, the Union army attempted to standardize and centralize anesthetization policy as part of an overall reorganization of the medical service aimed at regulating treatment regimens in general. On 30 October 1862, Jonathan Letterman, Medical Director of the Army of the Potomac, issued a circular letter that embodied a hospital reorganization plan that recommended that each of the 18 division hospitals appoint an assistant surgeon in charge of anesthesia. The circular letter specified who would make the decisions but not what those decisions would be. The individual doctor could still use his own discretion about anesthetization, "[b]ut the degree of centralization instituted by Letterman almost certainly did serve to minimize the extreme variations in military anesthetic use."[10(p183)]

Letterman's concern was propitious, considering the widespread use of anesthetics during the Civil War. The army medical service reported employing surgical anesthesia in no fewer than 80,000 cases. Surgeons preferred chloroform 76%[14(p887)] of the time, although a mixture of ether and chloroform, or ether alone, were popular in general hospitals. The average insensibility time for chloroform was 9 minutes, compared with 17 minutes for ether and chloroform and 16 minutes for ether alone.[14(p896)] Because of its ease of induction and the small amounts required, chloroform was the anesthetic of choice for field surgeons, who were surrounded by wounded soldiers in need of rapid relief.

Medical officers also liked the drug's nonflammability, its sweet smell, and its tendency to produce less vomiting and excitability among patients. Aware of its dangers—on occasion, patients inhaling the drug became convulsive and suffered cardiac arrest and sometimes liver damage—surgeons were careful to place time limits on the administration of chloroform and to ensure that the patient inhaled adequate amounts of air along with the anesthetic. In cases of exhaustion resulting from long-established injuries, when chloroform was considered too dangerous to use, ether became the preferred anesthetic agent.[7,14,15]

Despite the overwhelming use of anesthetics, the North reported, for cases studied, only 37 deaths due to the administration of chloroform; the South reported 2. One Confederate doctor exclaimed: "The safety of the substance was remarkable when you consider how loosely it was used!"[15(p95)] The Army Medical Department cited only 2 deaths from ether and 2 from chloroform and ether. The practice of cautious administration of anesthetics by surgeons of both armies may account for the good safety record. However, that chloroform anesthesia caused so few deaths in an era of little patient monitoring is difficult to believe. Many anesthesia deaths may have gone unrecorded or were incorrectly attributed to wounds. In March 1865, Surgeon General Joseph K. Barnes was sufficiently troubled by anesthesia deaths that he ordered U.S. Army surgeons to report on their experiences with these agents.[7,14,15]

The mode of administration of ether, chloroform, or a mixture of both remained quite simple during the Civil War. In a technique known as the *open* method, a liquid-soaked sponge, cloth, or handkerchief was placed over the patient's nose and mouth. For many operations in the open air, a funnel served as an inhaler to prevent excessive evaporation. Although less complicated than the elaborate systems used in modern gas anesthesia, the open method was an effective and relatively safe mode of achieving anesthesia on the battlefield.[14,15]

To prevent the waste of chloroform, a scarce commodity in the South, Confederate surgeon J. J. Chisolm employed a short, flattened cylinder with a plate on its broadest side and two nosepieces connected to the cover. Chloroform dripped through the plate of the Chisolm inhaler onto a sponge or folded cloth, which offered a broad area for evaporation, inside the cylinder. The patient's limpness, a rough but nevertheless quite reliable signal, let the surgeon know that the anesthetic was working and surgery could commence. Often the soldier received a premedication of whiskey to calm his nerves and desensitize him, which also reduced the amount of anesthetic needed.[14,15] A few fearless souls, who probably considered it cowardly to use an anesthetic, "would simply lean back and let the bloody operator saw away, telling the anesthetist to save his sweet-smelling potion for those who came in screaming."[15(p96)]

For the alleviation of pain, army surgeons also used analgesics such as alcohol and opiates. The widespread use of alcohol to relax a patient before the administration of an anesthetic caused some medical officers to worry about the masking of symptoms, but that problem never became significant during the Civil War. However, the possible overuse of opiates, especially opium in the treatment of diarrhea, was blamed for the many cases of drug addiction reported after the war. To reduce pain, army physicians also administered morphine and, on occasion, cannabis for tetanus and head injuries.[7]

The supply of anesthetic agents during the war remained more than adequate for the North but just marginal for the South. The drug manufacturer E. R. Squibb, the North's chief supplier, had perfected the method of mass production of drugs at Brooklyn's U.S. Naval Hospital laboratory a few years before the war started. Capturing medical supplies also augmented stocks. Supply trains of both sides got bogged down in mud or fell victim to enemy raiding parties. For example, Stonewall Jackson's men ran off with thousands of cases of chloroform at the Battle of Winchester. The South often used this form of supply replenishment.[15]

Anesthesia came into its own during the Civil War. Military surgeons demonstrated its usefulness beyond doubt and improved its safety through the knowledge acquired from thousands and thousands of administrations of ether and chloroform.[15]

Late–19th-Century Advancements

During the latter part of the 19th century, surgical anesthesia advanced to include new administrative techniques, other drugs with special properties, and innovative machines for the delivery of anesthetics. Closed inhalers, which had been improved since the Morton and Snow devices of the 1840s and 1850s, appeared in greater numbers. Noteworthy was the J.T. Clover inhaler, which regulated the flow of the anesthetic with air or with another anesthetic (Figure 31-7). Gardner Q. Colton popularized the use of pure nitrous oxide in dental operations in 1863. A mixture of nitrous oxide and oxygen appeared in anesthetic practice and led to the development of gas machines for surgical anesthesia. The latter were hardly used before World War I.[1–3]

The development of the hypodermic syringe (Figure 31-8) permitted the use of morphine during inhalational anesthesia and as a preanesthetic medication. The discovery of the anesthetic properties of cocaine led to the use of the drug topically in eye surgery, in nerve block anesthesia, by injection in or around the spinal canal to reduce pain, and in the first spinal anesthesia in man. (Spinal anesthesia became generally used in the Vietnam War.) Ethyl chloride became a local anesthetic agent late in the 19th century.[1–3]

William Stewart Halsted discovered conduction anesthesia by injecting the new drug cocaine into a nerve in 1885. The discovery's drawbacks made it controversial. Surgeons feared the lowering of blood pressure, especially in seriously injured patients; the psychic factor of the patient's being aware of his surroundings while undergoing surgery; and the poisonous effect of the drug, which could be habit-forming. With nerve block anesthesia as an option, however, surgeons began to choose the anesthetic to fit the patient rather than to select patients who were fit for anesthesia. The mid–19th-century practice of selective anesthetization was nearly over.[10,16]

The greatest influence on the development of anesthesia as a science was Joseph Lister's discovery of antisepsis during the latter part of the 19th century, which drastically reduced infection in surgery. Antisepsis and anesthesia together led to the advancement of surgery by making surgery less unhygienic and less dangerous. Also contributing to clean surgery at this time was the acceptance of the germ theory of disease in 1890, after developing gradually from the 1860s. Rubber gloves and operating coats began to appear in the operating room about 1900.[17] According to historian Martin S. Pernick:

> The gradual adoption of antiseptic surgery also helped end selective anesthetization.... The complex rituals of Lister's technique virtually demanded that all patients be immobilized with anesthesia.[10(p238)]

a

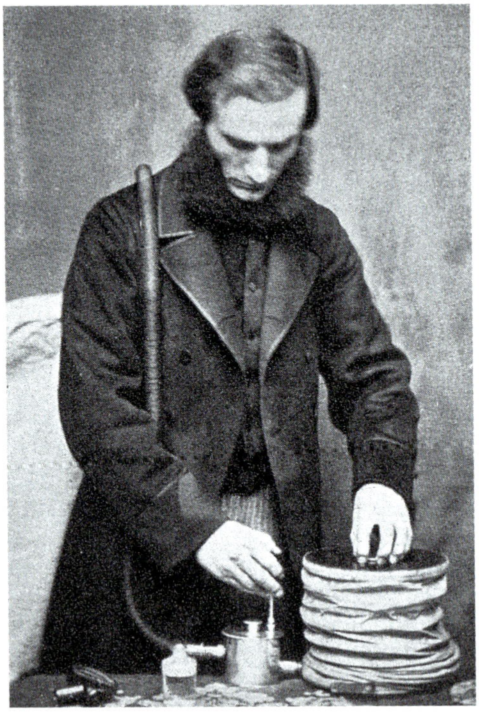

b

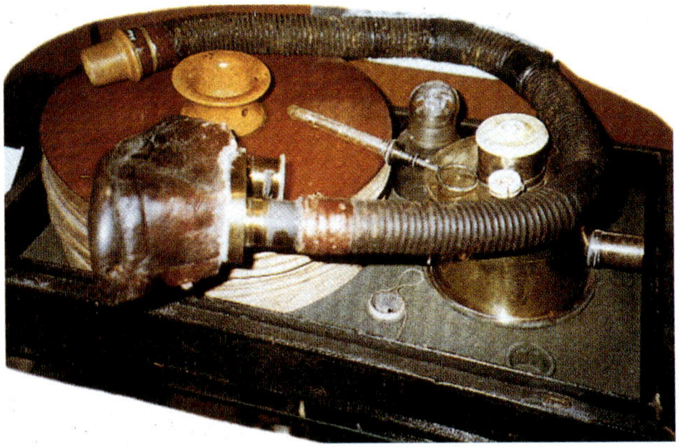

c

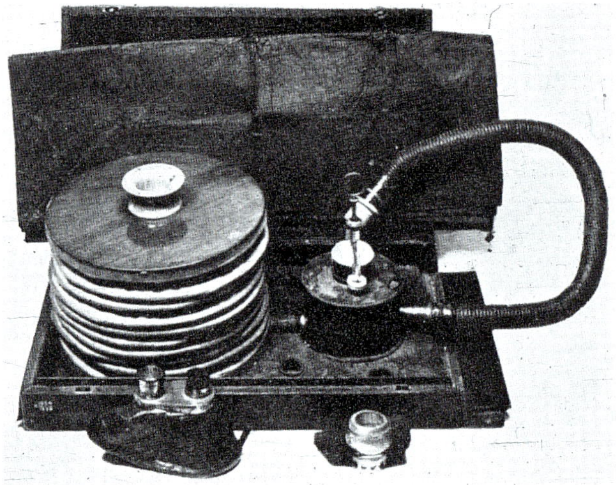

Fig. 31-7. (**a**) Joseph Thomas Clover, shown filling the reservoir bag of his chloroform apparatus with an accurate mixture of 4½% chloroform in air. (**b**) Clover's chloroform apparatus (ca 1860); the original is in the Wellcome Medical Exhibit, Science Museum London, England. A known quantity of chloroform was injected with a syringe onto a warmed metal surface inside the brass container (right). The concertina bag (left) was then filled with air, which was blown into a 7.2-L bag (not shown) with the chloroform. A large-diameter breathing hose and mask were connected to the bag to complete the nonrebreathing circuit. Dr. Clover is said to have given 7,000 anesthetics using 4½% chloroform without a death. (**c**) Clover's chloroform apparatus (ca 1870); the original is likewise in the Wellcome Historical Medical Museum.

The photograph shows the carrying case, folded reservoir bag made of impermeable material, hand bellows, chloroform vaporizing chamber with graduated glass syringe for injecting liquid chloroform, and connecting tube reinforced with a wire coil to prevent kinking. In the foreground, Clover's facepiece with an inflatable rubber rim, a feature that came into use with nitrous oxide anesthesia (ca 1870), and the metal junction, which has become detached from the filling tube and reservoir bag. Photograph (a): Reprinted with permission from Sykes WS. *Essays on the First Hundred Years of Anaesthesia*. Vol 3. Edinburgh, Scotland: Churchill Livingstone; 1982: 133. Sources for (b): (1) Sanson AE. *Chloroform, Its Action and Administration*. London, England: Churchill; 1865: 187. (2) Macintosh R, Mushin WW, Epstein HG. *Physics for the Anaesthetist*. 3rd ed. Oxford, England: Blackwell Scientific Publishers; 1963. Photograph (b): Reprinted with permission from *Wellcome Trends in Anesthesiology*. 1944;12(1):5. Photograph (c): Reprinted with permission from Duncum BM. *The Development of Inhalation Anaesthesia With Special Reference to the Years 1846–1900*. London, England: Oxford University Press, The Wellcome Historical Medical Museum; 1947: 246.

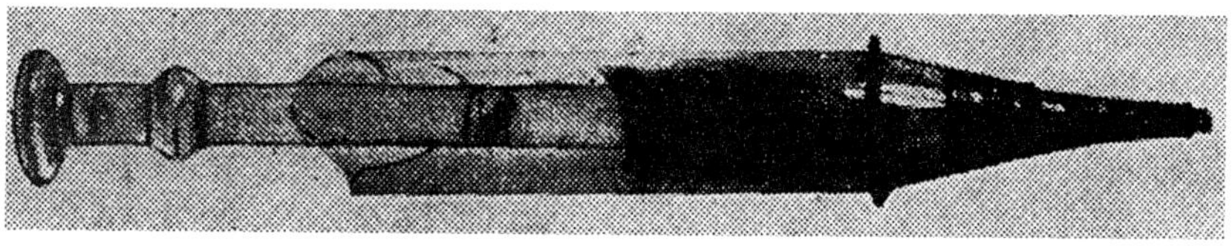

Fig. 31-8. Alexander Wood's syringe, which is displayed in the Royal College of Physicians in Edinburgh, Scotland. Intravenous anesthesia could not have been developed without the syringe, although Wood himself used his syringe to deliver anesthetic *locally*, not intravenously. His 1855 paper was titled *A New Method of Treating Painful Neuralgias by the Direct Application of Opiates to Painful Points*. Photograph: Reprinted with permission from Dundee JW, Wyant GM. *Intravenous Anaesthesia*. Edinburgh, Scotland: Churchill Livingstone; 1988: 1.

The almost universal practice of painless surgery eliminated objections to women becoming surgeons and operating room nurses. In the 1880s, increasing numbers of female personnel began administering anesthetics, under the guidance of surgeons. In the following decade, the U.S. Army had no objection to female nurses working alongside military surgeons in the care of the wounded.[10]

By 1902, both the army and the navy opened graduate schools of military medicine, where military surgeons studied the new science of bacteriology and sanitation mainly for public health work. Graduate medical education outside of the military at this time focused on learning specialized fields, such as antiseptic and aseptic surgery. Modern internship programs were just beginning in the major hospitals in Britain.[18]

The Spanish–American War

Antisepsis, of course, played an important role in the Spanish–American War, which was fought in the Caribbean and the Philippines at the end of the 19th century. During this conflict, antisepsis reduced the four greatest enemies of the wounded soldier: hospital gangrene, secondary hemorrhage, pyemia, and erysipelas. If the wounded survived the immediate effects of the injury—the explosive force of the small-caliber bullet had been greatly overestimated—the prospects of recovery were good.[19]

Actually, military surgeons performed fewer operations and administered less anesthesia per capita during the war with Spain than during the American Civil War. There were no stacks of amputated limbs as there had been during the Civil War. Tropical diseases, such as malaria and yellow fever, were the great killers during the Spanish–American War. To assist an inadequate number of skilled and trained medical officers, the medical department hired female contract nurses. Their help proved so beneficial that after the war, in 1901, they were organized into a female nurse corps under former contract nurse Dita H. Kinney.[19–21]

For surgical patients not seriously enfeebled by disease, chloroform administered by the drop method was the anesthetic of choice. (Drop chloroform was also used extensively during the Boer War [1899–1901] and the Russo-Japanese War [1904].) Soldiers considerably weakened by tropical ailments received ether, which was less potent and slower in onset of action than chloroform and therefore presumably less dangerous in the sick patient. During operations to incise and drain abscesses, surgeons preferred to work without an anesthetic, using only whiskey to relax the patient.[19]

Surgical procedures that posed great danger to the patient were avoided whenever possible. Bullets were allowed to remain in the body undisturbed unless they could readily be removed without additional risk. Some patients with penetrating wounds of the chest and abdomen did well without surgery. Conversely, to save the lives of patients suffering from empyema, surgeons opened chest cavities and extracted pus. A day or two before the operation, they aspirated the patient's pleural space to achieve partial pulmonary expansion before admitting air into the pleural cavity. They preferred to perform the surgery under partial anesthesia, using strychnia and alcohol to minimize the dangers of the anesthetic. In most cases of surgery for empyema, the patients completely recovered.[19]

Surgeons supervised other medical officers and corpsmen in the administration of anesthesia, as the discipline was relatively young and had few specialists. Antisepsis and conservatism helped to make surgery successful during the Spanish–American War.[19]

Although by the turn of the century individual practitioners with special skills were specializing, particularly in the new aseptic surgery—even naval hospitals at this time had the post of supervising surgeon—no formal courses existed in anesthesia. Anesthesia providers were usually medical students, interns, or nurses in metropolitan hospitals, and family practitioners in rural hospitals. They learned to administer anesthesia through observation or from gas machine manufacturers, who would teach the art to anyone who would buy a machine.[18,22]

On the eve of World War I, however, several hospitals in the United States offered to physicians 6 months of postgraduate courses in anesthesia, including instruction in anatomy, physiology of the respiratory tract, pharmacology of anesthetic agents, and training in the administration of the commonly used drugs. For nurses, several hospitals offered courses in the administration of anesthetics, lectures by physicians, and work on cadavers, including the passing of laryngeal tubes.[18,22] Hospital curricula reflected the growing interest in anesthesiology as it was about to enter an important era of its development.

World War I

While still an uncertain science, anesthesiology was forced prematurely into service in World War I (1914–1918). Military anesthesiologists Frederick Courington and Roderick Calverley described the state of the art of anesthesiology in 1914:

> Anesthesia machines were new and hardly widely accepted. There was no standardization of equipment; nothing fit together. Bottled gases were available but miserably cumbersome. Continuous-flow anesthesia with quantification of gas flow was scarce. Wire screen vaporizers, with names like Schimmelbusch, were simple, available, cheap, and "good enough." There were other vaporizers, but most were little improved since the time of Joseph T. Clover, 50 years before the war. Airways were sometimes available, but endotracheal intubation meant that a small, cuffless tube was inserted into the trachea through the glottis for insufflation of ether. Oxygen enrichment of air was uncommon. Nitrous oxide, known in England as "gas" and almost unknown in Europe, was frequently given in various pseudoscientific asphyxial mixtures. There were no muscle relaxants, nor was there an understanding of controlled ventilation or of the need for it. Venipuncture was a surgical cutdown. Rational fluid therapy would not become routine for decades, while blood transfusion was a near perfunctory act, rarely used. Trauma and shock, the unavoidable ingredients of war, were not understood, and therefore not effectively treated. Sir Frederick Hewitt had published a major text of anesthesia in England by 1893, and Dr. James Tayloe Gwathmey, a prominent New York anesthetist, published the first comprehensive American anesthesia text in 1914.[23(pp642–643)]

The *American Journal of Surgery* produced the first *Quarterly Supplement of Anesthesia and Analgesia* in October 1914, 2 months after the war in Europe started.[23]

Personnel

At the start of hostilities in 1914, few anesthesia providers were available to serve on the western front, and anesthesia was often left in the hands of inexperienced people. Early in the war, non-specialty-trained medical officers in the British casualty clearing stations, located at least 7 miles behind the front line and where initial surgery took place, administered anesthesia, often unsuccessfully. One British anesthesiologist remarked: "The bulk of preventable deaths at a casualty clearing station was due to improper anesthesia, giving the wrong anesthetic or giving the right anesthetic wrongly."[24(p103)]

To keep anesthesia out of inexpert hands, the British army appointed anesthesiologists to clearing station staffs in 1916. Even those proved too few to handle the casualties of an enemy push or offensive. After the Battle of the Somme in September 1916, one clearing station received 17,000 stretcher cases and experienced 700 deaths. A Canadian anesthetist lamented the lack of trained anesthetists at this battle:

> In a severe action, a [casualty clearing station] is very busy and I cannot imagine any place where the services of a skilled anesthetist would be more useful. A [casualty clearing station] cannot, however, afford to have too much cumbersome apparatus as when the army moves, it moves too. We had four operating tables going simultaneously. One day we had over 70 operations. A few days before we had admitted 760 wounded within 24 hours. There were a great many severe chest wounds.[23(p644)]

Responsibility for anesthesiology during the Great War rested mainly with reserve officers (both Allied and American) who came from civilian medicine into the armed forces for the duration of the war. Men like George Crile, a surgeon from the Cleveland (Ohio) Lakeside Unit, who volunteered to help the British Expeditionary Forces in France before the United States entered the war. He established an American Ambulance Hospital in Neuilly, bringing his own supplies and trained civilian nurse anesthetists with him. He and most of his staff served in the U.S. Army once the United States entered the war in April 1917. Dr. Crile helped shape the practice of surgery and anesthesiology during World War I.

In anticipation of the United States' entry into the war, the U.S. Army and the U.S. Navy appointed their first anesthesiologists (physician anesthetists) to the Medical Corps in 1916, with the rank of lieutenant. In April 1917, the army drafted dentists for anesthetic service, contracted for women physician anesthetists, and brought in nurse anesthetists to serve at base hospitals in England and France. They joined nurse anesthetists at American Ambulance Hospitals, such as the one run by Dr. Crile at Neuilly. Those women inspired the British army to train over 200 nursing sisters in anesthesia for service in France in 1918. The U.S. Army sent its own nurses to schools of anesthesia that had developed in the United States in response to the demands of war. After training, they returned to their bases to instruct others in anesthesia. (No records are available on the number of nurse anesthetists in the army during the war. On 11 November 1918, the U.S. Army Nurse Corps reached 21,480 nurses: 3,524 were regular nurses and 17,956 were reserve nurses.[22(pp22–23)]) To provide more anesthetists, Dr. Arthur Guedel, a physician anesthetist in charge of anesthesia for the U.S. Army, made daily rounds to base hospitals in the war zone, giving instruction in anesthesia. He administered open-drop ether at field hospitals, commuting between them by motorcycle. Guedel wrote a fundamental guide to inhalational anesthesia in 1937.[22,23,25,26]

To produce skilled combat surgeons, in 1918 the U.S. Army Medical Department's Division of Surgery arranged with some of the nation's finest medical schools to have medical officers receive intensive instruction in war surgery, including the treatment of wounds and the administration of anesthetics. Schools in New York; Boston, Massachusetts; Philadelphia and Pittsburgh, Pennsylvania; Chicago, Illinois; Cleveland, Ohio; New Orleans, Louisiana; and Rochester, Minnesota, participated in the program. On their return to army camps, the medical officers who took the courses instructed others in war surgery and anesthesia.[27]

Despite those efforts, there were never enough experienced anesthesia providers at the front. A nurse anesthetist, who administered anesthesia from June to November 1918, at a U.S. Army mobile hospital in the Chateau-Thierry area of France, recalled:

> How many anesthetics I gave during the World War, I cannot determine, except that when the big drives were on, lasting from a week to ten days, I averaged twenty-five to thirty a day.... During the drives patients came in so fast that all the surgeons could do was to remove bullets and shrapnel, stop hemorrhages and put iodoform packs in the wound and bandage it. As soon as they were through operating on one patient, I would have to have the next patient anesthetized.[22(p24)]

Another anesthetist, who treated 34 cases in 1 day, recalled: "While one patient was being operated on, another was being prepared for surgery, as the dressing was being applied to the third."[23(p645)] The operations during those drives were of necessity quick, deft, and light.

Equipment

Anesthesia providers needed to bring to the front supplies that were mobile and adequate for mass casualties. They also wanted to give the best anesthesia possible. Those wishes were usually contradictory, because the best anesthesia machines were often cumbersome and not easily transportable, and required experts to operate. Additionally, early in the war, certain machines, anesthetic equipment, and agents, as well as skilled anesthetists, were in short supply. For example, in 1917, the army's list of anesthesia supplies included ether, chloroform, and ethyl chloride only—but no anesthetic equipment.[23] World War I anesthetists, like medical men in every war, had to "make do," given the logistical constraints and the newness of the specialty.

The first anesthetists to feel the pinch were those of the British armed forces, who had been fighting since 1914. At the outbreak of war, these men had only chloroform and simple wire vaporizers known as the Schimmelbusch mask (Figure 31-9). Within a few months, ether became available, which they administered by the open method. In 1915, a Canadian medical team brought to England the new Ohio Monovalve anesthesia apparatus, which, unlike British machines, provided a steady flow of gas at a uniform pressure (Figure 31-10).[23,28]

In 1916, the new Shipway ether/chloroform apparatus, although not as advanced as the device from North America, became available. The machine of Dr. Francis Shipway, a British anesthetist, consisted of two bottles, one for chloroform and one for ether, and a three-way tap, which allowed air to be blown through one bottle at a time or through both in varying proportions as one wished. A tube

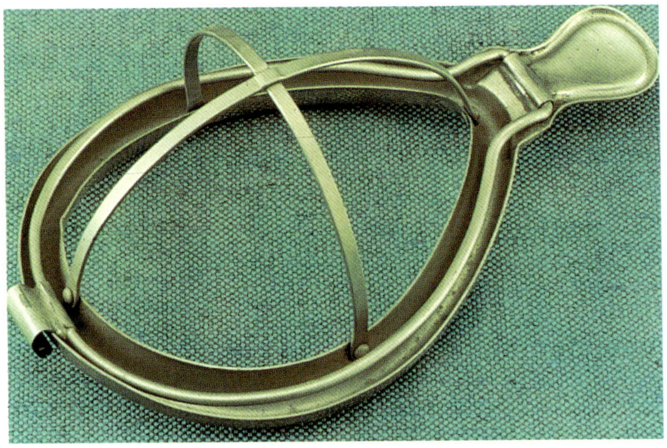

Fig. 31-9. The Schimmelbusch wire frame mask (ca 1890), the most widely known of all wire frame masks, was developed by Carl Schimmelbusch (1860–1895), a surgeon in Berlin, Germany. The lower rim of the mask, which collected surplus anesthetic liquid, is curved to allow air to be drawn under it during chloroform administration. With padding, this wire mask could be used for ether administration. Source: Thomas KB. *The Development of Anaesthetic Apparatus*. Oxford, England: Blackwell Scientific Publications; 1975: 252. Photograph: Reprinted with permission from the Charles King Collection of Historic Anaesthetic Apparatus (Colour Slide Collection), Association of Anaesthetists of Great Britain and Ireland, London, England.

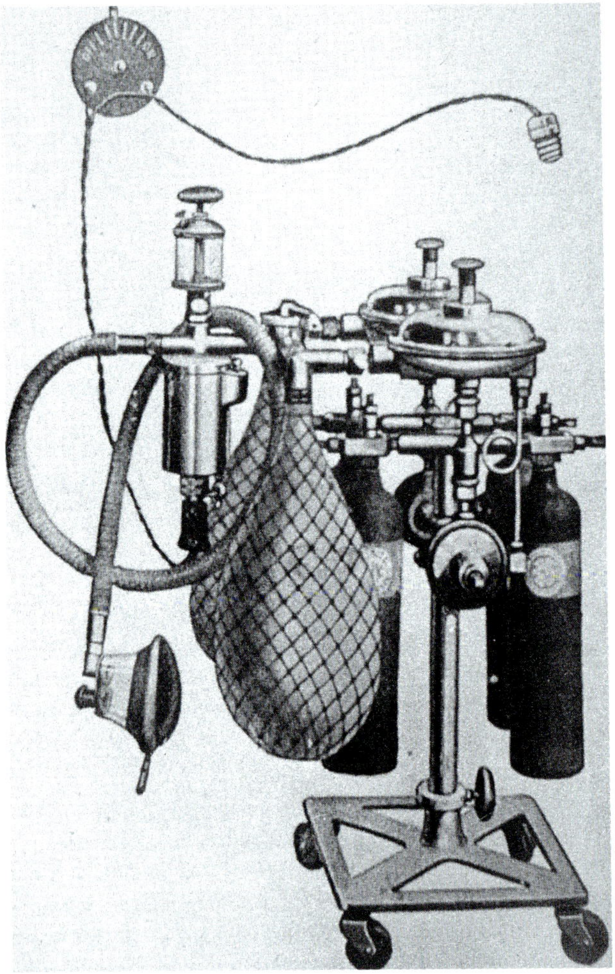

Fig. 31-10. The Ohio Monovalve anesthesia machine, an advanced apparatus from North America, with its continuous flow, multiple gases, and heated vaporizers, also became popular in Europe early in World War I. Photograph: Reprinted from Gwathmey JT. *Anesthesia*. New York, NY: Appleton; 1914.

from the device passed through a lint mask or directly into the patient's mouth or nose. The Shipway apparatus provided even and light administration of the anesthetic and was superior to the drop method. With the advent of the Shipway machine, warm ether vapor became the British anesthetic of choice when nitrous oxide and expert gas administrators were unavailable.[23,28] Shipway's nitrous oxide/oxygen/ether apparatus became available in 1920 (Figure 31-11).

For American anesthetists, the U.S. Army adopted the American Red Cross' nitrous oxide–oxygen machine, perfected by Captain James T. Gwathmey, an anesthetist from New York and a reserve officer who served on the western front (Figure 31-12). Gwathmey's machine provided an airtight mask that fitted closely to the face, an escape valve, a mixing bag close to the inhaler, and a rough gauge for measuring the proportion of the gases. Like the British army, the U.S. Army on the western front had gas machines but little nitrous oxide until a nitrous oxide plant from Cleveland, Ohio, opened in France in mid-1918, just a few months before the war ended. Dr. Crile, a great advocate of the use of gas, had, of course, brought his own supply with him to France. When nitrous oxide was unavailable, the Americans used ether, chloroform, or ethyl chloride, in that order.[29] Logistics became a determinant in the delivery of combat anesthesia.

Anesthetic and Delivery Method of Choice

Since Halsted's discovery of conduction anesthesia in the 1880s, surgeons had begun selecting the anesthetic agent and method of delivery that suited the patient's condition and the type of surgery he needed. This reasoning prevailed at the second session of the Inter-Allied Surgical Conference, held in Paris in 1917.

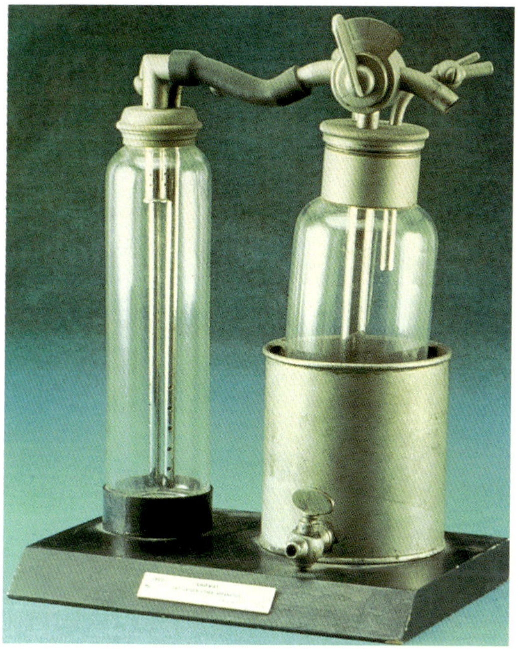

Fig. 31-11. Shipway's nitrous oxide/oxygen/ether apparatus (1920), a modification of earlier equipment, could be used in the draw-over mode if gases were unavailable by means of extra inlets into the ether jar and a complex control tap. Source: Thomas KB. *The Development of Anaesthetic Apparatus*. Oxford, England: Blackwell Scientific Publications; 1975: 152–153. Photograph: Reprinted with permission from the Charles King Collection of Historic Anaesthetic Apparatus (Colour Slide Collection), Association of Anaesthetists of Great Britain and Ireland, London, England.

The conference's conclusions about choice of anesthetic and treatment for war injuries confirmed the value of nitrous oxide in military surgery:

- *Treatment of gaseous gangrene.* Anesthesia by means of nitrous oxide with oxygen is considered the best; when this is not to be had, ether may be substituted.
- *Traumatic shock.* Local anesthesia combined with general anesthesia by means of nitrous oxide is the best. Next to this ether appears to be the least harmful. Spinal injections have produced varying results according to the surgeons employing them, especially in amputations of the lower limbs. The use of chloroform is dangerous.
- *Amputations.* In the case of serious shock, the use of nitrous oxide and oxygen is desirable; ether is the next best anesthetic. Only in the case of cerebral wounds is any other anesthetic method advised.
- *Cerebral wounds.* Local anesthesia is preferred for the operation. The sitting posture tends to diminish hemorrhage and is easily maintained in secondary or delayed operations.[29(p166)]

Allied armies, in general, followed the conclusions of the Paris conference of 1917.

Although healthy men with light wounds could receive any of a number of anesthetics, military surgeons in World War I preferred the advantages of nitrous oxide mixed with oxygen, when they could get it. The British considered the mixture,

> in experienced hands,...the ideal anesthetic for such patients, since it fulfilled the three essential conditions—safety, speed, and a rapid recovery. [The last permitted] immediate evacuation by ambulance and train.[28(p182)]

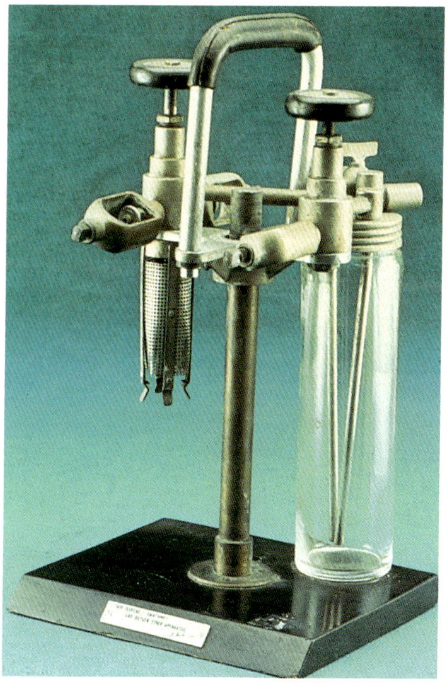

Fig. 31-12. Gwathmey's nitrous oxide/oxygen/ether apparatus (1913). This early apparatus utilized, for the first time in anesthesia, the water-sight flowmeter manufactured by Cotton and Boothby in 1912. The ether bottle is missing in this example of the apparatus, which shows only the flowmeter and cylinder yokes. Source: Thomas KB. *The Development of Anaesthetic Apparatus*. Oxford, England: Blackwell Scientific Publications; 1975: 139–142. Photograph: Reprinted with permission from the Charles King Collection of Historic Anaesthetic Apparatus (Colour Slide Collection), Association of Anaesthetists of Great Britain and Ireland, London, England.

But the ideal method was often unrealistic. Although the gas was beginning to become popular, it was not manufactured in great quantities. Hence, the short supply of nitrous oxide and of skilled administrators until late in the war led the British to use warm ether vapor more than any other anesthetic. For lightly wounded men, the French preferred ethyl chloride because of their "need to induce quickly, perform minimal surgery and transport [patients] sitting up in ambulances."[23(p650)] A vehicle could transport more casualties who were sitting rather than lying down. When the agent of choice was unavailable, the anesthetist made a judicious substitution of another drug and method.[23,28]

For chest surgery, U.S. Army anesthetists chose a light nitrous oxide–oxygen analgesia combined with local anesthesia. Using the results of animal experimentation and accounts from surgical teams at the front, Captain Gwathmey, working out of the U.S. Army's medical research laboratory in France, devised an effective anesthesia for chest surgery. Using a full preoperative dose of morphine to produce analgesia, he gradually

> administered 3:1 nitrous oxide and oxygen under 5–7 mm continuous positive pressure with a mask, adding light ether as required.[23(pp649–650)]
>
> . . . .
>
> During the operation, the proportions of the gas–oxygen mixture and the pressure transmitted to the trachea were varied to meet conditions.[29(p179)]

The Gwathmey method permitted intrathoracic surgery "without necessitating deep anesthesia for the introduction of intratracheal or endopharyngeal tubes."[29(p179)] Although greatly improved anesthesia permitted lifesaving thoracic surgery during World War I, chest surgery remained hazardous for all patients and, in general, "...anesthesia contributed significantly to surgical mortality."[23(pp649–650)]

For thoracic surgery, British anesthetists, in most cases, used chloroform or ether and oxygen with the Shipway apparatus. If the patient was of a placid temperament and sufficiently under the influence of morphia or omnopon, a few surgeons used "local infiltration combined with the administration of gas and oxygen."[28(p183)]

For abdominal operations, both American and British military surgeons established that regional anesthesia with novocaine to relax the abdominal muscles followed by general anesthesia with nitrous oxide–oxygen produced the best results. Warm ether vapor was the accepted substitute for nitrous oxide in those operations.[28,29]

Military surgeons also found nitrous oxide–oxygen, if properly administered, to be the best anesthetic for major amputations. When the gas was not available, surgeons substituted low spinal anesthesia, sometimes with a blood transfusion to overcome the anesthetic's tendency to lower the blood pressure.[28,29]

For operations on the severely wounded in shock, expert anesthetists, including many from the U.S. Army Nurse Corps, administered nitrous oxide–oxygen in the ratio of not more than 3 parts gas to one part oxygen to avoid deep anesthesia and cyanosis. (Future anesthetists would consider even this ratio too dangerous.) A higher ratio might have caused as great a fall in pressure as was produced by ether. When nitrous oxide was unavailable and ether was substituted, sometimes a blood transfusion or a gradual infusion of a gum–salt solution ("6 to 7 percent of gum acacia in 0.9 percent sodium chloride"[30(p194)]) accompanied ether administration for patients in shock to maintain or even raise the head of arterial pressure. Intravenous fluids or blood plasma did not receive widespread use, however, and physicians considered some hypovolemic patients simply inoperable.[28,30]

For gassed patients, anesthesia providers preferred nitrous oxide–oxygen. But if the anesthetic was not available, medical personnel used local, regional, or spinal anesthesia. Ether irritated the respiratory tracts of patients exposed to chlorine and other gases and was seldom used. Both British and American armies found that patients who had been gassed gave no special problem on the operating table.[28,29]

The Allies had differing opinions about the value of spinal anesthesia during World War I. Dr. Crile thought that spinal anesthesia was of value in all but rush periods, provided that the psychic factor of the wide-awake patient was eliminated by partial anesthesia, either morphine or light nitrous oxide, and that the fall in blood pressure was prevented by a blood transfusion. Most British surgeons did not favor spinal anesthesia because of its danger to hypovolemic or hemorrhaging patients. One French surgeon strongly advocated spinal anesthesia for all surgery below the 10th thoracic nerve. Most surgeons agreed that spinal and local anesthesia were preferred methods when respiratory disease made inhalational anesthesia difficult.[23,28,29]

Regarding local anesthesia, a survey of base hospitals in France by the American Red Cross, which was in charge of medical research for the American Army, revealed that anesthesia providers recommended local anesthesia in combination with morphine whenever possible. The technique suited the demands of war surgery, especially during "rush periods at the front"[29(p175)] when nitrous oxide–oxygen was unavailable and little time existed for the prolonged induction and recovery periods that normally followed the administration of ether or chloroform. Infiltration with novocaine was in common use alone or in combination with nitrous oxide–oxygen.[28,29]

Blood Transfusions and Other Treatments for Shock

Although the condition of shock had been known to military surgeons for 300 years, its causes, onset, and development remained a mystery. During World War I, British medical officers in the field, in conjunction with members of the Wound Shock Committee of the Medical Research Committee, studied the problem. American scientists, under the auspices of the National Research Council and the U.S. Army Surgical Research Laboratories, investigated shock during the war. Walter B. Cannon, U.S. Army Reserve officer and physiologist from Harvard University, studied shock and resuscitation with American and British forces in France and England and became a member of the British Shock Committee in 1917. He and allied scientists shared research findings and results in investigating the mysteries of shock.[31]

Cannon focused on treatments for shock when he became the director of a center for surgical research at the Central Medical Department Laboratory of the Army Expeditionary Force at Dijon, France, in 1918. He maintained a close relationship between the laboratory and the proving ground by establishing a network of resuscitation teams to treat soldiers in shock on or near the battlefield.

From May to November 1918, medical officers received instruction at weekly classes in Dijon on the nature of shock, onset theories, clinical symptoms, development circumstances, and treatment beliefs. They mastered methods of matching blood and giving blood transfusions. These officers went from the classroom to the shock wards at U.S. Army hospitals, where the seriously wounded received blood transfusions and other treatments in preparation for surgery later.[22,30–32]

The importance of blood volume in the treatment of shock was revealed during World War I. Medical officers had reported that "in cases of profound shock accompanied by loss of blood, excellent results are obtained from direct blood transfusion."[33(p42)] Because of the difficulties of giving transfusions at clearing stations during an attack, Captain (later Major) Oswald H. Robertson, U.S. Army, favored the collection, storage, and preservation of whole blood.[34] At his suggestion, small quantities of liquid blood had actually been preserved and transported considerable distances up to regimental aid posts. The addition of new red blood cells were, in Robertson's opinion, "the only means available of increasing the oxygen-carrying power of the blood....[T]his constitutes the unique value of blood transfusion."[33(p42)]

Robertson was a pioneer in establishing the concept of the world's first blood bank. He joined Cannon at the surgical research laboratory in Dijon, France, in August 1918, where he helped untangle the problem of "the efficacy of using gum acacia in the treatment of shock."[31(p243)] He concluded that there was an absence of convincing data as to gum acacia's usefulness in the treatment of shock.

At the end of World War I, William M. Bayliss, a distinguished British physiologist who had served on the Wound Shock Committee of the Medical Research Committee during the war, regretted "that so little positive evidence is forthcoming as to the superiority of blood transfusions. Statements are made on the basis of general impressions, rather than on convincing proof...."[33(p347)] Without convincing data, medical authorities might underestimate the importance of blood transfusions in the treatment of shock after the war.[33]

Also, the World War I Shock Committee's attempts to study shock were generally unsuccessful and led to fallacies. For example, the Committee had concluded at the end of the war "that the absorption of toxins from injured tissues was the primary cause of traumatic shock."[35(p29)] That belief led to misconceptions about the relationship of muscle injury to shock in the postwar years. Little progress was made on the relation of anesthesia to the development of shock. The Committee's great achievement, however, was in giving recognition to the complex problem of wound shock.

Other treatments for shock during World War I included restoration of lost body heat by surrounding the patient with blankets; injection of morphia to reduce pain and restlessness; and the return of blood from the large veins of the abdomen to the heart by raising the foot of the bed, a practice used for years in civilian hospitals, to permit gravity to aid the blood's return. Shock ward officers reported that the technique had no marked effect on either systolic or diastolic pressure. They also observed that the use of vasoconstrictor drugs to improve circulation in shock was futile, as clinical and experimental observations showed that the heart was not primarily affected in shock.[30]

Aftercare in World War I shock wards included monitoring of the patient's blood volume until it was restored to the normal level, a difficult procedure under field conditions, and the provision of fluids by either mouth or rectum until the urinary output equaled the water intake. Although military physicians stressed the need to watch for unfavorable developments and to treat them accordingly, postoperative care was not well developed in World War I.[30]

Despite its limitations, treatment of the seriously wounded during the war produced valuable lessons about shock and resuscitation. Cannon observed[30] that

- shock wards required two resuscitation teams, each consisting of a medical officer, a nurse, and an orderly;
- withdrawing 500 to 750 mL of blood did the slightly wounded man no harm, and saved the life of a soldier suffering from shock or severe hemorrhage;
- in preparation for shock cases, resuscitation officers needed to provide heating arrangements, transfusion equipment, and blood donors (and to determine their blood grouping); and
- resuscitation officers needed to perform or direct transfusions, give the surgeon their judgment of the optimum time for surgery, and do clinical work for the surgeon—so long as this work did not interfere with the resuscitation officer's important duties in the shock ward.

After a rocky start, military anesthesia greatly developed during the war to the benefit of the patient, the surgeon, and the war effort. For the first 2 years of the conflict, military anesthesia sorely lacked trained providers, advanced equipment, and supplies of nitrous oxide. Many soldiers' lives might have been saved had this not been the case. During the last 2 years of the war, the availability of improved apparatus, the employment of expert anesthetists, and the administration of warm ether vapor or nitrous oxide–oxygen instead of chloroform, whose potency could become dangerous, undoubtedly saved many lives.

Reserve officers from civilian medicine, who served as consultants to the armed forces, preferred nitrous oxide–oxygen anesthetic for most operations. The realization that this anesthetic required expert administration emphasized the need for trained anesthetists in the armed forces. As a result, the armed forces sent officers to study war surgery and anesthesia at medical schools throughout the country and nurses to schools of anesthesia that had developed in the United States in response to the demands of war. However, most of those students never made it overseas, as the war ended shortly after the buildup of American hospitals had begun.

Valuable information on the treatment of shock and resuscitation was produced during World War I, but the complex problem of shock remained shrouded in mystery. Nevertheless, the recognition of anesthesiology as a special field increased, as did the recognition of the anesthesia provider as a specialist rather than a technician. In 4 years, the state of the art of anesthesiology had vastly improved.[29] However, although anesthetists, like other specialists, found a home in the armed forces, decades would pass before the institution of residency programs in the U.S. Army.

After World War I, Dr. Crile wrote the chapter on anesthesiology for the official medical history of the war. His knowledge about anesthesia during the war led him to conclude[29] that

- nitrous oxide–oxygen, a light anesthetic, was the preferred anesthetic for the patient in shock; its administration required expert handling;
- in cases of profound exhaustion, spinal anesthesia would cause no serious fall in blood pressure if the patient first received an ordinary transfusion of blood;
- the psychic factor of being aware of the operating room and staff might be overcome by morphine or very light nitrous oxide anesthesia, or by light partial ether anesthesia; and
- ether, on the other hand, caused pneumonia in abdominal cases during the winter, was unsuitable in infections, and had a tendency to cause a fall in blood pressure after the operation; hence, ether should not be used in cases of shock.

Whether 20th-century medicine would substantiate these revelations remained to be seen.

Between the World Wars

The experiences of anesthesia providers in the Great War helped shape the revolution in anesthesiology that occurred during the 1920s and 1930s. As a result of the contribution of nurse anesthetists during the war, nurse anesthetist programs grew in number in both civilian and military medicine. Veteran physician anesthetists used their organizational skills and medical expertise to convince hospital personnel, mainly surgeons, across the country to establish divisions of anesthesia. As a result, departments of anesthesiology with residency programs began to appear. In 1939, the medical department of the U.S. Army began formal training of physicians in anesthesiology, one officer at a time, while increasing internships and postgraduate education in specialties in general. On the clinical side, transfusions, fluid therapy, intravenous anesthesia (revolutionized by the appearance of the barbiturates, especially pentothal, which is now known as sodium thiopental), and rebreathing anesthesia machines became more common (Figure 31-13).[1-3,22,36,37]

Anesthesiology grew as a profession during this period. Physician anesthetists founded the American Board of Anesthesiology in 1937 as an affiliate of the Board of Surgery and as an independent board to pass on the qualifications of trained anesthetists in 1941. The American Society of Anesthetists, a physician organization, grew out of the New York Society of Anesthetists and later became the American Society of Anesthesiologists. The American Association of Nurse Anesthetists, founded in 1931 to help guide the education of nurses in anesthesia, enhanced its power and helped cement the rivalry between nurse anesthetists and physician anesthetists, which had begun in the 1920s. Shortages of physician anesthetists meant that nurse anesthetists dominated most medical departments. New journals and books on anesthesia appeared in Europe and the United States, and an exhibit on anesthesia opened at the 1939 New York World's Fair. The roots of modern anesthesia were firmly planted between World War I and World War II.[36,37]

Other developments during this period included new techniques and agents. The improvement of the soft metal needle made continuous spinal anesthesia possible by permitting the use of very small doses and eliminating concern over the wearing off of the anesthetic. The endotracheal catheter, developed by British plastic surgeons Ivan Whiteside Magill and Edgar Stanley Rowbotham for use on wounded World War I veterans, gave anesthetists "direct control of the respiratory tract and its contents"[1(p286)] and provided the surgeon a quiet field in which to work. The combination of the new technique with the new anesthetic cyclopropane enabled the anesthetist to "synchronize the movements of the lung with the work of the surgeon."[1(p286)]

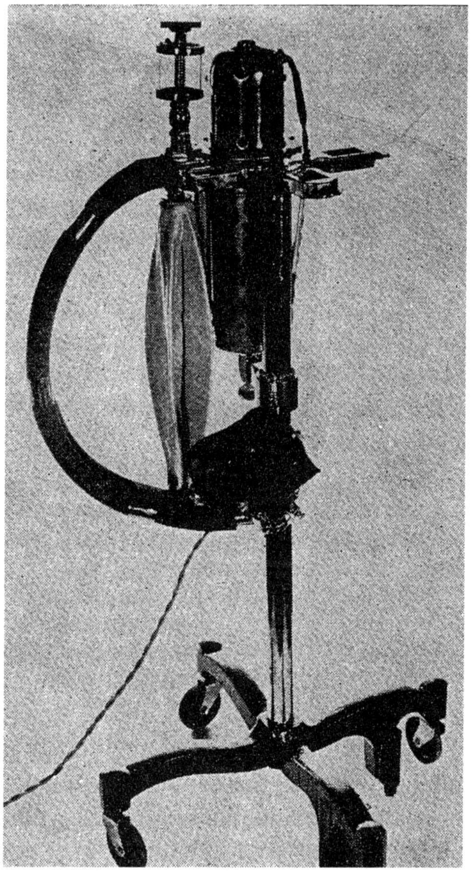

Fig. 31-13. This rebreathing anesthesia machine, made in 1918, was offered to the US Army in June 1918. Photograph: Reprinted with permission from Jackson DE. Anesthesia equipment from 1914 to 1954 and experiments leading to its development. *Anesthesiology*. 1955;16:962.

In the search for the ideal anesthetic, divinyl oxide, a cross of ether and ethylene (an anesthetic that was fast in action but weak), appeared. By producing a rapid and brief anesthesia, divinyl oxide, later replaced by sodium thiopental, put the patient to sleep before the ether was administered, rendering ether more pleasant. New anesthetics like Nembutal and the barbiturates—evipan and sodium thiopental—administered by the intravenous route came rapidly into favor. Man improved or produced machines for the administration of a variety of anesthetics. Those developments boded well for the future of anesthesia.

The development of the carbon dioxide–absorption technique made possible modern and efficient gas anesthesia machines (Figure 31-14). This technique permitted the patient to receive measured amounts of anesthetic gases and oxygen by adding ether to the mixture in small doses until the desired level of anesthesia was achieved. Expired gases passed through a soda lime canister that absorbed carbon dioxide before the gases entered a rebreathing bag, and the patient, on impulse, breathed in a warm blend of vapor and oxygen or of gases and oxygen. The containment of all gases in a closed circuit greatly reduced the chance of fire as well as the cost of anesthesia, since enclosed agents were not likely to escape. This technique also enabled the anesthetist to manage the patient's breathing and to maintain periodic positive-pressure anesthesia. This procedure was a boon to the anesthetist on the eve of World War II.[38]

Shock therapy, however, which is best studied in war, with its numerous casualties and major injuries, was an area that showed little improvement in the interwar years. After World War I, shock study took place in "experimental laboratories, in which attempts were made to [analyze shock] by physiologic and chemical techniques under a wide variety of experimentally induced conditions."[35(p29)]

Developments in shock therapy were understandably slow. The theory of toxemic shock persisted until the late 1920s, when A. Blalock, E. Parsons, and D. E. Phemister "demonstrated that shock produced by trauma to the limbs is not the result of toxemia but of a local loss of blood and fluid and of circulating blood volume."[35(p29)]

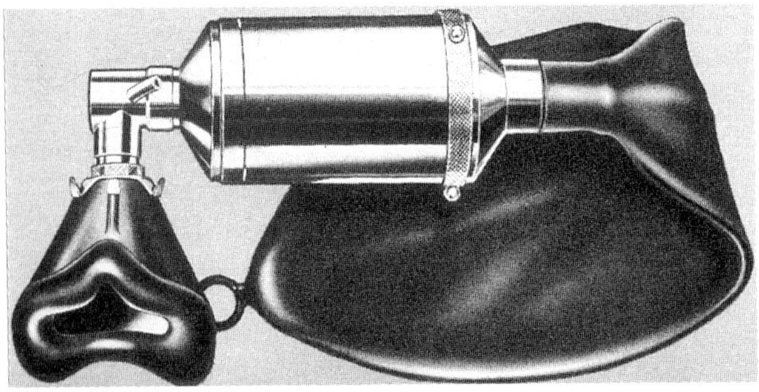

Fig. 31-14. The To-and-Fro Absorber was introduced by Ralph Waters, MD, in 1923 at the University of Wisconsin. Carbon dioxide–absorbent granules were placed in the canister; the patient was allowed to breathe "to and fro" through the canister. The device was accepted rapidly because it was simple and practical. Photograph: Courtesy of Ohmeda, Inc., Madison, Wis.

N. E. Freeman and his associates concluded from their observations "that the blood volume is a more reliable index of shock than the blood pressure," but the misconception persisted that "true shock [is] a generalized increase in capillary permeability."[35(p30)] Other fallacies also persisted, notably, that blood plasma is as effective as whole blood in the treatment of shock. Also, no practical way of determining blood volume under field conditions was developed during the years between World War I and World War II.

By 1940, the military, which had few medical specialists of any kind, depended largely on civilian medicine for specialized training of medical personnel and fulfillment of mobilization goals. Reserve medical officers and nurses entered the military in increasing numbers during the emergency buildup of 1940 and 1941. Specialists like Henry Swartley Ruth of the Philadelphia General Hospital taught young military physicians the values, concerns, and ideas of civilian medicine. The military started to respect specialization, accepting a civilian tenet that the "best care" for their patients "meant specialized care."[18(pp7–8)] The army took specialization into account when making assignments during the war. The navy established residency training in naval hospitals in 1944. Specialization was fast becoming an important factor in military medicine.[18]

World War II

Personnel

Even in World War II (1939–1945), however, there were never enough trained anesthetists to meet the needs of the military. At army hospitals in the United States, nurses gave inhalational anesthesia, while surgeons administered spinal, local, and regional anesthetics. At overseas theaters of operations, the military overcame shortages of skilled personnel and provided assistants for periods of peak loads by the continual training of nurse anesthetists, dentists, medical officers pressed into service, and corpsmen within the theater. Some dental officers learned drop ether and spinal anesthesia. Because surgery in forward-area hospitals taxed intelligence, judgment, resourcefulness, and technical ability, the army made every effort to assign its best-trained anesthesia providers to the combat zone. Anesthetists rendered great service in the forward areas of the North African Theater of Operations, where shortages of trained and experienced anesthesiologists persisted through 1943. By 1944, two skilled anesthesiologists served in each field and evacuation hospital sent to Europe, and one on each auxiliary surgical team on the front line (Figure 31-15).[38–41]

Anesthetics and Equipment

Shipping priorities and the need for simplicity at the front limited the choice of anesthetics and machines that accompanied frontline medics overseas, despite a wide range of agents and devices available at the start of the war. Combat anesthetists needed to have agents that could be hand carried and administered by improvised techniques and equipment. A scarcity of trained personnel narrowed the choice of drugs to those that people with limited experience could administer. Scarce shipping space and the need for forward-area hospitals to move quickly prohibited the employment of cumbersome equipment. The complex anesthesia apparatus, such as delicately adjusted gas machines, ran the risks of leakage and loss of serviceability due to rough handling during movement on short notice.[38] There was a need for portable gas machines in each platoon of the highly mobile (300-bed) field hospi-

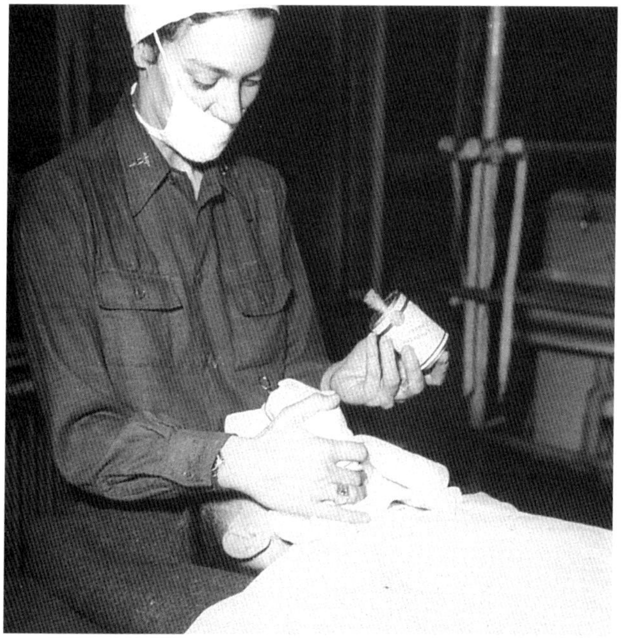

Fig. 31-15. Anesthesia as it was administered during World War II. Photograph: Courtesy of National Library of Medicine, Medical History Section, Bethesda, Md.

a

b

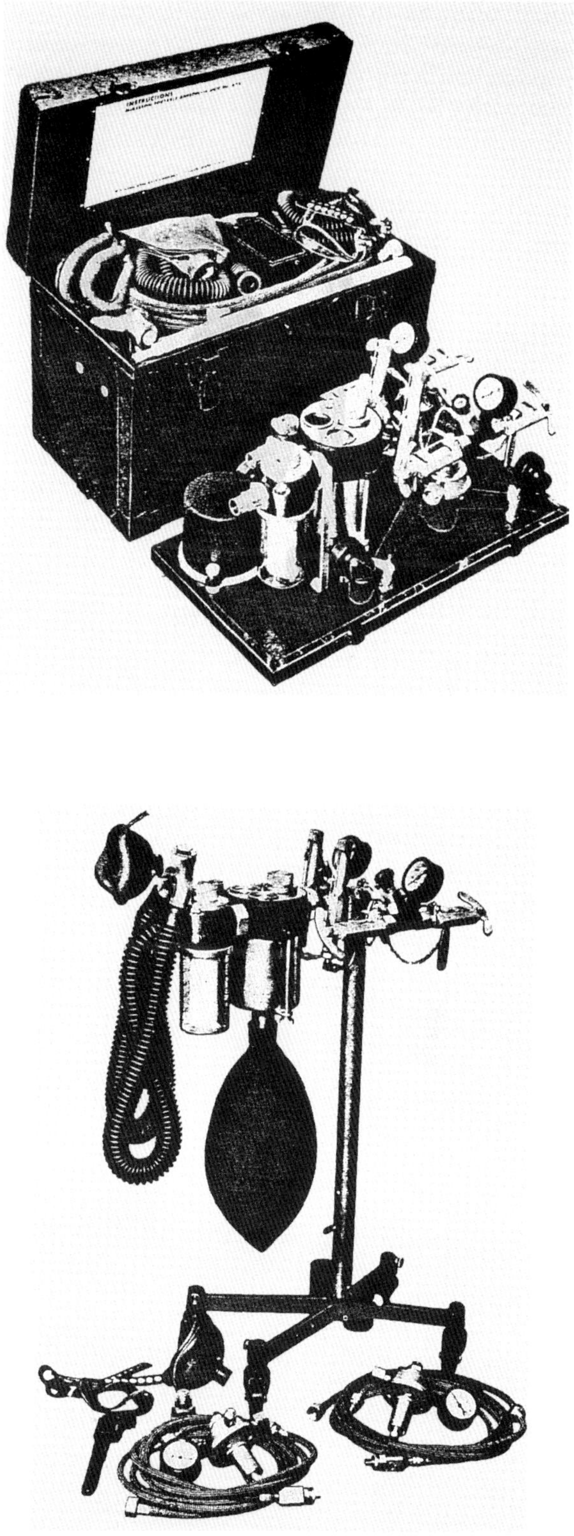

Fig. 31-16. Portable anesthesia apparatus, McKesson model 675, (**a**) packed in its carrying case and (**b**) assembled. Photographs: Reprinted from *Anesthesia Apparatus, Portable* (Item 9350000). Washington, DC: War Department; 1945: 4–5. Technical Manual 8-623.

tal or small (750- or 400-bed) evacuation hospital, "where intermittent positive pressure was essential for adequate care of nontransportables."[40(p600)]

The army issued four types of portable machines in World War II—the Ohio, McKesson, and Heidbrink (affectionately known as the "pig"), which were standard in civilian hospitals (Figures 31-16 and 31-17), and the Beecher machine, designed especially for active combat by Henry K. Beecher, reserve medical officer and Anesthesia

a

b

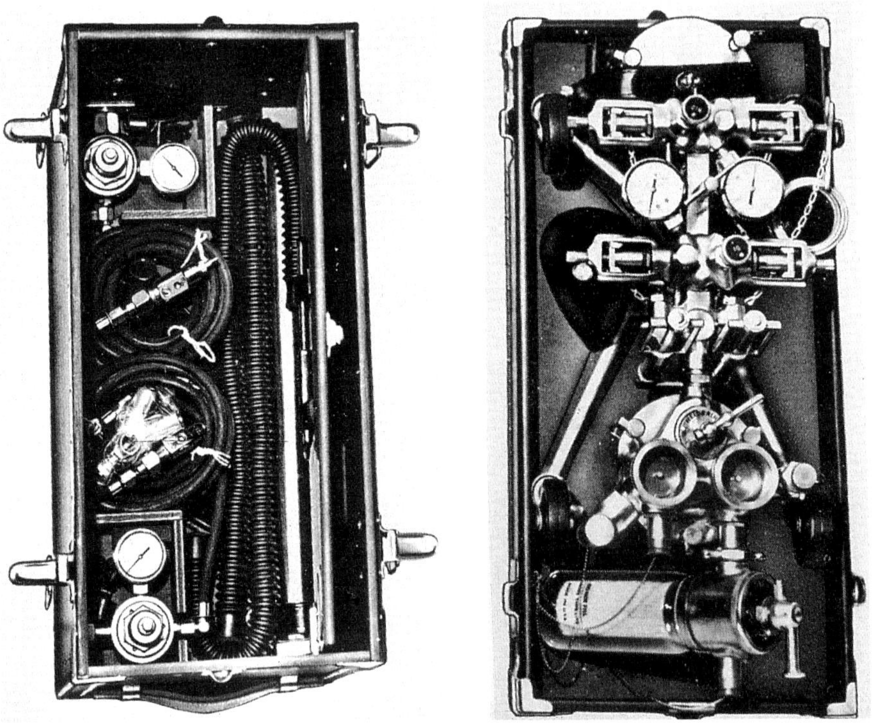

c

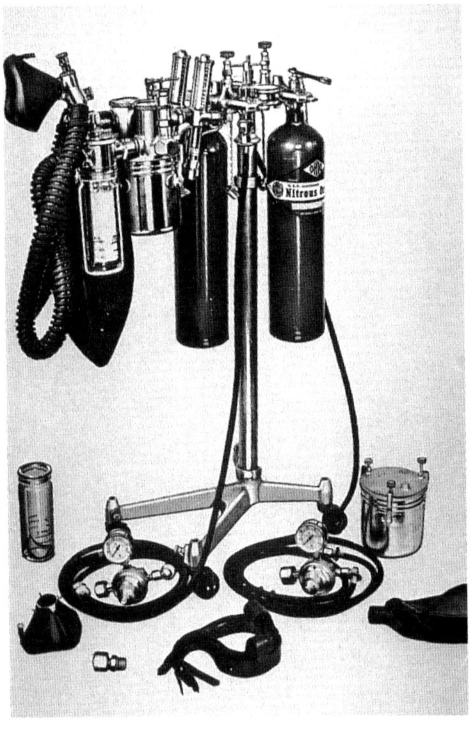

Fig. 31-17. Portable anesthesia apparatus, Heidbrink military model 685. (**a**) Upper half of storage case, (**b**) lower half of storage case, and (**c**) unit assembled. Photographs: Reprinted from *Anesthesia Apparatus, Portable* (Item 9350000). Washington, DC: War Department; 1945: 12, 13. Technical Manual 8-623.

Consultant to the North African–Mediterranean Theaters of Operation (October 1943–August 1945).

Light, compact, and easily hand carried, the Beecher machine could develop positive pressure in the airway without depending on tanks of oxygen, which were often unavailable at the front. Foot bellows were dispensed with when oxygen was on hand. The maintenance of a constant flow of room air through the apparatus allowed the system to continually flush, making the use of soda lime–carbon dioxide absorbent unnecessary. The device was encased in a compact container with enough capacity to hold a laryngoscope; intratracheal tubes; an aspiration bulb and catheter for emptying the bronchi; a packet of an induction agent, normally sodium thiopental; and two cans of ether, each weighing 1 lb. A fully loaded container weighed 25 lb.

Although designed specifically to make thoracic surgery possible without compressed air, the Beecher machine proved useful in combat for inhalational anesthesia, the administration of oxygen, and artifical respiration. This simplified machine became the apparatus that anesthetists used most often in World War II after mid-1944 and the buildup for Normandy. Before then, portable machines were in short supply, particularly in the North African theater. In the absence of portable machines, anesthetists relied on agents and methods that did not require movable devices, risking the lives of some patients.[25,38,39]

U.S. Army anesthetists had a wide variety of agents to choose from, including ether, chloroform, ethyl chloride, nitrous oxide, sodium thiopental, procaine, tetracaine hydrochloride, and cocaine. Cyclopropane and ethylene also were on hand, but military anesthesia machines were not equipped to handle those flammable bottled gases under pressure in cylinders. Hence, they were not used in combat.[38]

When machines were available, the choice of anesthetic usually depended on the experience of the anesthetist, the preference of the surgeon, and the problems of surgery. Ether anesthesia combined with oxygen, following induction with nitrous oxide, became popular because of its simplicity of administration, ready availability, easy tolerance by patients, and general safety. Ether's disadvantages, "irritat[ion] to the mucous membranes of the respiratory tract...[and] disturbance of metabolism, the blood sugar frequently being elevated from 100 to 200 percent,"[42(p69)] were outweighed by its advantages, particularly its margin of safety, since anesthetists were not equally trained, experienced, and capable.

Ether became the preferred anesthetic for casualties who were seriously wounded or in shock, which completely reversed the practice of World War I. By 1941, physicians knew that an impaired circulatory system took prolonged ether anesthesia well and that, according to Beecher, a man in shock tolerated ether far better than an animal in shock. Since trauma patients could take ether, then men less badly off could also take ether. In the Mediterranean Theater of Operations, where U.S. troops had been engaged in combat since November 1942, ether was the preferred anesthetic in more than 90% of cases.[25(p182)] In the European theater, inhalational anesthesia was used 86.2% of the time in Seventh U.S. Army field hospitals, compared to only 23.2% of the time in their evacuation hospitals, where fewer trauma cases were seen, and intravenous anesthesia with sodium thiopental became the preferred method.[39(p549)]

Nevertheless, the scarcity of portable machines, but more importantly, of fully experienced anesthesiologists, led to inexpert choices of agent and method for patients in critical condition. In the North African theater in 1943, for example, in the interest of time, inexpert anesthesiologists used spinal anesthesia or intravenous anesthesia with sodium thiopental when the poor condition of the patient dictated inhalational anesthesia. This trend was increased by the shortage of anesthesiologists trained in inhalational anesthesia using "carbon dioxide absorption and intermittent positive pressure administered through an endotracheal tube."[40(p603)] Shortfalls of machines and skilled personnel led to substandard combat anesthesia.

Sodium thiopental, a popular anesthetic, proved valuable as an induction agent preceding ether anesthesia of men in good condition, sometimes as an adjunct to spinal anesthesia, and as a sole agent for procedures of short duration. If the operation lasted longer than 30 to 45 minutes, the anesthesia provider switched to ether. Sodium thiopental had the advantages of being readily available; simply and compactly designed; easily and smoothly induced, even by inexperienced physicians; and with few undesirable aftereffects, all of which made it a good drug under combat conditions.

Medical personnel would not use sodium thiopental on patients suffering from shock, an impaired intake of oxygen, severe hemorrhage, inflammation "in the region of the carotid body or carotid sinus,"[38(p72)] gas gangrene, severe burns, when the operative position interfered with the airway or complicated artificial respiration, or when intracranial surgery was required. Bad-risk patients tolerated full barbiturate anesthesia poorly. Hence, sodium thiopental was used more often at evacuation hospitals, further back along the evacuation chain than in field hospitals, where more shock cases were observed. In Seventh U.S. Army hospitals, for example, intravenous anesthesia with sodium thiopental was used 53.1% of the time in evacuation hospitals and only 2.8% of the time in field hospitals.[39(p549)] Surgical problems influenced the anesthesia method chosen by combat medics.[25,38,39]

The medical department learned the hard way about the danger of using sodium thiopental on patients in shock. During the aftermath of the attack on Pearl Harbor on 7 December 1941, a number of patients suffering from traumatic shock and acute loss of blood experienced respiratory failure and died as a result of sodium thiopental anesthesia used intravenously. Those patients also did not receive a transfusion of blood or gum-salt solution, as the lessons of World War I regarding volume resuscitation were lost to medical practice between the wars. As a consequence of those deaths, anesthetists switched to open-drop ether, which proved safer for patients in shock. Casualties attended to later in Europe and the Pacific benefited from this new appreciation of the risks of sodium thiopental anesthesia on hypovolemic patients.[43]

A number of the other drugs supplied to the army received limited use. Since civilian practice discredited chloroform because of its intensely depressing effect on the circulatory system, it made little sense to use chloroform on wounded men suffering circulatory damage. Nitrous oxide became a routine induction agent but never the sole anesthetic. Oxygen concentrations of 21% or 30% or more always accompanied the gas. Ethyl chloride became a satisfactory induction agent if administered cautiously. In World War II, unlike in World War I, physicians understood the acceptability or unsuitability of most anesthetic agents.[25,38]

Methods of Choice

Medical officers considered the best method of anesthetic administration for military surgery to be closed-circuit anesthesia, either the closed-circle flow absorption method of the Heidbrink and McKesson machines, or the closed to-and-fro absorption technique of the Beecher machine. This system conserved body heat and moisture, maintained a high oxygen level while controlling the carbon dioxide volume in the blood, preserved desired degrees of anesthesia, regulated respiration, and maintained positive pressure. There was an increasing use of the closed-system technique as the war progressed.[25]

Although spinal anesthesia became an acceptable practice in World War I for wounds of the extremities and pulmonary trauma, the method was considered undesirable in World War II military surgery for a number of reasons: the technique caused a lowering of blood pressure in badly wounded men suffering from trauma and loss of blood, it made surgery lengthy and variable when other casualties were waiting for attention, and it allowed the undesirability of full consciousness in an apprehensive casualty fresh from the battlefield. Of 3,154 cases of abdominal injuries in the Mediterranean theater, anesthesia providers used spinal anesthesia on 3 patients only, each one in good condition and with minimal wounds.[25(p185)] Its limited use in combat reflected the belief that spinal anesthesia was a poor choice for badly wounded men at the front.[25,38]

Other regional or local anesthesia had limited use in combat. Early in the war, the English found that seriously wounded men tolerated poorly the moderate discomfort and psychological trauma of being conscious of their surroundings. The Allies therefore used local anesthesia for minor surgery on "easy-going" patients, who had exhibited a tolerance for occasional discomfort and other inconvenience. Local and regional block, normally with procaine, proved useful in certain neurosurgical and maxillofacial operations, but, in general, the method was not practical because of the multiplicity of wounds in each patient.[38,44] One anesthesiologist regretted not fully testing the combination of local anesthesia with a light inhalational anesthetic, which, he thought, might have had excellent potentialities in military surgery.[25(p185)]

Medical personnel performed topical anesthesia with tetracaine hydrochloride or cocaine. They used cocaine also for bronchoscopy or to ease a difficult intubation. Endotracheal intubation occurred routinely in intracranial, maxillofacial, and abdominal operations performed under general anesthesia; in all thoracic operations in which the pleura was involved; and in operations of more than 1 hour.[25,38]

Shock Therapy and Resuscitation

The anesthesia provider played an integral part in preoperative management, necessitating a knowledge of shock therapy and preanesthetic medication. Lessons of World War I regarding shock therapy and resuscitation were relearned, modified, and practiced in the North African theater by April 1943. When the flow of casualties was heavy and a shock team was unavailable, both anesthetists and surgeons worked in the resuscitation ward. Here patients received whole blood, pooled plasma, and 5% dextrose and water. If time allowed, the anesthetist conducted an examination of the patient before determining his presurgical medication. The anesthetist routinely used atropine (gr 1/100, equivalent to 0.6 mg), often in combination with morphine, given intravenously. The application of anesthetic care to trauma developed greatly during World War II, when evacuation from the front line to definitive care took 4 to 6 hours.[25]

Evacuation began shortly after an aid man gave the conscious casualty morphine and called for a litter squad. Depending on the wound, the medic administered plasma; dressed the wound; and filled out an emergency medical tag indicating the man's name, serial number from his dog tag, and the nature of the wound. The battalion aid station litter squad carried the wounded man back to the aid station, where he was examined for the first time by a medical officer, the battalion surgeon. The surgeon could administer more plasma and morphine and send the casualty to the collecting station for transfer by ambulance or litter bearer to the division clearing station, located 5 to 10 miles behind the front. Here, surgeons assigned to auxiliary teams performed acute surgical care, and, in the European and Mediterranean theaters, shock teams, including an anesthetist, saw the patient for the first time. When the patient was strong enough to be moved again, medical personnel transported him another 8 to 12 miles to an evacuation hospital, still under canvas and still in the combat zone. After the provision of definitive care, hospital authorities either evacuated the casualty to the rear or, if he was fully recovered, sent him forward for return to duty.[45]

Shock wards of field or evacuation hospitals were crucial to a patient's recovery during evacuation. Shock wards were headed by medical officers chosen from the internists or junior surgeons on the staff, or led by anesthetists and surgeons when the flow of casualties was heavy. Ideally, specific surgical or shock teams were assigned to the patient and stayed with him throughout his surgery to provide continuous care.[42]

The shock teams appraised the wounded man's therapy needs to enable him to tolerate surgery or evacuation to a rear hospital. A patient in shock did not remain in the same condition for any length of time. The team assessed the man's trends in both pulse rate and blood pressure (their quality and upward or downward trends were most important) to check the adverse forces at work. His degree of thirst and mental status, both of which medical officers paid little attention to in World War I, were found to be useful in evaluating the degree of shock. It was important to prevent a regression in the patient's condition in preparation for surgery.[42]

The anesthetist continued management of the hypovolemic patient in the operating room, administering high concentrations of oxygen to reestablish normal metabolism; anesthesia to abolish pain; blood transfusions to restore and maintain blood volume; dextrose and saline to rehydrate patients; and artificial respiration, if conditions indicated. The anesthesia providers did all they could to maintain a viable patient, while the surgeons worked as quickly as possible in light of the patient's needs.[42]

Casualties in shock or who had been in shock were usually easy to anesthetize, probably as a result of the resuscitation process practiced by military anesthetists. Military patients seldom experienced severe excitement—in contrast to patients in shock in civilian practice. Military anesthetists gave casualties in shock a light anesthesia compatible with their surgery because such patients tolerated deep anesthesia for brief periods only. Sometimes anesthetists authorized to administer curare used the agent as a muscle relaxant to facilitate intraperitoneal manipulations during periods of light anesthesia. Patients in shock, suffering thoracoabdominal wounds, or both, received nitrous oxide–ether anesthesia by the closed endotracheal technique and curare in various dosages and at various times during the operation. None of those cases suffered postoperative complications or deaths that could be attributed to the use of curare. Anesthesia providers stressed the importance of employing the endotracheal technique when using curare. Military anesthetists greatly expanded the role of the anesthesia provider in the care of the trauma patient during World War II.[42]

Volume resuscitation was pivotal in the treatment of patients in shock during the war. Early in the conflict, physicians relied on blood plasma because of the limited supply of whole blood, which resulted from general unpreparedness for war, and a myriad of theories about shock. Some experts considered blood plasma as effective as whole blood in the treatment of shock, easier to preserve and transport than whole blood and without the requirement of matching and typing. Shortages of blood for volume replacement, despite the use of blood donors in the field, meant a delay in surgery until the patient was stabilized. In February 1943, patients received treatment for shock in clearing stations for up to 24 hours before surgical therapy was even attempted. Medical officers did not give blood postoperatively to overcome anemia and promote wound healing or, for that matter, oxygen to improve circulation during this early period.[33,42]

The readier availability of whole blood in 1944, which followed the establishment of blood procurement centers in U.S. cities and refrigerated blood banks in rear combat hospitals, led to a change in the concept of stabilizing the casualty *first*, in favor of rapid preparation for surgery and a reduction in the time lag as compared with 1943. The concept of prompt operation required an understanding of what could be achieved by resuscitative measures and what was impossible. Medical officers came to realize that all that was needed was to make the patient safe for surgery. Since a seriously wounded man could slip back into shock once he had been brought out of it, surgery should not be delayed once he was resuscitated from shock. World War II anesthesiologist Lieutenant Colonel Henry K. Beecher stated that

> all military surgeons, no matter what their original point of view, eventually realized the importance of operating as soon as the patient had been brought to optimum status within a minimum period of time.[42(p21)]

The recognition of the essential unity of resuscitation and operation was an important surgical advance late in the war. The lessons learned about volume resuscitation in World War I had to be relearned in World War II.

Military surgeons also changed their minds about blood plasma's usefulness in the treatment of shock. The consideration of plasma as the ideal substitute for whole blood in the emergency treatment of shock and hemorrhage in war wounds was so entrenched early in the war that it handicapped the development of more effective measures for the management of shock. As the war progressed, however, experience proved the effects of plasma to be transient. Plasma brought men out of shock and maintained blood volume during transportation to the hospital, where a blood transfusion could be started. Plasma became a lifesaving stopgap measure only until the patient could receive whole blood.[42]

British anesthesiologists had concluded similarly about the transient nature of blood plasma. Of the 10% of all patients requiring resuscitation before surgery in British forward hospitals in March 1943, one out of five required whole blood.

> If treated with plasma alone, [remarked a medical officer of No. 1 Casualty Clearing Station in southern Tunisia,] the blood pressure [could] be brought back but [fell] again with operation and [did] not come back a second time. Patients treated with plasma remain[ed] pale, the pulse [was] rapid and the labile blood pressure [was] very sensitive to further operative procedures.[33(p36)]

In general, wounded American soldiers received one additional unit of plasma to three units of whole blood at the hospital. About two thirds of patients received another 500 mL of blood each, and about one third received 1,000 mL of blood each. Patients were considered ready for surgery when the systolic blood pressure was 80 mm Hg and tending upward, when the pulse volume was good and the rate tending downward, and when the skin was warm and the color good. Sometimes albumin, which was expensive in terms of the quantities of blood needed to prepare it but had small bulk (corpsmen could line their pockets with it), was used to elevate a low blood pressure in situations in which space and weight were at a premium.[42]

To establish effective resuscitation procedures based on scientific evidence, the medical department set up stationary research laboratories in the Mediterranean theater in late 1943 and early 1944 "to study by formal biochemic [*sic*] methods certain aspects of shock, hemorrhage, and dehydration,"[33(p348)] and a mobile laboratory in September 1944, called the Board for the Study of the Severely Wounded in the Mediterranean Theater of Operations, "to observe shock on a big scale"[33(p353)] and get insights into its nature. In the opinion of the Medical Research Committee of the theater,

> [i]t was essential...that the so-called impressions derived from experience be documented by hard, cold facts about the condition of a freshly wounded man.... The collection of data needed to be extended to a sufficient number of casualties to make the findings conclusive.[33(p349)]

The loss of lessons learned from World War I due to the absence of convincing data and the confusion over shock therapy early in World War II were the catalysts for this effort at documentation by scientific evidence of effective resuscitation procedures experienced during World War II.

Data collected from studies of thousands of badly wounded soldiers during the Italian campaign proved that the liberal use of whole blood transfusion was necessary for the success of reparative wound surgery. Extensive laboratory tests on at least 37 of those patients confirmed the absence of hemoconcentration in shock. The mobile research team, headed by Colonel Beecher, studied the physiological effects of blood loss in 186 severely wounded patients, concluding, in the broadest sense, that "wound surgery [was] inseparable from the management of wound shock."[46(p13)] Surgery became part of the continuous process of resuscitation. The team also determined that plasma, whole blood, penicillin, and sulfa drugs were not harmful to the kidneys, a question of concern in treating the severely wounded. Studies of wounded patients immediately after admission to forward hospitals helped to formulate procedure for the clinical management of the seriously impaired.[33,46]

Other resuscitative measures used in World War II included

- relief of physical and mental pain by sedation (barbiturate, usually sodium amytal) and administration of morphine,
- management of the local wound through control of hemorrhage and the application of splints,
- conservation of body heat,
- emptying of the stomach before anesthesia to avoid the risk of aspiration, and
- administration of oxygen to produce a lowered pulse rate and a better coloration of the blood.

Medical officers administered oxygen by nasal tube after it had been humidified by being bubbled through a water column. Patients usually tolerated well a gas flow of 4 to 5 L/min of 100% oxygen. A closed system with carbon dioxide absorption, usually by the Beecher machine, provided higher concentrations of oxygen, if needed. Vasoconstrictor and stimulating drugs were of no value in the management of battle casualties and were almost never used.[33]

Auxiliary Surgical Groups

To assure quality anesthesia and surgery, specialty consultants from Auxiliary Surgical Groups, each consisting of four surgical teams that performed frontline surgery in the absence of hospitals, visited forward units to check on patient supervision. Those consultants addressed relevant problems and recommended solutions.[47]

Statistics

Statistics from the Mediterranean theater reveal a record of safety in the prevention of anesthesia deaths. Surveys conducted in the Mediterranean theater in September 1943 and September 1944 show only 12 deaths attributed to anesthesia in 27,564 administrations of anesthetic agents.[38(p78)] Seventh U.S. Army hospitals attributed 11 deaths in 44,630 cases wholly or in part to anesthetic administration between 1 November 1944 and 30 April 1945.[39(p550)] One World War II anesthesiologist credited this safe record to more standardized methods and increased experience,[38(p78)] which made anesthesia safer for the seriously wounded man.[38] Statistics for World War II are sadly lacking, however, regarding numbers of physician and nurse anesthetists, anesthesia deaths in other theaters, and the frequency and place of employment of specific agents and techniques.

World War II Experience in Summary

World War II (1939–1945), like most wars, began with shortages of almost everything, including anesthesia providers. Continual training in anesthesia at home and overseas helped to provide the armed forces with skilled people, but never in the numbers needed. Although a variety of anesthetics were on hand during the war, ether's availability, ease of administration, and margin of safety made the agent most popular. Sodium thiopental given intravenously proved invaluable for preliminary anesthesia or as a sole agent. Sodium thiopental's compactness and ease of induction made it an ideal anesthetic for the good-risk patient under combat conditions.

Closed-circuit anesthesia with the simple Beecher machine gradually gained wide acceptance as a satisfactory method at forward area hospitals, where portable machines were needed. The apparatus proved useful in combat for inhalational anesthesia, the administration of oxygen, and artificial respiration.

The availability of whole blood in theaters of operation and the development of shock wards improved treatment and resuscitation of the patient in shock. Finally, medical departments in World War II officially recognized the administration of anesthetics as a highly skilled occupation and the anesthetist as a specialist.

Postwar Recruitment

After demobilization, the U.S. Army had to find ways to attract qualified physicians into military service. The army's acceptance of specialization, which resulted in the establishment of residency programs in 1947, helped. The army, like the navy, however, still depended on civilian reserve officers to serve as consultants to those programs. In 1948, to obtain specialists, the army began commissioning residents in civilian hospitals for service in the army. Most volunteers for this program had received some financial support from one of the military services during their medical school training. With specialization so popular and widespread in the country, the army began to develop graduate education programs that would maintain military medical standards while attracting and retaining skilled physicians in the service. By 1950, those programs were well on their way.[18]

The Korean War

Graduate medical education programs helped meet the needs of mobilization for the Korean War (1951–1953), which began with North Korea's invasion of South Korea in summer, 1950. The armed forces took young physicians who had recently finished residency programs in military hospitals and sent them to Korea. According to Howard D. Fading, Consultant in Neurology to The U.S. Army Surgeon General, the army's residency program "saved the bacon in the Korean War, and if it can never demonstrate another value, this alone proved its worth."[18(p12)]

When the numbers of medical officers were insufficient to meet the armed forces' needs, they began to draft young physicians from civilian hospitals and graduate education programs. The doctor draft in January 1951 helped relieve the critical shortage of medical officers, and courses given at general hospitals helped relieve the shortfall of nurse anesthetists, but specialists, including anesthesiologists, were in short supply throughout the war.[18]

At first notice, the treatment of the battle casualty in Korea seemed almost ideal. Personnel, equipment, and supplies, in most respects, were adequate. There were ample amounts of whole blood and prompt evacuation of the wounded from Korea. Casualty buildup did not pose a problem. Nor were new data gathered on the anesthetic management of the wounded during the Korean War.[48]

But this picture was deceiving. Casualty care in Korea was far from ideal. Frontline evacuations were less effective in Korea than in World War II. Korea's mountainous terrain meant a long evacuation from the front to the aid station and from the aid station to the mobile army surgical hospital (MASH). The helicopter helped, but there were never enough. At a meeting of the Armed Forces Medical Policy Council on 18 June 1951, Brigadier General Crawford F. Sams, head of SCAP's (Supreme Commander for the Allied Powers) Public Health and Welfare Section, said he did not doubt

> the quality of the front-line hospitals and the professional care available in them. [But, he lamented,] our death rate...is far higher than the last war because many do not reach the hospitals.... My impression is about 4,000 men [who have died] should be alive.[49(p189)]

Senior U.S. Army medical officers linked defective evacuation directly to medical specialization and professional development within the army to the detriment of military training. As army medicine became more professional, more expert, and more in line with civilian medicine, the army neglected to prepare physicians for field service. The army plucked young physicians straight from army hospitals and sent them to Korea without having had field medical experience. To meet immediate needs early in the war, medical officers in the civilian internship program also found themselves on the Korean front with no military training, and they suffered. Afteraction reports revealed that "some were captured, some were killed, [and] many performed ineffectively as officers."[18(p11)]

Additionally, the budget cuts of 1949 and 1950 had left the armed forces deficient in men, supplies, and training. Financial constraints had produced a paucity of medical personnel and hospital beds, with which a peacetime army could deal, but which became a problem once war began. The U.S. Army never had as many medical units in Korea as it needed; ambulance companies numbered about half of what was required, and the 750-bed evacuation hospital, which served as the backup unit to the 400-bed evacuation hospital and field and surgical facilities, was absent from Korea. Evacuation hospitals could not absorb sudden heavy casualty loads. Only U.S. air superiority and the presence of U.S. Army hospitals in Japan helped prevent a backlog of casualties awaiting evacuation from Korea. The

MASH worked well, and the blood program and combat psychiatry repeated the successes of World War II. But combat medics had to learn basic military surgical procedures "like wound debridement and delayed closure."[49(p363),50]

The lessons of World War II regarding anesthesia were also mostly forgotten. The limitation on the amount of anesthetic equipment and supplies that could be brought to the front made a variety of agents and techniques unavailable. Qualified anesthesiologists were scarce in forward units, such as surgical hospitals, where judgment and experience were highly necessary. Little standardization of anesthesia equipment made interchanges difficult among U.S. models, and among U.S. machines and those of other countries. There were national differences in terminology, electric current, and the coloring of gas cylinders. For example, a green U.S. cylinder contained oxygen and a green British cylinder contained carbon dioxide. Such practices led to letters of complaint to members of the U.S. Congress about the dismal anesthesia conditions in the war zone.[26]

Anesthesiology, like other medical specialties, was in a time of transition. The machines available to the armed forces were the World War II variety: the pig, the Foregger and McKesson machines, and the Beecher device. Some reserve officers brought their own anesthetic machines from civilian practice to Korea. An anesthesiologist from Massachusetts General Hospital, sent to the Far East Command to investigate anesthesia problems, brought with him a new compact anesthesia machine as well as methadone, a morphine substitute then undergoing clinical trials in the United States.[26,49]

The preferred agent and machine depended on the anesthetist's orientation and training. Some received training in sodium thiopental for the seriously wounded; others in nitrous oxide with adequate amounts of oxygen. One anesthesiologist reported using 50% to 60% nitrous oxide in oxygen (most likely with a relaxant and a narcotic) on the severely wounded patient, with satisfactory results. He wanted to spare the hypovolemic patient the consequences of a more potent depressant. Without definitive data to prove one agent or technique better than another, Robert D. Dripps, Civilian Consultant in Anesthesia to The U.S. Army Surgeon General, remarked, "[I]t seemed wise to permit anesthetists to apply those methods with which they [were] most familiar."[48(p119)] Regardless of which agent or machine was used, Dr. Dripps continued, the patient's susceptibility had to be kept in mind and his dosage carefully watched.[48]

Anesthesia providers reported using cyclopropane for the hypovolemic patient, and with good results. They also prepared a 0.5% solution of procaine for infiltration anesthesia and a 1% solution for nerve block. The muscle relaxant drugs, especially tubocurarine chloride and succinylcholine, proved useful in allowing rapid intubation of the trachea and providing muscular relaxation for varying periods of time. Patients in shock sometimes reacted to succinylcholine with exaggerated motor activity, resembling clonic convulsions. One anesthesiologist suggested that this represented a diminished amount of plasma cholinesterase. During the Korean War, anesthesiologists thought that shock exaggerated the motor activity associated with succinylcholine. Future anesthesia providers would know that motor activity resembling convulsions was a normal response to succinylcholine and not exaggerated by hypovolemia. For preoperative medication, anesthetists in Korea used morphine or sodium thiopental intravenously, as had been done in World War II.[48]

The lessons of World War II regarding resuscitation were retained for the Korean War, except that in Korea more information was available about the problem of homologous serum jaundice in untreated plasma. After World War II, plasma was subjected to ultraviolet sterilization as part of its processing to prevent serum hepatitis. But complete sterilization was never achieved, and hepatitis continued to follow the use of plasma no matter how it was treated. During the Korean War, the armed forces had to take the calculated risk of using plasma, even though it might cause hepatitis, because they needed an agent for resuscitation until the casualty could reach an installation and receive a transfusion of whole blood. The risk was considerable. Late in 1951, the incidence of hepatitis after plasma transfusion reached 21%, in sharp contrast to the reported World War II incidence of 7.5%. Part of the explanation was that much of the plasma used in Korea in the first months of the war had not been treated at all. Moreover, different diagnostic criteria were used in the two wars. In World War II, the diagnosis was chiefly clinical. In the Korean War, any elevation of the serum bilirubin was considered an indication of hepatitis. On 20 August 1953, Circular No. 73, Department of the Army, directed that because of the risk of serum hepatitis, the higher cost, and the need to use it for the production of specific globulins, plasma would not be used "to support blood volume" unless dextran was not available.[35]

The Korean War experience provided lessons for the future regarding equipment, organization, education, and training. Among the recommendations made were the following[48]:

- the standardization of equipment, fittings, and electrical current;
- the inclusion of equipment for infants and children in anesthesia kits (one seventh of the South Korean population were refugees at some time during the war);
- the provision of a field anesthesia record that would fit into the emergency medical tag jacket and accompany the casualty; and
- increases in numbers and varieties of drugs.

Also promoted were the following[48]:

- the employment of anesthesia consultants in forward surgical hospitals, in order for them to obtain first-hand knowledge of the problems involved so as to advise and train others more authoritatively;
- the collection of data on techniques used for various operations, deaths related to anesthesia, the anesthetics administered, and the physical condition of the patients;
- the preparation of manuals and training films for military anesthetists that would include the basic aspects of resuscitation, pharmacology, and physiology; and
- the study of problems associated with the management of battle casualties and nuclear and chemical warfare.

Many questions arose from the anesthesia experiences of World War II and the Korean War that required investigating.

Although the importance of anesthesia and combat care were appreciated in World War I, World War II, and the Korean War, only in 1954 did the U.S. Army institute a 3-year residency program in anesthesiology, following an internship. Also, after the Korean War, the appointment of a senior consultant in anesthesia to the Office of The Surgeon General helped initiate the correction of some of the anesthesia problems that had been revealed during the Korean War. In civilian medicine, university departments of anesthesiology had begun to break away from the surgical departmental structure and to emerge as separate departments.[47,48,51]

While anesthesia came into its own in civilian hospitals, the Selective Service Act of 1950 and the Cold War of the 1950s and 1960s produced a large peacetime military establishment. To support this establishment and keep pace with the standards of medical care provided in civilian life, the medical department needed to expand and improve its method of recruitment. The appointment of Dr. Frank Berry, a colonel in World War II and a New York surgeon, as Assistant Secretary of Defense for Health and Medicine was an important step in that direction. In 1954, the Berry Plan permitted physicians to postpone their military obligation under the draft until they completed their internship and residency programs: "This allowed for the continuous training of doctors (a pedagogical good) while at the same time providing the military services with completely qualified medical specialists."[18(p13)] Retention of physicians with only a 2-year military obligation under selective service, however, remained difficult, and the balance between specialists and general medical officers suffered.[18]

Another way the military acquired specialists was to make specialist training available to its medical officers. Twenty-four residency training programs in 8 army hospitals in 1959 grew to 28 programs in 17 hospitals a decade later, as the army built up for the Vietnam War. Expanding residency programs helped retain physicians through either military obligation or personal decision. Specialized training also permitted the military to meet the standards of civilian care.[18]

The new emphasis on specialized training benefited military anesthesia, which was fast becoming an important part of the structure of the U.S. Army Medical Department. The army acquired skilled anesthetists by offering members of the U.S. Army Nurse Corps 52 weeks of training in anesthesiology at six U.S. Army Medical Centers and Hospitals, namely, Brooke Army Medical Center, Walter Reed Army Medical Center, and Letterman, Fitzsimons, Beaumont, and Madigan Army Hospitals. Nurse anesthetists also attended anesthesia workshops at army hospitals. The training of U.S. Army nurse anesthetists met the requirements for certification by the American Association of Nurse Anesthetists.[52]

Besides offering internships and residencies in anesthesia, the U.S. Army Medical Department arranged for Medical Corps officers to take long courses in anesthesiology at civilian institutions, such as the University of Pennsylvania, and to attend review sessions in anesthesiology at Lackland Air Force Base, Texas. With the army's encouragement, military anesthesiologists in increasing numbers became board certified. No longer was the medical department dependent on civilian medicine for anesthesia consultants; it had its own professors of anesthesiology, although it still relied on skilled nurse anesthetists to augment hospital staffs.[52]

The Vietnam War

By the mid-1960s and the Vietnam War (1965–1972), military anesthesiologists were making the tough decisions, like what (people, agents, and machines) to bring to battle and what to leave home, and what level of care to provide. Civilian anesthesiologists had faced those issues during World War I and World War II. Incorporating lessons learned from previous wars regarding anesthesia care and evolving new concepts about critical care in Vietnam, the military

- deployed anesthesiologists to forward medical support hospitals;
- expanded the role of the anesthesiologist in the sustainment of life before, during, and after surgery;
- advanced the resuscitative process;
- introduced new anesthesia machines; and
- standardized anesthesia equipment.

These anesthesiologists also developed in Vietnam many of the ideas, particularly regarding critical care, subsequently used in civilian anesthesia in the United States. Developments in anesthesiology during the Vietnam War years have been well described elsewhere by Manfred ("Dutch") Lichtmann, an army anesthesiology professor who served in Vietnam and later as Consultant in Anesthesiology to The Surgeon General.[47]

The allocation of anesthesia providers to Vietnam followed the pattern of the deployment of regular troops. Early in the war, anesthesia personnel were sent as advisors and then as members of "K" teams assigned to fixed facilities and rotated to other hospitals according to casualty needs. After the military buildup of 1965, anesthesia personnel strength multiplied, with nurse anesthetists forming the bulk of the increase. Their numbers from 1968 until the phase-down began were about 65 but reached as high as 95 at one time. To obtain nurse anesthetists, the army fostered a move toward nurse anesthesia education at the master's degree level and upgraded the requirements for attaining such a degree.[47,53]

Anesthesiologists, trained to board-certification levels in military residency programs, were first deployed to forward surgical hospitals during the Vietnam War. Fully trained or board-certified anesthesiologists, however, were a luxury in Vietnam, as the residency training program, although growing, was still small. Of the 35 anesthesiologists covering 16 hospitals in 1967 through 1968, only 4 were board certified, 16 were fully trained, and 15 had learned on the job. The latter were sent directly to Vietnam following an internship and 14 weeks' instruction in anesthesiology. Although the army hoped that the physician trained on the job would work with another anesthesiologist, sometimes the former physician was the only anesthesiologist at the hospital. In those cases, the physician relied on an experienced nurse anesthetist to help and guide him. Together they formed a solid anesthesia care team. Lichtmann recalled:

> The severity of casualties, the austerity of the environment, and the continuous pressure and intensity of the care required molded physician and nurse anesthetist into a cohesive anesthesia care team.[47(p1300)]

The anesthesia care team that Lichtmann referred to was an ideal, brought about by the exigencies of war. The rivalry between nurse anesthetists and physician anesthesiologists was put aside to deal with the problems at hand. While nurse anesthetists played an important role in military medicine—the armed forces needed them—they played a less significant role in civilian medicine, where physician anesthesiologists reigned supreme.

This team helped care for many casualties during the Vietnam War. The U.S. armed forces suffered 46,000 killed in Vietnam and 300,000 wounded.[54(p410)] The wounds were usually multiple and devastating, the result of mine, high-velocity missile, and booby trap injuries. Yet casualties who would not have survived in other wars were salvaged here. Crucial to their survival were the immediate availability of whole blood, rapid resuscitation from shock, and helicopter transfer to hospitals. The latter brought the patient to definitive treatment faster than in any previous war. The time between wounding and effective treatment averaged 10 hours in World War I, 5 hours in World War II and Korea, and 1 hour in Vietnam. Rapid and effective air evacuation meant recovery for most of the wounded who reached definitive care.[54,55]

Speedy helicopter evacuation from the front in Vietnam also allowed continuous resuscitation. Initially the corpsmen, who were trained at the Medical Field Service School by noncommissioned officers and sometimes physicians, restored breathing (usually through mouth-to-mouth resuscitation) and occasionally started infusions of intravenous fluids. Helicopter evacuation medics continued the process. At the hospital, medical personnel started a 14-gauge intravenous line in the basilic or the external jugular vein and, under the supervision of or managed by an anesthetist, performed airway care, which sometimes required the use of an oropharyngeal tube, an endotracheal airway, or a tracheostomy. The triage officer selected those casualties who responded to resuscitation for anesthesia and surgery on the basis of severity of wounds. He informed anesthesia personnel which patient was next and the patient's condition. Well-functioning operating rooms had good coordination between the triage area and anesthesia providers.[47,56]

Anesthesia personnel continued resuscitation in the operating room and provided anesthesia. Those casualties who could not be resuscitated without surgical intervention received slight anesthesia with airway and ventilation control and continued "infusions of blood, colloids, and electrolytes."[56(p800)] While surgical teams operated on the patient to repair wounds, anesthesia personnel used all their skills to help keep the patient alive. John Jenicek, Consultant in Anesthesiology to The U.S. Army Surgeon General during the Vietnam War, described the expanding role of anesthetists in support of surgical procedures during that conflict.[47,56]

> It [became] the mission of the anesthesia team to support the circulating volume, the oxygen demand, and the anesthetic needs of the patient as well as to treat and correct all abnormal physiological and pharmacological responses of the casualty; all the while providing as near optimal surgical conditions as possible for the other equally busy surgical teams. It is this new concept of resuscitation-anesthesia-surgery, organized and functioning as a unit [and combined with speedy evacuation], which [produced] the highest survival rate seen in any conflict thus far.[56(p800)]

This new approach to field medicine—continuous resuscitation combined with speedy evacuation—resulted in lowered hospital mortality: 2.2% in Vietnam compared with 4.5% in World War II. Significantly more critically wounded survived to reach base hospitals in Vietnam than in World War II. Eighty-seven percent of those hospitalized in Vietnam returned to duty, another wartime record.[55]

Preoperative medication and induction techniques during the Vietnam War followed civilian practice. With no standardized policy on premedication established, anesthesia providers based their drug selection on their background and training. The most commonly used premedication drugs were the barbiturates (pentobarbital, secobarbital) and morphine with atropine or scopolamine. The induction agent of choice was sodium thiopental used with a relaxant.[47]

Problems associated with induction anesthesia included the reduction or elimination of the patient's protective responses to hypovolemia caused by too large a dose, the increased chance of tracheal aspiration of gastric contents because of soldiers eating immediately before being wounded, and cardiac arrest on induction of anesthesia by patients who received succinylcholine after suffering muscle injuries or severe burns. Finally, mismanagement of the airway or a short period of apnea during induction sometimes proved lethal. Gale Thompson, the first consultant in anesthesiology to be sent to Vietnam, reported that 76% of patients receiving general anesthesia received tracheal intubation. There are no statistics available for anesthesia deaths.[47]

Military anesthesiologists used a variety of agents and machinery in Vietnam because the war escalated slowly, allowing the U.S. Army Medical Department to establish in the combat zone large fixed hospitals (unlike in World War II, where mobile hospitals were the norm) with sophisticated equipment and skilled staffs. The chief anesthetic agents used included diethyl ether, halothane, methoxyflurane, nitrous oxide–oxygen, and spinal anesthetics. Of the 282 anesthetic administrations, mainly on civilians, given at the 8th Field Hospital from April 1962 to January 1963, 9% were diethyl ether, 15% halothane, and 39% spinal anesthetics, according to John Chase Daniels, the first U.S. Army anesthesiologist in Vietnam.[47]

Early in the war, halothane, which had widespread use in the United States, received limited use "because it caused hypotension and could prove lethal in the 'in-circuit' vaporizers that were on field machines," recalled Lichtmann.[47(p1302)] According to Brian F. Condon, a U.S. Army anesthesiologist in Vietnam and later Consultant in Anesthesiology to The U.S. Army Surgeon General:

> The "in-circuit" vaporizer or "number 8 jar" allowed the concentration of anesthetic to be varied by the pulmonary minute volume as well as the dial setting. This made prediction of anesthetic agent inspired concentration difficult. Therefore a hypovolemic, low–cardiac-output patient could easily be overdosed and hypotension could occur with little or no warning.[57]

After the U.S. Army equipped field machines with the Fluotec Mark 1 and 2 vaporizers in 1967, halothane replaced ether as the standard field anesthetic. As a trauma anesthetic, halothane's advantages included nonflammability, rapid recovery after brief operations, less nausea and vomiting than with ether, and good urinary production after fluid resuscitation. The drug, which could be given with oxygen alone, became the most frequently administered anesthetic from 1968 to 1971.[47]

Other anesthetic agents proved highly beneficial in Vietnam. Methoxyflurane served as an analgesic for short procedures or to augment muscle relaxation in prolonged abdominal operations. The drug could function in "large in-circuit vaporizers" and in "low-flow, high-oxygen systems."[47(p1302)] From 1970 on, nitrous oxide–oxygen with a relaxant, a narcotic, and, at times, a major tranquilizer added, became a popular general anesthetic as the use of halothane decreased. The literature of the time reported on hepatic injury due to halothane. Meperidine or morphine and later fentanyl became the most frequently used narcotics.

Innovar, a combination of droperidol, a major tranquilizer, and fentanyl, a synthetic high-potency narcotic, sold in a fixed ratio of one to the other, was found to be difficult to use (too much droperidol) and to cause patients to be sleepy and even catatonic in the recovery room. Anesthetists began using the drugs separately, with the droperidol, the longer-lasting drug, given near induction and fentanyl added as the patient required. This combination became the main anesthetic in the last years of the war.[47,57]

Ketamine proved valuable as a primary anesthetic agent for superficial wounds, "with the incorrect assumption that patients could protect their airways under its influence."[47(p1302)] Popular relaxants were succinylcholine used for induction, and curare used for maintenance. To avoid prominent hypotension, anesthesiologists administered curare in two or three incremental doses. Doses of neostigmine and atropine reversed the effect of competitive relaxants. Because field hospitals had no Wright respirometers or blockade monitors, anesthesia providers estimated reversal by observing the patient's cough, hand-grip strength, and head or arm lift.[47,57]

Various forms of regional anesthesia proved useful, as well. From February 1970 to May 1971, anesthesia providers at the 91st Evacuation Hospital performed spinal anesthesia in 15% of cases.

TABLE 31-1

ANESTHETIC ADMINISTRATION, U.S. ARMY 67TH EVACUATION HOSPITAL, DECEMBER 1970 TO JULY 1971

Anesthetic Administration	December 1970	February 1971	April 1971	June 1971	July 1971	Total	Percentage of Total
N_2O–O_2	28		5	4	6	43	4
N_2O–O_2-Halothane	86	71	40	34	32	263	26
N_2O–O_2-Methoxyflurane	51	74	102	19	11	257	26
N_2O–O_2-Meperidine	18	21	25	3	3	70	7
N_2O–O_2-Morphine	7	1	23	20	8	59	6
Axillary	10	2		6		18	2
Spinal	24	11	6	5	10	56	6
Caudal	3	1				4	—
Intravenous	6	49	37	64	40	196	19
Ketamine		27	35	52	32	146	
Innovar		21	2	12	8	43	
Diazepam		1				1	
Infiltration	17	11	10			38	4
						1,004	
Operative deaths	3	2					
Total number of cases	235	236	247	156	110	984	

N_2O: nitrous oxide; O_2: oxygen

Reprinted with permission from Lichtmann MW. Vietnam. In: Grande CM, ed. *Textbook of Trauma Anesthesia and Critical Care*. St. Louis, Mo: Mosby–Year Book; 1993: 1302.

TABLE 31-2

ANESTHETIC ADMINISTRATION IN EIGHT U.S. ARMY HOSPITALS IN JANUARY 1968

Anesthetic Administration	2nd Surg.	7th Surg.	8th Field	12th Evac.	24th Evac.	45th Surg.	67th Evac.	85th Evac.	93rd Evac.	Total	Percentage of Total
N_2O–O_2-Halothane	367	27	157	414	301	165	253	259	562	2,505	82
N_2O–O_2-Methoxyflurane		4	23	3	3	10	10	18	19	90	3
N_2O–O_2-Thiopental	16	1		7	18	4	7	5	7	62	2
N_2O–O_2-Ether			1								
O_2					5					5	
Regional	1	1	30	20	15	1	10	41	15	134	4
Spinal	11	10	30	74	67	14	27	19	26	<u>278</u>	9
										3,069	
Infiltration	138	8	85	88	77	11	66	91	66		
Total number of cases	539	90	431	629	501	164	371	431	636		
Personnel											
3115 B				1	1				1		
3115 C	1	2					1				
OJT			1	1	1	1		1	1		
3445	2	3	3	6	6	3	4	2	5		

N_2O: nitrous oxide; O_2: oxygen; 3115 B: board-certified anesthesiologist; 3115 C: fully trained anesthesiologist; OJT: on the job (ie, physician partially trained in anesthesia); 3445: certified nurse anesthetist

Reprinted with permission from Lichtmann MW. Vietnam. In: Grande CM, ed. *Textbook of Trauma Anesthesia and Critical Care*. St. Louis, Mo: Mosby–Year Book; 1993: 1303.

Epidural anesthesia evinced benefits in vascular repairs and grafts. When the casualty load was heavy, anesthesia personnel reinjected epidural catheters between cases in the operating room. Upper-extremity nerve blocks and Bier blocks (regional intravenous anesthesia) also proved valuable. The absence of double tourniquets sometimes caused local anesthetics to leak. Regional, especially spinal, anesthesia was more popular with anesthesia providers in the Vietnam War than in World War II. Spinal anesthesia's simplicity made it perfect for combat. The method had become more popular in the civilian sector by this time as well.[47]

In his essay on Vietnam titled "Military and Battlefield Anesthesia," Lichtmann constructed five tables (Tables 31-1 through 31-5) that

> give some temporal and geographic impressions of the anesthetics used. These reports are incomplete but do show trends over several years, as well as the impact of logistics, as in the case of the 67th Evacuation Hospital ([Table 31-1]), where methoxyflurane was used in 25 percent of cases primarily because that was the only anesthetic they had available.[47(p1302)]

In late 1971 and early 1972, in the 95th Evacuation Hospital in Da Nang, regional anesthesia was used in 23% of total cases done. Axillary and interscalene arm blocks as well as spinal and epidural blocks were popular. A regional anesthetic for an arm debridement in a stable patient would allow the procedure to be done in the holding area with minimal surgical equipment. This practice kept the patient from going to the operating room and therefore saved sterile equipment, drapes, and the time of skilled personnel for more serious cases. Two to four regional procedures per day were common at the 95th Evacuation Hospital.[57]

Recovery rooms in Vietnam resembled intensive care units in major civilian medical centers. Patients who could not be safely extubated immediately after surgery required "ventilatory, nutritional, and hemodynamic care in addition to wound care,"[47(p1302)] recalled Lichtmann. Recovery room

TABLE 31-3

ANESTHETIC ADMINISTRATION IN EIGHT U.S. ARMY HOSPITALS IN APRIL 1968

Anesthetic Administration	2nd Surg.	12th Evac.	17th Field	18th Surg.	27th Surg.	36th Evac.	45th Surg.	67th Evac.	71st Evac.	85th Evac.	93rd Evac.	Total	Percentage of Total
N_2O–O_2-Halothane	257	409	68		154	180	111	224	294	214	603	2,771	79
N_2O–O_2-Methoxyflurane	7	3	3	204	1	31	3	1	13	9	4	286	8
N_2O–O_2-Thiopental	16	11	16		7	2	1	3			6	78	2
O_2-Thiopental						1						1	
Thiopental						1						1	
Neurolept analgesia						1						1	
Meperidine-N_2O–O_2					1							1	
Relaxants													
Curare					22							22	
Succinylcholine drip					10							10	
Regional													
Block	4	4		3	5	6	2	1	14	29	33	107	3
Spinal	9	27	11	29	6	44	2	23	50	39	2	251	7
Epidural										2		2	
												3,499	
Infiltration	191	46	30	198		135	63	64	237	121	35		
Total number of cases	483	621	151	434	278	358	185	766	608	485	684		
Personnel													
3115 B		1									1		
3115 C	1			1	1		1	1					
OJT		1	1			1			1	1	1		
3445	2	6	2	3	3	4	4	4	4	2	5		

N_2O: nitrous oxide; O_2: oxygen; 3115 B: board-certified anesthesiologist; 3115 C: fully trained anesthesiologist; OJT: on the job (ie, physician partially trained in anesthesia); 3445: certified nurse anesthetist

Reprinted with permission from Lichtmann MW. Vietnam. In: Grande CM, ed. *Textbook of Trauma Anesthesia and Critical Care*. St. Louis, Mo: Mosby–Year Book; 1993: 1303.

staff, he stated, provided continuous nursing care, using electrocardioscopes, defibrillators, ventilators, and other respiratory techniques, often with the anesthesiologist in attendance.

Because there was no military occupation specialty for respiratory therapists, a system developed whereby personnel at Walter Reed Army Medical Center identified those skilled people as they came into service and coordinated their assignments, so that respiratory therapists were distributed throughout the hospitals in Vietnam. The military had plenty of opportunities to practice critical care medicine in Vietnam.[47] Declared Lichtmann: "The recovery rooms of those large field hospitals did not differ greatly from the busy intensive care unit of a large urban hospital…."[47(p1302)]

Early in the war, anesthesia equipment was adequate but antiquated. Anesthesia providers initially deployed brought with them the World War II–era 0400 and 0430 Heidbrink machines (the pig). These machines had 400-mL metal carbon dioxide absorbers but only a closed-circle vaporizer, which, as was stated above, was not readily adaptable for use with the newer potent inhalational agents such as halothane. In 1967, the army adopted the Ohio Model 785 Field Anesthesia Machine, which had undergone several design changes since production began in 1958, and or-

TABLE 31-4

ANESTHETIC ADMINISTRATION AT THE U.S. ARMY 91ST EVACUATION HOSPITAL, FEBRUARY 1970 TO MAY 1971

	1970										1971					
Anesthetic	**Feb**	**Mar**	**May**	**Jun**	**Jul**	**Aug**	**Sep**	**Oct**	**Nov**	**Dec**	**Jan**	**Feb**	**Mar**	**May**	**Total**	**Percentage of Total**
Halothane	240	248	311	239	247	235	177	162	163	189	156	165	117	65	2,714	52
Methoxyflurane	44	40	4	23	9	2			3	4		3	30	12	174	3
N_2O–O_2	18	13	26	10	28	62	110	91	68	72	107	147	118	104	974	19
Blocks	22	36	19	16	8	7	6	10	20	21	16	19	20	31	251	5
Spinals	93	105	65	44	37	60	68	48	62	58	49	39	47	30	805	15
Infiltration	22	15	17	7	7	6	12	10	12	15	2	8	6	11	150	3
Other		2	2	11	1	1	4	2	1			37	28	41	130	2
Ketamine										29	14				43	
															5,198	
Endotracheal	260	221	305	*	251	284	277	230	228	256	244	303	232	167	3,258	63
Total cases	439	459	444	343	337	373	483	313	329	403	404	428	*	291	5,046	

*Information missing
N_2O: nitrous oxide; O_2: oxygen
Reprinted with permission from Lichtmann MW. Vietnam. In: Grande CM, ed. *Textbook of Trauma Anesthesia and Critical Care*. St. Louis, Mo: Mosby–Year Book; 1993: 1304.

dered a number of these machines for issue to all medical units (Figures 31-18 through 31-21). The new anesthesia device weighed less than 95 lb; could be carried by one individual from surgery to vehicle; and could be air-dropped in one package, except for its four gas cylinders or pressure tanks.[26,47,57] The machine had a two-canister carbon dioxide absorber; was capable of accommodating cylinders of nitrous oxide–oxygen; had pressure regulators for those gases, a large in-circuit vaporizer, a heater rod

> to stabilize vaporization temperatures in all weather, [and was] capable of delivering anesthetic mixtures over a temperature range of 4°C to 38°C.... The era of administering ether with wet-drapes over the "ether screen" had ended.[26(pp66–67)]

TABLE 31-5

ACTIVITIES REPORT FOR THE U.S. ARMY 3RD FIELD HOSPITAL, 1967 THROUGH 1968

	Census Year 1967	Census Year 1968	Increase (%)
Total hospital admissions	6,747	11,382	69
Surgical procedures	2,857	6,406	124
Major	1,882	3,296	75
Minor	975	3,110	219
Deaths in hospital	148	150	1

1968 mortality rate for admissions: 1.3%
1968 mortality rate for surgical procedures: 2.3%
Adapted with permission from Lichtmann MW. Vietnam. In: Grande CM, ed. *Textbook of Trauma Anesthesia and Critical Care*. St. Louis, Mo: Mosby–Year Book; 1993: 1305. Numbers amended by the original author for this publication, 1995.

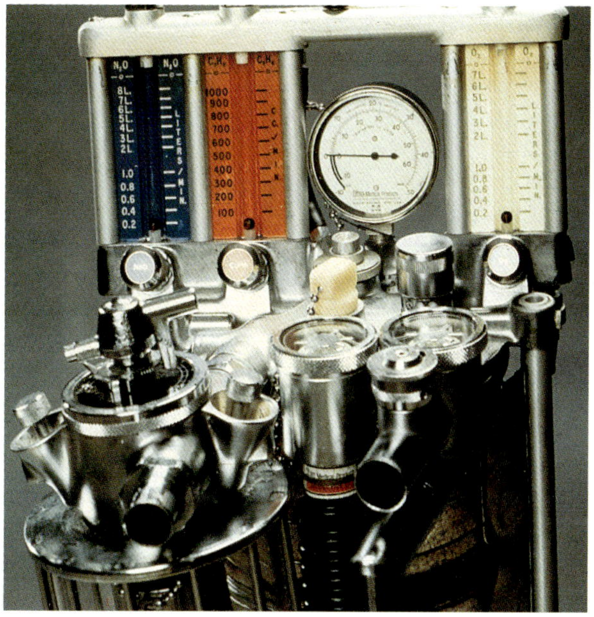

Fig. 31-18. Military Field Anesthesia Machine Model 785. The ether/chloroform in-circuit vaporizer is seen at bottom left. Flowmeters, seen left to right, are for nitrous oxide (blue), cyclopropane (orange), and oxygen (white, the international color for oxygen). A pressure gauge, calibrated in centimeters of water, monitors the pressure in the breathing circuit. Immediately below the pressure gauge is a round button, the oxygen flush valve. Two one-way valves for the breathing circuit can be seen at the bottom right. The white plug with a small chain attached, seen in the center of the photograph, can be removed and replaced by the hand-operated concertina bellows (also see Figs. 31-19 and 31-21). Photograph: Courtesy of William Clayton Petty, MD, Captain, Medical Corps, US Navy, Bethesda, Md.

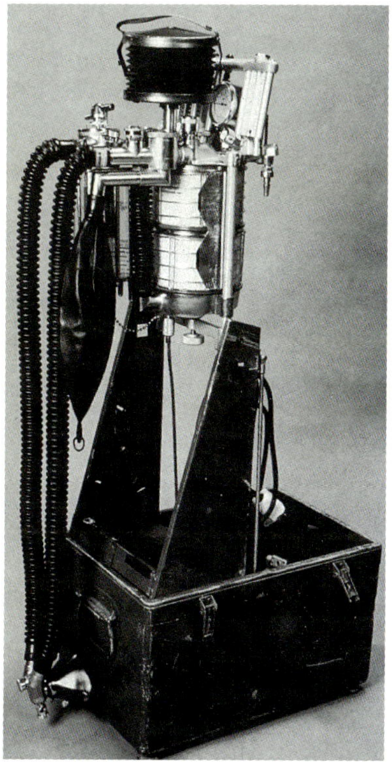

Fig. 31-19. Military Field Anesthesia Machine Model 785, with breathing hoses and rebreathing bag attached. Carbon dioxide–absorbent granules have been placed in the canisters. The hand-operated concertina bellows is in place. Photograph: Courtesy of William Clayton Petty, MD, Captain, Medical Corps, US Navy, Bethesda, Md.

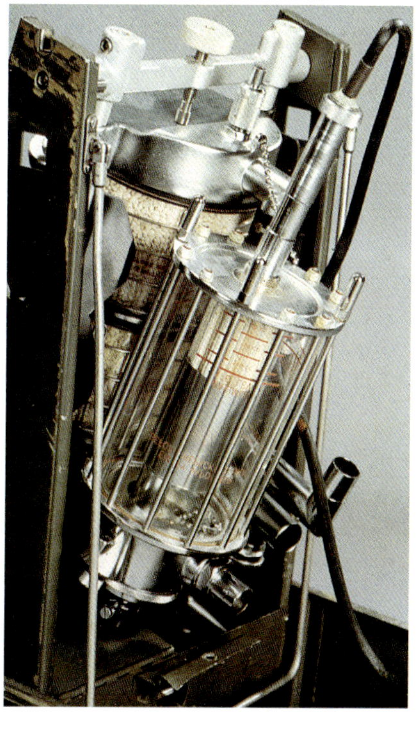

Fig. 31-20. A small, 110-volt cylindrical heater can be installed in the vaporizer to heat ether in cold climates and to stabilize its temperature during induction of anesthesia. A rapid ether induction can cause the outside walls of the vaporizer to coat with ice. The heater will maintain ether at a stable temperature, eliminating the marked reduction in vaporization of ether during induction. Photograph: Courtesy of William Clayton Petty, MD, Captain, Medical Corps, US Navy, Bethesda, Md.

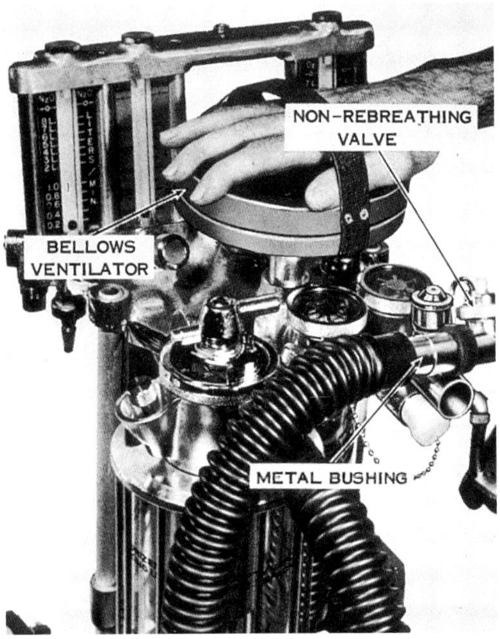

Fig. 31-21. The 1968 Ohio Model 785 Field Anesthesia Machine. Photograph: Reprinted with permission from Model 785 anesthesia apparatus, nitrous oxide, oxygen, ether, and cyclopropane, portable, 4-cylinder capacity. *Instruction and Service Manual.* Madison, Wis: Ohio Chemical and Surgical Equipment Company; Oct 1968: 11.

The Vietnam War was the first conflict in which anesthesia providers used equipment standardized to written specifications. The implements included endotracheal tubes, laryngoscopes, adapters, venotubes, carbon dioxide absorbents, vasopressors, and new relaxants. The capstone to the modernization effort was the regulation of a new field anesthesia chest. The chest weighed 110 lb when fully loaded with over 100 items and a 3-day supply of drugs, and could be air-dropped. Standardization provided the army with high-quality supplies and drugs in a medical specialty "where," according to John A. Jenicek, former Consultant in Anesthesiology to The U.S. Army Surgeon General, "the margin for error [did] not tolerate a substandard approach."[56(p801)]

Unlike that in any previous war, casualty care in the Vietnam War during the late 1960s and early 1970s was equal to, and in some respects better than, the treatment provided in the most sophisticated medical centers in the United States. There were two main reasons: (1) the gradual escalation of the war enabled the U.S. Army Medical Department (AMEDD; the acronym became established during the early 1970s) to establish fixed, well-equipped hospitals with highly trained staff; and (2) the air superiority enjoyed by the United States facilitated a rapid and effective evacuation system to those hospitals for definitive treatment. As a result, medical personnel were able to salvage most of the wounded who had not been killed outright on the battlefield.

The Vietnam War, more than any previous conflict, gave a new face and a new character to anesthesia providers. They played a pivotal role in preserving life before, during, and after surgery, redefining the meaning of intensive care. AMEDD's establishment of fixed, well-equipped hospitals, specially staffed with highly trained people, provided trauma treatment to rival that of any civilian trauma center in the world.

The Post–Vietnam War Era

The role of the anesthesiologist continued to expand in the post–Vietnam War era in the realm of resuscitation and critical care medicine. Advancements in anesthesiology as practiced in conflicts since the Vietnam War are well described elsewhere.[58–60] The anesthesiologist diagnosed and alleviated pain by simple and complex techniques, such as nerve block and intravenous anesthesia. In the operating room, the anesthesiologist used modern, sophisticated equipment to administer anesthesia and monitor blood pressure, central venous pressure, left atrial pressure, and so forth to make surgery safer for the patient at risk. In the recovery room, recalled Jenicek,

> a skilled staff, often trained and instructed by the anesthesiologist, provid[ed] immediate and continuous nursing care to protect the patient as far as possible from drug-induced respiratory depression, hyper or hypotension and a myriad of anesthetically or surgically induced occurrences that [might] beset the organ systems at [that] time.[61(p387)]

They used ventilators, antiarrhythmic drugs, cardiac monitors, or cardiopulmonary resuscitation, often with the anesthesiologist in attendance.[61]

The recognition by anesthesiologists, later joined by cardiologists and other specialists, of the possibility of saving patients by aggressive treatment in the early stages of a debilitating illness or acute trauma led to the discipline of critical care medicine, the successor to intensive care medicine. Enthusiasts of critical care designed curricula to enhance the skills of those wishing to work in this special field.[61]

The expanded knowledge and role of the anesthesiologist has led to more research in the field of anesthesiology and critical care, and increased and enlarged journals of anesthesiology and publications on the subject in major scientific periodicals. To John Jenicek, "Anesthesiology is art and science coexisting in the world of modern medicine, in a discipline that is demanding, exciting, and rewarding."[61(pp388–389)]

Because armed combat equates with trauma, Brian Condon, former Consultant in Anesthesiology to The U.S. Army Surgeon General, believes it is time for a natural alliance between military anesthesia and trauma anesthesia in the civilian sphere.[57] The military might help forge that alliance, especially since trauma anesthesia is receiving little national attention at present.[62]

SUMMARY

The military has shared man's eternal quest to alleviate pain and make possible the humane treatment of survivors. Military and civilian anesthesia providers have learned from each other strategies to promote the merciful treatment of the seriously impaired patient. The military has developed its own cadre of specialists, capable of independently solving complex medical problems. The military's vast and valuable experience in caring for combat casualties has advanced the field of critical care medicine and has led to a natural alliance of military and civilian anesthesiology in the treatment of trauma.

Acknowledgments

The author wishes to thank Dale Smith, Ph.D., Associate Professor of Medical History, and Colonel Robert J. T. Joy, M.D, Medical Corps, U.S. Army, (ret), Professor and Chairman, Section of Medical History, Uniformed Services University of the Health Sciences, for their helpful suggestions and review during the preparation of this chapter; and Captain William Clayton Petty, M.D., Medical Corps, U.S. Navy, Professor and Vice Chairman, Department of Anesthesiology, Uniformed Services University of the Health Sciences, 4301 Jones Bridge Road, Bethesda, Maryland 20814-4799, for his advice and for providing the illustrations.

REFERENCES

1. Robinson V. *Victory Over Pain, A History of Anesthesia.* London, England: Sigma Books; 1947: 7, 18, 19, 21, 33, 34, 44–80, 107, 117, 137, 171, 224, 261–264, 284, 286–313.

2. Trent JC. Surgical anesthesia, 1846–1946. *Journal of the History of Medicine and Allied Sciences.* 1946;1(4):505–514.

3. Keys TE. *The History of Surgical Anesthesia.* Huntington, NY: Robert E. Krieger; 1978: 15–19, 68, 108–118.

4. Horine EF. Episodes in the history of anesthesia. *Journal of the History of Medicine and Allied Sciences.* 1946;1(4): 524–525.

5. Faulconer A Jr, Keys TE. *Foundations of Anesthesiology.* Vol 1. Springfield, Ill: Charles C Thomas; 1965: 297–298.

6. Porter JB. Medical and surgical notes of campaigns in the war with Mexico, during the years 1845, 1846, 1847, and 1848. *American Journal of the Medical Sciences.* 1852;24:13–30.

7. Gillett MC. *The Army Medical Department 1818–1865.* Washington, DC: Center of Military History, US Army; 1987: 18–20, 125, 286, 287.

8. Aldrete JA, Marron GM, Wright AJ. The first administration of anesthesia in military surgery: On occasion of the Mexican-American War. *Anesthesiology.* 1984;61:585–587.

9. Duncan LC. Medical history of General Scott's campaign to the city of Mexico in 1847. *The Army Medical Bulletin.* 1939;50:72–73.

10. Pernick MS. *A Calculus of Suffering Pain Professionalism, and Anesthesia in Nineteenth-Century America*. New York, NY: Columbia University Press; 1985: 146, 150, 182, 183, 190–192, 219, 221, 223, 227, 237, 238.

11. Anonymous. *Western Lancet*. 1848;7(2):128.

12. Keys TE. John Snow, MD, anesthetist. *J Hist Med*. 1946:1(4):556–557.

13. Macleod GHB. *Notes on the Surgery of the War in the Crimea*. London, England: JB Lippincott & Co. 1862: 123–126.

14. The War Department, The Surgeon General's Office. *The Medical and Surgical History of the War of the Rebellion*. Part 3, vol 2. *Surgical History*. Washington, DC: War Department, Government Printing Office; 1883: 887–898.

15. Brooks S. *Civil War Medicine*. Springfield, Ill: Charles C Thomas; 1966: 72, 94–96, 123.

16. MacCallum WG. *William Stewart Halsted, Surgeon*. Baltimore, Md: The Johns Hopkins Press; 1930: 53, 55.

17. Sykes WS. *Essays on the First Hundred Years of Anesthesia*. Vol 1. Park Ridge, Ill: American Society of Anesthesiologists; 1982: 43, 44, 72.

18. Smith D. *Graduate Medical Education in the Military, An Historical Overview*. Bethesda, Md: The Uniformed Services University of the Health Sciences; n.d. Unpublished manuscript: 1–20.

19. Senn N. *Medico-Surgical Aspects of the Spanish–American War*. Chicago, Ill: American Medical Association Press; 1900: 89, 200, 224–226, 265, 278–282, 297, 341.

20. US Army Surgeon General. Annual Report to the Secretary of War. Washington, DC: Government Printing Office; 1899: 25.

21. Shields EA, ed. *Highlights in the History of the Army Nurse Corps*. Washington, DC: US Army Center of Military History; 1981: 13.

22. Harsch TL. *Nurse Anesthetists in the United States Army Nurse Corps During World War II*. Peoria, Ill: Bradley University; 1993. Thesis.

23. Courington FW, Calverley RK. Anesthesia on the western front: The Anglo-American experience of World War I. *Anesthesiology*. 1986;65:642–651.

24. Mousel LH. The present status of anesthesia and its practical application in the combat zone. *The Military Surgeon*. Aug 1939:103–113.

25. Donaghy GE, Doud EA, Hoeflich WF, Westerfield CW. Anesthesia. In: DeBakey ME, ed. *General Surgery*. Vol 2. In: Coates JB Jr, ed. *Surgery In World War II*. Washington, DC: US Army, Medical Department, Office of The Surgeon General; 1955: 181–189.

26. Petty WC. Historical perspectives on the evolution of today's military field anesthesia machine. *Milit Med*. 1990;155:66–71.

27. US Army Surgeon General. Annual Report to the Secretary of War. Washington, DC: Government Printing Office; 1918: 350.

28. Macpherson WG, Bowlby AA, Wallace C, English C, eds. Anesthesia. In: *Medical Services Surgery of the War*. In: *History of the Great War Based on Official Documents*. Vol 1. London, England: His Majesty's Stationery Office; 1922: 178–185.

29. Crile GW. Anesthesia. In: Weed FW, ed. *Surgery*. In: *The Medical Department of the United States Army in the World War*. Vol 11. Washington, DC: Government Printing Office; 1927: Chap 6: 166–184.

30. Cannon WB. Wound shock. In: Weed FW, ed. *Surgery*. In: *The Medical Department of the United States Army in the World War*. Vol 11. Washington, DC: Government Printing Office; 1927: Chap 7: 185–213.

31. Benison S, Barger A, Wolfe E. Walter B. Cannon and the mystery of shock: A study of Anglo-American co-operation in World War I. *Medical History*. 1991;35:217–249.

32. Hardaway RM. Wartime treatment of shock. *Milit Med*. 1982;147(12):1011.

33. Churchill ED. *Surgeon to Soldiers*. Philadelphia, Pa: JB Lippincott; 1972: 32–39, 42, 347–355.

34. Robertson OH. Transfusion with preserved blood cells. *British Medical Journal*. June 1918;691–692.

35. Kendrick DB. *Blood Program In World War II*. Washington, DC: US Army, Medical Department, Office of The Surgeon General; 1989: 29, 30, 776–782.

36. Bacon DR. A history of nurse anesthesia? *Anesth Analg*. 1991;72(3):412–413. Letter.

37. Axelrod HR. Henry Ruth: Pioneer of modern anesthesiology. *Anesthesiology*. 1993;78(1):178–183.

38. Beecher HK. Anesthesia for men wounded in battle. In: DeBakey ME, ed. *General Surgery*. In: Coates JB Jr, ed. *Surgery In World War II*. Vol 2. Washington, DC: US Army, Medical Department, Office of The Surgeon General; 1955: Chap 3: 53–78.

39. Berry FB. Seventh US Army. In: Carter BN, ed. *Activities of Surgical Consultants*. Vol 1. In: Coates JB Jr, ed. *Surgery in World War II*. Washington, DC: US Army, Medical Department, Office of The Surgeon General; 1962: Chap 18: 548–549.

40. Tovell RM. Anesthesia. In: Carter BN, ed. *Activities of Surgical Consultants*. Vol 2. In: Coates JB Jr, ed. *Surgery in World War II*. Washington, DC: US Army, Medical Department, Office of The Surgeon General; 1964: Chap 10: 600–603.

41. Condon-Rall ME, Cowdrey A. *The Medical Department: Medical Service in the War Against Japan, U.S. Army in World War II*. Washington, DC: The Center of Military History; 1996.

42. Beecher HK. Resuscitation of men severely wounded in battle. In: DeBakey ME, ed. *General Surgery*. Vol 2. In: Coates JB Jr, ed. *Surgery in World War II*. Washington, DC: US Army, Medical Department, Office of The Surgeon General; 1955: Chap 1: 3–39.

43. Condon-Rall ME. The U.S. Army Medical Department and the attack on Pearl Harbor. *The Journal of Military History*. 1989;53(1):75.

44. MacNalty AS, Mellor WF, eds. *Medical Services in War: The Principal Medical Lessons of the Second World War*. London, England: Her Majesty's Stationery Office; 1968: 439.

45. Wiltse CM. *The Medical Department: Medical Service in the Mediterranean and Minor Theaters*. In: *United States Army in World War II: The Technical Services*. Washington, DC: Office of the Chief of Military History; 1965: 1–4.

46. Beecher HK, ed. The Board for the Study of the Severely Wounded, North African–Mediterranean Theater of Operations. *The Physiologic Effects of Wounds*. Washington, DC: US Army, Medical Department, Office of The Surgeon General; 1952: 13, 45–59.

47. Lichtmann MW. Vietnam. In: Military and battlefield anesthesia. In: Trauma anesthesia and critical care under conditions of environmental and circumstantial extremes. In: Grande CM, ed. *Textbook of Trauma Anesthesia and Critical Care*. St. Louis, Mo: Mosby–Year Book; 1993: Part 13: Chap 107; Part 1: 1297–1306.

48. Dripps RD. Anesthesia for combat casualties on the basis of experience in Korea. In: *Recent Advances in Medicine and Surgery Based on Professional Medical Experiences in Japan and Korea, 1950–1953*. Washington, DC: US Army Medical Service Graduate School, Walter Reed Army Medical Center; 19–30 April 1954; 117–131. Proceedings.

49. Cowdrey AE. *The Medic's War*. In: United States Army in the Korean War. Washington, DC: Center of Military History, US Army; 1987: 32–35, 159, 188–189, 321–329, 362–364.

50. Lindsey D. Professional considerations of patient evacuation. In: *Recent Advances in Medicine and Surgery Based on Professional Medical Experiences in Japan and Korea, 1950–1953*. Washington, DC: Army Medical Service Graduate School, Walter Reed Army Medical Center; 19–30 April 1954; 89, 97. Proceedings.

51. Bowers JZ, Purcell EF, eds. *Advances In American Medicine: Essays At The Bicentennial.* Vol 2. New York, NY: Josiah Macy Jr Foundation; 1976: 674.

52. US Army Surgeon General. Annual Report to the Secretary of War. Washington, DC: Government Printing Office; 1959–1965.

53. Masters FL, Skidmore MD, Thibodeaux BL. US Army/Texas Wesleyan University program in anesthesia nursing. *AANA Journal*, Oct 1991;59(5):480–481.

54. Hardaway RM. Contributions of army medicine to civilian medicine. *Milit Med*. 1973;138(7):409–411.

55. Custis DL. Military medicine from World War II to Vietnam. *JAMA*. 1990;264(17):2261.

56. Jenicek JA. The new face of anesthesiology in Vietnam. *Milit Med*. 1967;132(10):799–802.

57. Condon BF. Colonel, Medical Corps, US Army; Consultant in Anesthesiology to The Surgeon General. Personal communication, May 1994.

58. Jowitt MD. Falklands campaign. In: Military and battlefield anesthesia. In: Trauma anesthesia and critical care under conditions of environmental and circumstantial extremes. In: Grande CM, ed. *Textbook of Trauma Anesthesia and Critical Care*. St. Louis, Mo: Mosby–Year Book; 1993: Part 13: Chap 107: Part 3: 1310–1317.

59. Jowitt MD, Knight RJ. Anesthesia during the Falklands campaign. *Anesthesia*. 1983;38:776–783.

60. Perkins D, Condon BF. Post Vietnam US conflicts: Grenada, Panama, and the Persian Gulf. In: Trauma anesthesia and critical care under conditions of environmental and circumstantial extremes. In: Grande CM, ed. *Textbook of Trauma Anesthesia and Critical Care*. St. Louis, Mo: Mosby–Year Book; 1993: Part 13: Chap 107: Part 4: 1318–1324.

61. Jenicek JA. The anesthesiologist. *Milit Med*. 1978;143(6):387–389.

62. Goldsmith M. Caring for all of those who fall in combat. *JAMA*. 1992;267(12):1583.

ACRONYMS AND ABBREVIATIONS

A

ABC: airway, breathing, and circulation
AC: assist control
acetyl-CoA: acetylcoenzyme A
ACTH: adrenocorticotropic hormone
ADH: antidiuretic hormone
ADSOL: adenine solution number 1
AFB: air force base
AIDS: acquired immunodeficiency syndrome
AIS: Abbreviated Injury Scale
AJBPO: Area Joint Blood Program Office
AMEDD: U.S. Army Medical Department
ANSI: American National Standards Institute
ARDS: adult respiratory distress syndrome
ARF: acute renal failure
ASBP: Armed Services Blood Program
ASBPO: Armed Services Blood Program Office
ASBPOSITREP: ASBPO situation report
ASIA: American Spinal Injury Association
ASTM: American Society for Testing and Materials
ASWBPL: Armed Services Whole Blood Processing Laboratory
ASWBPLSITREP: ASWBPL situation report
ATLS: Advanced Trauma Life Support
ATP: adenosine 5′-triphosphate
ATPase: adenosine triphosphatase
AVDO_2: arteriovenous oxygen contents
A–aDO_2: alveolar–arterial difference in partial pressure of oxygen

B

BAEP: brain stem auditory evoked potential
BDC: blood donor center
BLDREP: blood report
BLDSHIPREP: blood shipment report
BMR: basal metabolic rate
BPD: blood product depot
BSA: body surface area
BSU: blood supply unit
BTC: blood transshipment center
BUN: blood urea nitrogen

C

C.O.: cardiac output
CaCO_2: arterial carbon dioxide contents
CAM: chemical agent monitor
cAMP: adenosine 3′,5′-cyclic monophosphate
CaO_2: arterial oxygen contents
CAVH-D: continuous arteriovenous hemodiafiltration
CAVH: continuous arteriovenous hemofiltration
CBF: cerebral blood flow
CBPS: chemical biological protective shelter
cCBF: critical cerebral blood flow
CD: cluster of differentiation
CDC: Centers for Disease Control
CDO_2: cerebral oxygen delivery
CjvO_2: jugular venous oxygen contents
CK: creatine kinase
CMRO_2: cerebral metabolic rate for oxygen
CMV: controlled mechnical ventilation
CMV: cytomegalovirus
CNS: central nervous system
COHb: carboxyhemoglobin
CONUS: continental United States
CPAP: continuous positive airway pressure
CPDA-1: citrate phosphate dextrose adenine
CPE: collective protective ensemble
CPK: creatine phosphokinase
CPP: cerebral perfusion pressure
CPR: cardiopulmonary resuscitation
CRH: corticotrophin-releasing hormone
CRNA: certified registered nurse anesthetist
CSA: compressed spectral array
CSH: combat support hospital
CT: computed tomography
CvCO_2: venous carbon dioxide contents
CvO_2: venous oxygen contents
CZAR: Combat Zone Assessment and Requirements

D

DDAPV: desmopressin
DEPMEDS: Department of Defense's Deployable Medical Systems
DI: diabetes insipidus
DIC: disseminated intravascular coagulation
DNA: deoxyribonucleic acid
DO_2: oxygen delivery per unit time
DPL: diagnostic peritoneal lavage
DRASH: *d*eployable *r*apid *a*ssembly *sh*elter
DREZ: dorsal root entry zone
DSA: density spectral array

E

EBV: estimated blood volume
ECG: electrocardiogram
ED_{50}: median effective dose
EDP: expiratory distending pressure
EEA: energy expenditure of activity
EEG: electroencephalogram
ELISA: enzyme-linked immunosorbent assay
EMT: emergency medical treatment
EP: evoked potential
EPSP: excitatory postsynaptic potential
ETCO_2: end-tidal carbon dioxide

F

F: French (catheter)
FAM: field anesthesia machine
FDA: U.S. Food and Drug Administration
FEV_1: forced expiratory volume in 1 second
FEO_2: fraction of expired oxygen
FECO_2: fraction of expired carbon dioxide
FFP: fresh frozen plasma
FH: field hospital
FIO_2: fraction of inspired oxygen
FM: field manual
FRC: functional residual capacity
FSH: follicle-stimulating hormone
FST: forward surgical team
FVC: forced vital capacity

G

GABA: γ-aminobutyric acid
GB: sarin
GCS: Glasgow coma scale
GH: general hospital
GOS: Glasgow outcome scale
GPI: glucose phosphate isomerase
GPL: general-purpose, large tent

H

HAV: hepatitis A virus
Hb: hemoglobin
HBV: hepatitis B virus
HCV: hepatitis C virus
HIV: human immunodeficiency virus
HMMWV: high-mobility, multipurpose, wheeled vehicle
HUB: Hospital Unit, Base
HUH: Hospital Unit, Holding
HUM: Hospital Unit, Medical
HUS: Hospital Unit, Surgical

I

ICAD: individual chemical agent detector
ICD: International Classification of Disease
ICP: intracranial pressure
ICU: intensive care unit
Ig: immunoglobulin
IGF-1: insulinlike growth factor
IL: interleukin
IMV: intermittent, mandatory ventilation
IFN: interferon
IOP: intraocular pressure
IPE: individual protective ensemble
IPPB: intermittent positive-pressure breathing
IPPV: intermittent positive-pressure ventilation
IPSP: inhibitory postsynaptic potential
ISO: International Organization for Standardization, from the French
ISS: Injury Severity Score
IVOX/ECCOR: intravenacaval blood oxygen/carbon dioxide transfer device

J

JBPO: Joint Blood Program Office
JTF: Joint Task Forces

L

LH: luteinizing hormone
LMA: laryngeal mask airway
LVEDP: left ventricular end diastolic pressure
LVEDVI: left ventricular end diastolic volume index
LVSWI: left ventricular stroke work index

M

MAC: minimal alveolar concentration
MAP: mean arterial pressure
MASF: mobile aeromedical staging facility
MASH: mobile army surgical hospital
MEDSOM: Medical Supply, Optical, and Maintenance
MEP: motor evoked potential
MetHb: methemoglobin
MF2K: Medical Force 2000
MIAT: manual in-line axial traction
MIEMSS: Maryland Institute for Emergency Medical Services Systems
MMS: medical material sets
MODS: multiple organ dysfunction syndrome
MOPP: mission-oriented protective posture
MOS: military occupation specialty
MRE: meals ready to eat
MRI: magnetic resonance imaging
MRI: medical reengineering initiative
MSH: melanocyte-stimulating hormone
MSOF: multiple system organ failure
MTF: medical treatment facility
MUST: medical unit, self-contained, transportable
MVB: microvascular bleeding

N

NANB: non-A, non-B
NATO: North Atlantic Treaty Organization
NMDA: *N*-methyl-D-aspartate
NSAID: nonsteroidal antiinflammatory drug

O

O_2Hb: oxyhemoglobin
OCONUS: outside the continental United States
OMV: Oxford Miniature Vaporizers
OOTW: operations other than war

P

PAC: portable anesthesia circuit
$Paco_2$: arterial partial pressure of carbon dioxide
Pao_2: arterial partial pressure of oxygen
PAOP: pulmonary artery occlusion pressure
2-PAM Cl: 2-pyridine aldoxime methyl chloride, also pralidoxime chloride
PAP: peak airway pressure
PASG: pneumatic antishock garment
PCA: patient controlled anesthesia
PCP: phencyclidine
PCWP: pulmonary capillary wedge pressure
PEEP: positive end-expiratory pressure
PGE_2: prostaglandin E_2
PGI_2: prostacyclin
PISS: pin index safety system
PMN: polymorphonuclear leukocyte
Po_2: partial pressure of oxygen
POC: point of contact
POMCUS: prepositioned material configured in units and sets
PPN: peripheral parenteral nutrition
PRBCs: packed red blood cells
PRIMOB: primary mobilization stations
PRL: prolactin
PS: pressure support
PTH: posttransfusion hepatitis
PVR: pulmonary vascular resistance

R

RAE: Ring, Adair, and Elwyn endotracheal tube
RBC: red blood cell
RDA: recommended dietary allowances
REE: resting energy expenditure
RNA: ribonucleic acid
RQ: respiratory quotient
RVEF: right ventricular ejection fraction

S

SaO_2: oxygen saturation of arterial blood
SBPO: Service Blood Program Office
SCBF: spinal cord blood flow
SCUF: slow, continuous ultrafiltration
SIADH: syndrome of inappropriate antidiuretic hormone secretion
SIMV: synchronized, intermittent, mandatory ventilation
SIRS: systemic inflammatory response syndrome
$S_{mv}O_2$: mixed venous saturation
SpEP: spinal evoked potentials
SQRT: square root of time
SSEP: somatosensory evoked potential
STH: somatotropic hormone
succinyl-CoA: succinylcoenzyme A
SVI: systolic velocity integral
SvO_2: venous oxygen saturation
SVR: systemic vascular resistance
SWI: stroke work index

T

TBSA: total body surface area
TBTC: transportable blood transshipment center
TCA: tricarboxylic acid
TEE: total energy expenditure
TEF: thermic effect of food
TEMPER: *t*ents, *e*xtendable, *m*odular, *per*sonnel
TENS: transcutaneous electrical nerve stimulation
THBF: total hepatic blood flow
TNF: tumor necrosis factor
TOE: table of organization and equipment
TOF: train-of-four
TPN: total parenteral nutrition
TSH: thyroid-stimulating hormone
TV: tidal volume

U

UD: unit dose
USARIEM: U.S. Army Research Institute of Environmental Medicine
UUN: urinary urea nitrogen

V

V/Q: ventilation–perfusion
VA: alveolar ventilation
VCO_2: carbon dioxide consumption per unit time
VEP: visual evoked potential
VO_2: oxygen consumption per unit time

W

WDMET: Wound Data and Munitions Effectiveness Team
WRAIR: Walter Reed Army Institute of Research
WRAMC: Walter Reed Army Medical Center

INDEX

A

B

C

D

E

F

G

H

I

J

K

L

M

N

O

P

Q

R

S

T

U

V

W

N : 074180-000 ☆ U.S. GOVERNMENT PRINTING OFFICE : 1997 O - 430-973 (QL 1)